BMA

KT-438-797

Library

SECOND EDITION

APHASIA

and Related Neurogenic Communication Disorders

Ilias Papathanasiou, PhD, FRCSLT, ASHA Fellow

Associate Professor
Department of Speech and Language Therapy
Technological Educational Institute of Western Greece
Patras, Greece

Patrick Coppens, PhD, CCC-SLP

Professor
Department of Communication Disorders and Sciences
SUNY Plattsburgh
Plattsburgh, New York

WITHDRAWN FROM LIBRARY
BRITISH MEDICAL ASSOCIATION

JONES & BARTLETT
LEARNING

BRITISH MEDICAL ASSOCIATION

1006180

World Headquarters
Jones & Bartlett Learning
5 Wall Street
Burlington, MA 01803
978-443-5000
info@jblearning.com
www.jblearning.com

Jones & Bartlett Learning books and products are available through most bookstores and online booksellers. To contact Jones & Bartlett Learning directly, call 800-832-0034, fax 978-443-8000, or visit our website, www.jblearning.com.

Substantial discounts on bulk quantities of Jones & Bartlett Learning publications are available to corporations, professional associations, and other qualified organizations. For details and specific discount information, contact the special sales department at Jones & Bartlett Learning via the above contact information or send an email to specialsales@jblearning.com.

Copyright © 2017 by Jones & Bartlett Learning, LLC, an Ascend Learning Company

All rights reserved. No part of the material protected by this copyright may be reproduced or utilized in any form, electronic or mechanical, including photocopying, recording, or by any information storage and retrieval system, without written permission from the copyright owner.

The content, statements, views, and opinions herein are the sole expression of the respective authors and not that of Jones & Bartlett Learning, LLC. Reference herein to any specific commercial product, process, or service by trade name, trademark, manufacturer, or otherwise does not constitute or imply its endorsement or recommendation by Jones & Bartlett Learning, LLC and such reference shall not be used for advertising or product endorsement purposes. All trademarks displayed are the trademarks of the parties noted herein. *Aphasia and Related Neurogenic Communication Disorders, Second Edition* is an independent publication and has not been authorized, sponsored, or otherwise approved by the owners of the trademarks or service marks referenced in this product.

There may be images in this book that feature models; these models do not necessarily endorse, represent, or participate in the activities represented in the images. Any screenshots in this product are for educational and instructive purposes only. Any individuals and scenarios featured in the case studies throughout this product may be real or fictitious, but are used for instructional purposes only.

The authors, editor, and publisher have made every effort to provide accurate information. However, they are not responsible for errors, omissions, or for any outcomes related to the use of the contents of this book and take no responsibility for the use of the products and procedures described. Treatments and side effects described in this book may not be applicable to all people; likewise, some people may require a dose or experience a side effect that is not described herein. Drugs and medical devices are discussed that may have limited availability controlled by the Food and Drug Administration (FDA) for use only in a research study or clinical trial. Research, clinical practice, and government regulations often change the accepted standard in this field. When consideration is being given to use of any drug in the clinical setting, the health care provider or reader is responsible for determining FDA status of the drug, reading the package insert, and reviewing prescribing information for the most up-to-date recommendations on dose, precautions, and contraindications, and determining the appropriate usage for the product. This is especially important in the case of drugs that are new or seldom used.

09645-3

Production Credits
VP, Executive Publisher: David D. Cella
Executive Editor: Matt Kane
Acquisitions Editor: Laura Pagluica
Editorial Assistant: Taylor Ferracane
Associate Director of Production: Julie C. Bolduc
Production Manager: Tina Chen
Marketing Manager: Grace Richards
Composition: Cenveo® Publisher Services
Cover Design: Kristin E. Parker
Associate Director of Rights & Media: Joanna Lundeen
VP, Manufacturing and Inventory Control: Therese Connell
Rights & Media Specialist: Jamey O'Quinn
Media Development Editor: Troy Liston
Cover Image: © Involved Channel/ShutterStock, Inc.
Printing and Binding: Sheridan Books, Inc.
Cover Printing: Sheridan Books, Inc.

To order this product, use ISBN: 978-1-284-07731-5

Library of Congress Cataloging-in-Publication Data

Names: Papathanasiou, Ilias, author. | Coppens, Patrick, 1944- , author.
Title: Aphasia and related neurogenic communication disorders / Ilias Papathanasiou, Patrick Coppens.
Description: Second edition. | Burlington, MA : Jones & Bartlett Learning, [2017] | Includes bibliographical references and index.
Identifiers: LCCN 2015048789 | ISBN 9781284077315 (pbk. : alk. paper)
Subjects: | MESH: Aphasia | Apraxias | Brain Injuries | Dementia | Dysarthria
Classification: LCC RC425 | NLM WL 340.5 | DDC 616.85/52—dc23
LC record available at http://lccn.loc.gov/2015048789

6048

Printed in the United States of America
20 19 18   10 9 8 7 6 5 4

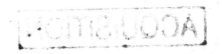

Contents

Introduction

Scientific fields constantly evolve. Keeping pace with the new developments in aphasiology and related neurogenic communication disorders is a challenge for clinicians and clinicians-in-training. The purpose of this text is to offer a state-of-the-art overview of our field by emphasizing important recent advances and presenting clinically relevant information. We trust that this volume provides a practical clinical resource for professionals as well as an informative learning tool for clinicians-in-training.

The contents of a text reflect, in part, the priorities of its editors. This volume is no exception and, as such, represents our attempt at an overview of neurogenic communication disorders with emphasis on the elements that we view as crucial for clinicians. Because we deem important that any analysis of a professional issue be illuminated by diverse points of view, we strive to include contributors from all over the world and encourage experts from different continents or countries to collaborate to offer an international perspective on all topics discussed. Because boundaries between disciplines blur and as technology facilitates exchanges between professionals worldwide, a true global perspective was a necessity in the development of this volume. The quality of a text is also a function of the expertise of its contributors. We are extremely grateful that each chapter is authored by expert clinicians and researchers who are able to present both theoretical information and clinical issues clearly and competently. We owe them a debt of gratitude.

Another important element in our view is to include the major recent developments in the area of neurogenic rehabilitation, such as the recent emphasis on psychosocial/functional approaches and evidence-based practice (EBP). The field of communication disorders and sciences has never been static. It is always in a state of flux because of theoretical, clinical, or technological innovations or even the occasional expansion of scope of practice. However, it seems that in the past few years, the winds of change have been blowing from a variety of directions, with a compounding effect. Among those, the World Health Organization developed a new disability scale, putting additional emphasis on social communication and quality of life.

Our specialty of neurogenic communication disorders has been naturally affected by these changes; for example, the concept of "functional therapy" (born in the 1960s and 1970s) recently blossomed into a full-blown philosophy of rehabilitation focusing on psychosocial issues and the person-centered approach to aphasia therapy. A recent publication (Martin, Thompson, & Worrall, 2008) contrasts the philosophical differences between expert clinicians applying the more traditional neurolinguistic (i.e., impairment-based) approach with those planning therapy from a more functional–social (i.e., consequence-based) perspective. The common thread in Martin et al. is that those two approaches share the same goals, and although they may differ in the means to achieve the goals, they are indeed complementary rather than antagonistic. It is with the same frame of mind that both the more traditional neurolinguistic approach of speech–language therapy as well as the more recently developed psychosocial–functional approach are covered in the present text.

Another major advance in the field is the clinical application of EBP. We believe that it is absolutely essential that future clinicians be exposed to EBP, both as a philosophy of rehabilitation and as a skill to apply in everyday clinical practice. In each chapter, the pertinent literature is reviewed critically, and its relevance for best clinical practices is addressed. Last, but not least, advances in the fields of neuroscience, neurophysiology, and neuroimaging have contributed to our knowledge of the dynamic mechanisms at work as the brain reorganizes language following an insult and have opened a window on how these mechanisms can be influenced by therapy processes.

Further, we tailored the depth of coverage to include a thorough literature review as well as practical clinical applications. This reflects our view that clinicians (and clinicians-in-training) not only need practical information but also must understand the underlying theoretical issues to provide therapy based on critical thinking and EBP. We also believe that the illustrative case studies included in all clinical chapters can facilitate readers' understanding of the concepts. Finally, the "Future Directions" section in each chapter provides a glimpse of where the field may be headed. Based on their thorough knowledge of their topic, the authors have anticipated the issues that are likely to be addressed in the near future so that readers are given a "heads-up" to follow the development of each topic area.

We purposefully avoided organizing chapters based on aphasia type. This should not be taken to imply that we find no value in aphasia classification per se, but rather that students should be trained to make symptom-specific clinical decisions rather than be influenced by a diagnostic label. The first part of the text covers aphasiology, and the second part addresses related disorders. In Chapter 1, a new chapter for this edition, Ilias Papathanasiou, Patrick Coppens, and Bronwyn Davidson include more details about issues related to the concept of aphasia and aphasia rehabilitation. Specifically, the authors discuss international challenges in service delivery, review a variety of aphasia management approaches, examine the efficacy of aphasia therapy, and present the international classification of functioning, disability, and health framework and how it has an impact on aphasia rehabilitation.

Chris Code provides an overview in Chapter 2 of the history of aphasiology. All the major contributions are highlighted, which should help the reader understand aphasiology and aphasia rehabilitation as an evolving area of study. In Chapter 3, Constantin Potagas, Dimitrios Kasselimis, and Ioannis Evdokimidis offer clinically relevant information on neuroanatomy and neurophysiology of stroke and describe the typical symptomatology and lesion location of the major aphasia types. Chapter 4 by Ilias Papathanasiou, Patrick Coppens, Edith Durand, and Ana Inés Ansaldo reviews the principles underlying poststroke language reorganization. This topic takes on renewed importance now that imaging technology allows us to observe firsthand the processing changes associated with speech–language pathology.

In Chapter 5, Laura Murray and Patrick Coppens provide theoretical and practical information about the linguistic, cognitive, and psychosocial measurement tools available; their properties and use; and the formal and informal assessment and baselining procedures. Chapter 6, by Linda Worrall, Sue Sherratt, and Ilias Papathanasiou, describes the therapy process and its context, such as the timing of therapy and the setting of clinical goals. They further emphasize the complementary character of the psychosocial and neurolinguistic rehabilitation approaches. In Chapter 7, also a new chapter in the second edition, Laura Murray and Jamie Mayer describe the extralinguistic cognitive factors important for understanding aphasia. The authors review important cognitive skills and their contribution to language processing, address assessment issues associated with these cognitive skills, and discuss their rehabilitation potential in the context of aphasia. In Chapter 8, Julie Morris and Sue Franklin address a specific aphasia symptom: impaired auditory comprehension. They review the language-decoding stages and pair each level with appropriate therapy options.

Nadine Martin discusses in Chapter 9 the ubiquitous aphasia symptom of anomia. She delineates the current models of word production and associates naming errors with specific stages of the model. This strategy allows clinicians to identify the underlying nature of the naming deficit and to develop clinical objectives accordingly.

In Chapter 10, Ellyn Riley, C. Elizabeth Brookshire, and Diane Kendall outline the various types of acquired alexias and analyze their respective symptomatology in light of the current dual-route model. They further critically review the therapy techniques available for each alexia type. Ilias Papathanasiou and Zsolt Cséfalvay provide the same thorough overview in Chapter 11 for the agraphias.

In Chapter 12, Jane Marshall presents the theoretical constructs underlying sentence production and the therapy strategies to remediate sentence-level disorders. Chapter 13, by Elizabeth Armstrong, Lucy Bryant, Alison Ferguson, and Nina Simmons-Mackie, examines language with yet a wider lens. They focus their analysis at the level of discourse, conversation, and narrative, which includes communicative context and psychosocial issues.

Katerina Hilari and Madeline Cruice provide an overview in Chapter 14 of the impact of aphasia on an individual's quality of life, review many specific measurement tools, and offer some strategies for clinicians to include quality-of-life concerns in clinical decisions. In Chapter 15, Bronwyn Davidson and Linda Worrall discuss client-centered aphasia assessment and intervention. This approach sensitizes clinicians to recognize that a traumatic event such as aphasia has an impact on a person's identity and has repercussions on a host of psychosocial issues.

In Chapter 16, José Centeno, Ladan Ghazi-Saidi, and Ana Inés Ansaldo address the important topics of not only bilingualism and multilingualism but also aphasia in a multicultural world. Because a majority of individuals around the globe speak more than one language, many clinicians will likely encounter bilingual individuals with aphasia in their practice. The remaining chapters cover associated populations, which required the authors to expertly summarize in one chapter a large body of work.

In Chapter 17, Connie Tompkins, Ekaterini Klepousniotou, and April Scott review the cognitive–linguistic symptomatology and the assessment tools and procedures for individuals who suffered a right hemisphere stroke. In Chapter 18, Connie Tompkins and April Scott outline in detail the best practices of rehabilitation for each major symptom in the population with right hemisphere disorders. Fofi Constantinidou and Mary Kennedy offer an overview in Chapter 19 of communication and neuropsychological disorders associated with traumatic brain injury. They discuss principles of rehabilitation as well as specific therapy techniques supported by EBP. In Chapter 20, Nidhi Mahendra and Tammy Hopper describe the cognitive and communicative difficulties in persons with dementia. They further detail the assessment process and the intervention principles and review the available rehabilitation techniques. Nick Miller and Julie Wambaugh present a similarly thorough overview in Chapter 21 of the symptomatology, differential diagnosis, assessment, and rehabilitation of individuals with acquired apraxia of speech. Finally, in the completely revised Chapter 22, Anja Lowit and Raymond Kent provide a thorough review of dysarthria. The authors describe the models of speech production, discuss the taxonomy of the dysarthria syndromes, and expand on practical clinical issues related to dysarthria assessment and rehabilitation.

ACKNOWLEDGMENTS

As the examples show, in the second edition of this text, our efforts focused on adding important updates and relevant information related to the clinical process. To identify these elements, we relied on the input of many individuals, who all are deserving of our thanks. We would like to express our gratitude to all the professionals who have relied on the first edition of the textbook for their professional needs, particularly those who have given us the constructive feedback needed to create an even better textbook. Your comments guided our discussions and decisions, and we sincerely hope that you will enjoy this new edition. We are also grateful to the team members at Jones & Bartlett Learning for their attention to detail and to the anonymous reviewers of both editions. Last, but not least, we thank all the chapter authors for their tremendous efforts to produce such outstanding contributions.

Ilias Papathanasiou
Patrick Coppens

REFERENCE

Martin, N., Thompson, C. K., & Worrall, L. (2008). *Aphasia rehabilitation: The impairment and its consequences*. San Diego, CA: Plural.

About the Authors

Ilias Papathanasiou, PhD, FRCSLT, ASHA Fellow, Associate Professor, Department of Speech and Language Therapy, Technological Educational Institute of Western Greece, Patras, Greece

Born in Greece, Dr. Papathanasiou trained in speech–language pathology at the University College London, University of London, England, and holds a master's degree in health sciences from St. George's Medical School, University of London. He completed his PhD at the Institute of Neurology, University College London, University of London, where he studied the mechanisms of recovery of writing in aphasia. His clinical and research interests include the study of the cognitive processes and neural substrates that support spoken and written language, as well as the nature and treatment of acquired impairments of language. Dr. Papathanasiou has contributed numerous scientific papers to refereed journals, written several book chapters, and organized a number of international meetings. He is the founder of the international series of conferences "The Sciences of Aphasia," which started in 2000. He is the editor of the book *Acquired Neurogenic Communication Disorders: A Clinical Perspective* and coeditor of the book *The Sciences of Aphasia: From Therapy to Theory.* He is on the editorial board of *Aphasiology* and *Communications Disorders Quarterly.* Currently, he is an associate professor in the Department of Speech and Language Therapy, Technological Educational Institute of Western Greece, and a research associate in the Department of ENT, Medical School, University of Athens, Greece, where he is actively involved in teaching, clinical research, and service delivery. Dr. Papathanasiou is a Fellow of the Royal College of Speech and Language Therapists (FRCSLT) in the United Kingdom and a Fellow of the American Speech-Language-Hearing Association (ASHA).

Patrick Coppens, PhD, CCC-SLP, Professor, Department of Communication Disorders and Sciences, State University of New York–Plattsburgh, Plattsburgh, New York

Dr. Patrick Coppens is professor in the Department of Communication Disorders and Sciences at SUNY Plattsburgh, where he teaches graduate neurogenics courses. Dr. Coppens was born and educated in Brussels, Belgium, where he acquired an undergraduate degree in Germanic linguistics and a master's degree in neurolinguistics under the mentorship of Yvan Lebrun. His doctorate in communication disorders and sciences was awarded at Southern Illinois University–Carbondale under the mentorship of Randall Robey. Dr. Coppens has 20 years of experience teaching and conducting research in the area of aphasia. He has published and presented extensively in his area of expertise and has edited and contributed to a prior volume, *Aphasia in Atypical Populations.* He sits on the editorial board of *Aphasiology.*

Contributors

Ana Inés Ansaldo
Centre de Recherche de l'Institut Universitaire de
  Gériatrie de Montréal and École d'Orthophonie et
  d'Audiologie
Faculté de Médecine
Université de Montréal
Montreal, Canada

Elizabeth Armstrong
Foundation Chair in Speech Pathology
Edith Cowan University
Perth, Australia

C. Elizabeth Brookshire
Department of Speech and Hearing Sciences
University of Washington
Seattle, Washington

Lucy Bryant
School of Humanities and Social Science
University of Newcastle
Newcastle, Australia

José G. Centeno
Department of Communication Sciences and Disorders
St. John's University
Queens, New York

Chris Code
School of Psychology
University of Exeter
Exeter, England

Fofi Constantinidou
Department of Psychology and Applied Neuroscience
  and Neurobehavioral Research Center
University of Cyprus
Nicosia, Cyprus

Patrick Coppens
Department of Communication Disorders
  and Sciences
State University of New York–Plattsburgh
Plattsburgh, New York

Madeline Cruice
Division of Language and Communication Science
School of Health Sciences
City University London
London, England

Zsolt Cséfalvay
Department of Communication Disorders
Comenius University
Bratislava, Slovakia

Bronwyn Davidson
Audiology, Hearing and Speech Sciences
University of Melbourne
Melbourne, Australia

Edith Durant
Centre de Recherche de l'Institut Universitaire de Gériatrie
    de Montréal and École d'Orthophonie et d'Audiologie
Faculté de Médecine
Université de Montréal
Montreal, Canada

Ioannis Evdokimidis
Department of Neurology
Medical School
National and Kapodistrian University of Athens
Athens, Greece

Alison Ferguson
School of Humanities and Social Science
University of Newcastle
Newcastle, Australia

Sue Franklin
Department of Speech and Language Therapy
University of Limerick
Limerick, Ireland

Ladan Ghazi-Saidi
Centre de Recherche de l'Institut Universitaire de Gériatrie
    de Montréal
Montreal, Canada

Katerina Hilari
Division of Language and Communication Science
School of Health Sciences
City University London
London, England

Tammy Hopper
Department of Speech Pathology and Audiology
Faculty of Rehabilitation Medicine
University of Alberta
Alberta, Canada

Dimitrios S. Kasselimis
Department of Neurology
Medical School
National and Kapodistrian University of Athens
Athens, Greece

Diane L. Kendall
Department of Speech and Hearing Sciences
University of Washington
Seattle, Washington

Mary Kennedy
Department of Communication Sciences and Disorders
Crean College of Health and Behavioral Sciences
Chapman University
Orange, California

Raymond (Ray) D. Kent
The Waisman Center
University of Wisconsin Madison
Madison, Wisconsin

Ekaterini Klepousniotou
Institute of Psychological Sciences
University of Leeds
Leeds, England

Anja Lowit
School of Psychological Sciences and Health
Strathclyde University
Glasgow, Scotland

Nidhi Mahendra
Department of Communicative Sciences and Disorders
California State University–East Bay
Hayward, California

Jane Marshall
Division of Language and Communication Science
School of Health Sciences
City University London
London, England

Nadine Martin
Department of Communication Sciences and Disorders
Temple University
Philadelphia, Pennsylvania

Jamie Mayer
School of Allied Health and Communicative Disorders
Northern Illinois University
DeKalb, Illinois

Nick Miller
Institute of Health and Society
Speech and Language Sciences
University of Newcastle upon Tyne
Newcastle upon Tyne, England

Julie Morris
School of Education, Communication, and Language
Sciences
University of Newcastle upon Tyne
Newcastle upon Tyne, England

Laura Murray
Department of Speech and Hearing Sciences
Indiana University
Bloomington, Indiana

Ilias Papathanasiou
Department of Speech and Language Therapy
Technological Educational Institute of Western Greece
Patras, Greece

Constantin Potagas
Department of Neurology
Medical School
National and Kapodistrian University of Athens
Athens, Greece

Ellyn A. Riley
Department of Communication Sciences and Disorders
Syracuse University
Syracuse, New York

April G. Scott
Speech, Hearing and Learning Services
Longwood University
Farmville, Virginia

Sue Sherratt
University of Newcastle
Newcastle, Australia, and
University of Queensland
Brisbane, Australia

Nina Simmons-Mackie
Department of Communication Sciences and Disorders
Southeastern Louisiana University
Hammond, Louisiana

Connie A. Tompkins
Department of Communication Sciences and Disorders
University of Pittsburgh
Pittsburgh, Pennsylvania

Julie Wambaugh
Department of Communication Sciences and Disorders
University of Utah
Salt Lake City, Utah

Linda Worrall
School of Health and Rehabilitation Sciences
University of Queensland
Brisbane, Australia

OBJECTIVES

The reader will be able to:

1. Define aphasia.
2. Describe the epidemiology of aphasia.
3. Understand the principles of care for people with aphasia.
4. Describe the basic concepts of the ICF framework.
5. Understand the basic issues of aphasia efficiency.
6. Describe the evidence supporting the efficacy of aphasia therapy.

Aphasia and Related Neurogenic Communication Disorders: Basic Concepts, Management, and Efficacy

Ilias Papathanasiou, Patrick Coppens, and
Bronwyn Davidson

INTRODUCTION

The main objective of this book is the study of aphasia and aphasia rehabilitation. Throughout this volume, aphasia is approached from a variety of perspectives, including neurological, linguistic, neuropsychological, and psychosocial. Each chapter further seeks to provide practical clinical applications supported by evidence-based practice (EBP) principles to link theoretical models to clinical practice for researchers, clinicians, and clinicians in training. Because these important basic concepts permeate all chapters, it is imperative that we define and explain them at the outset. This introduction, therefore, defines aphasia, outlines its management approaches and service delivery options, describes the basic EBP principles, and reviews the evidence on the efficacy of aphasia therapy.

WHAT IS APHASIA?

Many definitions of aphasia have been proposed during the history of aphasiology. These reflect the theoretical constructs and concerns of their time, and there is no reason to believe that any current definition will necessarily withstand further scientific developments. Still, generating an operational definition of aphasia is a necessary, albeit challenging, task because it is a multidimensional concept. From a neurological perspective, aphasia is an acquired language impairment resulting from a focal brain lesion in the absence of other cognitive, motor, or sensory impairments. This language impairment can be present in all language components (phonology, morphology, syntax, semantics, pragmatics), across all modalities (speaking, reading, writing, signing), and in the output (expression) and input (comprehension) modes. Describing the language symptoms of a given individual with aphasia may help identify a particular lesion location and possibly suggest a specific brain pathology (Damasio, 1992; Goodglass & Kaplan, 1983). From a neurolinguistic perspective, aphasia is a breakdown in specific language domains resulting from a focal lesion (Lesser, 1987). From a cognitive perspective, aphasia is considered the selective breakdown of language processing itself, of underlying cognitive skills, or of the necessary cognitive resources resulting from a focal lesion (Ellis & Young, 1988; McNeil, 1982). Finally, from a functional perspective, aphasia is a communication impairment masking inherent competence (Kagan, 1995). So, through the years, these different schools of thought have led researchers to generate many different definitions of aphasia.

Regardless of the perspective one espouses, most researchers agree on common elements in any definition of aphasia: Aphasia (a) is a mostly language-level problem, (b) includes receptive and expressive components, (c) is multimodal in nature, and (d) is caused by a central nervous system dysfunction. The first element seems obvious, but some authors do use the label *aphasia* to refer to acquired language impairment secondary to cognitive difficulties (following closed head injury or dementia, for example). Although it is possible for a closed head injury to cause damage to the language areas of the brain, the symptomatology is usually difficult to classify using the aphasia taxonomy because most of the communicative difficulties are caused by cognitive dysfunction (Wiig, Alexander, & Secord, 1988). On the other hand, it is not the case that the aphasic symptomatology displayed by a stroke victim is the consequence of cognitive impairments only, although cognitive processes can be involved. We argue in favor of using the term *aphasia* exclusively for acquired focal lesions in the language-dominant hemisphere. Therefore, the first part of this volume covers *aphasia*, and the second part addresses *related* disorders.

Whereas most definitions of aphasia center on the acquired neurological impairments impeding language function, the International Classification of Functioning, Disability, and Health (ICF; World Health Organization [WHO], 2001) focuses our attention on the consequences that these impairments have on the person's communicative and social functioning and quality of life (Martin, Thompson, & Worrall, 2008). Therefore, an up-to-date working definition of aphasia should include all these elements.

For the purpose of this book, we operationally define *aphasia* as *an acquired selective impairment of language modalities and functions resulting from a focal brain lesion in the language-dominant hemisphere that affects the person's communicative and social functioning, quality of life, and the quality of life of his or her relatives and caregivers.*

POPULATION AND PUBLIC HEALTH APPROACHES IN APHASIA

Approximately 30–35% of stroke survivors have aphasia on discharge from the hospital following a stroke, with the prevalence of speech (dysarthria) and language (aphasia) disability 6 months after stroke reported as 30–50/100,000 (Dickey et al., 2010; Enderby & Davies, 1989; Engelter et al., 2006). People with aphasia have higher health-care costs (8.5% or $1,700 attributable cost) and longer length of stays in the hospital (6.5%) compared with stroke survivors without aphasia (Ellis, Simpson, Bonilha, Mauldin, & Simpson, 2012). People with stroke-related aphasia may require additional services to address their communication disability in the hospital and also during community life, and such services might reduce their length of stay or incidence of adverse events (Bartlett, Blais, Tamblyn, Clermont, & MacGibbon, 2008; Hemsley, Werninck, & Worrall, 2013). However, the management of swallowing disorders (dysphagia) may be prioritized over aphasia services in acute hospital settings due to inadequate staffing ratios and lack of appropriate therapy space/resources (Foster, O'Halloran, Rose, & Worrall, 2015; Rose, Ferguson, Power, Togher, & Worrall, 2014). In addition, people with aphasia have poor long-term outcomes after stroke, including consequences such as social isolation, depression, and poor quality of life for themselves and their family members (Cruice, Worrall, & Hickson, 2006; Enderby & Davies, 1989; Grawburg, Howe, Worrall, & Scarinci, 2014; Hilari & Byng, 2009; Vickers, 2010). As a chronic disability, aphasia generates a number of long-term service needs, including therapy to enable functional and socially relevant communication (Worrall et al., 2011). Provision of quality, efficient, evidence-based care is critical for people with aphasia, their families, and health-care systems.

The study of aphasia and the service delivery systems for people with aphasia have traditionally centered on the individual with aphasia. Increasingly, the need for greater public awareness of aphasia has become apparent, as research has reported that people with aphasia and their families have identified barriers to social inclusion that exist due to a lack of community understanding of what aphasia is and how changes in spoken and written language have an impact on a person's daily functioning (Code et al., 2001, in press; Code & Petherham, 2011; Patterson et al., 2015; Worrall et al., 2013). Education programs to train communication partners of people with aphasia provide an example of interventions that seek to address communication access for those with communication disability (Simmons-Mackie, Raymer, Armstrong, Holland, & Cherney, 2010).

Thus, in addition to being responsive to the individual with aphasia, a need for public awareness and community interventions has been identified (McAllister, Wylie, Davidson, & Marshall, 2013). New models of public health highlight the promotion of health in the whole population, human rights, and the need to address health and social inequities, as discussed by the WHO (2013). Across the globe, there are many people with aphasia for whom services are unavailable or inaccessible. The term *underserved* specifies communities where the health and social services workforce is insufficient and also those in which people may experience barriers (e.g., distance, economic, cultural) to accessing services and participation in their community. Underserved communities exist in both minority and majority world countries (Wylie, McAllister, Davidson, & Marshall, 2013), and the demand for services relevant to the cultural and community context grows.

The *World Report on Disability* (WHO and the World Bank, 2011) provides a catalyst for an examination of how the needs of people with aphasia throughout the world are currently met. It offers an opportunity for the speech pathology profession to further its engagement with people with aphasia to ensure public awareness of aphasia and equitable access to care (Worrall et al., 2013).

CARE FOR PEOPLE WITH APHASIA

At no other time in the history of care of people with aphasia has the context in which clinicians work influenced the care that people with aphasia are receiving. Throughout the world, changes in health-care policies, insurance schemes, national health plans, political climate, clinical licensure and specialization, and professional training have a dramatic impact on the accessibility of services for people with aphasia as well as on the quality of the services provided. Also, advances in science and new technology have changed the focus of services and their delivery. However, even these developments are challenging the clinician as the focus of

therapy has moved from the management of the specific communication impairments of the person with aphasia to a broader, more holistic management of the person and his or her specific environment.

The ICF Framework

A worldwide framework was introduced by the WHO to redefine functioning and disability in an effort to increase awareness of the holistic components of health-care delivery and the interaction between impairment and environment that affects the participation and quality of life of the person with aphasia. The two primary levels within the most recent WHO ICF are (a) body structure and functioning and (b) activity and participation (WHO, 2001) (see Figure 1.1).

For a person with aphasia, *body functions and structure* refer to impairments of the brain and brain functions. *Activity* refers to tasks or actions that involve the four language modalities—listening, speaking, reading, and writing—as well as the daily functional communication tasks, such as conversing with family members and friends, reading a newspaper, writing an e-mail, and the like. These modalities have been the traditional focus of assessment and intervention.

The concepts of *activities and participation* add the notion of engagement in daily life and include immediate and long-term real-life goals. This might include shopping, going on a vacation, attending religious services, participating in local community organizations, and so on. For people with aphasia, these constructs represent the ability to use language in context to communicate. *Environment* is another key concept in the ICF. This includes relationships with others, policies and regulations, the use of assistive technology, physical environmental factors, and attitudes of individuals and society toward the person with aphasia.

The WHO-ICF framework broadens the classic biomedical models to a more holistic service delivery approach for people with aphasia. Viewing aphasia through this framework helps us consider social contacts as fundamental to the context in which people with aphasia communicate and engage in daily life activities and helps us realize that the communication partners are also responsible, in part, for the social consequences linked to aphasia. The framework highlights the dynamic interaction of all the important variables, such as risk factors, social support, etiologies, genetics, abilities, environmental factors, daily habits of social participation, and so on. Finally, this framework helps clinicians focus on the core features of health and well-being, to see aphasia within the context of real-life situations, and to encourage full

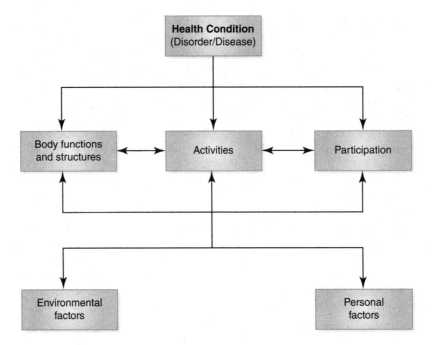

Figure 1.1   The World Health Organization's ICF model.

World Health Organization. (2001). International classification of functioning, disability and health. Geneva, Switzerland: Author. p.18.

life participation, culminating in an overall focus on quality of life with aphasia.

The Best Practice Recommendations

In 2015, the WHO reported that while health services have traditionally been nationally focused, the move toward globalization of health care is now apparent. This trend toward globalization to improve the health and well-being of people around the world entails the expectation that health-care services will follow similar quality standards and guidelines throughout the world (Schroth & Khawaja, 2007). It is anticipated that globalization will promote equality of services, improve health-care quality, decrease variations in practice, and stimulate research to support international health-care standards. Like other sectors of health care, rehabilitation, and more specifically aphasia rehabilitation, is moving toward increased sharing and equivalence of services internationally.

Power et al. (2015) developed and validated a national set of best practice statements for use in poststroke aphasia rehabilitation in Australia. They reported that a national community of practice of over 250 speech pathologists, researchers, consumers, and policy makers developed a framework consisting of eight areas of care in aphasia rehabilitation. This framework provided the structure for the development of a care pathway containing aphasia

rehabilitation best practice statements. The agreed areas of care were (a) receiving the right referrals, (b) optimizing initial contact, (c) setting goals and measuring outcomes, (d) assessing, (e) providing intervention, (f) enhancing the communicative environment, (g) enhancing personal factors, and (h) planning for transitions and discharges. The final outcome of this study was to develop a national set of 82 best practice statements across eight care areas for the rehabilitation of people with aphasia, which was the first to be validated by an expert panel. These best practice statements may require some adaptation for other regions; however, the majority of the data should be common and internationally applicable.

Subsequently, Aphasia United set up a working group to develop international best practice recommendations for aphasia. Aphasia United is an international umbrella organization founded in 2011 to advance aphasia services and science around the world. A key aim of Aphasia United has been to bring together international stakeholders (e.g., researchers, clinicians, consumers) to address global needs of aphasia rehabilitation (for more information, visit http://www.shrs.uq.edu.au/AphasiaUnited). The working group has developed the international best practice recommendations for aphasia (see the Appendix). Implementation of these recommendations worldwide, as well as ongoing revision and updating, will be required for people living with aphasia to obtain the best possible services.

WHAT IS APHASIA THERAPY?

Traditionally, aphasia rehabilitation has been behavioral in nature. That is, aphasia therapy is the supportive process designed to help people with aphasia modify their current communicative behaviors with practice to maximize their communication proficiency. This is true whether the service delivery model is one-on-one with a clinician, in group therapy, using a computer program, or through telepractice. However, nonbehavioral adjuvant therapy approaches for aphasia have also been recently investigated, such as pharmacotherapy and noninvasive brain stimulation protocols. It is believed that, in time, these procedures have the potential to be used clinically if deemed efficacious and safe. The main focus of this volume is to analyze the behavioral rehabilitation process of aphasia, emphasizing the clinician-client-family interaction based on the precepts of the ICF framework of the WHO. In the following sections, these adjuvant and alternative aphasia therapy delivery systems are briefly discussed.

Group Therapy

There are many types of approaches for group therapy in aphasia; they range from more didactic purposes to a focus on social and emotional support. However, most groups tend to be multipurpose (Kearns & Elman, 2008). Treatment efficacy has been shown to be overall positive (e.g., Wertz et al, 1981), even in patients in the chronic stages of recovery (e.g., Elman & Bernstein-Ellis, 1999). Based on a systematic review, Lanyon, Rose, and Worrall (2013) concluded that group therapy was efficacious for specific language processes, such as word finding, which translated into improved scores on formal assessment batteries. The authors further reported that group therapy effected positive changes on social networks, but could not evidence improvements in the activity/participation domain of the ICF because of lack of data.

Group therapy for aphasia was traditionally seen either as a transitional phase between individual therapy and dismissal or as an add-on technique to facilitate stimulus generalization. However, group therapy is now considered an essential component of aphasia therapy within the framework of the ICF (Kearns & Elman, 2008).

Computer-Based Therapy

Because of the time demands on clinicians, providing therapy via computer to people with aphasia seems a reasonable way to increase the amount and intensity of therapy in a cost-effective fashion. However, the data on the efficacy of this service delivery model is sparse. While acknowledging the lack of data, Zheng, Lynch, and Taylor (2014) concluded in a recent systematic review that computer therapy is better than no therapy and in some cases as good as therapy provided by a clinician. However, it may be that computer therapy still needs some clinician support to be fully effective. Unfortunately, no study has objectified the potential benefits of a combined (clinician + computer) approach.

Telepractice

The technological advances in various electronic devices and broadband availability now allow for reliable remote contacts between individuals. As a consequence, clinicians and clients do not need to be in the same physical location to accomplish a therapy session, a delivery means that is variously referred to as *telepractice, telerehabilitation, teletreatment, telehealth,* or *teletherapy*. This may be particularly useful when the person with aphasia is unable to travel to a clinic because of physical constraints or distance. However, the efficacy of such a service delivery model still has to be demonstrated, and some related issues are still being debated, such as necessary certification requirements, privacy, and third-party reimbursement (e.g., http://www.asha.org/PRPSpecificTopic.aspx?folderid= 8589934956&section=Key_Issues). Still, the American Speech-Language Hearing Association (ASHA) is interested in this recent service delivery as the association created a new special interest group (SIG 18) devoted to the subject.

Overall, the available (albeit still limited) data on the subject of telepractice efficacy are positive. Hall, Boisvert, and Steele (2013) performed a systematic review of the accumulated evidence and concluded that, for both assessment and therapy purposes, telepractice was equivalent to face-to-face sessions. The only concerns included technology and privacy issues, which the authors deemed easily surmountable.

Pharmacotherapy

The rationale for using pharmacological agents to improve aphasia symptoms relates to the manipulation of neurotransmitter levels with the intent of stimulating widespread cerebral activity. As such, these agents do not have an impact on language specifically but rather influence the widespread cognitive substrates of language processing, such as attention/concentration, short-term memory, or mood (Berthier, 2014). A wide variety of drugs have been investigated that act on an array of neurotransmitters (Berthier, Pulvermüller, Davila, Garcia Casares, & Gutierrez, 2011), with variable results. For example, in a review of dopaminergic therapy for aphasia, Gill and Leff (2014) noted that half the studies reviewed showed an effect and half did not, a discrepancy likely due to unspecified candidacy issues.

However, for some patients, the language improvements seem to be significant. Galling, Goorah, Berthier, and Sage (2014) treated a person with nonfluent aphasia with a combination of bromocriptine and language therapy. The client improved on all measures of language production but not comprehension. The authors concluded that, because bromocriptine affects mostly frontal brain regions, the best candidates would be patients with Broca or transcortical motor aphasia, particularly if adynamic characteristics predominate. Furthermore, they noted that only a concomitant regimen of language therapy and medication effected positive changes, an observation confirmed by other studies (e.g., de Boissezon, Peran, de Boysson, & Démonet, 2007). Interestingly, the intensity of the language therapy may also influence the amount of recovery. Berthier et al. (2014) compared massed-practice with distributed-practice language therapy in conjunction with donepezil (an acetylcholine agonist), and the more intensive therapy protocol yielded better results. In sum, the addition of neuropharmacological agents seems to enhance the effects of speech-language therapy to some degree. However, the actions of these substances are not on language per se but rather on the underlying cognitive support functions. In the best cases, these neurological changes facilitate or prime the brain to take advantage of behavioral language therapy because it is only when the two approaches are concomitant that the best results are observed. Finally, the benefits of pharmacological agents seem to depend on patient candidacy factors, such as lesion location or symptomatology, and on the intensity of the therapy delivery, but these factors are not well understood yet. It is only when researchers have a better grasp on these issues that pharmacological adjuvant therapy may be added to the existing behavioral therapy approaches for aphasia.

Noninvasive Brain Stimulation Approaches

Two noninvasive cortical stimulation approaches have been used in individuals with aphasia: repetitive transcranial magnetic stimulation (rTMS) and transcranial direct current stimulation (tDCS). Both techniques are able to inhibit or excite cortical areas, depending on the setting used; however, the majority of the research studies used inhibition of right hemisphere areas. Recent reviews have confirmed that both rTMS and tDCS showed increased language performance (Devlin & Watkins, 2007; Murdoch & Barwood, 2013; Torres, Drebing, & Hamilton, 2013), although the results mostly focused on individuals with chronic nonfluent aphasia and on language skills (e.g., naming) rather than language use (i.e., communication efficacy). Also, not all results were positive (e.g., Elsner, Kugler, Pohl, & Mehrholz, 2013; Seniow et al., 2013; Volpato et al., 2013), and many clinical questions still remain to be investigated.

In recent years, tDCS has received more attention than rTMS because it is believed to offer more advantages, such as cost, portability, and possibly safety (Murdoch & Barwood, 2013; Schlaug, Marchina, & Wan, 2011), but rTMS may be more efficacious (Murdoch & Barwood, 2013) and may effect more long-lasting changes (Murdoch & Barwood, 2013; Torres et al., 2013).

In sum, these cortical stimulation techniques seem to enhance the effects of language therapy for some, if not most, individuals with aphasia. However, before these can be used routinely in clinical situations, several candidacy issues require more investigation. Researchers need to determine which patients are most likely to benefit from which kind of stimulation.

WHAT IS EVIDENCE-BASED PRACTICE IN APHASIA THERAPY?

Clinicians have an ethical responsibility to treat their clients to the best of their ability using the best available rehabilitation approaches. EBP helps provide quality control. EBP is an approach to decision making in which the clinician uses the best evidence available, in consultation with the individual with aphasia, to select the best treatment option.

There are three prongs to EBP (Dollaghan, 2007): best available (external) evidence, client/family input and context, and clinical expertise. The clinician is required to integrate all three aspects of EBP to maximize quality of services (e.g., ASHA, 2005). It is beyond the scope of this volume to analyze each component of EBP in depth; however, because each subsequent chapter provides the best available evidence to support clinical approaches, we need to describe how good scientific information is developed and how professional peer-reviewed publications are evaluated.

The process of developing a novel therapy approach is a scientific endeavor that unfolds over time. This process, based on a medical model, is described as the "five-phase" model. In essence, it starts with a small-scale study testing a new treatment idea, but the proposed treatment needs to be investigated further in a larger sample with better control measures, applied to everyday clinical practice, and finally refined for maximal efficiency. In the context of speech-language pathology, *efficacy* refers to the fact that a treatment works in ideal conditions for a population; *effectiveness* refers to the fact that the treatment works in everyday clinical practice for individuals; and *efficiency* refers to the most efficient way to apply the treatment program. Any published study reporting results, regardless of what stage of the model it addresses, must be evaluated on its own merits. A "levels-of-evidence" scale was developed for this purpose. The five-stage model and the levels-of-evidence scale are described in detail next.

Five-Phase Model of Outcomes Research

In the five-phase model of outcomes research, phase I is designed to develop the research hypotheses, to establish the safety of the treatment, and to detect potential treatment effects in case studies, single-subject experiments, or small-group experiments (e.g., Robey & Schultz, 1998; Wertz, 2000).

Phase II is undertaken if the results of phase I are positive. This phase seeks to control variables more carefully, to optimize and standardize the treatment, to try to explain why the treatment works, to develop outcome measures, and so forth. Again, case studies, single-subject experiments, and small-group experiments with or without a control group are appropriate for phase II.

Phase III is the efficacy phase. This "clinical trial" phase requires a large sample size, strict experimental controls, and random group assignment. A multicenter research effort is often necessary to complete a phase III study.

Phase IV is the effectiveness phase. This phase applies an efficacious treatment (according to phase III) in clinical practice with typical patients under typical conditions. During this phase, the treatment may focus on a specific type of client (e.g., with Broca or Wernicke aphasia). A large sample size is again required, but control groups are not mandatory.

Phase V is the efficiency phase. This phase focuses on the cost-benefit ratio of the treatment as well as the general value of the treatment (e.g., consumer satisfaction, quality of life, value to society). Treatment variations are explored experimentally (intensity, length, delivery mode, cost, etc.) while maintaining the effectiveness level of phase IV.

Levels-of-Evidence Scale

There are several versions of the levels-of-evidence scale, but all are designed to evaluate the published evidence of a given topic. This implies that not all evidence is created equal, and that some publications should be given more weight than others when investigating a specific approach or treatment. The scale also uses Roman numerals but should not be confused with the preceding phase model.

Level I is used for meta-analyses or multiple randomized control trials (RCTs are considered the "gold standard" for medical evidence). Level Ia corresponds to one RCT. Levels II and IIa are quasi-experiments because groups are not randomized. Level III is used for nonexperimental studies, such as descriptive case studies or correlation studies. Level IV includes nonempirical information, such as expert opinion and committee reports.

It is important to realize that within each level of evidence there are good studies and poor studies. There are very good level III studies, as there are very poor level I studies. The study's experimental design should not be the only factor of quality; a clinician should also consider other factors, such as internal validity threats and significance of the hypothesis (Dollaghan, 2007).

DOES APHASIA THERAPY WORK?

Early group studies looking at aphasia therapy efficacy reported contradictory results, but in general, their research methods or designs were weak. Sarno, Silverman, and Sands (1970) reported no difference between treated and untreated individuals with severe aphasia, whereas several other group studies argued that speech-language therapy yielded significant improvement (Basso, Capitani, & Vignolo, 1979; Butfield & Zangwill, 1946; Poeck, Huber, & Willmes, 1989; Shewan & Kertesz, 1984; Vignolo, 1964; Wertz et al., 1981).

Although the positive results predominated then, an overall conclusion cannot be drawn confidently because of the weakness of the evidence. At that time, only two studies used random group assignment, and the results were again contradictory. Lincoln et al. (1984) observed no significant outcome differences between treatment and no-treatment groups, whereas Wertz et al. (1986) found that individuals with aphasia who were treated by a speech-language pathologist made significantly more improvement than did untreated individuals or individuals treated by a family member at home. When comparing the scientific value of these two studies, it is clear that the former had a much weaker design and weaker methods than the latter. For example, Lincoln et al. (1984) included individuals with multiple strokes, and fewer than 30% of the treatment group individuals received the prescribed amount of treatment. It is only more recently, with an increased awareness and understanding of statistical methods, that the weight of the evidence tipped the balance positively.

Single-subject designs cannot address efficacy (Robey & Schultz, 1998), and RCTs are difficult to design in our field because random assignment to groups is problematic (one cannot ethically assign an individual with aphasia to a no-treatment group). Therefore, researchers have recently started generating meta-analyses and computing effect size to provide more reliable evidence. A meta-analysis is a compilation of many similar studies for the purpose of combining the reported treatment effect in one large statistical analysis. An *effect size* is a simple computation of the magnitude of the effect observed (Schiavetti, Metz, & Orlikoff, 2011). Effect size can be calculated in single-subject or group designs and can also be combined into a meta-analysis for a specific therapy approach (Beeson & Robey, 2006).

Three meta-analyses (Robey, 1994, 1998; Whurr, Lorch, & Nye, 1992) of clinical outcomes in the treatment of aphasia have been reported. Whurr et al. (1992) concluded that there was not enough information in the literature to draw a definite conclusion on aphasia treatment efficacy. However, there were some statistical limitations to their analysis (Robey, 1994).

Robey (1994), on the other hand, concluded that when treatment was initiated in the acute stage, the treatment effect was medium to large, which was double that of spontaneous recovery, and that when treatment was started in the more chronic stage, the effect was small to medium. Robey (1998) essentially replicated the previous meta-analysis with a larger sample of studies, and the results were very similar. Therefore, we can reasonably conclude that the answer to the title question is "yes," and that "on average, treatment for aphasic persons is effective" (Robey, 1998, p. 181).

This positive (and reassuring) conclusion does not mean that we can rest on our laurels. However, now that we know that aphasia therapy works, we need to ascertain whether specific treatments work and for whom (Brady, Kelly, Godwin, & Enderby, 2012). ASHA and the Academy of Neurologic Communication Disorders and Sciences (ANCDS) have been spearheading this effort in recent years. ANCDS is developing and disseminating EBP guidelines for a range of neurological conditions, and ASHA is building the Compendium of EBP Guidelines and Systematic Reviews, which is a searchable repository of information on a wide variety of topics, including neurogenic communication disorders, as well as developing "evidence maps" that provide evidence for all three prongs of EBP given a specific topic. The interested reader is referred to these associations' respective websites for a perusal of this valuable information.

STUDY QUESTIONS

1. List and explain the important elements in a definition of aphasia.
2. Describe the main elements of the ICF framework.
3. How does the ICF change the service delivery approach for aphasia.
4. Explain the globalization process of the WHO regarding aphasia therapy.
5. Cite and discuss 2 types of service delivery models for aphasia therapy different than the traditional one-on-one approach.
6. Discuss the efficacy of pharmacotherapy for aphasia.
7. Define tDCS and rTMS and discuss their potential contributions to aphasia therapy.
8. Define and contrast the terms *efficacy*, *effectiveness*, and *efficiency* as related to aphasia therapy.
9. What are the 5 phases of outcome research?
10. What evidence do we have that aphasia therapy is efficacious?

REFERENCES

American Speech-Language-Hearing Association. (2005). *Evidence-based practice in communication disorders* [Position statement]. Retrieved from http://www.asha.org/docs/html/PS2005-00221.html

Bartlett, G., Blais, R., Tamblyn, R., Clermont, R. J., & MacGibbon, B. (2008). Impact of patient communication problems on the range of preventable adverse events in acute care settings. *Canadian Medical Association Journal*, 178, 1555–1562.

Basso, A., Capitani, E., & Vignolo, L. A. (1979). Influence of rehabilitation on language skills in aphasic patients: A controlled study. *Archives of Neurology*, 36, 190–196.

Beeson, P. M., & Robey, R. R. (2006). Evaluating single-subject treatment research: Lessons learned from the aphasia literature. *Neuropsychology Review*, 16, 161–169.

Berthier, M. L. (2014). Cognitive enhancing drugs in aphasia: A vote for hope. *Aphasiology*, 28(2), 128–132.

Berthier, M. L., Davila, G., Green-Heredia, C., Moreno Torres, I., Juarez y Ruiz de Mier, R., De-Torres, I., et al. (2014). Massed sentence repetition training can augment and speed up recovery of speech production deficits in patients with chronic conduction aphasia receiving donepezil treatment. *Aphasiology*, 28(2), 188–218.

Berthier, M. L., Pulvermüller, F., Davila, G., Garcia Casares, N., & Gutierrez, A. (2011). Drug therapy of post-stroke aphasia: A review of current evidence. *Neuropsychological Review*, 21, 302–317.

Brady, M. C., Kelly, H., Godwin, J., & Enderby, P. (2012). Speech and language therapy for aphasia following stroke. *Cochrane Database Systematic Review*, 16(5), CD000425. doi:10.1002/14651858.CD000425.pub3

Butfield, E., & Zangwill, O. (1946). Re-education in aphasia: A review of 70 cases. *Journal of Neurology, Neurosurgery, and Psychiatry*, 9, 75–79.

Code, C., & Petherham, B. (2011). Delivering for aphasia. *International Journal of Speech Language Pathology*, 13(3), 3–10.

Code, C., Papathanasiou, I., Rubio-Bruno, S., de la Paz Cabana, M., Villanueva, M.M., Haaland-Johansen, L., et al. (in press). International patterns of the public awareness of aphasia. *International Journal of Language and Communication Disorders*.

Code, C., Simmons-Mackie, N., Armstrong, E., Stiegler, L., Armstrong, J., Bushby, E., et al. (2001). The public awareness of aphasia: An international survey. *International Journal of Language and Communication Disorders*, 36(Suppl.), 1–6.

Cruice, M., Worrall, L., & Hickson, L. (2006). Quantifying aphasic people's social lives in the context of non-aphasic peers. *Aphasiology*, 20, 1210–1225.

Damasio, A. R. (1992). Aphasia. *New England Journal of Medicine*, 326, 531–539.

De Boissezon, X., Peran, P., de Boysson, C., & Démonet, J.-F. (2007). Pharmacotherapy of aphasia: Myth or reality? *Brain and Language*, 102, 114–125.

Devlin, J. T., & Watkins, K. E. (2007). Stimulating language: Insights from TMS. *Brain*, 130, 610–622.

Dickey, L., Kagan, A., Lindsay, M. P., Fang, J., Rowland, A., & Black, S. (2010). Incidence and profile of inpatient stroke-induced aphasia in Ontario, Canada. *Archives of Physical Medicine and Rehabilitation*, 91, 196–201.

Dollaghan, C. A. (2007). *The handbook for evidence-based practice in communication disorders*. Baltimore, MD: Brookes.

Ellis, A. W., & Young, A. W. (1988). *Human cognitive neuropsychology*. Hove, UK: Erlbaum.

Ellis, C., Simpson, A. N., Bonilha, H., Mauldin, P. D., & Simpson, K. N. (2012). The one-year attributable cost of poststroke aphasia. *Stroke*, 43, 1429–1431.

Elman, R. J., & Bernstein-Ellis, E. (1999). The efficacy of group communication treatment in adults with chronic aphasia. *Journal of Speech and Hearing Research*, 42, 411–419.

Elsner, B., Kugler, J., Pohl, M., & Mehrholz, J. (2013). Transcranial direct current stimulation (tDCS) for improving aphasia in patients after stroke [Review]. *The Cochrane Library*, 6, 1–45.

Enderby, P., & Davies, P. (1989), Communication disorders: Planning a service to meet the needs. *British Journal of Communication Disorders*, 24, 301–331.

Engelter, S. T., Gostynski, M., Papa, A., Frei, M., Born, C., Ajdacic-Gross, V., et al. (2006). Epidemiology of aphasia attributable to first ischemic stroke: Incidence, severity, fluency, etiology, and thrombolysis. *Stroke*, 37, 1379–1384.

Foster, A., O'Halloran, R., Rose, M., & Worrall, L. (2015). "Communication is taking a back seat": Speech pathologists' perceptions of aphasia management in acute hospital settings. *Aphasiology* [early online, 2015]. doi:10.1080/026870 38.2014.9851859

Galling, M. A., Goorah, N., Berthier, M. L., & Sage, K. (2014). A clinical study of the combined use of bromocriptine and speech and language therapy in the treatment of a person with aphasia. *Aphasiology*, 28(2), 171–187.

Gill, S. K., & Leff, A. P. (2014). Dopaminergic therapy in aphasia. *Aphasiology*, 28(2), 155–170.

Goodglass, H., & Kaplan, E. (1983). *The assessment of aphasia and related disorders* (2nd ed.). Philadelphia, PA: Lea & Febiger.

Grawburg, M., Howe, T., Worrall, L., & Scarinci, N. (2014). Describing the impact of aphasia on close family members using the ICF framework. *Disability and Rehabilitation*, 36, 1184–1195.

Hall, N., Boisvert, M., & Steele, R. (2013). Telepractice in the assessment and treratment of individuals with aphasia: A systematic review. *International Journal of Telerehabilitation*, 5(1), 27–38.

Hemsley, B., Werninck, M., & Worrall, L. (2013). "That really shouldn't have happened": People with aphasia and their spouses narrate adverse events in hospital. *Aphasiology*, 27, 706–722.

Hilari, K., & Byng, S. (2009). Health-related quality of life in people with severe aphasia. *International Journal of Language and Communication Disorders*, 44, 193–205.

Kagan, A. (1995). Revealing the competence of aphasic adults through conversation: A challenge to health care professionals. *Topics in Stroke Rehabilitation*, 2(1), 15–28.

Kearns, K. P., & Elman, R. J. (2008). Group therapy for aphasia: Theoretic and practical considerations. In R. Chapey (Ed.), *Language intervention strategies in aphasia and related neurogenic communication disorders* (5th ed., pp. 376–400). Baltimore, MD: Lippincott Williams & Wilkins.

Lanyon, L. E., Rose, M. L., & Worrall, L. (2013). The efficacy of outpatient and community-based aphasia group interventions: A systematic review. *International Journal of Speech-Language Pathology*, 15(4), 359–374.

Lesser, R. (1987). Cognitive neuropsychological influences on aphasia therapy. *Aphasiology*, 1, 189–200.

Lincoln, N. B., McGuirk, E., Mulley, G. P., Lendrem, W., Jones, A. C., & Mitchell, J. R. A. (1984). Effectiveness of speech therapy for aphasic stroke patients: A randomized controlled trial. *Lancet*, 1, 1197–1200.

Martin, N., Thompson, C. K., & Worrall, L. (2008). *Aphasia rehabilitation: The impairment and its consequences*. San Diego, CA: Plural.

McAllister, L., Wylie, K., Davidson, B., & Marshall, J. (2013). The World Report on Disability: An impetus to reconceptualise services for people with communication disability. *International Journal of Speech Language Pathology*, 15(1), 118–126.

McNeil, M. R. (1982). The nature of aphasia in adults. In N. J. Lass, L. V. McReynolds, J. L. Northern, & D. E. Yoder (Eds.), *Speech, language, and hearing: Volume III. Pathologies of speech and language* (pp. 692–740). Philadelphia, PA: Saunders.

Murdoch, B. E., & Barwood, C. H. S. (2013). Non-invasive brain stimulation: A new frontier in the treatment of neurogenic speech-language disorders. *International Journal of Speech-Language Pathology*, 15(3), 234–244.

Patterson, R., Robert, A., Berry, R., Cain, M., Iqbal, M., Code, C., et al. (2015). Raising public awareness of aphasia in southern Ontario, Canada: A survey. *International Journal of Speech-Language Pathology*, 17(2), 121–126

Poeck, K., Huber, W., & Willmes, K. (1989). Outcome of intensive language rehabilitation in aphasia. *Journal of Speech and Hearing Disorders, 54,* 471–479.

Power, E., Thomas, E., Worrall, L., Rose, M., Togher, L., Nickels, L., et al. (2015). Development and validation of Australian aphasia rehabilitation best practice statements using the RAND/UCLA appropriateness method. *British Medical Journal Open,* 5, e007641. doi:10.1136/ bmjopen-2015-007641

Robey, R. R. (1994). The efficacy of treatment for aphasic persons: A meta-analysis. *Brain and Language, 47,* 585–608.

Robey, R. R. (1998). A meta-analysis of clinical outcomes in the treatment of aphasia. *Journal of Speech, Language, and Hearing Research, 41,* 172–187.

Robey, R. R., & Schultz, M. C. (1998). A model for conducting clinical outcome research: An adaptation of the standard protocol for use in aphasiology. *Aphasiology, 12,* 787–810.

Rose, M., Ferguson, A., Power, E., Togher, L., & Worrall, L. (2014). Aphasia rehabilitation in Australia: Current practices, challenges and future directions. *International Journal of Speech Language Pathology, 16,* 169–180.

Sarno, M. T., Silverman, M., & Sands, E. (1970). Speech therapy and language recovery in severe aphasia. *Journal of Speech and Hearing Research, 13,* 607–623.

Schiavetti, N., Metz, D. E., & Orlikoff, R. F. (2011). *Evaluating research in communicative disorders* (6th ed.). Upper Saddle River, NJ: Pearson.

Schlaug, G., Marchina, S., & Wan, C. Y. (2011). The use of non-invasive brain stimulation techniques to facilitate recovery from post-stroke aphasia. *Neuropsychological Review, 21,* 299–301.

Schroth, L., Khawaja, R. (2007). Globalization of healthcare. *Frontiers of Health Services Management, 24*(2), 19–30.

Seniow, J., Waldowski, K., Lesniak, M., Iwanski, S., Czepiel, W., & Czlonkowska, A. (2013). Transcranial magnetic stimulation combined with speech and language training in early aphasia rehabilitation: A randomized double-blind controlled pilot study. *Topics in Stroke Rehabilitation, 20*(3), 250–261.

Shewan, C., & Kertesz, A. (1984). Effect of speech and language treatment on recovery from aphasia. *Brain and Language,* 23, 272–299.

Simmons-Mackie, N., Raymer, A., Armstrong, E., Holland, A., & Cherney, L. R. (2010). Communication partner training in aphasia: A systematic review. *Archives of Physical Medicine and Rehabilitation, 91*(12), 1814–1837.

Torres, J., Drebing, D., & Hamilton, R. (2013). TMS and tDCS in post-stroke aphasia: Integrating novel treatment approaches with mechanisms of plasticity. *Restorative Neurology and Neuroscience, 31,* 501–515.

Vickers, C. P. (2010). Social networks after the onset of aphasia: The impact of aphasia group attendance. *Aphasiology, 24,* 902–913.

Vignolo, L. (1964). Evolution of aphasia and language rehabilitation: A retrospective study. *Cortex, 1,* 344–367.

Volpato, C., Cavinato, M., Piccione, F., Garzon, M., Menenghello, F., & Birbaumer, N. (2013). Transcranial direct current stimulation (tDCS) of Broca's area in chronic aphasia: A controlled outcome study. *Behavioural Brain Research, 247,* 211–216.

Wertz, R. T. (2000). Aphasia therapy: A clinical framework. In I. Papathanasiou (Ed.), *Acquired neurogenic communication disorders: A clinical perspective* (pp. 3–27). London: Whurr.

Wertz, R. T., Collins, M. J., Weiss, D., Kurtzke, J. F., Friden, T., Brookshire, R. H., et al. (1981). Veterans Administration cooperative study on aphasia: A comparison of individual and group treatment. *Journal of Speech and Hearing Research, 24,* 580–594.

Wertz, R. T., Weiss, D. G., Aten, J. L., Brookshire, R. H., Garcia-Bunuel, L., Holland, A. L., et al. (1986). Comparison of clinic, home, and deferred language treatment for aphasia: A Veterans Administration cooperative study. *Archives of Neurology, 43,* 653–658.

Whurr, R., Lorch, M. P., & Nye, C. (1992). A meta-analysis of studies carried out between 1946 and 1988 concerned with the efficacy of speech and language therapy treatment for aphasic patients. *European Journal of Disorders of Communication, 27,* 1–17.

Wiig, E. H., Alexander, E. W., & Secord, W. (1988). Linguistic competence and level of cognitive functioning in adults with closed head injury. In H. A. Whitaker (Ed.), *Neuropsychological studies of nonfocal brain damage* (pp. 186–201). New York, NY: Springer-Verlag.

World Health Organization (WHO). (2001). *International classification of functioning, disability and health: ICF.* Geneva, Switzerland: Author.

World Health Organization (WHO). (2013). *Definition of public health.* WHO. Retrieved from http://www.who.int/trade/glossary/story076/en

World Health Organization (WHO). (2015). *Globalization of health.* Retrieved from http://www.who.int/trade/glossary/story045/en/

World Health Organization and the World Bank. (2011). *World report on disability.* Geneva, Switzerland: World Health Organization. Available online at http://www.who.int

Worrall, L., Howe, T., O'Callaghan, A., Hill, A.J., Rose, M., Wallace, S., et al. (2013). The *World Report on Disability* as a blueprint for international, national, and local aphasia services. *International Journal of Speech Language Pathology, 15*(1), 106–112.

Worrall, L., Sherratt, S., Rogers, P., Howe, T., Hersh, D., Ferguson, A., et al. (2011). What people with aphasia want: Their goals according to the ICF. *Aphasiology, 25,* 309–322.

Wylie, K., McAllister, L., Davidson, B., & Marshall, J. (2013). Changing practice: Implications of the *World Report on Disability* for responding to communication disability in underserved populations. *International Journal of Speech Language Pathology, 15*(1), 1–13.

Zheng, C., Lynch, L., & Taylor, N. (2014). Effect of computer therapy in aphasia: A systematic review. *Aphasiology* [published online January 3, 2015].

Aphasia United "Top 10" International Best Practice Recommendations for Aphasia*

1. All patients with brain damage or progressive brain disease should be screened for communication deficits.[1,2,3,5,7,8,9] (Level C)

2. People with suspected communication deficits should be assessed by a qualified professional (determined by country); Assessment should extend beyond the use of screening measures to determine the nature, severity, and personal consequences of the suspected communication deficit.[1,2,3,4,5,6,8,9] (Level B,C)

3. People with aphasia should receive information regarding aphasia, etiologies of aphasia (e.g., stroke) and options for treatment.[1,5,6,7,8,9] (Level A–C) This applies throughout all stages of health care from acute to chronic stages.

4. No one with aphasia should be discharged from services without some means of communicating his or her needs and wishes (e.g., using AAC, supports, trained partners) or a documented plan for how and when this will be achieved. (Level: Good Practice Point)

5. People with aphasia should be offered intensive and individualized aphasia therapy designed to have a meaningful impact on communication and life.[1,2,3,4,5,6,7,8,9] (Level A-GPP depending on approach, intensity, timing) This intervention should be designed and delivered under the supervision of a qualified professional.

   a. Intervention might consist of impairment-oriented therapy, compensatory training, conversation therapy, functional/participation oriented therapy, environmental intervention and/or training in communication supports or augmentative and alternative communication (AAC).

   b. Modes of delivery might include individual therapy, group therapy, telerehabilitation and/or computer-assisted treatment.

   c. Individuals with aphasia due to stable (e.g., stroke) as well as progressive forms of brain damage benefit from intervention.

   d. Individuals with aphasia due to stroke and other static forms of brain damage can benefit from intervention in both acute and chronic recovery phases.

6. Communication partner training should be provided to improve communication of the person with aphasia.[1,2,3,5,8] (Level A,B)

7. Families or caregivers of people with aphasia should be included in the rehabilitation process.[1,2,3,4,5,7,8,9] (Level A–C)

   • Families and caregivers should receive education and support regarding the causes and consequences of aphasia. (Level A)

   • Families and caregivers should learn to communicate with the person with aphasia. (Level B)

8. Services for people with aphasia should be culturally appropriate and personally relevant.[1,2,5,8] (Level: Good Practice Point)

9. All health and social care providers working with people with aphasia across the continuum of care

(i.e., acute care to end-of-life) should be educated about aphasia and trained to support communication in aphasia.[2,3] (Level C)

10. Information intended for use by people with aphasia should be available in aphasia-friendly/communicatively accessible formats.[1,3,5,7,8] (Level C)*Source:* http://www.shrs.uq.edu.au/docs/English-Best-Practices-Recommendations.pdf.

LEVELS OF RECOMMENDATION/ EVIDENCE

Level A: Body of research evidence can be trusted to guide practice

Level B: Body of research evidence can be trusted to guide practice in most situations

Level C: Body of research evidence provides some support for recommendation

Level D: Body of research evidence is weak

Good Practice Point: Recommendation is based on expert opinion or consensus

PRIMARY SOURCES FOR APHASIA UNITED BEST PRACTICE RECOMMENDATIONS FOR APHASIA

1. National Health and Medical Research Council Clinical Centre for Research Excellence in Aphasia Rehabilitation (CCRE) (2014). Australian Aphasia Rehabilitation Pathway. http://www.aphasiapathway.com.au/

2. Intercollegiate Stroke Working Party. National clinical guideline for stroke, 4th edition. London: Royal College of Physicians, 2012.

3. Lindsay MP, Gubitz G, Bayley M, Hill MD, Davies-Schinkel C, Singh S, and Phillips S. Canadian Best Practice Recommendations for Stroke Care (Update 2012). On behalf of the Canadian Stroke Strategy Best Practices and Standards Writing Group. Ottawa, Ontario Canada: Canadian Stroke Network.

4. Miller, E., Murray, L., Richards, L., Zorowitz R., Bakas, T., Clark, P. Billinger, S. (2010). Comprehensive Overview of Nursing and Interdisciplinary Rehabilitation Care of the Stroke Patient: A Scientific Statement from the American Heart Association. Stroke. 2010;41:2402–2448. Downloaded from http://stroke.ahajournals.org/

5. National Stroke Foundation Australia (2010). Clinical guidelines for stroke prevention and management. Melbourne Australia. http://strokefoundation.com.au/site/media/clinical_guidelines_stroke_managment_2010_interactive.pdf

6. Royal College of Speech & Language Therapists (2005). RCSLT Clinical Guidelines 4 Revised September, 2014.

7. Scottish Intercollegiate Guidelines Network (2010). Management of patients with stroke: Rehabilitation, prevention and management of complications, and discharge planning. A national clinical guideline. Edinburgh, Scotland. http://www.sign.ac.uk/pdf/sign118.pdf

8. Stroke Foundation of New Zealand and New Zealand Guidelines Group. Clinical Guidelines for Stroke Management 2010. Wellington: Stroke Foundation of New Zealand; 2010. http://www.stroke.org.nz/resources/NZClinicalGuidelinesStrokeManagement2010ActiveContents.pdf

9. US Veteran's Administration/Department of Defense (2010). Management of Stroke: VA/DoD Clinical Practice Guideline. http://www.healthquality.va.gov/guidelines/Rehab/stroke/online/

OBJECTIVES

The reader will be able to:

1. Understand the origins of different classifications of aphasia

2. Compare models of aphasia that have emerged in the history of aphasia

3. Appreciate that the history of aphasia is influenced by social and political developments in different countries

4. Name the main protagonists in the history of aphasia

5. Identify the main events in the history of aphasia

6. Identify the main shifts in approach to the treatment of aphasia throughout the history of aphasia

7. Understand where ideas about the nature of aphasia originated

Significant Landmarks in the History of Aphasia and Its Therapy

Chris Code

History doesn't repeat itself. At best it sometimes rhymes.
Mark Twain (1835-1910).

INTRODUCTION

In this chapter, we explore the origins of aphasia and attempts to treat it. Along the way, we can test Mark Twain's pithy aphorism. We start with a survey of how thought, language, and speech were represented in the body from ancient to modern times. The ancient Egyptians thought that the heart was the seat of the "soul" and mental life, and pre-Christian Greece and Rome developed a theory of "fluids." Plato's view that the mind was located in the head contrasted with Aristotle's idea that it was located in the heart. With early anatomical examinations of the brain, it was the ventricles of the brain, rather than the substance of the brain, where the soul was considered to reside. This view lasted well into the Middle Ages. It was not until the 15th century that basic treatments for aphasia began to develop based on the view that aphasia was a form of memory disorder. In the 18th century, Gall developed his language and speech localization theory, and Broca, Hughlings Jackson, and Bastian began to consider that recovery occurred because of some form of reorganization, and treatment could be beneficial. But, it was not until World War I that Goldstein, Luria, and the Viennese phoniatricians Hermann Gutzmann (1865–1922) ("the father of aphasia therapy") and Emil Froeschels developed the first systematic treatments.

Between the world wars, the focus shifted to North America, and a more behaviorist approach developed. Following World War II, there was a return to localization theory and an approach to treatment developed based on the Boston School and the "stimulation" approaches of Wepman and Schuell. In the latter part of the 20th century, approaches were developed based on linguistics, psycholinguistics, modular cognitive models, and psychosocial and social models. The history of aphasia is vast, and we cannot hope to cover it completely in a single chapter. There are more detailed treatments available, such as Eling's (1994) reader and the work of Tesak and Code (2008) and Howard and Hatfield (1987), whose focus was the history of aphasia treatment.

APHASIA IN THE ANCIENT PAST

An understanding of the past history of any field is essential to an appreciation of the present: The present, after all, is the realization of events in the past. St. Augustine (1,400 years before the present, henceforth BP) outlined a first understanding of what time past, time present, and time future might be. He contended that we can only really know the present because time past is only memory, even if it is recorded memory, and we know how unreliable memory can be, and time future is, by definition, impossible to know. For the history of anything, we are particularly reliant on the written records handed down to us from the past, and writing did not develop until 5,500 years before the present in the Middle East; even then, writing was limited to very few experts. But, the brain had no great importance in ancient Egyptian medicine and religion. For instance, in mummification all the organs were stored, but the brain was pulled out through the nose with a hook and discarded. This is a reflection of the cardiocentric view, where the heart was seen as the home of the soul, wherein resided a capacity for Good and Evil.

The oldest known reference to what we now call aphasia is in the Edwin Smith papyrus (5000 and 4200 years before the present), a medical record of a number of cases of brain damage (Breasted, 1930). One record referred to a man who was "speechless" and stated that the speechlessness was "an ailment not to be treated," but that the rubbing of ointment on the head and pouring a fatty liquid (possibly milk) into the ears was a beneficial therapy.

The Theory of Fluids

The causes of diseases in ancient times were thought to be due to some imbalance of the bodily fluids corresponding to the four basic elements from which all matter was considered to be made, a view that was to persist into the 18th century. This four-element theory was developed by different philosophers within natural philosophy (e.g., Empedocles, 2504–2433 BP), in an attempt to understand nature and the essence of human nature. The four bodily fluids and their corresponding elements were yellow bile (air), blood (fire), phlegm (earth), and black bile (water). Healing involved manipulating the balance of fluids: bloodletting, starvation, fluid deprivation, heat treatment, regurgitation, fecal evacuation, and sweating. Deficits following brain injuries were interpreted as an accumulation of undesirable life fluids. Cranial drillings (trepanations) were sometimes attempts at the evacuation of undesirable fluids and in some cases may have been effective.

The Greco-Roman Period

The connection between cognitive processing and a possible localization in the structure of the human body emerged in Greco-Roman times, and the following question was posed: Was the mind represented in the brain or in the heart? For Plato (2428–2347 BP), a tripartite soul corresponded to anatomically different parts of the body: Reason and mind were located in the head, but "higher" characteristics like pride, fear, and courage were in the heart; the lower characteristics of lust and desire were located in the liver or the abdomen. As human speech had been associated with the rational part of the soul since Pythagoras (2580–2428 BP), this was an important step for the examination of the relationship between speech, language, and brain.

Plato's pupil Aristotle (2384–2322 BP) had a particularly significant impact in subsequent centuries on philosophy and the development of medicine. He defined humans as speaking animals and language as innate, with the variety of languages in the world coming about through social factors. In contrast to his teacher Plato, he argued that the heart was the home of all cognitive, perceptual, and associated functions.

Ventricular Theory

The brain began to figure in Greco-Roman thought. Herophilos (2335–2280 BP), who is recognized as the "father of anatomy," described the cortex, the cerebellum, the ventricles of the brain, and the sensory and motor nerve trunks. It was with him that ventricular theory developed and where a connection was made between the "psyche" (soul) and the ventricles of the brain. Ventricular theory, or cell theory, to give it its other name, dominated into the Middle Ages.

Galen (2130–2200 BP) was the most significant brain anatomist until the 17th century. Galen was a physician to the gladiators and so had extensive experience of wounds to the head and the brain, although the dissection of human bodies was prohibited by Rome. He dissected cows, monkeys, pigs, dogs, cats, rodents, and at least one elephant. Although working in the tradition of Aristotle, he rejected Aristotle's theory.

THE MIDDLE AGES

The Middle Ages ran from the demise of the Roman Empire (400s) to the emergence of the Renaissance (1500s). During the Middle Ages, cell theory developed from ventricular theory (see Figure 2.1), but the ventricles were understood as theoretical concepts rather than as anatomical structures and simply depicted as circles. On the model, aphasic symptoms appear to result from damage to the third cell (the fourth ventricle) and were conceptualized as memory disorders. The idea that aphasia was a memory disorder was to dominate until well into the 19th century.

There were some references to aphasia during this time. Antonio Guainerio (died 1440) suggested that the cause of aphasia was damage to the fourth ventricle (the

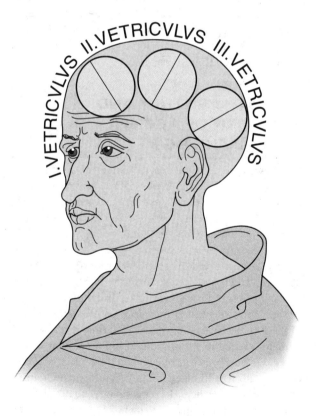

Figure 2.1 The ventricles of the brain according to medieval cell theory (adapted from Philosophia pauperum sive philosophia naturalis, 1490).

Source: From J. Tesak & C. Code. (2008). *Milestones in the History of Aphasia.* Hove, East Sussex: Psychology Press.

third cell), and memory was impaired because the ventricle contained too much phlegm. Nicolò Massa (1489–1569) described a man who lost his speech following a battle head wound and thought that a bone splinter was left in the brain. He located it and pulled it out, and immediately the patient called out (apparently in Latin!): "Ad Dei laudem, sum sanus!" (God be praised, I am healthy!). The Spaniard Francisco Arceo (1493–1573) described a worker hit on the head by a stone who was speechless for several days. Arceo remedied the fracture, and some days later the patient began to speak again and apparently recovered fully.

THE RENAISSANCE TO THE 17TH CENTURY

The Renaissance (the "rebirth") emerged and succeeded the darkness of the Middle Ages. It began in Italy in the 15th century and spread throughout Europe. It is associated with the beginnings of modern science and modern medicine. From the Renaissance to the 17th century, central advances were made in the anatomy and physiology of the brain, and there were increasing attempts to connect behavioral and cognitive functions to specific structures of the brain. Descriptions of aphasic symptoms became more precise, and early hypotheses on the causes began to emerge.

There were major advances in the development of medicine during the Renaissance, and a number of central personalities and their insights in medicine and philosophy stand out. Leonardo da Vinci (1472–1519) made significant contributions to anatomy. Da Vinci, the exemplary Renaissance man, used empirical methods, including sections on animal and human corpses, and produced exact anatomical sketches far superior to those of the earlier medieval tradition. For example, he noted that there was only an imprecise connection between the medieval drawings of ventricles and his own, although he did not question the belief in ventricular theory.

Two prominent Renaissance anatomists who dismissed Galean ventricular theory were Andreas Vesalius (1514–1564) and Thomas Willis (1621–1675). Vesalius published his famous and beautiful book *On the Fabric of the Human Body,* in 1543; the seventh and last volume was dedicated to the brain. This book was a major advance in anatomical detail and neurology, and it dismissed much of Galenian anatomy. The ventricles were described in detail, but memory was not localized there. It was in the cerebellum instead.

Thomas Willis (1621–1675) gained his knowledge of the brain from his observations of his patients with neurological conditions and was of great importance for the developing neuroscience of the 17th century. His great work, *Cerebri Anatome* (*Anatomy of the Brain and Nerves*, 1664/1965), benefitted from the anatomical drawings of the young Christopher Wren, later to design St. Paul's Cathedral in the center of London following the Great Fire of London. Willis dismissed ventricular theory, stating that mental life was essentially dependent on the cortex, thereby advancing probably the first cortical theory of the control of muscles and reflexes (Bennett & Hacker, 2003). He also suggested that the gyri or convolutions of the brain were responsible for memory and the will. He proposed a corporeal or physical soul present in humans and animals and associated with vital spirits, a kind of distilled liquor that was made in the brain and circulated in the blood. For Willis, the soul was immortal, nonmaterial, and separate from the brain, with interaction between body and soul.

During the Renaissance and the following centuries, because humans were thought to have been created in God's image, anatomical sectioning of the human body continued to be prohibited by the church: The body was not to be violated by the anatomist's knife. A solution to this problem came from the philosopher René Descartes (1596–1650) in the 17th century.

Each age has its dominant technology; for us in the latter part of the 20th and early 21st centuries, it is computer technology, and we tend to use the computer technology metaphor to explain the workings of the mind, among other things. Mechanics and hydraulics were the most highly developed technologies in the 17th century, and Descartes described humans as machines, a mechanical automaton, in his work *De Homine* (*On Man*). However, this automaton was a true human because it possessed a divine soul, and when the body died, the soul could live on. The difficult question remained regarding where the soul had its home, and Descartes suggested that it was in the pineal gland, a gland the size of a pea at the base of the brain, but crucially (for neuroanatomists at the time) just outside the brain proper. For Descartes, the unity between soul and body was only possible in humans, a position called Cartesian dualism, still influential in current thought. This Cartesian separation of body and soul permitted the church to lift its ban on anatomical sectioning, so the basis for further advances in medicine in the 18th and 19th centuries was established.

THE 18TH CENTURY ENLIGHTENMENT: REASON AND NATURE

Isaac Newton (1642–1727) supposed, based on Aristotle's teachings, that all human bodies contained a hidden, vibrating "ether" that moved through the nerves from sensory organs to brain and then to muscles, and it was under the command of the will. This was Newton's "vibration theory." The philosopher John Locke (1632–1704) considered the human mind a collecting point for sensory perceptions that were processed, connected, and associated with each other. David Hartley (1705–1757), most famous for his discovery of the circulation of the blood around the body, considered that the gyri were responsible for memory and the will and attempted to explain memory through association of ideas and Newton's vibration theory, which he combined in neurophysiology to produce *associationism*.

The idea that aphasia was an impairment of memory continued to dominate in the 17th and 18th centuries and indeed well into the 19th. For instance, Johannes Jakob Wepfer (1620–1695) described at least 13 clear cases of language disorder with brain injuries, which he attributed to memory loss. Johann Gesner (1738–1801) described his patient K.D. in the book *"The Language Amnesia,"* where he laid the foundation for the first real theory of aphasia, an impairment of memory caused by a congestion of the "nerve ducts," and according to Benton (1965), his was the first associationist aphasia theory. Gesner separated language from speech programming and laid the foundations for a separation of communicative competence, the latter apparently unimpaired in K.D.

THE 19TH CENTURY AND THE BIRTH OF A SCIENCE OF APHASIOLOGY

There was probably no real "science" of aphasiology until Gesner's work, but it was not really until the 19th century that the seriously systematic study of aphasia began. The 19th century is considered to be the foundation period of the modern history of aphasia, mainly because connections were made between the symptoms of aphasia and the localization of areas of brain damage, which emerged to form the basis for the later investigations of Broca, Wernicke, and others.

Napoleon's reign in France dominated the beginning of the 19th century in Europe. At that time, the scientific climate was notably more liberal in France than in the rest of Europe. This was one reason that Franz Josef Gall (1764–1828), a brilliant and highly significant anatomist, left Austria for France. His "organology" (better known as *phrenology*, the term coined by his student Spurzheim) had a massive influence on ideas about aphasia, neuroanatomy, and neuropsychology, even to the present day (see Figure 2.2). Organology considered that the inner form of the cranium was determined by the external form of the brain, and it was therefore possible to detect

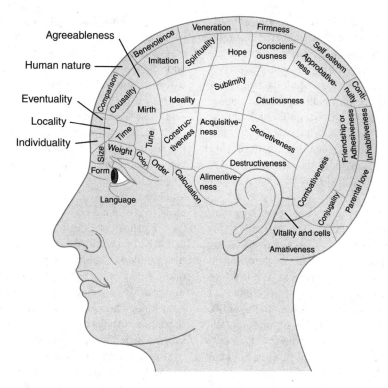

Figure 2.2 The 37 faculties, or phrenological organs, according to Johann Kaspar Spurzheim.
Source: J. Tesak and C. Code. (2008). *Milestones in the History of Aphasia*. Hove, East Sussex: Psychology Press.

the strength of particular human "faculties" from the shape and size of the cranium. Gall (1798) wrote: "The possibility of a theory of the psychological and mental functions of the brain presupposes: . . . that the brain was the organ of all tendencies, all emotions and all faculties . . . [and] that the brain was composed of as many individual organs as there are tendencies, emotions, faculties, which essentially differ from one another" (translated from Lesky, 1970, p. 73). With Gall, the foundations of cerebral localization of function began as a serious idea. He was a particularly skilled anatomist and the first to recognize the importance of the neocortex in localization, and he described mental faculties (or "organs") that were localized in specific parts of the brain. While Gall attributed no specific functions to the separate hemispheres of the brain, he did claim that the faculty for words, which was part of the faculty for language, was located in the frontal lobe, although this insight was tenuously based on an observation Gall made of a linguistically gifted school friend who could learn verbal material very well. His friend had strongly protruding eyes, suggesting to Gall that the boy's brain was particularly well developed behind the eyes, causing them to protrude, suggesting a large language organ situated in the frontal lobes. For Gall, the faculty of language

was innate, independent, and autonomous of reason and intelligence, and its primary purpose was as a means of expression. More recently, this has formed the basis for the idea that cognitive functions are organized into "modules," an important feature of modern cognitive neuropsychology.

The most important follower of Gall in Paris was Jean Baptiste Bouillaud (1796–1881), a founding member of the French Société Phrénologique, who was critical of most of the fanciful claims of phrenology in general, but he was a passionate supporter of Gall's language localization theory. He published studies until the 1840s, describing more than 500 cases that he claimed supported his view that language and speech were localized in the frontal lobes. He identified the connection between the separate loss of language and speech and frontal brain damage in significant numbers of patients he described, and divided the disorders into articulation (what we would now call apraxia of speech) and language disorders due to a memory problem. In the first, words are no longer correctly organized, retrievable, or usable, and in the other, the memory form of the word itself was damaged. But, phrenology was scorned on by most scientists at this time, and Bouillaud had few supporters.

In opposition to the localizationists, like Bouillaud, were the holists, most prominent being Pierre Flourens (1794–1867) (Finger, 1994), who carried out brain ablation and stimulation experiments, primitive by today's standards. He used "spoons" for ablations and often removed large parts of the brain so that the behavioral losses following ablations were often similar. In his stimulation studies, he observed that irritation of the cortex produced no reaction at all. He concluded that the cortex was not divided into functional regions but that functions were represented throughout the brain, what we now call cortical equipotentiality.

Bouillaud and other localizationists had difficulties getting their own views accepted by the scientific community. From Flourens's first publications in the 1820s until the 1870s, equipotentiality was the dominating paradigm of brain physiology. However, the dispute between the localizers and the equipotentialists was not restricted to the question of localization in the brain. First, it was a question of what was the right methodology: the clinical observation/case studies of the localizers or the repeatable experiment (e.g., animal brain ablations), the approach of Flourens's followers. In addition, the two groups took different basic political and philosophical positions that influenced the neurological debate. Following the revolution of 1848 in France instigated by Napoleon III, the localizationists took the role of progressive liberals and the equipotentialists the role of conservatives. Bouillaud's son-in-law, Ernest Auburtin (1825–1893), was the significant figure in the Paris Anthropology Society and in the Paris Language Localization Debates of 1861–1866. He argued strongly for the localization of speech to the frontal lobes.

On April 4, 1861, Auburtin presented a patient, Bache, who had lost his speech, was left with the automatism *Sacre Nom de Dieu,* but was said to understand everything and to be of sound mind. He was already very ill, and his demise was imminent. Auburtin announced that he would publicly revoke his views on localization if Bache's brain (or that of any other speech- or language-disordered patient) displayed *no* frontal brain damage in a postmortem autopsy. It was this public announcement by Auburtin that triggered the interest of Pierre-Paul Broca (1824–1880), and Auburtin's contribution has been overshadowed by the colleague he inspired. Anthropology played an essential role in the debates on localization at this time, and it was not a coincidence that questions of language localization were under discussion in the Anthropological Society in Paris in the 1860s (Broca, whose primary interest was anthropology, was cofounder and secretary).

By coincidence, on April 12, 1861, a patient named Leborgne was transferred to the clinic of Bicêtre Hospital, where Broca was working. Auburtin accompanied Broca, who had little experience of aphasia, in an examination of Broca's patient. The 51-year-old man had epilepsy since his youth, loss of speech 21 years earlier, and paralyses of the right arm for 10 years and of the leg for 4 years. Leborgne's comprehension was said to be intact, but for Broca comprehension was not part of language per se, but of intelligence and memory. Leborgne had almost no speech apart from the speech automatisms *tan tan* (/tā tā/ nonlexical) and Sacré Nom de Dieu (lexical). Following Leborgne's death on April 17 and brain autopsy, Broca described Leborgne the next day (April 18) at a meeting of the Anthropology Society (Broca, 1861). Leborgne had a massive frontal lesion centered on the third frontal gyrus (see Figure 2.3), and Broca called Leborgne's disorder *aphemia,* meaning loss of articulate speech, a term that is still in use, although now mainly called apraxia of speech. With this, modern aphasiology and neuropsychology were born, and Broca proclaimed that the third frontal convolution was the seat for articulated language.

The description of Leborgne by Broca is still regarded as the most significant event in the modern history of aphasia and was taken by most as confirmation that the views of Bouillaud, Gall, and Auburtin were correct, and that language and speech processing were indeed localized in this area of the brain. We have learned more about Leborgne the person recently (Domanski, 2013). We now know that Louis Victor Leborgne was born in 1809 in Moret, France. His father was Pierre Christophe Leborgne, a teacher, who married Margueritte Savard, the daughter of a guardsman, in 1801. They had six children, including Louis Victor. The family was educated and literate; one of his nephews became an official in one of the ministeries. The received opinion that Leborgne was an uneducated illiterate from the lower social orders is clearly false. He worked until he was 30 as a "formier"–a craftsman who produced forms for shoemakers.

Broca presented further cases of aphemia in 1863 (Broca, 1863); these individuals all had damage to the left hemisphere, and for all except one, the damage was to the third frontal convolution. While he noted that it was strange that the lesions were all in the left hemisphere, he made no issue of the fact. The beginnings of the idea that the left hemisphere was "dominant" for speech and language, and for most other useful functions, was formally crystallized in 1865, when Broca finally formulated a theory of language lateralization (Bogen, 1969), that is, that language was represented in the left hemisphere. It was in 1865 that he wrote his famous sentence "We speak with the left hemisphere" (*Nous parlons avec l'hémisphère gauche,* 1865, p. 384).

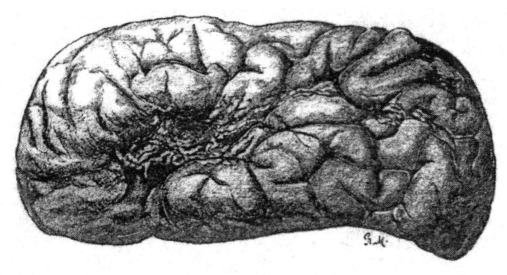

Figure 2.3 The brain of Leborgne (*Tan Tan*), the famous case presented by Broca in 1861.
Source: From J. Tesak and C. Code. (2008). *Milestones in the History of Aphasia*. Hove, East Sussex: Psychology Press.

He also discussed right hemisphere (RH) compensation in the case of damage to the left (Broca, 1865, p. 384) and that people with aphemia could actually be treated following the principles of child language acquisition under therapeutic guidance. These ideas appear to be the first to propose the possibility of reorganization of the brain and language following damage (Code, 1987).

However, the position of Broca as the originator of the idea of left hemisphere dominance remains controversial (Finger & Roe, 1996; Joynt & Benton, 1964; Schiller, 1992), with many contending that an unknown country doctor had already made the connection between left hemisphere damage and speech and language impairment in 1836. Marc Dax (1770–1837) had already written a paper for a regional physicians' meeting in 1836, a year before his death but nearly 30 years before Broca's paper wherein the connection between left hemisphere lesions and speech disorders was clearly stated: "There now remains a very interesting problem to solve: why does it happen that changes to the left cerebral hemisphere are followed by the loss of words, but not those of the right hemisphere?" (Dax, 1836–1865, p. 260). But, Marc Dax's work remained unpublished, and there is little evidence that he actually delivered the paper at the regional meeting, although it was submitted for publication to the Académie de Médecine by his son, Gustave Dax, together with his own contribution, as early as 1863, still 2 years before Broca's 1865 paper. But, the Dax contribution was not published until 1865, when Broca also argued in favor of left lateralization. This led to a bitter conflict, with Gustave Dax claiming that his father was the first to discover the role for

the left hemisphere in the control of speech production (Schiller, 1992). So it is Marc Dax who should be credited with the original finding that language is lateralized to the left, but he was just a country doctor and Broca was already famous.

Despite Broca's fame and influence, his preferred term for the disorder he had described, *aphemia*, was replaced with the term *aphasia*, mainly because of an article in 1864 by prominent physician Armand Trousseau (1801–1867); the article had the provocative title "On Aphasia, a Sickness Formerly Wrongly Referred to as Aphemia." He pointed out that the term *aphasia*, from the Greek meaning "without language," was more appropriate than aphemia (without speech). Trousseau believed that aphasia was a cognitive disorder that affects intellectual performance, a view also later expressed by John Hughlings Jackson. Of course, Broca's term referred to speech, as it still does today, and Trouseau's to language.

Henry Head (1926) noted that much of the great growth in German neurology and dominance in aphasiology was related to German victory in the Franco-Prussian War of 1870–1871. It was in this climate that universities in Germany and German-speaking countries became the world leaders for scientific research. A landmark development in neurology was "fiber theory," developed by Theodor von Meynert (1833–1892) in Vienna (Whitaker & Etlinger, 1993). Fiber theory described the important distinction between projection fibers, which connect subcortical to cortical regions, and association fibers, connecting cortical areas to one another. Thus, projection fibers communicated sensory information from the sensory organs to the cortex, and the association tracts transmitted perceptions, ideas, and memory contents between areas. Von Meynert was also responsible for determining that the anterior part of the brain was responsible for motor function and the posterior part for sensory function. His work with aphasic patients led him to describe a "sound-image system." This, and other aspects of fiber theory, form parts of the theory developed by von Meynert's student Wernicke.

In 1874, the young physician Carl Wernicke (1848–1905) completed his thesis, "The Symptom-Complex of Aphasia," in which he described cases with sensory aphasia due to lesions in the posterior left brain. With the anterior production aphasia of Broca (aphemia) and Wernicke's posterior sensory aphasia, the basis for a fuller

theory of language processing was developed. However, the impact of Wernicke's thesis went well beyond describing "sensory" aphasia, which had already been described by Bastian (Tesak & Code, 2008). Wernicke devised information-processing components to underlie the basic operations and pathways involved in the production and reception of speech, at least at the single-word level, from the highest cognitive center to the peripheral input and output levels. The model included a sound-image system and fiber connections and explained pathologies of speech and language; it predicted forms of aphasia that had not yet been discovered. In 1885, Lichtheim took Wernicke's model and expanded and refined it to produce what we now know as the Wernicke-Lichtheim model (Figure 2.4), which was to dominate aphasia theory in

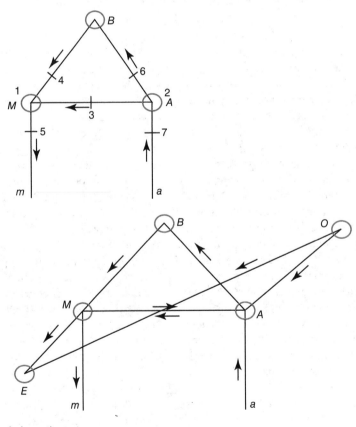

A: Acoustic center
M: Motor center
B: Concept center
O: Optical memory images for letters
E: Region from which writing movements are innervated
m: Motor pathway
a: Acoustic pathway

Figure 2.4 The Wernicke-Lichtheim models of language processing.
Source: From J. Tesak and C. Code. (2008). *Milestones in the History of Aphasia.* Hove, East Sussex: Psychology Press.

most of the world well into the 20th century. Because of its obvious similarity to the outline of a house, it is sometimes called the Wernicke-Lichtheim House.

However, not everyone was seduced by the localizationist agenda. During the 1874 Berlin language debate, the localizationist Hitzig took an opposing view to Steinthal, who was probably the first real psycholinguist (Eling, 2006). Heymann (Chajim) Steinthal (1871) complained that the physicians' descriptions of language and aphasia were too superficial and lacked the necessary linguistic detail, a complaint that still resonates. He stated, exasperatedly, "The clinical pictures have been recorded by far too incompletely and imprecisely; our physicians have not understood what the function of language is" (1871, p. 464). In England, John Hughlings Jackson (1835–1911) also was opposed to localization and proposed that reorganization of function could take place following damage. Hughlings Jackson was more than simply an antilocalizationist, however. Darwin's *Origin of Species* was published in 1859, and the impact that his evolutionary theory had on both scientific and public opinion is famous. Subsequently, Hughlings Jackson developed his highly significant theory of the evolution and organization of the nervous system, informed by his observations of aphasia and epilepsy and extensively influenced by the evolutionary ideas of Herbert Spencer (1820–1903). Head (1926) noted that: "Jackson derived all his psychological knowledge from Herbert Spencer, and adopted his phraseology almost completely" (p. 31). But, his work on aphasia had little impact outside Britain and remained relatively unrecognized until Head's writings led to its recognition in the early 20th century.

Hughlings Jackson had observed that people with aphasia can often produce complete phrases in particular contexts (curses, exclamations, stereotypies, etc.), even when they possessed little or no spontaneous speech, and he acknowledged Baillarger's (1865) earlier distinction between *voluntary* and *involuntary* speech. Hughlings Jackson (1878–1880, reproduced in Taylor, 1958), hypothesized that both the ontogenic (individual development) and phylogenic (species development over time) evolution of the nervous system entailed (a) a course from the most to the least organized, from the lowest, well-organized centers up to the highest, least organized, centers; (b) a course from the simplest to the most complex; and (c) a course from the most automatic to the most voluntary. *Dissolution* is a term he got from Spencer and Hughlings Jackson's model of the nervous system and mirrors closely Spencer's. Dissolution of the nervous system with a loss of function provides evidence of the reverse of evolution. Functions are organized hierarchically in the nervous system in Hughlings Jackson's theory at different *levels of representation* from the oldest to the most recently developed in evolution and individual development, from the lowest to the highest, from the most primitive to the most complex. Symptoms (e.g., aphasic speech automatisms, like Leborgne's *tan, Tan*) are the expression of lower levels released from the inhibition of higher levels caused by brain damage.

Many aphasiologists at this time were interested in clinical management and treatment of aphasia, Broca and Henry Charles Bastian (1837–1915), for instance. Bastian (1898) and Henry Head developed tests of aphasia, and their tests were used well into the second half of the 20th century.

The French suffered a military defeat at the hands of the Germans in 1870–1871, which resulted in the Germans marching into Paris. As a result, the French scientific community became rather closed to developments in German science and the revolution taking place in German aphasiology. French aphasiology remained staunchly devoted to Broca's mid-1860s findings (Gelfand, 1999). Jean-Martin Charcot (1825–1893) was a leading neurologist in Paris and holder of the chair for nervous diseases at the Hospice de la Salpêtrière. He was an advocate of a reactively patriotic competition with German science, and it was because of Charcot and his students that aphasia once again became an important topic in Paris, despite the fact that there had been a significant lack of enthusiasm for advances outside France since Broca. Charcot was interested in localization throughout his career, although a small, but important, part of his work was with aphasia. In a series of lectures (in 1883 and 1884), "on the different forms of aphasia" (Charcot, 1884), he developed his famous *bell diagram* (Figure 2.5), which was meant to allow a better understanding of normal and pathological language processing. His model contained four centers for *memory images* (speech, language, writing, reading) attributed to an association center. These centers were linked to the outside world by auditory and visual routes. Charcot, in common with many of his predecessors, thus saw aphasia as a memory disorder, with memory divided into subsystems. He also believed in submemories for language, understanding, writing, speaking, and reading, and the centers were linked to one another through many connections.

He attempted to localize aphasic disorders and went along with Broca's finding that aphemia was caused by a lesion of the third frontal gyrus, with a lesion in the second frontal gyrus as the cause of agraphia. Word deafness was caused by a lesion in the first temporal gyrus and word blindness from a lesion to the lower parietal gyrus.

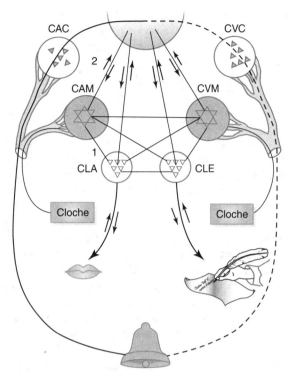

Cloche 'Bell'
IC *centre d'idéation*
Association center
CAC *centre auditif commun*
General auditory center
CAM *centre auditif des mots*
Hearing center for words
CLA *centre de language articulé*
Center for articulated speech
CVC *centre visuel commun*
General visual center
CVM *centre visuel des mots*
Visual center for words
CLE *centre du langage écrit*
Center for writing

Figure 2.5 Charcot's "bell" model.

Source: From J. Tesak and C. Code. (2008). *Milestones in the History of Aphasia.* Hove, East Sussex: Psychology Press.

Charcot's diagram became well known through the work of the young Pierre Marie (1853–1940), who joined Charcot at the Salpêtrière in 1885 and became one of his most famous students. With the work of the eminent Charcot, aphasia again became a topic of intense discussion in Paris.

In England, Hughlings Jackson published more on his evolutionary approach to aphasiology and was hardly influenced by the localization debates going on in Germany and France, although as an editor of the new journal *Brain* he published Lichtheim's work in English in 1885. Bateman's work, *On Aphasia, or Loss of Speech*,

appeared in 1890 in its second edition, in which Charcot, Kussmaul, and others were included, although Bateman was opposed to classifications and localization. At the end of the 1800s, Bastian (1898), in England, summarized his 30 years of work on aphasia.

Another important critic of connectionism and the Wernicke-Lichtheim model was Sigmund Freud (1891) in Vienna, a neurologist and aphasiologist before he founded psychoanalysis; Freud spent a few months with Charcot in 1885. Of course, he was to become far more famous for his work on the development of psychoanalysis. He published his short monograph on aphasia in 1891, but it was to have little impact at the time. However, an English translation was published in 1953, and more recently his contribution to aphasiology has been better appreciated (Buckingham, 2006). Henry Head (1926) was famously opposed to the proliferation of diagrammatic models of the representation of language in the brain and launched a bitter assault on what he called "the diagram makers."

The Swiss Jules Joseph Dejerine (1849–1917) was also working in Paris, and a student of Charcot, where he eventually became *Professeur de clinique des maladies du système nerveux* in 1910. Dejerine described a classification system of aphasia, but it was mainly through two case descriptions of isolated writing and reading disorders that his work became important. Dejerine (1891) described a 63-year-old man with word blindness (alexia) and total agraphia (Dejerine, 1892) and a 61-year-old educated woman with word blindness without agraphia, but who could write spontaneously and to dictation and had no difficulties with spontaneous speaking (Hanley & Kay, 2003). Autopsies showed a lesion in the angular gyrus on the left for the first case and a lesion in the area that separates the general language area from the angular gyrus in the second case (Dejerine, 1892). Dejerine suspected that visual word images were stored in the angular gyrus, which he assumed was necessary for reading and for writing. Thus, alexia and agraphia would therefore result from a lesion to the angular gyrus.

Three years later, Dejerine described a further form of alexia as it commonly occurs motor aphasia. This "third alexia" s explained with reference to Dejerine's language zone, containing Broca's area, Wernicke's area, and the angular gyrus, respectively responsible for production, auditory comprehension, and written language comprehension, and any disruption of the subcortical connecting pathways would lead to isolated phenomena. Cortical lesions of the language zone led to a disorder of "inner speech," and leads to disorders such as alexia in motor aphasia.

Also active in France in the later 1800s, Albert Pitres (1848–1928) is well known for his early work on *amnesic aphasia,* his term for impaired naming, and his book on aphasia in bi- and multilingual speakers. The concept of amnesic aphasia received a great deal of discussion from the 1860s, and Pitres attempted to establish it as an independent form of aphasia (Pitres, 1898). He described amnesic aphasia as "a form of aphasia in which the language difficulties consist in having forgotten the words that are necessary to express thoughts" (Pitres in Benton, 1988, p. 210), emphasizing that pure cases are rather rare. Amnesic aphasia would play an important role in Geschwind's reintroduction of the neoclassical model, developed in the 1960s in America, where it would reemerge as what we now call *anomia* (Benton, 1988).

Ribot (1881) had suggested that bilingual speakers with aphasia would recover their native language first. This idea was in general support of his theory that recent memories are more vulnerable to loss than earlier ones (Paradis, 1981). Pitres (1895) firmly believed that the most recently learned and most familiar language is the one that will recover first, and unlike Ribot, he based his perspective on a detailed review of the research and an analysis of eight new cases. Discussion continued for some years, with some supporting "Pitres's" rule," that the most recently used and familiar language would recover first, and some "Ribot's rule," that the first learned—the native language—would recover first (see Paradis, 1983, for relevant papers translated into English). Finally, Pitres strongly opposed the idea that different languages could occupy separate locations in the brain.

Pierre Marie followed Dejerine as professor of neurology at the University of Paris and was one of the most provocative figures in the history of aphasia. Head (1926) called him "the iconoclast." Marie was originally a localizationist like his mentor Charcot, but in 1906, he published a paper with the title "Révision de la Question sur l'Aphasie: La Troisième Circonvolution Frontale Gauche ne Joue Aucun Rôle Spécial dans la Fonction du Langage" (Revision of the Question of Aphasia: The Third Left Frontal Convolution Plays No Special Role in the Function of Language) that vehemently attacked Broca's model of aphasia. Marie reported cases where severe damage to this area did not result in aphasia and where Broca's aphasia could result without a lesion to the left third frontal convolution. He also stated that "l'anarthrie n'est pas de l'aphasie" (anarthria [Marie's term for aphemia] is not aphasia), and he coined the famous equation: Broca's aphasia = Wernicke's aphasia + Anarthria. Although an apparently unpleasant man, contemporary research tends to generally support his findings.

THE GROWTH OF LINGUISTIC APHASIOLOGY IN THE 19TH AND 20TH CENTURIES

There were attempts in the 19th and early 20th century from Steinthal, Freud, and the physician Arnold Pick to introduce linguistics as relevant in aphasiology. On the basis of a more exact linguistic examination, the early psycholinguist Steinthal (1871, p. 478) had described what he called *acataphasia,* which he contrasted with aphasia. He suggested that the problem in aphasia was at the lexical level (a word memory retrieval problem), whereas in acataphasia it is at the sentence level: an inability to make sentences rather than poor memory for words. Forty years later, Arnold Pick (1851–1924) took up the mantle with his work on the development of agrammatism. Indeed, most of this pioneering work came from German-speaking Europe. Pick (1913, p. 9) also believed that the developments in psychology and linguistics should form the basis for a new theory of aphasia:

> *Not only does the backwardness of the still authoritative psychology for aphasia theory urgently demand a revision, it is also the enormous progress that psychology itself has made. . . . The situation in terms of linguistic science presents itself similarly to that of psychology . . . of which even the most recent presentations of aphasia theory have not taken notice.*

In modern terms, Pick was advocating, as Steinthal had, a psycholinguistic perspective. In his monograph, *Agrammatic Language Disorders. Studies on the Psychological Foundation of Aphasia Theory* (1913), he developed a staged model of language production that shares many features with current models (e.g., the contemporary models of Garrett [1980] and Levelt [1989]).

In Pick's model, a *mental schema* develops that includes pragmatic and emotional components, which today we would call an intention to communicate or a preverbal message. Subsequently, a *sentence schema* is activated, which takes place before word choice. The choice of a word, Pick stated, is only determined by the position it takes in the sentence, so it must occur following sentence formulation. Likewise, word ordering and intonation precede word choice. Then, grammatical and lexical words are built into the sentence schema, where the specification of grammatical words (function words and inflections) precedes the specification of content words. Agrammatism for Pick was the core aphasic symptom, and he described separate forms associated with impairments to the different stages of production. To explain function word omissions in telegraphic speech, Pick supposed that the individual employs an *economy of effort* in the context of a severely impaired system—the word is omitted because it is the semantically least useful in the sentence. He also discussed the idea of "emergency language" in detail, a form of adaptation of the system to brain damage: "The whole mental language apparatus accommodates itself . . . extraordinarily fast with the situation created by the illnesses" (Pick, 1913, p. 156). Similar views would later also be developed by Isserlin (1922).

In 1914, Karl Kleist (1878–1960) described an impairment he called *paragrammatism*, a second word order disorder distinct from agrammatism. Kleist (1914, pp. 11–12) stated:

> *So far we have only spoken of agrammatism. We retain the term agrammatism for one of these two . . . word order disorders. The basic trait of agrammatism is the simplification and coarsening of word sequences. Complicated compound sentences (subordination of clauses) are not built. The patients only speak in small, primitive mini-sentences, if they continue to create sentences at all. All less necessary words, especially pronouns and particles, are reduced or eliminated. . . . Conjugation thereby also degenerates. . . . But also the changes occurring in the words themselves, through conjugation, declination, and comparison (flexions in the narrower sense), are more or less omitted.*

In contrast to this pattern, in paragrammatism

> *the ability to create word orders is not abolished, but phrases and sentences are often wrongly chosen and thereby amalgamate and contaminate each other . . . phrases and sentence constructions are not completed. . . . The spoken expression is not simplified overall; instead, also conditioned by a strong overproduction of word sequences, it swells to confused sentence monsters.*

Kleist considered a mixed agrammatic-paragrammatic symptom pattern to be the rule and pure cases to be rare. He was clear with regard to the anatomical basis (Kleist, 1914, p. 12): "We will not go wrong if, contrary to frontal agrammatism, we localize paragrammatism in the temporal lobe or its immediate neighborhood."

Later, Kleist (1916, p. 170) modified his position and concluded that the cause of agrammatism was "a loss or lowering of excitability of sentence and phrase formulae," which approximately corresponds to Pick's sentence schemata, and in paragrammatism "sentence and phrase formulae . . . are aroused incorrectly." So, for Kleist (1916, p. 198), paragrammatism was caused "by an incorrect arousal of acoustic sentence formulae." Kleist was another of Wernicke's many assistants, and Wernicke had a significant influence on him. Kleist was also the ultralocalizationist, and his brain map went beyond even the phrenological maps of Spurzheim in its detail.

Russian linguist Roman Jakobson (1896–1980) is sometimes considered the first to systematically apply linguistics in aphasiology. Jakobson was a founding member of the Prague Circle or School of phonology, established in 1926. When the Nazis entered Czechoslovakia, Jacobson fled, first to Denmark, Norway, and Sweden and then to the United States in 1941, where he eventually became a professor at Harvard and the Massachusetts Institute of Technology. In his 1941 monograph, *Child Language, Aphasia, and Phonological Universals* (English translation, 1968), Jakobson described parallels between language acquisition and aphasia and proposed a *regression hypothesis*, which stated that we can observe the same processes in both developing child speech and the impairments of speakers with aphasia, but in reverse: "The dissolution of the linguistic sound system in aphasics provides an exact mirror-image of the phonological development in child language" (Jakobson, 1968, p. 60), and "the order in which speech sounds are restored in the aphasic during the process of recovery corresponds directly to the development of child language" (p. 64).

For Jakobson, there was no doubt that aphasia should be understood in terms of linguistic theories, and aphasia could test the validity of linguistic theories. Jakobson (1964) also attempted to contrast Luria's six aphasia types (described in the next section) in terms of three linguistic dichotomies: encoding (combination, contiguity) impairments versus decoding (selection, similarity) impairments; limitation impairments versus disintegration; and sequence (syntagmatic, successivity) versus concurrence (paradigmatic, simultaneity). For instance, an encoding impairment, like Luria's dynamic aphasia or efferent motor aphasia, is characterized by problems with combination, whereas decoding impairments, like sensory or semantic aphasia, entail impairments in selection. Jakobson is admired as a pioneer of linguistic aphasiology, but his views had little mainstream impact and played little part in contemporary linguistic aphasiology.

It was not until the 1960s, when generative transformational grammar emerged, that a broad linguistic aphasiology developed. Chomsky's ideas were to have a revolutionary impact in linguistics, cognitive psychology, and philosophy. Noam Chomsky (born 1928) introduced *transformational generative grammar* (TG) at the turn of the 1950s and 1960s (Chomsky, 1957, 1957b, 1965), and linguistic science materialized as a dynamic enterprise. Chomsky (1957a, 1957) famously wrote a scathing critique of the behaviorist B. F. Skinner's book *Verbal Behavior,* in which Skinner claimed that language development is accountable in terms of stimulus–response learning. Chomsky dismissed the behaviorist account. For generative linguistics, children learn a set of rules and have an innate capacity for language acquisition; while learning is involved in language acquisition, they do not learn a set of utterances through imitation and reinforcement.

Chomsky proposed a partition between linguistic *competence* and linguistic *performance*. Competence is the abstract system of mental representations and processes that constitutes the basis of language, and performance is the actual realization of language through use. An important feature of TG is the powerful idea of a *universal grammar,* shared by all languages.

Chomsky regarded linguistics as a branch of cognitive psychology, where language is seen as a part of the mind and subject to scientific laws. Psycholinguistics advanced and the development of experimental investigations of language processing grew, and these emerged as a dynamic interchange on how the psychological reality of linguistic constructs might be tested (see, for instance, Miller, 1964). There was also a view developing that aphasia could be relevant for linguistics and psycholinguistics and vice versa. Linguistics has methods for describing aphasic language and might provide details to inform treatment planning, and aphasic data can act as "external" evidence for linguistic and psycholinguistic hypotheses. The separation of abstract phonological and concrete phonetic components in speech production has been a theoretical position since the origins of phonology and phonetics as disciplines, and dozens of studies have demonstrated that the distinction accounts well for separate phonological and apraxic speech errors occurring in different people with aphasia. A frequently observable double dissociation has been described between problems with *referential* or *modalizing* language that is differentially impaired across the broad range of aphasic types. This evidence supports a model of language that posits a referential and a modalizing form of language, which is taken to reflect certain linguistic and cognitive distinctions that cannot be accounted for by structurally motivated linguistic models (Nespoulous, Code, Virbel, & Lecours, 1998).

Another theory of language that was to become relevant in aphasiology from the 1970s is *systemic functional linguistics,* developed by M. A. K. Halliday (1961, 1985). At the heart of Halliday's model is the recognition that language has a fundamental social function as well as a cognitive–referential one. Language can be conversational and used to develop, cement, and maintain relationships using different registers and styles depending on whether the relationship is with the boss, loved ones, or friends, and paralinguistic features like facial expression, body language, and gesture are essential components of everyday communication. Systemic linguistics provided methods of analysis for all components of language and

several social contexts. This "functional" appreciation of language has been fully incorporated into contemporary psycholinguistic models (e.g., Tomasello, 2014).

APHASIOLOGY IN THE 20TH CENTURY

The devastation of war brings advances in science and technology, and aphasia and neuropsychology are no exceptions. The massive numbers of brain-injured soldiers of World War I resulted in new approaches to rehabilitation, many pioneered by Kurt Goldstein (1878–1965), who is often considered the major opponent to the classical localizationist approach (Geschwind, 1965). He took a holistic view of aphasia through his organismic approach and was deeply concerned with rehabilitation and the psychosocial impact of aphasia. World War I saw the development of aphasia therapy from what Howard and Hatfield (1987) called the "speech gymnastics" of the Viennese phoniatricians Hermann Gutzmann (1865–1922)—"the father of aphasia therapy"—and Emil Froeschels (1884–1973). They applied the techniques they knew from voice therapy, articulatory drills, and primary school teaching techniques. Also in Britain, treatment of aphasia was mainly developed by elocutionists and voice teachers. Bastian was an exception and introduced the still-influential division between *compensation* for lost functions and *restitution* of functions (Bastian, 1898). He described therapy for aphasia based on the potential of reorganization of the RH through functional compensation, which he distinguished from functional restitution. These processes have become axiomatic in neuropsychology and have a significant impact on how we plan and carry out therapy.

During World War II, A. R. Luria (1902–1977) in Russia collected a mass of data from brain-injured soldiers and developed a functional systems approach to the brain and language that resulted in a new perspective on the organization of cognition and language and a new classification of aphasia. Treatment involved the reorganization of function by which intact functional subsystems could be used to compensate for impaired ones in speech, language, reading, and writing. Luria's clinical approach had a major impact not only in Eastern Europe but also in the United Kingdom and Australia. He was influenced by the pioneering work of fellow Russian psychologists Pavlov and Vygotsky and has been called the "last giant" in the history of aphasia.

The essential foundations of Luria's approach are easily accessible in *The Working Brain* (1973) and in the work of Kagan and Saling (1992). His important early work, *Traumatic Aphasia*, was based on data gathered from

World War II; the English translation appeared in 1970. His general neuropsychology was extensively developed in *Higher Cortical Functions in Man* (1980), and a special issue of *Aphasiology* edited by Kaczmarek (1995) was devoted to Luria's contribution to aphasia.

Luria attempted to create a synthesis of the localizationist approach, as represented by Wernicke or Kleist, with the holistic approach. To Luria, neither approach seemed to be altogether appropriate to understand the functioning of the human brain. Central to his model is the notion of a *functional system*. Every single mental function (like thinking, writing, arithmetic) should be understood not as a single, simple function, "but as a complete functional system, embodying many components belonging to different levels of … motor and nervous apparatus" (Luria, 1973, p. 27). Therefore, "there can of course be no question of the localization of complex functional systems in limited areas of the brain or of its cortex" (Luria, 1973, p. 30).

Mental activity is a complex functional system "involving the participation of a group of concertedly working areas of the cortex" (Luria, 1973, p. 35). In addition, functional systems are characterized by the variability and mobility of the participating mechanisms. If we consider writing, for instance, then this can also be achieved using the feet or the mouth if circumstances require. For this reason also, rigid allocation of functions to specific brain areas cannot be assumed.

For Luria, language was also a functional system, and his classification of aphasia resulted from localized injuries and their relationship to the respective components of language processing. He outlined a classification that, on the surface and while using different terminology, is not dissimilar to classifications that others have produced. However, the underlying causes of symptoms can be different for Luria. In what follows, I have inserted Benson and Geschwind's (1971) equivalent "neoclassical" forms. Luria described *dynamic aphasia* (also called "frontal" aphasia), which is caused by a lesion of the left prefrontal lobe anterior to the premotor areas. The main features are an apparent lack of a *will* to speak and a disturbance of inner speech. The individual can no longer make predicative statements or propositions, and production is limited to empty phrases. He or she can understand well and can also name and repeat, although little speech is initiated without external stimulation. On the neoclassical model, this is transcortical motor aphasia.

Luria described two separate forms of "motor" aphasia. A lesion of the inferior frontal areas of the left premotor zone, which correspond to Broca's area, led to *efferent (kinetic) motor aphasia*. Individual sounds are not problematic, but the problems occur when the patient has to switch from one articulation to another. The individual

has a problem with the production of linear schemes, which also has effects in other domains, so writing is also impaired in a similar fashion. In later stages of the condition, agrammatism emerged. Neoclassically, this is Broca's aphasia. The second motor aphasia, *afferent (kinesthetic) motor aphasia,* is characterized by problems finding the positions of the articulators necessary for speech, and in milder forms, there is confusion between similar phonemes. Phonemic confusions also occur in reading and writing. The lesion is in the inferior region of the left postcentral parietal cortex, which, among other things, led to the impaired interpretation of kinesthetic feedback. The neoclassical model calls this form conduction aphasia.

Sensory aphasia, according to Luria, is caused by a lesion of the superior and posterior regions of the temporal lobe, which approximately corresponds to Wernicke's area, and indeed on the neoclassical model it would be called Wernicke's aphasia. Luria localized phonemic analysis in the secondary auditory cortex, and while the individuals have intact hearing, they cannot discriminate between, analyze, or synthesize similar phonemes, which leads to comprehension difficulties at the lexical level. Paraphasias and writing problems arose from impaired "phonemic hearing."

An injury to the middle gyrus of the temporal lobe is the underlying cause in *acoustic-amnestic aphasia,* which causes an impairment of verbal memory, the preservation of repetition, comprehension, with fluent speech but with paraphasic errors—a transcortical sensory aphasia in neoclassical terms. Finally, in *semantic aphasia* patients can understand the meaning of individual words, but they cannot grasp the meaning of the construction as a whole, and there is an impairment of what Luria called *logico-grammatical operations* with a disturbance of simultaneous (and spatial) synthesis that affects not only linguistic, but also spatial and praxic systems, and acalculia, and other problems can co-occur. The lesion covers most of the posterior left hemisphere in the parieto-temporo-occipital region. Benson and Geschwind (1971) considered this form of aphasia equivalent to anomia.

On the face of it, Luria's model seems similar to other major classifications, but Luria clearly had different views on the individual processes (analysis, synthesis, integration) engaged in language; his is a *process-model*. In addition, the possibility of aphasic symptoms being connected at different linguistic levels on the basis of abstract principles is implied; for instance, the disturbance of the linear scheme, which appear in sound production, sentence production, and in writing. Importantly, Luria's process model provided routes for the formulation of strategies for rehabilitation because the model is flexible and dynamic, in contrast to the static classical model and because the brain is conceptualized overall as a dynamic and interactive system. While Luria claimed not to be a localizationist but emphasized localizable "functional systems," his model helped to reintroduce localization and provide it with a more dynamic and multidimensional perspective rather than the two-dimensional connectionist view of the old or neo-classical model.

A historically significant study of the effectiveness of aphasia therapy was conducted in Edinburgh by psychologist Oliver Zangwill and speech therapist Edna Butfield and published in 1946 (Butfield & Zangwill, 1946). Howard and Hatfield (1987) suggested that the article "was the first published attempt to evaluate the efficacy of therapy properly, and to assess also the significance of specific factors, such as the form of aphasia and its aetiology" (p. 51). The short article described therapy for 66 cases of aphasia in individuals between the ages of 20 and 40 years, divided into Group 1, which received treatment within 6 months of the onset, and Group 2 whose treatment began after 6 months. The study examined the effects of spontaneous recovery in the second group. Treatment was mainly based on Goldstein's methods, and the amount varied between 5 and 290 sessions per individual. Progress was measured fairly grossly in ratings of *much improved, improved*, or *unchanged*. "Speech" was judged to be *much improved* in half of Group 1 and one third of Group 2, but improvement in the other modalities did not appear to be significant to the authors. Improvement did not appear to be related to spontaneous recovery.

The New World Takes the Lead

The decline in the massive influence of German aphasiology, neurology, and science in general was strongly related to the defeat of Germany in World War I and the shift in the focus of intellectual life to the English-speaking world. With Weisenburg and McBride (1935), there was a shift in focus across the Atlantic and a new, behavioral, psychometric, anticlassification, and antilocalizationist approach to aphasia developed in America. This was spearheaded by particular attention to assessment and rehabilitation. Many classifications of aphasia had developed in the previous century, but Weisenburg and McBride's own was the simple dichotomy of *expressive* or *receptive* aphasia (and mixed expressive–receptive).

The educational psychologist L. Granich (1947) developed therapy for 300 war veterans in Atlantic City Hospital, New Jersey, including 100 with aphasia and related disorders. Granich's therapy was also much influenced by

Goldstein's work, and he was not concerned with standardized testing or aphasic syndromes. He used drilling and believed in the beneficial effects of hard work by patients and in the value of the strategies that patients produced themselves, although his approach was mostly uneven and patchy (Howard & Hatfield, 1987).

Between 1940 and 1960 following World War II, Joseph Wepman (born 1907) and Hildred Schuell (1907–1970) developed assessment and treatment approaches for different aphasia types; these approaches were based heavily on significant auditory stimulation and repetition. For them, the person with aphasia has not lost language functions; the functions have become inaccessible. Language *competence* survived, and it was language *performance* that was impaired and that could be regained with the right kind of stimulation. Therapy essentially entailed facilitating and stimulating language use. Improvement, if it occurred, came because the patient facilitated and integrated what he or she already knew and did not learn new vocabulary or grammatical forms.

The principles of stimulation and repetition remain important ones in present-day approaches to therapy. Both Wepman and Schuell developed test batteries: Wepman developed the Language Modalities Test for Aphasia (LMTA) with Jones (Wepman & Jones, 1961). Schuell saw aphasia as a single unitary condition that could occur with additional complications and symptoms, and she attached great value to a detailed assessment in all modalities, as reflected in the Minnesota Test for Differential Diagnosis of Aphasia (MTDDA) (Schuell, 1955; Schuell, Jenkins, & Jiménez-Pabón, 1964), developed with detailed psychometric evaluation. This battery supported much clinical assessment for rehabilitation in the English-speaking world, well into the late 20th century.

Neoclassicism and the Return to Localization

Boston neurologist Norman Geschwind (1926–1984) was mainly responsible for the return of language localization as what is called neoconnectionism or neoclassicism. Geschwind resurrected the Wernicke–Lichtheim notion that certain areas of the left hemisphere have a narrowly specialized function in language processing, among them especially Broca's and Wernicke's areas (Geschwind, 1974), the connection between Broca's area and Wernicke's area via the arcuate fasciculus, and the angular gyrus mediating between visual and auditory information, which is important for written speech and for naming. Geschwind (1974) described language processing as a form of information processing. Visual information proceeds to the angular gyrus via the primary visual cortex, where the visual form is associated with a corresponding auditory pattern. When the word is required for speech, a representation is passed on to Broca's area via the arcuate fasciculus, where its production is implemented by the motor cortex. Neoclassicism dominated world aphasiology from the 1960s until the 1980s and still has a significant influence.

Wernicke's classification was repackaged as the Boston classification and became internationally known. In addition to considerable research activity in Boston, the influence of Boston was bolstered by the Boston Diagnostic Aphasia Examination (BDAE), developed by Harold Goodglass (1920–2002) and Edith Kaplan (Goodglass & Kaplan, 1972). It became probably the most popular and widely used aphasia battery ever produced, has been translated many times, and still appears to be a widely used clinical assessment in English-speaking countries (Katz et al., 2000). The main functions are the classification of aphasia into (neo) classical types on the basis of functional profiles that emerge from testing and the localization of damage on the basis of this classification. Brain imaging was in its infancy when the BDAE was developed, and localization of structural lesions from impaired functions was an important goal of aphasiological and neuropsychological testing. However, the ability of the BDAE to localize damage on the basis of aphasia classification was unreliable, at best, and the advent of brain-imaging methods made this goal mostly obsolete.

Cognitive Neuropsychology

New approaches were developing that would have a significant impact on how researchers and clinicians approached aphasia. These approaches were emerging from the growth of experimental psycholinguistics and developments in information-processing approaches to cognitive functioning. The cognitive neuropsychological model that was developed in the early 1980s pioneered a shift away from grouping and classifying aphasia. It advocated the development of single-case designs for therapy research (Coltheart, 1983; McReynolds & Kearns, 1983), and good success with well-selected individuals began to be demonstrated.

The development of the cognitive neuropsychological model emerged from the coming together of psycholinguistics, single-case methods, and the information-processing model, and a "theory-driven" and "hypothesis-testing" approach to investigation. This approach was claimed to be preferable to the comparison of mixed groups categorized according to the classical syndromes. Utilizing Jerry Fodor's (1983) ideas on *modularity*, an idea inspired by Gall's faculties,

the model assumed that components of cognition are organized in modules that are domain specific (computations performed by a module are specific to that module only), associated with circumscribed brain structures, genetically determined and computationally autonomous, and independent of other cognitive processes. The model became well known for its box-and-arrow diagrams to conceptualize processing; the diagrams were used to represent the stages and routes involved in activities like reading single words aloud, writing single words to dictation, and naming objects. The model can identify what is impaired and what is retained by detailed hypothesis-driven testing using psycholinguistically controlled tests. It shares some features with the Wernicke–Lichtheim model, not least its focus on single-word processing. Graves (1997) traced the evolution of the traditional Wernicke–Lichtheim model through the subsequent modeling of Dejerine (1892), Liepmann (1920), and Geschwind (1965) to the contemporary models of Marshall and Newcombe (1973) and Ellis and Young (1988). The model informs modern cognitive neuroscience and has had a substantial impact on approaches to assessment and treatment of aphasia.

Microgenetic Theory

While clearly dominant, the cognitive neuropsychological paradigm was not the only theoretical approach to emerge in the second half of the 20th century. Microgenetic theory also developed, although it has not had wide impact. The word *microgenesis* was first introduced in English by Heinz Werner (1956), who adapted the German *Aktualgenese* in an article, "Microgenesis and Aphasia," although Arnold Pick (1913) had explored the microgenetic idea in aphasia earlier. Jason Brown (1979, 1988) developed microgenic theory further. The theory is broadly in the tradition of Hughlings Jackson's evolutionary *levels of neural representation*, although distinct from it. "The idea of microgenesis developed in the Würburg school of psychology ... but the term was coined from the German ... for the microtemporal unfolding of object representations, conceived as a more or less instantaneous recapitulation in cognition of patterns laid down in phylo-ontogeny" (Brown, 1988, p.3).

For microgenesis, the basic assumption is that mental representations, actions, and affects emerge from a prehistory that shapes their major structure, where there is an "unfolding" in microtime (seconds or fractions of seconds) that leads to an idea or an action that unfolds from deep to surface structure. We are aware only of the surface events—ideas, actions—but not the deep prehistory. Measured in millions of years, the temporal unfolding process is evolutionary phylogenesis; measured over a lifetime, it is ontogenesis, and when over a second or less, the process is one of microgenesis, a kind of instantaneous evolution.

Although microgenic theory is in the tradition of Hughlings Jackson, explanations for the emergence of aphasic and other symptoms differs (Brown, 1988). For Hughlings Jackson, the earlier stages in evolution and individual development were released or disinhibited from the control of higher levels; in microgenesis, disinhibition appears to have less relevance. A symptom represents not only the result of a released lower, more primitive, level, but also a natural part of the prehistory of the surface behavior. For instance, the uncontrollable pathological laughing or crying that is a common symptom of pseudobulbar palsy are, on the Hughlings Jacksonian model, disinhibited primitive reactions that are out of higher control due to the upper motor neuron lesion, whereas in microgenic theory they are always there in the deep structure of the nervous system and part of the prehistory of the normal response that is shaped into a normal response by later stages in the unfolding of the response. Therefore, in microgenic theory symptoms are *errors* but are not *deficits*, and they are viewed as achievements of the cognitive processes underlying them. The significant claim is that a symptom represents a normal part of normal processing revealed by pathology (Brown, 1988).

THE TREATMENT OF APHASIA IN THE LATER 20TH CENTURY

Many treatments and therapies developed from often-opposing theoretical approaches during the latter half of the 20th century. It became increasingly clear that an aphasic language disability can result in significant emotional and psychosocial impact, can have a fundamental influence on relationships, and can set up socio-communicative barriers within the person's community.

At this time, treatment approaches and methods developed from a range of sources. There were principled treatments based on theoretical positions, and more symptomatic treatments aimed at reducing or eliminating specific aphasic features. In the 1970s, Frederick Darley (1918–1999) and his students emphasized the importance of the intensity, the duration, and the timing of therapy input (Darley, 1972). Data began to emerge on the best candidates for treatment; thus, the age, the educational background, the time since onset of the damage, and the severity of the aphasia began to emerge as important prognostic variables. A range of group-based randomized clinical trials (RCTs)

were conducted in the latter 20th century but proved difficult to design and carry out, mainly because of the heterogeneous nature of aphasia and the failure to specify and systematize therapy appropriately.

Howard and Hatfield (1987) classified most approaches into several main methodologies. There are didactic methods, which aim to reteach language utilizing traditional and intuitive educational methods from child and foreign language teaching. In common with didactic methods are established behavioral techniques, such as repetition, imitation, modeling, prompting, and cuing. They are utilized in some hierarchically organized therapy approaches for apraxia of speech, and contemporary computer-based methods use systematic behavioral methods (see chapters in Code & Müller, 1995, and Helm-Estabrooks & Albert, 1991). Treatments inspired by the Boston model were developed, mainly by Nancy Helm-Estabrooks and Martin Albert and colleagues (for review, see Helm-Estabrooks & Albert, 1991). Many of these approaches were designed for specific types of aphasia or impairment type, such as perseveration, and use systematic behavioral training hierarchies organized into steps and levels, like Melodic Intonation Therapy (MIT), which aims to reestablish some speech by reorganization of the speech production process using melodic intonation, and Visual Action Therapy (VAT) for Broca's or global impairments.

Schuell's language *stimulation* was a part of many treatments and universally utilized. Luria's (1970) functional systems model formed the basis for approaches to the reorganization of function. Intact functional subsystems could substitute for impaired subsystems. For instance, Luria suggested that letters made of sandpaper could aid a reading impairment via the tactile system, and drawn "articulograms" of the lips producing particular combinations of speech sounds were developed for severe apraxia of speech, with the speaker using his or her intact visual route to the speech production system.

The systematic nature of the cognitive neuropsychological approach had attractive features for clinical work with aphasia, and subsequently other aspects of impaired cognition, and began to have a significant impact on aphasia therapy. The model came with a model of assessment for treatment and an emphasis on the individual patient and their problems. Howard and Patterson (1990) outlined three strategies for therapy that could work with the model: reteaching of the missing information or missing rules or procedures based on detailed testing; teaching a different way to do the same task; and facilitating the use of impaired access routes. While these broad strategies for treatment were not new, the model's main contribution has been in systematizing assessment, allowing a clearer identification of the location of impairments within a hypothetical model.

The development of a cognitive neuropsychologically inspired single-case approach was much aided by the failure of RCTs to demonstrate that treatment was efficacious or effective. A similar disenchantment with medical-model, classification-based treatments was at least a partial cause for a parallel shift to more everyday functional communication at this time. Martha Taylor-Sarno (1969) and Audrey Holland (1980) were important in developing functional approaches to assessment and treatment. Approaches like promoting aphasics communicative effectiveness (PACE; Davis & Wilcox, 1985) emphasized successful communication, not precise oral naming or correct syntax. The main features of the approach are that the therapist and patient participate equally as sender and receiver of messages; interactions entail the exchange of new information; the person with aphasia chooses the modality or methods of communication; feedback is based on the person with aphasia's success in communicating the message and encourages writing, gesture, drawing, and pointing.

Reorganizational approaches developed based on surviving RH processing in the 1980s to 1990s. These include MIT, which claims to utilize intact RH musical processing. Artificial languages made up of visual arbitrary shapes or symbols were devised from work with chimpanzees, and remarkable success was reported, with globally impaired patients being able to use the systems propositionally. There were also attempts to directly influence cognitive processing in the RH and stimulate latent RH language processes using lateralization techniques like dichotic listening and hemifield viewing, although it was never clear that improvements observed were due to increased RH involvement (for review, see Code, 1987). In the 1980s, treatments began to be developed that were delivered by microcomputers using mainly behavioral methods (see the collection led by Katz, 1987). Intense stimulation and feedback on performance and control of the pace and level of difficulty by the user appeared to be clear advantages.

Also during the early 1980s, the relevance of the psychosocial impact of aphasia began to be better recognized, although Goldstein had pioneered its importance before World War II. Most of our happiness and sadness comes from our interactions with others. How we perceive our interactions with others is what determines the quality of our life experience, our psychosocial well-being. Our psychosocial life is grounded in our emotional experience, within a social context. The psychosocial impact of aphasia on people with aphasia and on their families began to be increasingly acknowledged, and approaches to improve the psychosocial state began to be developed (see the collection of papers in Code, 1999, and Code, Hemsley, & Herrmann, 1999). In 1980, the World Health Organization (WHO) introduced the terms *impairment, disability,* and *handicap* to describe and categorize disease. In this later part of the 20th century, the "disability movement" was successful in introducing a social model that contrasted significantly with the medical model's perspective of illness, and the social disability and social exclusion that accompany aphasia became increasingly acknowledged.

The more recent draft of the *International Classification of Impairments, Disabilities, and Health* (World Health Organization, 2001) proposed three dimensions: *Impairment* is a loss or abnormality of body structure or of a physiological or psychological function, whereas in an *activity limitation* the extent of functioning at the level of the person is reduced or limited. Activities may be limited in nature, duration, and quality. The term *disability* was replaced by *activity limitation*. Participation is the nature and extent of a person's involvement in life situations in relation to impairments, activities, health conditions, and contextual factors. *Handicap* was replaced by *participation restriction*. However, it may be some time before these rather awkward terms replace the familiar impairment, disability, and handicap.

This approach sees the problem lying not in the individual's impairments but in society's failure to accommodate their different needs, which lead to people with disabilities facing increased social barriers and oppression (Jordan, 1998). The main objective of the social approach to aphasic disability is to increase successful participation in authentic communication events, to focus on communication at the level of conversation, to provide communicative support systems within the speaker's own community, and to increase communicative confidence and empower speakers with aphasia (Simmons-Mackie, 1998).

In recent years, evidenced-based practice (EBP) has emerged as a concept and is essentially a principled and systematic approach to evaluating the relative strengths of a treatment for an individual. It combines clinical expertise, best current evidence, and client values with the aim of providing the highest quality service reflecting the needs and choices of the individual (Sackett, Strauss, Richardson, Rosenberg, & Haynes, 2000). This process of evaluation is aided in practice with the range of systematic reviews of therapy trials available, and there are a range of useful resources that can help with what could be time consuming for a busy clinician. The American Speech-Language-Hearing Association (ASHA) and Academy of Neurogenic Communication Disorders and Sciences (ANCDS) both provide detailed evaluations of evidence for the effectiveness of aphasia treatment that are freely available online (http://www.asha.org; http://www.ancds.org/evidence-based-practice-guidelines). SpeechBite is a free web resource that enables searching for approaches to therapy across the specialties of speech and language therapy and pathology, including aphasia and related conditions (http://www.speechbite.com/). It provides an online database established to gain fast access to evaluated relevant evidenced-based research for clinical decision making, contains references to more than 3,000 journal articles, and provides methodological reliably established ratings to help identify the research quality of therapy trials (Murray et al., 2013). The Aphasia Software Finder developed at Frenchay Hospital, Bristol, United Kingdom, and funded by the Tavistock Trust provides an online service for people with aphasia and their families as well as professionals for locating relevant computer treatment software packages and provides evaluation (http://www.aphasiatavistocktrust.org/aphasia/default/software.asp).

To end this brief sketch of the history of aphasia and its treatment, we might ask whether things got any better for people with aphasia in the 20th century. At the turn of the 21st century, Katz et al. (2000) conducted an international survey across the English-speaking world, with data collected from clinical aphasia departments in the United States, Canada, Australia, and the United Kingdom. Findings revealed that the mean amount of therapy per week received at the acute stage was just 30 minutes for Australia and the United Kingdom.

For North America, the mean was 60 minutes per week, but with a range of 16 to 20 sessions (the North American data included the Veterans Affairs hospital system). The figures for the United Kingdom and Australia in particular suggest that people with aphasia, even in the acute stage, can expect no more than 2.5 hours of therapy spread over 5 weeks. The amount of therapy someone with more long-term aphasia can expect is even less (see the collection of studies of the treatment of chronic aphasia edited by Code, 2010).

Yet, there is evidence that intensive therapy, even relatively short in duration, can improve outcome, especially, but not exclusively, in the early stages of recovery. Bhogal, Teasell, and Speechley (2003) conducted an analysis of the large-group trials that have been completed

over the years that examined the effectiveness of aphasia treatment. They found a significant treatment effect in studies that provided 8.8 hours of weekly therapy for 11.2 weeks; studies that did not show a significant treatment effect provided less than 2 hours for 23 weeks. The implication of these results seems clear: Intensive therapy over a relatively short duration can be more effective, and more cost-effective, than nonintensive therapy over twice the duration.

Methods of treatment have improved considerably over the centuries, and a great deal of research into rehabilitation demonstrated that it can be effective, as this volume demonstrates. People with aphasia do receive treatment for their impairments and their disabilities in modern times, but the gap between what we know about the effectiveness of treatment and the service we provide to people with aphasia does not appear to be narrowing.

What could a future history of aphasia look like? As noted elsewhere (Tesak & Code, 2008), predicting the future may well be imprudent given the obvious unpredictable nature of future events. However, trends in health care and public health suggest that the incidence of stroke in the 40- to 60-year age range will reduce—at least in the developed world—as improved medical interventions result in an increase in survival from stroke and improved awareness of the importance of diet, exercise, and life style make an impact. But, people are living longer, and this brings with it an increase in the incidence of progressive neurological conditions, including aphasia, so aphasia will be with us for many years yet, and the management of aphasia will continue to be a significant concern for the foreseeable future.

What might be the nature of this management of aphasia? Predictions suggest that pharmaceutical and neurophysiological interventions will emerge, but essentially coupled with behavioral assessment and treatment carried out by trained and experienced clinicians (Small, 2000, 2004).

Broca, Wernicke, Hughlings Jackson, and their contemporaries might be surprised and rather disappointed that aphasia still constitutes a significant problem for many in the early 21st century, but current developments in treatment and management, illustrated by this volume, should provide some optimism for the future.

STUDY QUESTIONS

1. When in the history of aphasia did thinkers associate damage to the brain with impairments in speech and language?
2. Describe the main forms of aphasia identified by the Wernicke–Lichtheim model.
3. What were the main trends that caused a shift of focus in aphasia research from Europe to North America?
4. What single event is often suggested to have heralded the beginnings of modern aphasiology?

5. Why was Gall's *organology* (Spurzheim's *phrenology*) so revolutionary, and in which ways is it an inadequate theory of the relationship between brain structure and brain function?

6. Who developed the so-called speech gymnastics approaches to aphasia treatment?

7. Writers in previous times have described aphasia as a memory disorder. Why, and does the idea that various aphasic impairments may be caused by some impairment in memory have relevance today?

8. In what ways did Arnold Pick describe and distinguish *agrammatism* from *paragrammatism*?

9. Who has been called the father of aphasia therapy?

10. Stimulation plays a particularly significant role in the history of the treatment of aphasia. With whom is the idea associated?

11. Who developed a more systematic and psychometric approach to testing for aphasia?

REFERENCES

Baillarger, J. G. F. (1865). *De l'aphasie au point de vie psychologique.* Paris: Masson.

Bastian, H. C. (1898). *A treatise on aphasia and other speech defects.* London: Lewis.

Bateman, F. (1890). *On aphasia, or loss of speech, and the localisation of the faculty of articulate language* (2nd ed.). London: Churchill.

Bennett, M. R., & Hacker, P. M. S. (2003). *Philosophical foundations of neuroscience.* Oxford, UK: Blackwell.

Benson, D. F., & Geschwind, N. (1971), Aphasia and related cortical disturbances. In A. B. Baker & L. H. Baker (Eds.), *Clinical neurology* (pp. 112–140). New York: Harper & Row.

Benton, A. L. (1965). Johann A. P. Gesner on aphasia. *Medical History, 1,* 54–60.

Benton, A. L. (1988). Pitres and amnesic aphasia. *Aphasiology, 2,* 209–214.

Bhogal, S. K., Teasell, R., & Speechley, M. (2003). Intensity of aphasia therapy, impact on recovery. *Stroke, 34,* 987–993.

Bogen, J. (1969). The other side of the brain II: An appositional mind. *Bulletin of the Los Angeles Neurological Societies, 34r,* 135–162.

Breasted, J. H. (1930). *The Edwin Smith surgical papyrus (2 vols.).* Chicago: University of Chicago Press.

Broca, P. (1861). Perte de la parole, ramollissement chronique de destruction partielle du lobe antérieur gauche du cerveau. *Bulletins de la Société d'Anthropologie de Paris* (séance du 18 avril), 235–238.

Broca, P. (1863). Localisation des fonctions cérébrales. Siège du langage articulé. *Bulletins de la Société Anthropologique de Paris* (séance du 2 avril), 200–204.

Broca, P. (1865). Sur le siège de la faculté du langage articulé. *Bulletins de la Société Anthropologique de Paris* (séance du 15 juin), 377–393.

Brown, J. W. (1979) *Language representation in the brain.* In: Steklis, H. & Raleigh, M. (Eds.) (1979) Neurobiology of Social Communication in Primates. New York: Academic Press.

Brown, J. W. (1988) *Life of the mind.* Mahwah, NJ: Erlbaum.

Buckingham, H. W. (2006). Was Sigmund Freud the first neogrammarian neurologist? *Aphasiology, 20,* 1085–1104.

Butfield, E., & Zangwill, O. (1946). Reeducation in aphasia: A review of 70 cases. *Journal of Neurology, Neurosurgery and Psychiatry, 9,* 75–79.

Charcot, J. M. (1884). *Differanti forme d'afasia.* Milan: Vallardi.

Chomsky, N. (1957a). A review of *Verbal Behavior,* by B. F. Skinner. *Language, 35,* 26–58.

Chomsky, N. (1957b). *Syntactic structures.* Hague: Mouton.

Chomsky, N. (1965). *Aspects of the theory of syntax.* Cambridge, MA: MIT Press.

Code, C. (1987). *Language, aphasia, and the right hemisphere.* London: Wiley.

Code, C. (Ed.). (1999). Management of psychosocial issues in aphasia. *Seminars in Speech and Language, 20,* 1–92.

Code, C. (Ed.). (2010). Treatment of chronic aphasia: International perspectives. *Seminars in Speech and Language, 31,* 3–75.

Code, C., Hemsley, G., & Herrmann, M. (1999). The emotional impact of aphasia. *Seminars in Speech and Language, 20,* 19–31.

Code, C., & Müller, D. J. (Eds.). (1995). *Treatment of aphasia: From theory to practice.* London: Whurr.

Coltheart, M. (1983). Aphasia therapy research: The single-case study approach. In C. Code & D. J. Müller (Eds.), *Aphasia therapy* (pp. 193–202). London: Arnold.

Darley, F. L. (1972). The efficacy of language rehabilitation in aphasia. *Journal of Speech and Hearing Research, 37,* 3–21.

Darwin, C. (1859). *On the origin of species by means of natural selection, or the preservation of favoured races in the struggle for life.* London: Murray.

Davis, G. A., & Wilcox, M. J. (1985). *Adult aphasia rehabilitation. Applied pragmatics.* San Diego, CA: College-Hill Press.

Dax, M. (1836–1865). Lésions de la moitié gauche de l'encéphale coincidant avec l'oubli des signes de la pensée—Lu au congrès méridional tenu à Montpellier en 1836. *Gazette Hebdomadaire de Médecine et de Chirurgie, 2* (2nd ser.), 259–260.

Dejerine, J. (1891). Sur un cas de cécité verbale avec agraphie suivi d'autopsie. *Mémoires de la Société de Biologie, 3,* 197–201.

Dejerine, J. (1892). Contribution a l'étude anatomo-pathologigue et clinique des différentes variétés de cécité verbale. *Comptes rendus hebdomadaires des séances et mémoires de la société de biologie et de ses filialies, 44,* 61–90.

Domanski, C. W. (2013). Mysterious *"Monsieur Leborgne"*: The mystery of the famous patient in the history of neuropsychology is explained. *Journal of the History of the Neurosciences: Basic and Clinical Perspectives,* 22(1), 47–52.

Eling, P. (Ed.). (1994). *Reader in the history of aphasia.* Amsterdam: Benjamins.

Eling, P. (2006). The psycholinguistic approach to aphasia of Chajim Steinthal. *Aphasiology, 20,* 1072–1084.

Ellis, A. W., & Young, A. W. (1988). *Cognitive neuropsychology.* Hove, UK: Erlbaum.

Finger, S. (1994). *Origins of neuroscience. A history of explorations into brain function.* Oxford: Oxford University Press.

Finger, S., & Roe, D. (1996). Gustave Dax and the early history of cerebral dominance. *Archives of Neurology, 53*, 806–813.

Fodor, J. A. (1983). *The modularity of mind*. Cambridge, MA: MIT Press.

Freud, S. (1891). *Zur Auffassung der Aphasien. Eine kritische Studie*. Leipzig, Germany: Deuticke.

Freud, S. (1953). *On aphasia. A critical study*. New York: International Universities Press. (Original work published 1891)

Gall, F. J. (1798). Des Herrn F. J. Gall Schreiben über seinen bereits geendigten Prodromus über die Verrichtungen des Gehirns der Menschen und der Thiere an Herrn Jos. Fr. von Retzer. *Der Neue Teutsche Merkur, 3*, 311–332. (Reprinted in Lesky, 1979[KB1]).

Garrett, M. F. (1980). Levels of processing in sentence production. In Butterworth, B. (Ed.), *Language production. Vol. 1: Speech and talk* (pp. 177–200). New York: Academic Press.

Gelfand, T. (1999). Charcot's brains. *Brain and Language, 69*, 31–55.

Geschwind, N. (1965). Disconnexion syndromes in animals and man. *Brain, 88*, 237–294, 585–644.

Geschwind, N. (1974). *Selected papers on language and the brain*. Dordrecht: Reidel.

Goodglass, H., & Kaplan, E. (1972). *The assessment of aphasia and related disorders*. Philadelphia: Lea & Febiger.

Granich, L. (1947). *Aphasia: A guide to retraining*. New York: Grune & Stratton.

Graves, R. E. (1997). The legacy of the Wernicke-Lichtheim model. *Journal of the History of Neurosciences, 6*, 3–20.

Halliday, M. A. K. (1961). Categories of the theory of grammar. *Word, 17*, 241–292.

Halliday, M. A. K. (1985). *An introduction to functional grammar*. London: Arnold.

Hanley, R., & Kay, J. (2003). Monsieur C: Dejerine's case of alexia without agraphia. In C. Code, C.-W. Wallesch, Y. Joanette, & A. R. Lecours (Eds.), *Classic cases in neuropsychology (Vol. 2*, pp. 57–74). Hove, UK: Psychology Press.

Head, H. (1926). *Aphasia and kindred disorders of speech (2 vols.)*. Cambridge, UK: Macmillan.

Helm-Estabrooks, N., & Albert, M. L. (1991). *Manual of aphasia therapy*. Austin, TX: Pro-Ed.

Holland, A. (1980). *Communicative abilities in daily living [CADL]. A test of functional communication for aphasic patients*. Baltimore: University Park Press.

Howard, D., & Hatfield, F. M. (1987). *Aphasia therapy: Historical and contemporary issues*. Hove, UK: Erlbaum.

Howard, D., & Patterson, K. (1990). Methodological issues in neuropsychological therapy. In X. Seron & G. Deloche (Eds.), (pp. 39-64) *Cognitive approaches in neuropsychological rehabilitation*. London: Erlbaum.

Hughlings Jackson, J. (1878–1880). In Taylor, J. (Ed.). (1958). *Selected writings of John Hughlings Jackson: Vol. 2: Evolution and dissolution of the nervous system, speech, various papers, addresses and lectures*. New York: Basic Books.

Isserlin, M. (1922). Über Agrammatismus. *Zeitschrift für die gesamte Neurologie und Psychiatrie, 75*, 332–410.

Jakobson, R. (1941). *Kindersprache, Aphasie und allgemeine Lautgesetze*. Uppsala, Sweden: Universitets Arsskrift.

Jakobson, R. (1964). Towards a linguistic typology of aphasic impairments. In A. de Reuck & M. O'Connor (Eds.), *Disorders of language* (pp. 223–246). London: Churchill.

Jakobson, R. (1968). *Child language, aphasia and phonological universals*. Hague: Mouton.

Jordan, L. (1998). Partners in care. *Bulletin of the Royal College of Speech & Language Therapists*, August, pp. 7–8.

Joynt, R., & Benton, A. (1964). The memoir of Marc Dax on aphasia. *Neurology, 14*, 851–854.

Kaczmarek, B. L. J. (Ed.). (1995). Special issue for A. R. Luria. *Aphasiology, 9*, 97–206.

Kagan, A., & Saling, M. (1992). *An introduction to Luria's aphasiology. Theory and application* (2nd ed.). Johannesburg: Witwatersrand University Press.

Katz, R. C. (1987). Efficacy of aphasia treatment using microcomputers. *Aphasiology, 1*, 141–175.

Katz, R. C., Hallowell, B., Code, C., Armstrong, E., Roberts, P., Pound, C., & Katz, L. (2000). A multi-national comparison of aphasia management practices. *International Journal of Language & Communication Disorders, 35*, 303–314.

Kleist, K. (1914). Aphasie und Geisteskrankheit. *Münchener Medizinische Wochenschrift, 61*(1), 8–12.

Kleist, K. (1916). Die Leitungsaphasie und grammatische Störungen. *Monatsschrift für Psychiatrie und Neurologie, 40*, 118–199.

Levelt, W. J. M. (1989). *Speaking: From intention to articulation*. Cambridge, MA: MIT Press.

Lesky, E. (1970). Structure and function in Gall. *Bulletin of the History of Medicine, 44*, 297–314.

Lichtheim, L. (1885). On aphasia. *Brain, 7*, 433–485.

Liepmann, H. (1920). Apraxie. *Ergebnisse der gesamten medizin, 1*, 516–543.

Luria, A. R. (1970). *Traumatic aphasia. Its syndromes, psychology and treatment*. Hague: Mouton.

Luria, A. R. (1973). *The working brain. An introduction to neuropsychology*. Harmondsworth, UK: Penguin.

Luria, A. R. (1980). *Higher cortical functions in man* (2nd ed.). New York: Basic Books.

Marie, P. (1906). Révision de la question sur l'aphasie: La troisième circonvolution frontale gauche ne joue aucun rôle spécial dans la fonction du langage. *La Semaine Médicale, 26*, 241–247.

McReynolds, L. V., & Kearns, K. P. (1983). *Single subject experimental designs in communicative disorders*. Baltimore: University Park Press.

Marshall, J. C., & Newcombe, F. (1973). Patterns of paralexia. *Journal of Psycholinguistic Research, 2*, 175–199.

Miller, G. A. (1964). The psycholinguistics. *Encounter, 23*, 29–37.

Murray, E., Power, E., Togher, L., McCabe, P., Munro, N., & Smith, K. (2013). The reliability of methodological ratings for speechBITE using the PEDro-P scale. *International Journal of Language & Communication Disorders, 48*, 297–306.

Nespoulous, J.-L., Code, C., Virbel, J., & Lecours, A.-R. (1998). Hypotheses on the dissociation between "referential" and "modalizing" verbal behaviour in aphasia. *Applied Psycholinguistics, 19*, 311–331.

Paradis, M. (1981). Acquired aphasia in bilingual speakers. In M. Taylor Sarno (Ed.), *Acquired aphasia* (3rd ed., pp. 531–549). San Diego: Academic Press.

Paradis, M. (Ed.). (1983). *Readings on aphasia in bilinguals and polyglots*. Montreal: Didier.

Pick, A. (1913). *Die agrammatischen Sprachstörungen*. Berlin: Springer.

Pitres, A. L. (1895). Etude sur l'aphasie chez les polyglottes. *Revue de Médecine, 15*, 873–899. (Translated in Paradis, 1983, 26–49)

Pitres, A. L. (1898). *L'aphasie amnésique et ses variétés cliniques*. Paris: Alcan.

Ribot, T. (1881). *Les maladies de la mémoire*. Paris: Baillère.

Sackett, D. L., Strauss, S. E., Richardson, W. S., Rosenberg, W., & Haynes, R. B. (2000). *Evidence-based medicine: How to practice and teach EBM* (2nd ed.). Edinburgh: Churchill Livingstone.

Schiller, F. (1992). *Paul Broca, founder of French anthropology, explorer of the brain.* New York: Oxford University Press.

Schuell, H. (1955). *Minnesota test for differential diagnosis of aphasia.* Minneapolis: University of Minnesota.

Schuell, H., Jenkins, J. J., & Jiménez-Pabón, E. (1964). *Aphasia in adults. Diagnosis, prognosis, and treatment.* New York: Harper & Row.

Simmons-Mackie, N. (1998). A solution to the discharge dilemma in aphasia: Social approaches to aphasia management. *Aphasiology, 12,* 231–239.

Small, S. L. (2000) The future of aphasia therapy. *Brain and Language, 71,* 227–232.

Small, S. L. (2004) A biological model of aphasia rehabilitation: Pharmacological perspectives. *Aphasiology, 18,* 473–492.

Steinthal, H. (1871). *Einleitung in die Psychologie und Sprachwissenschaft.* Berlin: Dümmler's Verlagsbuchhandlung.

Taylor, J. (Ed.). (1958). *Selected writings of John Hughlings Jackson: Vol. 2: Evolution and dissolution of the nervous system, speech, various papers, addresses and lectures.* New York: Basic Books.

Taylor-Sarno, M. (1969). *The functional communication profile: Manual of directions.* New York: Institute of Rehabilitation Medicine.

Tesak, J., & Code, C. (2008). *Milestones in the history of aphasia: Theories and protagonists.* Hove, UK: Psychology Press.

Tomasello, M. (2014). Introduction to the classic edition. In M. Tomasello (Ed.), *The new psychology of language: Cognitive and functional approaches to language structure* (Vol. 1, pp. vii–xii). Hove, UK: Psychology Press.

Trousseau, A. (1864). De l'aphasie, maladie décrite récemment sous le nom impropre d'aphémie. *Gazette des Hôpitaux Civils et Militaires, 37,* 13–14, 25–26, 37–39, 48–50.

Weisenburg, T. H., & McBride, K. E. (1935). *Aphasia: A clinical and psychological study.* New York: Commonwealth Fund.

Wepman, J., & Jones, L. (1961). *The language modalities test for aphasia.* Chicago: University of Chicago.

Werner, H. (1956) Microgenesis and aphasia. *Journal of Abnormal Social Psychology, 52,* 347–353.

Wernicke, C. (1874). *Der Aphasische Symptomencomplex. Eine psychologische Studie auf anatomischer Basis.* Breslau, Poland: Cohn & Weigert.

Whitaker, H., & Etlinger, S. (1993). Theodor Meynert's contribution to classical 19th century aphasia studies. *Brain and Language, 45,* 560–571.

Willis, T. (1965). *The anatomy of the brain and nerves.* Montreal: McGill University Press. (Original work published 1664)

World Health Organization (WHO). (2001). *International classification of functioning, disability and health.* Geneva: Author.

Elements of Neurology Essential for Understanding the Aphasias

Constantin Potagas, Dimitrios S. Kasselimis, and Ioannis Evdokimidis

INTRODUCTION

There is still much to be done to understand the nature of aphasia and to elucidate the organization of the brain relative to behavior. Nevertheless, since the time of Paul Broca, who was the first to show, in 1861, that a particular lesion of the cerebral cortex could lead to a disorder of language (Broca, 1861, as cited in Hécaen & Dubois, 1969), our knowledge of cerebral organization related to language has greatly advanced, and the clinical repercussions of cerebral lesions have been extensively described. In this chapter, we outline briefly the anatomy, physiology, and pathology of the nervous system, as well as the methods available for its study, and we then sketch the functional organization of the cerebral correlates of language. This brief overview concludes with the description of the clinical characteristics of the various forms of aphasia.

ELEMENTS OF THE NERVOUS SYSTEM

Language is a complex function involving substantial parts of the central nervous system; indeed, few brain sites could be destroyed without resulting in some language deficit. Speech, which is just one of the language outputs, is an extremely complex act: Consider, for example, the production of a single sound like the phoneme /a/. It involves the coordinated activity of several nerves and muscles for the air to be exhaled from the lungs, passing through the larynx, the pharynx, and the articulators (tongue, lips, teeth, cheeks), and multiple other actions, such as inspiration; expiration; opening and closing of the vocal cords; and movement of the larynx, pharynx, mouth, and so forth. Moreover, for their successful coordination, these actions need to be monitored, and monitoring requires sensory feedback to the brain from sensory nerves in the vocalization system, attesting to its correct configuration. Moreover, in real-life circumstances, speech sounds rarely, if ever, emerge as context-free productions: The phoneme /a/ in this example would sound different depending on the mood, on the intention, and on the physical condition of the speaker, as well as on the surrounding circumstances affecting the audibility of the sound produced. The speaker is therefore capable of modulating the sound to be produced, and this requires that its mode of production be decided first at a higher level, such as the frontal association cortex, and a signal transmitted to the "execution" part of the brain, the motor cortex. In the meantime, the auditory cortex of the temporal lobes informs the speaker about background sonority to modulate the voice, and the visual cortex informs the speaker about the relative position of his or her conversation partner. It is the purpose of the following section of this chapter to provide an outline of the nervous system, emphasizing those components that are necessary to support the processes of production and perception of speech and language.

Gross Anatomy

The two cerebral hemispheres, brain stem, and cerebellum together with the spinal cord form the central nervous system (CNS). Each hemisphere is divided into lobes: the frontal, the parietal, the temporal, and the occipital (Figure 3.1). On the surface of the brain are elevated convolutions called gyri separated by grooves called sulci. For example, the frontal lobe is divided into three convolutions: the superior, middle, and inferior frontal gyri. The two cerebral hemispheres are interconnected with commissures, the most massive of them being the corpus callosum. Behind and below them are located the brain stem and the spinal cord. The cerebellum consists of a central part, the vermis, and two cerebellar hemispheres. It is attached to the posterior part of the brain stem and resides under the cerebral hemispheres (Figure 3.1). All these structures are protected by three layers of meninges (i.e., dura mater, arachnoid membrane, pia mater) and the bony tube formed by the skull and the vertebrae that are part of the spinal column.

These structures are bathed in the cerebrospinal fluid (CSF), which absorbs noxious vibrations. The brain contains the ventricular system (Figure 3.1), also filled

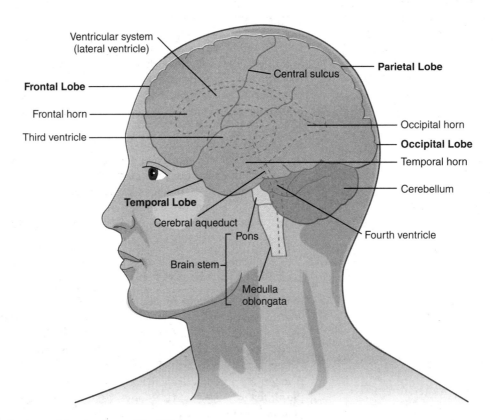

Figure 3.1 Anatomy of the structures of the CNS.

with CSF, which communicates with the spinal fluid surrounding the CNS. Two lateral ventricles, one in each hemisphere, with horns corresponding to each lobe (frontal, temporal, and occipital), communicate with a single third ventricle, above the brain stem, which continues through the cerebral aqueduct to the fourth ventricle, located between the back of the brain stem and the anterior surface of the cerebellum. Its extension is the small-diameter central canal that runs through the entire length of the spinal cord.

The content of CSF in cells, proteins, sugar, or other substances varies, normally only slightly. However, in various pathologic conditions its consistency or pressure is altered. For example, an infection and other conditions are characterized by the presence of particular types of leukocytes in the CSF or elevations in its pressure. Therefore, we can assess the condition of the CNS by analyzing CSF samples collected through insertion of a needle in the intrameningeal space between the last lumbar vertebras (where the spinal cord comes to its end, a procedure called lumbar puncture, LP). In neurosurgical settings, it is also possible to monitor the intracranial pressure, which usually increases after traumatic brain injury (TBI), by inserting pressure sensors directly in the brain's ventricular system.

The Vascular System of the Brain

The maintenance and the function of brain cells depend on arterial blood supply (see Figure 3.2). Blood arrives to the brain through two systems: the anterior or carotid circulation system and the posterior or vertebrobasilar circulation system. A communication system between the two carotids and the posterior system, the circle of Willis, allows arterial blood to circulate in both directions in case of disturbance of the normal inflow in either of the systems. For example, if one of the carotid arteries is obstructed by a blood clot, the corresponding anterior parts of the brain are supplied from the other carotid or from the posterior system. However, this system does not protect the areas irrigated from arteries beyond the circle of Willis.

Each of the two common carotid arteries divides into an exterior branch (external carotid), irrigating the face and meninges of the brain, and the internal carotid, which feeds the anterior two-thirds of the brain hemispheres. The first branch (the ophthalmic artery) irrigates the corresponding eye. The anterior cerebral artery emerges next (Figure 3.3b), directed to the front and curving backward, around the corpus callosum, at the internal surface of each hemisphere. It irrigates the anterior part of the frontal lobe, the corpus callosum, and the interior part of the frontal and parietal lobes, including the sensorimotor cortex part corresponding to the lower limb. The middle cerebral artery is the final branch of the internal carotid artery (Figure 3.3a), irrigating about two-thirds of the cerebral hemisphere, from the cortical surface to its depths. Specifically, it irrigates the basal ganglia, the posterior lateral part of the frontal lobe, and the lateral aspects of the temporal

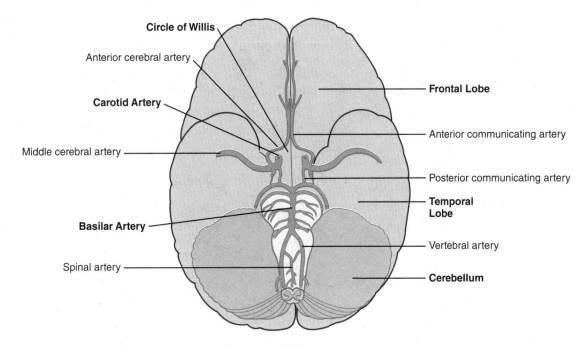

Figure 3.2 The vascular system of the brain and the circle of Willis.

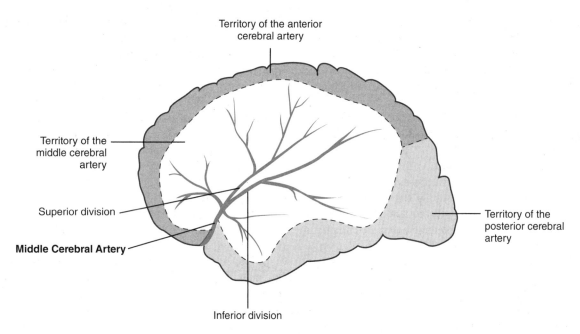

Territory of the anterior
cerebral artery

Territory of the
middle cerebral
artery

Superior division

Middle Cerebral Artery

Territory of the
posterior cerebral
artery

Inferior division

Figure 3.3a Irrigation areas of the brain's arteries. Schematic representation of irrigation territories of the cerebral arteries. External surface of the hemisphere.

and the parietal lobes, including the sensorimotor strip, except for the region corresponding to the lower limb, which is irrigated by the anterior cerebral artery.

The confluence of the two vertebral arteries forms the basilar artery, which irrigates the brain stem and the cerebellum; it is then divided in the two posterior cerebral arteries (Figure 3.3b), irrigating the corresponding occipital lobes, the posterior part of the temporal lobes, and some subcortical structures, such as the thalami.

Neurons and Synapses

The brain consists of about 100 billion neural cells, a supporting system of glial cells, and the cerebral

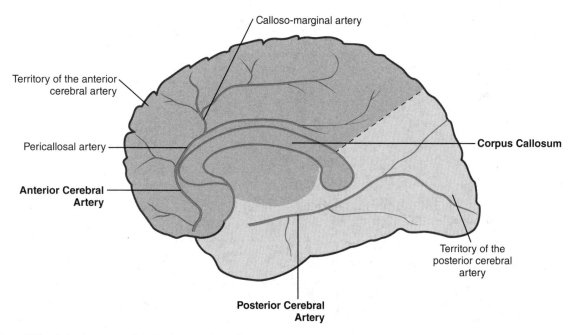

Calloso-marginal artery

Territory of the anterior
cerebral artery

Pericallosal artery

**Anterior Cerebral
Artery**

Corpus Callosum

Territory of the
posterior cerebral
artery

**Posterior Cerebral
Artery**

Figure 3.3b Irrigation areas of the brain's arteries. Schematic representation of irrigation territories of the cerebral arteries. Internal surface of the hemisphere.

vascular system. The neural cell, also called a *neuron*, includes a cell body and multiple extensions: one axon and one or more dendrites through which it establishes up to 10,000 connections with other neurons, the synapses. At the level of the synapse, chemical substances are exchanged and electric signals—positive (excitatory), negative (inhibitory)—are transmitted between the neurons. The several trillions of synapses within the brain form an immense network, which is the basis of the integrative function of the CNS, which may be understood through the analogy of the action of high-power computer systems. However, this analogy fails to capture many attributes of the nervous system, most importantly the lifelong capacity of neurons to continuously rearrange their synapses. This is the core element of the brain's capacity for functional reorganization, called *plasticity*. Rehabilitation techniques used for correcting many brain dysfunctions, such as spasticity control, or sensitivity enhancement to ameliorate reduced capacity for movement, are based on the principle of plasticity.

Gray and White Matter

We call *gray matter* the brownish tissue consisting of the bodies of neurons that constitute the cerebral cortex, that is, the surface of the cerebral hemispheres, and the cerebral nuclei, that is, the neural masses deep in the cerebral hemispheres (the basal ganglia, the thalamus, and the hypothalamus; see Figure 3.4), and the nuclei of the cranial nerves in the brain stem. A similar arrangement is found in the cerebellum. The gray matter occupies a central position in the spinal cord, forming the wall of the spinal canal. When seen in transverse sections, it has the shape of a capital *H*, with anterior and posterior horns. The bodies of the motor neurons are found in the anterior horns. Motor axons, which exit the spinal cord as the ventral root, and sensory axons, which enter the posterior horns as the dorsal root, together form the peripheral nervous system (PNS; see also the section "The Peripheral Nervous System: Peripheral Versus Central Paralysis").

The white matter fills the rest of the cerebral hemispheres, between cortex and basal ganglia, the brain stem, around the nuclei of cranial nerves, and the periphery of the spinal cord. White is the color of the sheath of myelin around the neural axons, and white matter consists of bundles of axons (fasciculi or tracts) that connect areas of the cortex with one another, the cortex with the nuclei in the hemispheres and the brain stem and with all levels of the spinal cord.[1]

The corpus callosum and other commissures (also white matter tracts) connect the two hemispheres and allow the communication and reciprocal control of cortical areas on both sides of the brain. Lesions that interrupt connections between areas of the cerebral cortex produce disconnection syndromes. A typical example of such a disconnection is the one resulting in pure alexia or alexia without agraphia. It consists of a lesion interrupting communication between visual areas of both occipital lobes with areas for language in the left hemisphere. Another example is the split-brain syndrome, caused by

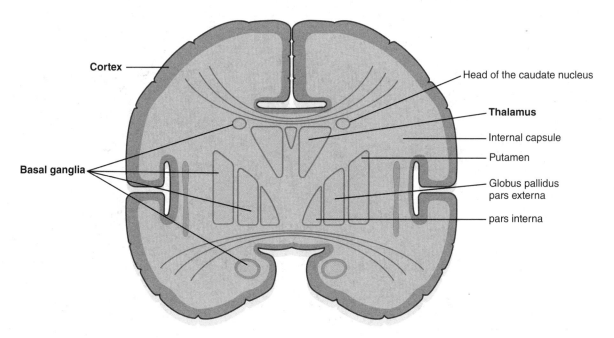

Figure 3.4 Coronal section of the cerebral hemispheres.

the section of the corpus callosum, which results in various disorders, such as the difficulty of naming objects palpated with the left (but not with the right) hand.

Long bundles of axons (i.e., tracts) connect the cortex, the brain stem, and the spinal cord, forming efferent and afferent tracts: An efferent, descending, motor pathway, the pyramidal tract, consists of the axons of neurons in the motor area of the cortex (first-order motor neuron), terminating in the motor nuclei of the brain stem (corticobulbar tract) and the anterior horns of the spinal cord (corticospinal tract). The pyramidal tract controls the motor cranial nerves exiting the brain stem and the motor neurons of the spinal cord (second-order motor neuron). Sensory axons form the afferent, ascending, or somatosensory tract, connecting sensory receptors all over the body to the somatosensory area of the cortex via the thalamus (one of the subcortical structures that functions as a relay station). Both the efferent and the afferent tracts spread out like a fan under the cortex, forming the corona radiata, which presents a narrow stem in the center of each hemisphere between the masses of gray matter, the internal capsule. The tracts continue beyond this level, along the brain stem and the spinal cord, crossing at midline (from left to right and conversely[2]) at various levels of the brain stem (see Figures 3.5a and 3.5b).

These anatomic details are useful to explain how a tiny lesion at the level of the internal capsule, such as a small lacunar infarct, is sufficient to completely interrupt these pathways, producing a hemiplegia with severely impaired motor and sensory function of the opposite half of the body, and also why a very large lesion would be necessary to produce a comparable effect at the level of the corona radiata and of the motor and somatosensory areas of the cortex.

The Extrapyramidal System

The basal ganglia, the thalamus, and the cerebellum form complex circuits, comprising the so-called extrapyramidal system. These circuits are connected to the direct motor pathway described previously, rendering control and coordination of movement possible. The basal ganglia[3] receive input from almost all regions of the cerebral cortex and send projections to some nuclei of the thalamus, which in turn are connected to the executive, premotor, and motor areas of the cortex. This system also involves two other loops, one through the pars compacta of the substantia nigra and another through the subthalamic nucleus of Luys (Figure 3.6). It is believed that this complex circuitry is mainly organized around the pars compacta of the substantia nigra and its production of dopamine.[4]

These circuits control the execution of overlearned and automated movement patterns, leaving control of voluntary activity to the premotor and motor cortex. For example, when we walk we do not have to think about the movements of our feet or the swinging of our arms, although they are indispensable to prevent falls. Also, highly elaborated movement patterns, such as dancing or piano playing, become possible because performers can concentrate on artistic expression, mediated by the cortex, while all the rest, such as maintenance of

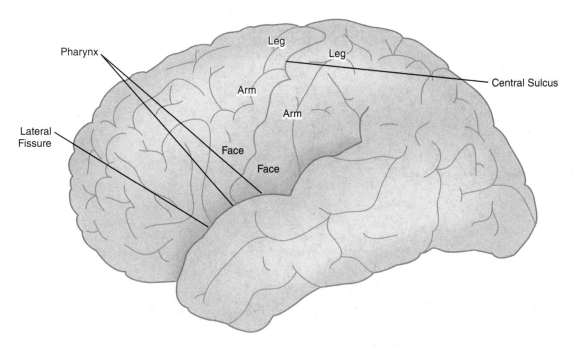

Figure 3.5a Representation of body parts on the motor and somatosensory areas of the cortex.

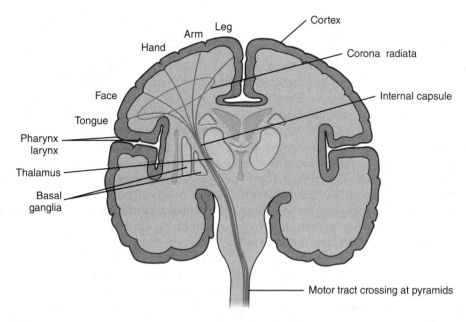

Figure 3.5b Coronal section of the brain showing the descending motor tract, forming the corona radiata, narrowing at the internal capsule.

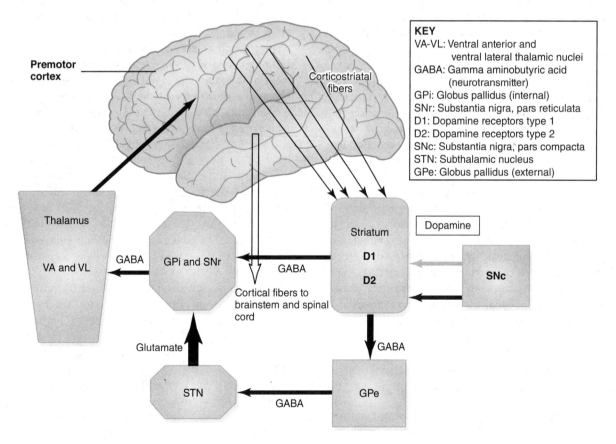

Figure 3.6 Schematic representation of basal ganglia circuits.

equilibrium and coordinated contractions of all the muscles involved, is automatically controlled by the basal ganglia.

Extrapyramidal disorders are described as hypokinetic or hyperkinetic syndromes. Hypokinesia is slow and effortful movement, with limited or absent automatic movements and rigidity of limbs and body.

Parkinson's disease is the most typical and most common hypokinetic condition, frequently accompanied by a characteristic rest tremor of the limbs. Hyperkinetic syndromes present with a variety of abnormal, involuntary, quick or slow movements.[5] Such syndromes bear such names as *Gilles de la Tourette syndrome, idiopathic tremor, Huntington's disease, generalized dystonia,* and many others.[6] Speech is more or less affected in all these conditions, and characteristic dysarthrias have been described. Parkinsonian or hypokinetic dysarthria consists of hypophonia, fainting of the voice at the end of the word or phrase, blurred articulation, fluctuations between slow and rapid speech, repetitions of syllables or words, and other signs and symptoms.

The cerebellum has rich connections to the brain, the brain stem, and the spinal cord and is responsible for body balance and the coordination of movements of hands and feet, head, eyes, and mouth. It ensures that each isolated movement and muscle contraction does not appear awkward or interrupted, but smooth, with precise start and end points, at intended and definite intervals. Moreover, it monitors the succession of movements necessary to achieve a precise action that consists of multiple movements, for example, clapping of hands that produces exactly the noise we desire, pointing our index finger to our nose, or walking. Absence of cerebellar control, on the other hand, produces defective movement patterns, such as the gait of a drunken person, who walks with his or her legs spread wider to reduce the risk of falling. The cerebellum also monitors speech movements. For a precise sound to be produced, each contraction of the lips, tongue, vocal cords, diaphragm, or intercostal muscles is precisely monitored to follow the intended speech production plan. Cerebellar lesions result in cerebellar (ataxic) dysarthria, a condition characterized by a more or less slow, blurred, and hesitating speech, with fluctuating intonation and either mute or explosive phonemes.

The Peripheral Nervous System: Peripheral Versus Central Paralysis

The nerves are bundles of axons of the motor or the sensory neurons. Sensory axons carry signals from receptors in all tissues and organs of the body to the brain. Those forming the cranial nerves enter the brain stem. The rest enter the posterior aspect of the spinal cord and are called spinal nerves. The information they convey varies according to their diameter. Thin, unmyelinated fibers inform about superficial sensitivity, that is, pain, temperature, and light touch. Thicker, myelinated fibers convey information about joint position, vibration, pressure, and discriminative (conscious) sensations. These kinds of sensation follow different tracts in the spinal cord. Motor nerves carry executive signals from the CNS to the striated muscles of the body, that is, muscles under voluntary control. They emerge from the brain stem (motor cranial nerves), innervating the region of the head and the neck, and from the spinal cord (spinal motor nerves), innervating the striated muscles of the body and limbs.

All spinal nerves are mixed in that they contain sensory and motor axons. Cranial nerves are of different kinds. Some, such as the olfactory and optic nerves (I and II cranial pairs) and the acoustic and vestibular nerves (together forming cranial nerve VIII), are purely sensory, transmitting olfactory, auditory, and visual information and information regarding the position of the head and body in space. The rest of the cranial nerves are either motor or mixed and innervate the face and the muscles necessary for speech production (articulators).

The trigeminal (cranial nerve V), although also controlling mastication movements, is mainly the sensory nerve of the face. The facial (cranial nerve VII) is the principal motor nerve of the face (including the lips and the chin). Paralysis of the facial nerve on one side results in asymmetry of the face (peripheral facial paralysis, i.e., Bell's palsy), involving difficulties in speech, drooling, and eye closure. Central facial paralysis is a different kind of paralysis caused by lesions in the central nervous system, such as stroke or other types of lesions in the trajectory of the motor tract from the motor cortex to the facial nucleus. It concerns mainly the lower part of the face and the voluntary movements of the face, and it may be part of the clinical picture of hemiplegia.[7]

The glossopharyngeal (IXth), the vagus (Xth), and the hypoglossal (XIIth) cranial nerves innervate the muscles of the pharynx, the larynx, the vocal cords, and the tongue. Their paralysis affects speech and voice in general. Hypophonia, whispering voice resulting from paralysis of one vocal fold caused by a lesion in the vagus nerve, prompted Galen to suggest that voice comes from the brain.

Nerves sustain lesions either in their axons (axonal lesions) or in the sheath of myelin (demyelinating lesions). These lesions have various etiologies and different prognoses. An axonal lesion is more or less definitive, whereas demyelinating processes often involve a continuous alternation of demyelination and remyelination,[8] finally resulting in axonal damage. These lesions produce motor and sensory paralysis, muscular weakness, and sensory deficits. The clinical pictures resulting from such lesions are variable (radiculopathies, plexopathies, or neuropathies), depending on the kind of fibers affected (motor, sensory, mixed, small fibers, etc.) and the location along the length of the nerve (from its root to its most distal point). It also depends on the number and location of the nerves affected (mononeuropathies, asymmetrical multifocal neuropathies, and symmetrical polyneuropathies). For instance, distal, symmetrical numbness and weakness in the feet slowly progressing to the hands is typical of polyneuropathies, one of the most common being diabetic neuropathy.

The Autonomic Nervous System

The smooth muscles of the internal organs, such as the heart, bowels, and bladder, function almost entirely unconsciously through the coordinated action of the sympathetic and parasympathetic divisions of the autonomic nervous system. The balance between these two divisions depends on internal and external conditions, including emotions and other psychological reactions. For instance, a chain reaction is initiated when we are frightened that includes reactions ranging from changes in heart rate to hair standing up and pupils dilating. The brain, mainly through the limbic system (a set of structures including the hypothalamus and the amygdala located in the medial aspect of the temporal lobes), controls and coordinates the autonomic system. The various parts of the nervous system function in close coordination with each other and with the rest of the body. The limbic system's activity may affect the capacities of a person to speak. This is true in the case of a student under the stress of examinations and in the case of a speaker with aphasia who performs differently when stressed or relaxed.

A MORE DETAILED VIEW OF THE CEREBRAL CORTEX

Primary Sensory and Motor Areas

The primary motor cortical area lies on the precentral gyrus, on the anterior bank of the central sulcus. Every part of the body that can be voluntarily moved is represented in this area, not proportionally to its size but to the complexity and accuracy of the movements that it can perform. The mouth and the fingers, for example, are represented by a vast area compared to that of the hip or the torso. This point-to-point correspondence is called somatotopy and is reversed in both directions, such that the right half of the body is represented on the left hemisphere and the foot is represented at the top of the motor strip, above the hip, torso, arm, hand, face, and mouth (Figures 3.5a and 3.7).

On the postcentral gyrus, on the posterior bank of the central sulcus, lies the primary somatosensory cortical area. It is also somatotopically organized, receiving sensory information from the different body regions, proportionally not to their size but to their sensitivity. Here again, the lips and the fingers represent an area proportionally more extensive than the hip or the torso. The motor and somatosensory areas work in close collaboration, and they are together referred to as the sensorimotor area of the cortex.

The temporal lobe, beneath the lateral sulcus (or Sylvian fissure) is divided into three convolutions. The primary auditory cortex is located on the middle portion of the superior temporal convolution (gyrus of Heschl) and is organized in a "tonotopical" way, that is, according to the frequency of sounds. Finally, at the posterior end of the hemispheres lies the primary visual cortex, around the calcarine sulcus (Figure 3.7); the right half of the visual field of *both* eyes is represented at the left visual cortex and vice versa. A lesion in this area (e.g., a stroke of the posterior cerebral artery) makes the person blind in the contralateral visual field.

Association Areas

The primary cortical areas described previously are surrounded by modality-specific, or unimodal, association cortical areas. Specifically, areas around the primary auditory area process information about sounds coming from the primary auditory area to recognize and identify these sounds. Areas around the primary visual area, in the anterior part of the occipital cortex and extending to (a) the temporal and (b) the parietal cortices, process the visual stimuli to identify and locate them in space.

The identification of the nature of a visual object involves the association cortex toward the inferior posterior temporal cortex (the "what" pathway), whereas, the location of the object in space involves regions toward the posterior parietal cortex (the "where" pathway). Finally, parietal regions immediately posterior to the somatosensory cortex process somatosensory stimuli. These unimodal association areas are not connected to each other so they avoid mixture of sensory information and ensure sensory fidelity. But,

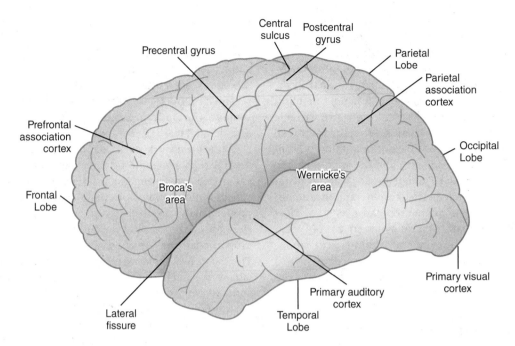

Figure 3.7 External surface of the left cerebral hemisphere.

recognition of an object, as a whole, requires convergence sensory information from multiple sources in the high-order multimodal association areas of the cortex. These areas include the prefrontal cortex, the perisylvian zone, posterior parietal cortex, lateral temporal cortex, and parahippocampal gyrus.

Lesions in the association areas of the cortex may produce selective perceptual deficits (e.g., erroneous perception of shapes, motion, colors) or agnosias, that is, bizarre situations where the patient cannot recognize things that he or she readily recognized before. For example, patients may not recognize common objects or familiar faces through vision (visual agnosia, prosopagnosia); pure sounds, words, or music through audition (acoustic or auditory agnosia, auditory verbal agnosia); or familiar objects through palpation. They may not be able to orient themselves or move in familiar surroundings (spatial agnosia).

The anterior multimodal association cortex, the prefrontal cortex, is dedicated to the executive functions, including working memory, planning and organizing of motor sequences, and monitoring and control of various behaviors, either motor or social. People with lesions in the frontal lobes present with dysexecutive syndrome, including awkward social behavior and many behavioral problems, such as apathy and passivity or disinhibition and aggressiveness, depending on which area of the frontal lobe (lateral or medial) is affected. These disorders are frequently encountered in closed TBIs, which are unfortunately frequent in younger individuals.

Finally, lesions in various parts of the association cortex may produce conditions known as apraxias, of which there are two basic types: ideomotor apraxias, wherein the patient finds it impossible to perform simple movements such as a military salute or waving goodbye, and ideational apraxias, which involve difficulty in executing a sequence of simple movements necessary to achieve a complex task, such as lighting a fire or addressing and mailing a letter.

Cortical Areas Related to Language

Language obeys the same principles as other cognitive functions, and its deficits (i.e., the *aphasias*) are the result of lesions of relevant multimodal association regions, usually of the left perisylvian regions of the cortex.[9] Note that the two hemispheres are not *equipotential* in this regard. That is, they are not responsible for the same functions. In the case of the cerebral organization for language, the left hemisphere is considered dominant in the great majority of people. Although we refer to the "dominant" or "left" hemisphere interchangeably in the following paragraphs, bear in mind that, in some people, there may be a different organization (see also the following section "Aphasia in Left-Handed Individuals"). The anterior brain regions are involved in language output, and the posterior brain regions are involved in reception of language. In the left inferior frontal gyrus, anterior to the motor area for the mouth and the face, lies Broca's area and in the left superior temporal gyrus lies Wernicke's area (Figure 3.7).

Cytoarchitectonic Organization of the Cortex

The cortex is obviously "doing" different things within its different regions. These regions have been thoroughly studied and microscopically compared to each other, showing histologic differences. "Cytoarchitectonic maps" of the cortex were introduced in the beginning of the 20th century, the most widely known being those by Brodmann and by Von Economo and Koskinas. Brodmann's 52 areas are more frequently used in scientific communications (see Figure 3.8). For instance, we refer to Broca's area as Brodmann's area (BA) 44 and 45, and Wernicke's area as BA22.

METHODS FOR THE STUDY OF THE NERVOUS SYSTEM AND THE BRAIN

The nervous system and the brain in particular can be studied in their normal condition or in pathologic situations. There are two main categories of methods: imaging methods, either structural or functional, and the clinical method, that is, the study of the effects of lesions on behavior. Lesions may be natural (e.g., resulting from stroke, TBI) or they may be experimental and reversible (e.g., resulting from the Wada test, transcranial magnetic stimulation [TMS], direct electrical stimulation of the cortex).

The clinical examination method is historically the first and still the most important method for the exploration of the nervous system. It enables us to relate particular areas of the brain to particular cognitive operations. Symptoms and combinations of symptoms (i.e., syndromes) are behavioral and psychological phenomena resulting from lesions in specific parts of the nervous system, and their presence enables us to localize lesions within the nervous system. Moreover, the temporal development of the clinical picture (as, for example, whether the signs and symptoms appear suddenly or progressively or whether they appear one by one or all together) and the necessary knowledge about the person affected (which is obtained through medical history) may guide us to discern the nature of the pathologic cause. For example, symptoms of disordered speech with sudden onset together with a right hemiplegia in an aged right-handed man are most likely caused by a stroke in the left cerebral hemisphere. A similar syndrome, but with progressive onset, also in an aged person might be caused by a growing lesion, such as a tumor or a chronic subdural hematoma. A complete medical history taken from the patient and from significant others (parents or friends) is therefore of great importance and forms an integral part of clinical assessment.

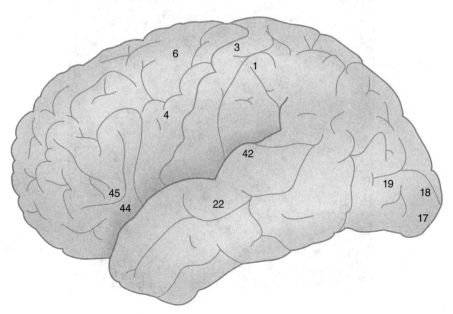

Figure 3.8 Brodmann's areas.

In view of the fact that all laboratory exploration furnishes additional elements to this assessment, we may proceed to explore the brain or the nervous system in two ways: first through the study of its anatomy and the localization and nature of lesions and second through the study of the electrochemical processes that mediate its various functions and their alterations resulting from pathology. Broca, Wernicke, and the other students of aphasia and neurology in general in the late 19th and the early 20th centuries reported anatomic lesion evidence linked to the syndromes they had observed. This anatomoclinical method provided the first strong argument in favor of an association between clinically observed disorders and their cerebral background. For a long time, physicians, based on the data collected through this method, had to rely on fine clinical semiology (i.e., a detailed description of signs and symptoms) to infer what the cause of those signs and symptoms were. A further refinement of this method was the development of objective and quantitative behavioral tests designed to assess particular psychological functions or subsidiary cognitive operations. These tests constitute the core of modern clinical neuropsychology.

Observation and testing were supplemented and, for the purpose of lesion identification, replaced with the advent of imaging, starting with computed tomography (CT) at the end of the 1970s and followed by magnetic resonance imaging (MRI) in the beginning of the 1980s. These techniques enabled the procurement of precise anatomic images of the brain in vivo. The CT scan (Figure 3.9) is still used as the first step of the diagnostic process in the case of strokes and reveals stroke-induced lesions. However, it is not accurate for small lesions, whether vascular or demyelinating, and it is not sensitive to brain stem lesions. These last lesions can be detected through MRI (Figure 3.10), which offers a variety of possibilities for identifying various structures and tissues, including the time of onset of a vascular lesion (how old it is). The vascular network of the brain can also be visualized and obstructed arteries or bleeding vascular lesions (such as aneurysms) identified either through magnetic resonance angiography (MRA) or through digital angiography, which requires the injection of a substance directly into the arterial system. All the preceding methods are part of "structural" imaging in the sense that they involve visualization of the structures of the brain, their physical appearance, the existence of lesions, and their location within the brain.

If, however, we are interested in the function—or malfunction—of particular structures rather than in their anatomy, *functional* imaging methods are needed. The oldest of these (since the 1930s), the electroencephalogram (EEG), is the recording of the electrical activity of the brain through the skull via electrodes placed on the scalp. It is always valuable as a method for diagnosing

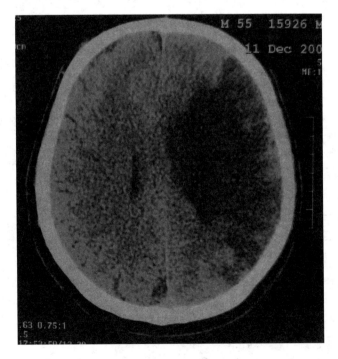

Figure 3.9a CT scan sample.

Courtesy of Constantin Potagas.

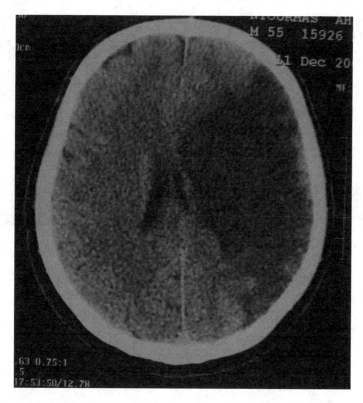

Figure 3.9b Computed tomographic scan sample.
Courtesy of Constantin Potagas.

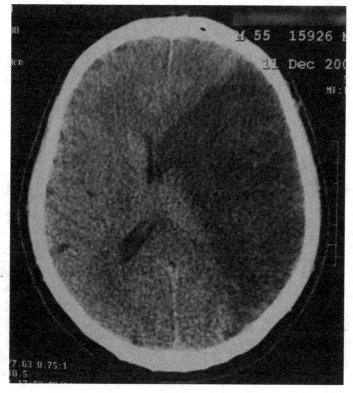

Figure 3.9c Computed tomographic scan sample.
Courtesy of Constantin Potagas.

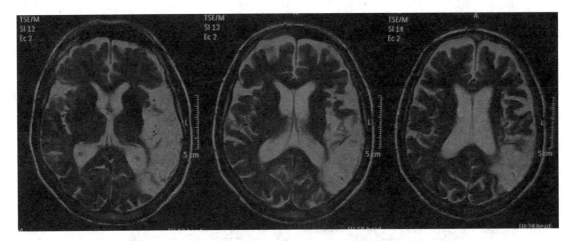

Figure 3.10a Magnetic resonance imaging samples.
Courtesy of Constantin Potagas.

epileptic conditions—not necessarily associated with anatomically visible lesions—and to differentiate the various stages of sleep and wakefulness.

Its counterpart within the PNS, electromyography (EMG), and electroneurography are techniques for recording the electrical activity of muscles when contracted and testing the integrity of nerves or localizing the possible site of their lesions. It is also possible to electrically stimulate nerves (whether motor or sensory) at various points of their trajectory and record their conduction velocity using the time interval between stimulation and responses.

Direct brain stimulation is limited to neurosurgical operations under local anesthesia. However, TMS is a method to stimulate brain regions through electromagnetic induction. It consists of applying very short magnetic pulses to the skull. These induce electrical currents that can depolarize or inhibit neurons of the brain and thus, activate or inhibit cortical functions. The application of TMS to the skull above a region of the motor strip results in the movement of the body part corresponding to this region, a response that we can precisely measure. The repetition of this stimulation (rTMS) at different frequencies results in enhancing or inhibiting activity of the brain regions to which it is applied, with seemingly longer-lasting changes. This is the reason rTMS is now experimentally applied for the treatment of various pathologic conditions.

Evoked potentials (EPs) and event-related potentials (ERPs) are based on the same principle as the EEG. They are records of the electrical activity of particular regions of the brain, showing the timing and the magnitude of responses of specific cerebral regions—mainly primary sensory areas—to particular stimuli, such as, for instance, the response of the primary auditory (temporal) cortex to a sound or the response of the posterior

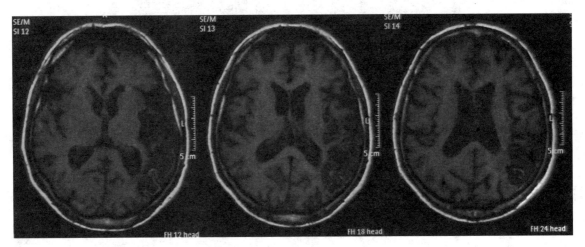

Figure 3.10b Magnetic resonance imaging samples.
Courtesy of Constantin Potagas.

(occipital) cortex to a light pattern. The latest version of the functional imaging methods is magnetoencephalography (MEG), which, through recording of the magnetic fields created by the electrical activity of the brain, reveals the response of the brain to various stimuli or the activation of cerebral regions during a variety of cognitive, linguistic, and affective tasks. A huge advantage of this method over positron emission tomography (PET) or functional magnetic resonance (described subsequently) is its temporal resolution, that is, its capacity for revealing the sequence of activation of brain regions within milliseconds. Various methods have also been developed to reveal brain function indirectly through indices of metabolism (such as variations of blood flow, glucose or oxygen consumption, or neurotransmitter binding). Functional magnetic resonance imaging (fMRI) shows the activation of particular brain regions through the rates of blood supply during performance of various tasks. Likewise, PET shows the activation of cerebral structures by visualizing the amount of glucose consumed or oxygen supplied to an area during performance of various tasks.

ELEMENTS OF CLINICAL NEUROLOGY

Overview

The brain is subject to various pathologies, such as infectious, vascular, demyelinating, neoplastic, and degenerative diseases, as well as trauma. Language disorders could be manifestations of any of these pathologies. Consequently, aphasia classification has been highly dependent on studied pathology. Aphasic syndromes can and have been classified differently, not only on the basis of characteristic symptoms and lesion loci but also on underlying pathology (see, for instance, descriptions of aphasias by the clinicians of the 19th century examining stroke patients compared to descriptions by A. Luria, who studied mainly TBIs).

Traumatic brain injuries are a frequent cause of fatalities and serious handicaps in younger individuals, and they have been extensively studied from a neuropsychological point of view because they often result in cognitive and behavioral deficits. The TBI lesions, although diffuse, are not random; they affect specific brain areas, such as the orbital and lateral surfaces of the frontal lobes, the inferior surface of the temporal lobes, and portions of the corpus callosum and brain stem. Frontotemporal lesions result in characteristic behavioral disorders, including apathy, fluctuating temper, disinhibition, sometimes aggressiveness, lack of initiative, and often, severe memory deficits.

Benign tumors developing from the brain's meninges and evolving slowly without evident signs and symptoms and, more frequently, malignant neoplasms originating from glial or other supporting cells and metastatic lesions from lung or breast cancer often interfere with specific cognitive functions. Symptoms of intracranial tumors may be diffuse or focal. Diffuse symptoms result from the pressure exerted by the tumor, brain swelling, or increase in intracranial pressure. Symptoms of impaired mental concentration and slow reaction time progressing into loss of consciousness may appear rapidly, depending on the tumor's position. For example, tumors of the midline (i.e., in the third ventricle) or in the posterior fossa (a small space in the skull containing the brain stem and cerebellum; a tumor growing there can block the flow of spinal fluid) may quickly produce hydrocephaly and increased intracranial pressure, headache, vomiting, papilledema (edema at the fundus of the eye), and the cognitive deficits mentioned previously. Signs and symptoms generally depend on the tumor's location. Frontal lobe tumors may result in behavioral disorders, including apathy, indifference, euphoria, facetiousness, lack of initiative (collectively referred to as the "frontal lobe syndrome"), motor impairments of the opposite part of the body, and often aphasic symptoms if located in the left hemisphere. Temporal lobe tumors may present with auditory and olfactory deficits, aphasic symptoms, memory impairment, and personality and mood changes or psychotic disorder. Agnosias, apraxias, and somatosensory and visuospatial deficits may be associated with neoplasms of the parietal lobe. Visual impairments are the main feature of occipital tumors. Lesions other than neoplastic (abscesses, hematomas, etc.) may cause similar signs and symptoms, caused by either their location or their size.

Degenerative diseases diffusely affecting the cerebral cortex also give rise to neuropsychological symptoms. Cortical degeneration early in Alzheimer's disease affects mainly the medial aspect of the temporal cortex, initially producing episodic memory-encoding deficits. Frontotemporal dementias may initially produce not only frontal lobe syndrome but also poor oral expression and word-finding difficulties. Vascular dementias resulting from multiple infarcts are characterized by sudden onset and escalating severity and give rise to various signs and symptoms depending on the location of the infarcts.

Vascular Pathology of the Brain

Irrigation of the brain, which is about 2% of total body weight, uses about 20% of the total cardiac supply, and the gray matter requires a sixfold quantity of blood compared to that of the white matter.

Eighty percent of all strokes are caused by a reduction or interruption of blood supply to brain areas resulting from a blood clot formed either in situ (thrombosis) or carried by the normal circulation of the blood from elsewhere, where it was initially formed (embolism), leading to ischemia of the cerebral tissue.[10] Bleeding within the brain is called *intracerebral hemorrhage* and represents 12% of strokes. But, blood can also drain into the subarachnoid space, causing acute and intense headache together with neck stiffness, an emergency condition, menacing life: Subarachnoid hemorrhages account for 8% of strokes. A very small percentage of strokes are caused by central venous thrombosis.

The risk of stroke depends on various factors: age (older people are mostly affected), gender (men are affected more than women are), race (African American and Asian individuals have higher incidence rates), and heredity (those with a family history of stroke are more likely to be affected). There are, however, other factors, such as hypertension, smoking, diabetes, heart disease, hyperlipidemia,[11] use of estrogens, use of alcohol, disorders of coagulation, and specific blood diseases, the influence of which may be controlled through preventive measures.

If the obstruction of the vessel persists, the ischemia of a region results in a sequence of modifications, the final consequence being the death or *necrosis* of the cerebral substance. The necrotic area progressively expands, and the surrounding zone, the *penumbra zone*, where cells are still partially functioning, in turn gradually narrows. The swelling (or edema) developing around the lesion compresses small vessels and blocks local circulation, thus worsening the situation. The extent to which the cells in the penumbra zone survive and recover their normal function contributes to the final outcome of the stroke. Together with the resorption of the edema, the survival of these cells partially explains spontaneous recovery that occurs within a few days poststroke.

Strokes have a sudden onset, and their clinical picture is established within minutes to hours. However, they may also evolve continuously within days from onset. The stroke is transient if its symptoms last minutes or hours and reversible if symptoms last up to some days, with subsequent recovery. Transient ischemic attacks (TIAs) are of great importance in that they are, most likely, precursors of another, more severe stroke, with permanent or established symptoms. However, even when established, the symptoms may partially recover over a 3- to 6-month period poststroke. Cerebral plasticity, a process that remains largely elusive, whether spontaneous or occasioned by rehabilitation, is considered to be the cause of recovery. It is hypothesized that this process includes a number of subsidiary events,

such as redistribution of impaired functions to healthy parts of the brain, reorganization of cerebral connections, perhaps even repair of certain injured structures. Thrombolysis, aimed at dissolving the obstructing blood clot, is the ideal emergency treatment of ischemic stroke, but it has to be performed within a very few hours following onset and involves potential risks.

Obstruction of the internal carotid may not produce any clinical signs if it progresses slowly enough to allow the collateral circulation to function. If sudden, a variety of symptoms may occur from the territories of the ophthalmic, anterior, and middle cerebral arteries, such as blindness of the corresponding eye and weakness and hemianesthesia of the opposite half of the body. Usually, however, carotid ischemia is associated with mild, transient symptoms, such as blindness of short duration (amaurosis fugax) of the corresponding eye, sometimes combined with weakness of an opposite limb. Occlusion of the first branch of the internal carotid, the ophthalmic artery, produces permanent or temporary blindness of the eye.

The relatively rare syndrome of anterior cerebral artery obstruction includes paralysis and sensory deficit of the opposite lower limb, urinary disorders, and behavior problems.

Obstruction of the middle cerebral artery—the final branch of the internal carotid artery—results in a severe clinical syndrome, sometimes including confusion or coma, with paralysis and sensory loss in the opposite limbs (hemiplegia and hemianesthesia, respectively); loss of vision in the opposite half of the visual field (hemianopia); and aphasia if the lesion is located in the dominant hemisphere for language (usually the left). If ischemia involves the "minor" hemisphere (usually the right), there may be agnosia of the opposite half of the body and agnosia or indifference for the left half of the space (hemispatial neglect, a condition different from hemianopia). Frequently, also, the patient may deny, ignore, or be indifferent to his or her own paralysis (anosognosia). If the superior branches of the artery are involved, there may be central facial paralysis with insensitivity and numbness of the opposite lower half of the face (i.e., a central VII) and of the opposite upper limb, together with Broca's aphasia if the lesion is in the left hemisphere. Ischemia in the territory of the inferior branches leads to contralateral hemianopia or superior quadrantanopia and to Wernicke's aphasia if the hemisphere dominant for language is affected. Ischemia in the territory of the penetrating branches (basal ganglia and part of the internal capsule) is associated with hemiplegia affecting both the contralateral upper and lower limbs and lower face. This capsular hemiplegia may be accompanied by hemianopia, dysarthria, or aphasia.

The vertebral arteries irrigate the inferior part of the brain stem (medulla oblongata), and the obstruction of one of them may remain asymptomatic if the other one is still functioning. Acute occlusion of the vertebral artery usually manifests with cerebellar symptoms (e.g., dysarthria, ataxia) and with lateral medullary ischemia (often resulting in ipsilateral sensory deficits in the face and contralateral sensory deficits in the body). Partial obstruction of the basilar artery may remain asymptomatic if gradual and if the collateral circulation is sufficient. However, it may result in a severe syndrome involving paralysis of the four limbs (quadriplegia) and profound coma and a multitude of pathologic signs involving eye movements and cranial nerve functions (strabismus, double vision or diplopia, enlargement or mydriasis of the pupil, ptosis of the upper eyelid, hypoesthesia [diminished sensation] and peripheral paralysis of one half of the face, dizziness, abnormal movements of the eyes, hoarse or whispering voice, and swallowing disorders), cerebellar symptoms all on the side of the lesion, and motor and sensory deficits involving the opposite side of the body. Many of these symptoms may be caused by obstruction of one of the thin arterial branches irrigating parts of the brain stem.

The *locked-in* syndrome, caused by a lesion in the upper part of the brain stem, is characterized by complete paralysis, including the head, only with the possibility of vertical movement of the eyes and eyelids. The most salient feature of this syndrome is that, whereas consciousness and sensation may be intact, they pass unnoticed by all observers because of the pervasive paucity of all capacity for movement.[12]

Ischemia in the territory of one posterior cerebral artery leads to hemianopia in the opposite visual field, which may be associated with hemiparesis and hypoesthesia or unilateral absence of movement coordination of the limbs (ataxia) resulting from the interruption of cerebellar circuits. Hemianopia may be the only symptom of the obstruction of the surface branches, associated with visual agnosia or alexia (loss of reading ability) when the lesion is located in the dominant hemisphere for language.

Sometimes, ischemia occurs *between* the previously mentioned major arterial territories, in their boundary zones and not within them. We then speak about "watershed infarction," and in some cases we suppose that the cause is not arterial occlusion but rather low flow of the blood caused by severe arterial hypotension, for example, in cases of cardiac arrest or cardiac surgery. This may happen either in the posterior boundary zones (between the territories of the middle cerebral artery and the posterior cerebral artery, in the conjunction of the parietal and the occipital cortex) or in the anterior boundary zones (between the territories of the middle cerebral artery and the anterior cerebral artery, in the frontal area close to the summit of the cerebral hemisphere). These infarcts may be unilateral or bilateral, and whenever they affect the dominant hemisphere, they cause aphasia.

CEREBRAL REPRESENTATION OF LANGUAGE

This section is not intended to be a historical account of notions regarding aphasia. We do, however, summarize the basic correlations between lesion location and aphasic deficits that emerged over the years from clinical observation. Paul Broca, a French surgeon, found on the postmortem examination of his "aphemic" patients (including his first patient, who uttered almost nothing but the syllable *tan*) a lesion involving "the third frontal convolution" (Broca, 1861, as cited in Hécaen & Dubois, 1969, p. 60), anterior to the motor area responsible for mouth and face movement, and speculated that this damaged region was the "seat of the faculty of articulate speech" (Broca, 1865, as cited in Hécaen & Dubois, 1969, p. 108).[13]

Some years later, Carl Wernicke (1874), a German neurologist, described a woman who spoke fluently, though erroneously, with distorted words, that is, *paraphasias*, but could not understand speech. He thought that the lesion had destroyed the "center for acoustic images of the words" in the superior temporal gyrus. This lesion was, according to Wernicke, the cause of her "sensory aphasia." He considered "Broca's region" as the "center for motor images of the words," and a lesion in it was the cause of a "motor aphasia." Lesions of the association fibers connecting these two "centers" were thought to produce "conduction aphasia" (fluent speech, good comprehension, but impossible repetition, with paraphasias).

Lichtheim (1885, cited in Compston, 2006) conceived an additional, not anatomically defined, "center of concepts." He, in fact, proposed a simple scheme for all aphasia known as the "Lichtheim's house." According to it, speech sounds arrive from the ears and the auditory regions of the brain and are identified as words in the center of acoustic images. Then, they are transmitted to the center of motor word images, both directly and indirectly, through the concept center. From there, they are transmitted to the nuclei of nerves innervating the speech apparatus. According to this scheme, "transcortical aphasias" (transcortical sensory, motor transcortical, and mixed transcortical aphasia) are caused by lesions in large cortical regions, outside Wernicke's and Broca's areas, and they affect connections between those areas and the concept center.

Table 3.1   Usual Characteristics of Aphasic Syndromes

Type of Aphasia	Fluency	Comprehension	Repetition	Naming
Global	Nonfluent	–	–	–
Broca	Nonfluent	+	–	–
Motor transcortical	Nonfluent	+	+	–
Mixed transcortical	Nonfluent	–	+	–
Wernicke	Fluent	–	–	–
Sensory transcortical	Fluent	–	+	–
Conduction	Fluent	+	–	–
Anomic aphasia	Fluent	+	+	–

Note: – = mostly impaired; + = mostly preserved.

Source: Data from J. R. Hodges, (1998). *Cognitive assessment for clinicians.* Oxford, England: Oxford Medical Publications.

Clinicians retained in practice Wernicke's and Lichtheim's schemes, using the criteria of fluency of speech, comprehension, and repetition (Table 3.1). Thanks to their simplicity and heuristic value, generations of neurologists (especially before the advent of structural brain imaging such as CT, MRI) were, and still are, able to deduce the existence and gross localization of brain lesions in aphasic patients from the type of aphasic symptoms.

Later, Dejerine (1892) described the case of a patient, a highly cultivated man, who suffered pure verbal blindness, also called pure alexia or alexia without agraphia, as a consequence of a stroke. This patient spoke readily and correctly, understood well what he was told, but when asked to read, he gave the impression of an illiterate individual. He could write perfectly well, but he could not read what he had just written. The lesion was located in the visual area (in the left occipital lobe) and included the posterior part of the corpus callosum called the *splenium*, consisting of axons coming from the visual area of the opposite hemisphere (Figure 3.11). Thus, no visual information whatsoever, from either hemisphere, could reach the language region in the left hemisphere (Dejerine, 1891/1977, pp. 94, 109). In this way, there would be no need for a specific center for reading besides the primary visual areas and a "language center." This associationist view could apply more generally in neuropsychology, explaining many pathologic situations as "disconnection syndromes." In general, a disconnection syndrome occurs because of rupture of connections between brain centers, which in theory are specific for a particular function (for example, Broca's area, the alleged speech center, as a part of the perisylvian language network).

The contemporary "neoassociationist" Wernicke-Geschwind model (Geschwind, 1965) was based on the preceding assumptions. Geschwind (1967) included most of Lichtheim's original formulation and suggested that semantic processing is mediated by a specific brain region, probably the inferior parietal cortex.

Meanwhile, many theorists have questioned the Wernicke–Geschwind model on various grounds. These theorists included Freud (1891/1953; who argued against Wernicke's model in his monograph "On Aphasias," in 1891), Pierre Marie,[14] and John Hughlings Jackson, who maintained that "to locate the damage that destroys speech and to locate speech are two different things" and that "to discuss the functions of the cortex as if they were based on abrupt geographical locations is logically absurd" (Finger, 1994, p. 379).

Hughlings Jackson and others—including, incidentally, Paul Broca[15]—observed some cases of patients with severe aphasia with large lesions of the left hemisphere who still uttered "automatic" speech, and they stated that language can be both automatic (swear words, poems, or prayers), supported by the right hemisphere, and "propositional" or "intentional," supported by the left hemisphere (Basso, 2003).[16] Thus, an important detail in studying aphasia is whether a patient can or cannot use language, a dissociation that constitutes evidence that language is not lost but only inaccessible under certain circumstances.[17] This notion is the basis of the stimulation approach in aphasia therapy (Basso, 2003).

Many clinicians adopting the holistic approach, such as Henry Head, Kurt Goldstein, and others, did not see language as localized in particular centers, but instead, they conceived the brain working as a whole (Lantéri-Laura, 1987; Riese, 1959) to mediate language.

There are now two supplementary kinds of evidence on which concepts of cerebral organization for language are based: First, some cases reported in the literature,

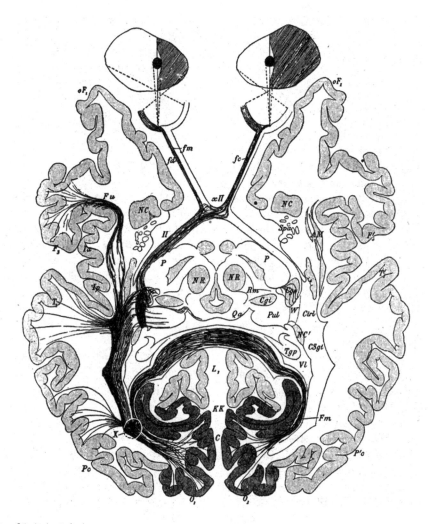

Figure 3.11 Design of Dejerine's lesion.

Source: Reproduced from Sémiologie des affections du système nerveux, J. Dejerine. Pure verbal blindness, p. 109, © Elsevier, 1914/1977.

but also some systematic studies of series of cases (e.g., Kreisler et al., 2000; Willmes & Poeck, 1993), have shown that there is no absolute one-to-one correspondence of symptoms or syndromes to localization of lesions. Second, functional studies with PET and fMRI in healthy persons showed the participation in language of many regions, varying according to the linguistic task (e.g., Hagoort, 2005; Hickok & Poeppel, 2004; Shalom & Poeppel, 2008); these studies also showed the activation of various brain structures along the recovery phases of aphasia after a stroke, in fact, the flexibility and plasticity of the brain (e.g., Breier, Maher, Schmadeke, Hasan, & Papanicolaou, 2007; Saur et al., 2006). Indeed, language processing is not dependent on Wernicke's and Broca's areas alone, but depends on many neural sites linked as systems and working in concert.

Broca's and Wernicke's areas may be "conceptualized as transmodal gateways [coordinating] reciprocal interactions between the sensory representations of word forms and the arbitrary (second-order or symbolic) associations that give them meaning." They would "constitute the two epicenters of a distributed language network" (Mesulam, 2000, p. 37). "They also provide 'neural bottlenecks' in the sense that they constitute regions of maximum vulnerability for lesion-induced deficits in the pertinent cognitive domain" (Mesulam, 2000, pp. 16–17). In other words, Broca's and Wernicke's areas play the role of epicenters or gateways of a network for language, which includes primary sensory and association cortical areas, as well as motor areas. Language is therefore distributed all over the left hemisphere, including even regions of the right hemisphere.

TYPES OF APHASIA, TYPICAL LESION LOCATIONS, AND TYPICAL SIGNS AND SYMPTOMS

As can be gathered from the preceding description, language disorders have been classified in several different ways, often based on different theoretical frameworks. The most typical classification is the so-called neoassociationist classification, which is based on the anatomic disconnection model (Geschwind, 1967). According to this model, a lesion in a specific brain area results in a more or less well-defined aphasic syndrome. In *Broca's aphasia*, speech is effortful, nonfluent, and consisting of short phrases or single words. However, the clinical picture may vary from a complete loss of speech to a mild deficit characterized simply by word-finding difficulties. For example, in the case of telegraphic speech (i.e., agrammatism), all small, function words (e.g., prepositions) are absent, and the patient communicates using mainly nouns and verbs. This pattern may also extend to written language. Automated verbal sequences, such as reciting the days of the week or counting, and occasionally cursing or emotional speech, are usually preserved. Comprehension is relatively spared. Nevertheless, thorough examination reveals specific comprehension deficits regarding complex syntactic structures. Repetition of words or sentences, reading aloud, naming, and writing are also affected. Phonemic paraphasias[18] are occasionally observed. Individuals with Broca's aphasia in general also suffer from apraxia of speech (Basso, 2003), ideomotor apraxia (D. F. Benson, 1993), and right hemiplegia of various degrees. Broca's aphasia is classically associated with a lesion in the posterior part of the inferior frontal gyrus, the insula, and the frontal operculum (the most posterior portion of the inferior frontal gyrus [i.e., of Broca's area] is part of the operculum). Premotor and prefrontal areas of the cortex, subcortical regions, and parts of the basal ganglia may also be affected.

An almost-reverse image, with difficulty in understanding language while the ability of verbal expression remains unaffected, is diagnosed as *Wernicke's aphasia*. The extent of comprehension problems may vary among patients, and moderate comprehension deficits are not uncommon (Basso, 2003). Verbal output is fluent, and it is characterized by the presence of phonemic and semantic paraphasias,[19] neologisms,[20] and empty speech,[21] while rich content words are reduced in frequency. When severe, this condition is called *jargon aphasia*. Because the persons with aphasia are unable to monitor their own verbal output because of the comprehension deficit, such patients are often unaware of

their language disorder (i.e., anosognosia), and this further affects communication difficulties and often hinders rehabilitation. Repetition, naming, reading aloud, and writing are impaired. Ideomotor apraxia and hemianopia (Basso, 2003) or superior right quadrantanopia (Adams, Victor, & Ropper, 1997) are common in Wernicke's aphasia, while motor disorders are rare. Wernicke's aphasia is usually associated with lesions of the posterior left perisylvian region, localized in particular at the posterior part of the superior temporal region traditionally referred to as Wernicke's area, and occasionally extending to the adjacent parietal and temporal areas.

In *conduction aphasia*, repetition is compromised, although speech remains relatively fluent, albeit characterized by phonemic paraphasias and word-finding difficulties. Patients are aware of their verbal paraphasias, and often, while trying to correct themselves, they produce several phonemic variations of the target word, a phenomenon called *conduite d'approche* (Alexander, 2000). Comprehension is generally spared, with some patients having problems understanding complex syntactic structures (Basso, 2003). Deficits in naming and writing are common. Reading aloud is impaired and contains semantic and phonemic paralexias.[22] Ideomotor apraxia and motor or sensory deficits may be present (Basso, 2003). The lesion associated with this aphasic syndrome is typically located in the left temporal-parietal junction. However, it has been proposed that conduction aphasia is the result of a more extensive lesion, including other structures, such as the insula, the primary auditory cortex, and the supramarginal gyrus (H. Damasio, 1998).

Global aphasia includes severe deficits in all aspects of language. Speech is nonfluent and often limited to stereotypic utterances ("ta-to," "to-po"). However, overlearned, automatized sequences (reciting the days of the week, for example) are sometimes preserved. Comprehension, naming, repetition, reading, and writing are severely impaired (Alexander, 2000). Such a condition is the result of a lesion covering a large portion of the perisylvian area, often caused by total occlusion of the left middle cerebral artery, therefore causing severe motor and sensory deficits involving the right half of the body and occasionally visual field defects, as well as oral, ideomotor, and ideational apraxias (Cummings & Mega, 2003).

Anomic aphasia is often referred to as *amnestic, amnesic*, or *nominal aphasia*. Anomia refers to the patient's inability to find names of people or objects. The patient, although aware of the nature of an object, is unable to name it on request. Verbal output is fluent, characterized by word-finding difficulties, frequent pauses, and circumlocutions, while phonemic and semantic paraphasias are rare. Repetition, comprehension, and reading aloud are spared. Anomic aphasia may be associated with lesions affecting posterior language areas, including the angular gyrus (in the parietal lobe, near the superior edge of the temporal lobe) or the middle temporal gyrus. However, it is frequently observed as the outcome of many recovered aphasics. Moreover, several brain regions are involved in confrontation naming, depending on the type and modality of the stimulus. Thus, anomic aphasia is considered to have little or no localization value (Basso, 2003).

Transcortical aphasias are characterized by a disproportionately preserved capacity of repetition. They result from a more or less complete isolation of the speech areas (i.e., the perisylvian language zone of the left hemisphere) from the rest of the cortex (Assal et al., 1983) caused by multiple cerebral infarcts or diffuse lesions (due to anoxia) in the border zones of irrigation of the arteries of the brain (i.e., the "watershed" area). Ischemic lesions in such cases may cover a hemicircular area from the convexity of the frontal lobe to the junction between parietal and occipital cortex, through the superior parietal cortex, or portions of this area, or deeper subcortical regions under this area.

Patients suffering from *transcortical motor aphasia* demonstrate nonfluent speech with preserved comprehension and relatively spared naming. Reading aloud and writing are impaired, and phonemic paraphasias are observed in some cases. There is a striking preservation of the repetition capacity that, in some cases, takes the form of passive, "parrot-like" echoing of everything heard (echolalia). Depending on the site and extent of the lesion, accompanying neurologic symptoms, such as mild dysarthria and sensory and motor disorders, may be present (Alexander, 2000). Transcortical motor aphasia may be the sequel of a recovered Broca's aphasia or part of the syndrome resulting from massive frontal lobe lesions, in which case it is accompanied by lack of initiative and akinetic mutism.[23] It corresponds to the "dynamic aphasia" described by Luria (Adams et al., 1997; Roch-Lecours & Lhermitte, 1979). Overall, the lesions that cause it have been found in various sites: in the frontal region anterior or superior to Broca's area (D. F. Benson, 1993), at the supplementary motor area, or at the cingulate gyrus (Cummings & Mega, 2003). In some cases, the lesion is subcortical, affecting white matter beneath the frontal lobe (A. Damasio & Geschwind, 1984).

In *transcortical sensory aphasia*, speech is fluent but in many cases meaningless or unintelligible (i.e., jargon), with many paraphasias and neologisms. Comprehension of oral and written language, naming, reading, and writing are severely impaired, while the most prominent characteristic is again the preserved ability of the patient to repeat words and sentences. Echolalia is present in some cases.[24] This type of aphasia is associated with lesions posterior to the perisylvian region, in the parietal-occipital region (Adams et al., 1997).

Mixed transcortical aphasia is a rare syndrome combining signs and symptoms of motor and sensory transcortical aphasias. Speech is nonfluent, and comprehension, naming, writing, and reading are severely impaired. Its salient feature is preserved repetition of words and sentences, often in the form of echolalia (Alexander, 2000). The lesion site is typically the watershed area.

Several other attempts of classification, made at various times in the history of aphasiology, have not been able to dislodge from its position of prominence the associationist classification based on the anatomic disconnection model. This model remains dominant and extensively used despite the fact that on its basis many aphasic patients are labeled "unclassified" and many symptoms are not clearly explained, as for instance, anomia, the comprehension deficits found in many individuals with Broca's and conduction aphasia. On the other hand, the utility of the associationist classification is doubtless the result of its inclusiveness and basic correctness, which facilitate the task of clinicians diagnosing and treating aphasic patients and of researchers studying aphasia in general. As stated by F. Benson and Ardila (1996), "The syndrome classification originally developed by the 19th century continental investigators remains basically accurate, replicable, and clinically useful" (pp. 111–112).

In any case, clinicians should follow a deficit-based assessment methodology. A careful and detailed analysis of language deficits is the best way to obtain a detailed patient profile and potentially a more efficient intervention strategy. Aiming to rehabilitate a single symptom and not the syndrome in its entirety would probably result in a better therapeutic outcome.

Subcortical Aphasia

Lesions of the white matter and the subcortical nuclei that do not affect the cortex can also result in various aphasic symptoms (Fasanaro et al., 1987; Hayashi, Ulatowska, & Sasanuma, 1985; Kreisler et al., 2000; Radanovic & Scaff, 2003; Willmes & Poeck, 1993; Yamadori, Ohira, Seriu, & Ogura, 1984). Thus, subcortical aphasia is not a homogeneous entity, and clinical manifestations often vary among patients. The syndrome related to lesions confined to the head of the left caudate nucleus and the anterior limb of the internal capsule (containing fibers from the frontal cortex to brain stem and from the thalamus to frontal lobes) includes deficits in comprehension, dysarthria, and motor impairments (A. Damasio, Damasio, Rizzo, Varney, & Gersh, 1982). Thalamic aphasia is characterized by nonfluent speech and rarely by comprehension deficits, sometimes complete suppression of speech at onset and later by low voice volume; by severe reduction of spontaneous speech, mainly restricted to responses to direct questions only; and by semantic paraphasias (Darby & Walsh, 2005).

Aphasia in Left-Handed Individuals

Hécaen and Ajuriaguerra (1963), who examined a population of 309 right-handed and 59 left-handed individuals with either left or right lesions, concluded that aphasic disorders are more frequent but less severe in left-handed individuals because of a hemispheric specialization that remains less strong. Other researchers suggested that aphasia in left-handed persons with left hemisphere dominance for language is clinically different from aphasia in right-handed individuals and has a better prognosis (Gloning et al., 1976, Luria, 1970, Subirana, 1969, all cited in Basso, 2003).

However, Basso, Farabola, Pia Grassi, Laiacona, and Zanobio (1990) stated that differences in type of aphasia and recovery between right-handed and non–right-handed individuals have been overemphasized and must be reconsidered. An invasive method used to address these questions, usually before surgical interventions for intractable epilepsies, is the intracarotid injection of sodium amytal, also known as the Wada test (Wada & Rasmussen, 1960). Left or right dominance for language is inferred from the presence of transient aphasic symptoms after injection of a barbiturate, typically sodium amytal, in the left or right internal carotid. If aphasia is present after both injections, language representation is considered to be bilateral. With this method, Rasmussen and Milner (1977) found left hemisphere dominance

in 96% of subjects and 4% of right dominance in 140 right-handed subjects; they found also 70% of left dominance, 15% of bilateral representation, and 15% of right dominance in 122 non–right-handed subjects (either left-handed persons or those with mixed manual preference). These numbers are still used as basic reference in the matter, but we have to keep in mind that the patients in this study had epilepsia, and that their repartition in left- and right-handed groups depended on the method used for the evaluation of manual preference (Dellatolas & Potagas, 2009).

Crossed Aphasia

Occasionally, there are cases of right-handed individuals suffering from aphasia after right hemisphere lesions. Since 1975, more than 180 such cases have been described (Coppens, Hungerford, Yamaguchi, & Yamadori, 2002; Mariën, Paghera, De Deyn, & Vignolo, 2004). Apart from these rare cases, patients with right hemisphere lesions will probably perform well in traditional aphasia tests, but they may present deficits in extralinguistic aspects of language, such as prosody and processing nonliteral verbal stimuli (e.g., metaphors, ironic or humorous phrases) and abstract concepts (Darby & Walsh, 2005).

Sign Language Aphasia

Deaf people who use a sign language can acquire aphasia in that language as a result of lesions in the left hemisphere, much in the same way as oral language users. Reported in the literature are cases of deaf patients with aphasia who could pantomime and understand an action such as "brushing of the teeth," whereas they were unable to produce or understand the sign for *toothbrush*, despite the similarity of the gesture and the sign (MacSweeney, Capek, Campbell, & Woll, 2008, p. 232). Such findings indicate that language is heavily dependent on the left hemisphere, whether the output is verbal (spoken language) or not (sign language).

STUDY QUESTIONS

1. Name the structures of the central nervous system.
2. Which are the important arteries supplying the brain with blood?
3. Which lesions of the cerebral hemispheres are related to aphasic signs and symptoms? In which arterial territories can ischemia cause aphasic symptoms?
4. Which cranial nerves are related to speech impairments?
5. What kind of speech disorders are caused by dysfunctions of the extrapyramidal system? In which way can a cerebellar lesion affect speech?
6. What are the symptoms of the main aphasic syndromes?

7. What deficits may accompany Broca's aphasia, beyond language deficits?
8. What are the fundamental characteristics of Wernicke's aphasia?
9. What is the usual localization of a cerebral lesion causing Broca's aphasia?
10. What is the usual localization of a cerebral lesion causing Wernicke's aphasia?
11. Can a deaf person become aphasic? In what sense is sign language aphasia similar to aphasia of patients with no hearing impairment?
12. What is the common characteristic of the three transcortical aphasic syndromes?

NOTES

1. Indeed, the vast majority of the connections between neurons are made within the brain, and only a very small number of the neurons connect with lower parts of the CNS, that is, the brain stem and the spinal cord.
2. The motor, or pyramidal, pathway crosses at the pyramids, at the level of the brain stem's medulla oblongata; the ascending posterior tract of the spinal cord, conveying the proprioceptive sensation, crosses a bit higher, at the interior lemniscus. The ascending fibers conveying superficial sensitivity (pain, temperature, light touch) go directly to the thalamus of the same side (spinothalamic tract) because they have already crossed at the level of their entry in the spinal cord.
3. The cortex is extensively connected to the external part of the basal ganglia, or neostriatum, consisting of the caudate, the putamen, and the pars externa of the globus palidus; these are, in turn, connected to the internal part of the ganglia, or paleostriatum, consisting of the pars interna of the globus palidus and the reticulate portion of the substantia nigra.
4. Dopamine (DA) is one of the neurotransmitters, the chemical substances serving the transmission of messages in the synapses of the nervous system.
5. *Myoclonus*, *tics*, *tremor*, *chorea*, *athetosis*, and *dystonic movements* or *positions* are the terms used to describe forms of involuntary movements seen in hyperkinetic extrapyramidal syndromes.
6. For the interested reader, clinical stories richly and vividly describing—and explaining—these and other conditions can be found in Oliver Sacks's books *The Man Who Mistook His Wife for a Hat and Other Clinical Stories*, *Awakenings*, and *Musicophilia*.
7. Paralysis of half of the body.
8. The same is also true in the frame of the CNS in cases of demyelinating diseases, including multiple sclerosis.
9. Lesion loci in the left perisylvian region are the most common cause of aphasia. However, several cases have been reported in the literature where aphasia was caused by a lesion in the right hemisphere or a lesion in the left hemisphere but outside the perisylvian zone.
10. Thrombus is usually the result of atherosclerosis of big or medium arteries of the brain; thrombi are formed of the atherosclerotic plaques on the artery's wall, thus gradually narrowing and finally obstructing the artery. Emboli of various sizes may be produced in other large arteries (usually in the common or the internal carotid artery) or the heart as a result of atherosclerosis or heart disease, and they migrate, obstructing smaller arteries. Stroke can also be the result of bleeding or hemorrhage caused by a lesion of some vessel.
11. Hyperlipedemia is abnormally elevated levels of any or all lipids in the blood.
12. This condition has been vividly illustrated in the first person by Jean-Dominique Bauby. On December 8, 1995, at the age of 43, Bauby suffered a stroke. When he woke up 20 days later, he was entirely speechless; most of his body was paralyzed, but his mental facilities were intact. He could only blink his left eyelid. Despite this condition—the locked-in syndrome—he wrote the book *The Diving Bell and the Butterfly* by blinking when the correct letter was reached by a person slowly reciting the alphabet over and over again. The book was published in France on March 7, 1997. Bauby died 10 days after the publication of his book.
13. The lesion was in fact much more important as "the frontal lobe of the left hemisphere was softened in the bigger part of its surface," extending to "the ascending fold of the parietal lobe . . . the marginal fold of the temporal lobe . . . the insula, and the corpus striatum" (P. Broca, 1861, cited in Hécaen & Dubois, 1969, p. 60).

14. Pierre Marie (1906) argued that there is only one true aphasia: Wernicke's aphasia, caused by a lesion in Wernicke's area and characterized by the loss of a specialized *form of intelligence*, a psychological construct referring to an integrated set of notions and procedures learned through instruction. However, in case of additional, coexistent lesions, this "true" aphasia can be accompanied by other symptoms, such as anarthria, which is caused by an anterior extension of the lesion into the deep white matter and the lenticular nucleus.

15. Paul Broca mentioned the complex swear of his aphasic patient Tan, the famous "Sacré Nom de D[ieu]!" (Broca, 1861, cited in Hécaen & Dubois, 1969, pp. 64, 75, 77).

16. This dissociation between voluntary or propositional versus automatic uses of language had already been described by Baillarger in 1865 as "automatic-voluntary dissociation" (Baillarger, 1890, cited in Hécaen & Dubois, 1969; Roch-Lecours & Lhermitte, 1979).

17. Alajouanine provided another example to illustrate the automatic–voluntary dissociation: He had asked an aphasic patient the name of her daughter, who was sitting beside her. After vainly struggling for her daughter's name, the lady turned toward her daughter and said in a very distressed voice, "Ma pauvre Jacqueline, voilà que je ne sais plus ton nom!" ("My poor Jacqueline, I don't even know your name!") (Alajouanine, 1968, p. 250, cited by Basso, 2003). As Basso (2003) commented: "Answering Alajouanine's question required an intentional search for her daughter's name, but addressing her by her name was automatic" (p. 13).

18. Phonemic paraphasia is the mispronunciation of a word as a result of deletion, substitution, transposition, or addition of one or several phonemes.

19. Semantic paraphasias involve substitution of a whole word with another one, usually semantically related.

20. Neologisms involve severe disturbance of the phonemic integrity of a word, resulting in a new, sometimes meaningless, word.

21. In empty speech, the patient speaks fluently, but the verbal output is of poor content.

22. Paralexia is the equivalent of paraphasia, when referring to reading aloud.

23. The patient does not initiate speaking or moving.

24. For example, during the aphasia assessment, the patient automatically repeats what the examiner says.

ACKNOWLEDGMENTS

We are grateful to Sotiris Filippakopoulos for his drawings and Professor Andrew Papanicolaou for revising the text.

REFERENCES

Adams, R., Victor, M., & Ropper, A. H. (1997). *Principles of neurology.* 6th ed. Columbus, OH: McGraw-Hill.

Alexander, M. P. (2000). Aphasia I: Clinical and anatomic issues. In M. J. Farah & T. E. Feinberg (Eds.), *Patient-based approaches to cognitive neuroscience* (pp. 165–181). Cambridge, MA: MIT Press.

Assal, G., Regli, F., Thuillard, F., Steck, A., Deruaz, J. P., & Perentes, E. (1983). Syndrome d'isolement de la zone du langage: Étude neuropsychologique et pathologique [Isolation syndrome of the language area: Neuropsychologic and pathologic study]. *Rev Neurol* (Paris), *139*, 417–424.

Basso, A. (2003). *Aphasia and its therapy.* New York: Oxford University Press.

Basso, A., Farabola, M., Pia Grassi, M., Laiacona, M., & Zanobio, M. E. (1990). Aphasia in left-handers: Comparison of aphasia profiles and language recovery in non-right-handed and matched right-handed patients. *Brain and Language, 38*(2), 233–252.

Benson, D. F. (1993). Aphasia. In K. M. Heilman & E. Valenstein (Eds.), *Clinical neuropsychology* (3rd ed., pp. 17–36). New York: Oxford University Press.

Benson, F., & Ardila, A. (1996). *Aphasia: A clinical perspective.* New York: Oxford University Press.

Breier, J., Maher, L., Schmadeke, S., Hasan, K., & Papanicolaou, A. (2007). Changes in language-specific brain activation after therapy for aphasia using magnetoencephalography: A case study. *Neurocase, 13*, 169–177.

Compston, A. (2006). On aphasia: By L. Lichtheim, MD, professor of medicine in the University of Berne. *Brain, 129*, 1347–1350.

Coppens, P., Hungerford, S., Yamaguchi, S., & Yamadori, A. (2002). Crossed aphasia: An analysis of the symptoms, their frequency, and a comparison with left-hemisphere aphasia symptomatology, *Brain and Language, 83*(3), 425-463.

Cummings, J. L., & Mega, M. S. (2003). *Neuropsychiatry and behavioral neuroscience.* New York: Oxford University Press.

Damasio, A., & Damasio, H. (2000). Aphasia and the neural basis of language. In M.-M. Mesulam (Ed.), *Principles of behavioral and cognitive neurology* (pp. 294–315). New York: Oxford University Press.

Damasio, A., Damasio, H., Rizzo, M., Varney, N., & Gersh, F. (1982). Aphasia with non-hemorrhagic lesions in the basal ganglia and internal capsule. *Archives of Neurology, 39*, 15–20.

Damasio, A., & Geschwind, N. (1984). The neural basis of language. *Annual Review of Neuroscience, 7*, 127–147.

Damasio, H. (1998). Neuroanatomical correlates of the aphasias. In M. T. Sarno (Ed.), *Acquired aphasia* (3rd ed., pp. 43–68). San Diego, CA: Academic Press.

Darby, D., & Walsh, K. (2005). *Walsh's neuropsychology: A clinical approach* (5th ed.). New York: Churchill Livingstone.

Dejerine, J. (1892). Contribution à l'étude anatomique et clinique des différentes variétés de cécité verbale. *Mémoires de la Société de Biologie, 4*, 61–90.

Dejerine, J. (1977). *Sémiologie des affections du système nerveux.* Paris: Masson. (Original work published 1891)

Dellatolas, G., & Potagas, C. (2009). Πλαγίωση, χειρονομίεσ και γλώσσα [Laterality, gestures, and language]. In C. Potagas & I. Evdokimidis (EdsΣυςζητήσεις για το λόγο: λόγος και κίνηση *Discussions on language: Language and movement*]. Athens, Greece: Synapseis. (In Greek)

Fasanaro, A. M., Spitaleri, D. L. A., Valiani, R., Postiglione, A., Soricelli, A., Mansi, L., & Grossi, D. (1987). Cerebral blood flow in thalamic aphasia. *Journal of Neurology, 234*, 421–423.

Finger, S. (1994). *Origins of neuroscience.* New York: Oxford University Press.

Freud, S. (1953). *Zur Auffassung der Aphasien* [*On aphasia: A critical study*] (E. Stengel, Trans.). London: Imago. (Original work published 1891)

Geschwind, N. (1965). Disconnection syndromes in animals and man. *Brain, 88*, 237–294.

Geschwind, N. (1967). Wernicke's contribution to the study of aphasia. *Cortex, 3*, 449–463.

Goldstein, K. (1995). *The organism: A holistic approach to biology derived from pathological data in man.* New York: Zone.

Hagoort, P. (2005). On Broca, brain, and binding: A new framework. *Trends in Cognitive Sciences, 9*, 416–423.

Hayashi, M. M., Ulatowska, H. K., & Sasanuma, S. (1985). Subcortical aphasia with deep dyslexia: A case study of a Japanese patient. *Brain and Language, 25*, 293–313.

Hécaen, H., & Ajuriaguerra, J. (1963). *Les gauchers: Prévalence manuelle et dominance cérébrale.* Paris: Presses Universitaires de France.

Hécaen, H., & Dubois, J. (1969). *La naissance de la neuropsychologie du langage (1825–1865).* Paris: Flammarion.

Hickok, G., & Poeppel, D. (2004). Dorsal and ventral streams: A framework for understanding aspects of the functional anatomy of language. *Cognition, 92*, 67–99.

Hodges, J. R. (1998). *Cognitive assessment for clinicians.* Oxford, UK: Oxford Medical.

Kreisler, A., Godefroy, O., Delmaire, C., Debachy, B., Leclercq, M., Pruvo, J. P., & Leys, D. (2000). The anatomy of aphasia revisited. *Neurology, 54*(5), 1117–1123.

Lantéri-Laura, G. (1987). *Le cerveau.* Paris: Seghers.

MacSweeney, M., Capek, C. M., Campbell, R., & Woll, B. (2008). The signing brain: The neurobiology of sign language. *Trends in Cognitive Sciences, 12*, 432–440.

Marie, P. (1906). Révision de la question de l'aphasie: La troisième circonvolution frontale gauche ne joue aucun rôle spécial dans la fonction du langage. *Semaine Médicale, 26*, 241–247.

Mariën, P., Paghera, B., De Deyn, P., & Vignolo L. A. (2004). Adult crossed aphasia in dextrals revisited. *Cortex, 40* 41–74.

Mesulam, M.-M. (2000). *Principles of behavioral and cognitive neurology.* New York: Oxford University Press.

Radanovic, M., & Scaff, M. (2003). Speech and language disturbances due to subcortical lesions. *Brain and Language, 84*, 337–352.

Rasmussen, T., & Milner, B. (1977). The role of early left-brain injury in determining lateralization of cerebral speech functions. *Annals of the New York Academy of Sciences, 199*, 355–369.

Riese, W. (1959). *A history of neurology.* New York: MD Publications.

Roch-Lecours, A., & Lhermitte, F. (1979). *L'aphasie.* Paris: Flammarion.

Saur, D., Lange, R., Baumgaertner, A., Schraknepper, V., Willmes, K., Rijntjes, M., & Weiller, C. (2006). Dynamics of language reorganization after stroke. *Brain, 129*, 1371–1384.

Shalom, D. B., & Poeppel, D. (2008). Functional anatomic models of language: Assembling the pieces. *Neuroscientist, 14*, 119–127.

Wada, J., & Rasmussen, T. (1960). Intracarotid injection of sodium amytal for the lateralization of cerebral speech dominance. *Journal of Neurosurgery, 17*, 242–282.

Wernicke, C. (1874). *Der Aphasische Symptomencomplex: Eine psychologische Studie auf anatomischer Basis.* Breslau, Poland: Cohn & Weigert.

Willmes, K., & Poeck, K. (1993). To what extent can aphasic syndromes be localized? *Brain, 116*, 1527–1540.

Yamadori, A., Ohira, T., Seriu, M., & Ogura, J. (1984). Transcortical sensory aphasia produced by lesions of the anterior basal ganglia area. *No To Shinkei, 36*(3), 261–266.

OBJECTIVES

The reader will be able to:

1. **Describe the concept of recovery and plasticity.**

2. **Understand the role of the physiologic and biochemical mechanisms in functional recovery.**

3. **Understand the role of the structural mechanisms in functional recovery.**

4. **Understand the role of the behavioral mechanisms in functional recovery.**

5. **Describe the patterns of language recovery in aphasia.**

6. **Associate the mechanisms of recovery and plasticity with language therapy in aphasia.**

Plasticity and Recovery in Aphasia

Ilias Papathanasiou, Patrick Coppens, Edith Durand, and Ana Inés Ansaldo

INTRODUCTION

Recovery is the overarching goal for clinicians working with individuals with aphasia. Observations of the patterns of clinical recovery have produced various hypotheses about the mechanisms underlying the recovery process. In this chapter, we attempt to synthesize the many different interpretations of functional recovery and to show how these different views have influenced the theory and practice of modern aphasia therapy.

Clinicians see aphasia as a breakdown in the functional system of communication. This concept of *function* representing an entire functional system is remarkably different from the *function* of a particular component of the system. According to Luria (1973), mental processes such as language are complex functional systems that are not localized in narrowly circumscribed areas of the brain. They take place through the participation of groups of brain structures working in concert, each making its own particular contribution to the organization of the functional system. Luria suggested that there are three principal functional systems in the brain whose participation is necessary for any type of mental activity: a unit for regulating tone or waking, a unit for obtaining and storing information, and a unit for programming, regulating, and verifying mental activity. The three units are hierarchical but work together as a dynamic and interactive system. Thus, according to Luria (1973), any complex mental process requires the synergistic cooperation of these units to take place.

Focusing on the functional language system, Westbury (1998) not only commented that a functional definition of language should include components organized in a structured hierarchy but also recognized that some of these elements are involved in all modalities of language input and output. The first major dichotomy of this hierarchical structure distinguishes between the two main language modalities: spoken and written. In each of these modalities, language breaks down into input and output functions or comprehension and expression, although these distinctions are more complex than it seems. In turn, the input (auditory comprehension and reading) and output (speaking and writing) mechanisms may be broken into two subhierarchies: semantics and modality-specific components. For example, in the written modality, these components include sentences, words, and letters, whereas in the auditory modality they consist of sentences, words, and phonemes. These components can function independently, interact with each other within a modality to facilitate input and output mechanisms, and interact with one another cross modally to integrate written and oral systems. Aspects of language influencing both written and oral modalities, such as affixes, word properties (e.g., frequency, concreteness), are not included in this hierarchical structure but affect the way the hierarchies are accessed and subsequently how language is realized.

In addition to the preceding linguistic concepts, we have to consider language use, that is, the environment in which language takes place and the behaviors associated with it. Language is a means of communication; thus, any functional linguistic system must successfully fulfill a communicative function. The principles underlying the dynamic organization of language and communication are regulated by networks of functional units forming a complex, yet synergistic, system supported by cortical and subcortical structures. Finally, changes in the communicative behavior of people with acquired aphasia are ultimately the result of changes at the level of the cellular and neuronal organization of the brain. All these concepts—be they at the level of the neuron or the level of the behavior—are important to understand the patterns of language recovery and plasticity seen in people with aphasia.

THE CONCEPTS OF PLASTICITY AND RECOVERY

In aphasia, recovery of language and communication ultimately involves brain alterations. These changes can be considered at two different levels, the microlevel and the macrolevel. Both levels are associated with the concepts of plasticity and recovery.

What Is Neuroplasticity?

According to Kolb (1995), neuroplasticity is considered to be the brain's capacity to change either at the microlevel (i.e., cellular/network level), known as *neural*

plasticity, or at the macrolevel (i.e., behavioral/system level), known as *behavioral plasticity*, allowing the brain to respond to environmental changes or changes in the organism itself. Plasticity can be adaptive or maladaptive. Adaptive brain plasticity consists of efficient rerouting, whereas maladaptive brain plasticity results in the persistence of aphasic symptoms and poor recovery resulting from inefficient rewiring (Ansaldo, 2004; Grafman, 2000; Kleim & Jones, 2008).

The mechanisms underlying neural plasticity are multiple and include biochemical, physiologic, and structural changes. The consequences of these changes, which express themselves in behavioral plasticity, are likewise multiple. Microlevel plasticity allows the brain to learn new behaviors and skills. By the same token, the behavior itself can alter the brain, which in turn reinforces that behavior. Thus, plasticity both results from and induces behavioral changes. Brain damage results in neurophysiologic changes in the brain that modify behaviors, and these behaviors, in turn, produce further changes in the brain. In a more empirical and functional approach to plasticity, which focuses at the macrosystemic level, Frackowiack (1997) argued that plasticity should be viewed as the changes of neural function over time or, more specifically, the changes effected by repeated behavior following an injury. Thus, plasticity represents the changes in brain activity associated with the tasks performed (e.g., action, perception, cognition) in an attempt to compensate for the impaired functions.

What Is Recovery?

The term *recovery* in its extended sense covers any and all behavioral changes, such as restoration, reorganization, compensation, habituation, restitution, substitution, new learning, and so on (Brant, Strupp, Arbusow, & Dieringer, 1997). In a sense, recovery is independent of the microlevel underlying structural changes because it refers to the macrolevel behaviors and functional systems. However, the two levels and their respective mechanisms do interact.

More recently, the definition of recovery has become more specific. Kleim and Schwerin (2010) made a distinction between recovery and compensation. They stated that both of these processes can be described at the microlevel (i.e., neural) and the macrolevel (i.e., behavioral), and both can be responsible for the observed improvement. However, at the behavioral level, recovery refers to the capacity to perform a previously impaired task in the same manner as before the injury, while compensation refers to the use of a new strategy to perform that same task. At the neurophysiologic level, recovery refers to the restoration of the function within an area of the cortex that was initially lost after the injury, while compensation occurs when a different neural tissue takes over the functions lost after injury.

Timeline and Patterns of Recovery

The loss of neural tissue associated with brain injury induces profound neurophysiologic changes throughout the brain, causing a wide range of behavioral impairments. Such impairments are not only a manifestation of the damaged brain region but also an expression of the attempts by the intact brain areas to remedy the decrease in function. The nature of these recovery mechanisms will vary according to time postonset. In cases of poststroke aphasia, unless the brain tissue is rapidly reperfused, lost abilities can only be restored by being rerouted through existing unimpaired pathways or by creating new connections. This is part of the evolution of recovery that takes place from the first hours until many years postonset.

Immediately after the trauma, there is a short period of shock in which many functions are affected. Within a few hours or days, there is a period of rapid recovery and then a steady improvement over several weeks, the rate of which gradually decreases as the months and years go by. Traditionally, these mechanisms are viewed as time-dependent phases: acute, subacute, and chronic (Hillis & Heidler, 2002; Teasell, Bayonna, & Bitensky, 2005).

Reperfusion happens within hours after stroke and consists of the restoration of blood flow to an organ or tissue. It can be spontaneous or induced by medical intervention. According to Powell (1981), three different plastic neuronal mechanisms are relevant to the timeline of the recovery process. First, the physical repair mechanism of the penumbra[1] area cells is important during the initial days as the wound and the body heal, the scar tissue forms, and the disturbed physiologic functions improve. Second, neural processing mechanisms reorganize impaired areas by taking advantage of intact brain regions spontaneously. Such adaptation takes place almost immediately and is sustained for a period of weeks; it then declines in importance as the limits of the reorganization are reached. Finally, new learning mechanisms govern the extent to which the person can be retrained to perform a specific skill. These last mechanisms are driven by rehabilitation and are separate from the improvements caused by the resolution of postinjury edema or inflammation (Kleim & Schwerin, 2010). The three phases described by Powell can be related to the three-stage model for the early, late subacute, and chronic phases of recovery

proposed by Saur and colleagues (Saur et al., 2006; Saur & Hartwigsen, 2012). In their longitudinal functional neuroimaging study examining recovery from aphasia from the acute to the chronic stages, the authors proposed that the left and right hemispheres play distinct roles according to recovery stage. Specifically, in the acute stage, there is a global breakdown of the entire language network, with weak left hemisphere activation. In the subacute stage, concurrent with a mild improvement in language function, bilateral cerebral activation is observed, with a stronger activation in the right hemisphere. Finally, a normalization of activation pattern in the last stage with a shift back to the left hemisphere is observed.

Kolb (1995) described the recovery timeline using behavioral concepts and identified three possible outcomes. Initially, compensation may occur, which may reflect a change in strategy or represent the substitution of a new behavior for the lost one. A second outcome might be a partial restitution of the original behavior, which could reflect the partial return of the function. Third, the original behavior could be completely restored. This happens because the structural properties of the brain allow plastic changes to take place, which allow recovery to occur. Powell (1981) suggested that the complexity of the recovery process cannot be overstated because it depends on so many variables. For example, individual differences in cerebral organization and learning strategies influence recovery. Specific mechanisms of recovery apply to some functions and are irrelevant to others. Thus, recovery is a multifaceted mechanism that varies across time, across functions, and across individuals themselves.

Powell (1981) suggested that once the physiologic repair and restitution have taken place and once the structural repair potential has been reached, the organism may still be functionally impaired. Then, the only option for further improvement is to use strategies that bypass the lesion site. Using new strategies may both prompt further physiologic changes (e.g., other connections are reinforced) and encourage further structural changes (e.g., an area is "coaxed" into contributing to a new function). Keefe (1995) suggested that combining our knowledge of the neural mechanisms underlying behavioral changes with our understanding of the mechanisms underlying language and communication impairments would result in more effective behavioral interventions for aphasia. Therefore, to reach the most effective treatment for the language and communication dysfunction associated with aphasia, we need to perform a neuropsychological analysis of the deficits based on the hierarchical cognitive processing approach and also a detailed neurophysiologic analysis focusing on the organic brain structures of the impaired functional system.

The Relationship Between Recovery and Plasticity

To understand how the recovery of language and communication takes place, we have to consider all the mechanisms involved in neural and behavioral plasticity. As stated previously, the mechanisms of plasticity can be classified as *biochemical/physiologic* at the cellular level, *structural* at the brain structure level, and *behavioral* at the function/behavior level. The first two mechanisms are known as *neural plasticity,* while the third one is referred to as *behavioral plasticity.* This distinction is rather arbitrary because there is a dynamic interaction between these mechanisms. According to Kolb (1995), neural plasticity drives behavioral plasticity, and the properties of this brain–behavior interactive relationship are as follows:

- Behavioral states and mind states correspond to brain states.
- The structural properties of the brain are important in understanding its function.
- Plasticity is a property of the synapse.
- Behavioral plasticity results from the summation of plasticity of individual neurons.
- Specific mechanisms of plasticity are likely to underlie more than one form of behavioral change.
- The cortex is the most likely locus for neural plasticity to take place.
- Behavior is difficult to study at a molecular level.

In contrast, Powell (1981) believed that behavioral changes drive brain plasticity. According to him, the properties of the language/brain dynamic relationship are as follows:

- A cognitive skill such as language may have more than one mode of expression.
- Superficially similar or functionally equivalent material may be analyzed or stored in distinct areas of the brain.
- In the damaged brain, intact areas can become involved in attempting to perform the lost function.
- Language tasks activate the right hemisphere as well as the left.
- Language, in a normal left hemisphere–dominant individual, is not sustained exclusively by the left hemisphere.
- Normal language processing is supported by specific pathways, although others may exist that, despite not being normally used, may come into play when primary routes are damaged.

PROGNOSTIC FACTORS OF RECOVERY

Clinicians who have treated individuals with aphasia have frequently sought to uncover indicators of recovery. Basso (1992) differentiated between neurologic factors and individual factors. Neurologic factors are related to the etiology of the injury, size and site of lesion, and severity and type of aphasia. Personal factors are characteristics such as age, education, handedness, and psychological and emotional issues. We discuss some of these factors in the following paragraphs.

The etiology of aphasia—hemorrhage versus ischemic stroke—has been related to the pattern of recovery. Holland, Greenhouse, Fromm, and Swindell (1989) reported that the type of stroke had a moderate influence on the recovery progress, with hemorrhage associated with a more favorable outcome than infarction. Also, Basso (1992), in her study of 46 patients with hemorrhage and 101 patients with infarction, reported that at 6 months and 12 months postonset, more patients with hemorrhage than infarction had experienced a substantial recovery. She suggested that this difference resulted from the fact that the hematoma displaced the fiber bundles without completely destroying them.

A basic assumption about recovery from aphasia has been that lesion size has a negative influence on recovery (Cherney & Robey, 2008). However, lesion size might have a different effect on expressive versus receptive skills. For example, Selnes, Knopman, Niccum, Rubens, and Larson (1983) reported a significant negative correlation (the larger the lesion, the smaller the recovery) between lesion volume and comprehension recovery for larger lesions only. Mazzoni et al. (1992) stated that patients with a smaller lesion demonstrated significant recovery in oral and written expression while they showed almost-intact comprehension skills, patients with a medium-size lesion made a good recovery in all language modalities except written expression, and patients with a large lesion demonstrated improvement only in auditory comprehension. On the other hand, Basso (1992) recognized the negative effect of lesion size on initial severity but stated that once initial severity is taken into account, the effect of lesion size on recovery was no longer clear, thereby suggesting that initial severity may be a more important predictor of recovery than lesion size is.

Furthermore, lesion size may be difficult to differentiate from lesion site and aphasia type. In a recent review of literature, Anglade, Thiel, and Ansaldo (2014) discussed the specific impact of lesion size on right hemisphere recruitment in the recovery from aphasia. In their theoretical model, the authors (Anglade et al., 2014), argued that right hemisphere recruitment is modulated by a number of factors, including the lesion's location, extent, and stability. Further, Anglade and collaborators (2014) argued that preservation of core language-processing areas results in minimal right hemisphere recruitment, as opposed to long-term right hemisphere recruitment in cases of permanent damage to core language left hemisphere processing areas.

A number of authors have explored the question of lesion site and its impact on aphasia recovery. The extent of damage to Wernicke's area was found to be correlated to auditory comprehension recovery at 6 months postonset, with better recovery observed when less than half of the temporal lobe was damaged (Naeser, Helm-Eastbrooks, Haas, Auerbach, & Shrinivasan, 1987). Similarly, Kertesz, Lau, and Polk (1993) suggested that the extent of damage within specific structures, rather than overall lesion size, contributed to the prediction of language recovery. They reported that, for patients with Wernicke's aphasia, the integrity of the angular gyrus and the anterior midtemporal gyrus seemed important for language recovery. Moreover, less angular gyrus involvement was related to recovery of auditory comprehension 1 year postonset. These authors further reported that involvement of the supramarginal gyrus was also correlated with poor recovery.

Naeser, Palumbo, Helm-Eastbrooks, Stiassny-Eder, and Albert (1989) reported that recovery of spontaneous speech in global aphasia was related to the involvement of subcortical white matter areas. In the same group of individuals, it was also reported that when Wernicke's area was spared, language recovery was better (Naeser, Gaddie, Palumbo, & Stiassny-Eder, 1990).

For Broca's aphasia, Kertesz and McCabe (1977) suggested that the best recovery was related to the intactness of subcortical areas. These authors also reported that transcortical aphasias tended to have a good prognosis in general, and that patients with anomic aphasia made slower progress but developed better functional communication skills overall. In conduction aphasia, they reported that progress seemed similar to that in Broca's aphasia. Bartha and Benke (2003) confirmed that conduction aphasia was not associated with a particularly good recovery, as was once thought.

Overall, it appears that individuals with expressive or nonfluent aphasia tend to have a better prognosis than those with receptive or fluent aphasias do. However, most of these studies were based on computed tomographic (CT) scans performed within the first year postonset and not after ultimate recovery, and most authors did not consider how these recovery factors may influence language therapy (Cherney & Robey, 2008). With the recent advances in functional neuroimaging techniques, we may be able to better understand how recovery occurs

in general, but the prognostic value of individual neurological factors remains undetermined. However, with a better understanding of the plasticity mechanisms, we are better placed to grasp how language is reorganized in the different parts of the brain, as discussed further in this chapter.

Although personal and biographical factors appear to play a minor role in recovery from aphasia compared to the neurological factors (Benson & Ardila, 1996), they should not be ignored. Younger patients were believed to have a more favorable outcome than older individuals were. However, age is correlated with etiology, aphasia type, and overall health. When those factors are controlled, age does not seem to contribute significantly to recovery (Basso, 1992; Plowman, Hentz, & Ellis, 2012). It was also reported that females have a better prognosis than males. For example, Basso, Capitani, and Moraschini (1982) followed 400 patients and reported that females did improve more than males in spoken language but not in auditory comprehension. In severe aphasia, however, women showed more improvement than men in auditory comprehension (Pizzamiglio, Mammucari, & Razzano, 1985). It was hypothesized that these differences might be attributed to possible gender differences in interhemispheric distribution of cognitive functions (Moir & Jessel, 1991).

Indeed, evidence with healthy populations (Cabeza, 2002) showed that brain activity during cognitive performance reflected distinct lateralization patterns in male and female subjects. Among others, activity in the inferior frontal gyrus during phonological processing was left lateralized in males, whereas it was bilateral in females.

A number of studies using diffusion tensor imaging supported the hypothesis of gender-related differences in brain organization (Catani et al., 2007; Hagmann et al., 2006). Specifically, the evidence showed that, in right-handed men, the cerebral cortex was characterized by a large intrahemispheric axonal connectivity between language areas and a sparse interhemispheric connectivity between homologous right hemisphere areas, whereas in right-handed women and left-handed men, there was a higher density of interhemispheric connections between left hemisphere language areas and their homologous right hemisphere areas. It has also further been shown that more symmetrical connections correlate with better semantic associations (Catani et al., 2007).

However, other studies have shown that gender in itself is not a predictor of prognosis (Kertesz & McCabe, 1977; Lendrem & Lincoln, 1985). Among these studies, Pedersen, Vinter, and Olsen (2004) followed 270 patients acute stroke patients with aphasia for 1 year and found that language recovery could not be predicted by gender.

The impact of anatomical connectivity patterns on aphasia recovery in right-handed and left-handed male and female individuals with aphasia needs to be further explored.

Handedness is also believed to influence recovery because of evidence that left-handed people have a more bilateral language representation in the brain (Springer & Deutsch, 1998). Therefore, there is the assumption that left-handed and ambidextrous individuals recover more rapidly from aphasia. However, several studies failed to identify differences in language recovery patterns between left-handed and right-handed individuals with aphasia (Basso, Farabola, Grassi, Laiacona, & Zanobio, 1990; Borod, Carper, & Naeser, 1990). Consequently, the prognostic value of handedness for recovery was not strongly supported.

Finally, the emotional and psychosocial changes that accompany aphasia may have an impact on prognosis. For example, depression has been reported in 25% of patients in the acute stages following a stroke (Astrom, Adolfsson, & Asplund, 1993). Although common sense would dictate that variables such as depression, motivation, and the like should affect prognosis, their purported influence has not yet been ascertained or quantified. The emotional and psychosocial adjustment over time in individuals with aphasia and their significant others also play a significant role in the chronic stage.

In conclusion, predicting prognosis is a complex task for which many neurological and personal factors must be considered. Because prognosis is multifactorial, clinicians must infer how each prognostic variable, as well as the interactions among those variables, is likely to influence language recovery. Importantly, whereas a clinician makes prognostic predictions for an individual, the influence of these variables has only been studied in groups of individuals, a procedure that stresses averages rather than individual results. Finally, recovery is influenced by time postonset, which in turn is related to neurophysiologic and behavioral mechanisms. In the following sections, we describe these mechanisms from the neuronal to the behavioral level.

BIOCHEMICAL AND PHYSIOLOGIC MECHANISMS OF RECOVERY

Injury in the brain following a stroke or other forms of neurological damage produces both primary and secondary changes. The primary changes occur within a few days postinjury and then stabilize. The secondary changes are set in motion as a consequence of the primary damage and continue to evolve over time (Carmichael, 2010; Keefe, 1995). Importantly, because these secondary processes develop over a longer timeline than the primary changes, the functional changes continue to take place. More than site of lesion, these secondary processes determine the residual deficits observed and contribute to the behavioral recovery (Keefe, 1995; Powell, 1981).

The primary changes (i.e., within a week after a cerebrovascular accident) include immediate necrosis (i.e., cell death), signs of inflammation in the cell, retrograde cell degeneration proximal to the lesion, and anterograde cell degeneration distal to the lesion. The secondary (indirect) changes are *transneuronal degeneration*, in which areas receiving neural input from, or providing input to, the infarcted area degenerate as a result of the loss of connections; *denervation supersensitivity*, in which neurons that have lost most of their input from the infarcted area become increasingly sensitive to any residual input received from that area; *development of diaschisis*, in which injury to a certain area temporarily inhibits connected noninjured areas remote from the infarcted tissue yet functionally connected to it; *vascular disruption*, which results in ischemia; and *collateral sprouting*, in which axons from nearby neurons grow new synaptic contacts with sites formerly innervated by the lesioned cells. As described previously, these secondary changes have a longer timeline and contribute to behavioral recovery and adult brain plasticity. These secondary changes can be further classified as structural or functional. Structural changes take place within the neurons themselves and include the following:

- *Regenerative sprouting* (Carmichael, 2010): This regeneration can be axonal or dendritic. The impaired process regenerates fibers from other branches that are capable of forming new working synapses.
- *Collateral regenerative sprouting* (Keefe, 1995; Powell, 1981): Nonlesioned cells grow new synaptic connections with neurons in the penumbra area, which are hypofunctional areas, in an attempt to reestablish lost input.

Functional changes, as follows, are related to the neuronal connections:

- *Relatively ineffective synapses* (Powell, 1981): The activation of preexisting connections that were originally unnecessary to execute a function and overshadowed by the main connections of the cell. This may be misinterpreted as the formation of new connections.
- *Denervation sensitivity* (Keefe, 1995; Powell, 1981): After the injury, the cell shows a lower response threshold to any remaining afferent fibers. Consequently, the activity potential of the target cell

remains the same, although the number of afferent connections may be reduced.

- *Synapse potentials* (Keefe, 1995; Leonard, 1998): Long-term potentiation (LTP) is the neuronal-level changes that explain learning and memory. It is a rapidly induced and sustained increase in the efficiency of neural transmission at a given synapse. This neuronal mechanism can cause long-term changes in synaptic transmission and subsequently to the functional systems involved.

The exact role of the physiologic mechanisms mentioned in the recovery of function in clinical (i.e., behavioral) terms may need further investigation. Some of these processes may be antagonistic. For example, the inhibitory character of diaschisis may not facilitate collateral spouting. However, because these mechanisms have been observed in experimental situations, the challenge is to find the correlations between neuronal and behavioral changes. Animal models provide a partial solution to the problem because they afford us the luxury of obtaining more specific neurobiological measures that may be more directly related to changes in behavior. The limitations of animal models of behavior, on the other hand, make studying the neural basis for improvements of complex behaviors such as language and cognition challenging.

STRUCTURAL MECHANISMS OF RECOVERY

The physiologic mechanisms discussed previously refer to what happens at the cellular level to repair affected connections. However, evidence of plasticity is available not only from the synaptic level but also from the examination of the connections in the brain as a whole (Keefe, 1995). Traditionally, various theories of structural mechanisms (which are caused by the physiologic changes) have been developed to provide an explanation for the reappearance of a lost function following a brain lesion (Blomert, 1998). Although neuroscientists have now established that the brain responds to damage by triggering complex processes that take place over long periods of time and produce changes throughout the entire nervous system (Stein & Glasier, 1992), the early theoretical accounts still provide a framework for current research. These theories include the following:

- *The resolution or regression of diaschisis* (Cappa, 1998; Powell, 1981): The initial diaschisis, which is considered to be an initial protective mechanism for the injury, tends to diminish or disappear, allowing brain areas to function again.

- *Restoration* (Kleim & Schwerin, 2010): Restoration refers to the reactivation of brain areas that are dysfunctional following the injury. This return of function in the neural tissue is related to the establishment of neural connectivity thanks to the physiologic mechanisms described previously.

- *Recruitment* (Kleim & Schwerin, 2010): Recruitment refers to the enlisting of brain areas that have the capacity to contribute to the lost function but that may not normally have been involved prior to the injury. These areas are asked to play a larger role in the performance of the impaired function but are not performing a new function (retraining).

- *Retraining* (Kleim & Schwerin, 2010): Brain areas perform novel or additional functions as a result of rehabilitation training. These brain areas usually do not lose their original premorbid functions, but they take over an additional role as a result of reorganization triggered by training.

- *Functional takeover* (Cappa, 1998): In the case of lateralized functions such as language, undamaged areas in the contralateral hemisphere can take over functions. This is considered to be the "unmasking" of a preexisting functional commitment, actively inhibited by the left hemisphere (Moscovitch, 1977). Another possibility includes a functional takeover by other brain areas in the same hemisphere.

It is evident that neural plasticity is the basic neural mechanism supporting functional improvement, be it for recovery or compensation (see the section "Language Recovery in the Brain"). These structural mechanisms of neural plasticity are not mutually exclusive and appear to be mediated by the physiologic and biochemical changes within cortical circuits. The ultimate goal is to develop a model of behavioral therapy based on specific neuronal plasticity mechanisms. With such a model, it would be possible to know the neuronal properties used in the therapy activities (i.e., neuronal organization of the therapy activity in Figure 4.1). Hence, the clinician would be able to choose the activity (i.e., "activities in therapy") based on its capacity to influence specific mechanisms of plasticity, which would alter the processing of the targeted function (i.e., "neural organization of function") and subsequently gain functional improvement (see Figure 4.1).

BEHAVIORAL MECHANISMS OF RECOVERY

The behavioral mechanisms of functional recovery rely on the brain's capacity to recover function beyond the limitations imposed by spontaneous physiologic and structural repair (Powell, 1981). Behavioral intervention

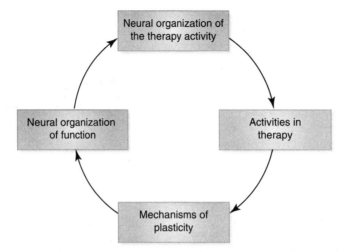

Figure 4.1 Plasticity and experience-driven therapy.

causes physiologic and structural alterations in the brain, and conversely, these neural modifications bring about further behavioral changes. The behavioral mechanisms of recovery of function are as follows:

- *Restitution–restoration–reactivation* (Blomert, 1998; Carlomagno & Iavarone, 1995; Huber, Springer, & Willmes, 1993; Lesser & Milroy, 1993): These three terms, which are often used interchangeably in the literature, refer to the mechanism of the total return of a behavior supported by the same premorbid functional system. Huber et al. (1993) described direct stimulation (e.g., repetition), indirect stimulation (e.g., cueing strategies), and deblocking (e.g., elicitation of the target response through a different task or modality first) as methods of treatment to reactivate temporarily impaired language function. They suggested that a detailed analysis of task demands used in a therapy activity in terms of input, output, and central processing in the impaired functional system is important to determine the activity used in therapy.
- *Reorganization–reconstitution–substitution within a functional system* (Edmundson & McIntosh, 1995; Howard & Hatfield, 1987; Lesser & Milroy, 1993): This mechanism, originally described by Luria, suggests that it is possible to reroute parts of a functional system without impeding the whole functional system. This can be accomplished by filling in the missing link of the functional system. The new route is different from the one that would normally be used, but the end result is the same. Bruce and Howard (1987) described a treatment approach by which word-finding problems were overcome with the use of a phonemic self-cueing strategy. This strategy provides access to the

phonological form of the word by using knowledge about grapheme–phoneme conversion rules. The grapheme–phoneme conversion is facilitated by teaching patients to use a voice output augmentative and alternative communication device. Patients type the first letter of the target word, listen to the computer-generated phonemic cue, and then attempt to produce it.

- *Relearning* (Edmundson & McIntosh, 1995; Howard & Hatfield, 1987): This mechanism implies the ability to relearn lost items or information or to reestablish lost rules or procedures in a functional system. De Partz (1986) reported using this mechanism in therapy to teach an individual with aphasia to relearn the phoneme–grapheme conversion rules for reading, for example, how the pronunciation of different consonants changes in the context of different vowels.
- *Facilitation* (Edmundson & McIntosh, 1995; Howard & Hatfield, 1987): This mechanism is usually employed as a therapy strategy in the case of difficulty accessing intact information in a functional system. Marshall, Pound, White-Thomson, and Pring (1990) used a facilitation strategy with a patient who experienced difficulties accessing the phonological output lexicon, although his semantic processing, his comprehension of pictures, and his reading skills were relatively intact. This approach reinforces the links between semantic representations and phonological output representations and thus, improves access to the phonological output lexicon.
- *Functional substitution–functional reorganization–functional compensation* (Blomert, 1998; Carlomagno & Iavarone, 1995; Lesser & Milroy, 1993; Powell, 1981): This mechanism implies that a specific function cannot recover within the original

functional system (as in *reorganization–reconstitu-tion–substitution within a functional system*). In this case, a different functional system supported by intact brain areas can substitute for the impaired original function. So, this mechanism is more one of adaptation than actual recovery of function because no attempt is made to restore the original function. Examples of this mechanism include the use of lip reading in acquired deafness; the use of gestures, computers, or other devices as means of communication following loss of oral language in individuals with aphasia; and the use of the left hand for writing when the right hand is paralyzed.

In conclusion, several key issues need to be raised. First, it is clear that, although time postonset may favor some of these recovery mechanisms over others, these processes do overlap significantly and are likely to interact. Second, the structural and biological mechanisms ultimately underlie all functional recovery, including language. Hence, the same basic behavioral mechanisms, such as relearning, facilitation, or reorganization, can be applied across all functional systems. Third, brain reorganization in individuals with aphasia is but one aspect of recovery. Communication can also be improved by manipulating external contextual factors, such as environmental changes, communication partner training, and so on. This is the basis of the *biopsychosocial* approach to aphasia therapy.

LANGUAGE RECOVERY IN THE BRAIN

Today, with the advances in neuroscience methodology and technology, our ability to understand brain functions and the process of recovery has increased significantly. Neuroimaging studies of the recovery from aphasia provide evidence for patterns of rerouting or functional reorganization, such as the recruitment of a neuronal network that was in existence before the stroke. The efficiency and success in language processing following rerouting depend on whether adaptive or maladaptive brain plasticity takes place. Adaptive brain plasticity leading to better aphasia recovery has been mostly related to the recruitment of perilesional areas in the left cerebral hemisphere (i.e., *map extension*; Grafman, 2000; Thompson, 2000), whereas the recruitment of right-hemispheric areas homologous to the damaged areas (i.e., *homologous area adaptation*) in the left hemisphere has been mainly associated with maladaptive brain plasticity and thus, poorer recovery (Thompson & Bart-den Ouden, 2008). Further, the former pattern is conceptualized as an intra-network

reorganization, whereas the latter has been associated with the use of a different strategy when performing the task (i.e., functional substitution; Kuest & Karbe, 2002). However, it is not always evident that the use of a different strategy could be limited to contralateral brain plasticity; ipsilateral compensation could also trigger the use of novel strategies as a result of brain damage in specific language-processing areas.

This dichotomy between left hemisphere–supported good recovery versus right hemisphere–supported poorer recovery has been challenged recently. However, there is evidence that efficient rerouting may include both ipsilateral and contralateral brain areas within a complex network that may be different from that observed in non–brain-damaged subjects (Marcotte & Ansaldo, 2010). Specifically, postintensive therapy recovery from severe and chronic naming deficits in both poststroke and primary progressive aphasia was found to be sustained by a bilateral network, including semantic processing and motor programming areas, as well as parietal areas, within the left and the right hemispheres (Marcotte & Ansaldo, 2010). Moreover, the type of approach used during therapy (e.g., semantic feature analysis [SFA]; Boyle & Coelho, 1995) appears to have an impact on posttherapy brain recruitment. Thus, therapy-induced recovery from anomia is sustained by the significant activation of semantic processing areas in the left and right cerebral hemispheres.

Furthermore, Kinsbourne (1971) noticed that two of his patients with aphasia who had somewhat recovered from speech production deficits showed complete speech arrest following an intracarotid amobarbital injection (Wada test) in the right hemisphere but no discernible change in language function following a left hemisphere injection. He concluded that language dominance had shifted poststroke and that the right hemisphere was solely supporting the remaining language abilities.

More recently, with the advent of modern imaging techniques, many authors have been able to confirm that, in many individuals with aphasia, increased right hemisphere activation during language tasks correlates with language improvement (e.g., Jodzio, Drumm, Nyka, Lass, & Gasecki, 2003). Thus, the brain shows the potential for long-term plasticity, an ability that can be triggered by specific and intensive language therapy. In summary, beyond controversies regarding the role of the right hemisphere versus the role of the perilesioned areas (Thompson & Bart-den Ouden, 2008), the evidence supporting that the right hemisphere can take over the processing of some linguistic functions after a left hemisphere stroke is considerable (Finger, Buckner, & Buckingham, 2003; Kuttner, 1930; Marcotte & Ansaldo, 2010; Marsh & Hillis, 2006).

The increased activation observed in the right hemisphere can be variously interpreted, however. First, its presence does not seem to guarantee a significant improvement in language skills. Buckner and Petersen (2000) reported that two individuals with aphasia can show a similar right-hemispheric activation increase, but one can manage to perform a task that the other is utterly incapable of completing. They concluded that the right hemisphere may be recruited rapidly after the cerebral insult, but with various degrees of success. This is in line with previous evidence from divided-visual-field studies showing that the right hemisphere can sustain the recovery of lexical semantic processing in the early stages of poststroke aphasia recovery (Ansaldo & Arguin, 2003). Second, it is possible that the right hemisphere activation observed in such cases corresponds to the activation of a route previously inhibited by the left hemisphere, released from inhibition by the left hemisphere damage. Third, widespread bilateral brain activation may represent an increase of effort to accomplish a task that used to be more automatic. Still, if increased activation in the right hemisphere correlates with improved performance, the link between the right hemisphere contribution and recovery becomes more evident. However, the nature of the right hemisphere contribution to recovery remains to be described.

The right hemisphere contribution to poststroke language processing has been related to an increase in perceived task complexity, in which case we can assume that cognitive as well as linguistic processing may be involved. Raboyeau et al. (2008) provided evidence of similar right inferior frontal activations in individuals with aphasia and normal control subjects following a training period of intensive learning of new lexical items. The authors concluded that the right hemisphere activity was related to learning and not merely an automatic reaction to a left hemisphere lesion. Still, such right hemisphere potential for learning or relearning lexical items supports adaptive brain plasticity in poststroke chronic aphasia. Interestingly, the fact that both healthy learners and individuals with brain damage showed similar activation patterns suggests that brain plasticity mechanisms involved in normal learning could also be triggered in aphasia recovery.

A fourth observation is that the recruitment of contralateral right-hemispheric circuits may represent the brain's attempt at compensation but at the cost of some level of efficacy, or it may represent a bypass mechanism that becomes maladaptive and hinders further improvements (Belin et al., 1996; Naeser et al., 2005; Rijntjes, 2006). In line with this claim, Naeser et al. (2005) showed that impeding the activity of the right inferior frontal area with repetitive transcranial

magnetic stimulation (rTMS) improved naming in an individual with chronic aphasia, an increase that was sustained for months. In this particular case, the reinstatement of left hemisphere activity combined with a decrease in right hemisphere activity led to a better outcome. However, the extent to which the right hemisphere contribution may either facilitate or hinder recovery could depend on the interaction between a number of variables, among which are left hemisphere lesion size and location and time postonset.

In another rTMS study, Winhuisen et al. (2007) showed that in the acute phase, the right inferior frontal gyrus is essential to language processing in nine nonfluent poststroke individuals. Eight weeks after a left hemisphere stroke, rTMS to the right inferior frontal gyrus inhibited speech in some of the individuals but not in others. These findings suggest that the right hemisphere contribution to aphasia recovery may be essential in the first stages following stroke, a process that may reflect short-term brain plasticity mechanisms based on available network integration. With time elapsed after the stroke, it is possible that the right hemisphere contribution varies according to the extent and location of permanent left hemisphere damage. Hence, in cases of permanent damage to core language-processing areas in the left hemisphere, aphasia recovery may rely exclusively on the significant activation of right hemisphere homologous areas (e.g., Thulborn, Carpenter, & Just, 1999; Weiller et al., 1995). These right-hemispheric areas typically are minimally active in normal individuals, which may indicate that this reorganization process may use preexisting pathways. Whether this increased activity also represents a release of inhibition from the left hemisphere is still under investigation. Regardless, the most frequent activation pattern observed consists of some level of increased bihemispheric activity (e.g., Calvert et al., 2000).

Further, although bilateral hemispheric activation during language tasks may be associated with better recovery as compared to mostly unilateral right-hemispheric activity (Cao, Vickingstad, George, & Welch, 1999), ipsilateral perilesional activity may also be important for recovery (e.g., Léger et al., 2002; Mimura et al., 1998; Warburton, Price, Swinburn, & Wise, 1999). Typically, a right-hemispheric increase in activity takes place before the left-hemispheric perilesional reactivation (e.g., Ansaldo, Arguin, & Lecours, 2002b; Fernandez et al., 2004). These observations lead to the conclusion that better recovery is associated with an eventual left hemisphere reorganization of language skills following a temporary right hemisphere increase in activity (Demeurisse & Capon, 1987; Heiss, Kessler, Thiel, Ghaemi, & Karbe, 1999; Karbe et al., 1998; Knopman, Rubens, Selnes, Klassen, & Meyer, 1984; Kuest & Karbe,

2002; Saur et al., 2006). Crinion and Leff's (2007) review article concluding that an early right frontal activation reflects a better recovery but that the correlation shifts to the left frontal areas in the more chronic stages also supports this observation.

Adaptive brain plasticity by right hemisphere recruitment may also vary as a function of language domain. In other words, it is possible that the right hemisphere may be more adept at taking over comprehension than expressive language skills. Therefore, the improvements in comprehension that are associated with increased right hemisphere activation may represent an acceptable compensatory mechanism (Heiss et al., 1999), whereas a better outcome for expressive language may require an eventual reutilization of left inferior frontal areas (e.g., Thomas, Altenmüller, Marckmann, Kahrs, & Dichgans, 1997). Hence, the typical picture reported is a progressive increase in left frontal activity with a remaining bilateral temporal activation (e.g., Ansaldo, Arguin, & Lecours, 2002a; Ansaldo et al., 2002b). This ultimate left hemisphere activity for expressive language may represent a reaction to the unsuccessful attempts at processing that ability through right hemisphere networks (Feagin Del Toro, 1997). Such a scenario implies that outcome depends on the availability of left hemisphere perilesional processing (and hence the importance of lesion size). However, this conclusion was tempered by Zahn et al. (2004), who noted that, even in some individuals with global aphasia with large perisylvian lesions, the improvement in comprehension was still modulated by left-hemispheric perilesional areas.

The gathering of language reorganization data and their interpretation are rendered more difficult by several variables. First, many authors concluded that there is an important element of individual variability in language recovery (e.g., Code, 2001; Thomas et al., 1997), particularly when it comes to the role of the right hemisphere (Gainotti, 1993). Second, the tasks used across neuroimaging studies to assess the extent of cortical reorganization were not identical. It is likely that the nature of the language-processing tasks translates into different activation patterns of compensation (Calvert et al., 2000). Some authors have used functional brain imaging in a rest condition (e.g., Demeurisse, Verhas, & Capon, 1981; Jodzio, Drumm, Nyka, Lass, & Gasecki, 2005), during word repetition (e.g., Heiss et al., 1999), pseudoword repetition (e.g., Weiller et al., 1995), word retrieval (e.g., Warburton et al., 1999), comprehension (e.g., Zahn et al., 2004), and so forth. Third, the types of aphasia investigated varied, which means that the language and cognitive skills that need to be reorganized were different. The noted differences in poststroke cortical language activation between individuals with Broca's and Wernicke's aphasia may be more the result of differences in receptive versus expressive language reorganization (Demeurisse & Capon, 1987; Gainotti, 1993). Fourth, lesion size was rarely controlled, and it is likely that language reorganization would be different depending on lesion size. For example, the activation of perilesional areas has been associated with a better recovery (Karbe et al., 1998; Warburton et al., 1999), and this is more likely to occur with a smaller lesion because the neurons neighboring a small lesion may have been contributing to the impaired skill in the first place (Crosson, 2008). In this regard, Vitali et al. (2007) reported on two individuals with Broca's aphasia. After a period of intensive naming treatment, the person with the smaller lesion showed left perilesional reactivation and better recovery, but the individual with the larger lesion demonstrated right inferior frontal compensation only, with recovery more limited.

THE LINK BETWEEN PLASTICITY, BEHAVIOR, AND THERAPY

So far, we have discussed that improvements in language abilities are associated with specific neurophysiologic changes. It can also further be demonstrated that language rehabilitation can be identified as the cause of some of these physiologic changes. Indeed, several studies showed that measurable physiologic changes were directly attributable to language therapy (e.g., Fridriksson, Morrow-Odom, Moser, Fridriksson, & Baylis, 2006; Musso et al., 1999; Wierenga et al., 2006). Not surprisingly, the nature of the therapy influenced the resulting changes in language reorganization. Thompson (2000) compared two aphasia rehabilitation studies, one focusing on comprehension and one focusing on syntactic processing (i.e., receptive versus expressive). The individuals exposed to an aural comprehension approach showed increased activity in the right hemisphere area homologous to Wernicke's, and the individuals subjected to expressive and receptive syntax therapy showed changes in the right frontal and temporal regions. The author concluded that the nature of the therapy approach affected the reorganization of language in the right hemisphere.

Most studies use an intensive therapy period preceded and followed by functional imaging measurements (i.e., treatment-induced recovery). Authors mostly reported bilateral changes following the rehabilitation period (C. H. Davis, Harrington, & Baynes, 2006; Fridriksson et al., 2006; Harnish, Neils-Strunjas, Lamy, & Eliassen, 2008; Musso et al., 1999; Pulvermüller, Hauk, Zohsel, Neininger, & Mohr, 2005). For example, Musso et al.

(1999) described metabolic increases in the right superior temporal gyrus and left precuneus in four individuals with chronic Wernicke's aphasia who underwent an intensive period of therapy focusing on language comprehension (Marcotte & Ansaldo, 2010). Meinzer et al. (2008) concluded that an intensive naming therapy program caused a significant increase in the left hemisphere perilesional areas in individuals with chronic aphasia, thereby confirming that left hemisphere reactivation was associated with positive symptomatic changes, even years after aphasia onset.

Marcotte and Ansaldo (2010) showed that intensive therapy with SFA (Boyle & Coelho, 1995) resulted in the recovery of noun and verb naming in two individuals with chronic and severe aphasia. In these two cases, noun and verb naming recovery was observed concurrently with the recruitment of a semantic processing area in the left hemisphere, namely, the left inferior parietal lobule (LIPL). These results suggested that the semantic nature of the approach may have triggered the contribution of preserved semantic processing networks. Moreover, because only correct responses were included in the functional magnetic resonance imaging data analysis, this study provided evidence for adaptive right hemisphere therapy-induced brain plasticity in chronic and severe aphasia.

Marcotte et al. (2012) applied the same approach to a group of nine persons with chronic aphasia and moderate-to-severe anomia. All participants benefited from SFA therapy, showing an improvement in noun and verb naming. Moreover, a positive correlation between a successful outcome following SFA and a significant activation of the left precentral gyrus was observed before therapy, thereby showing that an activation of the left precentral gyrus pretherapy may predict a good response to SFA. Finally, a significant activation of the LIPL was observed concurrently with naming recovery following SFA, which suggests that the semantic nature of the therapy triggered the recruitment of preserved components of the semantic network, such as the LIPL.

The studies mentioned clearly showed the potential of specific therapy approaches in triggering the recruitment of preserved components of the language circuit as well as that of functionally related cortical areas. An additional example was provided by Marcotte, Perlbarg, Marrelec, Benali, and Ansaldo (2013), who examined functional connectivity changes in the language network and the default-mode network (DMN) following SFA therapy in individuals with chronic aphasia and severe anomia. The DMN is a well-identified network that is active when the subject is at rest and has been related to preattentive processes and inner speech (Greicius et al., 2003). In the study by Marcotte et al. (2013), the connectivity within the DMN was identified for the first time in persons with

aphasia. Connectivity refers to the concept of integration, which reflects information exchange between the areas of a given network. In the study by Marcotte et al. (2013), language recovery following SFA was supported by the significant activation of the LIPL, but there was no improvement within the language network connectivity itself, probably because of the irreparable damage to this language-processing circuit by the stroke. However, SFA did have a positive impact on the DMN, as a normalization of DMN connectivity was observed after SFA therapy. This shows that language therapy may have an impact that goes beyond language itself, improving function in other domains than language. In this case, the fact that the therapy was of a semantic type had probably something to do with the recovery observed in DMN connectivity, as this recovery was sustained by increased integration between posterior DMN areas, all of which are also semantic processing areas.

In conclusion, we are starting to understand the neural mechanisms driving cerebral reorganization following an insult; however, many questions still need answering. Research studies showed that rehabilitation efforts do produce physiologic cortical reorganization, but the heterogeneity of the methods and of the research participants makes it difficult to compare the studies and draw robust conclusions (Crosson et al., 2007; Meinzer & Breitenstein, 2008). Mostly, we do not know enough about candidacy issues to be able to reach the level of "guided recovery" (Robertson & Murre, 1999), where one specific therapy approach can be suggested for a particular individual in an attempt to maximize recovery (similar to the process in Figure 4.1). Yet, it is unquestionable that positive physiologic and behavioral changes can be stimulated, usually with intensive therapy, even years postonset (Marcotte & Ansaldo, 2010).

These observations speak to the need to advocate for continued rehabilitative efforts beyond the traditionally short therapy programs.

RECONCEPTUALIZING APHASIA AND APHASIA THERAPY

Understanding these intricate mechanisms of functional recovery has implications for our conceptualization of aphasia and aphasia therapy. Aphasia is considered to be a dysfunction of language and communication resulting from a focal brain lesion. The course of recovery depends on a spectrum of biochemical, physiologic, structural, and behavioral mechanisms, which need to be in place to promote recovery. The fundamental question is how these mechanisms can be manipulated to enable individuals to achieve their full communicative potentials.

Some of the recovery mechanisms are time dependent. Clinicians are used to the terms *acute, subacute,* and *chronic* and understand that prognosis and therapy approaches may vary depending on time postonset (Powell, 1981). The difficulty, however, lies in the fact that the limits of these periods are poorly defined and that no therapy approach is exclusive to any one of these stages. On the other hand, Huber et al. (1993) suggested that all stages of aphasia therapy should include psychosocial support for the individual with aphasia and his or her family because clinical intervention should always combine impairment-based (neuropsychological) and consequence-oriented (psychosocial) components.

Huber et al. (1993) described three possible types of approaches to aphasia remediation: activation, symptom-specific training, and consolidation. These approaches may be associated with the three neuronal mechanisms described by Powell (1981): physical repair, neuronal adaptation to the deficit, and finally new learning. During activation (or physical repair), therapy should focus on enhancing temporarily impaired language functions. The therapeutic overall goal is to stimulate the patient by all available means to communicate as appropriately as possible. Techniques such as direct stimulation, indirect stimulation, and deblocking are typically used, which enable behavioral mechanisms in a functional system to recover.

The symptom-specific training (or neuronal adaptation) should start when the initial physical repair has been completed (although this point in time cannot be determined with precision). In theory, this approach could use existing synaptic connections that may or may not have been active premorbidly. This reorganization could be maladaptive, that is, the new processing paradigm is less efficient than the original one but becomes the norm and resists modification. Huber (1992) suggested that therapy focus on the relearning of degraded linguistic knowledge, the reactivation of impaired linguistic modalities, and the establishment of compensatory linguistic strategies. However, the issue of whether therapy should center on treating specific impairments or concentrate on residual skills remains unclear. It is assumed that both approaches, which represent substitution and functional compensation mechanisms, respectively, are contributing to the functional recovery of the entire system. Therapy approaches potentially applied at this stage include the language-oriented learning approaches such as those looking at linguistic structures, linguistic modalities, linguistic strategies, cognitive models of language processing, cognitive capacity processing, and so on.

During consolidation (or new learning), learning mechanisms are used to complement and maintain the linguistic skills learned in the previous phase, to enhance them, and to transfer them to everyday communicative situations (Huber et al., 1993). Subsequently, the functional system of language and communication is used at its full potential to enable the person to achieve communicative effectiveness. Potential therapeutic techniques to use include role playing, promoting aphasics communicative effectiveness therapy (PACE; G. A. Davis & Wilcox, 1985), conversation coaching, teaching caregivers communicative strategies, use of gestures or other nonverbal strategies, and so on. According to Powell (1981), many additional factors that influence therapy outcomes can intervene: the variables of the tasks used in therapy; patient parameters such as age, occupation, educational background, and so on; the patient's motivation to participate; and the environment in which therapy takes place.

It is clear that this partitioning of the language rehabilitation process in stages represents an artificial simplification. First, these time periods are not clearly defined; second, the three rehabilitation types defined by Huber et al. (1993) are too limiting; and third, the association between type of intervention and time period lacks flexibility. However, a potential association between specific neurophysiologic mechanisms and tailored intervention strategies may be a better avenue to explore.

Recently, some researchers started to adapt basic neuroscience findings to neurorehabilitation. This framework focuses on experience-dependent neuroplasticity and comprises a series of principles that—although initially derived from animal models (Kleim & Jones, 2008; see Table 4.1)—have been recently applied to neurorehabilitation in general and aphasia rehabilitation in particular (Raymer et al., 2008). This "translational research" approach may offer a potential road map for future investigations of aphasia treatment and recovery. Within this framework, principles and concepts that have emerged from basic neuroscience research are organized into categories of *dependent* or *independent* variables. The dependent variables include acquisition, generalization, interference, maintenance, and neural effects (plasticity), whereas independent variables include timing, intensity, quantity, salience of stimuli, any patient characteristics that could influence treatment outcome, neural conditions (e.g., lesion site and size), and treatment variables. The concept of treatment variables refers to any of the behavioral or neural manipulations taking place during the treatment to restore function (e.g., training a specific linguistic function with SFA; Boyle & Coelho, 1995) or to compensate for impaired functions (e.g., using gestures).

In addition to these two types of variables, a third dimension of this framework represents the variety of

Table 4.1 Principles of Experience-Dependent Plasticity

Principle	Description
1. Use it or lose it	Failure to drive specific brain functions can lead to functional degradation.
2. Use it and improve it	Training that drives a specific brain function can lead to an enhancement of that function.
3. Specificity	The nature of the training experience dictates the nature of the plasticity.
4. Repetition matters	Induction of plasticity requires sufficient repetition.
5. Intensity matters	Induction of plasticity requires sufficient training intensity.
6. Time matters	Different forms of plasticity occur at different times during training.
7. Salience matters	The training experience must be sufficiently salient to induce plasticity.
8. Age matters	Training-induced plasticity occurs more readily in younger brains.
9. Transference plasticity	Plasticity in response to one training experience can enhance the acquisition of similar behaviors.
10. Interference	Plasticity in response to one experience can interfere with the acquisition of other behaviors.

Reprinted with permission from Principles of experience-dependent neural plasticity: Implications for rehabilitation after brain damage by J.A. Kleim and T.A. Jones. *Journal of Speech-Language-Hearing Research*, 51, S225–S239. © 2008 by American Speech-Language-Hearing Association.

linguistic behaviors that can potentially be targeted during language treatment (phonology, syntax, etc.). Raymer et al. (2008) suggested that this framework provides an organizational scheme for systematically reviewing the literature and identifying areas of research lacking empirical support to bridge the gap between basic neuroscience and clinical trials.

In clinical practice, therapists observe, assess, and intervene at the behavioral level, while their knowledge of the neural mechanisms underlying behavioral changes remains theoretical. However, the evidence shows that behavioral manipulation can modify the neuronal organization. For example, LTP could represent the basic mechanism underlying the effects of intensive stimulation therapies. Thus, repeated use enhances synaptic effectiveness by reestablishing lost connections, reinforcing existing ones, or activating parallel pathways. However, applying this basic principle to language rehabilitation is no easy task. We still need to determine the type, intensity, and frequency of input required to trigger the neural mechanisms that will maximize functional recovery. Specifically, three important questions need to be answered. First, we need to understand why a function can be impaired by some lesions and not others. Second, we need to clearly determine the different recovery mechanisms that may contribute to the improvement of specific functional systems, in a specific individual, at a specific moment in the recovery process. Finally, we need to associate particular behavioral interventions

with specific recovery mechanisms to maximize functional outcome.

FUTURE DIRECTIONS

Research on the neural basis of aphasia recovery has progressed considerably during the last decade. The advent of sophisticated neuroimaging techniques has provided a new tool to examine therapy-induced brain plasticity; however, there is a need to find consensus on a number of methodological challenges, such as experimental designs, lesion and data analysis, and applications of neuroimaging research to clinical management aimed at improving functional communication in people with aphasia. Future studies with larger cohorts of homogeneous participants, who receive a specific type of therapy, may contribute to specify the various contributing factors in therapy-induced brain plasticity in aphasia recovery. The potential to trigger adaptive brain plasticity by means of specific therapy approaches should similarly be further explored. Thus, a better understanding of the neuroplasticity–therapy interface may contribute to optimize clinical management and the chances of recovery from aphasia.

Furthermore, as Raymer et al. (2008) suggested, studies in animal models of neurorehabilitation, computational simulations of aphasia, and the cognitive neuroscience work focusing on the acquisition of complex behaviors (i.e., skill acquisition theories and approaches) are all rich sources of translational interest to aphasiologists.

Questions, concerns, and problems encountered in human clinical interactions should then lead back to motivate further basic science investigations. A productive basic science and clinical science research process, then, is interactive, integrated, and complementary. More and more researchers are recognizing this critical need for increased cooperation and integration of research endeavors. Neurorehabilitation researchers, including aphasiologists, need to continue to build bridges among basic and clinical disciplines to promote a research agenda in which all researchers' treatment initiatives flourish.

STUDY QUESTIONS

1. Describe the concept of plasticity.
2. Describe the concept of recovery and how it differs from compensation.
3. Which prognostic factors are related to aphasia recovery?
4. Describe the different changes taking place in the brain during the first days postonset.
5. Explain the differences between restoration, recruitment, and retraining and how they relate to functional improvement in individuals with aphasia.
6. Explain the behavioral mechanisms of recovery and how they are applied to therapy for individuals with aphasia.
7. Explain how language reorganizes in the brain after stroke.
8. Differentiate between expressive and receptive language in poststroke language reorganization.
9. Explain the role of lesion size in poststroke language reorganization.
10. Associate the mechanisms of recovery with therapy planning for individuals with aphasia.

NOTE

1. Penumbra is the area surrounding the infarcted region, which can be affected by lack of oxygen. However, this area may shrink if the stroke is treated promptly, and cells that were hypofunctional can resume activity.

REFERENCES

Anglade, C., Thiel, A., & Ansaldo, A. I. (2014). The complementary role of the cerebral hemispheres in recovery from aphasia after stroke: A critical review of literature. *Brain Injury, 28*(2) 138–145.

Ansaldo, A. I. (2004) The right hemisphere contribution to recovery from aphasia: Examples of functional and dysfunctional plasticity and new avenues for speech and language therapy. *Rééducation orthophonique, 42*(219), 79–94.

Ansaldo, A. I., & Arguin, M. (2003). The recovery from aphasia depends on both the left and right hemispheres: Three longitudinal case studies on the dynamics of language function after aphasia. *Brain and Language, 87*, 177–178.

Ansaldo, A. I., Arguin, M., & Lecours, A. R. (2002a). The contribution of the right cerebral hemisphere to the recovery from aphasia: A single longitudinal case study. *Brain and Language, 82*, 206–222.

Ansaldo, A. I., Arguin, M., & Lecours, A. R. (2002b). Initial right hemisphere take-over and subsequent bilateral participation during recovery from aphasia. *Aphasiology, 16*(3), 287–304.

Astrom, M., Adolfsson, R., & Asplund, K. (1993). Major depression in stroke patients: A three year longitudinal study. *Stroke, 24*, 976–982.

Bartha, L., & Benke, T. (2003). Acute conduction aphasia: An analysis of 20 cases. *Brain and Language, 85*, 93–108.

Basso, A. (1992). Prognostic factors in aphasia. *Aphasiology, 6*, 337–348.

Basso, A., Capitani, E., & Moraschini, S. (1982). Sex differences in recovery from aphasia. *Cortex, 18*, 469–475.

Basso, A., Farabola, M., Grassi, M. P., Laiacona, M., & Zanobio, M. E. (1990). Aphasia in left handers: Comparison of aphasia profiles and language recovery in non-right handed and matched right handed patients. *Brain and Language, 38*, 233–252.

Belin, P., Van Eeckhout, P., Zilbovicius, M., Remy, P., François, C., Guillaume, S., et al. (1996). Recovery from nonfluent aphasia after melodic intonation therapy: A PET study. *Neurology, 47*, 1504–1511.

Benson, D. F., & Ardila, A. (1996). *Aphasia: A clinical perspective.* New York: Oxford University Press.

Blomert, L. (1998). Recovery from language disorders: Interactions between brain and rehabilitation. In B. Stemmer & H. A. Whitaker (Eds.), *Handbook of neurolinguistics* (pp. 547–557). San Diego, CA: Academic Press.

Borod, J. C., Carper, J. M., & Naeser, M. (1990). Long term recovery in left handed aphasic patients. *Aphasiology, 4*, 561–572.

Boyle, M., & Coelho, C. A. (1995). Application of semantic feature analysis as a treatment for aphasic dysnomia. *American Journal of Speech Language Pathology, 4*, 94–98.

Brant, T., Strupp, M., Arbusow, V., & Dieringer, N. (1997). Plasticity of the vestibular system: Central compensation and sensory substitution for vestibular deficits. In H. J. Freund, B. A. Sabel, & O. W. Witte (Eds.), *Advances in neurology: Brain plasticity* (Vol. 73) (pp. 297–309). Philadelphia, PA: Lippincott-Raven.

Bruce, C., & Howard, D. (1987). Computer-generated phonemic cues: An effective aid for naming in aphasia. *British Journal of Communication Disorders, 22*, 191–201.

Buckner, R. L., & Petersen, S. E. (2000). Neuroimaging of functional recovery. In H. S. Levin & J. Grafman (Eds.), *Cerebral reorganization of function after brain damage* (pp. 318–330). Oxford, England: Oxford University Press.

Cabeza, R. (2002). Hemispheric asymmetry reduction in older adults: the HAROLD model. *Psychology and Aging, 17*(1), 85.

Calvert, G. A., Brammer, M., Morris, R. G., Williams, S. C. R., King, N., & Matthews, P. M. (2000). Using fMRI to study recovery from acquired dysphasia. *Brain and Language, 71*, 391–399.

Cao, Y., Vickingstad, E. M., George, K. P., & Welch, K. M. (1999). Cortical language activation in stroke patients recovering from aphasia with functional MRI. *Stroke, 30*, 2331–2340.

Cappa, S. F. (1998). Spontaneous recovery in aphasia. In B. Stemmer & H. A. Whitaker (Eds.), *Handbook of neurolinguistics.* (pp 535-545) San Diego, CA: Academic Press.

Carlomagno, S., & Iavarone, A. (1995). Writing rehabilitation in aphasic patients. In C. Code & D. Muller (Eds.), *Treatment of aphasia: From theory to practice.* (pp 201-222) London: Whurr.

Carmichael, S. T. (2010). Molecular mechanisms of neural repair after stroke. In S. C. Cramer & R. J. Nudo (Eds.), *Brain repair after stroke.* (pp 11–21) Cambridge, England: Cambridge University Press.

Catani, M., Allin, M. P. G., Husain, M., Pugliese, L., Mesulam, M. M., Murray, R. M., et al. (2007). Symmetries in human brain language pathways correlate with verbal recall. *Proceedings of the National Academy of Sciences, 104*(43), 17163–17168.

Cherney, L., & Robey, R. (2008). Aphasia treatment: Recovery, prognosis, and clinical effectiveness. In R. Chapey (Ed.), *Language intervention strategies in aphasia and related neurogenic communication disorders* (5th ed., pp. 186–202). Philadelphia: Lippincott Williams & Wilkins.

Code, C. (2001). Multifactorial processes in recovery from aphasia: Developing the foundations for a multileveled framework. *Brain and Language, 77*, 25–44.

Crinion, J. T., & Leff, A. P. (2007). Recovery and treatment of aphasia after stroke: Functional imaging studies. *Current Opinion in Neurology, 20*, 667–673.

Crosson, B. (2008). An intention manipulation to change lateralization of word production in nonfluent aphasia: Current status. *Seminars in Speech and Language, 29*(3), 189–200.

Crosson, B., McGregor, K., Gopinath K. S., Conway T. W., Benjamin, M., Chang, Y.-L., et al. (2007). Functional MRI of language in aphasia: A review of the literature and the methodological challenges. *Neuropsychological Review, 17*, 157–177.

Davis, C. H., Harrington, G., & Baynes, K. (2006). Intensive semantic intervention in fluent aphasia: A pilot study with fMRI. *Aphasiology, 20*(1), 59–83.

Davis, G. A., & Wilcox, M. J. (1985). *Adult aphasia rehabilitation: Language pragmatics.* San Diego, CA: College Hill.

Demeurisse, G., & Capon, A. (1987). Language recovery in aphasic stroke patients: Clinical, CT and CBF studies. *Aphasiology, 1*(4), 301–315.

Demeurisse, G., Verhas, M., & Capon, A. (1981). Débit sanguins cérébraux et récupération du langage: Évolutions et relations. In X. Seron & C. Laterre (Eds.), *Rééduquer le cerveau* (pp. 45–60). Brussels, Belgium: Mardaga.

De Partz, M. P. (1986). Re-education of a deep dyslexic patient: Rationale of the methods and results. *Cognitive Neuropsychology, 3*, 149–177.

Edmundson, A., & McIntosh, J. (1995). Cognitive neuropsychology and aphasia therapy: Putting the theory into practice. In C. Code & D. Müller (Eds.), *Treatment of aphasia: From theory to practice* (pp. 137–163). London: Whurr.

Feagin Del Toro, J. (1997). Plasticity and recovery from brain damage in adulthood: What can recovery from aphasia teach us? *Perspectives on Neurophysiology and Neurogenic Speech and Language Disorders, 7*(3), 8–14.

Fernandez, B., Cardebat, D., Demonet, J.-F., Joseph, P. A., Mazaux, J.-M., Barat, M., et al. (2004). Functional MRI follow-up study of language processes in healthy subjects and during recovery in a case of aphasia. *Stroke, 35*, 2171–2176.

Finger, S., Buckner, R. L., & Buckingham, H. (2003). Does the right hemisphere take over after damage to Broca's area? The Barlow case of 1877 and its history. *Brain and Language, 85*, 385–395.

Frackowiack, R. S. J. (1997). The cerebral basis of functional recovery. In R. S. J. Frackowiack, K. J. Friston, C. D. Frith, R. J. Dolan, & J. C. Mazziotta (Eds.), *Human brain function* (pp. 275–300). London: Academic Press.

Fridriksson, J., Morrow-Odom, L., Moser, D., Fridriksson, A., & Baylis, G. (2006). Neural recruitment associated with anomia treatment in aphasia. *Neuroimage, 32*, 1403–1412.

Gainotti, G. (1993). The riddle of the right hemisphere's contribution to the recovery of language. *European Journal of Disorders of Communication, 28*, 227–246.

Grafman, J. (2000). Conceptualizing functional neuroplasticity. *Journal of Communication Disorders, 33*, 345–356.

Greicius, M. D., Krasnow, B., Reiss, A. L., & Menon, V. (2003). Functional connectivity in the resting state brain: A network analysis of the default-mode hypothesis. *Proceedings of the National Academy of Science of the U S A, 100*(1), 253–258.

Hagmann, P., Cammoun, L., Martuzzi, R., Maeder, P., Clarke, S., Thiran, J. P., et al. (2006). Hand preference and sex shape the architecture of language networks. *Human Brain Mapping, 27*(10), 828–835.

Harnish, S. N., Neils-Strunjas, J., Lamy, M., & Eliassen, J. (2008). Use of fMRI in the study of chronic aphasia recovery after therapy: A case study. *Topics in Stroke Rehabilitation, 15*(5), 468–483.

Heiss, W. D., Kessler, J., Thiel, A., Ghaemi, M., & Karbe, H. (1999). Differential capacity of left and right hemispheric areas for compensation of poststroke aphasia. *Annals of Neurology, 45*, 430–438.

Hillis, A., & Heidler, J. (2002). Mechanisms of early aphasia recovery. *Aphasiology, 16*(9), 885–895.

Holland, A. L., Greenhouse, L., Fromm, D., & Swindell, C. S. (1989). Predictors of language restitution following stroke: A multivariate analysis. *Journal of Speech and Hearing Research, 32*, 232–238.

Howard, D., & Hatfield, F. (1987). *Aphasia therapy: Historical and contemporary issues.* London: Erlbaum.

Huber, W. (1992). Therapy of aphasia: Comparison of various approaches. In N. V. Steinbuche, D. Y. von Cramon, & E. Poppel (Eds.), *Neuropsychological rehabilitation* (pp. 242–256). Heidelberg, Germany: Springer.

Huber, W., Springer, L., & Willmes, K. (1993). Approaches to aphasia therapy in Aachen. In A. L. Holland & M. M. Forbes (Eds.), *Aphasia treatment—world perspectives* (pp. 55–86). San Diego, CA: Singular.

Jodzio, K., Drumm, D., Nyka, W. M., Lass, P., & Gasecki, D. (2003, July). *Cerebral mechanisms of early recovery from aphasia:*

A SPECT prospective study. Paper presented at the meeting of the International Neuropsychological Society, Berlin, Germany.

Jodzio, K., Drumm, D., Nyka, W. M., Lass, P., & Gasecki, D. (2005). The contribution of the left and right hemispheres to early recovery from aphasia: A SPECT prospective study. *Neuropsychological Rehabilitation, 15*(5), 588–604.

Karbe, H., Thiel, A., Weber-Luxenburger, G., Herholtz, K., Kessler, J., & Heiss, W.-D. (1998). Brain plasticity in poststroke aphasia: What is the contribution of the right hemisphere? *Brain and Language, 64*, 215–230.

Keefe, K. (1995). Applying basic neurosciences to aphasia therapy: What the animal studies are telling us. *American Journal of Speech-Language Pathology, 4*, 88–93.

Kertesz, A., Lau, W. P., & Polk, M. (1993). The structural determinants of recovery in Wernicke's aphasia. *Brain and Language, 44*, 153–164.

Kertesz, A., & McCabe, P. (1977). Recovery patterns and prognosis in aphasia. *Brain, 100*, 1–18.

Kinsbourne, M. (1971). The minor cerebral hemisphere as a source of aphasic speech. *Archives of Neurology, 25*, 302–306.

Kleim, J. A., & Jones, T. (2008). Principles of experience dependent neural plasticity: Implications for rehabilitation after brain damage. *Journal of Speech, Language and Hearing Research, 51*, 225–239.

Kleim, J. A., & Schwerin, S. (2010). Motor map plasticity: A neural substrate for improving motor function after stroke. In S. C. Cramer & R. J. Nudo (Eds.), *Brain repair after stroke* (pp. 1–10). Cambridge, England: Cambridge University Press.

Knopman, D. S., Rubens, A. B., Selnes, O. A., Klassen, A. C., & Meyer, M. W. (1984). Mechanisms of recovery from aphasia: Evidence from serial Xenon 133 cerebral blood flow studies. *Annals of Neurology, 15*, 530–535.

Kolb, B. (1995). *Brain plasticity and behavior*. Hillsdale, NJ: Erlbaum.

Kuest, J., & Karbe, H. (2002). Cortical activation studies in aphasia. *Current Neurology and Neuroscience Reports, 2*, 511–515.

Kuttner, H. (1930). Über die Beteiligung der rechten Hirnhälfte ans der Sprachfunktion. *Archiv für Psychiatrie und Nervenkrankheiten, 91*, 691–693.

Léger, A., Démonet, J.-F., Ruff, S., Aithamon, B., Touyeras, B., Puel, M., et al. (2002). Neural substrates of spoken language rehabilitation in an aphasic patient: An fMRI study. *Neuroimage, 17*, 174–183.

Lendrem, W., & Lincoln, N. B. (1985). Spontaneous recovery of language in patients with aphasia between 4 and 34 weeks after stroke. *Journal of Neurology, Neurosurgery and Psychiatry, 48*, 743–748.

Leonard, C. T. (1998). *The neuroscience of human movement*. St. Louis, MO: Mosby.

Lesser, R., & Milroy, L. (1993). *Linguistics and aphasia: Psycholinguistic and pragmatic aspects of intervention*. London: Longman.

Luria, A. (1973). *The working brain*. Harmondsworth, England: Penguin.

Marcotte, K., Adrover-Roig, D., Damien, B., de Préaumont, M., Généreux, S., Hubert, M., et al. (2012). Therapy-induced neuroplasticity in chronic aphasia. *Neuropsychologia, 50*(8), 1776–1786. doi:10.1016/j.neuropsychologia.2012.04.001

Marcotte, K., & Ansaldo, A. I. (2010). The neural correlates of semantic feature analysis in Broca's aphasia: Discordant patterns according to etiology. *Seminars in Speech and Language. Special Issue on Treatment of Chronic Aphasia: International Perspectives, 31*(1), 52–63.

Marcotte, K., Perlbarg, V., Marrelec, G., Benali, H., & Ansaldo, A. I. (2013). Default-mode network functional connectivity in aphasia: Therapy-induced neuroplasticity. *Brain and Language, 124*(1), 45–55.

Marsh, E. B., & Hillis, A. E. (2006). Recovery from aphasia following brain injury: The role of reorganization. *Progress in Brain Research, 157*, 143–156.

Marshall, J., Pound, C., White-Thomson, M., & Pring, T. (1990). The use of picture/word matching tasks to assist word retrieval in aphasic patients. *Aphasiology, 4*, 167–184.

Mazzoni, M., Vista, M., Pardossi, L., Avila, L., Bianchi, F., & Moretti, P. (1992). Spontaneous evolution of aphasia after ischaemic stroke. *Aphasiology, 6*, 387–396.

Meinzer, M., & Breitenstein, C. (2008). Functional imaging studies of treatment-induced recovery in chronic aphasia. *Aphasiology, 22*(12), 1251–1268.

Meinzer, M., Flaisch, T., Breitenstein, C., Wienbruch, C., Elbert, T., & Rockstroh, B. (2008). Functional re-recruitment of dysfunctional brain areas predicts language recovery in chronic aphasia. *Neuroimage, 39*, 2138–2046.

Mimura, M., Kato, M., Kato, M., Sano, M., Sano, Y., Kojima, T., et al. (1998). Prospective and retrospective studies of recovery in aphasia. *Brain, 121*, 2083–2094.

Moir, A., & Jessel, D. (1991). *Brain sex: The real difference between men and women*. New York, NY: Laurel.

Moscovitch, M. (1977). The development of lateralisation of language and its relation to cognitive and linguistic development: A review of some theoretical speculations. In S. J. Segalowitz & F. A. Gruber (Eds.), *Language development and neurological theory* (pp. 193–211). New York: Academic Press.

Musso, M., Weiller, C., Kiebel, S., Müller, S. P., Bülau, P., & Rijntjes, M. (1999). Training-induced brain plasticity in aphasia. *Brain, 122*, 1781–1790.

Naeser, M. A., Gaddie, A., Palumbo, C. L., & Stiassny-Eder, D. (1990). Late recovery of auditory comprehension in global aphasia. *Archives of Neurology, 47*, 425–432.

Naeser, M. A., Helm-Eastbrooks, N., Haas, G., Auerbach, S., & Shrinivasan, M. (1987). Relationship between lesion extent in "Wernicke's area" on computed tomographic scan and predicting comprehension in Wernicke's aphasia. *Archives of Neurology, 44*, 73–82.

Naeser, M. A., Martin, P. I., Nicholas, M., Baker, E. H., Seekins, H., Kobayashi, M., et al. (2005). Improved picture naming in chronic aphasia after TMS to part of right Broca's area: An open-protocol study. *Brain and Language, 93*, 95–105.

Naeser, M. A., Palumbo, C. L., Helm-Eastbrooks, N., Stiassny-Eder, D., & Albert, M. L. (1989). Severe nonfluency in aphasia. *Brain, 112*, 1–38.

Pedersen, P., Vinter, K., & Olsen, T. S. (2004). Aphasia after stroke: Type, severity and prognosis. *Cerebrovascular Diseases, 17*(1), 35-43.

Pizzamiglio, L., Mammucari, A., & Razzano, C. (1985). Evidence for sex differences in brain organization in recovery in aphasia. *Brain and Language, 25*, 213–223.

Plowman, E., Hentz, B., & Ellis, C. (2012). Post-stroke aphasia prognosis: A review of patient-related and stroke-related factors. *Journal of Evaluation in Clinical Practice, 18*(3), 689–694.

Powell, G. (1981). *Brain function therapy*. London: Gower.

Pulvermüller, F., Hauk, O., Zohsel, K., Neininger, B., & Mohr, B. (2005). Therapy-related reorganization of language in both hemispheres of patients with chronic aphasia. *Neuroimage, 28,* 481–489.

Raboyeau, G., De Boissezon, X., Marie, N., Balduyck, S., Puel, M., Bézy, C., et al. (2008). Right hemisphere activation in recovery from aphasia. *Neurology, 70,* 290–298.

Raymer, A., Beeson, P., Holland, A., Kendall, D., Maher, L., Martin, N., et al. (2008). Translational research in aphasia: From neurosciences to neurorehabilitation. *Journal of Speech, Language and Hearing Research, 51,* 259–275.

Rijntjes, M. (2006). Mechanisms of recovery in stroke patients with hemiparesis or aphasia: New insights, old questions and the meaning of therapies. *Current Opinion in Neurology, 19,* 76–83.

Robertson, I. H., & Murre, J. M. (1999). Rehabilitation of brain damage: Brain plasticity and principles of guided recovery. *Psychological Bulletin, 125*(5), 544–575.

Saur, D., & Hartwigsen, G. (2012). Neurobiology of language recovery after stroke: Lessons from neuroimaging studies. *Archives of Physical Medicine and Rehabilitation, 93*(1), S15-S25.

Saur, D., Lange, R., Baumgaertner, A., Schraknepper, V., Wilmes, K., Rijntjes, M., et al. (2006). Dynamics of language reorganization after stroke. *Brain, 129,* 1371–1384.

Selnes, O. A., Knopman, D. S., Niccum, N., Rubens, A. B., & Larson, D. (1983). Computed tomographic scan correlates of auditory comprehension deficits in aphasia: A prospective recovery study. *Annals of Neurology, 5,* 558–566.

Springer, S. P., & Deutsch, G. (1998). *Left brain, right brain* (5th ed.). New York: Freeman.

Stein, D. G., & Glasier, M. M. (1992). An overview of developments in research on recovery from brain injury. *Advances in Experimental and Medical Biology, 325,* 1–22.

Teasell, R., Bayonna, N. A., & Bitensky, J. (2005). Plasticity and reorganization of the brain post stroke. *Topics in Stroke Rehabilitation, 12*(3), 11–26.

Thomas, C., Altenmüller, E., Marckmann, G., Kahrs, J., & Dichgans, J. (1997). Language processing in aphasia: Changes in lateralization patterns during recovery reflect cerebral plasticity in adults. *Electroencephalography and Clinical Neurophysiology, 102,* 86–97.

Thompson, C. (2000). Neuroplasticity: Evidence from aphasia. *Journal of Communication Disorders, 33,* 357–366.

Thompson, C. K., & Bart-den Ouden, D. (2008). Neuroimaging and recovery of language in aphasia. *Current Neurology and Neuroscience Reports, 8*(6), 475–483.

Thulborn, K. R., Carpenter, P. A., & Just, M. A. (1999). Plasticity of language-related brain function during recovery from stroke. *Stroke, 30,* 749–754.

Vitali, P., Abutalebi, J., Tettamanti, M., Danna, M., Ansaldo, A. I., Perani, D., et al. (2007). Training-induced brain remapping in chronic aphasia: A pilot study. *Neurorehabilitation and Neural Repair, 21,* 152–160.

Warburton, E., Price, C. J., Swinburn, K., & Wise, R. (1999). Mechanisms of recovery from aphasia: Evidence from positron emission tomography studies. *Journal of Neurology, Neurosurgery and Psychiatry, 66,* 155–161.

Weiller, C., Isensee, C., Rijntjes, M., Huber, W., Müller, S., Bier, D., et al. (1995). Recovery from Wernicke's aphasia: A positron emission tomographic study. *Annals of Neurology, 37,* 723–732.

Westbury, C. (1998). Research strategies: Psychological and psycholinguistic methods in neurolinguistics. In B. Stemmer & H. A. Whitaker (Eds.), *Handbook of neurolinguistics* (pp. 84–95). San Diego, CA: Academic Press.

Wierenga, C. E., Maher, L. M., Moore, A. B., White, K. D., McGregor, K., Soltysik, D. A., et al. (2006). Neural substrate of syntactic mapping treatment: An fMRI study of two cases. *Journal of the International Neuropsychological Society, 12,* 132–146.

Winhuisen, L., Thiel, A., Shumacher, B., Kesler, J., Ridolf, J., Haupt, W. F., et al. (2007). The right inferior frontal gyrus and post-stroke aphasia: A follow-up investigation. *Stroke, 38*(4), 1286–1292.

Zahn, R., Drews, E., Specht, K., Kemeny, S., Reith, W., Willmes, K., et al. (2004). Recovery of semantic word processing in global aphasia: A functional MRI study. *Cognitive Brain Research, 18,* 322–336.

Formal and Informal Assessment of Aphasia

Laura Murray and Patrick Coppens

INTRODUCTION

Assessment can be defined as the quantitative and qualitative data-gathering process for the purpose of circumscribing an individual's communicative function and activity limitations, understanding his or her participation restriction, and devising appropriate rehabilitation objectives. In addition, this process should include tools and procedures that allow (a) establishing a diagnosis and a prognosis; (b) describing and understanding all components of language functioning, as well as related functions that may positively or negatively influence language (e.g., cognitive and emotional status); (c) gathering background information regarding the individual with aphasia and the family; (d) seeking input from the person with aphasia and the family about rehabilitation goals; and (e) supporting initial communication interactions with the individual with aphasia, providing family and other health-care team members with an accurate description of the individual's current strengths and weaknesses. Carrying out the assessment process effectively also requires up-to-date background knowledge and sharp clinical skills. Inexperienced clinicians may think that administering a thorough aphasia battery leads to the golden path of successful therapy, but a quantification of communication behavior—be it as thorough as can be—will not translate into appropriate therapy objectives without a meticulous examination of additional information such as compensatory mechanisms, type of errors, family support, and so on.

No one set of tests or measures can be prescribed when assessing individuals with aphasia. Instead, clinicians must make the selection of an assessment approach and procedures on a case-by-case basis, taking into consideration a number of variables, such as the client's previous and current level of functioning, his or her unique current and future needs, and the amount and types of assessment resources available to the clinician. Accordingly, to guide planning and implementing the aphasia assessment process, the clinician should consider the organization frameworks presented next.

Formal Versus Informal Assessment Procedures

The assessment process is traditionally divided into formal and informal testing procedures. Although a clear separation between the two concepts is not easily drawn, formal assessment usually involves administering one or more commercially available tests, and the informal process encompasses all the strategies that the clinician employs to translate the symptomatology displayed by the person with a communication disorder into clinically useful information.

Formal assessment is commonly used as a synonym for *test*. Some authors limit the definition of formal tests to standardized and norm-referenced tools (i.e., tests that have detailed administration procedures and norms). We, however, purposefully adopt a wider definition of formal test to distinguish it effectively from any clinician-generated informal procedures. Thus, for this chapter, we define a formal test as any published quantification tool. Usually, clinicians purchase these tests or find them in the empirical literature. Formal tests vary along many variables, such as their length and breadth (e.g., battery versus screening), their purposes (e.g., neurolinguistic versus quality of life [QOL]), and the conclusions clinicians are able to draw from the results (e.g., norm versus criterion referenced). Typically, formal assessment results are quantitative and provide little guidance for the development of specific treatment procedures. *Informal assessment*, on the other hand, refers to the process of creating and manipulating stimuli for the purpose of making clinical decisions, usually by answering hypothesis questions (e.g., Does phonemic cueing help my client?). Logically, informal assessment also includes the essential process of gathering specific background information through record review and interviews with the person with aphasia and his or her family and caregivers.

Quantitative Versus Qualitative Results

Formal assessments usually yield quantitative results, whereas informal assessment procedures are more likely to yield qualitative information. Quantitative information is expressed in raw numbers or any mathematical transformation of the raw data (e.g., percentiles, stanines, Z scores). Qualitative information is gathered by observing the client's behaviors, either spontaneous or triggered by the clinician. Both formal and informal assessments, as defined previously, can yield quantitative and qualitative information. When a clinician administers an aphasia battery, the results are typically quantitative; however, the clinician may also record qualitative information, such as the individual's error types or spontaneous compensatory behaviors. Similarly, during the informal assessment process, the clinician may probe some specific abilities that were not covered by the formal aphasia battery. For example, the clinician may informally assess oral apraxia via a custom-made list of questions (i.e., the resulting number of successfully performed nonspeech articulator movements is quantitative data). The clinician can also attempt to improve the performance of the individual with aphasia by applying facilitating strategies (e.g., by providing articulatory placement cues), which will yield qualitative information. Finally, when the clinician baselines a specific clinical objective, the data are quantitative, but the process is informal.

International Classification of Functioning, Disability, and Health Model

Another important guiding framework with which clinicians and researchers must be familiar when evaluating individuals with aphasia is the International Classification of Functioning, Disability, and Health (ICF) model of the World Health Organization (WHO) (2001). The ICF system acknowledges not only the pathophysiologic processes that directly result from disease but also how the disease or health condition affects individuals in their daily lives and how other variables, such as caregiver attitudes, environmental barriers, and financial resources may influence how individuals deal with and recover from health conditions. Accordingly, the model has been found to foster a holistic approach to identifying and managing the needs of individuals with health conditions such as stroke (Tempest, Harries, Kilbride, & De Souza, 2013). Specifically, the model prescribes describing health conditions with respect to each of the following constructs (WHO, 2001):

- *Loss of Body Functions and Structures* refers to impairments that are a primary or secondary outcome of the health condition. For example, aphasia, cognitive deficits, hemiparesis, and visual field impairment would all fall under this ICF dimension in an individual with aphasia caused by stroke. Traditionally, most aphasia assessments and treatments have focused on this level of the ICF model.

- *Restrictions in Activity Participation* encompass problems individuals encounter when completing activities of daily living, relating to others in their environment, and attempting to maintain or reestablish life and societal activities and roles. For instance, many individuals with aphasia experience difficulties using a checkbook or a phone, resuming their premorbid occupation, sustaining their role or status in their family, or participating in previous or new leisure activities.
- *Personal Factors* include the internal attributes, such as attitude and feelings, that may influence how individuals experience and adapt to the consequences of their health condition.
- *Environmental Factors* include the attributes external to the individual, such as physical (e.g., architectural barriers, climate), social (e.g., degree of family and community support), and attitudinal variables (e.g., societal attitude toward disability). These factors can be barriers or facilitators.

In accord with the ICF model, assessment of individuals with aphasia should include measures that evaluate each component of the framework. Thus, aphasia assessment protocols must go beyond traditional aphasia tests that focus primarily or exclusively on the *losses of body function/structure* and instead involve additional formal and informal procedures, such as procuring input from caregivers and other health-care professionals, to identify *activity* and *participation* issues and influential *contextual factors* (Murray & Clark, 2015; Simmons-Mackie & Kagan, 2007). Relying solely on body function/structure measures assumes that there is a direct relationship among the different elements of the ICF model (e.g., severe impairments at the body function/structure level will lead to severe problems at the activity and participation level). Research, however, does not support this assumption and instead indicates that failure to consider all ICF components may result in under- or overestimation of how well individuals with disorders such as aphasia may function in their daily environments, relationships, and roles (Brown et al., 2006; Chaytor & Schmitter-Edgecombe, 2003; Irwin, Wertz, & Avent, 2002; Silverberg & Millis, 2009).

Evidence-Based Practice

Evidence-based practice (EBP) methods may also be useful in guiding selection and administration of aphasia assessment procedures. According to the position statement of the American Speech-Language-Hearing Association (ASHA) (2005), *evidence-based practice* "refers to an approach in which current, high-quality research evidence is integrated with practitioner expertise and client preferences and values into the process of making clinical decisions." Applied to aphasia assessment, EBP encourages clinicians not only to keep abreast of advances in tests and procedures for quantifying and qualifying aphasia but also to evaluate critically these advances in terms of their validity and applicability. More specifically, clinicians and researchers adhering to EBP guidelines should be:

- Utilizing aphasia test procedures that have been evaluated and found appropriate in the research literature.
- Administering aphasia test procedures in the manner with which they were empirically verified. This would include using tests only for their stated purpose (e.g., using an aphasia screening test to document the presence of aphasia, but not to quantify and qualify specific linguistic abilities) and with the client population and specific instructions, tasks, and scoring criteria with which they were developed and standardized (e.g., using a test standardized on individuals from northeastern sections of the United States may be inappropriate with clients from other geographic regions).
- Considering their own clinical knowledge and skills, the best available evidence in the professional literature, and their specific client's needs and preferences to help guide the selection of aphasia test procedures.

The purpose of this chapter is to review formal and informal assessment procedures that are suitable when evaluating individuals with aphasia in a variety of clinical and research settings. First, formal assessment is described in terms of its purposes, test constructs, and procedures. Next, informal assessment is reviewed in a similar manner. Subsequent sections of the chapter focus on issues pertinent to both formal and informal assessment procedures.

FORMAL ASSESSMENT: PURPOSES

Across work settings, formal assessment procedures are a common component of the aphasia evaluation process. *Formal assessment* refers to highly controlled observations garnered during the administration of one or more of the following: bedside or screening tests, test batteries, or tests of specific communicative or cognitive functions. The general purpose of formal assessment procedures is to establish the current level of communicative and cognitive functioning in the individual with aphasia, including identifying the presence, type, and severity of aphasia and delineating specific language and cognitive strengths and weaknesses. The data gleaned from a formal assessment can serve a variety of functions. First, formal assessment findings can be used to establish the pretherapy performance level of the individual with aphasia; such information is fundamental not only to decisions regarding the need for further diagnostic procedures and whether treatment should be initiated, but also to predictions regarding recovery and treatment outcomes. Second, when treatment is indicated, formal assessment results can contribute to distinguishing and prioritizing treatment goals. Third, when formal assessment procedures are administered during the treatment process, test data inform decisions regarding the need to continue, modify, or discontinue treatment.

Delineating more specific goals of a formal assessment can be achieved by considering patient-related factors, such as where within the care continuum the individual with aphasia is receiving services (Laska, Bartfai, Hellblom, Murray, & Kahan, 2007; Murray & Clark, 2015; Olness, Gyger, & Thomas, 2012). For instance, in acute care settings, a formal aphasia assessment should focus on identifying the presence and type of communication problem (e.g., aphasia vs. dysarthria) and determining basic communication needs (e.g., expressing yes/no responses via verbal vs. written vs. gestural means) (Duffy, Fossett, & Thomas, 2011). With reference to the ICF system, assessments of individuals in the acute stages of aphasia recovery concentrate on quantifying impairments and a small set of daily activity limitations because these individuals are often too fatigued or sick to complete lengthy test batteries. Furthermore, the impact of the communicative symptoms on the individuals' social activities and roles is difficult to appreciate given the structure of acute care settings and the limited experiences these individuals (and their significant others) possess in dealing with these symptoms. In contrast, when individuals with aphasia progress to other levels of the care continuum, formal assessment procedures should be more comprehensive to allow examining communication and cognitive status in terms of all levels of the ICF model (i.e., body functions and structures, activity participation, and personal and environmental factors).

When utilizing a team approach to health-care delivery, the role and responsibilities of each team member should be established before administering formal assessment procedures, particularly in settings in which all team members do not work within the same facility. Such organization and communication among team members are necessary to prevent superfluous testing. For example, several health-care professions have interest and experience in identifying language disorders, including speech–language pathologists, neuropsychologists, nurses, and neurologists (Poslawsky, Schuurmans, Lindeman, & Hafsteinsdottir, 2010); similarly, emotional status and sensory skills (i.e., audition, vision) may be screened by professionals from various disciplines. Accordingly, it must be established which professional will conduct these types of assessments.

FORMAL ASSESSMENT: TEST CONSTRUCTS AND PROCEDURES

Numerous formal tests have been developed to identify aphasia and, more generally, to assess linguistic and cognitive abilities. These tests vary in terms of their length (e.g., aphasia screening test vs. aphasia test battery), scope (e.g., a test of auditory comprehension vs. a test of spoken and written language comprehension and production), and target population (e.g., elderly adults vs. young adults; monolingual vs. bilingual individuals). To help identify which test or set of tests will be most appropriate for a given individual with aphasia, the clinician must consider the specific goals of the assessment (e.g., identify a disorder vs. identify potential treatment targets) and review the psychometric characteristics of each test. Importantly, it is more useful to develop an understanding about effectively evaluating the strengths and weaknesses of a formal test than to be exposed to an exhaustive list of all the tools available. In addition, critically evaluating assessment instruments is an intrinsic part of EBP as defined by ASHA (2005).

Psychometric Properties

An important consideration when selecting a formal test is the quality of its psychometric properties because these provide information pertaining to how and to whom the test should be administered as well as how the test results should be interpreted (Mitrushina, Boone, Razani, & D'Elia, 2005). Review of a test's psychometric characteristics is also consistent with a tenet of EBP, in which critical appraisal of assessment procedures is recommended (ASHA, 2005; Frattali & Worrall, 2001). The fundamental psychometric properties that require discussion in the test manual include standardization, reliability, and validity.

Standardization

Standardization refers to the process of administering a test to an, ideally, extensive sample of individuals who represent the population segment with whom the test will be used (Cronbach, 1990; Lezak, Howieson, & Loring, 2004). This process yields standardized test administration procedures that, in turn, minimize measurement error and permit comparing an individual client's performance to those in the normative sample. Over time, most tests need to be revised to update their normative sample so that it remains representative of the target population's demographic characteristics or so that their sampling procedures can be enhanced (e.g., obtain a larger normative sample or include more diverse reference groups in terms of age, gender, education, language background, or ethnocultural representation). Whereas revised versions of tests are often commercially published (e.g., Examining for Aphasia—III vs. Examining for Aphasia—IV), sometimes these updates are only published in the research literature. For instance, Rami and colleagues (2008) provided normative data for Spanish-speaking elderly adults for several tests frequently used with individuals with aphasia, including the Pyramids and Palm Trees (Howard & Patterson, 1992) and the Boston Naming Test (BNT; Kaplan, Goodglass, & Weintraub, 2001).

A test administrator must ensure that the standardization sample of a selected test reflects the demographic characteristics (e.g., age, sociocultural background, education level) of the test examinee (Marquez de la Plata et al., 2009; Molrine & Pierce, 2002). A mismatch in these characteristics could result in inaccurate interpretation of that individual's test scores because both the reliability and the validity of the test may be compromised, leading to test bias (Marquez de la Plata et al., 2009; Pedraza & Mungas, 2008). That is, just because a test has been found to have appropriate reliability and validity for a particular segment of the population, it may not necessarily yield fair test data for the rest of the population.

Reliability

The psychometric property that provides information pertaining to the degree with which a test yields similar data across repeated administrations in similar testing circumstances is *reliability* (Cronbach, 1990; Mitrushina et al., 2005). If the results vary substantially across repeated administrations, the test has poor or questionable reliability; more specifically, when reliability coefficients fall below .80, test reliability is suspect. A test should offer detailed directions for administering tasks, scoring responses, and interpreting test outcomes to help minimize intra- (i.e., repeated test use by the same examiner) and interexaminer (i.e., repeated

test use across different examiners) measurement error, both of which can compromise test reliability. In addition, overall test as well as subtest reliability should be reported, particularly if only select subtests can be administered. When a test is used to monitor linguistic changes over time, the *test–retest reliability* should also be considered. Poor test–retest reliability indicates that performance changes resulting from practice or chance are likely when the test is administered more than once.

Validity

In general, *validity* refers to the degree of theoretical and empirical support a test has (Lezak et al., 2004). Several types of validity, such as content, construct, ecological, and criterion-related (or predictive) validity, should be considered when evaluating a test (Mitrushina et al., 2005; Sbordone, 1996). The *content validity* of a test provides information regarding how well a test measures the skills or functions that it contends to measure. Therefore, an aphasia test should evaluate those linguistic abilities that theoretical and applied research have found essential to successful communication.

Construct validity refers to the degree to which a test corresponds with other tests designed to measure the same function or construct. A reading comprehension test, for example, would be deemed to have poor construct validity if clients' performances on that test did not correlate well with their performances on other reading comprehension tests.

Ecological validity is a type of criterion-related validity that indicates how well clients' test scores reflect their behavior in their typical environments during their daily activities and interactions. For example, to determine the ecological validity of a confrontation naming test, test developers need to demonstrate that their test's scores correspond well with word retrieval abilities during conversations or other types of daily communication activities.

Criterion-related validity (also known as predictive validity) reflects the accuracy with which a test determines a client has a deficit. In the case of an aphasia test, it should be able to distinguish clients with aphasia from those with other types of communication difficulties (e.g., dementia) or from those with intact communication abilities. Terms related to this type of validity include *sensitivity* and *specificity* (Pedraza & Mungas, 2008). Sensitivity reflects the proportion of individuals with a given deficit who are correctly identified by the test to have that deficit, whereas specificity reflects the proportion of individuals without a deficit who are correctly identified by the test not to have a deficit. Accordingly, tests with high sensitivity help with confident exclusion of a deficit diagnosis, and tests with high specificity help with confident identification of a deficit diagnosis.

Aphasia Batteries

Often, the first formal assessment procedure during a comprehensive aphasia evaluation is the administration of an aphasia test battery. Aphasia test batteries assess a number of linguistic skills (e.g., lexical-semantic retrieval, syntactic comprehension) and communication modalities (i.e., listening, speaking, reading, writing, and sometimes gesturing) via tasks and stimuli that vary in complexity (Murray & Chapey, 2001). There are several commonalities as well as differences among the currently available aphasia test batteries (see Table 5.1 for examples).

Most aphasia batteries were designed to identify the presence and type of aphasia. For example, the *Western Aphasia Battery—Revised* (WAB-R; Kertesz, 2007) includes subtests for evaluating spoken and written language comprehension and production, praxis, calculation, and construction skills. Subtest scores can be used not only to calculate an Aphasia Quotient, which provides information pertaining to aphasia severity, but also to determine aphasia type according to the connectionist aphasia syndromes (e.g., Broca's, Wernicke's, conduction).

A more recently developed option, the *Scales of Cognitive and Communicative Ability for Neurorehabilitation* (SCCAN; Milman & Holland, 2012), allows determining the presence and severity of neurogenic language and cognitive disorders, including aphasia. That is, this test was normed on individuals with aphasia as well as those with cognitive–communication disorders due to right hemisphere brain damage, traumatic brain injury, or progressive neurological disease. Designed for use in both rehabilitation and long-term care settings, the SCCAN has subtests that evaluate not only spoken and written language comprehension and production but also cognitive abilities (i.e., attention, memory, and executive functions).

The choice of which battery to use depends on many factors, such as local availability, personal choice, geographic location, and language. In the United States, Canada, and New Zealand, the WAB-R and the older *Boston Diagnostic Aphasia Examination–3* (BDAE-3; Goodglass, Kaplan, & Barresi, 2001) are more prevalent, whereas the *Aachen Aphasia Test* (Huber, Poeck, Weniger, & Willmes, 1983; N. Miller, Willmes, & De Bleser, 2000) is used more often in western European countries.

Despite many similarities across aphasia batteries, there are also some important differences. For example, with respect to the WHO ICF model, some batteries, such as the WAB-R, provide evaluation of the Body Functions level, aiming to identify the presence and type of aphasia and language deficits. Others such as the *American Speech-Language-Hearing Association Functional Assessment of Communication Skills for Adults* (ASHA FACS; Frattali, Thompson, Holland, Wohl, & Ferketic, 1995), the SCCAN, and the Scenario Test (van der Meulen, van de Sandt-Koenderman, Duivenvoorden, & Ribbers, 2010) focus more on the Activity Participation level. That is, these tests aim to identify daily communication activities with which individuals with aphasia may require assistance as well as activities they can complete independently.

The target client population also may differ across aphasia batteries. Whereas many batteries are only appropriate for monolingual English-speaking clients (e.g., WAB-R), a few were initially or subsequently modified for administration to monolingual clients who speak a language other than or in addition to English (e.g., Calis, On, & Durmaz, 2013; Huber et al., 1983; van der Meulen et al., 2010; for a list of aphasia tests in the world's 20 most widely spoken languages, see Ivanova & Hallowell, 2013). For instance, the Aachen Aphasia Test (Huber et al., 1983), which was originally developed to identify the presence, type, and severity of aphasia in German, has since been adapted for English, Dutch, Italian, Thai, and Portuguese (e.g., Lauterbach et al., 2008; N. Miller et al., 2000), taking into consideration the linguistic properties of each language (i.e., not translated literally) while maintaining the psychometric qualities of the original German version.

Direct translations of formal tests are not preferred because linguistic or cultural differences tend to be disregarded, which could result in inclusion of inappropriate stimuli or tasks as well as omission of crucial stimuli or tasks (Barratt, Khoza-Shangase, & Msimang, 2012; Calis et al., 2013; Ivanova & Hallowell, 2013; Paradis, 2011). For example, a repetition subtest arranged to increase from monosyllabic words to long sentences in English may have a different length hierarchy when translated to another language. Likewise, an English repetition subtest translated into a highly inflectional language such as Greek may fail to include a diverse enough sample of morphemes.

Other aphasia batteries, such as the Scenario Test (van der Meulen et al., 2010) and the Assessment of Communicative Effectiveness in Severe Aphasia (Cunningham, Farrow, Davies, & Lincoln, 1995), were developed for clients with more severe language impairments. These test batteries have modified tasks, stimuli,

Table 5.1 Examples of Aphasia Test Batteries and Screening Tools

Aphasia Batteries	ICF Level(s)	Auditory comp.	Spoken lang.	Reading	Writing	Gesture	Cognitive functions
ASHA FACS (Frattali et al., 1995)	Act. Part.	X	X	X	X		
Aphasia Check List (Kalbe et al., 2005)	Body Function	X	X	X	X		X
Bilingual Aphasia Examination[1] (Paradis & Libben, 1987)	Body Function	X	X	X	X		
Boston Assessment of Severe Aphasia (Helm-Estabrooks et al., 1989)	Body Function/ Act. Part.	X	X	X	X	X	
Boston Diagnostic Aphasia Examination – 3rd Ed. (Goodglass et al., 2001)	Body Function	X	X	X	X	X	
Communication Activities of Daily Living – II (Holland et al., 1999)	Body Function/ Act. Part.	X	X	X	X		
Comprehensive Aphasia Test (Swinburn et al., 2004)	Body Function/ Act. Part.	X	X	X	X	X	X
Examining for Aphasia – IV (Eisenson & LaPointe, 2008)	Body Function	X	X	X	X		
Scales of Cognitive and Communicative Ability for Neurorehabilitation (Milman & Holland, 2012)	Body Function/ Act. Part.	X	X	X	X		X
Scenario Test (van der Meulen et al., 2010)	Act. Part.		X		X	X	
Western Aphasia Battery – Revised (Kertesz, 2007)	Body Function	X	X	X	X	X	X
Aachen Aphasia Test (Miller et al., 2000- English version)	Body Function	X	X	X	X		
Aphasia Screening Tests							
Aphasia Rapid Test (Azuar et al., 2013)	Body Function	X	X				
Frenchay Aphasia Screening Test – II (Enderby et al., 2006)	Body Function	X	X	X	X		
In-Patient Functional Communication Interview (O'Halloran et al., 2004)	Body Function/ Act. Part.	X	X	X	X		
Language Screening Test (Flamand-Roze et al., 2011)	Body Function	X	X				
Mississippi Aphasia Screening Test (Nakase-Thompson et al., 2005)	Body Function	X	X	X	X		
The Aphasia Screening Test – 3 (Whurr, 2011)	Body Function	X	X	X	X		

Note: Act. Part. = ICF Level of Activity Participation.

[1] Available for free at www.mcgill.ca/linguistics/research/bat/ (Paradis, 2011)

and scoring procedures so that more subtle, spared communication abilities in both verbal and nonverbal modalities, which are often missed when more traditional aphasia batteries are administered, can be uncovered. The Scenario Test, for example, has a scoring system based on the amount of information, regardless of the modality in which it was conveyed and the amount of assistance needed from the communication partner (van der Meulen et al., 2010); this test also requires a qualitative analysis of the client's responses (e.g., most frequent communication modality; facility in switching from one communication modality to another). In contrast, most traditional aphasia test batteries only give credit for fully complete and accurate verbal responses.

Still other batteries were designed for screening or quickly ascertaining the presence or absence of aphasia (i.e., administration time of typically less than 30 minutes), determining the need for further testing, and identifying initial treatment targets (Flamand-Roze et al., 2011; Salter, Jutai, Foley, Hellings, & Teasell, 2006). These screening tests, most of which have been adapted for bedside administration and for use by not only speech–language pathologists but also other health-care professionals, are typically used in acute care settings because of (a) the brief length of stay in acute care facilities, (b) significant pressure to contain costs in these facilities, and (c) poor stamina and alertness among many patients in this health-care setting.

Several aphasia screening instruments are available (see Table 5.1), some of which are included when longer aphasia batteries are purchased. For instance, both the WAB-R (Kertesz, 2007) and the BDAE-3 (Goodglass et al., 2001) include shortened forms to be used for bedside administration or screening purposes. Alternately, shortened versions of a few comprehensive aphasia batteries can be found in the research literature, such as the SPICA, a screening version of the *Porch Index of Communicative Ability* (Porch, 1981) developed by Holtzapple, Pohlman, LaPointe, and Graham (1989).

Tests of Specific Linguistic Skills

Whereas aphasia batteries appear comprehensive because they evaluate a number of language abilities and modalities, most are inadequate at identifying the specific linguistic or cognitive problems that may contribute to impaired language skills and at discriminating motor speech disorders such as apraxia of speech and dysarthria. Accordingly, prior to crafting aphasia treatment goals and activities, administration of one or more tests of specific linguistic skills may be necessary. Further evaluation beyond an administration of an aphasia battery or screening is particularly crucial when an individual has performed at a ceiling or basal level and thus, little is known about the nature of the suspected language disorder (Ross & Wertz, 2004).

Before discussing tests designed to evaluate specific linguistic abilities, it is important to acknowledge that most language tests place demands on a number of perceptual, motor, and cognitive abilities (Ivanova & Hallowell, 2013; Murray, 2012a). Take for example, a reading comprehension test, which requires the individual with aphasia to read a paragraph and then read and answer multiple-choice questions pertaining to the paragraph. A slow-and-inaccurate performance on this test could indicate a text-level reading problem, but could also (or instead) reflect visuoperceptual problems (e.g., visual scanning difficulties that impede staying on a line of text or skipping down to the next line of text) or cognitive impairments (e.g., visual neglect that decreases attention to words on the right side of each line of text; a verbal memory deficit that impairs retention of the paragraph). Consequently, prerequisites to using one of these tests include familiarity with the specific task and response demands of the test and establishing whether such demands will be feasible or problematic for a given client.

Table 5.2 presents examples of the many formal tests available to examine each linguistic process, including phonological, orthographic, lexical–semantic, morphosyntactic, and discourse and pragmatic processes. Some of these tests evaluate only one or a restricted number of linguistic processes. For example, the BNT (Kaplan et al., 2001) examines spoken retrieval of nouns only, and the *Northwestern Assessment of Verb and Sentences* (Cho-Reyes & Thompson, 2012; Thompson, 2011) assesses production and understanding of verbs and a variety of canonical and noncanonical syntactic constructions.

In contrast, other tests evaluate a broader range of linguistic abilities. For instance, the *Psycholinguistic Assessments of Language Processing in Aphasia* (PALPA; Kay, Lesser, & Coltheart, 1997) is composed of 60 stimulus sets that allow determining whether one or a number of linguistic functions (e.g., phonemic perception, phonemic-to-graphemic conversion, grammatical morpheme recognition) contribute to the language difficulties of an individual with aphasia. Rather than administering the entire PALPA, clinicians should utilize data from other assessment procedures to help them select which subtests will be most appropriate for each client. Currently, the PALPA requires updating given previously raised concerns regarding the validity of several subtests, the size and characteristics of the normative

Table 5.2 Examples of Tests of Specific Language Functions

	ICF Level(s)	Phonologic/ Orthographic	Lexical- Semantic	Morpho- Syntactic	Pragmatics/ Discourse	Gesture
Boston Naming Test (Kaplan et al., 2001)	Body Function		Production			
Comprehensive Receptive and Expressive Vocabulary Test – 3 (Wallace & Hammill, 2013)	Body Function		Production/Compr.			
Controlled Oral Word Association Test (Benton et al., 2001)	Body Function		Production			
Discourse Comprehension Test (Brookshire & Nicholas, 1997)	Body Function/ Act. Part.				Compr.	
Gray Oral Reading Tests – 5 (Wiederholt & Bryant, 2012)	Body Function	Production	Compr.		Compr.	
NIH Toolbox Oral Reading Recognition Test (NIH & Northwestern University, 2006-2012)	Body Function	Production				
Northwestern Assessment of Verbs and Sentences (Thompson, 2011)	Body Function		Production/Compr.	Production/ Compr.		
Psycholinguistic Assessments of Language Processing in Aphasia (Kay et al., 1997)	Body Function	Production/ Compr.	Production/Compr.	Production/ Compr.		
Pyramids and Palm Trees (Howard & Patterson, 1992)	Body Function		Compr.			
Revised Token Test (McNeil & Prescott, 1978)	Body Function		Compr.	Compr.		
Sentence Production Test (Wilshire et al., 2014)	Body Function		Production	Production		
Test for Reception of Grammar – II (Bishop, 2003)	Body Function			Compr.		
Test for Upper Limb Apraxia (Vanbellingen et al., 2010)	Body Function					Production

Note: Compr. = Comprehension; Act. Part. = Activity Participation ICF domain.

samples, and some outdated stimuli (Bate, Kay, Code, Haslam, & Hallowell, 2010; Cole-Virtue & Nickels, 2004; Murray & Clark, 2015).

For at least some tests of specific linguistic functions, versions have been developed for individuals with aphasia who speak a language other than or in addition to English (Ivanova & Hallowell, 2013). For example, the Pontón-Satz Boston Naming Test (Pontón et al., 1992) was developed to evaluate confrontation naming in Spanish speakers, ensuring that culturally loaded items (e.g., "pretzel," "beaver") from the original BNT were excluded. Similarly, Tallberg (2005) adapted the stimuli and scoring rules of the BNT for use with Swedish speakers.

Discourse Sampling and Analyses

In addition to using one or more of the commercially available aphasia batteries or tests of specific linguistic functions, discourse sampling and analyses are also recommended for several reasons. First, connected speech or discourse is examined either minimally or not at all by most formal aphasia or language tests. Instead, structured tests tend to evaluate language processing at the sound, word, or sentence level in a decontextualized manner. This is of concern because only a weak relationship between these levels of language processing and discourse skills has been identified (Beeke, Maxim, & Wilkinson, 2008; Herbert, Hickin, Howard, Osborne, & Best, 2008; Mayer & Murray, 2003). Second, most structured aphasia and language tests were developed to document impairments at the Body Functions level of the ICF model. In contrast, analysis of discourse provides information pertaining to the Activity Participation level (Armstrong & Feguson, 2010; Olness et al., 2012; Simmons-Mackie & Kagan, 2007); if the discourse sample involves conversations between the client and a frequent communication partner, discourse analysis may also yield information regarding Environmental Factors (i.e., positive or negative communication strategies used by the partner without aphasia). Third, certain language skills (e.g., turn-taking, topic management) can be assessed only through discourse sampling and analyses. Finally, discourse analysis can be sensitive and thus, useful for quantifying more modest treatment-related improvements that may be missed on aphasia and language tests (Hussmann et al., 2012).

Ideally, when eliciting spoken and written discourse samples, the clinician should evaluate a number of discourse genres. Possible elicitation methods include description of a picture or picture sequence, role-playing, storytelling or retelling, video narration, interviewing, conversation, and description of a procedure. Utilizing just one discourse task will likely result in a sample with a restricted number and variety of phonological/orthographic, lexical–semantic, morphosyntactic, and pragmatic behaviors (Armstrong & Ferguson, 2010; Beeke et al., 2008; Rousseaux, Delacourt, Wyrzykowski, & Lefeuvre, 2001; Shadden, 1998). Furthermore, utilizing just one discourse task will often result in an inadequate sample size. Brookshire and Nicholas (1994) recommended samples at least 300 to 400 words in length to ensure acceptable test–retest stability of discourse analysis measures.

Numerous discourse analysis protocols have been developed to quantify and qualify a broad range of linguistic abilities (e.g., Kong, 2011; Lind, Kristoffersen, Moen, & Simonsen, 2009; Olness et al., 2012). Computer software programs are also available to facilitate quantitative analysis of samples collected in a number of languages (e.g., Hussmann et al., 2012; MacWhinney, 2000). Because a comprehensive review of these protocols is well beyond the scope of this chapter, we provide only a few examples, and readers interested further in discourse analysis procedures and issues should consult Cherney, Shadden, and Coelho (1998) or MacWhinney (2000).

To evaluate morphosyntactic abilities, spoken or written discourse samples can be analyzed in terms of the number, accuracy, and types of form words, grammatical morphemes, and syntactic structures. Scoring systems for fluent aphasia (e.g., S. Edwards, 1995), nonfluent aphasia (e.g., Rochon, Saffran, Berndt, & Schwartz, 2000), or any type of aphasia profile (e.g., Lind et al., 2009) have been developed and found to have adequate levels of intra- and interjudge reliability (Prins & Bastiaanse, 2004; Rochon et al., 2000).

Of the several measures created to analyze the lexical–semantic content of spoken or written discourse samples, those quantifying discourse informativeness, such as the correct information unit (CIU; Nicholas & Brookshire, 1993) and main concepts (Kong, 2011), are most common. As an example, Nicholas and Brookshire (1993) defined CIUs as words that are "accurate, relevant and informative relative to the eliciting stimulus" (p. 340) and provided a set of rules for differentiating CIUs from uninformative words and other output (e.g., nonword fillers, part-word repetitions). Several researchers have documented the reliability of the CIU measure and established that it is indicative of unfamiliar listeners' ratings of informativeness and of socially relevant changes in the verbal output of individuals with aphasia (Doyle, Goda, & Spencer, 1995; Doyle, Tsironas, Goda, & Kalinyak, 1996; Ross & Wertz, 1999).

Analyses at the pragmatic levels might include documenting the number and types of speech acts (e.g., greetings, assertions, requests for information); topic management skills (e.g., topic initiation, coherence); story grammar or components (e.g., specification of characters or agents, number, accuracy, and sequence of story events); or repair or revision strategies (e.g., repetition, request for revision). Whereas several rating scales and analysis protocols have been developed to quantify these types of pragmatic skills (e.g., Lille Communication Test, Rousseaux et al., 2001; Pragmatic Protocol, Prutting & Kirchner, 1987), the psychometric qualities of some scales and protocols are either not specified or have been found inadequate (Murray & Clark, 2015; Prins & Bastiaanse, 2004). In addition, the variety and frequency of these pragmatic behaviors and strategies can vary significantly among adults, depending on their ethnocultural background (Molrine & Pierce, 2002; Ulatowska, Olness, Hill, Roberts, & Keebler, 2000). Consequently, there is a need to refine existing pragmatic analysis systems to strengthen their psychometric characteristics, including obtaining normative data for individuals from diverse ethnocultural backgrounds.

Tests of Cognitive Skills

A comprehensive aphasia evaluation should extend beyond the domain of language and also include procedures for determining the integrity of other cognitive skills (Milman et al., 2008; Murray & Clark, 2015). Cognitive measures should be included because a growing literature has documented that not only do individuals with aphasia frequently have concomitant cognitive deficits (Hachioui et al., 2014; Murray, 2012b; Zinn, Bosworth, Hoenig, & Swartzwelder, 2007), but also these cognitive deficits may negatively affect their language abilities, treatment outcomes, and caregivers' level of burden (Bakas, Kroenke, Plue, Perkins, & Williams, 2006; Brownsett et al., 2014; Murray, 2000; van de Sandt-Koenderman et al., 2008). Furthermore, the cognitive test performances of individuals with aphasia cannot always be predicted based on their aphasia severity (Helm-Estabrooks, 2002; Murray, 2012b). Finally, a formal cognitive assessment is necessary because research with the stroke patient population has found that informal evaluation alone will miss a significant number of cognitive symptoms (D. Edwards et al., 2006; Fure, Bruun Wyller, Engedal, & Thommessen, 2006). Therefore, each individual with aphasia should receive a cognitive evaluation, which minimally includes formal screening procedures,

particularly because cognitive test results may provide important information regarding prognosis and the length and type of treatment.

A cognitive evaluation should assess attention, memory, and executive function abilities because each of these cognitive domains may be compromised in individuals with aphasia (Kalbe, Reinhold, Brand, Markowitsch, & Kessler, 2005; Murray, 2004, 2012a). Although a plethora of cognitive tests is available for each cognitive domain (for a comprehensive listing, see Lezak et al., 2004), many are inappropriate for individuals with aphasia because of the significant language demands of traditional cognitive tests. Likewise, as with language tests, a smaller set of cognitive tests has been developed for individuals who do not speak English or who are from ethnocultural minorities, and often clinicians must look to the empirical literature to identify cognitive tools (e.g., Common Objects Memory Test; Kempler, Teng, Taussig & Dick, 2010) or norms (e.g., Lucas et al., 2005; Messinis, Malegiannaki, Christodoulou, Panagiotopoulos, & Papathanasopoulos, 2011) for this segment of their caseload. As discussed with aphasia and language tests, failure to use culturally and linguistically appropriate cognitive tests and normative data can negatively affect diagnostic accuracy (Marquez de la Plata et al., 2009; Pedraza & Mungas, 2008). Table 5.3 lists some examples of cognitive test batteries as well as tests for each cognitive domain, some of which have been developed specifically for individuals with language impairments, have relatively reduced language demands, or both.

INFORMAL ASSESSMENT: LOGIC, PURPOSES, AND PROCEDURES

The overarching purpose of the informal assessment process is to distill the most appropriate clinical goals from the analysis of the abilities and behaviors of the individual with aphasia at any level of the ICF model. This is the crucial intermediary step between formal testing and therapy without which clinical objectives cannot be properly articulated. Muma (1978) contrasted the *ability* assessment that is exclusively quantitative and diagnostic with the *clinical* assessment and further stated that there is no such thing as a "quick-and-easy" clinical assessment (p. 216). The process leading to the development of appropriate clinical objectives hinges heavily on informal assessment. However, the procedures to devise an effective informal assessment have not been clearly operationalized because they cannot be reduced to a series of discrete steps. Many authors have indeed described informal assessment

Table 5.3 Examples of Cognitive Tests Developed for Individuals with Language Impairments or That Have Relatively Low Language Demands

Test Batteries with Language and Cognitive Subtests

Aphasia Check List	Kalbe et al. (2005)
Brief Neuropsychological Screening	Lunardelli et al. (2009)
Cognitive Linguistic Quick Test	Helm-Estabrooks (2001)
Global Aphasic Neuropsychological Battery	Van Mourik et al. (1992)
Scales of Cognitive and Communicative Ability for Neurorehabilitation	Milman et al. (2008)

Tests of More Specific Cognitive Functions

Attention	
Behavioral Inattention Test	Wilson et al. (1987)
Color Trails Test	D'Elia et al. (1996)
Test of Everyday Attention	Robertson et al. (1994)
Memory	
Continuous Visual Memory Test	Trahan & Larrabee (1988)
Design Memory	Weschler (2009)
Spatial Addition	Weschler (2009)
Executive Functioning	
Colored Progressive Matrices	Raven (1998)
Ruff Figural Fluency Test	Ruff (1996)
Modified Wisconsin Card Sorting Task	Schretlen (2011)

as a process of seeking answers rather than a process of steps (Haynes & Pindzola, 2004; Kamhi, 1994; Lidz & Peña, 1996; Muma, 1978; Rosenbek, Lapointe, & Wertz, 1989; Tomblin, Morris, & Spriestersbach, 2000; Whitworth, Webster, & Howard, 2005; Whurr, 1988). For example, ASHA (2004) explicitly included the notion of hypothesis testing in its description of the informal clinical process.

In the ICF domain of Body Function, the formal assessment process yields a quantification of the abilities the individual with aphasia displays. The clinician can now draw the appropriate conclusions depending on the battery of tests administered. For example, the test results may yield an overall level of aphasia severity, the relative severity levels of specific language skills (e.g., naming, repetition), a diagnosis based on the distribution of test scores, and a comparison point with a sample of subjects. However, knowing that an individual with aphasia has scored 42/60 on a naming task does not contribute to the development of clinical objectives. As stated previously, it provides at best a general rank ordering of therapy targets based on the respective severity levels of the various communicative

and cognitive areas tested. To circumscribe appropriate therapy approaches and procedures, clinicians must also devote time and thought to the informal assessment process. In the other ICF domains, the use of formal tests is not as prevalent, in part because fewer formal tests have been developed for these domains. In the domain of Activity Participation, more functional tests (e.g., the Scenario Test; van der Meulen et al., 2010) or questionnaires (e.g., Communicative Effectiveness Index, CETI; Lomas et al., 1989) can be used. For the Personal Factors domain, some assessment tools are available to analyze attitudes toward communication. Finally, in the domain of Environmental Factors, some conversation analysis checklists may be used. However, in a clinical setting, the assessment of these domains is much more likely to be informal in nature.

The informal assessment process is a fluid exercise in critical thinking. Clinicians must constantly generate pertinent hypotheses (e.g., Does the person with aphasia have apraxia of speech that interferes with production? Are concrete words easier to understand? Can the person communicate basic needs or call for help? Does the written modality facilitate communication? Is the naming difficulty related to the phonological output mechanism?). The clinician must then design tasks and probes that answer these questions effectively. Lidz and Peña (1996) referred to a "mini-experiment in intervention" (p. 368), Rosenbek et al. (1989) urged "clinicians to make the clinic a laboratory" (p. 187), Tomblin et al. (2000) conceptualized assessment as a "problem-solving process" (p. 5), and Whitworth et al. (2005) asserted that "a hypothesis-testing approach should be taken in the assessment process" (p. 25). Furthermore, clinicians must exercise their observation skills and search for clues in the behaviors the individual with aphasia displays. The way the person answers a question, the types of errors committed, and the slightest hint of a spontaneous compensatory strategy must be noted and must trigger further hypothesis questions.

To be sure, functional tests, such as the Scenario Test (van der Meulen et al., 2010), offer a richer source of informal qualitative observations because they are contextualized in nature, in contradistinction to aphasia batteries (e.g., WAB-R, BDAE-3), which are purposefully decontextualized. Experienced clinicians have undoubtedly noticed that our view of the informal assessment process includes the concept of *dynamic assessment* as described in the child language development literature. Successful informal assessment, then, requires answering pertinent fact-seeking questions (i.e., hypothesis-testing questions), the ultimate purpose of which is to generate the most appropriate objectives for therapy.

We recommend that the following four questions always be considered during informal assessment: (a) What is the extent of the problem? (b) Where does the behavior break down? (c) What helps the behavior? and (d) What is/are the underlying mechanism(s) for the behavior? These questions are not necessarily sequential in the process because any information can be gleaned from observation during any activity related to informal as well as formal testing procedures. However, we list them in order of progressive difficulty. That is, the hypothesis questions needed to answer the first of these questions are more obvious to generate and easier to answer than those for the last question.

What Is the Extent of the Problem?

When assessing an individual with aphasia, not all affected abilities can realistically be measured using formal tests. Although formal tests are available that measure written language impairments, apraxias, dysarthria, and associated cognitive impairments, such a lengthy formal assessment process would be overwhelming. It is up to the clinician to determine which of these abilities should be assessed formally because a precise quantification is necessary and which need to be circumscribed informally. Regardless, the clinician needs to ascertain the presence of these impairments and understand their impact on the clinical picture.

Measuring additional behaviors informally should provide a better picture of the breadth of functional difficulties facing the individual with aphasia at all levels of the ICF model. However, the behaviors measured should yield clinically useful information in addition to a basic quantification. For example, the informal quantification of attention skills should help determine whether they contribute to comprehension difficulties, measuring writing skills may help determine the potential use of writing as a cue or a compensatory mechanism, and measuring social connectivity (Simmons-Mackie, 2008) provides an indication of the psychosocial consequences of the communicative impairment. Table 5.4 presents examples of abilities to analyze, along with the clinical information such a measurement may provide. Usually, informal measurement of these behaviors requires generating a set of stimuli or adapting tasks from other sources. The data gathered are typically quantitative.

Where Does the Communicative Behavior Break Down?

To develop tailored clinical objectives, the clinician must determine a precise level of competence for each individual skill that will be targeted in therapy. That is, the precise area where the person with aphasia is starting to show difficulty must be delineated so that treatment progress can come from building on remaining skills. The point at which any given ability breaks down may be gleaned from a formal tool assessing a specific linguistic skill (e.g., BNT). However, the clinician can also rely on informal assessment. For example, for comprehension skills: How many pieces of information can the person understand? Are single concrete and abstract words equally well understood? For syntax: What type of morpheme is always absent, sometimes present, or always present in utterances? What is the average and maximal length of utterance? In the ICF domain of Activity Participation, how limited is the person's amount and quality of social relationships? The answer to these questions may come from observation, or in a more controlled method, the stimuli may be clinician generated. In the former case, the data will be qualitative and in the latter instance, quantitative.

Table 5.4 Examples of Skills Often Measured Informally and Their Clinical Use

Skill Measured	Clinical Information
Attention	Potential impact on comprehension, conversation
Writing	Potential compensatory mechanism
	Potential as a multimodal cue
Reading	Potential as a multimodal cue
Limb apraxia	Potential compensatory mechanism (gesture)
Apraxia of speech	Contribution to expressive difficulties
Dysarthria	Contribution to expressive difficulties
Conversation analysis	Identification of potential repair mechanisms
Short-term memory	Contribution to comprehension difficulties
Social diagram	Impact on psychosocial well-being

What Helps the Communicative Behavior?

Affected communicative behaviors should be observed and manipulated to identify facilitating strategies. Sometimes, the individual with aphasia relies on spontaneous adaptations that facilitate communication; in this case, clinicians must rely on their clinical observation skills and note these behaviors for potential use in therapy. Some of these behaviors may already be noticeable during the formal assessment. For example, the person may trace the first letter to help word finding or speak more slowly to ease language output. Most often, clinicians exploit their experience and clinical acumen to generate hypothesis-testing questions to assist the individual with aphasia increase performance. Essentially, this approach is reminiscent of the concept of dynamic assessment (Coelho, Ylvisaker, & Turkstra, 2005; Haywood & Lidz, 2007; Lidz & Elliott, 2000), in which clinicians manipulate context to scaffold the individual's responses. By definition, such an interaction is contextualized, and the clinician switches roles from observer to active participant. Essentially, informal assessment becomes a collaborative effort between the clinician and the person with aphasia to maximize communication, and the process becomes viewed as "relationship centered" (Worrall et al., 2010). Hersh et al. (2013) argued that dynamic assessment should take place also during the rehabilitation period. This collaborative process between client and clinician helps the clinician identify the best communicative strategies (for both members of the dyad) as well as expose the individual with aphasia to successful communicative exchanges.

There are many possible strategies in any given specific communicative or cognitive domain—too many to provide an exhaustive list here. For example, does background noise hinder language processing in the clinic or at home? Which cues are the most helpful? Can the person benefit from using the written form of the word? Can the individual point to the appropriate depiction among an array of action pictures? Does decreasing speech rate or syntax complexity maximize comprehension? Ultimately, these strategies can become clinically useful in two ways. First, by providing easier production of the target response, it can be deblocked and practiced, in which case the facilitating strategy can be phased out. Second, the facilitating strategy can be internalized by the individual with aphasia and become an alternate way to reach the same communicative goal.

What Is the Underlying Mechanism for the Communicative Behavior?

The question of underlying mechanism for the communicative behavior is the most difficult element of the informal testing process—but also possibly the most important.

In the words of Luria, Naydin, Tsvetkova, and Vinarskaya (1969):

> Before beginning the retraining of a patient, it is essential to make a detailed neuropsychological analysis of the disturbance, to identify the primary defects responsible for it, to describe its neurophysiological structure accurately, and only when this has been done, to outline the plan of the necessary measures of rehabilitation. (p. 383)

Indeed, the clinician must attempt to pinpoint with precision the causal origin(s) of the difficulty, and this kind of information can be difficult to obtain solely from the administration of formal tests (Muma, 1978). Passive observation may provide some basic clues; the type of naming errors, for example, may suggest semantic-based rather than phonologically based anomia. But, in most cases, mere observation does not reveal the nature of the impairment. The clinician also has to rule out specific hypotheses by interacting actively with the individual. For instance, short utterance length can be explained by various mechanisms (e.g., motor speech issues, productive syntax problems, preexisting passive communicative style), and an individual with aphasia may have difficulties following requests for many reasons (e.g., poor attention, memory, or language comprehension skills). If careful dynamic assessment based on hypothesis testing is not performed, rehabilitation efforts may be directed at the wrong underlying problem. To carry out this process successfully, the clinician must use critical thinking skills to generate and test a hypothesis that isolates one possibility at a time.

Identifying the underlying nature of the impairment can be conceptually facilitated by relying on an existing theoretical model. Any language-processing model offers discrete receptive and production stages that can be subject to informal testing. Whitworth et al. (2005) described the strategies available to clinicians to identify which element of a language-processing model might be affected. They further logically recommended to test from general (i.e., whole model) to more specific aspects of the model (i.e., separate routes followed by progressively narrower components of the model), depending on the errors exhibited. For example, naming, in general, tests the whole-word retrieval model, using nonwords assesses the intactness of the nonsemantic route, and a length effect may indicate a difficulty in phonological assembly. In the ICF Activity Participation domain, the clinician should analyze communicative interactions between the person with aphasia and several conversational partners in different functional settings to identify the nature of the communicative breakdowns. Dynamic assessment is likely to involve manipulation of the communicative output of the person with aphasia as well as the communicative style of his or her partner in an attempt to maximize successful exchanges.

To summarize, informal testing is the crucial element of the assessment process leading to appropriate clinical decisions. Clinicians must possess good observation skills to glean as much information as possible from the behaviors and responses of the individual being assessed, both in the clinical setting and in social environments. In addition, clinicians must generate, test, and answer relevant hypothesis questions to reach a thorough understanding of the extent, depth, and nature of the clinical difficulties the person with aphasia experiences.

ASSESSING THE PERSON WITH APHASIA

Commensurate with the ICF model (WHO, 2001), assessment of individuals with aphasia should extend beyond quantifying and qualifying their communication and cognitive abilities to examining how aphasia and other concomitant impairments affect these individuals' perceptions of themselves and their overall QOL or well-being. Such QOL information can help guide selection of intervention targets (e.g., treating first symptoms that are perceived to compromise QOL significantly) as well as evaluate the success of an aphasia intervention. A comprehensive aphasia assessment should also extend to include evaluation of the family or close caregivers. Family and caregivers can provide valuable information pertaining not only to changes in the individual with aphasia subsequent to its onset but also to the identification of potent Contextual Factors, another component of the ICF model, that may be hindering or facilitating the recovery of the individual with aphasia.

Quality-of-Life Measurement

Quality-of-life measures are designed to evaluate feelings, experiences, attitudes, and beliefs that may positively or negatively influence an individual's ability to participate and take pleasure and satisfaction in life (Glozman, 2004). Typically, QOL measures are disease or disorder specific because they are developed to focus on the effects of that disease or disorder that are most likely to influence QOL. Although many QOL measures have been developed for the variety of disorders that cause aphasia (e.g., stroke, traumatic brain injury), few of these are appropriate for most individuals with aphasia because either individuals with aphasia cannot complete the QOL measure because of its language or cognitive demands or the QOL measure focuses more on physical or cognitive rather than communication issues.

Currently, only a few QOL measures have been developed specifically for individuals with communication limitations such as aphasia (see Table 5.5). For example, the *Stroke and Aphasia Quality of Life Scale–39* (SAQOL-39; Hilari, Byng, Lamping, & Smith, 2003) requires the individual with aphasia to rate 39 items

Table 5.5 Examples of Tests to Assess Quality of Life and Related Constructs in Individuals with Aphasia or Their Caregivers

	Target Population	Target Area(s)	Mode of Response
ASHA Quality of Communication Life (Paul-Brown et al., 2004)	Individuals with communication difficulties	Communication skills/activities	5-point scale
Assessment for Living with Aphasia (Aphasia Institute; 2010)	Individuals with aphasia	Communication skills/activities, environment issues	9-point visual analogue scale
Bakas Caregiving Outcomes Scale (Bakas, Champion, et al., 2006)	Caregivers of stroke survivors	Caregiver social, well-being, and physical health changes	7-point scale
Burden of Stroke Scale (Doyle et al., 2004)	Individuals with stroke	Mobility, self-care cognition, communication, swallowing, social relations, energy/ sleep, mood	5-point scale
Carer Communication Outcome After Stroke (Long et al., 2009)	Caregivers of stroke survivors	Caregivers' perception of stroke survivor's communication skills, caregiver well-being	5-point scale
Communicative Effectiveness Index (Lomas et al., 1989)	Individuals with aphasia and/ or caregivers	Communication skills/activities	100 mm visual analogue scale
Communication Outcome After Stroke (Long et al., 2008)	Individuals with stroke	Communication skills/activities, well-being	5-point scale
Scale of Quality of Life of Caregivers (Glozman et al., 1997)	Caregivers	Preservation of caregiver's professional and social/leisure activities, and responsibilities	yes/no and 7-point scale
Stroke and Aphasia Quality of Life Scale – 39 (Hilari et al., 2003)	Individuals with aphasia	Physical, energy, psychosocial, communication domains	5-point scale

pertaining to physical (e.g., trouble with walking), psychosocial (e.g., feeling irritable), communication (e.g., trouble with finding words), and energy domains (e.g., feeling tired often); furthermore, the SAQOL-39 is available in several additional languages, such as Spanish (Lata-Caneda et al., 2009), Italian (Posteraro et al., 2006), and Greek (Efstratiadou et al., 2012). The *Quality of Communication Life Scale* (QCLS; Paul-Brown et al., 2004) is more specific to communication issues. It consists of 18 statements that reflect social participation (e.g., "I stay in touch with family and friends") and QOL matters (e.g., "I am confident that I can communicate") that are rated on a 5-point vertical scale. The individual with aphasia is instructed to ask himself or herself, "Even though I have difficulty communicating..." before reading and then rate each statement so that the focus is on the quality of the individual's communication life. It should also be noted that some items in the Disability Questionnaire of the *Comprehensive Aphasia Test* (Swinburn et al., 2004) pertain to QOL issues (e.g., "Does it [communication] make you dissatisfied with life?").

Despite the development of these tools, some individuals with aphasia will still be unable to provide their own QOL ratings because severe linguistic or cognitive impairments confound their comprehension of test items or their awareness of their symptoms, respectively. For these individuals, a spouse, family member, or other person who knows them well will need to serve as a proxy rater. Proxy ratings must, however, be interpreted cautiously because mismatches between proxy ratings and those of the individuals with the disorder have been identified: Some researchers have found proxies to rate the individuals with a disorder as more severely affected than these individuals would rate themselves, with greatest disagreement on items pertaining to less concrete domains (Cruice, Worrall, Hickson, & Murison, 2005; Doyle et al., 2013; Hilari, Owen, & Farrelly, 2007), and the inverse pattern has also been reported (proxies' ratings indicated less impairment than those of the individuals with aphasia; Doyle et al., 2013). Importantly, proxy raters and individuals with disorders are more likely to agree during the chronic phases of recovery when the couples have had more experience with the disorder and its symptoms (Pickard et al., 2004); agreement between proxy raters and individuals with aphasia is also more likely when ratings pertain to directly observable communication modalities, such as writing ability (Doyle et al., 2013).

Caregiver Evaluation

The majority of assessment tools reviewed in previous sections of this chapter focus on administering tests to or observing the behavior of individuals with aphasia. Considering the perspective of family, caregivers, and other daily communication partners, however, is essential, particularly when attempting to determine the impact of aphasia on the Activity Participation domain and the Environmental Factors of the ICF model (WHO, 2001) because these individuals are most familiar with the premorbid communication style and ability of the individual with aphasia. Likewise, family and caregiver perspectives may be fundamental when evaluating individuals with aphasia who have more severe comprehension impairments or decreased insight. Caregivers' views of aphasia and its impact on daily interactions and activities are also valuable for treatment planning. For example, such information can be used to set reciprocally agreed-on therapy goals (i.e., the third prong of EBP).

Both formal and informal methods are available when gathering information from family and caregivers regarding their views of the communicative and cognitive strengths and weaknesses of the individual with aphasia. For example, the CETI (Lomas et al., 1989) consists of 16 items pertaining to important daily communication activities (e.g., "Being part of a conversation when it is fast and there are a number of people involved"); the caregiver rates the individual with aphasia for each item using a visual analogue scale that varies from "not at all able" to "as able" as before the onset of aphasia. The CETI's validity and reliability have been established, and CETI scores were found to correlate significantly with WAB scores in individuals with aphasia during the acute and subacute recovery phases (Bakheit, Carrington, Griffiths, & Searle, 2005).

In addition to documenting the caregivers' perspectives regarding the communicative abilities of the individual with aphasia, clinicians should collect information pertaining to the caregivers' communication skills and overall well-being. Such information can assist in identifying treatment goals and activities. For example, it has been well documented that caring for individuals with aphasia and other acquired cognitive or communicative disorders can negatively affect the caregiver's physical and emotional health (Bakas, Kroenke, et al., 2006;

Draper et al., 2007; E. Miller et al., 2010). For caregivers experiencing significant burden, an aphasia treatment protocol that requires substantial caregiver involvement would be contraindicated. Alternately, some caregivers, via their own communicative behaviors (e.g., speaking too quickly, acknowledging only spoken responses), may be inadvertently exacerbating the communication difficulties of the individual with aphasia (Murray, 1998; Turner & Whitworth, 2006). Therefore, measures of both caregiver burden and communication skills should be considered important components of a comprehensive aphasia assessment.

To evaluate caregiver stress or burden, several valid and reliable scales have been developed for the caregiver population as a whole (e.g., Caregiver Strain Index; Robinson, 1983) as well as for more specific segments of the caregiver population, such as those caring for stroke survivors (e.g., Bakas Caregiving Outcomes Scales; Bakas, Champion, Perkins, Farran, & Williams, 2006) (see also Table 5.5). Relatedly, QOL measures expressly for caregivers have been developed (for a review, see Glozman, 2004). To determine whether the communication style and behaviors of caregivers are facilitating or impeding the aphasia recovery of their significant others, the clinician can use conversational sampling and analysis procedures already described in this chapter, focusing on the output of the caregiver rather than or in addition to that of the individual with aphasia (Armstrong & Ferguson, 2010). Analysis protocols specific to caregivers have also been designed. For example, the Measure of Skill in Supported Conversation (Kagan et al., 2004) allows rating how well conversational partners acknowledge (e.g., use appropriate emotional tone and humor) and support (e.g., modify output to ensure understanding by the individual with aphasia) the communicative competence of individuals with aphasia (or other communicative disorders).

ONGOING DATA COLLECTION

In many clinical and research settings, ongoing data collection is needed to monitor the stability or progress of individuals with aphasia. More specifically, repeatedly assessing individuals with aphasia may allow determining if they (a) have sufficient stamina and stability to begin regular treatment sessions; (b) are continuing to respond positively to treatment; (c) are reaching a plateau, suggesting a need to change treatment procedures or to discharge from treatment; or (4) are maintaining treatment-related gains beyond discharge from treatment. Likewise, the status of caregivers can change over time as well; therefore, ongoing consideration of their perceptions and communicative style and strategies is recommended. Both formal and informal assessment procedures may be used for ongoing data collection.

Ongoing Formal Assessment

When formal tests are used to document change over time in a given individual, the clinician should select tests that have been designed for multiple administrations. For example, tests that offer multiple forms are appropriate because they minimize practice effects that can influence client performance when the same test items are repeatedly administered. Whereas several cognitive tests offer multiple forms (e.g., *Test of Everyday Attention*; Robertson, Ward, Ridgeway, & Nimmo-Smith, 1994), few aphasia or, more broadly, language tests offer this feature. Consequently, another approach to repeated administrations of the same test is to identify the test's standard error of measurement (SEM). This statistic indicates how much an examinee's score may vary if the test is repeatedly administered to that same examinee (Mitrushina et al., 2005). The clinician can use SEM to plot a confidence interval or range in which the examinee's "true" score lies; if on subsequent administrations the examinee's score falls outside this range, it is likely this subsequent score indicates a performance change rather than one reflecting measurement error.

Ongoing Informal Assessment

Alternately or in addition to the use of formal test procedures, informal probe tasks may be developed to monitor the communication functioning of individuals with aphasia over time. Ideally, a set of probe tasks should be developed. First, at least one probe task should assess the behavior being targeted in treatment. For example, if picture-naming activities are being used during therapy sessions to improve written word retrieval, possible probe tasks include written fluency (e.g., write as many words as possible in 1 minute that begin with the letter *s*), written phrase completion, or written picture naming. Preferably, these probes should include stimuli and tasks that were not used in treatment activities so that the evaluation extends beyond measuring task-specific effects. Note, however, that sometimes treatment has been designed to target a limited set of stimuli (e.g., writing checks to increase independence in paying bills); in this case, just one probe task that is similar to the treatment activity may be needed. Second, at least one probe task should be designed to assess a control behavior, that is, a behavior that the treatment is not

expected to modify. Given the previous example, a sentence verification listening task might be used to probe the control behavior, auditory comprehension, which would not be expected to benefit from a written naming treatment. Including this type of probe task, which is logically similar to the multiple-baseline method, helps document that changes in the trained behavior were the result of the treatment and not because of general effects (e.g., an affinity for the clinician). Third, a probe task that evaluates generalization to an untrained, related language behavior may be included. For instance, given that written word retrieval is the target of treatment, a probe task evaluating spoken word retrieval might be designed to document cross-modal generalization.

The schedule of informal probes should also be considered. All probe tasks should be completed prior to treatment onset to baseline the performance level of the individual with aphasia. Next, once treatment has begun, the probes can be administered periodically (e.g., every third treatment session) to evaluate progress and identify whether treatment activities or goals require modification; importantly, when probing during a phase of intervention, the probe tasks should be administered at the beginning of the treatment session so that training conducted that day does not influence probe task performance. Finally, probe tasks should also be administered immediately and several weeks following the termination of treatment.

These probes quantify patterns of change since the baseline measurements and determine whether the individual with aphasia can maintain treatment gains when direct training is no longer provided.

ASSESSMENT PROCEDURES: SOME ADDITIONAL DOS AND DON'TS

Feedback and Reinforcement

Clinicians are taught to provide reinforcement and feedback fairly systematically during therapy interactions. However, during the assessment process, reinforcement and feedback cannot be dispensed in the same manner, and in some instances, clinicians must learn to counter the tendency to praise and to provide information on the quality of the responses.

Reinforcement refers to the overall qualitative judgment of a response provided by the clinician. With adults with neurogenic communicative disorders, reinforcement is usually verbal. Although the impact of reinforcement on linguistic performance is doubtful (Brookshire, 2007), it understandably may increase motivation.

Therefore, it is not surprising that clinicians use verbal praise much more than negative statements in therapy interactions, even if the response is incorrect.

Feedback refers to the specific information that clinicians provide the individual with aphasia describing how or why a particular response was or was not successful. Feedback following an error should specify how to modify the response to produce the desired target (i.e., corrective feedback). However, during most of the assessment process, feedback and specific reinforcement should not be used at all. The assessment stimuli have the potential to be used again in the future; therefore, no information can be provided on the correctness of responses. This applies to formal tests (which have standard administration procedures, including what can and cannot be said to the test taker), any informal materials used to quantify a behavior, and baseline stimuli or probes. Instead, the clinician should instruct the person with aphasia that the results will be discussed at the end of the exercise but not during the task. During assessment, praise should be limited to occasional general statements, such as "You are giving it your best; that's great" or "that's exactly what I want you to do, keep going." Feedback, however, should not be used at all.

Testing Versus Baselining

As defined previously, testing (i.e., assessing) is the process of providing quantitative and qualitative information about the abilities of an individual with a communication disorder. As such, testing can be performed before and after a rehabilitation period to measure change over time. Usually, pre- and posttherapy testing are performed with formal tests and measure an overall skill. For example, the BNT may be used to establish the amount of improvement in naming ability. *Baselining* refers to the pretherapy measurement or probing of clinical objectives. In that sense, baselining is more specific than testing because it quantifies a particular objective associated with specific methods. For example, after having carefully assessed an individual with aphasia, the clinician decides to target spoken word retrieval in therapy, among other things. That behavior has already been quantified with the BNT during the formal assessment process. Now, the clinician develops several specific objectives, such as practicing naming as many tools or kitchen utensils as possible. The clinician must now baseline these objectives individually prior to the start of therapy.

Regardless of the assessment tool employed (formal or informal), the items contained in the testing material must never be used in treatment tasks because this practice would amount to "teaching to the test." Similarly, the stimuli used for baseline probes cannot be used during therapy unless the clinical objective targets a closed set of stimuli. In the preceding clinical example, the overall goal is to improve spoken word retrieval. Therefore, generalization is expected, and the baseline items should not be practiced in therapy so that generalization can be examined. However, if the objective is for the individual with aphasia to master naming a set of 20 highly functional items, treatment activities, pretreatment baseline, and posttreatment probe tasks will all include the same 20 items. In this case, though, no generalization is expected.

Bilingual Individuals and Use of Interpreters

When evaluating individuals with aphasia who use more than one language, it is essential to assess each of their languages (Lorenzen & Murray, 2008; Paradis, 2004, 2011). Such an extensive evaluation is necessary to understand the relative types and severities of deficits across languages and because, depending on the structure of the languages used, some deficits may be detectable only in one language. Consequently, assessing a bi- or multilingual person involves two difficult issues: selecting the assessment tools and identifying the best person to perform the assessment. We have already discussed the psychometric pitfalls and the cultural inaccuracies associated with translated tests (Barratt et al., 2012; Ivanova & Hallowell, 2013; Roger & Code, 2011; see also Battle, 2012, and Roberts, 2008). Essentially, unless there is a formal test battery in a target language, all assessment will be informal in nature.

The second important issue concerns the use of translators/interpreters during the assessment process. In an ideal situation, the clinician him- or herself is bilingual and bicultural; otherwise, the only alternative is to assess the person indirectly by recruiting the help of a translator/interpreter. In such a case, bilingual assistance should preferably be sought from outside the family and social circles of the person with aphasia. In a position statement, ASHA (1985) suggested how to access bilingual speech–language pathologists, such as trying to develop partnerships with local university programs. If there are professional interpreter programs in the community, interpreters with an emphasis on health-care interpreting may be available who have received additional training in confidentiality issues. Finally, large hospitals maintain a network of bilingual volunteers, but their competence in foreign languages and with assessment procedures naturally varies.

Regardless of how the bilingual person is recruited, clinicians should be prepared to train the interpreter in speech–language pathology assessment techniques in general (e.g., when clarification questions can be posed to the client with aphasia) and in issues related to neurogenic communication disorders in particular (Roger & Code, 2011).

If the clinician cannot find bilingual assistance, a member of the individual's larger community or more immediate family may be used. However, the former may bring about family resistance because of confidentiality issues (Tomblin et al., 2000), and the latter may impede objectivity (Roberts, 2008). In both cases, a much more extensive training period with the interpreter should precede assessment.

Regardless of the qualification of the interpreter/translator, licensing bodies (ASHA, 1985) and researchers (Roger & Code, 2011) recommend a period of training to familiarize the person with the specific assessment tools and the characteristics of the clinical interaction. Both ASHA (n.d.) and Roger and Code (2011) provided some additional, useful tips about working with interpreters. Other guides on the subject are also available (e.g., Langdon & Cheng, 2002).

FUTURE DIRECTIONS

Formal tests currently available for evaluating linguistic and cognitive abilities in individuals with aphasia require further development in several areas. First, the psychometric qualities of many tests require substantial improvements (Ivanova & Hallowell, 2013). For example, although large and diverse normative samples help reduce test variance related to confounding factors (e.g., age, education) and thus enhance test specificity (Pedraza & Mungas, 2008), most language and cognitive assessment tools suitable for individuals with aphasia have been standardized with small normative samples or have not been created or validated for diverse cultural groups (Ivanova & Hallowell, 2013). Relatedly, even though substantial research has confirmed that demographic variables such as age, education level, and ethnocultural background may significantly influence performance on language tests (Murray & Clark, 2015; Roberts & Doucet, 2011; Zec, Burkett, Markwell, & Larsen, 2007), few aphasia tests have been examined for the potential of these test score biases or have provided adjusted scores to offset these biases (Salter et al., 2006).

Both researchers and clinicians have identified psychometric issues with many aphasia screening tests used in acute care settings (Flamand-Roze et al., 2011; Salter et al., 2006; Vogel, Maruff, & Morgan, 2010).

In particular, few of these screening instruments have been submitted to investigations exploring their sensitivity to language changes (especially among individuals with milder forms of aphasia) or their prognostic capabilities (e.g., does good performance on the screening tool suggest good aphasia recovery?); whereas the recently developed Aphasia Rapid Test (Azuar et al., 2013) addresses some of these issues, it was not designed to identify or discriminate aphasia from other communication disorders.

Additional psychometric concerns relate to several forms of validity. For instance, the content and construct validity of several aphasia and language tests have been questioned because they fail either to specify the language model on which the test was constructed or to define operationally what communicative functions are being evaluated (Byng, Kay, Edmundson, & Scott, 1990; Ivanova & Hallowell, 2013; Murray & Chapey, 2001). Furthermore, the ecological validity of many linguistic and cognitive tests is either substandard or not reported (Ross & Wertz, 1999). To address these psychometric limitations, existing tests for individuals with aphasia could be updated or undergo more rigorous psychometric evaluation; alternately, new tests could be developed. As another option, the usefulness of tests designed for other clinical populations (e.g., *Listening Comprehension Test—Adolescent*; Bowers, Huisingh, & LoGiudice, 2009) should be examined and adapted if needed.

A second assessment matter in need of further investigation relates to the ICF model (WHO, 2001): Most currently available aphasia tests assess language impairment or loss of body function. It should not be surprising, then, that clinicians reported infrequent use of more functional and qualitative measures (Klippi, Sellman, Heikkinen, & Laine, 2012). Thus, more tools that can identify daily language activity challenges, evaluate language for societal participation, and discern influential personal and environmental factors should be developed (Eadie et al., 2006; Milman et al., 2008; Simmons-Mackie & Kagan, 2007); clinicians have also voiced the need for such tools to use as treatment outcome measures (Klippi et al., 2012). In fact, in 2008, Dalemans, de Witte, Lemmens, van den Heuvel, and Wade reviewed currently available measures of participation and concluded that only two (Community Integration Questionnaire, Nottingham Extended Activities of Daily Living) appeared suitable for use with individuals with aphasia. They cautioned, however, that even these two instruments were less than ideal because of the content of some items, the language demands associated with completing the measures, or the lack of psychometric property data pertaining to using the measures with individuals with aphasia.

Encouragingly, Tucker, Edwards, Kirchner Mathews, Baum, and Tabor Connor (2012) developed a set of modifications that could be applied to self-report QOL and participation outcome measures routinely used with nonaphasic populations (e.g., Stroke Impact Scale; Duncan et al., 1999). The modifications included changes to test administration (e.g., use of uncomplicated font) and response format (e.g., ensuring a consistent response scale across items) as well as the provision of examiner support techniques (i.e., specification of steps an examiner could apply if the client's response was unclear or the client failed to respond to an item; e.g., simplifying and restating an item). Tucker et al. found that with these modifications clients with a variety of aphasia profiles were able to complete the outcome measures, and results from statistical analyses also supported the use of the test and the administration modifications.

A third issue that must be addressed in the near future, particularly in the United States, is the limited time available for assessing individuals with aphasia and other neurogenic communication disorders. For example, in 2006, ASHA reported that clinicians had only approximately 60 minutes to complete all aspects of a cognitive-communication assessment (i.e., chart review, administration and scoring of formal and informal cognitive and linguistic assessment procedures, writing chart notes and reports). It is quite suspect whether such restricted assessment times allow accurate and reliable decisions regarding the nature and extent of cognitive and communicative disorders (including the impact of such disorders on daily activities and social participation), prognosis, or the length and type of treatment needed. Thus, two lines of research need to be pursued to address this time issue: (a) identifying test procedures that can afford

evaluation of a broad number of cognitive and linguistic abilities in a prompt and efficient manner and (b) empirically documenting the negative consequences of rushed evaluations and, perhaps, identifying a minimum time limit that will still afford the information necessary for treatment planning.

Finally, given the significant advances in technology over the past decade, telerehabilitation is emerging as a viable service delivery model to foster access to speech–language pathology services, not only for individuals living in rural or remote areas but also for those using languages that their local clinicians cannot speak. Initial research indicated that when videoconferencing and face-to-face assessment sessions are compared, they yield similar aphasia findings (Palsbo, 2007; Theodoros, Hill, Russell, Ward, & Wootton, 2008), even when individuals with severe aphasia are evaluated (Hill, Theodoros, Russell, Ward, & Wootton, 2009). Newton, Acres, and Bruce (2013), however, recently compared the scores of individuals with aphasia when they completed language tests alone on a computer, on a computer with the clinician present, or in a traditional testing format. The language scores of the participants with aphasia were significantly lower when tests were completed alone on the computer but were still correlated with their scores from the traditional testing format. Such data highlight the influence of test format on language test outcomes, which could confound comparing scores collected in a traditional versus a computerized or telerehabilitation format. To extend these initial findings, future studies of the feasibility, reliability, and validity of telerehabilitation must evaluate a broad range of aphasia assessment procedures (e.g., formal and informal measures) and include study participants who represent diverse communicative and cognitive profiles (e.g., aphasia with concomitant apraxia of speech) and language and ethnocultural backgrounds.

Case Illustration 5.1

As a clinician working in an outpatient rehabilitation facility, you have just received a referral to assess a client, Mrs. H. As the first step of the assessment process, you request and review her medical records and also send intake forms to Mrs. H. and her husband to collect background information that will help you select formal and informal assessment procedures prior to your first session with Mrs. H. Review of these records indicates that Mrs. H. is a 78-year-old retired librarian who, prior to a left hemisphere hemorrhagic stroke 4 weeks ago, was relatively healthy except for a history of hypertension. Subsequent to this stroke, she presented with right hemiparesis, right visual field cut, and aphasia. While an inpatient, Mrs. H. was seen by a speech–language

(continues)

pathologist, who administered the Bedside Evaluation Screening Test–II (West, Sands, & Ross-Swain, 1998) and a hearing screening. Findings from these formal tests confirmed that Mrs. H. presented with aphasia, described by the speech–language pathologist as moderately severe in terms of both production and comprehension impairments, and that Mrs. H. passed the hearing screening. There was little information pertaining to whether aphasia treatment had been provided during her 2-week stay in the acute care hospital. It is noted on the intake forms completed by her husband that Mrs. H. was an avid reader prior to her stroke and that her current reading difficulties are a primary area of concern.

Based on this background information, you administer the following formal measures at your first session with Mrs. H.: the subtests of the WAB-R that allow you to calculate Aphasia and Language Quotients and in turn determine aphasia severity and type, and Symbol Cancellation, Clock Drawing, Symbol Trails, Design Memory and Generation, and Mazes subtests of the *Cognitive Linguistic Quick Test* (CLQT; Helm-Estabrooks, 2001) to screen for the presence and types of cognitive impairment. In addition, Mr. H. is asked to take home and complete the ASHA FACS (Frattali et al., 1995) to identify and quantify the communication strengths and weaknesses of Mrs. H. at the Activity Participation level of the ICF model.

Based on data collected from these formal tests, you determine that Mrs. H. is currently presenting with moderate (i.e., WAB-R Aphasia Quotient = 52, Language Quotient = 66.5) conduction aphasia, characterized by frequent spoken word retrieval errors and attempts at self-correction (i.e., *conduites d'approche*), reduced spoken utterance length, significant repetition difficulties, and mild auditory comprehension problems, particularly when attempting to understand lengthy and syntactically complex sentences and, as observed by you and reported by her husband, when in group settings or noisy listening conditions. Written language testing revealed mild alexia and agraphia. Reading out loud was significantly worse than reading comprehension. ASHA FACS findings were consistent with those of the WAB-R and further indicated that the language production and comprehension difficulties of Mrs. H. were negatively influencing her completion of everyday activities and social interactions in her home and other settings. She did not demonstrate cognitive problems on the CLQT; however, you note that these subtests evaluate cognitive skills only in the visual modality, and given her reported difficulties with comprehension in noisy environments, you still have some concerns regarding auditory attention skills.

Informal testing focused on addressing the four questions described previously. First, to circumscribe *the extent of the problem,* you need to probe behaviors not measured during the formal assessment. You decide to test praxis to see if gestural communication can be used and to rule out apraxia of speech. The language sample from the WAB-R indicated that her speech contains phonemic paraphasias and does not seem to include phonetic errors. Mrs. H. scored 8/8 on ideomotor praxis tasks. These results exclude praxic difficulties. Next, you decide to assess short-term memory (STM) because it may affect comprehension in individuals with conduction aphasia because of anatomic proximity (Baldo & Dronkers, 2006). Indeed, the results of the digits forward test show that Mrs. H has a verbal span of 2 and a nonverbal span within normal limits. Because of the repetition problems, you decide to readminister the task with a pointing response (Martin & Saffran, 1992), which brings her verbal span performance to within normal limits. You conclude that her STM is normal. In terms of attention, you assume that focused (sustained) attention is functional because Mrs. H. has been able to finish the formal testing session without breaks. However, you decide to test selective attention because of the reported difficulty with background noise. You prepare two similar language comprehension tasks, but you play the radio at 40 dB in the background during half of the test. Her performance is significantly decreased when the background sound is present. Finally, you decide to ask Mr. H. to help you draw a premorbid and a current social network diagram (Simmons-Mackie, 2008) because of the psychosocial impact of the stroke noted on the ASHA FACS. These diagrams will illustrate the difference in social contacts before and after the stroke and can be used as a baseline.

Second, you want to identify *the level at which the communicative behaviors break down.* For repetition, you test one-, two-, and three-syllable low- and high-frequency words and nonwords. You note that there is a clear word length effect, a lexicality effect, but no word frequency effect. Because Mrs. H. performed better on the WAB-R naming task than on word finding in spontaneous speech, you decide to administer the BNT (Kaplan et al., 2001). She obtained 45/60, which confirms mild-to-moderate anomia, and you note that errors are mostly phonemic, no response, or circumlocutions. For reading, you already noticed that reading comprehension was significantly better than oral reading.

(continues)

Third, you want to determine *what improves the communicative behaviors.* You already know that a quiet background will help comprehension, and the BNT results showed that phonemic cueing—but not semantic cueing—helps word finding. Further, you decide to investigate the effect of speed on language reception and production. You prepare two similar lists of words to repeat and two similar sentence comprehension tasks with increasingly complex syntax. In both cases, Mrs. H.'s performance is dramatically improved when the stimuli are presented more slowly. You also decide to probe unison speech to see if it could be used as a cue in therapy, and it works. Because of Mrs. H.'s concern about reading, you give her a reading comprehension task. For half the items, you instruct her to read it silently more slowly than she is used to, and for the other half, you instruct her to read it again a second time before answering the questions. Both strategies improve her performance as compared to the test results.

Fourth, you need to understand as well as possible *the underlying mechanism of the language symptoms.* In naming tasks, Mrs. H makes mostly no response, phonemic paraphasias, and circumlocutions, but few semantic paraphasias. In spontaneous speech, the errors are similar but more numerous. Phonemic cueing works, and semantic cueing does not. Also, the WAB-R showed that written production is somewhat better than oral production. In repetition, there is a word length and a lexicality effect but no word frequency effect. All these elements point to a difficulty centered on accessing the phonological output lexicon from the semantic system and a difficulty with phonological assembly (Whitworth et al., 2005). In comprehension, her difficulty seems to be related to processing speed rather than a true syntactic difficulty because slowing down the stimuli normalizes the performance.

In conclusion, you decide that your therapy will focus on (a) word finding, possibly using a phonological strategy (e.g., the Phonological Components Analysis method; Leonard, Rochon, & Laird, 2008); (b) slowing down expressive language to practice phonological assembly; (c) progressively increasing processing speed in reading and receptive language; (d) training family members to slow down their speech temporarily and to minimize auditory distractions while therapy is ongoing to facilitate comprehension; and (e) stimulating social networking by training conversational partners.

STUDY QUESTIONS

1. Define formal and informal assessment.
2. Explain the four main constructs of the ICF model as applied to aphasia assessment.
3. What can clinicians do to apply evidence-based practice to the assessment process?
4. What are the purposes of the formal assessment process?
5. What is the difference between a standardized and a normed test?
6. What is the difference between test reliability and validity?
7. Define the four main types of test validity.
8. Compare and contrast the purposes of the WAB-R and the ASHA FACS.
9. What are the differences between an aphasia battery and an aphasia screening test?
10. What are the benefits of analyzing discourse in an individual with aphasia?
11. What is the rationale for assessing cognition in aphasia?
12. Explain the four main purposes of the informal assessment process.
13. Explain how conducting a caregiver evaluation fits in the ICF model.
14. Describe how you would use generalization probes in clinical practice.
15. Explain how feedback and reinforcement differ between therapy and assessment.
16. What is "training to the test," and how do you avoid it?

REFERENCES

American Speech-Language-Hearing Association. (1985). *Clinical management of communicatively handicapped minority language populations (Position statement).* Rockville, MD: Author.

American Speech-Language-Hearing Association. (2004). *Preferred practice patterns for the profession of speech-language pathology.* Rockville, MD: Author.

American Speech-Language-Hearing Association. (2005). *Evidence-based practice in communication disorders* [Position statement]. Retrieved July 2, 2015 from http://www.asha.org/policy

American Speech-Language Hearing Association. (2006). [National Outcome Measurement System (NOMS): Average evaluation time for cognitive-communicative disorders in healthcare settings 2000–2006]. Unpublished raw data.

American Speech-Language Hearing Association. (n.d.). *Tips for working with an interpreter.* Retrieved May 19, 2009, from http://www.asha.org/practice/multicultural/issues/interpret.htm

Aphasia Institute. (2010). *Assessment for Living with Aphasia.* Toronto, Canada: Author.

Armstrong, E., & Ferguson, A. (2010). Language, meaning, context, and functional communication. *Aphasiology, 24*(4), 480–496.

Azuar, C., Leger, A., Arbizu, C., Henry-Amar, F., Chomel-Guillaume, S., & Samson, Y. (2013). The Aphasia Rapid Test: An NIHSS-like aphasia test. *Journal of Neurology, 260*(8), 2110–2117.

Bakas, T., Champion, V., Perkins, S. M., Farran, C. J., & Williams, L. S. (2006). Psychometric testing of the revised 15-item Bakas Caregiving Outcomes Scale. *Nursing Research, 55*(5), 346–355.

Bakas, T., Kroenke, K., Plue, L. D., Perkins, S. M., & Williams, L. S. (2006). Outcomes among family caregivers of aphasic versus nonaphasic stroke survivors. *Rehabilitation Nursing, 31*(1), 33–42.

Bakheit, A., Carrington, S., Griffiths, S., & Searle, K. (2005). High scores on the Western Aphasia Battery correlate with good functional communication skills (as measured with the Communicative Effectiveness Index) in aphasic stroke patients. *Disability and Rehabilitation, 27*(6), 287–291.

Baldo, J. V., & Dronkers, N. F. (2006). The role of the inferior parietal and inferior frontal cortex in working memory. *Neuropsychology, 20*(5), 529–538.

Barratt, J., Khoza-Shangase, K., & Msimang, K. (2012). Speech-language assessment in a linguistically diverse setting: Preliminary exploration of the possible impact of informal "solutions" within the South African context. *South African Journal of Communication Disorders, 59*(1), 34–44.

Bate, S., Kay, J., Code, C., Haslam, C., & Hallowell, B. (2010). Eighteen years on: What next for the PALPA? *International Journal of Speech-Language Pathology, 12*(3), 190–202.

Battle, D. E. (2012). *Communication disorders in multicultural populations* (4th ed.). St. Louis, MO: Elsevier Mosby.

Beeke, S., Maxim, J., & Wilkinson, R. (2008). Rethinking agrammatism: Factors affecting the form of language elicited via clinical test procedures. *Clinical Linguistics and Phonetics, 22*(4–5), 317–323.

Benton, A. L., Hamsher, K., & Sivan, A. B. (2001). *Multilingual aphasia examination* (3rd ed.). Lutz, FL: Psychological Assessment Resources.

Bishop, D. (2003). *Test for reception of grammar* (2nd ed.). San Antonio, TX: Pearson.

Bowers, L., Huisingh, R., & LoGiudice, C. (2009). *Listening Comprehension Test: Adolescent.* East Moline, IL: Linguisystems.

Brookshire, R. H. (2007). *Introduction to neurogenic communication disorders.* St. Louis, MO: Mosby.

Brookshire, R. H., & Nicholas, L. E. (1994). Speech sample size and test-retest stability of connected speech measures for adults with aphasia. *Journal of Speech and Hearing Research, 37*, 399–407.

Brookshire, R. H., & Nicholas, L. E. (1997). *The Discourse Comprehension Test* (Rev. ed.). Minneapolis, MN: BRK.

Brown, K., McGahan, L., Alkhaledi, M., Seah, D., Howe, T., & Worrall, L. (2006). Environmental factors that influence the community participation of adults with aphasia: The perspective of service industry workers. *Aphasiology, 20*(7), 595–615.

Brownsett, S. L. E., Warren, J. E., Geranmayeh, F., Woodhead, Z., Leech, R., & Wise, R. J. (2014). Cognitive control and its impact on recovery from aphasic stroke. *Brain, 137*, 242–254.

Byng, S., Kay, J., Edmundson, A., & Scott, C. (1990). Aphasia tests reconsidered. *Aphasiology, 4*, 67–91.

Calis, F. A., On, A. Y., Durmaz, B. (2013). Validity and reliability of a new test for Turkish-speaking aphasic patients: Ege Aphasia Test. *NeuroRehabilitation, 32*, 157–163.

Chaytor, N., & Schmitter-Edgecombe, M. (2003). The ecological validity of neuropsychological tests: A review of the literature on everyday cognitive skills. *Neuropsychological Review, 13*, 181–197.

Cherney, B., Shadden, B., & Coelho, C. A. (Eds.). (1998). *Analyzing discourse in communicatively impaired adults.* Gaithersburg, MD: Aspen.

Cho-Reyes, S., & Thompson, C. K. (2012). Verb and sentence production and comprehension in aphasia: Northwestern Assessment of Verbs and Sentences (NAVS). *Aphasiology, 26*(10), 1250–1277.

Coelho, C., Ylvisaker, M., & Turkstra, L. S. (2005). Nonstandardized assessment approaches for individuals with traumatic brain injuries. *Seminars in Speech and Language, 26*(4), 223–241.

Cole-Virtue, J., & Nickels, L. (2004). Spoken word to picture matching from PALPA: A critique and some new matched sets. *Aphasiology, 18*, 77–102.

Cronbach, L. J. (1990). *Essentials of psychological testing* (4th ed.). New York: Harper and Row.

Cruice, M., Worrall, L., Hickson, L., & Murison, R. (2005). Measuring quality of life: Comparing family members' and friends' ratings with those of their aphasic partners. *Aphasiology, 19*, 111–129.

Cunningham, R., Farrow, V., Davies, C., & Lincoln, N. (1995). Reliability of the assessment of communicative effectiveness in severe aphasia. *European Journal of Disorders of Communication, 30*, 1–16.

Dalemans, R., de Witte, L., Lemmens, J., van den Heuvel, W., & Wade, D. (2008). Measures for rating social participation in people with aphasia: A systematic review. *Clinical Rehabilitation, 22*, 542–555.

D'Elia, L. F., Satz, P., Uchiyama, C. L., & White, T. (1996). *Color Trails Test.* Lutz, FL: Psychological Assessment Resources.

Doyle, P. J., Goda, A. J., & Spencer, K. A. (1995). The communicative informativeness and efficiency of connected discourse by adults with aphasia under structured and conversational sampling conditions. *American Journal of Speech-Language Pathology, 4*, 130–134.

Doyle, P. J., Hula, W., Austermann Hula, S., Stone, C., Wambaugh, J., Ross, K., & Schumacher, J. (2013). Self- and surrogate-reported communication functioning in aphasia. *Quality of Life Research, 22*, 957–967.

Doyle, P. J., McNeil, M. R., Mikolic, J. M., Prieto, L., Hula, W. D., Lustig, A. P., Elman, R. J. (2004). The burden of stroke scale (BOSS) provides valid and reliable score estimates of functioning and well-being in stroke survivors with and without communication disorders. *Journal of Clinical Epidemiology, 57*, 997–1007.

Doyle, P. J., Tsironas, D., Goda, A. J., & Kalinyak, M. (1996). The relationship between objective measures and listeners' judgments of the communicative informativeness of the connected discourse of adults with aphasia. *American Journal of Speech-Language Pathology, 5*, 53–60.

Draper, B., Bowring, G., Thompson, C., Van Heyst, J., Conroy, P., & Thompson, J. (2007). Stress in caregivers of aphasic stroke patients: A randomized controlled trial. *Clinical Rehabilitation, 21*, 122–130.

Duffy, J., Fossett, T. R., & Thomas, J. E. (2011). Clinical practice in acute care hospital settings. In L. L. La Pointe (Ed.), *Aphasia and related neurogenic language disorders* (pp. 38–58). New York: Thieme.

Duncan, P. W., Wallace, D., Lai, S. M., Johnson, D., Embretson, S., & Laster, L. J. (1999). The Stroke Impact Scale Version 2.0: Evaluation of reliability, validity, and sensitivity to change. *Stroke, 30*, 2131–2140.

Eadie, T. L., Yorkston, K. M., Klasner, E. R., Dudgeon, B. J., Deitz, J. C., Baylor, C. R., et al. (2006). Measuring communicative participation: A review of self-report instruments in speech-language pathology. *American Journal of Speech-Language Pathology, 15*, 307–320.

Edwards, D., Hahn, M., Baum, C., Perlmutter, M., Sheedy, C., & Dromerick, A. (2006). Screening patients with stroke for rehabilitation needs: Validation of the Post-Stroke Rehabilitation Guidelines. *Neurorehabilitation and Neural Repair, 20*, 42–48.

Edwards, S. (1995). Profiling fluent aphasic spontaneous speech: A comparison of two methodologies. *European Journal of Disorders of Communication, 30*, 333–345.

Efstratiadou, E. A., Chelas, E. N., Ignatiou, M., Christaki, V., Papathanasiou, I., & Hilari, K. (2012). Quality of life after stroke: Evaluation of the Greek SAQOL-39g. *Folia Phoniatrica et Logopaedica, 64*(4), 179–186.

Eisenson, J., & LaPointe, L. L. (2008). *Examining for aphasia* (4th ed.). Austin, TX: Pro-Ed.

Enderby, P., Wood, V., & Wade, D. (2006). *The Frenchay Aphasia Screening Test* (2nd ed.). Hoboken, NJ: Wiley.

Flamand-Roze, C., Falssard, B., Roze, E., Maintigneux, L., Beziz, J., Chacon, A., et al. (2011). Validation of a new language screening tool for patients with acute stroke: The Language Screening Test. *Stroke, 42*, 1224–1229.

Frattali, C. M., Thompson, C., Holland, A., Wohl, A., & Ferketic, M. (1995). *American Speech-Language-Hearing Association Functional Assessment of Communication Skills for Adults*. Rockville, MD: American Speech-Language-Hearing Association.

Frattali, C. M., & Worrall, L. E. (2001). Evidence-based practice: Applying science to the art of clinical care. *Journal of Medical Speech Language Pathology, 9*, ix–xiv.

Fure, B., Bruun Wyller, T., Engedal, K., & Thommessen, B. (2006). Cognitive impairments in acute lacunar stroke. *Acta Neurologica Scandinavia, 114*(1), 17–22.

Glozman, J. M. (2004). Quality of life of caregivers. *Neuropsychology Review, 14*(4), 183–196.

Glozman, J. M., Bicheva, K., & Fedorova, N. (1997). Scale of Quality of Life of Care-Givers (SQLC). *Journal of Neurology, 245*(5), 539–541.

Goodglass, H., Kaplan, E., & Barresi, B. (2001). *Boston Diagnostic Aphasia Examination* (3rd ed.). New York: Lippincott Williams & Wilkins.

Hachioui, H., Visch-Brink, E. G., Lingsma, H. F., van de Sandt-Koenderman, M. W., Dippel, D. W., Koudstaal, P. J., et al. (2014). Nonlinguistic cognitive impairment in post-stroke aphasia A prospective study. *Neurorehabilitation and Neural Repair, 28*(3), 273–281.

Haynes, W. O., & Pindzola, R. H. (2004). *Diagnosis and evaluation in speech pathology*. Boston: Pearson.

Haywood, H. C., & Lidz, C. S. (2007). *Dynamic assessment in practice: Clinical and educational applications*. Cambridge, England: Cambridge University Press.

Helm-Estabrooks, N. (2001). *Cognitive Linguistic Quick Test*. San Antonio, TX: Psychological Corporation.

Helm-Estabrooks, N. (2002). Cognition and aphasia: A discussion and a study. *Journal of Communication Disorders, 35*, 171–186.

Helm-Estabrooks, N., Ramsberger, G., Morgan, A. R., & Nicholas, M. (1989). *Boston Assessment of Severe Aphasia*. Austin, TX: Pro-Ed.

Herbert, R., Hickin, J., Howard, D., Osborne, F., & Best, W. (2008). Do picture-naming tests provide a valid assessment of lexical retrieval in conversation in aphasia. *Aphasiology, 22*(2), 184–204.

Hersh, D., Worrall, L., O'Halloran, R., Brown, K., Grohn, B., & Rodriguez, A. D. (2013). Assess for success. In N. Simmons-Mackie, J. M. King, & D. R. Beukelman (Eds.), *Supporting communication for adults with acute and chronic aphasia* (pp. 145–164). Baltimore: Brookes.

Hilari, K., Byng, S., Lamping, D. L., & Smith, S. C. (2003). Stroke and Aphasia Quality of Life Scale–39 (SAQOL-39): Evaluation of acceptability, reliability, and validity. *Stroke, 34*, 1944–1950.

Hilari, K., Owen, S., & Farrelly, S. (2007). Proxy and self-report agreement on the Stroke and Aphasia Quality of Life Scale–39. *Journal of Neurology, Neurosurgery and Psychiatry, 78*, 1072–1075.

Hill, A. J., Theodoros, D. G., Russell, T. G., Ward, E. C., & Wootton, R. (2009). The effects of aphasia severity on the ability to assess language disorders via telerehabilitation. *Aphasiology, 23*(5), 627–642.

Holland, A., Frattali, C., & Fromm, D. (1999). *Communication Activities of Daily Living* (2nd ed.). Austin, TX: Pro-Ed.

Holtzapple, P., Pohlman, K., LaPointe, L. L., & Graham, L. F. (1989). Does SPICA mean PICA? *Clinical Aphasiology, 18*, 131–144.

Howard, D., & Patterson, K. E. (1992). *Pyramids and palm trees*. Bury St. Edmunds, England: Thames Valley Test.

Huber, W., Poeck, K., Weniger, D., & Willmes, K. (1983). *Der Aachener Aphasie Test*. Göttingen, Germany: Hogrefe.

Hussmann, K., Grande, M., Meffert, E., Christoph, S., Piefke, M., Willmes, K., et al. (2012). Computer-assisted analysis of spontaneous speech: Quantification of basic parameters in aphasic and unimpaired language. *Clinical Linguistics and Phonetics, 26*(8), 661–680.

Irwin, W., Wertz, R., & Avent, J. (2002). Relationships among language impairment, functional communication, and pragmatic performance in aphasia. *Aphasiology, 16*, 823–835.

Ivanova, M., & Hallowell, B. (2013). A tutorial on aphasia test development in any language: Key substantive and psychometric considerations. *Aphasiology, 27*(8), 891–920.

Kagan, A., Winckel, J., Black, S., Duchan, J., Simmons-Mackie, N., & Square, P. (2004). A set of observational measures for rating support and participation in conversation between adults with aphasia and their conversation partners. *Topics in Stroke Rehabilitation, 11*(1), 67–83.

Kalbe, E., Reinhold, N., Brand, M., Markowitsch, J. J., & Kessler, J. (2005). A new test battery to assess aphasic disturbances and associated cognitive dysfunctions—German normative data on the Aphasia Check List. *Journal of Clinical and Experimental Neuropsychology, 27,* 779–794.

Kamhi, A. G. (1994). Research to practice. Toward a theory of clinical expertise in speech-language pathology. *Language, Speech, Hearing Services in Schools, 25,* 115–118.

Kaplan, E., Goodglass, H., & Weintraub, S. (2001). *Boston Naming Test* (2nd ed.). Philadelphia: Lippincott Williams & Wilkins.

Kay, J., Lesser, R., & Coltheart, M. (1997). *Psycholinguistic assessments of language processing in aphasia.* Hove, England: Psychology Press.

Kempler, D., Teng, E. L., Taussig, M., & Dick, M. B. (2010). The Common Objects Memory Test (COMT): A simple test with cross-cultural applicability. *Journal of the International Neuropsychology Society, 16*(3), 537–545.

Kertesz, A. (2007). *Western Aphasia Battery—Revised.* San Antonio, TX: Psychological Corporation.

Klippi, A., Sellman, J., Heikkinen, P., & Laine, M. (2012). Current clinical practices in aphasia therapy in Finland: Challenges in moving towards national best practice. *Folia Phoniatrica et Logopaedica, 64,* 169–178.

Kong, A. (2011). The main concept analysis in Cantonese aphasic oral discourse: External validation and monitoring chronic aphasia. *Journal of Speech, Language, and Hearing Research, 54,* 148–159

Langdon, H. W., & Cheng, L. L. (2002). *Collaborating with interpreters and translators: A guide for communication disorders professionals.* Austin, TX: Pro-Ed.

Laska, A. C., Bartfai, A., Hellblom, A., Murray, V., & Kahan, T. (2007). Clinical and prognostic properties of standardized and functional aphasia assessments. *Journal of Rehabilitation Medicine, 39,* 387–392.

Lata-Caneda, M. C., Pineiro-Temprano, M., Garcia-Fraga, I., Garcia-Armesto, I., Barrueco-Egido, J., & Meijide-Failde, R. (2009). Spanish adaptation of the Stroke and Aphasia Quality of Life Scale–39 (SAQOL-39). *European Journal of Physical and Rehabilitation Medicine, 45,* 1–6.

Lauterbach, M., Martins, I., Garcia, P., Cabeca, J., Ferreira, A., & Willmes, K. (2008). Cross linguistic aphasia testing: The Portuguese version of the Aachen Aphasia Test. *Journal of the International Neuropsychological Society, 14,* 1046–1056.

Leonard, C., Rochon, E., & Laird, L. (2008). Training naming impairments in aphasia: Findings from a phonological components analysis treatment. *Aphasiology, 22*(9), 923–947.

Lezak, M. D., Howieson, D., & Loring, D. (2004). *Neuropsychological assessment* (4th ed.). New York: Oxford University Press.

Lidz, C., & Elliott, J. G. (2000). *Dynamic assessment: Prevailing models and applications.* Amsterdam: JAI.

Lidz, C. S., & Peña, E. D. (1996). Dynamic assessment: The model, its relevance as a nonbiased approach, and its application to Latino American preschool children. *Language, Speech, and Hearing Services in Schools, 27,* 367–372.

Lind, M., Kristoffersen, K., Moen, I., & Simonsen, H. (2009). Semi-spontaneous oral text production: Measurements in clinical practice. *Clinical Linguistics and Phonetics, 23*(12), 872–886.

Lomas, J., Pickard, L., Bester, S., Elbard, H., Finlayson, A., & Zoghaib, C. (1989). The Communicative Effectiveness Index: Development and psychometric evaluation of functional communication measure for adult aphasia. *Journal of Speech and Hearing Disorders, 54,* 113–124.

Long, A. F., Hesketh, A., Paszek, G., Booth, M., & Bowen, A. (2008). Development of a reliable self-report outcome measure for pragmatic trials of communication therapy following stroke: The Communication Outcome After Stroke (COAST) scale. *Clinical Rehabilitation, 22,* 1083–1094.

Long, A. F., Hesketh, A., & Bowen, A. (2009). Communication outcome after stroke: A new measure of the carer's perspective. *Clinical Rehabilitation, 23,* 846–856.

Lorenzen, B., & Murray, L. L. (2008). Bilingual aphasia: A theoretical and clinical review. *American Journal of Speech-Language Pathology, 17,* 1–19.

Lucas, J. A., Ivnik, R. J., Smith, G. E., Ferman, T., Willis, F., Petersen, R., et al. (2005). Mayo's older African Americans normative studies: Norms for Boston Naming Test, Controlled Oral Word Association, category fluency, animal naming, Token Test, WRAT-3 Reading, Trail Making Test, Stroop Test, and Judgment of Line Orientation. *Clinical Neuropsychologist, 19,* 243–269.

Lunardelli, A., Mengotti, P., Pesavento, V., Sverzut, A., & Zadini, A. (2009). The Brief Neuropsychological Screening (BNS): Valuation of its clinical validity. *European Journal of Physical and Rehabilitation Medicine, 45,* 85–91.

Luria, A. R., Naydin, V. L., Tsvetkova, L. S., & Vinarskaya, E. N. (1969). Restoration of higher cortical function following local brain damage. In P. J. Vinken & G. W. Bruyn (Eds.), *Handbook of clinical neurology: Vol. 3. Disorders of higher nervous activity* (pp. 368–433). Amsterdam: North Holland.

MacWhinney, B. (2000). *The CHILDES Project: Tools for analysing talk* (3rd ed.) Mahwah, NJ: Erlbaum.

Marquez de la Plata, C., Arango-Lasprilla, J. C., Alegret, M., Moreno, A., Tarraga, L., Lara, M., et al. (2009). Item analysis of three Spanish naming tests: A cross-cultural investigation. *NeuroRehabilitation, 24,* 75–85.

Martin, N., & Saffran, E. M. (1992). A computational account of deep dysphasia: Evidence from a single case study. *Brain and Language, 43,* 240–274.

Mayer, J. F., & Murray, L. L. (2003). Functional measures of naming in aphasia: Word-retrieval in confrontation naming versus connected speech. *Aphasiology, 17,* 481–498.

McNeil, M. R., & Prescott, T. E. (1978). *Revised Token Test.* Baltimore: University Park Press.

Messinis, L., Malegiannaki, A., Christodoulou, T., Panagiotopoulos, V., & Papathanasopoulos, P. (2011). Color Trails Test: Normative data and criterion validity for the Greek adult population. *Archives of Clinical Neuropsychology, 26*(4), 322–330.

Miller, E., Murray, L., Richards, L., Zorowitz, R., Bakas, T., Clark, P., et al. (2010). Comprehensive overview of nursing and interdisciplinary rehabilitation care of the stroke patient. *Stroke, 41*(10), 2402–2448.

Miller, N., Willmes, K. & De Bleser, R. (2000). The psychometric properties of the English language version of the Aachen Aphasia Test (EAAT). *Aphasiology, 14*(7), 683–722.

Milman, L. & Holland, A. (2012). *Scales of Cognitive and Communicative Ability for Neurorehabilitation.* Austin, TX: Pro-Ed.

Milman, L., Holland, A., Kaszniak, A., D'Agostino, J., Garrett, M., & Rapcsak, S. (2008). Initial validity and reliability of the SCCAN using tailored testing to assess adult cognition and communication. *Journal of Speech, Language, and Hearing Research, 51,* 49–69.

Mitrushina, M., Boone, K. B., Razani, J., & D'Elia, L. F. (2005). *Handbook of normative data for neuropsychological assessment* (2nd ed.). New York: Oxford University Press.

Molrine, C. J., & Pierce, R. S. (2002). Black and white adults' expressive language performance on three tests of aphasia. *American Journal of Speech-Language Pathology*, 11, 139–150.

Muma, J. R. (1978). *Language handbook: Concepts, assessment, intervention.* Englewood Cliffs, NJ: Prentice Hall.

Murray, L. L. (1998). Longitudinal treatment of primary progressive aphasia: A case study. *Aphasiology*, 12, 651–672.

Murray, L. L. (2000). The effects of varying attentional demands on the word-retrieval skills of adults with aphasia, right hemisphere brain-damage or no brain-damage. *Brain and Language*, 72, 40–72.

Murray, L. L. (2004). Cognitive treatments for aphasia: Should we and can we help attention and working memory problems? *Journal of Medical Speech-Language Pathology*, 12, xxi–xxxviii.

Murray, L. L. (2012a). Assessing cognitive functioning in older patients: The why, who, what, and how. *Perspectives on Gerontology*, 17(1), 17–26.

Murray, L. L. (2012b). Attention and other cognitive deficits in aphasia: Presence and relation to language and communication measures. *American Journal of Speech-Language Pathology*, 21, 167–179.

Murray, L. L., & Chapey, R. (2001). Assessment of language disorders in adults. In R. Chapey (Ed.), *Language intervention strategies in adult aphasia* (4th ed., pp. 55–126). New York: Lippincott Williams & Wilkins.

Murray, L. L., & Clark, H. M. (2015). *Neurogenic disorders of language and cognition: Evidence-based clinical practice.* Austin, TX: Pro-Ed.

Nakase-Thompson, R., Manning, E., Sherer, M., Yablon, S. A., Gontkovsky, S., & Vickery, C. (2005). Brief assessment of severe language impairments: Initial validation of the Mississippi Aphasia Screening Test. *Brain Injury*, 19, 685–691.

National Institutes of Health & Northwestern University. (2006–2012). NIH Toolbox Reading Recognition Test. Retrieved May 25, 2015 from http://www.nihtoolbox.org/WhatAndWhy/Cognition/Language/Pages/NIH-Toolbox-Oral-Reading-Recognition-Test.aspx

Newton, C., Acres, K., & Bruce, C. (2013). A comparison of computerized and paper-based language tests with adults with aphasia. *American Journal of Speech-Language Pathology*, 22, 185–197.

Nicholas, L. E., & Brookshire, R. H. (1993). A system for quantifying the informativeness and efficiency of the connected speech of adults with aphasia. *Journal of Speech and Hearing Research*, 36, 338–350.

O'Halloran, R., Worrall, L., Toffolo, D., Code, C., & Hickson, L. (2004). *In-Patient Functional Communication Interview.* Oxen, UK: Speechmark.

Olness, G. S., Gyger, J., & Thomas, K. (2012). Analysis of narrative functionality: Toward evidence-based approaches in managed care settings. *Seminars in Speech and Language*, 33, 55–67.

Palsbo, S. E. (2007). Equivalence of functional communication assessment in speech pathology using videoconferencing. *Journal of Telemedicine and Telecare*, 13, 40–43.

Paradis, M. (2004). *A neurolinguistic theory of bilingualism.* Amsterdam: Benjamins.

Paradis, M. (2011). Principles underlying the Bilingual Aphasia Test (BAT) and its uses. *Clinical Linguistics and Phonetics*, 25(6–7), 427–443.

Paradis, M., & Libben, G. (1987). *The assessment of bilingual aphasia.* Hillsdale, NJ: Erlbaum.

Paul-Brown, D., Frattali, C. M., Holland, A. L., Thompson, C. K., Caperton, C. J., & Slater, S. C. (2004). *Quality of Communication Life Scale.* Rockville, MD: American Speech-Language-Hearing Association.

Pedraza, O., & Mungas, D. (2008). Measurement in cross-cultural neuropsychology. *Neuropsychology Review*, 18, 184–193.

Pickard, A. S., Johnson, J., Feeney, D., Shuaib, A., Carriere, K. C., & Nasser, A. M. (2004). Agreement between patient and proxy assessments of health-related quality of life after stroke using the EQ-5D and health utilities index. *Stroke*, 35, 607–612.

Pontón, M. L., Satz, P., Herrera, L., Young, R., Ortiz, F., D'Elia, L., et al. (1992). Modified Spanish version of the Boston Naming Test. *Clinical Neuropsychologist*, 3(6), 334.

Porch, B. E. (1981). *Porch Index of Communicative Ability: Vol. 2: Administration, scoring, and interpretation* (3rd ed.). Palo Alto, CA: Consulting Psychologists Press.

Poslawsky, I., Schuurmans, M., Lindeman, E., & Hafsteinsdottir, T. (2010). A systematic review of nursing rehabilitation of stroke patients with aphasia. *Journal of Clinical Nursing*, 19, 17–32.

Posteraro, L., Formis, A., Grassi, E., Bighi, M., Nati, P., Proietti Bocchini, C., et al. (2006). Quality of life and aphasia. Multicentric standardization of a questionnaire. *Europa Medicophysica*, 42(3), 227–230.

Prins, R., & Bastiaanse, R. (2004). Analysing the spontaneous speech of aphasic speakers. *Aphasiology*, 18, 1075–1091.

Prutting, C., & Kirchner, D. M. (1987). A clinical appraisal of the pragmatic aspects of language. *Journal of Speech and Hearing Disorders*, 52, 105–119.

Rami, L., Serradell, M., Bosch, B., Caprile, C., Sekler, A., Villar, A., et al. (2008). Normative data for the Boston Naming Test and the Pyramids and Palm Trees Test in the elderly Spanish population. *Journal of Clinical and Experimental Neuropsychology*, 30(1), 1–6.

Raven, J. C. (2003). *Raven's Progressive Matrices.* San Antonio, TX: Pearson.

Roberts, P. (2008). Aphasia assessment and treatment for bilingual and culturally diverse patients. In R. Chapey (Ed.), *Language intervention strategies in aphasia and related neurogenic disorders* (pp. 245–275). Baltimore: Lippincott Williams & Wilkins.

Roberts, P., & Doucet, N. (2011). Performance of French-speaking Quebec adults on the Boston Naming Test. *Canadian Journal of Speech-Language Pathology and Audiology*, 35(3), 254–264.

Robertson, I. H., Ward, T., Ridgeway, V., & Nimmo-Smith, I. (1994). *The Test of Everyday Attention.* Gaylord, MI: Northern Speech Services.

Robinson, B. C. (1983). Validation of a caregiver strain index. *Journal of Gerontology*, 38, 344–348.

Rochon, E., Saffran, E. M., Berndt, R. S., & Schwartz, M. F. (2000). Quantitative analysis on aphasic sentence production: Further development and new data. *Brain and Language*, 72, 193–218.

Roger, P., & Code, C. (2011). Lost in translation? Issues of content validity in interpreter-mediated aphasia assessments. *International Journal of Speech-Language Pathology*, 13(1), 61–73.

Rosenbek, J. C., Lapointe, L. L., & Wertz, R. T. (1989). *Aphasia: A clinical approach.* Austin, TX: Pro-Ed.

Ross, K. B., & Wertz, R. T. (1999). Comparison of impairment and disability measures for assessing severity of, and improvement in, aphasia. *Aphasiology, 13*, 113–124.

Ross, K. B., & Wertz, R. T. (2004). Accuracy of formal tests for diagnosing mild aphasia: An application of evidence-based medicine. *Aphasiology, 18*, 337–355.

Rousseaux, M., Delacourt, A., Wyrzykowski, N., & Lefeuvre, M. (2001). *TLC: Test Lillois de Communication*. Isbergues, France: Orthoédition.

Ruff, R. (1996). *Ruff Figural Fluency Test*. Lutz, FL: Psychological Assessment Resources.

Salter, K., Jutai, J., Foley, N., Hellings, C., & Teasell, R. (2006). Identification of aphasia post stroke: A review of screening assessment tools. *Brain Injury, 20*(6), 559–568.

Sbordone, R. J. (1996). Ecological validity: Some critical issues for the neuro-psychologist. In R. J. Sbordone & C. J. Long (Eds.), *Ecological validity of neuropsychological testing* (pp. 15–41). Delray Beach, FL: St. Lucie Press.

Schretlen, D. (2011). *Modified Wisconsin Card Sorting Test*. Lutz, FL: PAR.

Shadden, B. (1998). Obtaining the discourse sample. In L. R. Cherney, B. Shadden, & C. A. Coelho (Eds.), *Analyzing discourse in communicatively impaired adults* (pp. 35–64). Gaithersburg, MD: Aspen.

Silverberg, N. D., & Millis, S. R. (2009). Impairment versus deficiency in neuropsychological assessment: Implications for ecological validity. *Journal of the International Neuropsychological Society, 15*, 94–102.

Simmons-Mackie, N. (2008). Intervention for a case of severe apraxia of speech and aphasia: A functional-social perspective. In N. Martin, C. Thompson, & L. Worrall (Eds.), *Aphasia rehabilitation: The impairment and its consequences* (pp. 75–108). San Diego, CA: Plural.

Simmons-Mackie, N., & Kagan, A. (2007). Application of the ICF in aphasia. *Seminars in Speech and Language, 28*, 244–253.

Swinburn, K., Porter, G., & Howard, D. (2004). *Comprehensive Aphasia Test*. East Sussex, England: Psychology Press.

Tallberg, I. M. (2005). The Boston Naming Test in Swedish: Normative data. *Brain and Language, 94*, 19–31.

Tempest, S., Harries, P., Kilbride, C., & De Souza, L. (2013). Enhanced clarity and holism: The outcome of implementing the ICF with an acute stroke multidisciplinary team in England. *Disability and Rehabilitation, 35*(22), 1921–1925.

Theodoros, D., Hill, A., Russell, T., Ward, E., & Wootton, R. (2008). Assessing acquired language disorders in adults via the Internet. *Telemedicine and e-Health, 14*(6), 552–559.

Thompson, C. K. (2011). *Northwestern Assessment of Verbs and Sentences*. Evanston, IL: Northwesten University.

Tomblin, J. B., Morris, H. L., & Spriestersbach, D. C. (2000). *Diagnosis in speech-language pathology*. San Diego, CA: Singular.

Trahan, D. E., & Larrabee, G. J. (1988). *Continuous Visual Memory Test*. Lutz, FL: Psychological Assessment Resources.

Tucker, F., Edwards, D., Kirchner Mathews, L., Baum, C., & Tabor Connor, L. (2012). *American Journal of Occupational Therapy, 66*, 42–50.

Turner, S., & Whitworth, A. (2006). Conversational partner training programmes in aphasia: A review of key themes and participants' roles. *Aphasiology, 20*(6), 483–510.

Ulatowska, H. K., Olness, G., Hill, C., Roberts, J., & Keebler, M. (2000). Repetition in narrative of African Americans: The effect of aphasia. *Discourse Processes, 30*, 265–283.

Vanbellingen, T., Kersten, B., Van Hemelrijk, B., Van de Winckel, A., Bertschi, M., Muri, R., et al. (2010). Comprehensive assessment of gesture production: A new test of upper limb apraxia (TULIA). *European Journal of Neurology, 17*, 59–66.

van der Meulen, I., van de Sandt-Koenderman, W., Duivenvoorden, H. J., & Ribbers, G. (2010). Measuring verbal and non-verbal communication in aphasia: Reliability, validity, and sensitivity to change of the Scenario Test. *International Journal of Rehabilitation Research, 45*, 424–435.

van de Sandt-Koenderman, W., van Harskamp, F., Duivenvoorden, H. J., Remerie, S., van der Voort-Klees, Y., Wielaert, S., et al. (2008). MAAS (Multi-axial Aphasia System): Realistic goal setting in aphasia rehabilitation. *International Journal of Rehabilitation Research, 31*, 314–320.

Van Mourik, M., Verschaeve, M., Boon, P., Paquier, P., & Van Harskamp, F. (1992). Cognition in global aphasia: Indicators for therapy. *Aphasiology, 6*, 491–499.

Vogel, A., Maruff, P., & Morgan, A. (2010). Evaluation of communication assessment practices during the acute stages post stroke. *Journal of Evaluation in Clinical Practice, 16*, 1183–1188.

Wallace, G., & Hammill, D. D. (2013). *Comprehensive Receptive and Expressive Vocabulary Test* (3rd ed.). Austin, TX: Pro-Ed.

Weschler, D. (2009). *Weschler Memory Scale* (4th ed.). San Antonio, TX: Pearson.

West, J., Sands, E., & Ross-Swain, D. (1998). *Bedside Evaluation Screening Test of Aphasia* (2nd ed.). Austin, TX: Pro-Ed.

Whitworth, A., Webster, J., & Howard, D. (2005). *A cognitive neuropsychological approach to assessment and intervention in aphasia*. Hove, England: Psychology Press.

Whurr, R. (1988). The speech therapist's assessment of aphasia. In F. Clifford Rose, R. Whurr, & M. A. Wyke (Eds.), *Aphasia* (pp. 445–470). London: Whurr.

Whurr, R. (2011). *The Aphasia Screening Test* (3rd ed.). Milton Keynes, UK: Speechmark.

Wiederholt, J. L., & Bryant, B. R. (2012). *Gray Oral Reading Tests* (5th ed.). Austin, TX: Pro-Ed.

Wilshire, C., Lukkien, C., & Burmester, B. (2014). The sentence production test for aphasia. *Aphasiology, 28*(6), 658–691.

Wilson, B. A., Cockburn, J., & Halligan, P. (1987). *The Behavioral Inattention Test*. Bury St. Edmunds, England: Thames Valley Test.

World Health Organization. (2001). *ICF: International classification of functioning, disability, and health*. Geneva, Switzerland: Author.

Worrall, L., Davidson, B., Hersh, D., Howe, T., Sherratt, S., & Ferguson, A. (2010). The evidence for relationship-centered practice in aphasia rehabilitation. *Journal of Interactional Research in Communication Disorders, 1*, 277–300.

Zec, R. F., Burkett, N. R., Markwell, S. J., & Larsen, D. L. (2007). Normative data stratified for age, education, and gender on the Boston Naming Test. *Clinical Neuropsychology, 21*(4), 617–637.

Zinn, S., Bosworth, H., Hoenig, H., & Swartzwelder, H. (2007). Executive function deficits in acute stroke. *Archives of Physical Medicine and Rehabilitation, 88*(2), 173–180.

OBJECTIVES

The reader will be able to:

1. **Describe what therapy is and what it encompasses.**

2. **Distinguish among the International Classification of Functioning, Disability, and Health (ICF) disability components.**

3. **Determine who the target of therapy is and who determines the type of therapy provided.**

4. **Outline when therapy should start and finish and how often it should take place.**

5. **Broadly distinguish between the different therapy approaches.**

6. **Gain an understanding of the process of therapy using the cycle of five steps at each stage of rehabilitation.**

7. **Delineate the usual course of rehabilitation experienced by a person with aphasia and his or her family members.**

Therapy Approaches to Aphasia

Linda Worrall, Sue Sherratt, and Ilias Papathanasiou

INTRODUCTION

This chapter aims to provide clinicians a broad overview of therapy for aphasia. The first part of the chapter establishes the overarching context of therapy—the who, what, when, and why of therapy. This discussion shows that there are many different therapy approaches. Each approach should be guided by a strong rationale. A good clinician can provide a strong rationale for the approach taken with each and every client. The rationale not only integrates the needs of the client but also the research literature and the therapist's experience and constraints. When all three sources of practice knowledge are integrated, evidence-based practice is realized. The second part of the chapter provides more detail about therapy, in particular the process of therapy. This is illustrated in the final section by a case study of therapy for a person with aphasia.

WHAT IS THERAPY?

Most students and clinicians describe therapy in terms of one-on-one, face-to-face treatment of the communication deficit associated with aphasia. This is often termed *direct therapy*. Although direct therapy is the focus of this chapter because it is the mainstay of aphasia rehabilitation, clinicians could first consider other indirect ways that a speech–language pathologist can help a person with aphasia. Many interventions can and should be conducted in parallel to one-on-one direct communication therapy and so should be considered as an essential part of comprehensive service delivery. The indirect approaches are sometimes not considered "aphasia treatment," but the scope of therapy cannot be considered in isolation from the aspect of aphasia that therapy is seeking to change. The International Classification of Functioning, Disability, and Health (ICF) or a biopyschosocial approach is a useful and widely accepted conceptual framework for considering questions about both what therapy is and which aspects of aphasia should be the targets of intervention. The ICF provides a useful framework for aphasia rehabilitation. It combines both the medical and social models of disability, so it is often termed a "biopsychosocial" approach. This combined or holistic approach is well suited to aphasia rehabilitation because historically both the medical and social models have been considered as separate and distinct approaches in aphasia rehabilitation. Hillis, Worrall, and Thompson (2008) concluded that the approaches only differ in their relative emphasis, but both approaches cover all domains.

The ICF primarily consists of two main parts: the functioning or disability of the person with the health condition and the contextual factors that can affect the person to either improve or worsen the disability. The disability associated with aphasia is described in terms of impairments, activity limitations, and participation restrictions. A person with aphasia therefore has *language impairments* (e.g., comprehension difficulties, lexical access difficulties, syntactic difficulties); *communication activity limitations* (e.g., conversation difficulties, difficulty using the phone, difficulty reading a newspaper); and *participation restrictions* (e.g., employment restrictions, relationship restrictions). The difference between the impairment component and the participation restriction component is the increasing effect of context (Davidson & Worrall, 2000). Contextual factors for the disability are considered to act as either barriers or facilitators of the disability. Both environmental factors (i.e., external to the person) and personal factors (i.e., internal preaphasia factors such as age, gender, and coping style) are considered to affect the level of disability.

Stucki, Ewert, and Cieza (2003) considered the ICF as a framework that spans the broadest spectrum of health from the cell to society. In the same way, the ICF system conceptualizes aphasia from the behavioral effects of cell damage in the language pathways of the brain all the way to the effect this has on the person's functioning in society and, in turn, society's effect on the functioning or disability of the person.

The living with aphasia: Framework for outcome measurement (A-FROM; Kagan et al., 2008) (see Figure 6.1) is a diagrammatic representation of the ICF domains that are particularly relevant to aphasia. Therapy can therefore intervene in any component of this dynamic process. Therapy should aim to reduce the overall disability (impairment, activity limitations, or participation restrictions) associated with aphasia. Direct therapy can achieve this by improving language function (e.g., better comprehension, word retrieval, or sentence structure); everyday communication activities (e.g., conversation, writing shopping lists, paying bus fares); or social participation (e.g., maintaining and developing friendships, facilitating voting in elections). Reducing the communication disability of aphasia can also be achieved by optimizing contextual factors. Environmental barriers and facilitators for people with aphasia include communicative behavior of other people and aphasia-friendly information (Howe, Worrall, & Hickson, 2008; Le Dorze, Salois-Bellerose, Alepins, Croteau, & Hallé, 2014). There is a dynamic interaction between disability and the environment so that the environment needs to accommodate a person's disability so that the person can access society. For example, in the same way that wheelchair ramps facilitate physical access to buildings, communication access can be facilitated through the use of iconic symbols instead of words. Therapists can therefore create an aphasia-friendly environment by implementing the following techniques:

- Write information with aphasia-friendly formatting (e.g., simplified sentences, larger font, white space, appropriate illustrations) (T. A. Rose, Worrall, & McKenna, 2003)
- Facilitate group therapy in which barriers and facilitators are discussed (Elman, 2007).
- Implement communication partner training (i.e., training the family members or friends of the person with aphasia to communicate well with people with aphasia) (Simmons-Mackie, Raymer, Armstrong, Holland, & Cherney, 2010)
- Support and routinely refer clients to advocacy or support organizations (e.g., National Aphasia Association, Speakability, Australian Aphasia Association, Connect, Aphasia Institute)
- Improve societal attitudes toward and public awareness of aphasia (e.g., by talking to hospital staff about aphasia, talking to the media about aphasia).

Speech and language pathologists can also help create an enriched communicative environment to stimulate communication for people with aphasia with the following strategies:

- Providing them with many opportunities to communicate (e.g., ensuring that visitors to patients with aphasia continue to visit by facilitating good communication practices; group therapy at all stages of rehabilitation, including the early stages) (Brown, Davidson, Worrall, & Howe, 2013; Lanyon, Rose, & Worrall, 2013; Simmons-Mackie & Kagan, 1999)

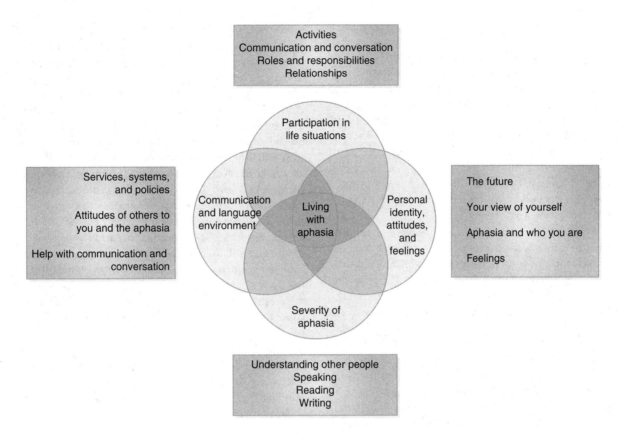

Figure 6.1 A-FROM domains.
Courtesy of The Aphasia Institute.

- Providing challenging communicative opportunities (e.g., public speaking, radio interviews)
- Encouraging people with aphasia to write their story for newsletters, websites, or their own family (Hinckley, 2006) or express their experiences through painting, drawing, or other media
- Forming a book club so that people are challenged to read (Bernstein-Ellis & Elman, 2007)
- Modifying personal preaphasia factors such as coping styles, aspects of feelings, and personal identity (Le Dorze et al., 2014; Shadden, 2005; Shadden & Koski, 2007).

Speech and language pathologists can optimize the effect of personal factors in the following ways:

- Counseling and optimizing daily well-being. For example, speech and language pathologists can refer to professional counselors who are trained by them to communicate with people with aphasia. They can ensure that staff and family maintain positive communication patterns, such as by reinforcing what they have achieved at the end of a therapy session and what the next goal is and by giving regular feedback on progress (Ryff & Singer, 1998, 2000; Simmons-Mackie & Damico, 2011).
- Referring clients to self-management programs that improve a person's ability to solve problems that occur in everyday life (Jones, Riazi, & Norris, 2013).

In summary, therapy can be direct or indirect, depending on which aspect of functioning the person with aphasia and the treatment team wishes to target with therapy. The ICF provides a conceptual framework for human functioning and can therefore be used to map a treatment plan for people with aphasia. A recent and unique aphasia rehabilitation pathway, the Australian Aphasia Rehabilitation Pathway (NHMRC CCRE in Aphasia Rehabilitation, 2014) has been designed for speech–language pathologists to help guide person-centered, evidence-based care across all stages of the aphasia rehabilitation journey. This pathway, divided into eight key areas, includes 82 best practice statements together with supporting information, resources, and references.

WHO IS THE TARGET OF THERAPY?

As discussed previously, the person with aphasia should be the central focus of the rehabilitation process. However, family members, friends, colleagues, and health-care workers are all affected by aphasia and need to be able to communicate with the person with aphasia. Family members in particular are essential to the success of rehabilitation. They also have suffered the loss of communication brought about by the aphasia (Draper et al., 2007; Hilari & Northcott, 2006) but are in a position to support the person with aphasia throughout the rehabilitation period and beyond. Social isolation and activity limitation is an all-too-frequent sequela of aphasia, sometimes for the spouse as well as for the person with aphasia, and as a consequence needs to be targeted early (Grawburg, Howe, Worrall, & Scarinci, 2013). Depression is another unwanted, possibly preventable, consequence of aphasia and is correlated with poorer quality of life and well-being (Cruice, Worrall, Hickson, & Murison, 2003; Hilari, Needle, & Harrison, 2012). The development and maintenance of social networks that include family members, friends, organizations, and groups therefore play a key role in maintaining well-being in aphasia and possibly preventing depression (Thomas & Lincoln, 2008; Thomas, Walker, Macniven, Haworth, & Lincoln, 2012). In addition to the strategies outlined previously, therapists can optimize the maintenance of social networks for people with aphasia with the following strategies:

- Offering communication partner training to family members and friends at all stages of rehabilitation, but particularly in the early stages (Kagan, Black, Duchan, Simmons-Mackie, & Square, 2001; Simmons-Mackie et al., 2010).
- Offering information and resources to existing friends and family (Aphasia Institute, 2003; Berens, 2006; Byng, Duchan, & Pound, 2007; Byng, Pound, & Swinburn, 2001).
- Recruiting experienced people with aphasia as volunteers to connect new patients with existing networks (Worrall, Davidson, Howe, & Rose, 2007).

What Is the Target of Therapy?

The traditional impairment-based or medical approach suggests that the goal of therapy is to focus on the language impairment of the person with aphasia. The goal of an impairment-based intervention is to provide treatments for the aspects of language that are impaired. Impairment-based treatments use models of normal language and cognitive processing to determine components and processes of language and communication systems that have been disrupted by brain damage. The main target of treatment is to improve them. Generalization and subsequent improvement in communicative functions, reduction of the disability, and an ability to participate in social activities should be the results of the treatment. However, intervention with the person with aphasia requires ongoing assessment of the impact of treatment on functional communication. Thus, although predictions can be made about the learning, generalization, and skills to be acquired by the person with aphasia, nothing can be assumed. If generalization and transfer of the language skills necessary for functional communication are not achieved in everyday life situations, then the target of treatment should be shifted to other and different cognitive and language structures and processes or focused directly on language use in everyday life skills.

Transfer and generalization of the language and communication skills targeted in therapy in everyday situations are key concepts for aphasia treatment to be effective. Byng (1995) stated the steps to encourage generalization are as follows:

- Outline the uses of language of the person with aphasia prior to the onset of aphasia.
- Facilitate accommodation to change in communication skills.
- Investigate the nature and effects of the language deficits with respect to the whole language system.
- Remediate the language deficit.
- Increase the use of all other potential means of communication to support, facilitate, and compensate for the impaired language.
- Enhance the use of the remaining language.
- Provide opportunities to use newly acquired and emerging language and communication skills in familiar communicative situations.

Who Decides What Therapy to Give?

The predominant paradigm in aphasia rehabilitation has been the speech and language pathologists as experts. Speech–language pathologists are educated in the complexity of language processing and the symptoms of aphasia so that they can diagnose, assess, and treat aphasia. They have therefore led the aphasia rehabilitation process in terms of when and where the service can be delivered as well as what the focus of the service and therapy should be. While taking the individual needs of the patient into account, the predominant paradigm has been a therapist-led approach (Leach, Cornwell, Fleming, & Haines, 2010).

An emerging trend is the client-as-expert paradigm. This client-led approach has appeared following several key qualitative studies that took a phenomenological (insider's) perspective (Byng, Pound, & Hewitt, 2004; Parr, Duchan, & Pound, 2003). This research provided greater understanding of the experiences of people with aphasia in the health-care system and showed that they and their families harbor some degree of dissatisfaction with speech–language pathology services (Worrall, 2006). Although some clients with aphasia are willing for the therapist to take the lead and some clients wish to dictate the direction of rehabilitation, many prefer a collaborative approach. A good clinician is able to negotiate the decision-making process with skill and expertise. There is some high-level evidence that clients who select their own goals in collaboration with the therapist have better outcomes (Levack, Dean, McPherson, & Siegert, 2006). The subsequent section on goal setting describes in more detail the process of negotiating goals with clients.

WHEN?

When Do People With Aphasia Need Help?

People with aphasia and their families may need help within days of onset, and if the aphasia persists, rehabilitation may be ongoing for many years; many individuals continue to improve and significant language gains can be made, even at relatively long times postonset (Allen, Mehta, McClure, & Teasell, 2012; El Hachioui et al., 2013). A large number (43%) of people diagnosed with aphasia at onset still had significant aphasia after 18 months (Laska, Hellblom, Murray, Kahan, & Von Arbin, 2001) and residual deficits up to 3 years postonset (El Hachioui, van de Sandt-Koenderman, Dippel, Koudstaal, & Visch-Brink, 2011). Hence, although many recover their language in that period, a significant proportion has aphasia for the rest of their life. Their need for therapy may vary according to the severity of the disorder and their integration back into the community, among other factors.

Usually, the demand for therapy outstrips the supply of speech–language pathology services. Although the amount of available aphasia therapy varies internationally, speech–language pathologists are committed to beneficence through a professional code of ethics and therefore aim to optimize service to their clients. If ongoing individual therapy is not an option, it is even more important for the therapist to connect the person with aphasia and his or her family to community supports such as aphasia or stroke groups and organizations.

The stages of rehabilitation are sometimes referred to as acute, rehabilitation, and community. Speech–language pathology services in countries like Australia, the United Kingdom, and the United States are mostly provided in the earlier acute and rehabilitation stages (Verna, Davidson, & Rose, 2009), but there continues to be a strong demand for services in the community after hospital rehabilitation has finished (M. Rose, Ferguson, Power, Togher, & Worrall, 2014). Therapy in these post spontaneous recovery periods has shown to be efficacious (Allen et al., 2012; Code, 2012; Goodman, 2013), so there is evidence to link successful outcomes to providing therapy many months or years after onset. Therapy should therefore be offered along the entire continuum of care.

When to Start?

Speech–language pathologists usually diagnose the presence of aphasia in the very early acute stages following a stroke. In the early emotional days after a stroke, however, other conditions, such as dysphagia, take precedence. The early days poststroke are also critical for a person with aphasia and the family. Not only is the person with aphasia coping with the sudden trauma of a stroke but also he or she is unable to use language to understand what is happening or to express basic health-care needs or turbulent emotions. The speech–language pathologist's role in these early stages following a stroke is therefore as follows:

- Attend to the immediate health-care needs that dysphagia often presents.
- Diagnose the presence or absence of aphasia and other communication disorders using professional judgment, informal assessments, or more formal screening assessments.
- Monitor the rapid changes that usually occur in the first few days by charting these in the medical notes, communicating these to anxious family and friends, as well as reassuring the patient.
- Inform and educate hospital staff and family and friends about the best way to communicate with the person with aphasia.
- Inform, support, and counsel the person with aphasia as well as his or her family and friends.

- Ensure that the person with aphasia is able to communicate health-care needs to hospital staff.
- Establish a communicatively accessible environment for the person with aphasia (Simmons-Mackie, 2013; Weissling & Harvey, 2013).
- Ensure that adequate supports and referrals to groups or support organizations are in place post-discharge.

Once a patient is alert and medically stable, a program of intervention that aims to rehabilitate the communicative functions that have been lost can begin. It is probable that the main goal of the patient and his or her family will simply be to return home from the hospital as soon as possible. Although physical function often determines whether a patient can safely return home, any added communicative deficits brought about by the aphasia can complicate hospital discharge. This may include the ability of the person with aphasia to seek help in an emergency so that he or she can be left at home alone. Speech–language pathologists may wish to prioritize for therapy the communicative functions required for safe discharge.

The transition from hospital to home is one of the most difficult phases for people with aphasia and their family. The speech–language pathologist must support them through this transition stage. It is critical that the speech–language pathologist provide information about available services, assist in establishing links with the community to prevent isolation and depression, and help the patient and family maintain a sense of hope and well-being. Practical examples of how this can be achieved include routinely offering a support organization visit to patients and their family in the hospital prior to discharge or once they are at home, introducing patients to a group that includes patients and families who have experienced aphasia for several years (Worrall et al., 2007), and answering the "Will I get better?" question with positivity and hope (i.e., "We don't know how much progress you will make, but together we hope to achieve a good outcome for you").

It is recommended that language therapy starts as early as possible to capitalize on spontaneous recovery (Godecke, Hird, & Lalor, 2008; Holland & Fridriksson, 2001). Scientific evidence also supports starting therapy early. Robey (1998) examined the magnitude of treatment effect sizes relative to the timing of treatment and found that treatment begun during the acute period (first 3 months postonset) resulted in almost twice the effect size of spontaneous and long-term recovery, and that the effect size of the treatment initiated during the subacute period (3 to 12 months postonset) was small but greater than in the untreated individuals. In addition, treatment started in the chronic period (after 1 year postonset) showed an effect size similar to that of the subacute period but still larger than in untreated individuals. Godecke and colleagues (Godecke et al., 2014; Godecke, Hird, Lalor, Rai, & Phillips, 2012) demonstrated that early-stage therapy results in improved communication outcomes compared to spontaneous recovery and in significantly greater communication gains compared to clients receiving usual care at both treatment termination and at 6 months. This shows that early treatment may be maximally beneficial but that later treatment also has some impact on language ability and use (e.g., Moss & Nicholas, 2006).

The following caveats, however, may affect an early start to language therapy: (a) The patient and the family should want language therapy; (b) the patient should be able to participate in and learn from language tasks; (c) health and well-being matter (e.g., depression) and should take precedence over language therapy; and (d) language therapy should be presented using a positive but realistic approach (Holland, 2007). The process of what to do in therapy is explained subsequently.

How Often?

The notion that providing intense treatment enhances recovery to a greater degree than distributed practice (e.g., once a week) was a basic principle of Schuell's approach to treatment in the 1960s (Schuell, Jenkins, & Jiminez-Pabon, 1964). Today, the intensity or dosage of therapy has been shown to be a factor affecting the efficacy of therapy. The principles of neuroplasticity (Raymer et al., 2008; Winstein & Kay, 2015), particularly the principle of "use it or lose it,", suggest that more intensive therapy promotes greater recovery. Robey (1998) reported that the more intense the treatment, the greater the change. In general, it appears that two or more hours of treatment per week result in greater change than treatment delivered at lower intensity. The optimal "dose" of therapy, however, is still not known.

Review articles (Brady, Kelly, Godwin, & Enderby, 2012; Cherney, Patterson, Raymer, Frymark, & Schooling, 2008) suggested that in chronic cases more intensive therapy is associated with better communication outcomes. Furthermore, there is some evidence that intensive therapy in chronic cases also yields better outcomes on measures of communication activity/participation (Pulvermuller et al., 2001; Winans-Mitrik et al., 2014).

All these authors suggested that there is modest evidence to support intensive treatment for people with aphasia, and that treatment decisions should be considered within the framework of evidence-based practice; that is, they should be made in conjunction with clinical expertise, the client's individual values, and service financial constraints (Code, 2012). However, none of these studies measured the effect of therapy intensity on quality-of-life measurements.

When to Finish?

The question of when to finish primarily emerges in hospital-based rehabilitation programs after some months of rehabilitation. Hospitals "discharge" patients, and hence speech–language pathologists are required to conform to hospital policies and discharge patients with aphasia. In addition, it was previously proposed that all recovery would occur in the first 6 to 12 months poststroke; therefore, when patients reached a plateau in language abilities, they were to be discharged. Two recent advances have challenged this common practice. First, neuroplasticity research contends that recovery of function through neuroplasticity of the brain may occur for years after a stroke (Meinzer, Djundja, Barthel, Elbert, & Rockstroh, 2005; Nadeau, 2014). Second, a chronic disease model in stroke and in health services recognizes that the effects of stroke cannot be rehabilitated completely in the first 6 to 12 months poststroke, and that ongoing issues will exist (Code, 2012; Epping-Jordan, Pruitt, Bengoa, & Wagner, 2004); this model is becoming more widely adopted. Indeed, often when the person with aphasia goes home and discovers the restrictions that aphasia imposes, he or she needs professional help to fend off depression and to facilitate community integration.

Hersh (1998) and others (Pound, 1998; Simmons-Mackie, 1998) challenged the professional concept of a plateau. This concept of language that will not improve with further therapy emerged when the sole purpose of speech pathology services was to improve language, that is, when the focus was on the language impairment only. The use of the term *plateau* is outdated, inaccurate, and potentially harmful; there is increasing evidence that language can improve with therapy many months and years after onset (Allen et al., 2012). Furthermore, the broader biopsychosocial approach predominates in modern rehabilitation, and Hersh's narratives of people with aphasia and their families tell of the significant negative impact of the use of this term.

This is not to say that people with aphasia cannot be discharged from a service. Health services operate under policy and funding constraints, and many services cannot provide aphasia rehabilitation beyond 6 to 12 months postonset. However, it is important that clients who are discharged have other services to go to. If these are not available, speech and language pathologists should make every effort to advocate for these services in partnership with people with aphasia and their families.

If a speech and language pathologist and the surrounding community and rehabilitation team have done their work well, the majority of clients with aphasia will self-discharge from community-based rehabilitation. The person with aphasia may have returned to former roles or will accept new roles and activities and will continue satisfying relationships or form new ones as well as accept the new language system that they have worked hard to achieve.

WHY?

What is the purpose of therapy? In the last few decades, there has been continuing debate about whether the purpose of therapy is to improve language skills, improve overall communication skills, or help the person live well with aphasia (Martin, Thompson, & Worrall, 2008). This debate stems from various interpretations of the nature of aphasia symptoms and gave rise to different schools of thought or approaches to therapy, which are still evolving (see Figure 6.2). Aphasia therapy is still challenged by different approaches and still lacks a single universally accepted aphasia therapy theory. Recent Cochrane reviews of speech and language therapy for aphasia following stroke (Brady et al., 2012; Kelly, Brady, & Enderby, 2010) concluded that currently available evidence suggests that there may be a benefit from speech and language therapy; however, there is currently no evidence that any therapy approach is superior to any other (Brady et al., 2012).

Current research in the domain of cognitive neurosciences shows that many early ideas about the brain and language were not completely correct. The most insightful finding is that language is subserved by a highly interactive neural network, which includes parts of the brain that were previously identified as language areas. Therefore, classic aphasia syndromes do not always coincide with specific brain lesions, and the symptomatology presented by specific individuals with aphasia does not always coincide with the description of classic aphasia

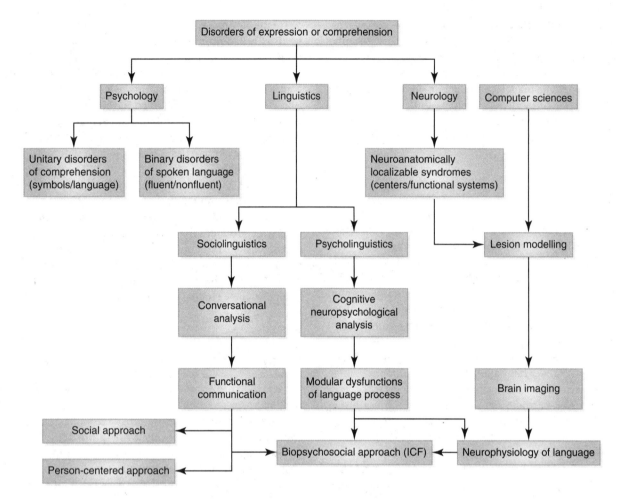

Figure 6.2 The developments of interpretations of aphasia.

This article was published in F. Fabbro (Ed.), *The Concise Encyclopedia Of Language Pathology* (pp. 294–304); Copyright Elsevier Science 1999.

types. This challenges some of the notions supported by the syndrome–site of lesion approach. In addition, research in neuroscience affects thinking about the mechanisms of recovery and the role of the environment in shaping recovery. Finally, psychoneurolinguistics research influences thinking of aphasia and its treatment, especially the mechanisms of sentence processing, while cognitive neuropsychological models of words and sentence processing have a significant effect on how assessment and intervention are planned. The most currently accepted approaches to aphasia therapy are presented in Table 6.1.

Although there are crucial philosophical differences among the approaches, which influence the targets of intervention to some extent, there are also similarities. All use mechanisms of learning and cognitive processes related to communication within a context of interaction that aims to improve the quality of life of a person with aphasia and his or her family by intervening with either the person or the environment. Further, these approaches take the person with aphasia through the same processes of therapy (as described further here) within each individual environment. The critical difference among them is the focus of therapy. Today, the term *biopsychosocial approach to therapy* is used to indicate that therapy should take into account the biological impairment-based factors and the psycholinguistic and cognitive processes of language and communication within the social context of the person with aphasia and his or her family. A *biopsychosocial approach* refers to treatment of a health condition such as aphasia following stroke,

Table 6.1 Theory Approaches

Approach	Aphasia as	Process of Therapy	Hypothesized Mechanism of Change	Examples of Influential Therapy Technique
Stimulation approach: Schuell	An obstacle to access language processing; a general problem varying only in severity	Intensive stimulation of disrupted language processes, then reeducation or correcting language	Restoration	Intensive auditory stimulation
Localization: Boston school	Syndrome based, classified according to grouping of symptoms and lesion sites	Stimulation with specific therapies for specific syndromes	Restoration Reconstitution Compensation	• Melodic intonation therapy • Visual action therapy • Voluntary control of involuntary utterances
Neurolinguistics	Neurologically caused language disorder that can be described using linguistic concepts	Reteaching of linguistic rules and processes	Restoration	Training of grammatical structures (e.g., wh- movements)
Cognitive neuropsychological	A collection of information-processing impairments that can be modality specific (components of the language-processing system are selectively impaired)	Explicit teaching of language-processing knowledge or alternative methods of achieving a language function	Restoration Reconstitution Compensation	• Mapping therapy • Naming facilitation techniques
Pragmatic/functional	A communication disability that primarily affects the ability of a person to engage in social interaction and everyday communication activities	Teaching of conversational principles; training of compensational strategies in the clients and/or the conversation partner	Rehearsal in everyday contexts Compensation in the client Learning for the partner	• Conversational coaching and training • Total communication • PACE (Promoting Aphasics Communicative Effectiveness) • Script training
Social	A communication disability within disabling environmental factors	Holistic and client directed; may include changing the barriers by communication training of partners and educating others in the community	Problem-based learning in partner, community, society	• Living with aphasia approach • Community aphasia groups • Information in aphasia-friendly formatting • Aphasia organizations
Biopsychosocial (ICF)	A disability resulting from a health condition (stroke/brain injury) that results in language impairment, activity limitations, and participation restrictions and influenced by environmental and personal contextual factors	Client-directed or therapist-directed choice of goals across the biopsychosocial spectrum	Restoration of language function; participation in communication activities and roles; enabling environments; optimizing personal factors	• All of the above

and sometimes the overarching aim of this approach is termed *health-related quality of life* (HRQL). The World Health Organization does not conceptualize quality of life within the ICF framework; however, there is clearly some overlap, as illustrated in the A-FROM (see Figure 6.1). Health-related quality of life, quality of life, life satisfaction, well-being, and life participation are all constructs that have arisen as potential terms for the overarching goal of therapy; however, there is a lack of consensus on the best construct or measure to use for people with aphasia.

Many approaches have been researcher or theory driven (e.g., Coelho, Sinotte, & Duffy, 2008; Schuell et al., 1964), but what do people with aphasia and their families want from aphasia rehabilitation? In a recent investigation (Sherratt, Worrall, Hersh, Howe, & Davidson, 2014; Worrall et al., 2011), 50 people with aphasia expressed nine broad categories of personal rehabilitation goals. They wanted to return to their prestroke life and to communicate not only their basic needs but also their opinions and feelings. They also wanted information about aphasia, stroke, and available services; more speech and language pathology services; greater autonomy; to regain their physical health; and dignity and respect. They highlighted the importance of being engaged in social, leisure, and work activities, as well as helping others. Their 49 family members identified six goals for themselves: they wanted information about aphasia, stroke, prognosis, and recovery and ways to communicate with the person with aphasia (Howe et al., 2012). They highlighted their desire to be included in the rehabilitation process and the need for hope. They expressed the need for general support and counseling and to have some space and time for themselves. First and foremost, family members wanted their relative with aphasia to survive and then to become independent, particularly in emergencies. Family members wanted their relative with aphasia to be able to communicate, to be involved in stimulating and meaningful activities, and to be socially engaged. Speech–language pathologists must be cognizant of these issues, listen to their clients' needs, and strive to meet these challenges (Rohde, Townley-O'Neill, Trendall, Worrall, & Cornwell, 2012; Sherratt et al., 2011, 2014).

HOW?

The Process of Therapy

Many students or novice clinicians ask, "But what do you actually do with clients with aphasia?" Most therapists reply, "It varies with each client!" Most clinicians, however, use a common process or set of steps (Worrall,

1999). There may be subtle variations depending on the context of the rehabilitation (e.g., acute versus rehabilitation vs. community). This section describes this process, and then presents a case study to show how these steps are translated into real therapy.

The five steps of therapy (Worrall, 1999) are as follows:

Step 1: Information Gathering and Sharing
Step 2: Collaborative Goal Setting
Step 3: Pretherapy Assessment (i.e., baselining)
Step 4: Therapy
Step 5: Reassessment

These steps are then repeated in as many cycles as required.

Step 1: Information Gathering and Sharing

Depending on the setting, information gathering may require reading the medical chart and conferring with the referring health professional. Information gathering should also refer to obtaining information about the person as a person (conversational style, preferred topics of conversation, conversational partners, regular communication activities, current concerns) from his or her family and from the person with aphasia. Although some tools are available for this (e.g., Worrall, 1999), a semistructured interview with the person with aphasia and his or her family that starts with, "Tell me about yourself," and then, "Tell me about your stroke and aphasia" will usually prompt clients to tell their story. The essence of this step is to obtain sufficient information prior to collaborative goal setting with the client. Hence, the clinician requires information from the client and the referring agencies about all aspects of the ICF, their health condition (stroke), the language impairment (aphasia), as well as other impairments that have occurred following the stroke, the everyday activities (particularly communicative) they need to or like to engage in, participation in life, and the context of the person with aphasia and the family.

Ideally, prior to collaborative goal setting the person with aphasia and family members should be informed about aphasia, stroke, and potential services. They should certainly know the term *aphasia* and what it means, what the likely consequences are in the long term, and what services can be provided to help. This information can be acquired from a number of sources, and the speech–language pathologist can enlist the help of volunteers with aphasia as well as provide accessible verbal and written information for both the person with aphasia and family members. Toward the end of this step, both the clinician and the client (the person with aphasia and the family) should have a shared knowledge of aphasia and current concerns. At this time, some clinicians prefer to take a baseline measure of the client's communicative functioning using standardized measures. This enables the clinician to provide feedback to the client about the severity of the aphasia and allows progress to be monitored throughout therapy. Other clinicians prefer to assess the patient fully once they know the client better and both parties have agreed on the overall goals of therapy.

Step 2: Collaborative Goal Setting

Goal setting is an important step that should occur early in the therapeutic process as well as at strategic points along the journey. It is an important component of evidence-based practice; identifying the clients' rehabilitation goals allows meaningful and effective treatment to occur (McPherson & Siegert, 2007; Winstein & Kay, 2015). Collaborative goal setting assumes that both the therapist and the client have a shared understanding of the problem and contribute equally to the process of setting goals. In the early stage of aphasia, family members may take on a greater share of this collaborative process than the person with aphasia, but as the person with aphasia begins to understand the nature of aphasia, he or she is usually willing to be more involved in establishing priorities.

The process begins with the client and speech–language pathologist identifying the major priorities at that time, and then these are converted into written goals. The conversation might start with the clinician requesting the client to tell the story of the stroke. This may lead into a discussion of how aphasia has affected the client. It should prompt some discussion of what long-term or life goals the client still has. Actively listening to the client (both the person with aphasia and his or her family) is an important component of collaborative goal setting. Allowing plenty of time and providing a quiet, private environment if possible are also highly desirable. Choosing important and relevant goals is one of the most crucial aspects of therapy; therefore, allocating enough time to this task is vital. As Thompson (2007) said: "If your ladder is leaning against the wrong wall, you'll find yourself expending your energy and effort faithfully, only to reach the top and realize it's not where you [or your client] desire to be."

In this process, the clinician and the client usually set both longer-term goals (e.g., to read a book) and shorter-term goals (e.g., to achieve 90% word–picture matching for verbs). The linking phrase in order to can be used to translate specific linguistic goals into everyday activity goals that the person with aphasia may have. For example, "We will achieve 90% word–picture matching for verbs in order to read a book."

Step 3: Pretherapy Assessment

Once specific goals are established, the therapist establishes a baseline for the task. Depending on the goal, this may mean that the client matches a set of 30 verbs and pictures, or if increased initiation of communication is the goal, then the number of times a client is observed initiating communication within a group therapy setting is recorded. Hence, the baseline task is tailored to the individual's goals. At this stage, therapists may complete a standardized assessment.

Therapists may wish to explore the language capabilities of the person with aphasia to determine the level of breakdown in the language-processing system. Assessments such as the PALPA (Psycholinguistic Assessments of Language Processing in Aphasia; Kay, Lesser, & Coltheart, 1992) or Comprehensive Aphasia Test (Swinburn, Porter, & Howard, 2004) are often used for this purpose. Assessment informs the therapist about the best type of language therapy for the individual client (e.g., naming therapy using semantic cues, syntax training). Therapists can use other standardized assessments (e.g., Western Aphasia Battery; Kertesz, 1982, 2006); functional assessments (e.g., American Speech-Language-Hearing Association Functional Assessment of Communication Skills for Adults [ASHA FACS]; Frattali, Thompson, Holland, Wohl, & Ferketic, 1995); or Communication Activities of Daily Living (Holland, 1980; Holland, Frattali, & Fromm, 1998), measures of quality of life (e.g., Quality of Communication Life; Paul et al., 2004), or assessments focusing on a number of aspects of living with aphasia (e.g., A-FROM; Kagan et al., 2010), depending on the primary focus of rehabilitation at that time. The choice to postpone standardized assessment until after the client and the therapist have had an opportunity to collaborate on shared goals is a deliberate strategy to enlist the client's participation in and ownership of the rehabilitation process.

Baselining serves to provide the client and speech-language pathologist with test scores that can measure progress over time. Tasks can be individually designed to baseline performance prior to therapy for specific items (e.g., number of verbs named, time taken to compose an e-mail message).

Step 4: Therapy

So far, the process of planning therapy should ensure that it is client focused, goal directed, and outcome oriented. The tasks of therapy should be aligned to goals so that, for example, the long-term goal of reading a book (an activity within the ICF framework) can be achieved through different strategies:

- By relearning component skills such as orthographic decoding and word recognition (impairment-level tasks)
- By practicing smaller chunks of the task, for example, reading headlines of newspapers (activity-level task)
- By modifying the environment by reading a simplified version of the book or listening to the audio version of the book at the same time as reading the book (environmental factor task)
- By participating in an aphasia book club that discusses the book after a modified version is read (participation-level task)

People with aphasia value therapy that is positive, that gives them hope, and that contributes to their well-being. This suggests that a strengths perspective (Worrall, 2000) is useful in that it focuses and builds on what the person can do rather than what he or she cannot do. It incorporates positive affirmations and frequent reports of positive progress as well as a "you-can-do-it" attitude. Furthermore, treatment that is salient, meaningful, motivating, and engaging for the client enhances the possibility of neuroplastic changes (Winstein & Kay, 2015).

The actual interaction taking place during the treatment session can be very structured (e.g., in the preceding example, the component skills of orthographic decoding) or more casual and can serve as an opportunity to maintain the relationship, motivate and enable the person with aphasia within the environment, and check connected speech and the changing needs of the client. Indirect therapy (as opposed to direct therapy described here) may also target environments (e.g., modifying the environment by providing a simpler version of the book), including conversational partners (Simmons-Mackie, 2013). Indirect therapy does not typically include a structured session. The speech-language pathologist communicates to the client (including the family members) clear objectives to achieve the short- and long-term goals with the overriding objective of facilitating maximal return of the communication abilities of the person with aphasia and subsequently his or her ability to participate in everyday life activities. This goal encompasses all modalities, linguistic processes, and levels of severity, as well as the contexts in which communication takes place.

The following general treatment sequence is an adaptation of the LaPointe (1982) impairment-based therapy sequence. It describes a typical clinical interaction or treatment sequence for many, but not all, tasks used in therapy:

1. Identify the change required in the performance of the person with aphasia.
2. Discuss the nature of the change required of the person with aphasia.
3. The person with aphasia produces the desired target spontaneously or with the help of the clinician through the use of a cueing hierarchy (e.g., phonologic cueing, repetition) or prompts to facilitate the response (reinforce).
4. Repetition stabilization (reinforce), first immediately and then with delay.
5. The person with aphasia transitions to volitional control (laddering: changing instructions; increasing length, complexity, and/or naturalness) (reinforce).
6. Check that the target is being performed in the clinic and then in real life.

Therapy does not need to be all direct therapy provided by the therapist. Group therapy and participation in community groups, activities, and events are important communication opportunities. (For further information on group therapy, see Elman, 1999, 2007; Kearns & Elman, 2001; Lanyon et al., 2013).

There are a number of recent and rapidly developing therapy approaches and supplements that hold promise for clients with aphasia. One current approach is constraint-induced aphasia therapy; in this intensive treatment, clients are not permitted to use compensatory strategies to communicate. The evidence thus far has shown that there is limited support for constraining clients' communication (M. Rose, 2013). Noninvasive brain stimulation to stimulate either the lesional or contralesional parts of the brain may provide additional applications in aphasia treatment (Brewer, Horgan, Hickey, & Williams, 2012; Galletta & Barrett, 2014). The use of drugs (e.g., piracetam) in combination with speech–language therapy has provided a moderate level of evidence for better communication outcomes (Berthier, Pulvermüller, Dávila, Casares, & Gutiérrez, 2011; Salter, Teasell, Foley, & Allen, 2013). Aphasia rehabilitation has not been slow to incorporate technology (King, 2013). Most programs using computers, tablets, or smartphones (usually impairment- or functionally based treatment) have had a beneficial effect on language skills (van de Sandt-Koenderman, 2011; Zheng, Lynch, & Taylor, 2015).

Step 5: Reassessment

Reassessment of the baseline tasks is part of the continuous cycle of therapy. Again, this can be overall progress measurement or baselining. Reassessment provides evidence of progress and may lead the clinician and client to negotiate a new goal either because the original goal has been achieved or because the client wants to set a different goal. The feedback loop is important for both the therapist and the client, so it is important to share and translate results for the client with aphasia and his or her family.

This cycle of five steps can continue throughout the entire rehabilitation process. The goals at onset are likely to change over time. For example, a common goal early poststroke is for the client to understand stroke and aphasia, whereas toward the end, a common goal is to help other people, including newly diagnosed people, understand stroke and aphasia. The pupil becomes the teacher. Another common early goal stated by people with aphasia is to recover completely from aphasia. Careful communication of prognosis is required to ensure that they have hope, but with the understanding that full recovery may not be possible. Later, people with aphasia have learned to live with it, and their goals turn to life goals, such as traveling or helping to raise grandchildren.

CONCLUSIONS AND FUTURE DIRECTIONS

Aphasia rehabilitation is fascinating, complex, challenging, and boundless; ultimately, it can be a lifeline for clients with aphasia and, on a personal level, can be one of the most rewarding roles for a speech–language pathologist. This chapter outlines the answers to the main questions surrounding the what, who, when, why, and how of aphasia therapy. It reminds the reader of the many approaches to aphasia therapy and condenses these into a common five-step process.

The case illustration that follows represents the ideal aphasia service that the next generation of speech–language pathologists could aspire to.

The future challenge for speech–language pathologists is to continue to work in partnership with people with aphasia, their families, and policy makers toward best practice in rehabilitation across the continuum of care; a person-centered, evidence-based rehabilitation pathway has already been initiated (NHMRC CCRE in Aphasia Rehabilitation, 2014). A consensus between these stakeholders on what constitutes best practice will propel aphasia therapy forward and yield maximum outcomes for the majority of people living with aphasia.

Case Illustration 6.1

Peter, a 69-year-old retired English-speaking teacher, was admitted to the stroke unit of the local hospital after suffering a left frontal-temporal infarct. From the clinical notes, Kate (the stroke unit speech–language pathologist) established that he had no history of previous strokes but had poorly controlled hypertension and mild arthritis. The nurses on duty report that Peter is responding appropriately to commands but seems unable to speak.

When Kate reaches his bedside, she introduces herself to Peter and his wife and explains why she is there. Peter is alert and cooperative but becomes tearful when he tries to talk. He has a moderate hemiplegia affecting his right arm and leg. Kate concludes that he has aphasia and discusses with both of them the basic effects of a stroke on swallowing and communication. She uses aphasia-friendly written information about stroke and aphasia to guide this discussion and leaves the information for Peter and his wife to refer to. She then assesses his swallowing ability; fortunately, although he has mild facial weakness, he has no dysphagia and is able to swallow a normal diet.

In the next few days, Kate continues to interact with and provide support for Peter and his wife. She asks Peter if he is having any difficulties communicating his health-care needs while in the hospital (O'Halloran, Worrall, Toffolo, Code, & Hickson, 2004). She then establishes whether he can indicate "yes" and "no," for example, by using head nodding/shaking, thumbs up/down, pointing to yes/no pictures, and so forth and alerts the staff regarding the most effective way of interacting with him. She also encourages his wife and family to bring in photos so that Peter can refer to these when talking about people and places in his life. Kate follows up on the information about stroke and aphasia she provided previously and discusses it further with Peter and his wife. Kate encourages

(continues)

Peter to share this and the communication guidelines with his two daughters and his friends and leaves her name and contact number for the family to contact her if they wish. With Peter's permission, Kate organizes a volunteer with aphasia to visit him in the hospital to provide support and insight into living with aphasia.

Because Peter is medically stable and alert, the stroke unit staff are keen for him to move rapidly to rehabilitation. Kate makes sure that Peter, his wife, and family are provided with relevant information regarding their options for rehabilitation and ensures that they are included in the family meeting to discuss Peter's transition to rehabilitation. Because transitions to the next stage of care can occur rapidly, Kate decides to perform the Comprehensive Aphasia Test on Peter; this provides him, his family, and his rehabilitation clinician with additional information regarding his strengths and weaknesses. Kate then writes a full report on Peter, including his swallowing and communication status and social situation. She gives him a copy of this report to take to the rehabilitation facility.

Peter is transferred to the local rehabilitation center, where he remains an inpatient for a few weeks. The speech–language pathologist based there, Jenny, meets Peter and his family and uses the five-step process of therapy outlined in this chapter. Jenny gathers information from Peter's previous speech–language pathologist and then schedules a meeting with Peter and as many of his family members who wish to participate.

During this meeting, she finds out about who Peter was and what his life was like before the stroke. Jenny answers questions about stroke and aphasia and determines Peter's needs and priorities. Jenny then discusses the proposed goals with Peter and his family. Peter indicates that he wants to be able to say his family members' names and also to ask them questions. His family adds that he also wants to be able to drive again.

Jenny informally determines that Peter appears to have good comprehension skills and his spontaneous speech is halting, labored, monotonous, and characterized by articulatory groping and frequent pauses. She chooses to conduct a baseline assessment of the Western Aphasia Battery (WAB) with Peter and asks his wife to complete the Communicative Effectiveness Index (CETI; Lomas et al., 1989). Jenny then asks for named photos of all his family members and also uses this as a baseline assessment. She records the time it takes Peter to say the name and transcribes the utterance (hence recording the accuracy of the name and the presence of any paraphasic errors). His next goal is to ask his family questions. The baseline assessment is his use of questions during visiting hours. He and his wife write down in a diary the questions he is able to ask during each visiting time. Jenny measures at baseline the goal of returning to driving in terms of component skills such as road sign recognition and interpretation of road rules.

Jenny begins daily individual therapy but also arranges for Peter to attend group therapy. Peter's wife attends some individual and group sessions. While Peter is at a group therapy session, Jenny arranges to meet Peter's wife, Patricia, and ask her about her needs. Patricia indicates that she has found the last few weeks very stressful and that she is struggling to cope. Jenny offers her an appointment with a counselor and also puts her in touch with a support group for spouses of people with aphasia. Patricia also asks for advice on the best way to communicate with her husband, and Jenny gives her some hints and tells her about a class on this topic that the support group is running in a few weeks' time. Jenny and Patricia agree to meet again in 2 weeks to review her situation.

Individual therapy with Peter begins with discussing what he wants to work on or achieve during treatment. Peter's priorities are still to say his family members' names and to ask questions. He also states that he would like to be able to read a book again; at the present moment, he can read only single words and short sentences. Later that day, a three-way conversation, including his wife confirms these treatment goals are relevant to Peter. Initially, therapy sessions incorporate intensive naming therapy using labeled family photos. To improve his ability to retrieve these names, Jenny first uses comprehension tasks, including matching auditory word–family photo and written word–family photo. Jenny and Peter also work on tasks to facilitate his naming ability; these use initial phonemes, rhyming, and repetition cues, as well as semantic or meaning cues (e.g., "my wife's name is …"). Jenny uses a similar approach for developing Peter's questioning. Peter practices responding to Jenny's questions (e.g., "Where are your glasses?") using written question cues (e.g., "Who?" "Where?"). As Peter's comprehension of questions improves, he is encouraged to begin producing the questions himself, using the written question cues. Because he would like more practice in naming and other communication skills, Jenny provides him with appropriate therapy apps that he can use on his tablet (Kurland, Wilkins, & Stokes, 2014).

(continues)

Jenny also spends some time conversing informally with Peter on topics of interest to him using total communication strategies. After 2 weeks, Jenny introduces reading tasks into the therapy sessions. Initially, Jenny reinforces Peter's ability to read single words by presenting him with written-word-to-picture matching tasks (using pictures of practical items, such as bread, milk). Jenny then introduces the reading of short sentences on topical news items presented in an aphasia-friendly format (i.e., larger type, well spaced, and with pictures). Peter demonstrates good progress on his reading ability, which enables him to begin reading newspaper headlines. Jenny also provides a written summary of communication strategies for Peter's frequent visitors to use. The aphasia volunteer who had visited Peter in the hospital continues to visit him during his inpatient stay.

Peter attends weekly inpatient group therapy, which provides him with an opportunity for conversation as well as support. Volunteers with aphasia often attend the groups to provide information, strategies, and encouragement.

After 4 weeks, Peter is sufficiently mobile and independent in activities of daily living to be discharged home. A reassessment using the WAB indicates that although he has improved substantially, his aphasia remains moderately severe. He and his wife are provided with information regarding community services for people with aphasia and stroke as well as additional details on aphasia and strategies others could use to facilitate communication. A twice-weekly outpatient therapy program with a new therapist, Emma, is set up for Peter; he will travel with patient transport to the rehabilitation center for physiotherapy (physical therapy), occupational therapy, and speech–language therapy.

During the first outpatient therapy session, Emma, Peter, and Patricia discuss Peter's progress and difficulties he is facing at home and in the community and review his therapy goals. His goals are revised to include an increased emphasis on conversational participation strategies so that he can become more involved during visits by his friends and grandchildren and engage more fully at his bowling club. Emma and Peter continue to focus on naming and naming strategies and also on acquiring useful carrier phrases during the therapy sessions. Although Peter's wife no longer attends therapy frequently, she and Emma speak often on the phone regarding progress and therapy. Emma also provides reading tasks and other relevant computer programs that Peter and his wife complete at home. The local aphasia support association proves to be a good source of advice, information, and support for both Peter and his wife, and they participate regularly in the association's social and educational events.

After 3 months and discussions with Emma, Peter is referred to the weekly community aphasia group. He wants to increase his conversational skills and also to offer and receive support. He begins attending the aphasia group immediately, with the understanding that he can reaccess individual therapy again at a later time. He is assessed by the group therapists on his communication effectiveness and quality of life, and his wife completes the CETI. The aphasia groups provide a supportive environment for practicing communication strategies and trying out new ones, social support, negotiating self-identity, and advocacy. The groups are conversation focused and include a discussion of news and current affairs, conversation on particular topics, and discussions about living with stroke and aphasia. The group also produces brochures, posters, news articles, and videos to fulfill various needs in the community.

Peter and his wife are satisfied with the group therapy, and Peter's confidence during conversation increases. Because the aphasia group has a no-discharge policy, Peter can continue to attend as long as he feels he is benefitting from participation there. He is also reassessed by the group's therapists every 6 months to monitor his progress and provide him with feedback. He is referred back to outpatient therapy for periods of individual therapy focusing on specific communication deficits (e.g., reading, money management skills). Since his discharge home, the aphasia volunteer continues to visit him. With the support of this volunteer and the two group speech–language pathologists, Peter returns to bowling and shopping at his local shopping center. He also is referred to an occupational therapist for assistance in regaining his driver's license. Via the aphasia group speech–language pathologists, Peter and his wife access counseling, stroke education, exercise programs, and art therapy groups. They both contribute to research projects about aphasia. Patricia finds her carer group to be a source of considerable support. Peter participates in a training program for volunteers with aphasia, and he begins visiting people with newly acquired aphasia in the hospital, traveling independently to the hospital via public transportation.

(continues)

Despite remaining moderately communicatively disabled, Peter reclaims a fulfilling and socially engaged life in the community.

Peter and his wife have had an unexpected journey learning to live with aphasia. It has been facilitated by several speech–language pathologists and a supportive aphasia community. Although this description may be considered ideal in many health service contexts, it is aspirational. Each novice speech–language pathologist should understand what could and should be provided for clients living with aphasia and work toward this, rather than be constrained by the realities of everyday service provision.

STUDY QUESTIONS

1. Which factors would you take into account when deciding on a particular therapy approach?
2. How would you explain to a person with aphasia and his or her family the usual rehabilitation pathway?
3. What is the set of steps commonly used at each stage of treatment?
4. How can you address the needs of family members at each stage of rehabilitation?
5. How would you decide when to begin and end therapy with a person with aphasia?
6. What are the benefits of group therapy for the person with aphasia living in the community?
7. How could you facilitate the reintegration of a lone-living older man with aphasia into the community?
8. What issues would arise and how could you deal with them when treating a person with aphasia who comes from a culturally or linguistically diverse community?
9. What steps could you take to make a hospital ward more communicatively accessible for a person with aphasia?
10. As an advocate for people with aphasia, how would you describe aphasia and explain supported communication to the congregation of a church that your client with aphasia regularly attends?

REFERENCES

Allen, L., Mehta, S., McClure, J. A., & Teasell, R. (2012). Therapeutic interventions for aphasia initiated more than six months post stroke: A review of the evidence. *Topics in Stroke Rehabilitation, 19*(6), 523–535. doi:10.1310/tsr1906-523

Aphasia Institute. (2003). *What is aphasia? An interactive resource for adults with aphasia, their families and their caregivers.* Toronto, Canada: Aphasia Institute.

Berens, A. (2006). *The Australian aphasia guide.* St. Lucia, QLD, Australia: AAA.

Bernstein-Ellis, E., & Elman, R. J. (2007). Aphasia group communication treatment: The Aphasia Center of California Approach. In R. J. Elman (Ed.), *Group treatment of neurogenic communication disorders: The expert clinician's approach* (2nd ed., pp. 71–94). San Diego, CA: Plural.

Berthier, M., Pulvermüller, F., Dávila, G., Casares, N., & Gutiérrez, A. (2011). Drug therapy of post-stroke aphasia: A review of current evidence. *Neuropsychology Review, 21*(3), 302–317. doi:10.1007/s11065-011-9177-7

Brady, M. C., Kelly, H., Godwin, J., & Enderby, P. (2012). Speech and language therapy for aphasia following stroke (Review). *Cochrane Database System Review, 5,* CD000425.

Brewer, L., Horgan, F., Hickey, A., & Williams, D. (2013). Stroke rehabilitation: Recent advances and future therapies. *QJM, 106*(1), 11–25.

Brown, K., Davidson, B., Worrall, L. E., & Howe, T. (2013). "Making a good time": The role of friendship in living successfully with aphasia. *International Journal of Speech-Language Pathology, 15*(2), 165–175.

Byng, S. (1995). What is aphasia therapy? In C. Code & D. Muller (Eds.), *Treatment of aphasia: From theory to practice* (pp. 3–17). London: Whurr.

Byng, S., Duchan, J., & Pound, C. (2007). *The aphasia therapy file* (Vol. 2). Hove, UK: Psychology Press.

Byng, S., Pound, C., & Hewitt, A. (2004). *Living with severe aphasia: The experience of communication impairment after stroke.* Brighton, UK: Pavilion.

Byng, S., Pound, C., & Swinburn, K. (2001). *The aphasia therapy file* (Vol. 1). Hove, UK: Psychology Press.

Cherney, L., R., Patterson, J., P., Raymer, A., Frymark, T., & Schooling, T. (2008). Evidence-based systematic review: Effects of intensity of treatment and constraint-induced language therapy for individuals with stroke-induced aphasia. *Journal of Speech, Language, and Hearing Research, 51*(5), 1282–1299.

Code, C. (2012). Apportioning time for aphasia rehabilitation. *Aphasiology, 26*(5), 729–735. doi:10.1080/02687038.2012.676892

Coelho, C., Sinotte, M., & Duffy, J. R. (2008). Schuell's stimulation approach to rehabilitation. In R. Chapey (Ed.), *Language intervention strategies in aphasia and related neurogenic communication disorders* (5th ed., pp. 403–449). Philadelphia: Lippincott, Williams and Wilkins.

Cruice, M., Worrall, L., Hickson, L., & Murison, R. (2003). Finding a focus for quality of life with aphasia: Social and emotional health, and psychological well-being. *Aphasiology, 17*(4), 333–353.

Davidson, B., & Worrall, L. (2000). The assessment of activity limitation in functional communication: Challenges and choices. In L. Worrall & C. Frattali (Eds.), *Neurogenic communication disorders: A functional approach* (pp. 19–33). New York: Thieme.

Draper, B., Bowring, G., Thompson, C., Van Heyst, J., Conroy, P., & Thompson, J. (2007). Stress in caregivers of aphasic stroke patients: A randomized controlled trial. *Clinical Rehabilitation, 21,* 122–130.

El Hachioui, H., Lingsma, H. F., van de Sandt-Koenderman, M. E., Dippel, D. W., Koudstaal, P. J., & Visch-Brink, E. G. (2013). Recovery of aphasia after stroke: A 1-year follow-up study. *Journal of Neurology, 260*(1), 166–171.

El Hachioui, H., van de Sandt-Koenderman, M. W., Dippel, D. W., Koudstaal, P. J., & Visch-Brink, E. G. (2011). A 3-year evolution of linguistic disorders in aphasia after stroke. *International Journal of Rehabilitation Research, 34*(3), 215–221.

Elman, R. J. (Ed.). (1999). *Group treatment of neurogenic communication disorders: The expert clinician's approach.* Boston: Butterworth Heinemann.

Elman, R. J. (Ed.). (2007). *Group treatment of neurogenic communication disorders: The expert clinician's approach* (2nd ed.). San Diego, CA: Plural.

Epping-Jordan, J. E., Pruitt, S. D., Bengoa, R., & Wagner, E. H. (2004). Improving the quality of health care for chronic conditions. *Quality and Safety in Healthcare, 13*(4), 299–305. doi:10.1136/qshc.2004.010744

Frattali, C. M., Thompson, C. K., Holland, A. L., Wohl, C. B., & Ferketic, M. M. (1995). *The American Speech-Language-Hearing Association Functional Assessment of Communication Skills for Adults (ASHA FACS).* Rockville, MD: American Speech-Language-Hearing Association.

Galletta, E., & Barrett, A. M. (2014). Impairment and functional interventions for aphasia: Having it all. *Current Physical Medicine and Rehabilitation Reports, 2*(2), 114–120. doi:10.1007/s40141-014-0050-5

Godecke, E., Ciccone, N. A., Granger, A. S., Rai, T., West, D., Cream, A., et al. (2014). A comparison of aphasia therapy outcomes before and after a very early rehabilitation programme following stroke. *International Journal of Language & Communication Disorders, 49*(2), 149–161. doi:10.1111/1460-6984.12074

Godecke, E., Hird, K., & Lalor, E. (2008). Aphasia therapy in the acute hospital setting: Is it justified? *Internal Medicine Journal, 38*(s4), A88.

Godecke, E., Hird, K., Lalor, E. E., Rai, T., & Phillips, M. R. (2012). Very early poststroke aphasia therapy: A pilot randomized controlled efficacy trial. *International Journal of Stroke, 7*(8), 635–644. doi:10.1111/j.1747-4949.2011.00631.x

Goodman, M. L. (2013). *Long-term recovery outcomes in aphasia.* Honors Thesis, University of Arizona, Tucson.

Grawburg, M., Howe, T., Worrall, L., & Scarinci, N. (2013). Describing the impact of aphasia on close family members using the ICF framework. *Disability & Rehabilitation, 36*(14), 1184–1195.

Hersh, D. (1998). Beyond the "plateau": Discharge dilemmas in chronic aphasia. *Aphasiology, 12*(3), 207–218.

Hilari, K., Needle, J. J., & Harrison, K. L. (2012). What are the important factors in health-related quality of life for people with aphasia? A systematic review. *Archives of Physical Medicine and Rehabilitation, 93*(1, Supplement), S86–S95.e84.

Hilari, K., & Northcott, S. (2006). Social support in people with chronic aphasia. *Aphasiology, 20*(1), 17–36.

Hillis, A. E., Worrall, L., & Thompson, C. K. (2008). The state of impairment- and consequences-based approaches to treatment for aphasia: Final commentary. In N. Martin, C. K. Thompson, & L. Worrall (Eds.), *Aphasia rehabilitation: The impairment and its consequences* (pp. 261–269). San Diego, CA: Plural.

Hinckley, J. J. (2006). Finding messages in bottles: Living successfully with stroke and aphasia. *Topics in Stroke Rehabilitation, 13*(1), 25–36.

Holland, A. L. (1980). *Communicative Abilities in Daily Living.* Austin, TX: Pro-Ed.

Holland, A. L. (2007). *Counseling in communication disorders: A wellness perspective.* San Diego, CA: Plural.

Holland, A. L., Frattali, C., & Fromm, D. (1998). *Communicative Abilities in Daily Living (CADL 2).* Austin, Texas: Pro-Ed.

Holland, A. L., & Fridriksson, J. (2001). Aphasia management during the early phases of recovery following stroke. *American Journal of Speech-Language Pathology, 10*(1), 19–29.

Howe, T., Davidson, B., Worrall, L., Hersh, D., Ferguson, A., Sherratt, S., et al. (2012). "You needed to rehab … families as well": Family members' own goals for aphasia rehabilitation *International Journal of Language & Communication Disorders, 47*(5), 511–521.

Howe, T., Worrall, L., & Hickson, L. M. H. (2008). Interviews with people with aphasia: Environmental factors that influence their community participation. *Aphasiology, 22*(10), 1–29.

Jones, F., Riazi, A., & Norris, M. (2013). Self-management after stroke: Time for some more questions? *Disability and Rehabilitation, 35*(3), 257–264.

Kagan, A., Black, S. E., Duchan, J. F., Simmons-Mackie, N. N., & Square, P. (2001). Training volunteers as conversation partners using "supported conversation for adults with aphasia" (SCA): A controlled trial. *Journal of Speech, Language and Hearing Research, 44*(3), 624–638.

Kagan, A., Simmons-Mackie, N., Rowland, A., Huijbregts, M., Shumway, E., McEwen, S., et al. (2010). *Assessment for living with aphasia.* Toronto: Aphasia Institute.

Kagan, A., Simmons-Mackie, N., Rowland, A., Huijbregts, M., Shumway, E., McEwen, S., et al. (2008). Counting what counts: A framework for capturing real-life outcomes of aphasia intervention. *Aphasiology, 22*(3), 258–280.

Kay, J., Lesser, R., & Coltheart, M. (1992). *Psycholinguistic Assessments of Language Processing in Aphasia (PALPA).* Hove, UK: Erlbaum.

Kearns, K. P., & Elman, R. J. (2001). Group therapy for aphasia: Theoretical and practical considerations. In R. Chapey (Ed.), *Language intervention strategies in aphasia and related neurogenic communication disorders* (pp. 316–337). Baltimore: Lippincott Williams and Wilkins.

Kelly, H., Brady, M. C., & Enderby, P. (2012). Speech and language therapy for aphasia following stroke. *Cochrane Database of Systematic Reviews, 5,* CD000425.pub3.

Kertesz, A. (1982). *Western Aphasia Battery.* New York: Grune and Stratton.

Kertesz, A. (2006). *Western Aphasia Battery–Revised.* San Antonio, TX: Pearson

King, J. M. (2013). Supporting communication with technology. In N. Simmons-Mackie, J. M. King, & D. R. Beukelman (Eds.), *Supporting communication for adults with acute and chronic aphasia* (pp. 73–97). Baltimore: Brookes.

Kurland, J., Wilkins, A. R., & Stokes, P. (2014). Practice: Piloting the effectiveness of a tablet-based home practice program in aphasia treatment. *Seminars in Speech and Language, 35*(1), 51-63.

Lanyon, L. E., Rose, M. L., & Worrall, L. (2013). The efficacy of outpatient and community-based aphasia group interventions: A systematic review. *International Journal of Speech-Language Pathology, 15*(4), 359–374.

LaPointe, L. L. (1982, May). *Movement toward volitional control in aphasia treatment: Laddering and self-cueing strategies.* Paper presented at the Assessment and Diagnosis Based Treatments for Aphasia, University of Wisconsin, Madison.

Laska, A. C., Hellblom, A., Murray, V., Kahan, T., & Von Arbin, M. (2001). Aphasia in acute stroke and relation to outcome. *Journal of Internal Medicine, 249*(5), 413–422.

Leach, E., Cornwell, P., Fleming, J., & Haines, T. (2010). Patient centered goal-setting in a subacute rehabilitation setting. *Disability and Rehabilitation, 32*(2), 159–172.

Le Dorze, G., Salois-Bellerose, É., Alepins, M., Croteau, C., & Hallé, M.-C. (2014). A description of the personal and environmental determinants of participation several years post-stroke according to the views of people who have aphasia. *Aphasiology, 28*(4), 421–439. doi:10.1080/02687038.2013.869305

Levack, W. M. M., Dean, S. G., McPherson, K. M., & Siegert, R. J. (2006). How clinicians talk about the application of goal planning to rehabilitation for people with brain injury: Variable interpretations of value and purpose. *Brain Injury, 20*(13), 1439–1449.

Lomas, J., Pickard, L., Bester, S., Elbard, H., Finlayson, A., & Zoghaib, C. (1989). The Communicative Effectiveness Index: Development and psychometric evaluation of a functional communication measure for adults aphasia. *Journal of Speech and Hearing Disorders, 54*, 113–124.

Martin, N., Thompson, C. K., & Worrall, L. (2008). *Aphasia rehabilitation: The impairment and its consequences.* San Diego, CA: Plural.

McPherson, K. M., & Siegert, R. J. (2007). Person-centred rehabilitation: Rhetoric or reality? *Disability and Rehabilitation, 29*(20), 1551–1554.

Meinzer, M., Djundja, D., Barthel, G., Elbert, T., & Rockstroh, B. (2005). Long-term stability of improved language functions in chronic aphasia after constraint-induced aphasia therapy. *Stroke, 36*(7), 1462–1466.

Moss, A., & Nicholas, M. (2006). Language rehabilitation in chronic aphasia and time postonset: A review of single-subject data. *Stroke, 12*, 3043–3051.

Nadeau, S. E. (2014). Neuroplastic mechanisms of language recovery after stroke. In: J. I. Tracy, B. M. Hampstead, & K. Sathian K. (Eds.), Cognitive plasticity in neurologic disorders (pp. 61-84). Oxford, England: Oxford University Press.

NHMRC CCRE in Aphasia Rehabilitation. (2014). Australian Aphasia Rehabilitation Pathway. Retrieved March 3, 2015, from http://www.aphasiapathway.com.au

O'Halloran, R., Worrall, L., Toffolo, D., Code, C., & Hickson, L. (2004). *Inpatient Functional Communication Interview.* Bicester, UK: Speechmark.

Parr, S., Duchan, J., & Pound, C. (Eds.). (2003). *Aphasia inside out: Reflections on communication disability.* Maidenhead, UK: Open University Press.

Paul, D. R., Frattali, C. M., Holland, A. L., Thompson, C. K., Caperton, C. J., & Slater, S. C. (2004). *Quality of Communication Life Scale.* Rockville, MD: American Speech-Language-Hearing Association.

Pound, C. (1998). Therapy for life: Finding new paths across the plateau. *Aphasiology, 12*(3), 222–227.

Pulvermuller, F., Neininger, B., Elbert, T., Mohr, B., Rockstroh, B., Koebbel, P., et al. (2001). Constraint-induced therapy of chronic aphasia after stroke. *Stroke, 32*(7), 1621–1626.

Raymer, A. M., Beeson, P., Holland, A., Kendall, D., Maher, L. M., Martin, N., et al. (2008). Translational research in aphasia: From neuroscience to neurorehabilitation. *Journal of Speech, Language, and Hearing Research, 51*(1), S259–S275. doi:10.1044/1092-4388(2008/020)

Robey, R. R. (1998). A meta-analysis of clinical outcomes in the treatment of aphasia. *Journal of Speech, Language, and Hearing Research, 41*, 172–187.

Rohde, A., Townley-O'Neill, K., Trendall, K., Worrall, L., & Cornwell, P. (2012). A comparison of client and therapist goals for people with aphasia: A qualitative exploratory study. *Aphasiology, 26*(10), 1298–1315.

Rose, M. (2013). Releasing the constraints on aphasia therapy: The positive impact of gesture and multimodality treatments. *American Journal of Speech-Language Pathology (Online), 22*(2), S227–S239.

Rose, M., Ferguson, A., Power, E., Togher, L., & Worrall, L. (2014). Aphasia rehabilitation in Australia: Current practices, challenges and future directions. *International Journal of Speech-Language Pathology, 16*(2), 169–180. doi:10.3109/17549507.2013.794474

Rose, T. A., Worrall, L., & McKenna, K. T. (2003). The effectiveness of aphasia-friendly principles for printed health education materials for people with aphasia following stroke. *Aphasiology, 17*(10), 947–963.

Ryff, C. D., & Singer, B. (1998). The contours of positive human health. *Psychological Inquiry, 9*(1), 1–28.

Ryff, C. D., & Singer, B. (2000). Interpersonal flourishing: A positive health agenda for the new millenium. *Personality and Social Psychology Review, 4*(1), 30–44.

Salter, K., Teasell, R., Foley, N., & Allen, L. (Eds.). (2013). *Aphasia* (16th ed.). London, ON, Canada: Western University.

Schuell, H., Jenkins, J. J., & Jiminez-Pabon, E. (1964). *Aphasia in adults.* New York: Harper and Row.

Shadden, B. B. (2005). Aphasia as identity theft. *Aphasiology, 19*(3), 211–223.

Shadden, B. B., & Koski, P. R. (2007). Social construction of self for persons with aphasia. *Journal of Medical Speech-Language Pathology, 15*(2), 99–105.

Sherratt, S., Worrall, L., Hersh, D., Howe, T., & Davidson, B. (2014). Goals and goal setting for people with aphasia, their family members and clinicians. In R. J. Siegert & W. M. Levack (Eds.), *Rehabilitation goal setting: Theory, practice and evidence* (pp. 325–344). Boca Raton, FL: CRC Press.

Sherratt, S., Worrall, L., Pearson, C., Howe, T., Hersh, D., & Davidson, B. (2011). "Well it has to be language-related": Speech-language pathologists' goals for people with aphasia and their families. *International Journal of Speech-Language Pathology, 13*(4), 317–328. doi:10.3109/17549507.2011.584632

Simmons-Mackie, N. (1998). A solution to the discharge dilemma in aphasia: Social approaches to aphasia management. *Aphasiology, 12*(3), 231–239.

Simmons-Mackie, N. (2013). Staging communication supports across the health continuum. In N. Simmons-Mackie, J. M.

King, & D. R. Beukelman (Eds.), *Supporting communication for adults with acute and chronic aphasia* (pp. 99–144). Baltimore: Brookes.

Simmons-Mackie, N., & Damico, J. S. (2011). Counseling and aphasia treatment: Missed opportunities. *Topics in Language Disorders October/December, 31*(4), 336–351.

Simmons-Mackie, N., & Kagan, A. (1999). Communication strategies used by "good" versus "poor" speaking partners of individuals with aphasia. *Aphasiology, 13*(9–11), 807–820.

Simmons-Mackie, N., Raymer, A., Armstrong, E., Holland, A., & Cherney, L. R. (2010). Communication partner training in aphasia: A systematic review. *Archives of Physical Medicine and Rehabilitation, 91*(12), 1814–1837.

Stucki, G., Ewert, T., & Cieza, A. (2003). Value and application of the ICF in rehabilitation medicine. *Disability and Rehabilitation, 25*, 628–634.

Swinburn, K., Porter, G., & Howard, D. (2004). *Comprehensive Aphasia Test (CAT)*. Hove, UK: Psychology Press.

Thomas, S. A., & Lincoln, N. B. (2008). Predictors of emotional distress after stroke. *Stroke, 39*(4), 1240–1245.

Thomas, S. A., Walker, M. F., Macniven, J. A., Haworth, H., & Lincoln, N. B. (2013). Communication and Low Mood (CALM): A randomized controlled trial of behavioural therapy for stroke patients with aphasia. *Clinical Rehabilitation, 27*(5), 398–408. doi:10.1177/0269215512462227

Thompson, K. (2007). Which wall is your ladder leaning against? Retrieved from http://www.eslteachersboard.com/cgi-bin/motivation/index.pl?page = 4;read = 798

van de Sandt-Koenderman, W. M. E. (2011). Aphasia rehabilitation and the role of computer technology: Can we keep up with modern times? *International Journal of Speech-Language Pathology, 13*(1), 21–27. doi:10.3109/17549507.2010.502973

Verna, A., Davidson, B., & Rose, T. (2009). Speech-language pathology services for people with aphasia: A survey of current practice in Australia. *International Journal of Speech-Language Pathology, 11*(3), 191–205.

Weissling, K. S. E., & Harvey, J. (2013). Integrating communication supports into aphasia intervention in inpatient and outpatient rehabilitation. In N. Simmons-Mackie, J. M. King, & D. R. Beukelman (Eds.), *Supporting communication for adults with acute and chronic aphasia* (pp. 165–188). Baltimore: Brookes.

Winans-Mitrik, R. L., Hula, W. D., Dickey, M. W., Schumacher, J. G., Swoyer, B., & Doyle, P. J. (2014). Description of an intensive residential aphasia treatment program: Rationale, clinical processes, and outcomes. *American Journal of Speech-Language Pathology (Online), 23*, S330–S342.

Winstein, C. J., & Kay, D. B. (2015). Translating the science into practice: Shaping rehabilitation practice to enhance recovery after brain damage. *Progress in Brain Research, 218*, 331–360.

Worrall, L. (1999). *FCTP—Functional Communication Therapy Planner*. Oxon, UK: Winslow Press.

Worrall, L. (2000). The influence of professional values on the functional communication approach in aphasia. In L. Worrall & C. Frattali (Eds.), *Neurogenic communication disorders: A functional approach*. New York: Thieme Medical Publishers.

Worrall, L. (2006). Professionalism and functional outcomes. *Journal of Communication Disorders, 39*(4), 320–327.

Worrall, L., Davidson, B., Howe, T., & Rose, T. (2007). Clients as teachers: Two aphasia groups at the University of Queensland. In R. J. Elman (Ed.), *Group treatment of neurogenic communication disorders: The expert clinician's approach* (pp. 127–144). San Diego, CA: Plural.

Worrall, L., Sherratt, S., Rogers, P., Howe, T., Hersh, D., Ferguson, A., et al. (2011). What people with aphasia want: Their goals according to the ICF. *Aphasiology, 25*(3), 309–322.

Zheng, C., Lynch, L., & Taylor, N. (2015). Effect of computer therapy in aphasia: A systematic review. *Aphasiology*, 1–34. doi:10.1080/02687038.2014.996521

OBJECTIVES

The reader will be able to:

1. Summarize the rationale for addressing extralinguistic cognitive factors as part of aphasia management.

2. Define the cognitive domains of attention, memory, and executive functioning.

3. List attention, memory, and executive functioning impairments that commonly co-occur with aphasia.

4. Describe how extralinguistic cognitive impairments may underlie or exacerbate specific aphasia symptoms.

5. Identify assessment procedures suitable for evaluating extralinguistic cognitive abilities in individuals with aphasia.

6. Summarize treatment approaches that may be used to manage directly or indirectly the extralinguistic cognitive impairments of individuals with aphasia.

Extralinguistic Cognitive Consideration in Aphasia Management

Laura Murray and Jamie Mayer

INTRODUCTION

Aphasia is a disorder affecting the comprehension and production of spoken and written language. It is an acquired disorder indicating that it is a consequence of brain damage and disease affecting the neural structures and circuits that support language abilities. However, the neural circuitry supporting language also subserves other extralinguistic cognitive skills (Brownsett et al., 2014; Meyer, Cunitz, Obleser, & Friederici, 2014). For example, Broca's area has been associated not only with aspects of syntactic processing and spoken language production, but also with working memory. Consequently, extralinguistic cognitive impairments, including attention, memory, and executive function deficits, frequently co-occur with aphasia (Hachioui et al., 2014; Pulsipher, Stricker, Sadek, & Haaland, 2013). Likewise, language is viewed as a part of cognition with active ties to other cognitive domains. Identifying concomitant cognitive impairments is therefore an important component of aphasia management given that such impairments may underlie or exacerbate aphasia symptoms (Frankel, Penn, & Ormond-Brown, 2007; Meteyard, Bruce, Edmundson, & Oakhill, 2015), as well as hamper reacquiring language skills and learning strategies to support communication (Hachioui et al., 2014; Nicholas, Sinotte, M., & Helm-Estabrooks, 2011). Furthermore, the description of extralinguistic cognitive abilities is an essential component of the assessment process when attempting to distinguish variants of primary progressive aphasia (Piguet, Leyton, Gleeson, Hoon, & Hodges, 2015). Therefore, fundamental to aphasia management is an understanding of possible extralinguistic cognitive disorders.

This chapter summarizes the extralinguistic cognitive deficits that individuals with aphasia may experience. Procedures for identifying and addressing these cognitive deficits within the aphasic patient population are also reviewed.

COGNITIVE DOMAINS AND CONSTRUCTS

Our cognitive abilities allow us to process, store, and utilize incoming information and thus serve as our interface with our external and internal environments (Guilford & Hoepfner, 1971). Most models of cognition identify perception, attention, memory, executive functioning, and language domains; however, because management of perceptual abilities falls outside the scope of speech–language pathology, this chapter only focuses on the extralinguistic cognitive domains of attention, memory, and executive functioning.

Attention

Attention is often viewed as the foundation of the other cognitive domains. Most attention models identify a set of skills that uphold distribution of our limited capacity of processing resources (Murray & Kean, 2004; Norman & Shallice, 1986). These skills include the more basic function of sustained attention or vigilance, which allows us to maintain attention and stable performance over long periods of time. Selective or focused attention enables concentrating on and prioritizing certain elements within our environment, both external and internal, even when there are competing stimuli or elements. Another aspect of attention allows us to move our attentional focus, in an accurate and timely fashion, from one stimulus, stimulus feature, or task to another. One of the most advanced attention functions is divided attention, which permits attending to and performing more than one task or concurrently attending to and processing numerous stimuli.

Memory

Memory is not a unitary process. One important differentiation is based on storage duration, which can vary from seconds (*short-term memory,* STM) to a lifetime (*long-term memory,* LTM). Within LTM, a distinction is made between *declarative* memories that are consciously acquired and can be verbalized (e.g., recalling a life event) and *nondeclarative memories* that are acquired and retrieved unconsciously and can be demonstrated but not easily verbalized (e.g., skill-based memories such as riding a bike).

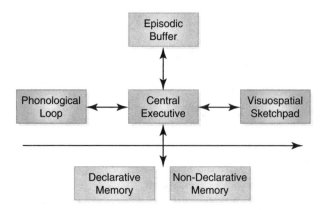

Figure 7.1 Theoretical structure of memory. The horizontal line marks the theoretical divide between working memory (WM) and its component processes, above, from long-term memory (LTM), divided into its components, below.

Given the known roles of attention and executive control in acquiring and manipulating information, Baddeley and Hitch (1974) proposed the concept of *working memory* (WM), which incorporates a limited-capacity attentional controller, the *central executive,* aided by two domain-specific subsystems designed for temporary storage: a *phonological loop* for verbal information and a *visuospatial sketchpad* for nonlinguistic information. More recently, Baddeley (2012) proposed an *episodic buffer* to account for the multimodal and chronological nature of some memories. Thus, WM incorporates the temporary storage functions of STM with the manipulation and integration of information to achieve a cognitive goal (Jarrold & Towse, 2006). Working memory is viewed by many cognitive neuropsychologists as the gateway to and from LTM (Figure 7.1).

Executive Functioning

The cognitive domain of executive functioning encompasses those high-level, interrelated, supervisory skills responsible for generating, selecting, organizing, and monitoring goal-directed and premeditated responses (Mueller & Dollaghan, 2013; Toplak, West, & Stanovich, 2013). Accordingly, executive functions (EFs) enable independent, purposeful, or novel behavior and flexible and efficient behavior adaptation to changes in circumstance or the environment. The EFs support such complex skills by engaging, coordinating, and amalgamating more basic cognitive processes. Although debate persists regarding theoretical models of executive functioning, including the number and level of independence among skills considered "executive," cognitive processes frequently viewed as EFs include problem solving and reasoning, planning and prioritizing, organizing or categorizing, inhibition, cognitive flexibility, and self-regulation and monitoring.

EXTRALINGUISTIC COGNITIVE IMPAIRMENTS IN APHASIA

Attention Impairments

A variety of attention profiles has been identified in the aphasia literature, ranging from relatively intact attention skills to the more common profile of difficulties in a number of attention functions (Murray, 2012; Villard & Kiran, 2015). That is, when compared to healthy age-matched peers, many individuals with aphasia due to static or progressive brain damage perform less accurately, more slowly, or both on sustained attention (Oron, Szymaszek, & Szelag, 2015; Villard & Kiran, 2015), attention switching (Frankel et al., 2007; Murray, 2012), and selective and divided attention tasks (Murray, 2012; Villard & Kiran, 2015). There are also reports of more impaired attention abilities among individuals with left hemisphere brain damage who have aphasia versus those who do not have aphasia (Lee & Pyun, 2014; Pulsipher et al., 2013). Importantly, such attention difficulties have been identified regardless of whether the attention tasks have relatively high or low language demands or are in the auditory or visual modality.

A particularly problematic attention deficit that can co-occur with aphasia is neglect syndrome. Neglect syndrome is a collection of attention problems that affect the speed or accuracy of attending to information presented contralateral to the side of brain damage (Kortte & Hillis, 2011). Although typically more severe and persistent following nondominant, right hemisphere lesions, neglect can also be caused by left hemisphere brain damage. Because aphasia is most commonly associated with left hemisphere lesions, neglect, if present, will affect attention to the right hemispace. The most overt signs of right neglect include (a) hemiinattention, which is a difficulty finding, responding to, or reporting information presented on the right side that cannot be ascribed to sensory or motor deficits (e.g., failing to describe items on the right side of a pictured scene; reacting more slowly to sounds presented to the right versus left ear); and (b) hemiakinesia or motor neglect, which is the inconsistent or lack of use of the right side of the body, including inadequate exploration of the right hemispace with the right side of the body (e.g., greater difficulties using the right hand to point to objects on the right versus left side). Neglect can manifest in any modality (e.g., visual, auditory, tactile, olfactory). Research indicated that following left hemisphere brain damage, between 15% and 65% of survivors will present with right-sided neglect (Barker-Collo, Feigin, Lawes, Parag, & Senior, 2010; Ihori, Kashiwagi, & Kashiwagi, 2015; Wee & Hopman, 2008); neglect has also been reported in primary progressive aphasia (Zilli & Heilman, 2015). Importantly, both the frequency and clinical consequences of neglect following left hemisphere lesions are similar to those reported among individuals with right hemisphere damage.

Evidence has accumulated to indicate that attention impairments may instigate or intensify language symptoms in individuals with aphasia. In fact, all levels of language processing (i.e., morphosyntax, lexical-semantic, pragmatic, and discourse skills) may be affected by attention problems. As an example, Ziegler, Kerkhoff, Cate, Artinger, and Zierdt (2001) had individuals with aphasia complete a word discrimination task by listening to word pairs presented in different locations within their right or left spatial field. Regardless of aphasia severity, their participants were less accurate when responding to word pairs in their right spatial field; in addition, a tonal cue regarding the spatial sound location improved the participants' response accuracy. Other researchers have identified potent relationships between attention abilities or demanding attention conditions (e.g., presence of noise or a competing task) and performance of tasks involving word retrieval and identification, grammatical processing, and discourse comprehension and production (Ihori et al., 2015; Kok, van Doorn, & Kolk, 2007; Murray, 2000, 2012; Oron et al., 2015; Petroi, Koul, & Corwin, 2014; Rogalski, Altmann, Plummer-D'Amato, Behrman, & Marsiske, 2010). The integrity of attention may also be an important predictor of language recovery and functional outcomes among individuals with aphasia (Goldenberg, Dettmers, Grothe, & Spatt 1994; Hachioui et al., 2014). For example, Ramsing, Blomstrand, and Sullivan (1991) found that attention ability more so than severity of language impairment predicted return to work among individuals with aphasia. As with other patient populations (Kortte & Hillis, 2011), presence of neglect is a negative prognostic indicator of functional outcome for individuals with aphasia, including longer stays in rehabilitation and a decreased likelihood of home discharge (Wee & Hopman, 2008).

Memory Impairments

Memory problems are one of the most frequently reported cognitive changes following left hemisphere stroke (Visser-Keizer, Jong, Deelman, Berg, & Gerritsen, 2002). These subjective reports by stroke survivors have been corroborated by a large literature demonstrating deficits for individuals with aphasia across multiple memory subtypes, including nonverbal and verbal declarative memory (Beeson, Bayles, &

Kaszniak, 1993; Vukovic, Vuksanovic, & Vukovic, 2008); nonverbal learning/encoding (Valilla-Rohter & Kiran, 2013); nonverbal and verbal STM (Baldo, Katseff, & Dronkers, 2012; Fucetola, Connor, Strube, & Corbetta, 2009; Laures-Gore, Marshall, & Verner, 2011); and nonverbal and verbal WM (Friedmann & Gvion, 2003; Jee et al., 2009; Mayer & Murray, 2012; Potagas, Kasselimis, & Evdokimidis, 2011). Whereas some researchers have reported a correlation between aphasia severity and memory impairment (Kasselimis et al., 2013; Potagas et al., 2011), others have downplayed or constrained this association to particular aphasia types. For example, Ivanova, Dragoy, Kuptsova, Ullcheva, and Laurinavichyute (2015) found WM correlated with language skills among persons with nonfluent, but not fluent, aphasia. Moreover, a number of researchers have found that even for individuals with aphasia in whom memory is negatively affected, the direct consequences for language are only apparent in specific situations (Friedmann & Gvion, 2003, 2007; Papagno, Cecchetto, Reati, & Bello, 2007). For example, studies of conduction aphasia have led to proposals that verbal STM (i.e., the phonological loop in Baddeley's WM model) is critical primarily for processing syntactically complex sentences (Friedmann & Gvion, 2007), or alternatively, that it does not contribute to spoken language comprehension unless some aspect of a sentence requires revision (e.g., lexical-semantics; Papagno et al., 2007).

Despite the heterogeneity of viewpoints regarding the nature, direction, and strength of the association, there is general agreement that reported links between memory and language in aphasia likely reflect the central role of WM in language processing: Language processing takes place over time, and therefore requires a mechanism for maintaining and manipulating linguistic representations (Martin, Kohen, Kalinyak-Fliszar, Soveri, & Laine, 2012). Researchers have suggested that the well-known variability in language performance often associated with aphasia (e.g., in response to particular cueing procedures or linguistic stimuli) reflects that WM for language processes is at the root of the disorder, rather than loss of linguistic representations themselves (Kolk, 2006; Martin, Saffran, & Dell, 1996). For example, Linebarger, McCall, Virata, and Berndt (2007) observed that when individuals with aphasia were given the opportunity to "refresh working memory" for language (by utilizing a system that can record words/phrases for later playback or rearrangement), the grammatical structure of their utterances improved (without provision of any new linguistic information by the device).

Memory impairments in aphasia have been shown to have an impact on not only linguistic function (Caplan, Michaud, & Hufford, 2013; Martin et al., 2012) but also functional communication as well as social, academic, and vocational outcomes (Fillingham, Sage, & Lambon Ralph, 2005; Murray, 2004, 2012). Notably, interactions between STM, WM, and LTM appear crucial for successful language rehabilitation (Helm-Estabrooks, 2002). Take, for example, the therapeutic practice of conversational coaching, which involves practicing scripts for various social interactions (e.g., ordering food in a restaurant). In this language treatment, individuals with aphasia must attend to the clinician's utterances and construct mental representations thereof, recall their own use of language and detect differences, and store the new linguistic stimuli in such a way that enables retrieval. Moreover, when they subsequently find themselves in the relevant setting, the new language knowledge and skill must be retrieved. From this perspective, it is clear that intact memory processes are crucial to successful aphasia rehabilitation.

Executive Function Impairments

Early investigations regarding the integrity of EFs in aphasia focused on attempting to determine if intelligence was or was not compromised in aphasia and typically used only nonverbal reasoning tests (e.g., Kertesz & McCabe, 1975). Contemporary researchers have acknowledged the multidimensional nature of executive functioning and sought to evaluate a broader range of EFs (e.g., Purdy, 2002). Collectively, the research indicated that the onset of aphasia can be accompanied by difficulties in one or a combination of EFs, including planning and problem-solving difficulties, disinhibition, problems detecting and following rules, and poor error awareness or detection. These difficulties may be more persistent compared to other cognitive problems (Fucetola et al., 2009; Hachioui et al., 2014; Murray, 2012; Nicholas et al., 2011; Vukovic et al., 2008). Furthermore, among individuals with left hemisphere brain damage, those with aphasia demonstrated more impaired EF than those without aphasia (Lee & Pyun, 2014; Pulsipher et al., 2013). However, there were conflicting reports regarding the presence and strength of the relationship between EF deficits and aphasia or lesion variables (e.g., Kalbe, Reinhold, Brand, Markowitsch, & Kessler, 2005, versus Helm-Estabrooks, 2002).

A growing literature indicates that EF deficits can negatively affect not only language symptoms and recovery among individuals with aphasia, but also their overall rehabilitation and functional outcomes (Brownsett et al., 2014; Hachioui et al., 2014; Nicholas et al., 2011). Whereas connections between EF and most levels of language processing have been identified (Fridriksson, Nettles, Davis, Morrow, & Montgomery, 2006; Nys et al., 2005), EFs appear most closely tied to the pragmatic abilities and discourse production and comprehension of individuals with aphasia (Frankel et al., 2007; Meteyard et al., 2015; Penn, Frankel, Watermeyer, & Russell, 2010). For instance, several investigators have identified that difficulties with topic management skills (e.g., difficulties with topic initiation or switching), spoken discourse informativeness and efficiency, and monitoring and repairing communication breakdowns are more likely if the individual with aphasia has concomitant EF deficits. Furthermore, aphasia studies have identified that EF rather than language ability predicted word retrieval treatment outcomes, including generalization and maintenance (Fillingham, Sage, & Lambon Ralph, 2006; Lambon Ralph, Snell, Fillingham, Conroy, & Sage, 2010; Yeung & Law, 2010), and that EFs are closely related to acquisition and use of compensatory, communication strategies, including augmentative and alternative communication devices (Nicholas et al., 2011; Purdy & Koch, 2006). With respect to broader rehabilitation outcomes, Rasquin, Welter, and van Heugten (2013) found that among the participants with stroke who demonstrated little response to their rehabilitation services, 40% had EF deficits, a percentage higher than that for other cognitive impairments. A similar relationship between EFs and functional outcomes has been reported by other aphasia researchers (Hachioui et al., 2014). Thus, the integrity of EFs appears to be a particularly potent prognostic indicator for individuals with aphasia.

ASSESSMENT

Given the presence and effects of cognitive impairments that co-occur with aphasia, a comprehensive aphasia evaluation should include assessment of attention, memory, and EF abilities (Milman & Holland, 2012; Murray & Clark, 2015). Because many health-care professions have training in and regularly utilize cognitive assessment procedures (e.g., occupational therapy, nursing, neuropsychology), an important first step is to clarify which health-care team member(s) will be responsible for the cognitive evaluation to avoid superfluous or, contrariwise, insufficient testing. Another consideration is to confirm which, if any, cognitive measures each health-care team member may administer. That is, in some locations, professional organizations or test publishers mandate which cognitive tests

may be used or purchased by which health-care professional. Nonetheless, cognitive testing does fall within the scope of practice for speech–language pathologists (American Speech-Language-Hearing Association, 2007). The involvement of speech–language pathologists is thus, recommended given their expertise in aphasia management and their insight pertaining to (a) which cognitive testing procedures are most suitable and (b) how to interpret cognitive test results in light of a given aphasic individual's language profile.

Similar to the aphasia assessment process, a cognitive evaluation should involve reviewing data from a case history and observations to inform the selection of subsequent formal and informal test procedures. Cognitive assessment tools vary widely from those that broadly screen general cognitive status to those designed to provide an in-depth characterization of a particular cognitive function (e.g., a test that evaluates visuospatial STM). They also vary in how they address the International Classification of Functioning, Disability, and Health framework (ICF) of the World Health Organization's (WHO, 2001): Where as, most focus on the ICF level of *Loss of Body Functions and Structures* (e.g., line bisection task to document visual neglect), some instead focus on determining if cognitive issues are leading to *Restrictions in Activity Participation* (e.g., use of a questionnaire to determine if visual neglect is affecting daily hygiene activities). A brief description of general cognitive, attention, memory, and EF measures follows, with an emphasis on those that may be most suitable for use with the aphasic population (i.e., designed for individuals with aphasia or other language disorders or who have limited language demands).

General Cognitive Status Screening Measures

General cognitive status screening tests establish the presence or absence of a cognitive problem or dementia and thus, assist in determining the need for additional cognitive evaluation. Despite the number of cognitive screening tests available, their formats are quite similar: They have a brief administration time and only include a restricted number of items to evaluate a variety of cognitive skills (Table 7.1). In fact, not all cognitive domains are necessarily screened on these tests (e.g., the *Mini-Mental Status Examination* [Folstein, Folstein, & McHugh, 2001] has no EF items). Some aphasia test batteries include subtests to screen cognitive abilities (Table 7.1). For example, the *Comprehensive Aphasia Test* (Swinburn, Porter, & Howard, 2004) includes attention (i.e., Line Bisection)

Table 7.1 Examples of General Cognitive Assessment Tools

General Cognitive Status Screening Tools

	ICF Level(s)	Attention		Memory		Executive Functioning	
		Verbal	Nonverbal	Verbal	Nonverbal	Verbal	Nonverbal
Burden of Stroke Scale Cognitive Domain (Doyle et al., 2004)	Activity Part.	X		X		X	
Cognitive Assessment Scale for Stroke Patients (Barnay et al., 2014)	Body Function		X	X			X
Cognitive Behavioral Rating Scale (Sasaki et al., 2014)	Body Function/ Activity Part.		X	X		X	X
Montreal Cognitive Assessment (Nasreddine et al., 2005)	Body Function	X		X		X	
General Cognitive Test Batteries							
Cognitive-Linguistic Quick Test (Helm-Estabrooks, 2001)	Body Function	X	X	X	X	X	X
Repeatable Battery for the Assessment of Neuropsychological Status Update (Randolph, 2012)	Body Function	X	X	X	X		
Scales of Cognitive and Communicative Ability for Neurorehabilitation (Milman & Holland, 2012)	Body Function/ Activity Part.		X	X		X	X
Aphasia Tests with Cognitive Subtests							
Aphasia Check List (Kalbe et al., 2005)	Body Function	X	X	X			X
Comprehensive Aphasia Test (Swinburn et al., 2004)	Body Function		X	X			

Note: Activity Part. refers to the ICF Level of Activity Participation.

and memory (e.g., Semantic and Recognition Memory) subtests.

Given their brevity, data from general cognitive status screening tests are, by themselves, inappropriate for formulating treatment plans or documenting treatment outcomes (Murray & Clark, 2015; Tate, 2010). Concerns have also been raised that these tests are insensitive to mild cognitive difficulties and single-domain deficits (Melkas, Jokinen, Hietanen, & Erkinjuntti, 2014; Wolf & Rognstad, 2013). Furthermore, such tests may overestimate the presence and severity of cognitive problems in individuals with aphasia (Barnay et al., 2014; Vigliecca, Peñalva, Molina, Voos, & Vigliecca, 2012). Consequently, if a general cognitive status screening test is administered to an individual with aphasia, the results must be interpreted cautiously and always in concert with other assessment data, such as clinician observations or ratings (e.g., Cognitive Behavioral Rating Scale; Sasaki et al., 2014) and patient and caregiver feedback collected via interviews or self-report scales (e.g., Burden of Stroke Scale Cognitive Domain; Doyle et al., 2004).

General Cognitive Functioning Test Batteries

Psychology and neuropsychology regularly utilize comprehensive cognitive test batteries such as the *Wechsler Assessment Intelligence Scales–IV* (WAIS-IV; Wechsler, 2008), but the purchase of these tests, at least in the United States, is typically limited to professionals with a clinical license in these fields of health care. Other test batteries, however, are more widely available to other health-care professions; in some cases, these batteries are more suitable for administration to individuals with aphasia given that they have been designed for populations with neurogenic disorders and include subtests with nominal language demands (Table 7.1). For example, the *Repeatable Battery for the Assessment of Neuropsychological Status Update* (Randolph, 2012) has Immediate Memory, Visuospatial/Constructional, Language, Attention, and Delayed Memory cognitive domain subtests; offers parallel forms and normative data for individuals aged 12 to 90; and can be administered in its entirety or via select cognitive domain subtests (e.g., Immediate and Delayed Memory only). Because these general cognitive test batteries, compared to the WAIS-IV, tend to evaluate a narrower range of cognitive abilities and provide a more shallow description of individual cognitive functions, additional assessment is typically needed to characterize specific attention, memory, or EF abilities.

Attention Measures

Attention skills may be assessed using a test battery designed to evaluate the spectrum of attention functions or tests designed to evaluate one or a limited set of attention functions (Table 7.2). Among the few currently available attention test batteries, the *Test of*

Table 7.2 Examples of attention assessment tools

	ICF Level(s)	Sustained Attention	Selective Attention	Divided Attention	Attention Switching	Neglect
Balloons Test (Edgeworth et al., 1998)	Body Function					X
Behavioral Inattention Test (Wilson et al., 1987)	Body Function/ Activity Part.					X
Color Trails Test (D'Elia et al., 1996)	Body Function		X		X	
Moss Attention Rating Scale (Whyte et al., 2008)	Activity Part.	X	X		X	
Rating Scale of Attentional Behavior (Ponsford & Kinsella, 1991)	Activity Part.	X	X	X		
Test of Everyday Attention (Robertson et al., 1994)	Body Function/ Activity Part.	X	X	X	X	
Test of Variables of Attention – 8 (Greenberg, 2011)	Body Function	X	X			

Note: Activity Part = Activity Participation ICF domain

Everyday Attention (TEA; Robertson, Ward, Ridgeway, & Nimmo-Smith, 1994) has been used in prior aphasia research (e.g., Murray, 2012) and offers subtests for measuring sustained, selective, and divided attention as well as attention switching in both auditory and visual modalities. The TEA strengths include offering parallel forms and incorporating everyday life materials and activities into its tasks (e.g., a map search for target symbols); a weakness is the need to update the two-decade-old normative data and certain aspects of the test materials.

A limited number of patient- or caregiver-reported measures are also available to provide a broad view of attention abilities and their impact on daily activities. For example, the Moss Attention Rating Scale (Whyte, Hart, Ellis, & Chervoneva, 2008) has 22 items, which a caregiver rates on a 5-point scale (1 = definitely false; 2 = false, for the most part; 3 = sometimes true, sometimes false; 4 = true, for the most part; 5 = definitely true). Items pertain to behaviors indicative of intact (e.g., persists at a task or conversation for several minutes without stopping or "drifting off") or impaired attention (e.g., fails to return to a task after an interruption unless prompted to do so). Whereas the scale has proven reliable and sensitive in inpatient settings, Whyte and colleagues have noted that additional research is needed to determine if the scale will catch the more subtle attention deficits that are common in more chronic stages of recovery.

Tests that examine in greater depth more circumscribed aspects of attention are also available (Table 7.2), albeit there are limited options for evaluating divided attention. Many of these tests are suitable for individuals with aphasia because of their relatively low language demands (e.g., simple instructions, nonverbal responses). For instance, the *Test of Variables of Attention-8* (Greenberg, 2011) is computerized, assesses auditory (simple tone stimuli) and visual (geometric figure stimuli) sustained and selective attention abilities, and provides both response speed (e.g., response time consistency) and accuracy (e.g., errors of omission vs. commission) data. The *Behavioral Inattention Test* (BIT; Wilson, Cockburn, & Halligan, 1987) is a compilation of conventional paper-and-pencil (e.g., symbol cancellation, line bisection) and more functional tasks (e.g., telling and setting the time) designed to identify visual neglect. Whereas the BIT has been used with individuals with aphasia (e.g., Murray, 2012), its normative data and some test materials are in need of an update. Researchers have warned that conventional neglect measures (e.g., line bisection, figure copying), particularly if only one type of task is used on only one occasion, may fail to identify neglect, particularly in mild

cases (e.g., Shiraishi, Yamakawa, Itou, Muraki, & Asada, 2008). Thus, using multiple tasks, including observing performance of daily activities with many external stimuli, is recommended.

Memory Measures

A number of memory test batteries are available, although some of the most commonly used, such as the *Weschler Memory Scale-IV* (Wechsler, 2009), have restricted access in the United States (i.e., most speech–language pathologists do not have the educational/licensure qualifications to purchase them). A more widely available option, the *Rivermead Behavioral Memory Test-III* (RBMT; Wilson et al., 2008), like other memory batteries, examines verbal and nonverbal STM and LTM skills (Table 7.3). Unlike many other memory batteries, however, the RBMT utilizes tasks more akin to daily activities (e.g., remembering the name of a person and a short route), and its use with aphasic patient populations has been examined (Cockburn, Wilson, Baddeley, & Hiorns, 1990).

Despite a multitude of tests for examining more specific aspects of memory, many have both language comprehension and production demands that will confound their completion by individuals with aphasia (e.g., a story recall task used to evaluate verbal LTM). That is, if the individual with aphasia obtains a poor score on one of these tests, impaired verbal memory, aphasic symptoms, or both may be the source of the deficient performance. There are, however, tests with reduced language requirements that evaluate the immediate or delayed recall of objects, symbols, or patterns or the location of objects, symbols, or patterns (Table 7.3). To evaluate STM, DeDe, Ricca, Knilans, and Trubl (2014) developed a Picture Span task that involves an array of nine pictured items (e.g., fish, car, chair). Like other span tests, the patient must recall a gradually longer list of items. Rather than verbally responding, the patient points to the pictures in the same order spoken by the examiner (i.e., forward span) or in the reverse order (i.e., backward span). DeDe and colleagues determined that their Picture Span task had both acceptable validity and reliability, and that individuals with a range of aphasia severity profiles could complete the task.

Rather than a pointing response, the *Rey Complex Figure Test* (Meyers & Meyers, 1995) involves copying an intricate, abstract design and then recalling it immediately (via drawing) and then again after a 20- to 30-minute delay. Various versions of this task are available to evaluate visual STM and LTM (for a description of various complex figure test and scoring protocols, see Knight &

Table 7.3 Examples of Memory Assessment Tools

	ICF Level(s)	Short-term/Working Memory		Long-term Memory	
		Verbal	Nonverbal	Verbal	Nonverbal
Cambridge Test of Prospective Memory (Wilson et al., 2005)	Body Function/ Activity Part.			X	X
Continuous Visual Memory Test (Trahan & Larrabee, 1988)	Body Function				X
Picture Span (DeDe et al., 2014)	Body Function	X			
Rey Complex Figure Test (Meyers & Meyers, 1995)	Body Function		X		X
Rivermead Behavioral Memory Test - 3 (Wilson et al., 2008)	Body Function/ Activity Part.	X	X	X	X
Test of Memory and Learning – Senior Edition (Reynolds & Voress, 2012)	Body Function	X	X	X	X
Working Memory Questionnaire (Vallat-Azouvi et al., 2012)	Activity Part.	X			

Note: Activity Part = Activity Participation ICF domain

Kaplan, 2003) and have been used in the aphasia literature (e.g., Vukovic et al., 2008).

Patient- and caregiver-reported measures of memory abilities are also available. Most of these have been developed for identifying memory issues in individuals with traumatic brain injury or dementing diseases and have a predominance of items pertaining to episodic memory issues (e.g., Evaluation of Everyday Memory; Tropp, Lundqvist, Persson, Samuelsson, & Levander, 2015). There are some that focus on other aspects of memory such as WM (e.g., Working Memory Questionnaire; Vallat-Azouvi, Pradat-Diehl, & Azouvi 2012) and memory strategy use (Hutchens et al., 2012), but the language demands of many of these (particularly in terms of reading the questionnaire items), again because designed for other patient populations, are such that they may only be suitable for individuals with mild aphasia or those who have a caregiver who can serve as a proxy.

Executive Function Measures

Given the multidimensional nature of EF and its close connection with rehabilitation and, more broadly, functional outcomes (e.g., Hachioui et al., 2014), assessing an array of EFs is recommended (Constantinidou, Werthmeier, Tsanadis, Evans, & Paul, 2012; MacNeill Horton, Soper, & Reynolds, 2010). Accordingly, use of an EF test battery should be considered if other assessment procedures have not suggested a particular EF problem

(Table 7.4). One battery, the *Behavioral Assessment of Dysexecutive Syndrome* (BADS; Wilson, Alderman, Burgess, Emslie, & Evans, 1996) consists of seven subtests, some of which involve tasks like those you might encounter in daily activities (e.g., drawing a search plan for finding a lost set of keys within a large field depicted on a piece of paper). The strengths of the BADS include (a) normative data for healthy adults and those with brain damage; (b) some tasks reflective of the ICF level of Activity Participation and thus, compared to many other EF batteries and tests, superior ecological validity (Norris & Tate, 2000); (c) inclusion of patient and caregiver forms of the Dysexecutive Questionnaire, which allows rating the presence and frequency of behaviors indicative of EF problems (e.g., "Has trouble making decisions, or deciding what she/he wants to do"); and (d) research establishing its use in a number of languages and cultures (e.g., Canali, Brucki, Bertolucci, & Bueno, 2011). However, the BADS is now almost 20 years old; thus, a revision with updated normative data would be useful. In addition, the language demands of some subtests, particularly in terms of task instructions, may be challenging for individuals with aphasia and moderately severe (or worse) comprehension deficits.

A number of tests designed to assess one or a limited set of EFs are suitable for individuals with aphasia (Table 7.4); these tests place nominal demands on language abilities in terms of their task instructions, procedures, or stimuli. As an example, the *Comprehensive*

Table 7.4 Examples of Executive Function Assessment Tools

	ICF Level(s)	Planning/ Organizing		Reasoning/ Problem Solving		Inhibition		Self-Monitoring		Cognitive Flexibility	
		Vb	Nvb	Vb	Nvb	Vb	Nvb	Vb	Nvb	Vb	Nvb
Behavioral Assessment of the Dysexecutive Syndrome (Wilson et al., 1996)	Body Function/ Activity Part.	X	X	X	X	X		X	X	X	X
Calibrated Ideational Fluency Assessment (Schrelten & Vannorsdall, 2011)	Body Function	X	X					X	X	X	X
Comprehensive Test of Nonverbal Intelligence – 2 (Hammill et al., 2009)	Body Function			X	X						
Modified Wisconsin Card Sorting (Schretlen, 2011)	Body Function				X						X
NAB Mazes Test (Stern & White, 2009)	Body Function		X				X				
Raven's Progressive Matrices (Raven, 2003)	Body Function				X						
Tower of London Dx – 2 (Culbertson & Zillmer, 2012)	Body Function		X		X		X				
Visual-Analogue Test Assessing Anosognosia for Language Impairment (Cocchini et al., 2010)	Body Function/ Activity Part.							X			

Note: Activity Part. = Activity Participation ICF domain.

Test of Nonverbal Intelligence–2 (CTONI-2; Hammill, Pearson, & Weiderholt, 2009) assesses problem solving and reasoning. Patients are shown a series of pictured items or geometric designs and must select from an array of choices, which pictured item or geometric design, respectively, fits best with the series. The pictorial and geometric series vary as some depict analogies, some categories, and some sequences to examine a number of types of reasoning.

A relatively novel EF measure is the *Visual-Analogue Test Assessing Anosognosia for Language* (VATA-L; Cocchini, Gregg, Beschin, Dean, & Della Sala, 2010), a patient- and caregiver-reported measure designed to examine awareness of language strengths and weaknesses in aphasia. Individuals with aphasia and their caregivers each rate how well the individual with aphasia completes daily communication tasks depicted in a set of drawings. The VATA-L yields scores to compare awareness of language production versus comprehension abilities and a discrepancy score (via comparing patient versus caregiver ratings), for which a positive value indicates that the patient is underrating daily language difficulties.

Additional Cognitive Assessment Considerations

Informal assessment procedures can augment formal cognitive tests or replace them if formal measures cannot be accessed or are not suitable for a given individual with aphasia (e.g., language symptoms or other deficits confound test performance, language or cultural issues negate use of tests or normative data). For instance, the interview or case history segment of an aphasia evaluation should include questions pertaining to cognitive abilities (e.g., Have you noticed changes in your short-term memory since your stroke?). During any component of a language evaluation, the clinician can also watch for the occurrence of behaviors suggestive of cognitive impairments. Attention problems should be suspected if patients are easily distracted (i.e., impaired sustained or selective attention impairments), their performance wanes on longer tasks (i.e., impaired sustained attention), their performance suffers with a switch in tasks (i.e., impaired attention shifting), they demonstrate difficulty on tasks requiring processing of more than one modality or information source or simultaneous completion of multiple components (i.e., impaired divided attention), or they fail to or infrequently attend or respond to stimuli on their right side (i.e., neglect). Memory impairments

may manifest as a need for multiple prompts regarding task instructions or a pattern in which language performance appears more sensitive to the length of the material to be produced or comprehended rather than the linguistic complexity of that material. Behaviors suggestive of EF impairments include impulsivity, perseveration, or decreased awareness or appreciation of one's language or other symptoms; in contrast, relatively intact problem-solving and planning skills are suggested when individuals with aphasia have developed independently positive compensatory strategies to deal with their aphasia or other neurologic symptoms. Self-monitoring can be explored by asking patients to predict their performance on language tasks or to judge how well they did after completing a language task; such predictions and judgments can then be compared to the patients' actual performance to examine if they are over- or underestimating their language abilities.

Another option is to administer language tests or probes in formats that vary the cognitive load of the language tasks or evaluation environment. For instance, selective attention demands of a confrontation naming probe task could be manipulated by adding or minimizing visual clutter or noise. The memory demands of that same naming task could be increased by imposing a delay between when the picture is shown and when the patient with aphasia may respond. The EF demands of a language probe task can be varied by adjusting the level of novelty and structure. When comparing language performance under conditions of high versus low cognitive load, it is crucial to maintain the linguistic complexity and language response demands. If linguistic variables also vary, it will be impossible to parse out the impact of the cognitive manipulations.

TREATMENT

Attention Intervention

Attention rehabilitation has been evaluated extensively in the traumatic brain injury literature (e.g., Rohling, Faust, Beverly, & Demakis, 2009), with two primary approaches emerging: (a) direct attention training (DAT) and (b) metacognitive strategy training. In the aphasia literature, these two approaches have been utilized in a small number of single-case and controlled, single-subject studies; preliminary evidence has shown some promise for improvement in both attention/related cognitive processes and language skills.

Direct Attention Training

Direct attention training presumes that recovery of the impaired attentional network can be achieved by activating and stimulating specific attentional processes through repetitive drills (Ponsford et al., 2014). Such training is available in published packages such as *Attention Process Training* (Sohlberg & Mateer, 2013) designed for patient populations and online computerized cognitive exercises (e.g., Lumosity.com) designed for the general population. Whereas the language demands of many activities in these programs will exceed the capabilities of individuals with aphasia, initial data support feasibility of program use, given periodic support, for those with mild language deficits in the chronic stage (Mayer, 2013). A limited set of aphasia studies has provided evidence for improved attention, WM, or executive control following DAT that corresponds to improved auditory comprehension (Helm-Estabrooks, Connor, & Albert, 2000) or reading skills (Coelho, 2005; Sinotte & Coelho, 2007). Other researchers, however, have reported DAT improvements limited to trained skills (e.g., trained attention tasks and tests of closely related cognitive skills), with nominal improvements in language or broader attention skills (Murray, Keeton, & Karcher, 2006). These last results are consistent with previous findings in brain-injured populations that DAT produces improvements in only specific, trained attention skills rather than global cognitive or linguistic functioning (Sturm, Willmes, Orgass, & Hartje, 1997; Zickefoose, Hux, Brown, & Wulf 2013).

Metacognitive Strategy Training

In contrast to DAT, there is wider empirical support for explicit, metacognitive strategy training in the context of functional treatment tasks that more closely resemble patients' everyday cognitive-communicative activities (Ponsford et al., 2014). To date, one aphasia study (Lee & Sohlberg, 2013) has utilized this approach: Individuals with aphasia and alexia received DAT in conjunction with metacognitive strategy training, with the goal of increasing reading comprehension. In this pilot study, six individuals with aphasia and alexia received DAT in tandem with (a) consistent visual feedback (i.e., line graphs that captured performance on each exercise) and encouragement of self-reflection for monitoring, goal-setting, and awareness and (b) strategy training for transferring improved attention or executive control to daily living tasks. Results were mixed: The protocol appeared to improve attentional skills and generalize to reading comprehension (as measured by a maze reading task) for three of the six participants. The authors suggested that the efficacy of DAT plus strategy training for improving language-related skills in individuals with aphasia may be most robust for those who are able to actively transfer trained metacognitive strategies to daily activities.

Memory Intervention

Thus far in the aphasia treatment literature, researchers have examined two areas pertaining to memory: (a) interventions to address STM or WM impairments and (b) spaced retrieval and errorless learning training protocols to foster learning and recall of language targets. For other patient populations, the evidence base and consequently treatment guidelines endorse training compensatory strategies to support memory, particularly LTM skills (e.g., Velikonja et al., 2014); however, our review of the empirical literature yielded no aphasia studies examining treatments that focused on such external or internal memory strategies.

Short-Term and Working Memory Treatments

A number of treatments have been developed to improve verbal STM or WM and, in turn, language abilities in individuals with aphasia. In most studies to date, the treatment has involved sentence (Francis, Clark, & Humphreys, 2003), word and nonword (Harris, Olson, & Humphreys, 2014; Kalinyak-Fliszar, Kohen, & Martin, 2011), or a combination of word and sentence (Berthier et al., 2014; Koenig-Bruhin & Studer-Eichenberger, 2007) repetition tasks. Whereas some of these treatments involved the immediate repetition of the verbal stimulus (e.g., Francis et al., 2003), others instead or in addition required repetition after a delay, the length of which was increased as the participant's performance improved (e.g., Kalinyak-Fliszar et al., 2011). Following these repetition treatments, study participants, most of whom had conduction aphasia profiles, demonstrated improvements on cognitive–linguistic tests, but only those closely related to the training tasks (e.g., repetition tests, verbal span tasks). Some modest generalization to untrained language tasks was observed in some studies (e.g., improved auditory comprehension [Francis et al., 2003]; longer sentence length in a spoken language sample [Koenig-Bruhin & Studer-Eichenberger, 2007]); however, study design limitations (e.g., case study design, failure to establish a stable baseline) necessitate further research to determine the reliability of such generalization effects.

Similar treatment effects have been reported when different memory training tasks have been utilized. Salis (2012) developed a listening span task during which his participant with transcortical motor aphasia had to decide if two lists of words were the same or different. As the participant improved, the number of words per list and the number of syllables per word were increased. Gains on a verbal span task were observed with some modest generalization to a sentence comprehension test.

In a study by Mayer and Murray (2002), an individual with anomic aphasia completed a memory treatment that involved reading a set of sentences; after each sentence, the individual had to report if the sentence was grammatical or not and then, after the individual had read the set of sentences, had to generate a semantic category that would apply to the final word in each sentence. Although the participant demonstrated gains on WM and reading tests, the study had an alternating treatment design, making it difficult to attribute such gains to just the memory treatment (versus the oral reading treatment also provided).

Finally, Vallat and colleagues (2005) created a treatment for their participant with mild conduction aphasia; the treatment involved eight different tasks with auditory stimuli. Examples of the tasks included listening to a set of words and then saying them back in alphabetical order and listening to some scrambled syllables and then naming what word those syllables form. Treatment outcomes included improvement on memory tests similar (e.g., digit span) as well as not similar (e.g., arithmetic problem solving) to the training tasks. Importantly, these researchers also included some patient-reported outcome measures, on which their participant reported improved participation in several everyday activities (e.g., in person and phone conversations).

Spaced Retrieval and Errorless Learning

Both spaced retrieval and errorless learning are instructional approaches in which automatic, implicit memory functions are capitalized on to support learning and recalling (Murray & Clark, 2015; Piras, Borella, Incoccia, & Carlesimo, 2011). In spaced retrieval training, patients practice recalling to-be-learned material or a strategy with a progressively increasing recall delay. That is, each time the patient correctly recalls the target, the length of the time interval between when the clinician presents the target and when the patient is cued to recall that target is doubled. If the patient recalls incorrectly, the time interval is reduced. In errorless learning, patients' errors are minimized by providing maximal cues and asking patients to respond only if they are certain they are correct. As the patient demonstrates stable recall accuracy, the extent of cueing is decreased (e.g., a patient might move from direct repetition of a to-be-remembered person's name when shown that person's picture, to being provided a cue of the person's name minus the first sound). Both instructional approaches, which can be used in concert, require extensive training, and only gains in trained items or strategies are expected.

In the aphasia literature, both spaced retrieval (Fridriksson, Holland, Beeson, & Morrow, 2005; Morrow & Fridriksson, 2006) and errorless learning (Fillingham et al., 2005, 2006) have been examined as part of word retrieval treatments. Errorless learning has also been investigated as part of a treatment to improve sentence processing (Wierenga et al., 2006) and use of an augmentative communication device (Wallace & Hux, 2014). Across these studies, participants with aphasia have made gains on their language targets. However, it has not yet been confirmed that these instructional approaches are any more effective or efficient than more traditional, effortful learning techniques. Likewise, future investigations should examine whether individuals with certain aphasia or cognitive profiles are more or less responsive to these implicit memory approaches.

Executive Function Intervention

To date, EF treatments have been inadequately examined in the aphasia literature. This may be due in part to the extensive overlap among attention, WM, and EF skills (e.g., Mayer & Murray, 2012); therefore, many of the treatments reviewed previously as targeting high-level attention and WM simultaneously target EFs as well (Sohlberg & Mateer, 2013).

Perseveration (i.e., inappropriate continuation or disinhibited use of a previous response), experienced to various degrees by the majority of individuals with aphasia (Rodrigues & Castro-Caldas, 2014), has been targeted directly in a handful of case studies (Helm-Estabrooks, Emery, & Albert, 1987; Muñoz, 2011). Treatment consisted of either (a) increasing awareness of the perseverative response(s), in the presence of graded cueing procedures to increase naming accuracy and decrease perseveration, or (b) systematically increasing interstimulus intervals based on perseverative responses, within the context of confrontation naming. Both approaches yielded various degrees of success in decreasing perseveration; Muñoz (2011) also reported generalization of treatment gains to increased verbal output, albeit there were nominal gains in confrontation naming of trained or untrained stimuli. For some individuals with aphasia, initial treatment to explicitly reduce perseveration may then pave the way for lexical retrieval intervention.

Accommodations for Cognitive Limitations in Language Interventions

Rather than or in addition to treating directly the cognitive deficits that co-occur with aphasia, clinicians may modify language-focused therapy to indirectly address or accommodate for cognitive limitations. For example, Dotson and colleagues (2008) reported improved naming for some individuals with fluent aphasia following manipulation of spatial attention (i.e., confrontation naming 45 degrees left of midline), based on the idea that orienting individuals' attention to their ipsilesional hemispace recruits intact, right hemisphere mechanisms for language processing. Crosson and colleagues (Altmann et al., 2014; Crosson et al., 2007) similarly examined engaging right hemisphere mechanisms by utilizing intentional but unrelated left-hand gestures during anomia treatment. Compared to anomia treatment alone, this intention manipulation was more effective at improving picture naming of trained and untrained items as well as generalizing these skills to discourse.

Another option is to select language interventions that support cognitive limitations. For aphasic individuals with significant deficits across cognitive domains, clinicians might consider training caregiver- versus patient-implemented strategies (Murray & Clark, 2015; Nys et al., 2005). That is, learning and transferring use of compensatory communication strategies to everyday contexts place substantial demands on attention, memory, and EF abilities; thus, aphasic individuals who are deficient in these cognitive supports are unlikely to achieve independent communication strategy use. In these cases, a more efficient treatment approach may be to train caregivers to utilize communication strategies (e.g., their use of multimodality communication) or to be responsible for strategy use by the individual with aphasia (e.g., request that the individual with aphasia use a gesture during a word retrieval failure).

Similarly, language intervention approaches integrated into an individual's everyday communicative context, such as script therapy (Cherney, Kaye, & van Vuuren, 2014) or conversational coaching (Hopper, Holland, & Rewega, 2002), can accommodate for cognitive deficits, particularly EF problems, that impede transferring learned behaviors to untrained contexts (e.g., Ponsford et al., 2014). These language approaches

provide scaffolding for the cognitively demanding communicative environments within which many individuals with aphasia are unable to generalize skills learned in the rather unnatural, contrived context typical within therapy sessions; such language approaches are also consistent with the focus of the ICF (WHO, 2001) on the functional consequences of language and cognitive impairments.

A few additional options include (a) environmental modifications such as minimizing distractions, limiting response choices, and in the case of neglect, drawing attention to the right hemispace, during language therapy activities and (b) extensively training language behaviors or strategies so that their use is completely automatic and thus, does not draw on limited cognitive resources (Murray, 2004; Murray & Clark, 2015). However, these as well as the other cognitive accommodations require empirical verification, particularly to help determine whether certain patient characteristics (e.g., aphasia profile) might assist in identifying the most appropriate accommodation for a given individual with aphasia.

FUTURE DIRECTIONS

Consideration of extralinguistic cognitive factors in aphasia management, in both empirical literature and clinical practice, has grown considerably compared to just a few decades ago. Despite this increased awareness of the complex interactions between linguistic and cognitive factors in aphasia, there is an appreciable need for more research into addressing these cognitive factors in aphasia assessment and treatment. For example, individuals with severe aphasia profiles have been infrequently included in studies examining aphasia and cognition; thus, it is unknown whether any of the assessment and treatment strategies discussed in this chapter are directly applicable to this subset of individuals.

Clinicians need further guidance to assist in predicting which individuals with aphasia are at greatest risk for concomitant cognitive impairments. That is, there has been little exploration of variables influencing the individual differences so frequently observed in the existing aphasia and cognition literature. Possible variables to examine include aphasia profile (e.g., overall severity, degree of comprehension difficulties); lesion characteristics (e.g., site, size); and participant characteristics (e.g., age, education level, premorbid cardiovascular health). In particular, future studies should aim to recruit larger and more diverse aphasic participant samples to ensure sufficient statistical power to identify such relationships.

With respect to the assessment process, specification of whether individuals with aphasia were or were not included in normative test samples is needed, and when included, some description of their aphasia profiles is critical (e.g., overall severity). For example, Tropp et al. (2015) specified that they involved participants with left hemisphere brain damage to develop their self-ratings of everyday memory problems but provided no tests for, nor mention of, aphasia in their normative sample. Given the central role for contextually based treatment strategies in rehabilitation (e.g., Ponsford et al., 2014), development of cognitive tests aimed at the ICF level of Activity Participation that are suitable for individuals with aphasia is critical both for treatment planning and measurement of treatment effects. Finally, there is a need to identify cognitive measures with test–retest responsiveness for individuals with aphasia (i.e., a given cognitive measure has been used in treatment research and has proven sensitive to the effects of the cognitive treatment; Mueller & Dollaghan, 2013).

Rehabilitation of aphasia in the context of concomitant cognitive deficits requires research examining the utility of and methodology for metacognitive strategy instruction in conjunction with realistic communicative interactions and functional tasks. Whereas the aphasia literature has explored communication training in naturalistic conditions (e.g., Hopper et al., 2002), and the traumatic brain injury literature advocates compensatory strategy training within functional, task-based contexts (e.g., Ponsford et al., 2014), we found only one study that considered specifically the role of metacognitive strategy training in conjunction with aspects of aphasia rehabilitation (Lee & Sohlberg, 2013). Finally, the management of neglect and certain aspects of EF dysfunction (e.g., impaired deficit/error awareness) in people with aphasia are untapped areas. Research is needed to assess whether and how empirically supported strategies for managing such deficits in other patient populations can apply to those with aphasia (e.g., Kortte & Hillis, 2011).

Case Illustration 7.1

Michelle is a 28-year-old right-handed female who was completing an intense MD–PhD program when she suffered a series of strokes in the distribution of the left middle cerebral and anterior communicating arteries, resulting in left frontal and temporal ischemic infarcts. As soon as medical stability was achieved, Michelle was enrolled in intensive speech–language therapy, first as an inpatient (1 to 4 weeks postonset), then at a day rehabilitation center (1 to 6 months postonset), and later as an outpatient (6 to 12 months postonset). She initially demonstrated severely impaired linguistic and oral–motor modalities, with severe verbal and oral apraxia, dysphagia, and aphasia. The apraxia and dysphagia resolved by 3 months postonset, at which time she was described as having moderate-to-severe fluent aphasia, "significant memory and attention deficits," and moderately impaired pragmatic skills. Her therapy sessions after that point focused primarily on word retrieval practice and a variety of compensatory strategies to supplement her expressive and receptive oral and written language skills and her memory and attention for completing basic activities of daily living.

Michelle desperately wanted to return to school in some capacity and, as such, sought additional therapy in an outpatient setting at 12 months postonset. Language testing at this time revealed mild fluent aphasia characterized primarily by anomia, decreased verbal fluency, and mildly impaired auditory comprehension (especially for sequential commands), in addition to moderate alexia. Given previous reports of cognitive deficits as well as Michelle's difficulty with the more cognitive demanding aspects of language tests (e.g., verbal fluency taps EFs; following sequential commands requires WM), she was also administered the CTONI-2 to measure problem solving, the RBMT-3 to measure functional visual and verbal learning and memory, and the *Calibrated Ideational Fluency Assessment* (CIFA; Schretlen & Vannorsdall, 2011) to examine the EF skills of planning, organizing, self-regulation, and monitoring.

Michelle's aphasia, although mild, was a confounding factor during testing. On the RBMT-3, she scored within normal limits on subtests involving primarily visual memory (e.g., picture and face recognition [immediate and delayed]), but poorly on subtests requiring verbal memory (e.g., story retelling [immediate and delayed], name recall). On the CIFA verbal fluency subtest, she demonstrated significantly impaired scores due to anomia and

(continues)

significant perseveration. However, Michelle also demonstrated a number of deficits during cognitive testing that did not appear related to language skills. On the CTONI-2, she scored at the first percentile on subtests involving geometric patterns. Michelle was noted to complete this test at a rapid rate and to impulsively choose answers; thus, it was questionable whether her scores truly reflected her problem-solving skills versus her ability to selectively attend to a complex task. Michelle completed the design fluency subtest of the CIFA in a similarly rapid, impulsive manner and demonstrated significant perseveration: Of 67 attempted designs total, 47 were repeated (i.e., 70% perseveration).

Michelle's speech and language pathologist, Karyn, noted informally that Michelle also demonstrated poor self-awareness, rarely if ever correcting errors during reading or other assessment tasks. She had trouble selectively attending to any task for more than a few minutes if external distractors (e.g., noise outside the therapy room) were present. Finally, Michelle's time management was a concern; she would often arrive 15–20 minutes late to therapy sessions without explanation (and on occasion arrived over an hour early—similarly without explanation).

At the completion of Michelle's diagnostic, Karyn was left with a dilemma. Michelle clearly demonstrated mild aphasia and moderate alexia and repeatedly voiced her singular goal of improving reading fluency and comprehension for eventual return to academia; prevailing therapy approaches would involve stimulation for her continued anomia and poor verbal fluency, in addition to phonological (Brookshire, Conway, Pompon, Oelke, & Kendall, 2014) and text-level training (Cherney, 2010) for her alexia. However, Michelle's additional cognitive deficits appeared to be impacting both her linguistic performance and her ability to successfully complete instrumental activities of daily living; Karyn was worried about Michelle's ability to attend consistently to (and thus, benefit from) language therapy tasks.

Therefore, Karyn developed a three-prong approach to remediating Michelle's deficits. Based on the literature, Karyn knew that direct attention/WM training in conjunction with consistent and supported practice reading aloud had facilitated reading improvement for several individuals with mild alexia and attention/WM deficits (Coelho, 2005; Lee & Sohlberg, 2013; Mayer & Murray, 2002; Sinotte & Coelho, 2007). She also knew that context-based strategy training and metacognitive instruction had been shown to be effective for addressing functional deficits associated with EF dysfunction (Ponsford et al., 2014). Accordingly, Michelle's treatment sessions consisted of DAT, utilizing Attention Process Training–III (Sohlberg & Mateer, 2013), with concurrent metacognitive training and collaborative strategy development based on Michelle's performance (Lee & Sohlberg, 2013). Michelle also spent a portion of each session reading aloud paragraph-level stimuli utilizing a repeated, errorless learning format (Cherney, 2010). Although sessions were conducted just once per week, Michelle completed daily home practice, including reading text-level material aloud in unison with a trained communication partner; she also reviewed strategies developed during treatment for use during everyday activities (e.g., the strategy of consciously redirecting attention midtask, used during DAT, was also assigned for use during meal preparation).

Therapy lasted 4 months (90-minute session/week). Posttreatment assessment revealed only nominal changes on formal cognitive tests; however, on written language tasks, Michelle demonstrated improved single-word and sentence-/paragraph-level reading accuracy in conjunction with a slower reading rate (reflecting a more deliberate approach to the task). At that point, Michelle's reading and functional language skills were sufficient to begin utilizing a compensatory tool (i.e., smartphone) to support memory for daily routines. Although Michelle was unable to return to her MD–PhD program, her cognitive and written language gains allowed her to successfully secure employment through a local vocational rehabilitation agency and to hold down a volunteer position in a physical therapy department. This case illustrates the deep intertwining of cognitive and linguistic skills at both the impairment level as well as in affecting functional outcomes.

STUDY QUESTIONS

1. Describe three reasons for considering extralinguistic cognitive factors as part of aphasia management.
2. Provide a definition for each of the cognitive domains reviewed in this chapter.
3. What is the difference between a general cognitive status screening measure and general cognitive status test battery?
4. Explain why patient- or caregiver-reported measures of cognitive abilities might be used instead of or in addition to standardized cognitive tests.
5. Provide one direct and one indirect treatment protocol for each of the extralinguistic cognitive domains reviewed in this chapter.

REFERENCES

Altmann, L. J. P., Hazamy, A. A., Carvajal, P. J., Benjamin, M., Rosenbek, J. C., & Crosson, B. (2014). Delayed stimulus-specific improvements in discourse following anomia treatment using an intentional gesture. *Journal of Speech, Language, and Hearing Research, 57*, 439–454.

American Speech-Language-Hearing Association. (2007). *Scope of practice in speech-language pathology* [Scope of Practice]. Retrieved July 3, 2015 from http://www.asha.org/policy

Baddeley, A. (2012). Working memory: Theories, models, and controversies. *Annual Review of Psychology, 63*, 1–29.

Baddeley, A. D., & Hitch, G. J. (1974). Working memory. In G. A. Bower (Ed.), *The psychology of learning and motivation: Advances in research and theory* (Vol. 8, pp. 47–89). Philadelphia: Academic Press.

Baldo, J. V., Katseff, S., & Dronkers, N. F. (2012). Brain regions underlying repetition and auditory-verbal short-term memory deficits in aphasia: Evidence from voxel-based lesion symptom mapping. *Aphasiology, 26*(3–4), 338–354.

Barker-Collo, S. L., Feigin, V. L., Lawes, C. M., Parag, V., & Senior, H. (2010). Attention deficits after incident stroke in the acute period: Frequency across types of attention and relationships to patient characteristics and functional outcomes. *Topics in Stroke Rehabilitation, 17*(6), 463–476.

Barnay, J., Wauquiez, G., Bonnin-Koang, H., Anquetil, C., Pérennou, D., Piscicelli, C., et al. (2014). Feasibility of the Cognitive Assessment scale for Stroke Patients (CASP) vs. MMSE and MoCA in aphasic left hemispheric stroke patients. *Annals of Physical and Rehabilitation Medicine, 57*, 422–435.

Beeson, P. M. Bayles, K., & Kaszniak, A. W. (1993). Memory impairment and executive control in individuals with stroke-induced aphasia. *Brain and Language, 45*, 253–275.

Berthier, M., L., Davila, G., Green-Heredia, C., Moreno Torres, I., De Mier, R., & De-Torres, I. (2014). Massed sentence repetition training can augment and speed up recovery of speech production deficits in patients with chronic conduction aphasia receiving donepezil treatment. *Aphasiology, 28*, 188–218.

Brookshire, C. E., Conway, T., Pompon, R. H., Oelke, M., & Kendall, D. L. (2014). Effects of intensive phonomotor treatment on reading in eight individuals with aphasia and phonological alexia. *American Journal of Speech-Language Pathology, 23*(2), S300–S311.

Brownsett, S. L. E., Warren, J. E., Geranmayeh, F., Woodhead, Z., Leech, R., & Wise, R. J. (2014). Cognitive control and its impact on recovery from aphasic stroke. *Brain, 137*, 242–254.

Canali, F., Brucki, S., Bertolucci, P. H., & Bueno, O. F. (2011). Reliability study of the Behavioral Assessment of the Dysexecutive Syndrome adapted for a Brazilian sample of older-adult controls and probable early Alzheimer's disease patients. *Revista Brasileira de Psiquiatria, 33*(4), 338–346.

Caplan, D., Michaud, J., & Hufford, R. (2013). Short term memory, working memory, and syntactic comprehension in aphasia. *Cognitive Neuropsychology, 30*(2), 77–109.

Cherney, L. R. (2010). Oral Reading for Language in Aphasia (ORLA): Evaluating the efficacy of computer-delivered therapy in chronic nonfluent aphasia. *Topics in Stroke Rehabilitation, 17*(6), 423–431.

Cherney, L. R., Kaye, R. C., & van Vuuren, S. (2014). Acquisition and maintenance of scripts in aphasia: A comparison of two cueing conditions. *American Journal of Speech-Language Pathology, 23*, S343–S360.

Cocchini, G., Gregg, N., Beschin, N., Dean, M., & Della Sala, S. (2010). VATA-L: Visual analogue test assessing anosagnosia for language impairment. *The Clinical Neuropsychologist, 24*, 1379–1399.

Cockburn, J., Wilson, B., Baddeley, A., & Hiorns, R. (1990). Assessing everyday memory in patients with dysphasia. *British Journal of Clinical Psychology, 29*(4), 353–360.

Coelho, C. (2005). Direct attention training as a treatment for reading impairment in mild aphasia. *Aphasiology, 19*(3–5), 275–283.

Constantinidou, F., Werthmeier, J., Tsanadis, J., Evans, C., & Paul, D. (2012). Assessment of executive functioning in brain injury: Collaboration between speech-language pathology and neuropsychology for an integrative neuropsychological perspective. *Brain Injury, 26*(13–14), 1549–1563.

Crosson, B., Fabrizio, K. S., Singletary, F., Cato, M. A., Wierenga, C. E., Parkinson, R. B., et al. (2007). Treatment of naming in nonfluent aphasia through manipulation of intention and attention: A phase I comparison of two novel treatments. *Journal of the International Neuropsychological Society, 13*, 582–594.

Culbertson, W. C., & Zillmer, E. A. (2012). *Tower of LondonDX–2nd Edition*. North Tonawanda, NY: Multi-Health Systems.

DeDe, G., Ricca, M., Knilans, J., & Trubl, B. (2014). Construct validity and reliability of working memory tasks for people with aphasia. *Aphasiology, 28*(6), 692–712.

D'Elia, L. F., Satz, P., Uchiyama, C. L., & White, T. (1996). *Color Trails Test*. Lutz, FL: Psychological Assessment Resources.

Dotson, V. M., Singletary, F., Koehler, S., Bacon Moore, A., Gonzalez Rothi, L. J., & Crosson, B. (2008). Treatment of word-finding deficits in fluent aphasia through the manipulation of spatial attention: Preliminary findings. *Aphasiology, 22*(1), 103–113.

Doyle, P. J., McNeil, M. R., Mikolic, J. M., Prieto, L., Hula, W. D., Lustig, A. P., et al. (2004). The Burden of Stroke Scale (BOSS) provides valid and reliable score estimates of functioning and well-being in stroke survivors with and without communication disorders. *Journal of Clinical Epidemiology, 57*, 997–1007.

Edgeworth, J., Robertson, I. H., & MacMillan, T. (1998). *The Balloons Test*. Bury St. Edmunds, UK: Thames Valley Test.

Fillingham, J., Sage, K., & Lambon Ralph, A. (2005). Further explorations and an overview of errorless and errorful therapy for aphasic word-finding difficulties: The number of naming attempts during therapy affects outcome. *Aphasiology, 19*, 597–614.

Fillingham, J. K., Sage, K., & Lambon Ralph, M. A. (2006). The treatment of anomia using errorless learning. *Neuropsychological Rehabilitation, 16*, 129–154.

Folstein, M. F., Folstein, S. E., & McHugh, P. R. (2001). *Mini-Mental State Examination*. Lutz, FL: Psychological Assessment Resources.

Francis, D. R., Clark, N., & Humphreys, G. W. (2003). The treatment of an auditory working memory deficit and the implications for sentence comprehension abilities in mild receptive aphasia. *Aphasiology, 17*, 723–750.

Frankel, T., Penn, C., & Ormond-Brown, D. (2007). Executive dysfunction as an explanatory basis for conversation symptoms of aphasia: A pilot study. *Aphasiology, 21*(6–8), 814–828.

Fridriksson, J., Holland, A. L., Beeson, P., & Morrow, L. (2005). Spaced retrieval treatment of anomia. *Aphasiology, 19*, 99–109.

Fridriksson, J., Nettles, C., Davis, M., Morrow, L., & Montgomery, A. (2006). Functional communication and executive function in aphasia. *Clinical Linguistics & Phonetics, 20*(6), 401–410.

Friedmann, N., & Gvion, A. (2003). Sentence comprehension and working memory limitations in aphasia: A dissociation between semantic-syntactic and phonological reactivation. *Brain and Language, 86*, 23–29.

Friedmann, N., & Gvion, A. (2007). As far as individuals with conduction aphasia understood these sentences were ungrammatical: Garden path in conduction aphasia. *Aphasiology, 21*(6/7/8), 570–586.

Fucetola, R., Connor, L. T., Strube, M., & Corbetta, M. (2009). Unraveling nonverbal cognitive performance in acquired aphasia. *Aphasiology, 23*(12), 1418–1426.

Goldenberg, G., Dettmers, H., Grothe, C., & Spatt, J. (1994). Influence of linguistic and non-linguistic capacities on spontaneous recovery of aphasia and on success of language therapy. *Aphasiology, 8*, 443–456.

Greenberg, L. (2011). *Test of Variables of Attention, Version 8*. Los Alamitos, CA: TOVA.

Guilford, J. P., & Hoepfner, R. (1971). *The analysis of intelligence*. New York: McGraw-Hill.

Hachioui, H., Visch-Brink, E. G., Lingsma, H. F., van de Sandt-Koenderman, M. W., Dippel, D. W., Koudstaal, P. J., et al. (2014). Nonlinguistic cognitive impairment in post-stroke aphasia: A prospective study. *Neurorehabilitation and Neural Repair, 28*(3), 273–281.

Hammill, D. D., Pearson, N. A., & Weiderholt, J. L. (2009). *Comprehensive Test of Nonverbal Intelligence–2nd Ed*. Austin, TX: Pro-Ed.

Harris, L., Olson, A., & Humphreys, G. (2014). The link between STM and sentence comprehension: A neuropsychological rehabilitation study. *Neuropsychological Rehabilitation, 24*(5), 678–720.

Helm-Estabrooks, N. (2001). *Cognitive Linguistic Quick Test*. San Antonio, TX: Psychological Corporation.

Helm-Estabrooks, N. (2002). Cognition and aphasia: A discussion and a study. *Journal of Communication Disorders, 35*, 171–186.

Helm-Estabrooks, N., Connor, L. T., & Albert, M. L. (2000). Treating attention to improve auditory comprehension in aphasia. *Brain and Language, 74*, 469–472.

Helm-Estabrooks, N., Emery, P., & Albert, M. L. (1987). Treatment of aphasic perseveration (TAP) program: A new approach to aphasia therapy. *Archives of Neurology, 44*, 1253–1255.

Hopper, T., Holland, A., & Rewega, M. (2002). Conversational coaching: Treatment outcomes and future directions. *Aphasiology, 16*(7), 745–761.

Hutchens, R. L., Kinsella, G. J., Ong, B., Pike, K. E., Parsons, S., Storey, E., et al. (2012). Knowledge and use of memory strategies in amnestic mild cognitive impairment. *Psychology and Aging, 27*(3), 768–777.

Ihori, N., Kashiwagi, A., & Kashiwagi, T. (2015). Right unilateral spatial neglect in aphasic patients. *Brain and Language, 147*, 21–29.

Ivanova, M. V., Dragoy, O. V., Kuptsova, S. V., Ullcheva, A. S., & Laurinavichyute, A. K. (2015). The contribution of working memory to language comprehension: Differential effects of aphasia type. *Aphasiology, 29*(6), 645–664.

Jarrold, C., & Towse, J. N. (2006). Individual differences in working memory. *Neuroscience, 139*, 39–50.

Jee, E. S., McNeil, M. R., Pratt, S. R., Dickey, M. W., Hula, W. D., Szuminsky, N. J., et al. (2009). Verbal working memory and its relationship to sentence-level reading and listening comprehension in persons with aphasia. *Aphasiology, 23*(7–8), 1040–1052.

Kalbe, E., Reinhold, N., Brand, M., Markowitsch, J. J., & Kessler, J. (2005). A new test battery to assess aphasic disturbances and associated cognitive dysfunctions—German normative data on the Aphasia Check List. *Journal of Clinical and Experimental Neuropsychology, 27*, 779–794.

Kalinyak-Fliszar, M., Kohen, F., & Martin, N. (2011). Remediation of language processing in aphasia: Improving activation and maintenance of linguistic representations in (verbal) short-term memory. *Aphasiology, 25*(10), 1095–1131.

Kasselimis, D. S., Simos, P. G., Economou, A., Peppas, C., Evdokimidis, I., & Potagas, C. (2013). Are memory deficits dependent on the presence of aphasia in left brain-damaged patients? *Neuropsychologia, 51*, 1773–1776.

Kertesz, A., & McCabe, P. (1975). Intelligence and aphasia: Performance of aphasics on Raven's Coloured Progressive Matrices (RCPM). *Brain and Language, 2*, 387–395.

Knight, J., & Kaplan, E. (Eds.) (2003). *The handbook of Rey-Osterrieth Complex Figure usage: Clinical and research applications*. Lutz, FL: PAR.

Koenig-Bruhin, M., & Studer-Eichenberger, F. (2007). Therapy of short-term memory disorders in fluent aphasia: A single case study. *Aphasiology, 21*(5), 448–458.

Kok, P., van Doorn, A., & Kolk, H. (2007). Inflection and computational load in agrammatic speech. *Brain and Language, 102*(3), 273–283.

Kolk, H. H. J. (2006). How language adapts to the brain: An analysis of agrammatic aphasia. In L. Progovac, K. Paesani, E. Casielles, & E. Barton (Eds.), *The syntax of nonessentials: Multi-disciplinary perspectives* (pp. 229–258). London: Benjamins.

Kortte, K., & Hillis, A. E. (2011). Recent trends in rehabilitation interventions for visual neglect and anosognosia for hemiplegia following right hemisphere stroke. *Future Neurology, 6*(1), 33–44.

Lambon Ralph, M., Snell, C., Fillingham, J., Conroy, P., & Sage, K. (2010). Predicting the outcome of anomia therapy for people with aphasia post CVA: Both language and cognitive status are key predictors. *Neuropsychological Rehabilitation, 20*(2), 289–305.

Laures-Gore, J., Marshall, R., & Verner, E. (2011). Performance of individuals with left-hemisphere stroke and aphasia and individuals with right brain damage and forward and backward digit span tasks. *Aphasiology, 25*(1), 43–56.

Lee, B., & Pyun, S. B. (2014). Characteristics of cognitive impairment in patients with post-stroke aphasia. *Annals of Rehabilitation Medicine, 38*(6), 759–765.

Lee, J. B., & Sohlberg, M. M. (2013). Evaluation of attention training and metacognitive facilitation to improve reading comprehension in aphasia. *American Journal of Speech-Language Pathology, 22*(2), 318–333.

Linebarger, M., McCall, D., Virata, T., & Berndt, R. S. (2007). Widening the temporal window: Processing support in the treatment of aphasic language production. *Brain and Language, 100*, 53–68.

MacNeill Horton, A., Soper, H., & Reynolds, C. (2010). Executive functions in children with traumatic brain injury. *Applied Neuropsychology, 17*, 99–103.

Martin, N., Kohen, F., Kalinyak-Fliszar, M., Soveri, A., & Laine, M. (2012). Effects of working memory load on processing of sounds and meanings of words in aphasia. *Aphasiology, 26*(3–4), 462–493.

Martin, N., Saffran, E. M., & Dell, G. S. (1996). Recovery in deep dysphasia: Evidence for a relation between auditory-verbal STM capacity and lexical errors in repetition. *Brain and Language, 52*, 83–113.

Mayer, J. F. (2013). Updates in evidence-based practice and intervention for adult neurogenic communication disorders. *NSSLHA Mid-Tennessee Conference on Communication Disorders*, Murfreesboro, TN.

Mayer, J. F., & Murray, L. L. (2002). Approaches to the treatment of alexia in chronic aphasia. *Aphasiology, 16*(7), 727–743.

Mayer, J. F., & Murray, L. L. (2012). Measuring working memory deficits in aphasia. *Journal of Communication Disorders, 45*(5), 325–339.

Melkas, S., Jokinen, H., Hietanen, M., & Erkinjuntti, T. (2014). Poststroke cognitive impairment and dementia: prevalence, diagnosis, and treatment. *Degenerative Neurological & Neuromuscular Disease, 4*, 21–27.

Meteyard, L., Bruce, C., Edmundson, A., & Oakhill, J. (2015). Profiling text comprehension impairments in aphasia. *Aphasiology, 29*(1), 1–28.

Meyer, L., Cunitz, K., Obleser, J., & Friederici, A. D. (2014). Sentence processing and verbal working memory in a white-matter-disconnection patient. *Neuropsychologia, 61*, 190–196.

Meyers, J. E., & Meyers, K. R. (1995). *Rey Complex Figure Test and Recognition Trial*. Odessa, FL: Psychological Assessment Resources.

Milman, L., & Holland, A. (2012). *Scales of cognitive and communicative ability for neurorehabilitation*. Austin, TX: Pro-Ed.

Morrow, K. L., & Fridriksson, J. (2006). Comparing fixed- and randomized-interval spaced retrieval in anomia treatment. *Journal of Communication Disorders, 39*, 2–11.

Mueller, J., & Dollaghan, C. (2013). A systematic review of assessments for identifying executive function impairment in adults with acquired brain injury. *Journal of Speech, Language and Hearing Research, 56*, 1051–1064.

Muñoz, M. (2011). Reducing aphasic perseverations: A case study. *Perspectives on Neurophysiology & Neurogenic Speech and Language Disorders, 21*, 176–183.

Murray, L. L. (2000). The effects of varying attentional demands on the word-retrieval skills of adults with aphasia, right hemisphere brain-damage or no brain-damage. *Brain and Language, 72*, 40–72.

Murray, L. L. (2004). Cognitive treatments for aphasia: Should we and can we help attention and working memory problems? *Journal of Medical Speech-Language Pathology, 12*, xxi–xxxviii.

Murray, L. L. (2012). Attention and other cognitive deficits in aphasia: Presence and relation to language and communication measures. *American Journal of Speech-Language Pathology, 21*, 167–179.

Murray, L. L., & Clark, H. M. (2015). *Neurogenic disorders of language and cognition: Evidence-based clinical practice*. Austin, TX: Pro-Ed.

Murray, L. L., & Kean, J. (2004). Resource theory and aphasia: Time to abandon or time to revise? *Aphasiology, 18*, 830–835.

Murray, L. L., Keeton, R. J., & Karcher, L. (2006). Treating attention in mild aphasia: Evaluation of Attention Process Training-II. *Journal of Communication Disorders, 39*, 37–61.

Nasreddine, Z. S., Phillips, N. A., Bedirian, V., Charbonneau, S., Whitehead, V., Collin, I., et al. (2005). The Montreal Cognitive Assessment, MoCA: A brief screening tool for mild cognitive impairment. *Journal of the American Geriatric Society, 53*, 695– 699.

Nicholas, M., Sinotte, M., & Helm-Estabrooks, N. (2011). C-Speak Aphasia alternative communication program for people with severe aphasia: Importance of executive functioning and semantic knowledge. *Neuropsychological Rehabilitation, 21*(3), 322–366.

Norman, D. A., & Shallice, T. (1986). Attention to action: Willed and automatic control of behavior. In R. J. Davidson, G. E. Schwartz, & D. Shapiro (Eds.), *Consciousness and self-regulation* (pp. 1–18). New York: Plenum Press.

Norris, G., & Tate, R. L. (2000). The Behavioural Assessment of the Dysexecutive Syndrome (BADS): Ecological, concurrent and construct validity. *Neuropsychological Rehabilitation, 10*(1), 33–45.

Nys, G., M., Van Zandvoort, M., De Kort, P., Jansen, B., Van Der Worp, H., Kappelle, L., et al. (2005). Domain-specific cognitive recovery after first-ever stroke: A follow-up study of 111 cases. *Journal of the International Neuropsychological Society, 11*, 795–806.

Oron, A., Szymaszek, A., & Szelag, E. (2015). Temporal information processing as a basis for auditory comprehension: Clinical evidence from aphasic patients. *International Journal of Language & Communication Disorders, 50*(5), 569–720. doi:10.1111/1460-6984.12160

Papagno, C., Cecchetto, C., Reati, F., & Bello, L. (2007). Processing of syntactically complex sentences relies on verbal short-term memory: Evidence from a short-term memory patient. *Cognitive Neuropsychology, 24*(3), 292–311.

Penn, C., Frankel, T., Watermeyer, J., & Russell, N. (2010). Executive function and conversational strategies in bilingual aphasia. *Aphasiology, 24*(2), 288–308.

Petroi, D., Koul, R., & Corwin, M. (2014). Effect of number of graphic symbols, levels, and listening conditions on symbol identification and latency in persons with aphasia. *Augmentative and Alternative Communication, 30*(1) 40–54.

Piguet, O., Leyton, C. E., Gleeson, L. D., Hoon, C., & Hodges, J. R. (2015). Memory and emotion processing performance contributes to the diagnosis of non-semantic primary progressive aphasia syndromes. *Journal of Alzheimer's Disease, 44*(2), 541–547.

Piras, F., Borella, E., Incoccia, C., & Carlesimo, G. (2011). Evidence-based practice recommendations for memory rehabilitation. *European Journal of Physical Rehabilitation and Medicine, 47*, 149–175.

Ponsford, J., & Kinsella, G. (1991). The use of a rating scale of attentional behavior. *Neuropsychological Rehabilitation, 1*, 241–257.

Ponsford, J., Bayley, M., Wiseman-Hakes, C., Togher, L., Velikonja, D., McIntyre, A., et al. (2014). INCOG recommendations for management of cognition following traumatic brain injury, part II: Attention and information processing speed. *The Journal of Head Trauma Rehabilitation, 29*(4), 321–337.

Potagas, C., Kasselimis, D., & Evdokimidis, I. (2011). Short-term and working memory impairments in aphasia. *Neuropsychologia, 49*(10), 2874–2878.

Pulsipher, D. T., Stricker, N. H., Sadek, J. R., & Haaland, K. Y. (2013). Clinical utility of the Neuropsychological Assessment Battery (NAB) after unilateral stroke. *The Clinical Neuropsychologist, 27*(6), 924–945.

Purdy, M. (2002). Executive function ability in persons with aphasia. *Aphasiology, 16*, 549–557.

Purdy, M., & Koch, A. (2006). Prediction of strategy usage by adults with aphasia. *Aphasiology, 20*(2–4), 337–348.

Ramsing, S., Blomstrand, C., & Sullivan, M. (1991). Prognostic factors for return to work in stroke patients with aphasia. *Aphasiology, 5*, 583–588.

Randolph, C. (2012). *Repeatable Battery for the Assessment of Neuropsychological Status Update*. San Antonio, TX: Pearson.

Rasquin, S., Welter, J., & van Heugten, C. (2013). Course of cognitive functioning during stroke rehabilitation. *Neuropsychological Rehabilitation, 23*(6), 811–823.

Raven, J. C. (2003). *Raven's Progressive Matrices*. San Antonio, TX: Pearson.

Reynolds, C., & Voress, J. (2012). *Test of Memory and Learning—Senior Edition*. Austin, TX: Pro-Ed.

Robertson, I. H., Ward, T., Ridgeway, V., & Nimmo-Smith, I. (1994). *The Test of Everyday Attention*. Gaylord, MI: Northern Speech Services.

Rodrigues, I. T., & Castro-Caldas, A. (2014). Aphasia with recurring utterances: Old syndrome, new perspectives. *Aphasiology, 28*(11), 1350–1363.

Rogalski, Y., Altmann, L. J., Plummer-D'Amato, P., Behrman, A. L., & Marsiske, M. (2010). Discourse coherence and cognition after stroke: A dual task study. *Journal of Communication Disorders, 43*(3), 212–224.

Rohling, M. L., Faust, M. E., Beverly, B., & Demakis, G. (2009). Effectiveness of cognitive rehabilitation following acquired brain injury: A meta-analytic re-examination of Cicerone et al. (2000, 2005) systematic reviews. *Neuropsychology, 23*(1), 20–39.

Salis, C. (2012). Short-term memory treatment: Patterns of learning and generalisation to sentence comprehension in a person with aphasia. *Neuropsychological Rehabilitation, 22*, 428–448.

Sasaki, T., Kojima, T., Kanaya, K., Yamada, K., Shibahara, M., Oikawa, N., et al. (2014). Reliability, validity, and factor structure of the cognitive behavioral rating scale for stroke patients. *International Journal of Rehabilitation Research, 37*(4), 343–348.

Schretlen, D. (2011). *Modified Wisconsin Card Sorting Test*. Lutz, FL: Psychological Assessment Resources.

Schretlen, D. J., & Vannorsdall, T. D. (2011). *Calibrated Ideational Fluency Assessment*. Lutz, FL: Psychological Assessment Resources.

Shiraishi, H., Yamakawa, Y., Itou, A., Muraki, T., & Asada, T. (2008). Long-term effects of prism adaptation on chronic neglect after stroke. *NeuroRehabilitation, 23*, 137–151.

Sinotte, M. P., & Coelho, C. A. (2007). Attention training for reading impairment in mild aphasia: A follow-up study. *NeuroRehabilitation, 22*(4), 303–310.

Sohlberg, M. M., & Mateer, C. A. (2013). *Attention Process Training-III*. Wake Forest, NC: Lash & Associates.

Stern, R. A., & White, T. (2009). *NAB Mazes Test*. Lutz, FL: Psychological Assessment Resources.

Sturm, W., Willmes, K., Orgass, B., & Hartje, W. (1997). Do specific attention deficits need specific training? *Neuropsychological Rehabilitation, 7*(2), 81–103.

Swinburn, K., Porter, G., & Howard, D. (2004). *Comprehensive Aphasia Test*. East Sussex, UK: Psychology Press.

Tate, R. (2010). *A compendium of tests, scales, and questionnaires: The practitioner's guide to measuring outcomes after acquired brain impairment*. New York: Psychology Press.

Toplak, M. E., West, R. F., & Stanovich, K. E. (2013). Practitioner review: Do performance-based measures and ratings of executive function assess the same construct? *Journal of Child Psychology and Psychiatry, 54*(2), 131–143.

Trahan, D. E., & Larrabee, G. J. (1988). *Continuous Visual Memory Test*. Lutz, FL: Psychological Assessment Resources.

Tropp, M., Lundqvist, A., Persson, C., Samuelsson, K., & Levander, S. (2015). Self-ratings of everyday memory problems in patients with acquired brain injury—A tool for rehabilitation. *International Journal of Physical Medicine and Rehabilitation, 3*(2), 258. doi:10.4172/2329-9096.1000258

Valilla-Rohter, S., & Kiran, S. (2013). Non-linguistic learning and aphasia: Evidence from a paired-associate and feedback-based task. *Neuropsychologia, 51*, 79–90.

Vallat, C., Azouvi, P., Hardisson, H., Meffert, R., Tessier, C., & Pradat-Diehl, P. (2005). Rehabilitation of verbal working memory after left hemisphere stroke. *Brain Injury, 19*(3), 1157–1164.

Vallat-Azouvi, C., Pradat-Diehl, P., & Azouvi, P. (2012). The Working Memory Questionnaire: A scale to assess everyday life problems related to deficits of working memory in brain injured patients. *Neuropsychological Rehabilitation, 22*, 634–649.

Velikonja, D., Tate, R., Ponsford, J., McIntyre, A., Janzen, S., & Bayley, M. (2014). INCOG recommendations for management of cognition following traumatic brain injury, part V: Memory. *The Journal of Head Trauma Rehabilitation, 29*(4), 369–386.

Vigliecca, N. S., Peñalva, M. C., Molina, S. C., Voos, J. A., & Vigliecca, M. R. (2012). Is the Folstein's Mini-Mental test an aphasia test? *Applied Neuropsychology: Adult, 19*(3), 221–228.

Villard, S., & Kiran, S. (2015). Between-session intra-individual variability in sustained, selective, and integrational non-linguistic attention in aphasia. *Neuropsychologia, 66*, 204–212.

Visser-Keizer, A.C., Jong, B., Deelman, B. G., Berg, I. J., & Gerritsen, M. J. J. (2002). Subjective change in emotive, cognition, and behaviour after stroke: Factors affecting perception of patients and partners. *Journal of Clinical and Experimental Neuropsychology, 24*(8), 1032–1045.

Vukovic, M., Vuksanovic, J., & Vukovic, I. (2008). Comparison of recovery patterns of language and cognitive functions in patients with post-traumatic language processing deficits and in patients with aphasia following stroke. *Journal of Communication Disorders, 41*, 531–552.

Wallace, S. E., & Hux, K. (2014). Effect of two layouts on high technology AAC navigation and content location by people with aphasia. *Disability and Rehabilitation: Assistive Technology, 9*(2), 173–182.

Wechsler, D. (2008). *Wechsler Adult Intelligence Scales IV*. San Antonio, TX: Pearson.

Wechsler, D. (2009). *Wechsler Memory Scale IV*. San Antonio, TX: Pearson.

Wee, J., & Hopman, W. (2008). Comparing consequences of right and left unilateral neglect in a stroke rehabilitation population. *American Journal of Physical Medicine Rehabilitation, 87*(11), 910–920.

Whyte, J., Hart, T., Ellis, C., & Chervoneva, I. (2008). The Moss Attention Rating Scale for traumatic brain injury: Further explorations of reliability and sensitivity to change. *Archives of Physical Medicine and Rehabilitation, 89*(5), 966–973.

Wierenga, C., Maher, L., Moore, A., White, K., McGregor, K., Soltysik, D., et al. (2006). Neural substrates of syntactic mapping treatment: An fMRI study of two cases. *Journal of the International Neuropsychological Society, 12*, 132–146.

Wilson, B. A., Alderman, N., Burgess, P., Emslie, H., & Evans, J. J. (1996). *Behavioral Assessment of the Dysexecutive Syndrome*. Bury St. Edmunds, UK: Thames Valley Test.

Wilson, B. A., Cockburn, J., & Halligan, P. (1987). *The Behavioral Inattention Test*. Bury St. Edmunds, UK: Thames Valley Test.

Wilson, B. A., Greenfield, E., Clare, L., Baddeley, A., Cockburn, J., Watson, P., et al. (2008). *The Rivermead Behavioral Memory Test-3rd Ed*. Bury St. Edmunds, UK: Thames Valley Test.

Wilson, B. A., Shiel, A., Foley, J., Emslie, H., Groot, Y., Hawkins, K., & Watson, P. (2005). *Cambridge Test of Prospective Memory*. Bury St. Edmunds, UK: Thames Valley Test.

Wolf, T. J., & Rognstad, M. C. (2013). Changes in cognition following mild stroke. *Neuropsychological Rehabilitation, 23*(2), 256–266.

World Health Organization. (2001). *ICF: International classification of functioning, disability, and health*. Geneva, Switzerland: Author.

Yeung, O., & Law, S.-P. (2010). Executive functions and aphasia treatment outcomes: Data from ortho-phonological cueing therapy for anomia in Chinese. *International Journal of Speech-Language Pathology, 12*(6), 529–544.

Zickefoose, S., Hux, K., Brown, J., & Wulf, K. (2013). Let the games begin: A preliminary study using Attention Process Training-3 and Lumosity! brain games to remediate attention deficits following traumatic brain injury. *Brain Injury, 27*(6), 707–716.

Ziegler, W., Kerkhoff, G., Cate, D., Artinger, F., & Zierdt, A. (2001). Spatial processing of spoken words in aphasia and in neglect. *Cortex, 37*, 754–756.

Zilli, E. M., & Heilman, K. M. (2015). Spatial neglect in a patient with logopenic progressive aphasia. *Neurocase*. doi:10.1080/13554794.2015.1031254

Disorders of Auditory Comprehension

Julie Morris and Sue Franklin

INTRODUCTION

Auditory comprehension in aphasia[1] is a fascinating, but somewhat neglected, area of study. Many people with aphasia do have some difficulty understanding spoken language, but this is not always investigated in depth. Yet, auditory comprehension disorders can be the most debilitating symptoms of aphasia. The lack of focus on auditory comprehension may result from several factors: underreporting, possible spontaneous recovery (e.g., see the section "Pure Word Deafness/Word Sound Deafness" in the "Disorders of Auditory Comprehension" section in this chapter), and co-occurring and evident spoken output difficulties. In addition, most standard aphasia batteries do not include subtests that allow for differential diagnosis of different levels of deficit in comprehension, and many research papers in the area are concerned only with "pure" forms of the disorders. Despite the topic being underresearched, there are some key findings in the area. This chapter discusses disorders of auditory comprehension and models that are used to shed light on the processes involved in auditory comprehension. Approaches to assessment and treatment are then discussed.

MODELS OF NORMAL AUDITORY PROCESSING

The model of auditory comprehension that prevails in the literature is one based on Morton's logogen model (Morton & Patterson, 1980) and is discussed in detail by Ellis and Young (1996). This is shown in Figure 8.1. The logogen model describes three levels of processing

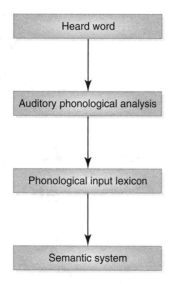

Figure 8.1   A model of auditory comprehension.

for comprehension: an auditory/speech level, a lexical level, and a semantic level. So, in this model, the spoken word is heard and then the auditory/phonological aspects are analyzed. This is then used to access the representation in a phonological input lexicon (a store of known words), and subsequently the meaning is accessed within the semantic system. Items not recognized as lexical (nonsense words, new words, words from a foreign language) can be heard and analyzed but do not access a representation within the lexicon. This is clearly an underspecified model, and there has been and continues to be debate about the processes involved (as discussed further in this chapter). In addition, this model presents auditory comprehension as linear, and authors such as McClelland and Elman (1986) and Marslen-Wilson and Warren (1994) have proposed models that allow for more interaction between levels of processing.

The exact way in which individuals process heard words continues to be controversial with respect to the levels and types of processing required to understand a word successfully. For many decades, theorists have argued whether there is a speech-specific level of prelexical processing or whether lexical forms are accessed on the basis of nonspecific acoustic processes. If there is a speech-sound-specific level of comprehension, is it specific to input, or is it also used for speaking? An area of study in psycholinguistics is how speakers use context and their knowledge of language to interact with perceptual information. To what extent are processes driven only by the input they receive, feeding information forward to subsequent levels, and to what extent is there

interaction (two way) between levels of processing? Early experiments such as the phoneme restoration effect (Kashino, 2006) strongly demonstrate that people do use top-down processing, but at what levels? We briefly consider some of the more recent evidence about prelexical and lexical processing before considering how these processes might break down (i.e., disorders of auditory comprehension).

Prelexical Processing

Recent developments in the understanding of the neuroanatomy of the temporal lobes, in addition to neuroimaging studies, suggest that auditory prelexical processing goes through a series of stages once the acoustic information is analyzed in the primary auditory cortex (Scott & Wise, 2004). Auditory analysis is carried out bilaterally for all complex sounds, which is consistent with the notion that word sound deafness often coexists with auditory agnosia and that this pattern generally results from bilateral temporal lobe damage. However, imaging studies that compare speech sounds with complex stimuli composed of transformed speech stimuli, such as vocoded speech (Scott, 2012), suggest the existence of a left lateralized speech-specific processing in addition to a right lateralized processing associated with music recognition. This again is consistent with the word deafness literature, where a small number of studies report word deafness following left hemisphere damage only.

Imaging studies that show activation of the primary motor cortex during auditory comprehension resurrected the motor theory of speech perception (Lieberman & Mattingly, 1985). A repetitive transcranial magnetic stimulation (rTMS) study found that when the lip representation in the left primary motor cortex was temporarily disrupted by electromagnetic induction, categorical perception was affected (Mottonen & Watkins, 2009). However, some of these effects may have resulted because of the experimental tasks used; that is, tasks were used for which conscious decision making was required rather than online tasks that require only auditory input processing. Hickok, Costanzo, Capasso, and Miceli (2011) and Rogalsky, Love, Driscoll, Anderson, and Hickok (2011) assessed people whose aphasia was due to anterior lesions but who did not necessarily have any problems in speech sound comprehension and concluded that speech production and perception processes do overlap but are nonidentical.

A wealth of cognitive experimentation demonstrates that lip-read information is integrated with auditory information at an early stage of processing (Schwartz, Berthommier, & Savariaux, 2004). Localization studies suggest that this integration happens at multiple levels of the auditory cortex (Besle et al., 2008).

Lexical Processing

The majority of cognitive models of auditory comprehension include a level of lexical as well as phonological processing (Cutler, 2008). An important feature of the auditory lexicon is the notion of neighborliness. That is, some words have many other words that are phonologically similar (many neighbors), whereas other words are phonologically distinctive (few neighbors). Neighborhood density has been shown to interact with word frequency in auditory lexical decision tasks (Goh, Suarez, Yap, & Tan, 2009). Given that longer words tend to have fewer phonological neighbors and therefore are more phonologically distinctive, this may explain why a patient with a lexical access deficit, M.K. (Howard & Franklin, 1988), was more likely to comprehend words if they were long.

Another concern, important in the consideration of deficits in comprehension, is how the levels interact, specifically how top-down processing works with bottom-up processing of the incoming acoustic information. An interactive activation model such as that classically described by McClelland and Elman (1986) suggests that all levels are highly interactive. Norris (1994), through a mixture of word-priming experiments and computer modeling, suggests that top-down processing has its effect only at the point where the acoustic information has been sufficiently processed to contact the lexical level. This is important because it suggests that, for example, an enrichment of semantic processing will not help word deafness (see further discussion in this chapter of treatment study by Woolf, Panton, Rosen, Best, & Marshall, 2014).

The parallel distributed processing (PDP) model of Seidenberg and McClelland (1989) differs radically in that it comprises phonological, orthographic, and conceptual semantic layers, with no lexical level (the layers are connected via a layer of hidden units). Although this no-lexicon model has not been used specifically to look at auditory comprehension, it has been applied to anomia (Lambon-Ralph, Moriarty, & Sage, 2002) and, if applied to comprehension, would, for example, predict no deficit at the level of the word form. Coltheart (2004) and Borman and Weiller (2011) argued against the notion of no lexical level, largely on the basis of single-subject neuropsychological data. The PDP model also contains a single phonological layer, common to input and output, which is challenged by Hanley and Nickels (2009), who found no correlation between the strength of impairment of input and output phonology in a group of people with aphasia.

Almost every aspect of auditory comprehension is controversial despite an explosion of research in cognition, computer modeling, and neuroscience. This is perhaps unsurprising considering the uniquely human nature of language, meaning that the animal models that have, for example, been so useful in our understanding of object recognition are not available. There is also an increased challenge in studying processes involved in comprehension rather than production, where impairment can be more directly observed.

DISORDERS OF AUDITORY COMPREHENSION

We consider historical accounts of auditory comprehension disorders before describing the three specific forms of deficit predicted by models such as the one shown in Figure 8.1. Two contrasting "pure" auditory comprehension deficits were identified in the 19th century and were further developed from the 1960s onward by the Boston School (Geschwind, 1971). The first, pure word deafness, was a syndrome where the patient was unable to understand, repeat, or write to dictation the words heard (Goldstein, 1974). This was a kind of deafness because speech and reading were not significantly impaired. However, patients were not literally deaf because they could hear sounds. In contrast, Bramwell (1897, reprinted in Ellis, 1984) describes a patient who could repeat and write heard words to dictation but could not understand them. Bramwell referred to this as "word meaning deafness." In this case, the patient could process the word's sounds as demonstrated by intact repetition, but they were in some way disconnected from the meaning. Reading comprehension was intact; once the patient wrote down the word he or she could not understand, the patient was able to read and comprehend it.

More commonly, poor word comprehension is associated with the syndrome of Wernicke's aphasia (Geschwind, 1971). In this aphasia syndrome, both impaired naming and impaired comprehension occur, with phonological and semantic errors in both modalities. This is demonstrated by impaired single-word comprehension, naming, and word repetition. Errors in naming range from semantic errors to jargon. The semantic deficit may be a central one, with reading comprehension also impaired. A somewhat rarer syndrome, where comprehension is poor but repetition is intact, is transcortical sensory aphasia. This is potentially an impure form of word meaning deafness. For example, although reading comprehension is also impaired, naming is intact, which suggests semantic processing is also intact (Berthier, 1995).

Applying the logogen model described at the beginning of this chapter, Franklin (1989) assessed a number of people with impaired auditory comprehension and found that this model predicted their contrasting patterns of impairment. Using this information-processing approach resulted in three advances on the classical descriptions of comprehension disorder: greater specification of the features of each deficit, an extra level of potential deficit, and the possibility of defining the level of impairment even when the deficit is not pure. Thus, Franklin describes patients with a deficit corresponding to pure word deafness (word sound deafness); a lexical-level deficit (word form deafness, but also see Kohn and Friedman's [1986] description of "pre-access word meaning deafness"); word meaning deafness; and a central semantic deficit by which reading comprehension and naming are also impaired. In this approach, these terms are used to describe symptoms, not a syndrome, and therefore it is possible, for example, to establish word sound deafness concomitant with a central semantic deficit (Grayson, Franklin, & Hilton, 1997; Morris, Franklin, Ellis, Turner, & Bailey, 1996) or a word meaning deafness concomitant with a repetition deficit (Franklin, Howard, & Patterson, 1994).

Pure Word Deafness/Word Sound Deafness

Although a rare disorder, particularly in its pure form, there have been a large number of reports throughout the 20th century of pure word deafness/word sound deafness. Its rarity has been attributed to two causes, one that it may require bilateral damage to the temporal lobes, the other to the fact that in its pure form there tends to be good spontaneous recovery so that it may be evident only in the acute phase. The question of bilateral representation is still somewhat controversial and is bound up with the question of whether word deafness always co-occurs with an auditory agnosia (an inability to recognize familiar nonspeech sounds). Although many cases of pure word deafness do have both bilateral damage and auditory agnosia, there are some accounts of pure word deafness alone, associated with left temporal lobe damage (Griffiths, Rees, & Green, 1999; Slevc, Martin, Hamilton, & Joanisse, 2011).

A deficit at the speech sound level of auditory comprehension, whether the syndrome or the symptom, is demonstrated functionally by someone appearing to be deaf when hearing speech although the individual is normally aware of any kind of sound occurring in the environment. The latter is demonstrated experimentally by normal performance on audiometric testing.

Patients with this condition are invariably impaired at repetition and at any test that requires the specific recognition of sounds, such as minimal pair tests or pointing to words in the presence of phonologically related distracters. Functionally, comprehension is particularly difficult when the individual with word sound deafness is unable to use context to aid comprehension, for example, when there is a change of subject. Word sound deafness is almost always ameliorated by the individual being allowed to lip-read (Morris et al., 1996).

A number of studies have suggested that word sound deafness may actually be caused by an earlier deficit, for example, of temporal processing (Albert, 1974; Slevc et al., 2011). Morris et al. (1996) describe a patient they tested on both temporal and frequency sensitivity processing, and both were impaired.

Word sound deafness as a symptom, rather than a syndrome, may be much more common; Robson and her colleagues (Robson, Grube, Lambon Ralph, Griffiths, & Sage, 2013) found that people with Wernicke's aphasia, as a group, had deficits in speech sound comprehension. Moreover, similar to the Morris et al. (1996) patient, the deficit seemed to be in complex auditory processing of stimuli that varied in both time and frequency. People with Wernicke's aphasia can have difficulties with phonological and semantic distracters in comprehension. Robson found that the severity of their comprehension impairments could be predicted through a combination of speech sound difficulty and central semantic impairment (Robson, Sage, & Ralph, 2012).

Word Form Deafness

Word form deafness is even more rarely reported than is pure word deafness, with the number of reports in English at around six (e.g., case A.P.; Martin, Breedin, & Damian, 1999). Word form deafness is differentiated from pure word deafness because these individuals can make minimal pair discriminations but still have a comprehension deficit that is specific to the auditory modality and is phonological in nature; for example, word-to-picture matching is especially difficult when distracters are phonologically rather than semantically related. Patient M.K. (Howard & Franklin, 1988), when asked to give one-word definitions for words he heard, clearly "misheard" some as other, phonologically related words, for example, defining *myth* as "spinster" (presumably having heard *miss*).

The key assessments to demonstrate word form deafness are auditory discrimination of minimal pairs (intact), auditory lexical decision (significantly impaired), and written lexical decision (intact). Good performance on written lexical decision demonstrates that the impairment is specific to the auditory modality. Good phoneme discrimination suggests speech sound processing is not severely impaired, but the poor lexical decision suggests an impairment at the lexical level because the individual cannot differentiate between unknown and nonsense words. An interesting feature of M.K.'s word form deafness was that he was better at comprehending longer than shorter words. This apparently rather unusual reverse length effect becomes explicable when understood in terms of phonological distinctiveness. That is, a long word does not have to be so perfectly processed because there are fewer phonological neighbors competing to be accessed (e.g., consider *crocodile* as opposed to *cat*).

In addition to being rarely reported, it is notable that in no case of word form deafness is repetition and auditory short-term memory shown to be normal. This begs the question of whether word form deafness is actually just a milder form of word sound deafness. Better testing of these individuals is required, but we must point out that these individuals are as impaired at lexical decision as are the individuals with word sound deafness, which argues against this being merely a less severe impairment. Also, note that the signature test for word form deafness, lexical decision, is rarely carried out in a routine aphasia assessment.

Word Meaning Deafness

Word meaning deafness is also rarely reported (about five cases). In such cases, the impairment appears more semantic in nature, with performance worse for abstract words in at least two cases (D.R.B: Franklin et al., 1994; Dr.O.: Franklin et al., 1996). However, written comprehension is unimpaired, demonstrating an effect specific to the auditory modality. Some individuals with word meaning deafness are able to discriminate minimal pairs and perform well on auditory lexical decision tests but are unable to understand words they are able to repeat (such as the original Bramwell case)—a convincing demonstration that the phonology of the word is available. For example, patient Dr.O. was asked to define heard words, and this is an example of his trouble with comprehension of the word *mature*:

> *Mature, mature, mature, what's a mature? I don't know I missed it. [The written word was given at this point.] Oh mature, mature, that it somebody who is very wise and usually older.*

Word meaning deafness, using a cognitive neuropsychological model, is an inability to access semantic

information from the correctly accessed lexical form. Functionally, when a patient is unable to understand speech, writing down the key words helps. This deficit specific to the auditory modality contrasts with a central semantic deficit for which all input and output modalities are impaired.

Summary

Word sound deafness is a well-described syndrome, although its underlying deficit(s) are yet to be agreed on. Despite its rarity, the fact that some individuals with word meaning deafness can repeat words that they are at the same time unable to understand convincingly differentiates word meaning deafness from word sound deafness. The status of word form deafness is more questionable, and more in-depth tests of auditory processing and phoneme discrimination need to be carried out in these cases.

ASSESSMENT OF AUDITORY COMPREHENSION

Assessment of auditory comprehension should aim to differentially diagnose the impairment and, importantly, consider the person, his or her perception of any difficulties, and the person's communicative needs. This section discusses all of these aspects, although there is a focus within the literature and in testing material on the differential diagnosis of the underlying impairment.

How we approach assessment depends on our rationale for doing it. If it is to inform treatment options for someone with aphasia, then it should be multifaceted and consider all relevant factors. A framework such as Living with Aphasia: Framework for Outcome Measurement (A-FROM; Kagan et al.,2008), based closely on the International Classification of Functioning, Disability, and Health (ICF; World Health Organization, 2001), reminds us to consider the aphasia itself, the activity and participation needs of the person, his or her communication environment, and factors relevant to the person. In considering each of these important areas, assessment may then comprise a combination of formal and informal assessment of linguistic performance, assessment of conversational behaviors, observation of behavior, and self or others' reports. It is clear, then, that the assessment will go beyond traditional formal assessments of language functioning and may include interview data, questionnaires, and observation. Assessment of auditory comprehension would, of course, be part of a wider remit of assessing communication more holistically. It is also important to note that assessment of auditory comprehension may be more or less relevant depending on the individual's views and needs. For example, if the person perceives he or she has no difficulty understanding speech, yet an assessment shows a mild difficulty, it may not be appropriate to explore further. Conversely, the person with aphasia or a family member may express concern. If the individual is hoping to return to work or further study, it may be crucial to intervene at this high level.

It may be clear that comprehension of speech is compromised in the everyday setting and warrants further investigation. Rankin, Newton, Parker, and Bruce (2014) made the important point that while people with aphasia frequently report difficulties understanding conversation, we should not simply attribute this to the aphasia alone. Rankin et al. discuss the possible contribution (to a reported difficulty in understanding) of cognitive and emotional problems, alongside hearing acuity. Information on hearing acuity may be available from audiological assessment or may need to be requested should there be any suggestion of hearing difficulty. People in the older age group may have age-related hearing loss that particularly affects the higher frequencies (presbycusis), but this should not have a significant effect on comprehension, unless under demanding conditions. In terms of cognitive factors, Rankin et al. also discuss needing to consider attention and memory given findings from the literature of increased difficulty processing speech when attentional demands are high.

In considering the aphasia itself (in ICF terms, the impairment), a cognitive neuropsychological approach is often used (e.g., Whitworth, Webster, & Howard, 2014). This aims to delineate strengths and weaknesses (relative intact and impaired processes) and compare modalities of input. If we accept the four levels of breakdown put forward by Franklin (1989), clear indications for assessment are provided. Assessment need not be worked through in sequential order of these four levels. The choice of particular assessments is motivated by hypotheses that may result from observation or from test results. A useful starting point is in fact a relatively broad test of "auditory comprehension," such as spoken word-to-picture matching. From the patterns of results on such a test, combined with already-known information, hypotheses can be made that would direct future assessment.

Predominantly, assessment is of single words, although it is important to recognize that spoken word understanding happens in connected speech situations, usually with rich contextual cues. Because of

this, comprehension is often described at an observational level as *functional*. That is, the person is able to understand simple everyday conversation in the context in which it occurs and with the redundancy present in normal conversation. However, in more demanding situations, comprehension problems can occur. Further investigation of these can inform both treatment options for the person with aphasia and possibly our knowledge of the processes involved in auditory comprehension. Assessment of auditory comprehension takes place at multiple levels and involves a comparison between modalities of presentation. It is important to look at strengths and weaknesses, relatively impaired and intact processes. This informs both diagnosis and treatment options.

The processes or stages involved in auditory comprehension (discussed previously) are addressed in relation to possible assessment approaches in the next section.

Breakdown at the Level of Auditory Analysis (Word Sound Deafness)

The simplest way to assess auditory analysis is through repetition. For English speakers, there are a number of word and nonword repetition tests in the Psycholinguistic Assessments of Language Processing in Aphasia (PALPA; Kay, Lesser, & Coltheart, 1992) or screening tests in the Comprehensive Aphasia Test (CAT; Swinburn, Porter, & Howard, 2004). However, an impaired ability to repeat items does not necessarily imply a problem with auditory processing; it may result from impaired processes in spoken output. If the person is able to repeat, then this does suggest that the ability to analyze the auditory input is intact.

Assessments designed to tap this level of processing, and which do not require output, mainly consist of the clinician asking the person to compare two syllables (usually consonant/vowel/consonant [CVC] items) and decide whether they sound the same or different. These have been called minimal pairs in that the two words differ minimally, usually with one phoneme differing by only one or two distinctive features, for example, *but* and *bud*. Examples of these tests exist within the PALPA and Action for Dysphasic Adults (ADA; Franklin, Turner, & Ellis, 1992) test batteries. Tests containing word pairs or nonword pairs are provided. These are contrasted because the word pairs (lexical items) may benefit from lexical-level knowledge in a way that the nonword items cannot.

To supplement these tests, Morris et al. (1996) present a maximal pairs format in which pairs differ more widely along a continuum to allow for detection of level of breakdown. Thus, for someone who is at or near chance on traditional minimal pairs, maximal pairs could be used to demonstrate whether, given sufficient difference between items, the person is able to hear the difference. This allows one not only to rule out that the individual is misunderstanding the task, but also gives an idea of the point of similarity at which the person's ability breaks down, which may be of use therapeutically.

Whereas the published assessments available use CVC stimuli, some authors have looked at minimal pair discrimination of longer items (e.g., Howard & Nickels, 2005; Morris, 1997). Others have looked at discrimination under more demanding conditions (e.g., with background noise; e.g., Morris, 1997).

In interpreting assessment results, the clinician should use appropriate control data (matched for age). It may also be important to consider whether the auditory processing problem is part of a more general difficulty not specific to speech sounds. In this instance, tests of environmental sound processing have frequently been used. These are often based on available materials (e.g., sound–picture matching resources) or are research materials rather than published tests. Although these provide a gross assessment of nonspeech sound processing, it is important to recognize that the discriminations involved are often less specific than in the speech sound minimal pair–type tasks. Some research papers describe finer-grained analysis and assessment of auditory processing (e.g., temporal change, gap detection, frequency, and pitch changes). However, these types of tests remain within the research domain.

Breakdown at the Level of Phonological Input (Word Form Deafness)

In a traditional cognitive neuropsychological approach to assessment, the next level of consideration is the phonological input lexicon itself or its access. If the person has already been shown to have word sound deafness, then he or she will necessarily also be impaired at tests for this level of processing because lexical access follows auditory analysis. However, if repetition or minimal pair discrimination is normal, then word form deafness is usually assessed using a lexical decision task, by which a word or nonword item is presented and the person has to decide whether it is a real word. Nonword items are closely related to the real word, usually differing by one phoneme in tests such as the PALPA lexical decision. Rogers, Lambon-Ralph, Hodges, and Patterson (2004) discuss the fact that performance on the lexical decision task can be manipulated by changing the nature of the difference between items,

including whether items are orthographically legal, or in their study by manipulating the bigram and trigram frequencies within items. The tests typically used in clinical settings are not controlled for bigram frequency and are restricted to items that are orthographically legal and that differ only slightly (i.e., the tests are relatively difficult).

A verification task has also been used (e.g., Howard & Franklin, 1988) in which people are shown a picture and then given the correct name or a phonologically related word or nonword to accept or reject. The question here is how effectively the person recognizes the item (correct or phonologically distorted) as the pictured word. Can it be accessed in the person's lexicon? A similar useful test is the PALPA test with phonologically related distracters. Finally, if this level of deficit is suspected, it may be useful for the clinician to have the person give words for definition. A person with word form deafness gives definitions for phonologically related words and may find it easier to define longer words (see previous discussion of M.K.).

Breakdown at the Level of Semantic Access (Word Meaning Deafness)

To investigate whether word meaning deafness is present (i.e., if it is a problem of semantic access), comprehension of spoken items in contrast to written presentation is assessed (looking at access to word meaning from the spoken modality). The PALPA and ADA batteries both provide assessments that allow a direct comparison across spoken and written versions of tests (e.g., synonym judgment, word–picture matching). In the ADA and PALPA batteries, the items are identical across the spoken and written versions to facilitate this comparison; only the mode of presentation differs. In addition, the CAT has word–picture matching subtests that broadly examine response delays as well as response accuracy. The written and spoken comparison is important because, if the difficulty is with auditory comprehension rather than comprehension (or semantics) per se, the person will be more impaired with auditory presentation than with written presentation. Indeed, in a pure case, written comprehension would be preserved. Word–picture matching is the task of choice to examine this. The person sees a choice of usually four to six pictures and has to select the one that matches the heard word. Pictures presented as distracters may be semantically, phonologically, or visually related to the target, depending on the test. It is important to recognize the limits of this assessment. The person can operate a process of elimination: He or she may not know with certainty which picture is correct but knows which ones are incorrect and so deduces the correct choice. Equally, in word–picture matching tests, it is rare to have any information about what subjects think when they see a picture; if they do not interpret the distracters as they are intended, the distracters may no longer be effective.

Thus, people may perform well on this assessment but still have difficulties with auditory comprehension. A test format that does not use picture stimuli and includes lower imageability items is the test of synonym judgment (see ADA/PALPA batteries). In this subtest, the person hears two words and has to decide if the words have the same or different meanings (e.g., *marriage–wedding*). Some subjects who are within normal limits on word–picture matching may have difficulty with this task. There may be effects of imageability, with lower-imageability items producing more errors. D.R.B., described by Franklin et al. (1994), presented with particular difficulties with the comprehension of spoken abstract words, termed *abstract word meaning deafness*.

Franklin et al. (1996) use a combined task of repetition followed by definition to examine auditory processing. In a case of pure word meaning deafness, the person is able to accurately repeat a word that he or she cannot then define. The person can, however, define the word when it is written down rather than heard (as described for Dr.O. previously).

Performance on the preceding tasks can distinguish a person with word meaning deafness from someone with a central semantic problem, where comprehension of items is affected whether presentation is via the auditory or written modality. Other authors would call this type of difficulty with semantics an impairment of lexical semantics and contrast this with conceptual semantic difficulty, for which the understanding of the item is affected at the level of the concept (usually assessed via picture processing). The Pyramids and Palm Trees Test (Howard & Patterson, 1992) is frequently used to assess this semantic level. The test allows contrasting presentations with combinations of pictures, spoken words, and written words. Contrasting performance on the different versions can provide evidence to test hypotheses about comprehension across modalities.

While having their place, the assessments described here are limited in that they present items as single short units, devoid of any context. Other assessments examine auditory comprehension at the sentence and discourse levels (described further in the chapter), but it is important to recognize that a gap generally exists with comprehension of words not examined in a progressive way. There may be a role for assessing comprehension of linguistic units within a simple sentence context. The earlier work of Naeser, Hass, Mazurski, and Laughlin (1986; see the section "Word Sound Deafness" in the "Impairment-Based Approaches and Strategies" section in this chapter) provides some suggestions, but these have not been developed further.

Assessment often leaps to the sentence level, with understanding of sentence structure/syntax confounded. A test that has dominated at this level is the Test for Reception of Grammar (TROG-2; Bishop, 2003), which assesses comprehension from the single word (so-called vocabulary check) and then via a progression in grammatical complexity. This tool is a picture-matching test, with the focus on understanding of certain grammatical constructions. Within batteries such as the CAT assessment, sentence-level comprehension is also assessed in this way. The Reversible Sentences Test (J. Marshall, Black, & Byng, 1999) assesses one particular aspect of sentence processing, usually done to inform about sentence processing rather than auditory processing per se. The Revised Token Test (McNeil & Prescott, 1978) is another test allowing sentences of increasing complexity to be assessed. This test uses tokens, and verbal contextual redundancy is reduced to a minimum. However, the relationship between comprehension of this type of stimuli and everyday comprehension is not clear.

The Discourse Comprehension Test (Brookshire & Nicholas, 1993) and the Measure of Cognitive-Linguistic Abilities (Ellmo, Graser, Krchnavek, Calabrese, & Hauck, 1995) allow assessment of understanding of longer pieces of discourse with information of increasing length read aloud to the person, followed by a series of questions that test comprehension of the material. As Brookshire and Nicholas (1993) discuss in the rationale for the Discourse Comprehension Test, the relationship between sentence comprehension and discourse comprehension may be weak. They suggest that assessing single-word and sentence comprehension has its role but does not usually predict a person's ability to understand discourse more typical of everyday life.

There are of course several test batteries that assess auditory comprehension at some level. Assessment within these batteries tends to give an indication of a broad level of functioning rather than information about the underlying impairment. The Western Aphasia Battery—Revised (WAB-R; Kertesz, 2007) uses a series of questions beginning with questions relevant to the person, and then to those regarding the environment, and finally ones assessing more general information. Linguistic complexity increases over the 20 questions used. The battery also contains a section assessing the comprehension of single items within a category (the task is word–picture matching), and finally there is a set of sequential commands that increase in terms of the number of commands involved.

The Boston Diagnostic Aphasia Examination (BDAE-3; Goodglass, Kaplan, & Barresi, 2001) contains similar subtests that examine single-word understanding (via word–picture matching), understanding of increasingly complex commands, and understanding of extended discourse (short stories). This again gives a broad picture of level of functioning but not the underlying difficulty. Each subtest contains a limited number of items.

The CAT assessment also provides a series of subtests that examine auditory comprehension. Single-word, sentence-level, and paragraph-level comprehension are all considered. However, the CAT has an extended number of items (although still relatively short) and, importantly, carefully controls stimuli and distracters, taking into account important word variables known to influence performance in aphasia. The CAT does not include minimal pair or lexical decision tests.

In assessing auditory comprehension, it is important to consider factors that may affect comprehension positively or negatively. A key one is the effect of context. As stated previously, someone who has difficulty on an assessment may actually perform well in everyday life because of the effect of context on comprehension. There is little systematic investigation of this within any formal assessment.

People with auditory comprehension difficulties have also been reported to benefit from lip-read information, which is the information they gain from watching the speaker's face. This has been demonstrated by several people (e.g., Campbell, 1988; Morris et al., 1996; Shindo, Kaga, & Tanaka, 1991). The ADA comprehension battery was initially presented on tape to control for possible presenter bias and allows contrast between this form of presentation and that where the speaker is visible. Although tests generally do not assess the utility of lip-reading information to the individual, it is straightforward to do this. Clinicians can present an assessment where the speaker's face is visible for half the questions and nonvisible for the other half (e.g., the person with aphasia is asked to look down).

With the preceding assessments, it can still be the case that people perform well yet report difficulties with auditory comprehension. Morris, Franklin, and Menger (2011) report the case of G.D. that demonstrates this: G.D. reported difficulties understanding people, but tests revealed little difficulty. His understanding broke down when his system was "pushed" in some way, such as with the presence of background noise. Morris (1997) describes a subject, J.D., who showed superior performance when presentation was at regular timed intervals (via taped presentation) rather than from natural speech production. One possible explanation for this is that J.D. benefited from the predictability or regularity of the timing of presentation of items. Assessment might therefore consider the presence of background noise, the relationship between comprehension, and multiple speakers.

Assessment in a Wider Sense

Consideration of the influence of factors such as background noise and multiple speakers begins to lead into other areas, notably participation and communication and language environment. Where, why, and in what situations is the person trying to understand spoken language? Is it in a quiet home environment, with friends in a public place, in a train station with poor-quality announcements? These different listening situations place different demands on the listener. What is the topic matter? Is it a conversation about the day where some information is already known, a work meeting with fast-moving topics and lower-frequency words? Is the speaker in view, is there competing noise, is the content rapidly changing? All these factors interact in complex ways. In assessment, it may become important to tease out the relevant factors. Questions about the person's participation and about the environment can be useful, as can observation.

Clearly, observation can contribute, but there is a need for self-report (and perhaps other reports). Self-report can be done via interview, and there are several tools that may help elicit information or measure whether there are changes in perception over time. The Communication Disability Profile (Swinburn & Byng, 2006) is a tool to use during an interview to look at perceptions of communication and barriers and facilitators to communication. It includes items about comprehension. Within the Comprehensive Aphasia Test (Disability Questionnaire), there is also a set of questions that looks at the impact of auditory comprehension. Within the Communication Outcome After Stroke scale (Long, Hesketh, Paszek, Booth, & Bowen, 2008) are three questions relating to the person's perception of his or her auditory comprehension and a parallel form of questions for the caregiver to answer. Indeed, the Functional Communication Profile (Sarno, 1963) includes a large set of questions related to understanding, from environmental sounds to rapid complex conversation. In this profile, the clinician is asked to rate each area as poor, fair, good, or normal, providing a profile of ability.

Although a range of assessments assess auditory comprehension, there remain some important gaps. Any formal assessment needs to be combined with observation, interview information, and self/other report. In the future, auditory comprehension assessments need to broaden or extend in focus to examine these other aspects. We also need to consider measures that tap everyday understanding. Some of the subtests within the aphasia batteries (WAB-R, BDAE-3) do look at everyday understanding; Tessier, Weill-Chounlamountry, Michelot, and Pradat-Diehl (2007), for example, used a communication scale that questions communicative behavior and includes items about telephone communication. Woolf et al. (2014) describe a telephone listening task that attempts to examine everyday understanding. Filling these gaps will help inform treatment choices and may inform our understanding of auditory comprehension.

In investigating auditory comprehension with a view to planning intervention, it is important to investigate strengths and possible support for auditory processing. The potential usefulness of lip-reading information has been discussed. The written word may provide invaluable assistance in therapy; for example, consider the power of the written word for Dr.O. (and see the "Case Illustration" in this chapter). For both diagnostic and therapy-planning reasons, assessment should, therefore, investigate written word comprehension.

As discussed, it is also the case that particular patterns of performance can co-occur, for example, word sound deafness with semantic difficulties. Clearly, assessment needs to consider the possibility of other language-processing difficulties and the fact that we rarely see pure deficits.

INTERVENTION APPROACHES

Application of the ICF Model

Few therapy studies focus on auditory comprehension. Whitworth et al. (2014) argue that this is for two reasons: First, "most people with aphasia show substantial recovery in understanding single words during the first few months postonset. As a result, there are few good candidates for therapy aimed at this level in the chronic stages" (p. 102). Second, therapy (generally) draws on intact processes to support the impaired ones. Whereas, comprehension can support production, the reverse, they argue, is not true: Word production cannot aid comprehension. Note, however, that written word processing may be a contender as an intact or superior process that can offer support in therapy.

Therapy for auditory comprehension difficulties can be informed by one of the same frameworks that we used previously to inform assessment, that is, the ICF or the A-FROM framework. Clinicians can aim for treatment to involve or have an impact on the aphasia itself, the person's activity and participation, the environment, or the person's feelings and attitudes. Of course, these four aspects are interwoven and cannot (or should not) be considered in isolation. However, using a framework can ensure that we at least consider all these aspects in treatment. It is possible that what is perceived as a narrow linguistic therapy, with focus on the impairment, does in fact affect participation as well as the person. However, this cannot be assumed; it needs to be investigated and demonstrated. For example, if we improve somebody's ability to process pairs of minimally different items (minimal pairs), what does this mean for that person? Does this have an impact on his or her everyday communication?

Broadly, therapy approaches may be reactivation (aiming to improve the impaired process) or strategic (harnessing compensatory strategies to improve comprehension). The best may well combine both.

Impairment-Based Approaches and Strategies

In the area of impairment-based approaches and strategies, therapy aimed at the aphasia (the impairment) dominates, but even that is limited in comparison with other areas of therapy research, such as therapy for spoken output.

Word Sound Deafness

A group of studies focus on the earlier stages of auditory processing, auditory analysis. In these studies, the person is identified as having a word sound deafness, and therapy focuses at this level. The approach is to improve the person's ability to discriminate between similar-sounding words using a limited range of therapy tasks. An earlier reported study describes a therapy procedure using an illustrative case study to demonstrate its application (Gielewski, 1989). As such, it is not a robust demonstration of treatment effectiveness but does provide the foundation for later studies. Gielewski's therapy program uses lip-reading information and mouth drawings, with an aim of providing extra information about the differences between phonemes. Therapy is structured, progressing by increasing the similarity between phonemes being discriminated and their position (initial position, moving to medial or final position) in conjunction with reducing support provided (lip-reading and mouth-drawing information).

Morris et al. (1996) take Gielewski's ideas forward in a tightly controlled single-case study with client J.S. Assessment with the maximal pairs test (see the section "Assessment of Auditory Comprehension" discussed previously in this chapter) revealed that, provided the difference between items was great enough, J.S. was able to detect a difference. Morris et al. used this as the basis for where to start in therapy, and they built a task progression with items becoming increasingly phonologically similar, with lip-reading information used and then removed, and with the use of cued articulation (Passy, 1990) for added support. Tasks within therapy included phoneme and consonant-vowel (CV) discrimination, word-to-picture matching, auditory-written phoneme, or word matching. (Therapy materials based closely on this work are available from the Newcastle Aphasia Therapy Resources [Morris, Webster, Whitworth, & Howard, 2009], which provide a structured and extensive set of resources for therapy.) Posttherapy assessment revealed that J.S. had improved significantly at discrimination tasks and that there was a nonsignificant trend toward improvement on other auditorily presented tasks (lexical decision, synonym judgment, and TROG). However, it is not clearly demonstrated that an improvement at this level translated to an improvement in J.S.'s everyday communication.

Hessler and Stadie (2006) replicate the work of Morris et al. (1996) with their client M.T.R. They used a well-controlled set of stimuli, which allowed examination of improvement across treated and untreated items. Hessler and Stadie demonstrate that M.T.R. improved on both treated and untreated items, including more complex material. However, no change was seen on related tasks (lexical decision, auditory word-to-picture matching, synonym judgment). Hessler and Stadie argue that although they were unable to demonstrate an improvement on other auditory comprehension tasks, therapy was an essential precursor to subsequent treatment. They hypothesized that the next stage of therapy should be semantic, and that it was M.T.R.'s additional semantic deficit that led to the lack of change in other tasks. However, this was not tested within the research study. Hessler and Stadie reinforce the findings of Morris et al., but it is clear that questions remain about the relationship between change on these discrimination measures with change in other auditorily presented tasks and ultimately with everyday auditory comprehension.

Maneta, Marshall, and Lindsay (2001) report the same overall type of therapy for P.K. However, in this study, therapy did not produce improvement at any level in auditory processing or comprehension. One likely reason is the severity of deficit in phoneme discrimination tasks

in P.K. Tessier et al. (2007) point this out and suggest that P.K.'s impairment was simply too severe to benefit from this particular therapy.

In contrast, Grayson et al. (1997) combined auditory and semantic therapy with client L.R. Like J.S. and M.T.R., L.R. suffered from word sound deafness and had a semantic deficit affecting both spoken and written words. Following semantic therapy only, only written word comprehension improved. The next therapy episode included both semantic and auditory therapy. Auditory therapy consisted of spoken word-to-picture matching with phonological foils. L.R. was encouraged to lip-read and not repeat. Following therapy, L.R. improved on a minimal pair discrimination task (where the items were different from those used in therapy) and on spoken word-to-picture matching. Grayson and colleagues argue that L.R.'s auditory comprehension benefited from both semantic therapy and auditory discrimination training.

In the study by Tessier et al. (2007), elements of the previous therapies were developed. However, Tessier and associates' study differs in that it harnesses computer delivery to allow systematic presentation and the use of a different sort of visual cue within therapy. Therapy involved phoneme discrimination and phoneme recognition. Tessier et al. demonstrate improvement for their subject not only in phoneme discrimination and recognition but also in sentence-level auditory comprehension, syllable repetition, and a telephone conversation activity (more everyday life measure). Thus, therapy can be deemed successful, and this reinforces the findings of Morris et al. (1996) and Hessler and Stadie (2006). Tessier et al. (2007) postulate that the difference in generalization of treatment effects may result (in part) from the fact that J.S. (Morris et al., 1996) had other language/aphasia difficulties, whereas their subject is described as having "word deafness but no aphasia and had no other language disorder reasons to be impaired in oral repetition or comprehension" (p. 1172).

An early study by Naeser et al. (1986) extended the discrimination-type training into structured sentence contexts. Therapy began with traditional CVC discrimination, but then the CVC items were put into sentence contexts. The second level involved a simple sentence frame, for example, "The word is (*pill*)"; the third level of therapy involved sentence contexts with semantic information, for example, "It's time to take your (*pill*)." Interestingly, Naeser and associates (1986) presented this as a therapy that took advantage of retained phoneme discrimination ability and aimed to improve sentence comprehension. Presentation was auditory alone, with the aim to "train the auditory modality to focus on verbal information without visual cues" (p. 394).

In this respect, the study differed from others presented, where visual cues were used to support auditory processing. Of the seven subjects in the main study, five showed what was described as a "good response" with increased scores on the Token Test. This study at least offers some ideas of how to extend discrimination training into sentential contexts.

Woolf et al. (2014) report a study with eight participants who they describe as having word sound deafness, although not (as is in the case in some of the previous studies) in its pure form. Woolf et al. contrast phonological therapy with a combined phonological and semantic therapy, which aimed to exploit semantic context to support speech processing. The phonological therapy was based closely on the previous reports described, with judgments in the semantic-phonological therapy primarily based on meaning (although also involving phonological processing). Unlike many of the studies reported previously here, Woolf et al. did not find, either at group or individual level, evidence that discrimination skills improved as a result of either therapy. Woolf et al. carefully discuss these findings and offer possible explanations for this null effect, including a possible influence of number of items, therapy dosage, aphasia profile, hearing acuity, and type of assessment tools. Of these, the assessment tools used are perhaps the most likely factor; all involved computer delivery of stimuli, whereas therapy was delivered "live" by a therapist. This may be an important factor to consider. Milman (2014), in a commentary on this research, suggested that methodological issues contributed to the null finding, discussing dosage, outcome measures, and choice of statistical analysis.

Bastianse, Nijboer, and Taconis (1993) present a program for improving auditory comprehension (the Auditory Language Comprehension Program). This program contains phonological, semantic, and combined levels, based on word–picture matching tasks. The subject improved across a range of tasks, making it difficult to attribute improvement directly to the program. The authors argued that this effect was seen because training had its effect at the semantic level (therefore, auditory comprehension, written comprehension, and naming improved).

Szelag and colleagues (2014) report an experimental paradigm, taking this forward into rehabilitation training. Szelag et al. aimed to improve auditory comprehension (as measured by the Token Test) by training rapid auditory processing. They contrasted training involving either temporal order processing or nontemporal processing (loudness judgment). The authors report that the rapid auditory processing training led to comprehension improvement, in contrast to the control

condition. They suggest therefore, that the training may have a role in future clinical practice. However, results can be considered tentative given the small numbers involved and particularly the possible role of spontaneous recovery, given that participants' performance changed further even after therapy had ended. In an earlier study with N.L., a participant with pure word deafness, Slevc et al. (2011) reported a similar training study, involving temporal and spectral changes in speech and nonspeech stimuli. They demonstrate convincingly that while N.L.'s ability to process temporal changes in nonspeech stimuli does show change, there was no impact for speech stimuli.

We can conclude that specific theoretically motivated therapy can improve auditory discrimination skills and therefore improve auditory analysis. In earlier studies, although improvement on discrimination was robustly demonstrated, it is less clear what the impact of this is on comprehension in a wider sense. However, the Tessier et al. (2007) study demonstrates clear generalization of effects to untreated items and, more important, across a range of auditory tasks, showing a clear impact of therapy. It appears that the presence of additional semantic deficits may affect generalization. Studies have yet to demonstrate whether, for people with additional semantic impairments, therapy focusing on auditory discrimination is an important precursor to subsequent semantic therapy (Hessler & Stadie's [2006] argument). The Grayson et al. (1997) study with L.R. provides some evidence that, for a patient with word sound deafness and semantic impairment, working on both minimal pairs and semantics results in improvement. While improvement in temporal processing may be seen (e.g., Slevc et al., 2011; Szelag et al., 2014), it remains to be demonstrated that this has any impact on speech processing.

There remain important questions and challenges of measurement of the impact of changes occurring at the impairment level. Woolf and colleagues (2014) report an innovative task in their treatment study, where impact of therapy was examined using a telephone listening task. Participants listened to recorded messages and had to select from a choice the final word heard. At the group level, there was improvement on this task, but this was not reflected in analysis at the individual level.

Although there have been a number of studies in this area, no clear picture regarding therapy emerges, with often-conflicting findings between studies. On the whole, discrimination training does result in improvement, although there are exceptions. The Maneta et al. (2001) study suggests that the clinicians must consider severity of deficit and that the point at which therapy begins may be crucial. The study by Woolf and colleagues (2014), carefully designed, also raises questions, perhaps concerning measurement.

Word Form Deafness

Whereas questions remain about word sound deafness, word form deafness is an entirely neglected area. Franklin (1989) hypothesizes that the patient with word sound deafness in her study, M.K., required therapy to be focused at the word level. Clearly, the use of written words supports the individual's processing. The findings of effects of distinctiveness also suggest that therapy with such a client start with distinctive words (with few phonological neighbors) and move to less distinctive items.

Word Meaning Deafness

Francis, Riddoch, and Humphreys (2001) discuss the dearth of studies in the area of word meaning deafness. They discuss whether treatment for word meaning deafness should target the impaired modality (the auditory processing) or perhaps use the strengths of the written processing system (a suggestion from Franklin, 1989). In their study with K.W., a patient with word meaning deafness, Francis and colleagues compare two different therapies: a semantic therapy that used silent reading tasks (no direct focus on auditory processing; described as "implicit") and an "auditory access therapy," with a more direct or "explicit" focus on the auditory access difficulty. The implicit access therapy consisted of silent reading of definitions and written semantic judgments. The auditory access (explicit) therapy consisted of the same tasks, but both auditory and written presentation were used. The majority of the therapy was conducted with K.W. at home. Both types of treatment showed item-specific improvement, but the researchers found that improvement from the explicit auditory access treatment was more durable. The authors argue that treatment for word meaning deafness should involve use of the impaired and unimpaired routes. The implications of an item-specific treatment effect also need to be considered; clearly, if this is the case, then selection of items for therapy becomes crucial.

We do not discuss therapy for central semantic deficits here. However, it also remains a neglected area in the study of treatment effectiveness and efficacy. Nickels (2000) and Morris and Franklin (2012) provide good summaries of the relevant studies in this area. As Nickels discusses, there are many semantic tasks within therapy, but often these are employed to effect change in spoken output. Studies rarely examine the effect of these semantic tasks on comprehension itself.

Auditory Comprehension Therapy (General)

Some therapy studies aim to improve auditory comprehension in a wider sense and where diagnosis and treatment have not been informed by the language-processing model and levels of deficit discussed previously. These are variably described as auditory comprehension therapy or sentence therapy. In a study by West (1973), therapy worked on the types of structures tested within the Token Test. Therapy progressed through a series of levels of comprehension difficulty, akin to the test itself. Participants in the study showed improvement on the Token Test, and there were some subjective reports of improvement in auditory comprehension in a wider sense. Burger, Wertz, and Woods (1983) describe a similar approach, as do Holland and Sonderman (1974).

Approaches Involving the Communication and Language Environment

This section considers therapies that focus on modifications to the physical or communication environment and to the behaviors of others. Maneta and associates (2001) report on a second phase in their study, using an indirect therapy approach, building on work in training conversational partners rather than working directly on the language impairment with the person with aphasia (see Turner & Whitworth, 2006, for a review of conversational partner training). This phase of therapy aimed to change the communicative behaviors of P.K.'s wife so that P.K. was better able to understand her during their conversations. Assessment had shown that P.K.'s written comprehension was a strength, and this was harnessed in therapy by demonstrating the utility of writing key information down during conversation. In addition, P.K.'s wife was encouraged to simplify sentences to contain one key message and to check understanding. Therapy used these strategies and was based on communicating the type of information they might want to use in their conversations. Following therapy, P.K.'s ability to answer questions in a structured task improved, demonstrating that his wife had modified her communication to support him. Maneta and colleagues argued that P.K.'s wife needed structured help and feedback to modify her communication, and that the therapy was effective in achieving this objective.

Conversational partner training generally focuses on the repair and turn-taking behaviors of the conversational partners. However, as Maneta et al. (2001) demonstrate, this type of approach (working with the conversational partner) can be used to facilitate the comprehension of the person with aphasia. The Supporting Partners of People With Aphasia in Relationships and Conversation (SPPARC) program (Lock, Wilkinson, & Bryan, 2001) includes advice and activities related to comprehension. General advice is provided, including minimizing noise, ensuring appropriate seating and lighting, gaining the person's attention before speaking, emphasizing key words, simplifying sentences, using concrete words, avoiding topic change, using appropriate rate and pauses, and using gesture, facial expression, intonation, and writing. A useful handout for the conversational partner is provided. It is important to note that the advice listed in the program is excellent for family members or friends even if conversational partner training is not the focus of therapy. SPPARC also discusses possible strategies for dealing with comprehension problems, including repeating, using gesture, and writing key words, and discusses how the person with aphasia may demonstrate that he or she has not understood. Although only briefly discussed, the information is presented in a clear and helpful way for the conversational partner.

Ferguson (2000) lists a set of communicative strategies that the person with aphasia or the conversational partner might employ to maximize communicative effectiveness. These are therefore potential targets for therapy or advice. They include, for the person with aphasia, repeating to aid processing and to indicate trouble understanding, requesting repetition or clarification, and asking others to slow down or to write. For the conversational partner, this includes using gesture, pausing, slowing down, exaggerating stress, altering word choice, repeating, chunking, reducing complexity, writing, using verbal introducers, touching or using the person's name to alert, and seeking feedback. This type of approach is also seen within the notion of conversational ramps and of training conversational partners to support the person with aphasia (e.g., Kagan, 1998). Support is provided with the aim of allowing the person with aphasia to communicate and have conversations and to reveal his or her competence.

In the preceding therapy approaches, although therapy is indirect in the sense that it primarily involves the conversational partner, there is still direct training, discussion, and practice of communicative strategies with the person with aphasia. General advice is often provided about environmental modifications to aid comprehension (reducing background noise, ensuring the speaker is visible, etc.). The context may also contribute to facilitating comprehension; Wallace, Dietz, Hux, and Weissling (2012) report a study that aimed to investigate the effect of different types of visual support on comprehension of narrative. Overall, they did not find an effect of visual support but suggest that, clinically, the potential impact of visual support should be evaluated. There are also specific examples of advice giving related to auditory comprehension, including Personalised Advice Booklets for Aphasia (PABA; Booth & Wilson, 1999), which allowed for customization, with a set of options selected by the clinician in terms of the specific strategies that support the individual's comprehension.

Previously in the chapter, we discussed how the syndrome of Wernicke's aphasia involves disrupted auditory comprehension (with relatively fluent speech). R. C. Marshall (2001) discusses management of Wernicke's aphasia and advocates "context-based intervention," which allows the person to maximize use of context and of personally relevant information and emphasizes functional outcomes. Marshall advocates manipulation of key linguistic and timing variables by the clinician and teaching relevant others to do the same. This includes message length, syntactic plausibility, vocabulary, personal relevance, level of redundancy, rate, pause, stress, and alerting signals.

FUTURE DIRECTIONS

Clearly, auditory comprehension and the therapeutic approaches available are a much neglected area of research. Recent advances, particularly from brain-imaging research, include more knowledge about the early auditory processing involved. The challenge is to advance our assessment techniques to probe further into the difficulties people experience. Does word form deafness exist? What does this tell us about the models of auditory comprehension we have been considering?

Importantly, future work is needed in therapy for auditory comprehension disorders. The evidence base is weak, particularly for word form and word meaning deafness. Even with word sound deafness, further work is needed to study the impact of specific linguistic therapy on wider communication. What is the most efficacious therapy? Is it a combination of work focusing on the impairment alongside strategic compensatory work? Is it important to improve auditory analysis before embarking on therapy with a different focus (e.g., semantic therapy)? Can we do more to harness the semantic context effect within therapy? This is a rich and exciting area. We look forward to new developments.

Case Illustration 8.1

J. is a 61-year-old woman, married with two children. She was retired at the time of her stroke but had previously worked as a school principal. She reported her hearing to be good. She had a left anterior parietal circulation infarct 11 months prior to the assessments reported here. J. reported difficulties understanding people at times and particularly feeling that people spoke "too fast," and that it helped if they slowed down. She frequently tried to write down what she heard to maximize her understanding.

In terms of overall communication, J. was able to get her message across effectively, producing sentence-level output, but experienced word-finding difficulties, using circumlocution and finger spelling as strategies. On a test of verb and noun naming, she scored 59% and 52%, respectively.

Assessment and Interpretation

The difficulties J. reported with auditory comprehension were confirmed by assessment. She made errors on both single-word and sentence-level auditory comprehension tests, requiring repetitions of items on some occasions before responding. On spoken word-to-picture matching (from the CAT), she performed well (100%), but on a test of auditory synonym judgments (PALPA), she scored 48/60. At sentence level (again from the CAT), J. scored 11/16, requiring some repetitions, and was frequently delayed in her response.

In contrast to her performance with auditorily presented stimuli, performance was better when items were presented in written form. At a single-word level, on the PALPA written word-to-picture matching test she scored 40/40. When assessed on written synonyms, she scored 55/60, with performance superior to when presentation had been auditory. J. did report some problems with reading everyday text, and this was confirmed by an assessment of text-level comprehension that revealed some difficulty.

To examine whether her problems understanding spoken words reflected an earlier level of deficit, she was assessed on the PALPA word minimal pairs test and scored 69/72. She was also able to repeat words correctly. She did not therefore appear to have problems with auditory analysis. On auditory lexical decision, she scored 77/80, requesting repetition of the stimuli for the three incorrect items and being correct on a further two following repetition. This result suggests that she was able to access the word form.

Like in the Franklin et al. (1996) study, J. was asked to repeat and then define a set of words. She was able to repeat the word but then frequently failed to define it from auditory presentation. Her ability to provide a definition improved once the item had been written down. Examples of her errors include the following:

- *Character:* Given auditorily, J. asked for the word to be repeated but was unable to define. Once the word was written down, she said, "Could be someone that's on the television, acting, a character, a person."
- *Bonus:* J. repeated the word but asked for it to be written down, and then said, "If you [were] in a bank you would get more money or something like that—an extra thing."

In this assessment, her performance was better once the word was written down, but her abilities were not intact, replicating the findings from the synonym judgment task.

In summary, J. clearly had difficulties with auditory comprehension, but this was in the presence of superior (though not intact) written word comprehension. The diagnosis is of word meaning deafness, although in the presence of probable difficulty with lexical semantic processing. Assessment results showed that her difficulties were not the result of word sound or word form deafness; she was able to analyze the auditory input and to recognize the word in the phonological input lexicon. However, J.'s word meaning deafness was not pure. Written word comprehension was superior but not intact, and she had some spoken output difficulties; her word retrieval was impaired in contrast to good reading aloud and repetition skills.

Therapy

J. had been seen by her community clinician and was identified as a good candidate for rehabilitation. She was then referred to an intensive treatment facility for individual and group therapy, in combination. It immediately

(continues)

became apparent that J. experienced difficulty in the group setting in particular, finding it difficult to follow activities. She used writing as a strategy and found it helpful if others used this. Her writing strategy facilitated comprehension of the particular words involved but was also counterproductive at times because she then missed what was being said next. She was also prepared to ask for repetitions or rewording if she did not understand.

Goals were negotiated with J., via interview, and a set of real-life goals was established. These included talking and understanding in groups, reading for meaning for everyday text, and spoken production of people and place names. It can be seen then that therapy for this woman had a wider focus than the auditory comprehension difficulties. However, this was one important element. One aspect of therapy involved the auditory and written (explicit) definition task discussed by Francis et al. (2001) and used with their client with word meaning deafness. This used a set of functional words for J. because Francis et al. reported effects of therapy to be specific to those items used in treatment.

Strategies were discussed with J.'s husband in terms of the most effective ways of supporting understanding, and written guidelines were also provided. At the point data were collected, intervention with J. was ongoing.

STUDY QUESTIONS

1. Define the terms *word sound deafness*, *word form deafness*, and *word meaning deafness*.
2. What models might you consider in looking at auditory comprehension in aphasia?
3. Consider what the following assessments reveal about auditory comprehension: auditory word–picture matching, repetition, lexical decision, and minimal pair discrimination.
4. If someone has pure word sound, form, or meaning deafness, what would you predict their written word comprehension to be?
5. If repetition ability is intact, what does this tell you?
6. How strong do you consider the evidence base for therapy for word sound deafness?
7. What possible therapeutic approaches could be used with a client with word meaning deafness?
8. What frameworks can inform your thinking when considering a client's functional auditory comprehension?
9. How does speech sound processing relate to nonverbal sound processing?

NOTE

1. We consider disorders of auditory comprehension, which are specific to the auditory modality; central semantic disorders are beyond the scope of this chapter.

REFERENCES

Albert, M. L. (1974). Time to understand: A case study of word deafness with reference to the role of time in auditory comprehension. *Brain, 97*, 373–384.

Basti-anse, R., Nijboer, S., & Taconis, M. (1993). The Auditory Language Comprehension Programme: A description and case study. *European Journal of Disorders of Communication, 28*(4), 415–433.

Berthier, M. L. (1995). Transcortical sensory aphasia: Dissociation between naming and comprehension. *Aphasiology, 9*, 431–451.

Besle, J., Fischer, C., Bidet-Caulet, A., Lecaignard, F., Bertrand, O., & Giard, M.-H. (2008). Visual activation and audiovisual interactions in the auditory cortex during speech perception: Intracranial recording in humans. *Journal of Neuroscience, 28*, 14301–14310.

Bishop, D. V. M. (2003). *Test for Reception of Grammar version 2*. London: Psychological Corporation.

Booth, S., & Wilson, G. (1999). *PABA: Personalised Advice Booklet for Aphasia*. Glasgow: Glasgow Royal Infirmary University NHS Trust.

Bormann, T., & Weiller, C. (2012). "Are there lexicons?" A study of lexical and semantic processing in word-meaning deafness suggests "yes." *Cortex, 48*(3), 294–307.

Brookshire, R. H., & Nicholas, L. E. (1993). *Discourse Comprehension Test*. Tucson, AZ: Communication Skill Builders.

Burger, L. H., Wertz, R. T., & Woods, D. (1983, May 29–June 2). *A response to treatment in a case of cortical deafness*. Paper presented at the Clinical Aphasiology Conference, Minneapolis, MN.

Campbell, R. (1988). *Visible language: A special issue on lip-reading.* Providence, RI: Brown University Press.

Coltheart, M. (2004). Are there lexicons? *Quarterly Journal of Experimental Psychology, 57,* 1153–1171.

Cutler, A. (2008). The abstract representations in speech processing. *Quarterly Journal of Experimental Psychology, 61,* 1601–1619.

Ellis, A. W. (1984). Introduction to Byrom Bramwell's Word Meaning Deafness. *Cognitive Neuropsychology, 1,* 245–258.

Ellis, A. W., & Young, A. W. (1996). *Human cognitive neuropsychology: A textbook with readings.* Hove, UK: Psychology Press.

Ellmo, W. J., Graser, J. M., Krchnavek, E. A., Calabrese, D. B., & Hauck, K. (1995). *MCLA: Measure of Cognitive Linguistic Abilities.* Vero Beach, FL: Speech Bin.

Ferguson, A. (2000). Maximising communication effectiveness. In N. Muller (Ed.), *Pragmatics and language pathology: Studies in clinical applications* (pp. 53–87). Amsterdam, Netherlands: Benjamins.

Francis, D. R., Riddoch, M. J., & Humphreys, G. W. (2001). Cognitive rehabilitation of word meaning deafness. *Aphasiology, 15*(8), 749–766.

Franklin, S. (1989). Dissociations in auditory word comprehension: Evidence from nine fluent aphasic patients. *Aphasiology, 3,* 189–207.

Franklin, S., Howard, D., & Patterson, K. (1994). Abstract word meaning deafness. *Cognitive Neuropsychology, 11*(1), 1–34.

Franklin, S., Turner, J. E., & Ellis, A. W. (1992). *ADA Comprehension Battery: Action for dysphasic adults.* London: Action for Dysphasic Adults.

Franklin, S., Turner, J., Lambon Ralph, M. A., Morris, J., Ellis, A. W., & Bailey, P. J. (1996). A distinctive case of word meaning deafness? *Cognitive Neuropsychology, 13*(8), 1139–1162.

Geschwind, N. (1971). Current concepts: Aphasia. *New England Journal of Medicine, 284,* 654–656.

Gielewski, E. (1989). Acoustic analysis and auditory retraining in the remediation of sensory aphasia. In C. Code & D. J. Muller (Eds.), *Aphasia therapy* (pp. 138–145). London: Whurr.

Goh, W. D., Suarez, L., Yap, M. J., & Tan, S. H. (2009). Distributional analysis in auditory lexical decision: Neighbourhood density and word frequency effect. *Psychonomic Bulletin and Review, 16,* 882–887.

Goldstein, M. N. (1974). Auditory agnosia for speech ("pure word deafness"): A historical review with current implications. *Brain and Language, 1,* 195–204.

Goodglass, H., Kaplan, E., & Barresi, B. (2001). *BDAE-3: Boston Diagnostic Aphasia Examination* (3rd ed.). Baltimore: Lippincott, Williams & Wilkins.

Grayson, E., Franklin, S., & Hilton, R. (1997). Early intervention in a case of jargon aphasia: Efficacy of language comprehension therapy. *European Journal of Disorders of Communication, 32*(3), 257–276.

Griffiths, T. D., Rees, A., & Green, G. G. R. (1999). Disorders of complex sound processing. *Neurocase, 5,* 365–378.

Hanley, J. R., & Nickels, L. (2009). Are the same phoneme and lexical layers used in speech production and comprehension? A case-series test of Foygel and Dell's (2000) model of aphasic speech production. *Cortex, 45*(6), 784–790.

Hessler, D., & Stadie, N. (2006, September 4–5). *Treatment of word sound deafness with an aphasia patient—Was it effective?* Paper presented at the British Aphasiology Society Therapy Symposium, Plymouth, UK.

Hickok, G., Costanzo, M., Capasso, R., & Miceli, G. (2011). The role of Broca's area in speech perception: Evidence from aphasia revisited. *Brain and Language, 119*(3), 214–220.

Holland, A. L., & Sonderman, J. C. (1974). Effects of a program based on the Token test for teaching comprehension skills to aphasics. *Journal of Speech & Hearing Research, 17,* 589–598.

Howard, D., & Franklin, S. (1988). *Missing the meaning? A cognitive neuropsychological study of the processing of heard words.* Cambridge, MA: MIT Press.

Howard, D., & Nickels, L. (2005). Separating input and output phonology: Semantic, phonological, and orthographic effects in short-term memory impairment. *Cognitive Neuropsychology, 22*(1), 42–77.

Howard, D., & Patterson, K. (1992). *The Pyramids and Palm Trees Test: A test of semantics from words and pictures.* Bury St. Edmunds, UK: Thames Valley Test Company.

Kagan, A. (1998). Supported conversation for adults with aphasia: Methods and resources for training conversation partners. *Aphasiology, 12*(9), 816–830.

Kagan, A., Simmons-Mackie, N. S., Rowland, A., Huijbregts, M., Shumway, E., McEwen, S., et al. (2008). Counting what counts: A framework for capturing real-life outcomes of aphasia intervention. *Aphasiology, 22*(3), 258–280.

Kashino, M. (2006). Phonemic restoration: The brain recreates missing speech sounds. *Acoustic Science and Technology, 27,* 318–321.

Kay, J., Lesser, R., & Coltheart, M. (1992). *Psycholinguistic Assessments of Language Processing in Aphasia (PALPA).* Hove, UK: Erlbaum.

Kertesz, A. (2007). *Western Aphasia Battery—Revised.* San Antonio, TX: Pearson.

Kohn, S. E., & Friedman, R. B. (1986). Word-meaning deafness: A phonological-semantic dissociation. *Cognitive Neuropsychology, 3,* 291–308.

Lambon-Ralph, M. A., Moriarty, L., & Sage, K. (2002). Anomia is simply a reflection of semantic and phonological impairments: Evidence from a case series study. *Aphasiology, 16,* 56–82.

Lieberman, A. M., & Mattingly, I. G. (1985). The motor theory of speech perception, revised. *Cognition, 21,* 1–36.

Lock, S., Wilkinson, R., & Bryan, K. (2001). *SPPARC: Supporting Partners of People with Aphasia in Relationships and Conversation.* Milton Keynes, UK: Speechmark.

Long, A. F., Hesketh, A., Paszek, G., Booth, M., & Bowen, A. (2008). Development of a reliable, self-report outcome measure for pragmatic trials of communication therapy following stroke: The Communication Outcome After Stroke (COAST) scale. *Clinical Rehabilitation, 22,* 1083–1094.

Maneta, A., Marshall, J., & Lindsay, J. (2001). Direct and indirect therapy for word sound deafness. *International Journal of Language & Communication Disorders, 36*(1), 91–106.

Marshall, J., Black, M., & Byng, S. (1999). *The sentence processing resource pack.* Bicester, UK: Winslow Press.

Marshall, R. C. (2001). Management of Wernicke's aphasia: A context-based approach. In R. Chapey (Ed.), *Language intervention strategies in aphasia and related neurogenic communication disorders* (4th ed., pp. 435–456). Philadelphia: Lippincott Williams & Wilkins.

Marslen-Wilson, W. D., & Warren, P. (1994). Levels of perceptual representation and process in lexical access: Words, phonemes and features. *Psychological Review, 101,* 653–675.

Martin, R. C., Breedin, S. D., & Damian, M. F. (1999). The relation of phoneme discrimination, lexical access, and short-term memory: A case study and interactive activation account. *Brain and Language, 70*, 437–482.

McClelland, J. L., & Elman, J. L. (1986). The TRACE model of speech perception. *Cognitive Psychology, 18*, 1–86.

McNeil, M., & Prescott, T. (1978). *The Revised Token Test*. Austin, TX: Pro-Ed.

Milman, L. H. (2014). Therapy for auditory processing impairment in aphasia: More data revealed, more questions to ask. *Evidence-Based Communication Assessment and Intervention, 8*(4), 163–170.

Morris, J. (1997). *Word deafness: A comparison of auditory and semantic treatments*. Unpublished doctoral dissertation, University of York, York, UK.

Morris, J., & Franklin, S. (2012). Investigating the effect of a semantic therapy on comprehension in aphasia. *Aphasiology, 26*(12), 1461–1480.

Morris, J., Franklin, S., Ellis, A. W., Turner, J., & Bailey, P. J. (1996). Remediating a speech perception deficit in an aphasic patient. *Aphasiology, 10*(2), 137–158.

Morris, J., Franklin, S., & Menger, F. (2011). Returning to work with aphasia: A case study. *Aphasiology, 25*(8), 890–907.

Morris, J., Webster, J., Whitworth, A., & Howard, D. (2009). *Newcastle University aphasia therapy resources: Auditory processing*. Newcastle Upon Tyne, UK: Newcastle University.

Morton, J., & Patterson, K. (1980). A new attempt at an interpretation, or, an attempt at a new interpretation. In M. Coltheart, K. Patterson, & J. C. Marshall (Eds.), *Deep dyslexia* (pp. 91–118). London: Routledge and Kegan Paul.

Mottonen, R., & Watkins, K. E. (2009). Motor representations of articulators contribute to categorical perception of speech sounds. *Journal of Neuroscience, 29*, 9819–9825.

Naeser, M. A., Haas, G., Mazurski, P., & Laughlin, S. (1986). Sentence level auditory comprehension treatment programme for aphasia adults. *Archives of Physical Medicine and Rehabilitation, 67*, 393–399.

Nickels, L. (2000). Semantics and therapy in aphasia. In W. Best, K. Bryan, & J. Maxim (Eds.), *Semantic processing: Theory and practice*. (pp 108-124)London, England: Whurr.

Norris, D. (1994). Shortlist: A connectionist model of continuous speech recognition. *Cognition, 52*, 189–234.

Passy, J. (1990). *Cued articulation*. Northumberland, UK: STASS.

Rankin, E., Newton, C., Parker, A., & Bruce, C. (2014). Hearing loss and auditory processing ability in people with aphasia. *Aphasiology, 28*(5), 576–595

Robson, H., Grube, M., Lambon Ralph, M. A. L., Griffiths, T. D., & Sage, K. (2013). Fundamental deficits of auditory perception in Wernicke's aphasia. *Cortex, 49*(7), 1808–1822.

Robson, H., Sage, K., & Ralph, M. A. (2012). Wernicke's aphasia reflects a combination of acoustic-phonological and semantic control deficits: A case-series comparison of Wernicke's aphasia, semantic dementia and semantic aphasia. *Neuropsychologia, 50*(2), 266–275.

Rogalsky, C., Love, T., Driscoll, D., Anderson, S. W., & Hickok, G. (2011). Are mirror neurons the basis of speech perception? Evidence from five cases with damage to the purported human mirror system. *Neurocase, 17*(2), 178–187.

Rogers, T. T., Lambon-Ralph, M. A., Hodges, J. R., & Patterson, K. (2004). Natural selection: The impact of semantic impairment on lexical and object decision. *Cognitive Neuropsychology, 21*(2/3/4), 331–352.

Sarno, M. T. (1963). *Functional Communication Profile*. New York: Institute of Rehabilitation Medicine, New York University Medical Center.

Schwartz, J. L., Berthommier, F., & Savariaux, C. (2004). Seeing to hear better: Evidence for early audio-visual interactions in speech identification. *Cognition, 93*, B69–B78.

Scott, S. K. (2012). The neurobiology of speech perception and production—Can functional imaging tell us anything we did not already know? *Journal of Communication Disorders, 45*(6), 419–425.

Scott, S. K., & Wise, R. J. S. (2004). The functional neuroanatomy of pre-lexical processing in speech perception. *Cognition, 92*, 13–45.

Seidenberg, M. S., & McClelland, J. L. (1989). A distributed, developmental model of word recognition and naming. *Psychological Review, 96*, 523–568.

Shindo, M., Kaga, K., & Tanaka, Y. (1991). Speech-discrimination and lip reading in patients with word deafness or auditory agnosia. *Brain and Language, 40*(2), 153–161.

Slevc, L. R., Martin, R. C., Hamilton, A. C., & Joanisse, M. F. (2011). Speech perception, rapid temporal processing, and the left hemisphere: A case study of unilateral pure word deafness. *Neuropsychologia, 49*(2), 216–230.

Swinburn, K., & Byng, S. (2006). *The Communication Disability Profile*. London: Connect.

Swinburn, K., Porter, G., & Howard, D. (2004). *The Comprehensive Aphasia Test*. Hove, UK: Psychology Press.

Szelag, E., Lewandowska, M., Wolak, T., Seniow, J., Poniatowska, R., Pöppel, E., et al. (2014). Training in rapid auditory processing ameliorates auditory comprehension in aphasic patients: A randomized controlled pilot study. *Journal of the Neurological Sciences, 338*(1–2), 77–86.

Tessier, C., Weill-Chounlamountry, A., Michelot, N., & Pradat-Diehl, P. (2007). Rehabilitation of word deafness due to auditory analysis disorder. *Brain Injury, 21*, 1165–1174.

Turner, S., & Whitworth, A. (2006). Conversational partner training programmes in aphasia: A review of key themes and participants' roles. *Aphasiology, 20*(6), 483–510.

Wallace, S. E., Dietz, A., Hux, K., & Weissling, K. (2012). Augmented input: The effect of visuographic supports on the auditory comprehension of people with chronic aphasia. *Aphasiology, 26*(2), 162–176.

West, J. A. (1973). Auditory comprehension in aphasic adults: Improvement through training. *Archives of Physical Medical Rehabilitation, 54*, 78–86.

Whitworth, A., Webster, J., & Howard, D. (2014). *A cognitive neuropsychological approach to assessment and intervention in aphasia* (2nd ed.). Hove, UK: Psychology Press.

Woolf, C., Panton, A., Rosen, S., Best, W., & Marshall, J. (2014). Therapy for auditory processing impairment in aphasia: An evaluation of two approaches. *Aphasiology, 28*(12,) 1481–1505.

World Health Organization. (2001). *International classification of functioning, disability and health: ICF*. Geneva, Switzerland: Author.

OBJECTIVES

The reader will be able to:

1. **Understand the ways in which research on speech errors that occur in everyday speech helped theorists develop cognitive models of word production.**

2. **Describe how cognitive models of word production are used to understand the nature of word production disorders in aphasia.**

3. **Explain a streamlined approach to determining the locus of a word production disorder in a two-step interactive activation model of word production.**

4. **Understand current approaches to rehabilitation of word production disorders and how they address issues of generalization and endurance of treatment effects.**

Disorders of Word Production

Nadine Martin

INTRODUCTION

In aphasia, impairment of word retrieval is common and is the primary difficulty in one subtype of aphasia, anomic aphasia. Words comprise meaning and sounds, and retrieval of either or both of these aspects can be affected by aphasia. Thus, although word-finding difficulties are common in aphasia, the nature of the impairment is not uniform across aphasia types. People without aphasia or language disorder also have word retrieval difficulties from time to time, so-called slips of the tongue. These are similar in many ways to the word retrieval difficulties that occur in aphasia but are far less numerous. The study of speech errors committed by speakers with and without aphasia has contributed much to the understanding of the cognitive organization of language and, in turn, has guided approaches to the diagnosis and rehabilitation of word production disorders in aphasia.

This chapter is divided into three sections. The first section reviews cognitive and psycholinguistic models of stages and processes involved in word production and research that validates those models. The second section focuses on diagnosis of word retrieval impairments in the context of a cognitive model of word production. A diagnostic approach that uses two tasks, naming and repetition, and varies stimulus characteristics (e.g., frequency) is proposed. The third section reviews some current impairment-based treatment approaches for word retrieval disorders and some current issues addressed in aphasia rehabilitation research.

MODELS OF WORD PRODUCTION: THEORETICAL AND EMPIRICAL FOUNDATIONS

What Are the Fundamental Steps in Word Production?

Models of word production are meant to depict how a word's meaning and its sounds (or form) are retrieved. There is general agreement that these two aspects of words are retrieved, but some theorists propose discrete stages of retrieval, and others propose that there is interaction between meaning and sound levels of representation during the word retrieval process. The process of producing a word (e.g., a picture name.) begins with an image in mind and ends with the articulation of a sound sequence that makes up the word a person has learned to associate with that image. What happens between these two points? Figure 9.1a shows a discrete-stage model of the steps involved in retrieving a word. The term *discrete stage* means that the steps involved in producing a word occur independently of each other. Once a word's meaning is retrieved, that stage is complete and the next stage, word form retrieval, begins. Levelt and colleagues advocate this type of model (see Levelt, Roelofs, & Meyer, 1999, for review).

The process of producing a word begins at the conceptual level. A concept is stimulated by intention of the speaker or by some sensory input (e.g., seeing a cat, hearing bells chime, smelling a pie baking). A concept is not linguistic in nature. Rather, it is a network of knowledge about something tangible (e.g., a person, thing, or action) or something abstract, such as emotions (e.g., joy) or topics (e.g., peace). The first stage of the word retrieval process begins with conceptually driven activation of the semantic features of a word. If the word to be spoken is *cat*, semantic features specific to cat (e.g., animal, furry, domestic) would be activated. The second stage is selection of the word form in the lexicon (the mental dictionary) that is associated with these semantic features. At this stage, activation from these semantic features also makes contact with other words in the lexicon that overlap in meaning with the target word. These semantically related words could be synonyms of the target (e.g., *dog–canine*), associated words (*dog–bone*), super- or subordinates (*dog–animal, dog–poodle*), or category coordinates (*dog–cat*). One of the many activated word forms is selected to be spoken. If all goes well, this should be the target word *cat*. However, it could be one of the semantically related lexical neighbors that were made active by the spread of activation from the semantic feature level.

Once the word form is retrieved, the third stage, phonological encoding, begins, and the sounds of the word are retrieved and ordered.

Figure 9.1b shows another version of a word production model that not only holds a similar view of the stages involved in retrieving a word but also maintains that the stages interact with and influence each other during word production. What does it mean to say there is *interaction* between stages? In this model, as activation spreads forward from one stage to another, there is also feedback activation between stages that keeps semantic, word form, and phonemes stable during the time it takes to select and produce the intended word. Dell and colleagues advocate this interactive activation (IA) model (Dell, 1986; Dell & Reich, 1981; Foygel & Dell, 2000; Harley, 1984). Further in this chapter, different types of word production disorders are discussed in the context of the IA model of word production (Foygel & Dell, 2000; Schwartz, Dell, Martin, Gahl, & Sobel, 2006). This model has proved successful as an account of word retrieval patterns in aphasia (Dell, Schwartz, Martin, Saffran, & Gagnon, 1997; Schwartz et al., 2006). Like other production models (e.g., Fromkin, 1971; Garrett, 1975, 1976, 1982; Harley, 1984, 1990, 1995; Stemberger, 1985), it was originally developed to account for speech errors made in everyday speaking contexts (slips of the tongue). Before discussing its account of word production impairments in aphasia, I review the evidence from speech errors and other sources that word production occurs in several stages reflecting retrieval of a word's meaning (semantic), its word form (lexical), and its sounds (phonology).

Research on the Properties of Language Production and Its Breakdown in Everyday Speech Contexts

In the latter part of the 20th century, a number of theorists proposed models of word and language production (e.g., Caramazza, 1997; Dell, 1986; Fromkin, 1971; Garrett, 1975; Harley, 1984; Levelt, 1989; Stemberger, 1985). Some of these models were used later as frameworks to evaluate and understand disorders of word retrieval (e.g., Caramazza, 1997; Dell et al., 1997). Most of these early models were developed through analysis of speech errors made in everyday conversations and other speaking contexts. The data from everyday speaking errors are rich in the information they provide about the units of language and how those units are ordered into the words and sentences people speak. Speech

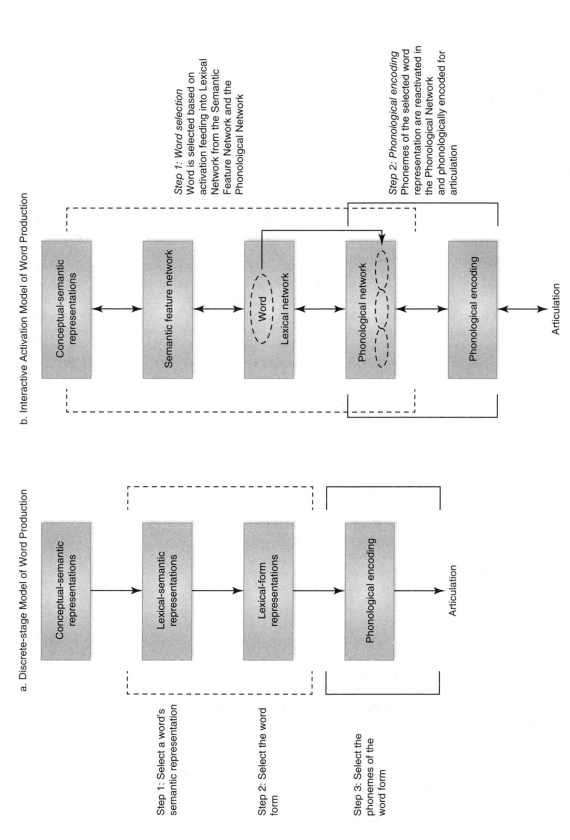

Figure 9.1 Comparison of a discrete-stage model of word production and an interactive activation (IA) model of word production. Bidirectional arrows in the IA model indicate interaction between stages of production. Also, dotted and solid line brackets indicate overlap between Step 1 and Step 2 in the IA model but not in the discrete-stage model.

errors are not random in character or in the contexts in which they occur. Rather, units that are involved in an error (the target sound or word and the erroneous sound or word) tend to be systematically related in form (sounds or words) or meaning (words) or in the linguistic context in which they occur. Studies of speech errors reveal patterns that suggest rules that govern their occurrence. The term *rule* as used here refers to probabilities of certain patterns of error or influences on errors that are interpreted as a reflection of rules that govern successful production of words and sentences. It was proposed (e.g., Fromkin,1971) that speech errors indicate the psychological reality of sounds, syllables, words, and other linguistic units in language.

What Everyday Speech Errors Indicate About the Organization of Language Production

Speech production errors involve all types of language units, including phonetic features, phonemes, syllables, morphemes, words, and even sentences. Some errors are syntagmatic, involving sequential relations between linguistics units. These so-called movement errors include anticipations, perseverations, or exchanges of two sounds, morphemes, or words. Other errors involve paradigmatic relations with other units and include additions or deletions of units or substitution of one unit for another. Table 9.1 shows a list of speech error types and examples.

Once classified by type of error, speech errors can be analyzed further with respect to their relationship with the target sound or word and the context in which they occur.

These analyses provide further evidence of how the language system organizes and processes its output. Word substitution errors can be related to the target word phonologically (e.g., *cantaloupe* → *candlelight*), semantically (e.g., *cantaloupe* → *watermelon*), or both phonologically and semantically (*cantaloupe* → *cucumber*). Semantically related and phonologically related errors are evidence that at some point in the word retrieval process the meaning of a word is retrieved and at another point in time the word form or sounds of the word are retrieved. The occurrence of errors that are both semantically and phonologically related to the intended word suggests that there is some interaction

---

Table 9.1 Examples of Speech Errors That Occur in Everyday Speaking Situations and in Aphasia

I. Phoneme and phonetic stages

  Substitutions: *bat* → *mat*, *bat* → *lat*

  Additions: *bake* → *brake*

  Deletions: *brake* → *bake*

  Phoneme movement errors:

    Anticipatory: John dropped his *cup of coffee.* → John dropped his *cuff of coffee.*

    Perseverative: John gave the boy ... → John **g**ave the **g**oy ...

    Full exchange: **K**eep a **t**ape → **T**eep a **k**ape

  Phonetic feature movement errors: **b**ig and **f**at → **p**ig and **v**at

  Errors that are seen in aphasia but rarely in normal speech:

  Neologisms: *chicken* → /tlpko/

II. Word-level errors

  Semantic: *elbow* → *knee*

  Phonological: *mustache* → *mushroom*

  Semantic + phonological (mixed): *penguin* → *pelican*

  Blends (word- and phoneme-level error): *lecture + session* → *sessure* or *lecsion*; *athlete/player* → *athler*

  Word movement errors (samples from Garrett, 1975, 1980, 1988):

    Exchange errors: This **seat** has a **spring** in it. → This **spring** has a **seat** in it.

    They **forgot** it and **left** it behind. → They **left** it and **forgot** it behind.

    Stranding errors: I thought the **truck** was **park**ed. → I thought the **park** was **truck**ed.

    They were **talking Turkish**. → They were **turking Talkish**. (Garrett, 1988)

  Errors that are seen in aphasia but rarely in normal speech:

    Unrelated: *donkey* → *chair*

    Double errors: *unicorn* → *house* (*horse* → *house*)

    Decomposition errors on compounds: *waterfall* → *ice fall*, *ice farm*

between stages of retrieving the meaning and sounds of a word. Although that apparent interaction could be a chance event, studies have shown that these so-called mixed errors occur more often than would be expected by chance (N. Martin, Gagnon, Schwartz, Dell, & Saffran, 1996; N. Martin, Weisberg, & Saffran, 1989). Thus, characteristics of word substitution errors indicate two features of the word retrieval system: distinct semantic and phonological retrieval stages and interaction or cross talk between these stages.

The linguistic context in which errors occur is also informative about the organization of word retrieval processes. One relevant pattern is that speech errors do not violate the phonotactic rules of one's language. That is, sound sequences may be in error, but sound combinations that are not part of a language (e.g., *fs* at the beginning of a word) are not produced as errors. This observation indicates that the speaker has an implicit knowledge of the phonotactic rules of the language (Walker & Dell, 2006).

Speech errors involve linguistic units of similar type. For example, consonants exchange with or replace other consonants, not vowels (and vice versa). Content words (nouns, verbs, modifiers) do not exchange with or replace function words (e.g., determiners, prepositions). Content word exchanges tend to respect syntactic category (Example 1, which follows) and exchange across phrases. In contrast, phoneme exchanges (Example 2) tend to occur within a phrase.

1. The *ticket* that she bought for the *concert* was left on the table. → The *concert* that she bought for the *ticket* was left on the table.

2. The *tr*ick *qu*estion stumped us all. → The *qu*ick *tr*estion stumped us all.

Another informative error type involves the movement of morphemes, as in Example 3:

3. The *truck* is *back*ing out. → The *back* is *truck*ing out (from Garrett, 1975).

The free morphemes exchange and the bound morpheme *-ing* is stranded in its place within the sentence. This pattern of error indicates a stage in which free and bound morphemes are represented separately. Garrett (1975) proposes that the patterns of movement errors illustrated in Examples 1 through 3 indicate two stages of word retrieval in the context of sentence production. In the first stage, the functional level of representation, content words are retrieved on the basis of the functional argument structure of a sentence. In the second stage, the positional level of representation, the content words are inserted into a sentence frame and phonologically specified.

Several constraints on phoneme movement errors relate to the position of sounds within a word. Phoneme anticipations, perseverations, and exchanges all involve movement of sounds from one word to another. First, movement errors involve initial phonemes more than any other position of the word (80% of all sound errors, as estimated by Stemberger, 1982). Second, the positions of the phonemes within a word or syllable involved in the movement errors are nearly always the same (as in Example 4, which follows). A third influence on phoneme movement errors is a phenomenon called the *repeated phoneme* effect. Phoneme exchanges are more common when each phoneme has a similar phoneme next to it, especially vowels. Example 4 demonstrates the initial phoneme bias, positional constraint, and the repeated phoneme effect:

4. left hemisphere → heft lemisphere (from Dell, 1986)

The exchanging phonemes come from the same position within their respective words, they are in the initial position, and each is followed by the vowel /ɛ/.

Another important pattern of error with implications for cognitive models of word production is the *lexical bias* effect: Phonological errors (substitutions, deletions, additions, and movement errors) are more likely to occur if the outcome is a word rather than a nonword (Baars, Motley, & MacKay, 1975). This bias implies that the language system is effective at editing out flawed productions, and that these are harder to detect, when the potential error is a word. In addition, this finding indicates that the study of monitoring behaviors could provide useful insights about word production.

Other Methods Used to Investigate Word Production Processes

The preceding review of speech error research is not meant to be exhaustive but should give an idea of how so-called slips of the tongue can be used to infer the processes and linguistic units that compose the language system. The study of everyday speech errors is only one approach to understanding the stages and processes involved in producing a word. Researchers also constructed experiments to induce speech errors in normal speakers (e.g., Baars et al., 1975; Bredart & Valentine, 1992; N. Martin et al., 1989). By this method, they could control the linguistic context in which a word was spoken. A typical approach to inducing errors, especially movement errors, was to present pairs of words that set up a context that would increase the probability of a substitution or movement error (e.g., Baars et al., 1975).

Other researchers examined normal breakdowns in the flow of speech that are not errors, but momentary blocks or hesitations. The most studied of these is the *tip-of-the-tongue* phenomenon (e.g., Brown & McNeill, 1966; Burke, MacKay, Worthley, & Wade, 1991; Jones & Langford, 1987). Everyone has experienced this feeling of knowing there is a certain word we want to say to express something, but not being able to retrieve that word. This kind of experience is perhaps most similar to what a person with anomic aphasia experiences when he or she cannot retrieve a word. The tip-of-the-tongue state is evidence that retrieval of meaning and form of a word are somewhat separable events.

Levelt and colleagues (1999) argue that speech errors represent a breakdown in the language system and as such may not be reliable indicators of the organization of the language system. They introduced a different approach to the study of the word production system using a paradigm that involves picture naming in the context of a second task, lexical decision, or listening to an auditory probe (Levelt et al., 1991; Schriefers, Meyer, & Levelt, 1990). They identified variations in the time it takes to name a picture by presenting probe words that are related to the target word (name of the picture) semantically or phonologically. The probes were presented auditorily at different points in time that coincided with presumed stages of semantic and phonological retrieval. Interference or facilitation effects at these points would verify that semantic or phonological processing was occurring at that moment (Levelt et al., 1991; Schriefers et al., 1990). By tracking the interference of the probes at these different points in time, they were able to identify with some reliability the semantic and phonological stages of word retrieval.

Summary of the Foundations of Word Production Research

The use of word production models to understand language impairments in aphasia stems from a foundation of research on speech errors and speech production processes in speakers without aphasia. In turn, data from speakers with aphasia have further informed cognitive models of word processing (e.g., Dell, Martin, & Schwartz, 2007; Dell et al., 1997; Laine & Martin, 1996; N. Martin, Dell, Saffran, & Schwartz, 1994; Schwartz et al., 2006; Schwartz, Saffran, Bloch, & Dell, 1994). The early research on speech errors informed our understanding of the cognitive representations and stages involved in word production. Current models focus

more on the dynamics of language processing, a shift that was sparked in part by the development of computer instantiations of language-processing models (e.g., Dell, 1986; McClelland & Rumelhart, 1988; Plaut & Shallice 1991). One source of behavioral evidence to confirm these models of processing dynamics comes from studies of changing error patterns in aphasia after recovery (e.g., N. Martin et al., 1994; N. Martin, Saffran, & Dell, 1996; Schwartz & Brecher, 2000) or after treatment (e.g., Abel, Wilmes, & Huber, 2007). These and other such studies represent an exciting direction in research on word production disorders.

APPLICATION OF COGNITIVE/PSYCHOLINGUISTIC MODELS OF WORD PRODUCTION TO THE DIAGNOSIS OF WORD PRODUCTION DISORDERS IN APHASIA

As noted, models of word production identify three major stages of word production that follow the conceptual level of representation: access to word-specific semantic features (semantic network), retrieval of the word form (lexical network), and encoding the corresponding phonemes of that word. In this respect, both the discrete-stage and IA models can serve as guides to diagnosing the source of word production disorders in aphasia. As a framework for diagnosis of word production disorders in aphasia, I use the IA model to illustrate how a model can help identify the stages of production that are affected in a word production disorder. As depicted in Figure 9.1b, the stages are not modular but rather interact or cross talk during the process of retrieving semantic and phonological representations of the word and encoding its phonology. Figure 9.1b shows a simplified version of the IA model intended to facilitate a comparison with a discrete-stage model.

A more typical sketch of the IA model of word retrieval (Dell & O'Seaghdha, 1992) is shown in Figure 9.2. This depiction includes representations of the semantic features in a semantic network, word representations (also called word nodes) in a lexical network, and phonemes in a phonological network. It also shows two distinct retrieval events: retrieval of the word representation, which involves interactive feed-forward and feedback activation into the lexicon, and a second event when the

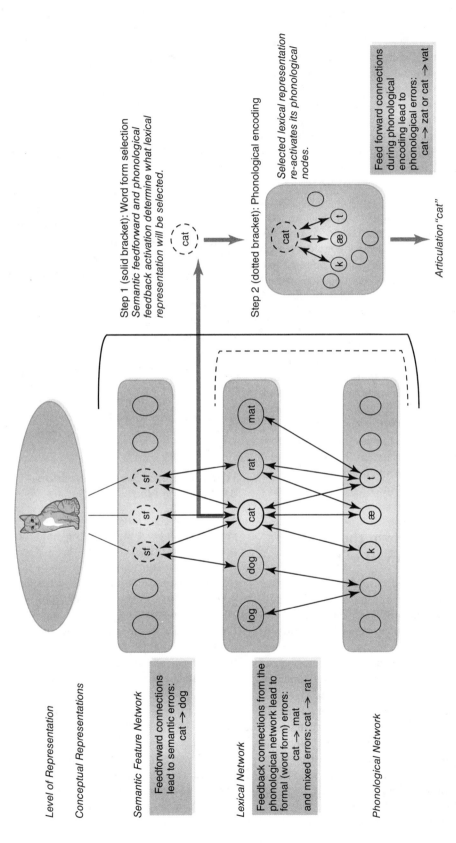

Figure 9.2 A more typical depiction of the IA model of word retrieval with contents of each level of representation shown (semantic features, word nodes, phonemes). The two stages of retrieval, word selection, and phonological encoding, are shown, and their overlap is indicated by the dotted and solid line brackets.

phonemes of the selected word are selected and encoded. The connections between semantic lexical and phonological networks are interactive, which means that when activation from semantic features spreads to the corresponding word representations, it feeds back to the semantic level to keep these features active until a word is produced. In the same manner, when activation from a word node spreads forward to its corresponding phonemes, it also feeds back to the lexicon to keep that representation active until a word is produced. For a more detailed discussion of this model, refer to the work of Laine and Martin (1996).

An important assumption of the IA model is that at each level of representation, multiple candidates are activated by feed-forward and feedback activation. Although the intended word is usually selected, conditions such as priming, characteristics of the word to be retrieved, and integrity of semantic and phonological processes can alter the dynamics of the activation in the network such that one of the competing words is retrieved. In aphasia, all of these factors can influence activation dynamics. Potential semantic substitutions (e.g., *cat* → *dog*) are activated by feed-forward activation between the semantic and lexical networks. Potential form-related word substitutions (*cat* → *mat*) are activated by feedback activation between the phonological and lexical networks. And, potential mixed errors (both semantically and phonologically related, e.g., *cat* → *rat*) are activated by feed-forward activation between the semantic and lexical networks and feedback activation between the phonological and lexical networks.

Major Types of Anomia in the Context of the Interactive Activation Model

Although discrete-stage models and IA models differ in the assumptions about processing in word production, they do agree that the process involves access and retrieval of three representations: semantic, phonological form (word form), and the constituent phonemes. Three major types of word production disorders reflect impairment of each of these stages: semantic anomia, word form anomia, and disordered phoneme assembly. In the discrete-stage model of word production depicted in Figure 9.1a, semantic anomia has been attributed to impaired spread of activation between conceptual and semantic representations (e.g., Laine & Martin, 1996), word form anomia to impaired activation of word forms by semantic activation, and phoneme assembly disorders to impaired activation of phonemes. Word production disorders in the context of the IA model are

described somewhat differently. As Figures 9.1b and 9.2 show, beginning with a message from conceptual knowledge, activation of the semantic network initiates two steps of word production: retrieval of the word node (Step 1) and phonological encoding (Step 2). The following sections describe the activities of these stages of word production.

Conceptual Activation of the Semantic Network

Stroke-based aphasia does not involve impairment of connections between conceptual knowledge and the semantic network. However, progressive semantic dementia is based on a breakdown of these connections. Semantic dementia involves a progressive degradation of conceptual knowledge that supports the language system (the long-term knowledge and memories to be expressed in language or other forms of communication or action). In language, a breakdown of this kind results in anomia but is distinguished from the anomia associated with stroke-based aphasia in several ways. First, the errors that are made can be semantic (as occur in aphasia), but they are more often superordinate errors (e.g., *knife* → *kitchen tool*) or visually related (*knife* → *flat stick*). The errors tend to reflect loss of the conceptual representations of the objects being named.

Word Retrieval Step 1: Selection of the Word Node

There is much activity in Step 1, in which a word node is selected from the lexical network. There are two potential points of breakdown: (a) interactive activation between the semantic and lexical networks and (b) interactive activation between the lexical and phonological levels. When the impairment affects the connections between the semantic and lexical networks, the pattern of error is one typically described as follows: The semantic activation is too weak or unstable to effectively activate the target lexical entry. This does not mean there is a *loss* of semantic features or conceptual knowledge as in semantic dementia described previously. Rather, the spread of activation from those features is weak. When the activation of the target is weak or unstable, other words that have been activated through the spreading activation process may be selected in error. The word substitutions that occur in this stage are semantically related to the intended word and are typically categorically related (*cat* → *dog*; *knife* → *fork*) or associated in some way (*cat* → *meow*; *knife* →

cut). These semantic substitutions are called *semantic paraphasias*. Also at this stage would be no responses (also called *omissions*), when no word node is active enough to be retrieved.

Other error types occur in Step 1 during the spread of activation between the lexical and phonological networks. Phonologically related word errors (also called *formal paraphasias*) result from phonological feedback activating phonologically related word nodes in the lexical network during the Step 1 word-priming process. Unrelated word errors also result from phonological feedback, but from primed phonemes of semantically related words primed in the first part of Step 1. For example, if *dog* is activated in the lexical network (when *cat* is intended), its activation will spread to phonemes of the word *dog* and feed back to the lexicon to support activation of *dog*, but at that point the word node for *log* is activated (Figure 9.2). Finally, mixed errors that are semantically and phonologically related to the target word (e.g., *cat → rat*) occur when feed-forward activation from the semantic network and feedback activation from the phonological network converge on a lexical representation that is both semantically and phonologically related and increases the possibility that this competing lexical node will be selected in error in a system that suffers from weakened activation spread.

Word Retrieval Step 2: Phonological Encoding

Thus far, mechanisms for word substitutions have been discussed. These occur in Step 1 and, as described, are related to the target word in ways that reflect the source of activation into the lexicon (semantic feed-forward activation, phonological feedback activation). Sound errors occur in the second stage of word retrieval, phonological encoding. The end stage of Step 1 is the selection of a word representation. This could be the target word or one of the word error types described previously. This selected word is then phonologically encoded via the same connections that link the lexical and phonological networks in Step 1. If these connections are impaired, the likelihood of phoneme selection errors increases, and the resulting output is a phonologically related nonword error (*cat → dat*) or a phonological substitution that by chance creates a word (*cat → bat*). The latter error type is called a *sublexical* phonologically related word error because it occurs in the phonological encoding stage, not the lexical stage. As noted, phonologically related word errors also occur at the Step 1 lexical selection stage and are called formal paraphasias. Thus, there are two sources of a phonologically related word error: Step 1 (a lexical selection error) and Step 2 (a phoneme selection error that by chance creates a word).

How do we distinguish the sources of phonological word errors? The lexical-level word form errors tend to share fewer phonemes with the target word (e.g., *population → pollution*) than phonological slips that create words (e.g., *cattle → battle*). Also, it has been shown that lexical-level phonological word errors tend to share the same grammatical category as the target word (Gagnon, Schwartz, Martin, Dell, & Saffran, 1997), making them distinct from phonological errors that create words by chance.

The description of the major forms of anomia in the context of Dell's IA model might seem a bit different from the traditional classification scheme shown in Figure 9.1a. And yet, three predominant types of anomia still affect (a) activation of the word form from semantics, (b) stability of the phonological aspects of the word form in the lexical network, and (c) encoding and ordering of a word's phonemes. The description of the nature of these deficits may change again as it has in the past, as our understanding of the processes and representations underlying word retrieval evolves and our tools to investigate and characterize the deficits become more sophisticated. For diagnostic purposes, it is still useful to divide word production difficulties into these three types. This classification guides our interpretation of test results from diagnostic batteries designed to probe each of these stages of production.

Diagnosing the Word Production Disorder

There are three things to consider in assessment of word retrieval: the task, the characteristics of the words being probed in a particular task, and the levels of processing involved in performance of that task. The objective of an assessment of word production is to determine which levels of processing are available to support word retrieval and which are not. This is accomplished in more ways than simply testing the ability to name a picture, although production tasks would certainly play an important role in the evaluation. A word production disorder does not typically occur in isolation but rather is one symptom of a word-processing disorder that may affect input and output processing. Other tasks can provide critical information about the locus of impairment in the word-processing system that underlies the production disorder.

Clinicians can use many tasks to probe word-processing ability, including picture naming; word recognition;

phoneme discrimination tests; semantic processing tests (comparison of features, meanings of words); repetition of words; and pseudowords. The approach I describe here includes two tasks: word production (picture naming and naming words in response to a definition) and repetition of words and nonwords. The analysis of error types in each task also is informative. With these two tasks and careful variation of stimulus characteristics, enough information can be gained to determine the locus (or loci) of a word retrieval deficit. Once this is determined, other tests sensitive to functions of the impaired and spared parts of the language system can be administered to obtain a more refined profile of the word-processing impairment.

There are many ways to vary stimulus characteristics, but four are discussed here: word frequency, word imageability, word length, and lexicality (whether a phoneme string is a real word or a pseudoword). The first two variables reflect lexical and semantic properties (words and their meanings) and are sensitive to impairments in Step 1 (word selection) in the IA model. The last two reflect lexical and phonological properties (word forms, Step 1, and their corresponding phonemes, Step 2 phonological encoding). Other variables of interest can provide added information about the nature of a word-processing deficit, for example, category-specific naming deficits or differences in ability to retrieve nouns versus verbs.

The four variables reviewed here, however, can be used in combination with the naming and repetition tasks to determine whether the underlying mechanism of the word retrieval deficit is lexical–semantic (affecting activation spreading from semantics to the lexicon), lexical–phonological (affecting stability of activated word forms in the lexicon), or phonological encoding (retrieving or ordering of phonemes).

For this discussion, refer to Figure 9.3, another simplified depiction of the IA model that includes *both* word production and word repetition pathways. The model includes all of the assumptions of Dell's IA model of word production as in Figure 9.2 except that it adds a repetition component and depicts this as separate but interactive input and output phonological networks (see Dell et al., 2007, and Schwartz et al., 2006, for details of this repetition component of the IA model). Most models assume a single semantic network subserving input and output word processing, but there is disagreement about whether there is a single phonological network (N. Martin et al., 1994) or separate input and output phonological networks (e.g., R. Martin & Lesch, 1996). Discussion of the details of that controversy is beyond the scope of this chapter, but refer to the work of N. Martin and Saffran

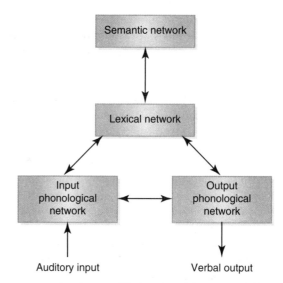

Figure 9.3 Another simplified version of the IA model of naming that also includes pathways that mediate repetition of a word. Bidirectional arrows indicate interaction between phonological, lexical, and semantic networks and between input phonological and output phonological networks.

(2002) for more information. Briefly, there is evidence of separate networks from reports of aphasia profiles that include output phonological difficulties without evidence of input phonological disturbance (R. Martin, Lesch, & Bartha, 1999). Evidence of interaction between input and output phonological networks comes from studies showing that performance on input and output phonological processing tasks is strongly correlated (N. Martin & Saffran, 2002; N. Martin, Schwartz, & Kohen, 2005). It is the latter model (separate but interactive input and output phonological networks) that is used to guide the diagnosis of word-processing disorders.

Lexical–Semantic Variables, Frequency, and Imageability

High-frequency words are easier to retrieve than are low-frequency words, and words of high imageability are easier to retrieve than are words of low imageability. It is important to note that word frequency and imageability effects are normal effects. That is, people without language impairment show differences in retrieval ability relative to these factors, but this difference is only seen in a sensitive measure such as reaction time. In aphasia, frequency and imageability effects can be exaggerated depending on the level of processing that is impaired. If either of these variables *does* affect performance on word production or repetition tasks, the differences are evident in accuracy of performance. The following material discusses each of these variables and how they inform us about the locus of word production impairment in aphasia.

Frequency. Word frequency is considered to be a lexical variable (Jescheniak & Levelt, 1994), but numerous studies of frequency effects in normal speakers and people with aphasia indicate that word frequency reflects processing at all levels in word production (see Kittredge, Dell, Verkuilen, & Schwartz, 2008, for a review). *Frequency* refers to how common a word is compared to other words in the language. Frequency counts based on sampling of written and spoken language of many speakers are available (e.g., Francis & Kucera, 1982). Apart from this general frequency account of words, it is important to consider that speakers have unique differences in familiarity of words related to their individual experiences. Someone who is a carpenter, for example, may have a vocabulary that reflects a facility with tool names that others may not have.

The frequency effect is a powerful effect and is present in many tasks, including naming and repetition. Frequency is also confounded with length; more frequent words tend to be shorter (Harley, 2001). Thus, care must be taken to control for length when choosing stimuli for a task. In word production tasks and repetition tasks, it is important to include words of high, medium, and low frequency and words of different syllable length within each of the frequency groups.

The frequency effect can be seen in word production and word repetition:

- *Frequency effects in word production.* The more frequent a word is in the English language or in a person's individual vocabulary, the stronger is its representation in the lexicon. This means that all else being equal, words of high frequency are easier to access and retrieve than are words of lower frequency. If frequency effects are present in word production tasks, this indicates that the word production disorder involves the Step 1 word retrieval process. It does not narrow the diagnosis any further to involvement of lexical–semantic or lexical–phonological connections. However, the word repetition task can provide some insight into the source of the Step 1 retrieval impairment.
- *Frequency effects in word repetition.* If connections between lexical and phonological representations are compromised, performance on repetition of a word depends on lexical and semantic representations that remain viable (Figure 9.3). Phonological input is more successful at activating high-frequency words than low-frequency words, and these are better able to support the output response. This pattern does not indicate damage at the level of lexical representations. Rather, the spread of activation from phonological to lexical levels is impaired and unmasks the normal differences in accessibility of high versus low frequency. Unimpaired speakers and speakers with aphasia whose phonological processing is intact can repeat words accurately with support just from the activated phonemes of the words. Thus, when frequency effects in word repetition are present, they indicate phonological processing impairment and a reliance on lexical representations to repeat.

Imageability Imageability of a word is a semantic variable meaning that it reflects the integrity of semantic processing. It refers to the degree to which a concept denoted by a word can be mentally pictured. *Hammer* and *chair* and the verb *jump* can be imaged easily. Even though there are different types or sizes of these objects and different manners of jumping, these concepts have certain fixed characteristics that can be brought to mind. Abstract words, in contrast, are not fixed objects. They are principles, ideas, or themes. Words such as *justice*, *integrity*, or *transpire* are not imageable as single entities but are understood in the context of a scenario (e.g., *justice* may invoke an image of a courtroom proceeding).

Imageability effects can be seen in word production and word repetition:

- *Imageability effects in word production.* Imageability effects are not apparent in a picture naming task because pictureable words are also highly imageable (but see Nickels & Howard, 1995). However, other word production tasks, such as providing a name in response to a definition, are sensitive to this variable. If someone has more difficulty retrieving word names of abstract concepts than concrete, imageable concepts, this indicates impaired spread of activation between the semantic and lexical networks. Such activation is weaker for abstract concepts in the normal case, but when compromised further by brain damage, the difference in ease of retrieval between high- and low-imageable concepts is even more apparent.
- *Imageability effects in word repetition.* The presence or absence of an imageability effect in word repetition reveals the integrity of the phonological route for repetition in the same way as the presence or absence of the frequency effect does. It provides evidence that the speaker is dependent on

lexical–semantic processes to repeat the word and implies that, in this case, phonological processing (spread of activation between the phonological networks [input and output]) is impaired. An absence of this effect implies that the phonological route is available to support performance on the repetition task. This pattern has been termed *phonological dysphasia*, an auditory–verbal version of the reading disorder phonological dyslexia.

Some patients not only present with imageability in repetition but also produce semantic errors. For example, when asked to repeat the word *horse*, they say *cow*. This pattern is thought to reflect impaired phonological processing and a reliance on semantic processing to repeat, as in phonological dysphasia. However, there is also an impairment in activating semantic representations of words, thus the presence of semantic errors. In terms of the IA model discussed previously, this pattern has been attributed to an overly rapid decay of a word's phonological and semantic representations over the course of the repetition task (N. Martin et al., 1994). A spoken word activates the word's phonemes, which in turn activate the lexical representation and its corresponding semantics, but all of these representations decay before the output processes of repetition begin. Semantically related words are activated by feedback from the semantic activation (feedback before it decays), and these are retrieved instead of the intended word. The term for this pattern is *deep dysphasia*, the auditory–verbal version of the reading disorder deep dyslexia.

Lexical–Phonological Variables: Word Length and Lexicality

Word Length Effect. Word length is sensitive to the integrity of phonological processing. In Figure 9.3, separate input and output phonological networks connect with the lexical network, and an interactive passage is between them. The input phonological network mediates word recognition and word repetition (via its connections to the lexical network). The lexical network and output phonological network mediate word production and the output stage of word repetition. The route between input and output phonological networks mediates the repetition of nonwords.

Word length effects can be seen in production and repetition tasks:

- *Word length and production.* Performance on word production tasks is affected if there is damage affecting the lexical–phonological output pathway and phonological encoding. Longer words are harder to produce than are shorter words, so a word production test, whether it be a picture-naming test or naming to definition, should include words that are one to four syllables in length. Errors will include phonological substitutions, additions, omissions, and misordering of phonemes.

- *Word length and repetition.* Word length also affects repetition performance, but in two different ways, depending on whether the input or output phonological network is damaged. Impaired activation of phonemes in the output phonological network affects repetition in the same way that it affects production tasks. Longer words are more difficult than shorter words, and errors will be phonological.

Impairment of activation in the input phonological network has a different effect on repetition than production. In this instance, the phonological route cannot be used to repeat a word, and to repeat the word the listener must rely on activation of the word form corresponding to the phonological input. Phonological activation spreads to the lexical network and activates the corresponding word, which in turn activates the corresponding phonemes in the output phonological network. This route not only can lead to successful repetition but also increases the probability of errors on shorter words. This phenomenon has been termed the *reverse length effect.* Shorter words have many more neighbors (i.e., phonologically related words) in the lexicon than do longer words. When activation spreads from the phonological network to the lexicon, it activates the target word as well as other words related to it. With many more neighbors, there is more competition, and if that spread of activation to the lexicon is impaired, there is a greater probability of error. The type of error in this case is a phonologically related word. Target-related nonword errors occur if the output lexical–phonological connections are impaired.

In summary, then, various word length in production or repetition tasks demonstrates the integrity of input and output phonological networks and their connections with the lexicon and the integrity of the route between the input and output phonological networks. More errors on longer words than shorter words in word production and repetition indicate a problem in activating the phonemes in the output phonological network. If shorter words are more difficult than longer words, this indicates impairment of the input phonological network and a reliance or partial reliance on activation of the lexical network to repeat words. If the repetition errors include phonologically related words, this indicates lexical involvement in the repetition process and suggests further that the phonological route to the output phonological network is compromised. This pattern is discussed further in the next section.

Lexicality Effects I have suggested that the presence or absence of imageability or frequency effects in word repetition provides some indication that the speaker is relying on lexical and semantic processes to repeat and suggests that phonological processing is compromised. A thorough evaluation, however, should include direct tests of the integrity of the connections between the input and output phonological networks. For this, clinicians can turn once more to the task of repetition and choose for the test stimuli words and pseudowords. *Lexicality* refers to whether or not a phoneme string is a real word in a speaker's language. Strings of phonemes that resemble words in the speaker's language and respect all of the phonotactic characteristics of that language are called *pseudowords*.

To repeat a pseudoword accurately, the connections between input and output phonological processes must be intact. A comparison of word and nonword repetition can provide information about what route is being used in repetition. If pseudowords cannot be repeated accurately, there is damage to the input or output phonological networks. If errors that are made in repetition of pseudowords are phonologically related nonword errors, this indicates that the damage is affecting the output phonological network. The speaker is trying to repeat the pseudoword that was spoken using the input–output phonological network connections. If errors include phonologically related real words, this suggests that there is damage to the input phonological network and that the speaker is relying on the lexical network to drive the repetition response. That is, phonological input of a nonword stimulus will spread to the lexicon in an attempt to access a representation corresponding to that phoneme string. Nonwords are not present in the lexicon, but phonologically similar real words are present. One of these words will become activated and be produced as a response. This type of error is known as a *lexicalization error*. Sometimes, the speaker is aware of the error and sometimes not. This pattern indicates at least partial reliance on the lexical route to repeat as a result of impaired activation at the level of the phonological input network.

Word Production Errors: How the Type of Error Informs About the Nature of the Word-Processing Deficit

The most obvious test to administer to determine whether someone has a word retrieval deficit is a picture-naming task. This is one of the most common methods used to assess naming ability. An analysis of the error types made in a picture-naming task, for example, can be used to determine whether the word production disorder is a Step 1 (word selection) or Step 2 (phonological encoding) error. As noted in the discussion of Dell's IA model, if an error pattern includes some semantic paraphasias and a relatively higher rate of phonologically related word errors and no responses, this suggests that the lexical–semantic connections in the Step 1 word retrieval process are impaired. If the error pattern includes some semantic substitutions and target related nonword errors, but few phonological word errors and no responses, this suggests that the connections between the lexical and phonological networks are impaired, and this affects Step 1 and Step 2 of the naming process.

Summary of Diagnosing a Word Production Disorder

This section offers a streamlined approach to identification of the locus of a word production impairment in aphasia. By using two tasks, naming and repetition, and varying the stimuli in these tasks in ways that probe semantic, lexical, and phonological levels of representation, clinicians can locate impairment(s) to the production system that affect Step 1 word selection processes (semantic–lexical connections and lexical–phonological connections) and Step 2 phonological encoding processes. Several commercially available tests and test batteries can be used to complete this assessment. The Boston Naming Test (BNT; Kaplan, Goodglass, & Weintraub, 2001), which is used widely to assess naming, includes items that vary in frequency and length. Several aphasia test batteries include naming-to-definition tasks (e.g., the Boston Diagnostic Aphasia Examination–3 [BDAE-3]; Goodglass, Kaplan, & Barresi, 2000). The repetition subtests from the Psycholinguistics Assessments of Language Processing in Aphasia (PALPA; Kay, Lesser, & Coltheart, 1992) that vary imageability, frequency, word length, and lexicality are ideal for the diagnostic protocol outlined here. Alternatively, clinicians can create their own informal battery of tasks by selecting stimuli that are varied as presented here and, if possible, using the same items in repetition and naming tasks. This option allows clinicians to create a screening test that takes less time to administer than does a more comprehensive aphasia battery yet still obtains a profile of the client's word production deficit to guide further in-depth assessment.

There are three caveats to consider when clinicians choose to use this streamlined approach to assessment of word production disorders in aphasia. First, it is important to know that, if time allows, further testing beyond the streamlined protocol described here is highly recommended. Once the locus (or loci) of the word production impairment has (have) been identified, more tests can and should be carried out to fully reveal the underlying mechanism of that particular deficit. For example, if the clinician determines that input phonological processing is compromised on the basis of the types of errors made in repetition (more trouble with short words than long words and a tendency to lexicalize nonword stimuli), more testing of input processing should be conducted. This could include tests of phoneme discrimination, rhyme recognition, word recognition, and word comprehension, all of which are available in the PALPA battery.

The second caveat is that not all word production deficits fit cleanly into one of the three loci of deficits described here. The word production system is highly interconnected. Even if a deficit involves primarily lexical–semantic connections or primarily lexical–phonological connections, all levels of representation are affected to some extent. For example, if representations and connections from semantic to lexical nodes are intact and the breakdown involves lexical-to-phonological encoding, the intact part of the system must function in the context of its relations with the damaged part of the system. In addition, an individual could have impairments throughout the semantic–lexical–phonological network. Thus, when evaluating the patterns of performance on the naming and repetition tasks described here, it is important for the clinician to know how these reveal functioning at each level and what components of the language system are still available to support word production.

The third caveat regarding the approach outlined here is that many other interesting aspects of word production are captured in other assessments, and these can inform the clinician about details of a particular deficit. For example, category-specific naming impairments are studied to help us understand more about lexical and semantic processing more generally. Dissociations in the ability to retrieve nouns versus verbs or proper names versus object names, for example, can tell us much about the cognitive–linguistic organization of the language system. It is important for clinicians to be familiar with research describing the implications of these patterns of dissociation observed in aphasia. A discussion of the category-specific naming impairments is beyond the scope of this chapter, but the reader is referred to several review papers on the topic that cover cognitive, neural, and rehabilitation implications of category-specific disorders: Berndt (1988); Laws, Adlington,

Gale, Moreno-Martínez, and Sartori (2007); and Lambon Ralph, Lowe, and Rogers (2007).

As a starting point to plan treatment for a client with word production difficulties, the tasks and stimuli that have been described here can provide much information about the nature of the production deficit in a reasonably short period of time.

TREATMENT OF WORD RETRIEVAL DISORDERS

General Considerations

There are several issues to consider regarding research on treatment of word production disorders and treatment of aphasia more generally. One issue concerns the objective of treatment. Should the treatment focus on the impairment itself (hereafter, the direct treatment approach) or on the consequences of the impairment for a person's quality of life? This issue is not discussed at length here (see Chapters 14 and 15). Most clinicians and theorists advocate a combination of both approaches, and that is the assumption here.

A second issue has to do with generalization of improvements from words that are trained to those that are untrained and generalization of improved naming abilities from the clinic to speaking situations outside the clinic in the context of the person's daily life. This issue has consequences for the efficacy of treatment and the well-being of the person with aphasia. Health-care programs in the United States typically do not support an extensive period of treatment. Thus, a major objective of treatment research is to identify principles of treatment and specific methods that maximize generalization from trained to untrained words and from a training context to other environments. This means that research investigating factors that influence learning and relearning are highly relevant to development of effective treatment approaches in aphasia.

Another important consideration is that both language processing and treatments of language impairment are dynamic processes. As we choose or design our treatment methods, we must consider more than *which* language representations to address. We need to be cognizant of how treatment methods affect language processing so that we choose methods that *manipulate* processing of language in ways that facilitate access to language representations and do not unintentionally interfere with access. Priming, for example, is a technique used in many forms of therapy (repetition priming, semantic priming, syntactic priming, and so on). A person hears or says a word in one context (e.g., repeating) and then is asked to retrieve the word in another (naming a picture). This technique can make sound and word representations more accessible by raising their activation levels for a short time. However, it also can interfere with accessibility of a sound or word because priming a word also primes other semantically or phonologically related words. If the activation of words in the lexical network is unstable, this could make retrieval more difficult (N. Martin, Fink, Laine, & Ayala, 2004). Thus, it is important to appreciate the dynamics of activation in normal and disordered word production and how a particular treatment technique will alter those dynamics.

With these considerations in mind, I review a few recent approaches to the treatment of word production disorders that target Step 1, selection of the word, and Step 2, phonological encoding. This is not an exhaustive review because the history of research on treatment methods for word retrieval disorders is long and has yielded many studies. The reader is referred to a website of the Academy of Neurologic Communication Disorders and Sciences (aphasia treatment website: http://aphasiatx.arizona.edu/) that has a current and fairly comprehensive list of published articles about treatment of word retrieval and other language disorders in aphasia. In this brief review, I focus on studies that exemplify current approaches and considerations in treating word production disorders.

Treatments That Aim to Improve Access and Retrieval of Words From the Lexical Network

Treatments that target Step 1 of word production aim to increase the strength of connections between the semantic and lexical networks or between the phonological and lexical networks. Some of the treatments described here aim to strengthen semantic–lexical connections; others aim to strengthen lexical–phonological connections.

Semantic Feature Analysis

Semantic feature analysis has been used to improve word retrieval abilities associated with aphasia (Boyle, 2004; Boyle & Coelho, 1995; Coelho, McHugh, & Boyle, 2000) and with traumatic brain injury (Haarbauer-Krupa, Moser, Smith, Sulliivan, & Szekeres, 1985; Massaro & Tompkins, 1992). The person with aphasia and the clinician work together to develop a chart that lists semantic attributes of a particular concept. This is

intended to help facilitate retrieval of the word associated with that concept. To help elicit features, the clinician poses questions or provides partial sentences to be completed by the client (e.g., "You use this for . . ."). If the elusive word were *cat*, for example, the clinician and client would explore features such as superordinate category, associated words, physical appearance, and so on. The semantic feature analysis approach has proved to be somewhat successful in improving the ability to retrieve words that are directly treated as well as untreated items that were probed during and after training. Some generalization to discourse production has also been observed (Boyle, 2004).

Verb Network Strengthening Treatment

Verb network strengthening treatment, developed by Edmonds, Nadeau, and Kiran (2009), aims to strengthen semantic–lexical connections to improve word retrieval. As in the semantic feature analysis approach, it aims for improved word retrieval to generalize to discourse contexts. In this treatment, three-word utterances are elicited by presenting a card with a verb written on it along with other cards with nouns that could be agents of the verbs and nouns that could be patients of the verb. Through a series of five steps, the client is asked to identify and generate agents (e.g., *chef?*) and patients (e.g., *flour*) that go with each verb (e.g., *measure*). These agent–patient pairings are elicited with the help of *wh-* questions from the clinician. Some of the agents and patients are provided with pictures, and some are generated by the client. Also included in this protocol is an exercise involving semantic plausibility judgments of sentences with correct and incorrect agent–verb–patient combinations. In the study reported by Edmonds et al. (2009), this treatment approach proved to be successful. Retrieval of content words in association with trained and untrained verbs was observed in all four participants. In addition, three of the four participants showed generalization of word retrieval to connected speech.

The semantic feature analysis approach and the verb network strengthening treatment each include methods to involve the participant in the generation of words to be practiced and used in subsequent tasks. Self-generation of their own words is one factor that likely contributed to the generalization of treatment effects to spontaneous connected speech.

Cueing Hierarchies

A therapy approach with perhaps the longest history in aphasia rehabilitation is the cueing hierarchy

(Linebaugh & Lehrner, 1977). There are semantic cueing hierarchies and phonological cueing hierarchies. Initial phoneme cues and sentence completion cues are most effective in facilitating the retrieval of an elusive word (Pease & Goodglass, 1978). Linebaugh (1983) notes several principles to follow in cueing hierarchies, whether they are phonological or semantic in nature. He recommends that cueing begin with the least amount of facilitation possible, and once a response is facilitated, it should be faded as soon as possible. Thus, cueing hierarchies begin with the least powerful cue and provide increasingly more information in the cues that follow. This hierarchy is then followed in reverse, gradually decreasing the facilitative power of the cues. Linebaugh also recommends that clinicians help their clients develop internal cueing strategies.

Raymer, Thompson, Jacobs, and Le Grand (1993) and others (Greenwald, Raymer, Richardson, & Rothi, 1995; Hillis, 1993, 1998) have used phonological cueing hierarchies with some success, observing especially improvement on trained items. As with all treatments, generalization is a consideration when evaluating the effectiveness of cueing hierarchies. Patterson (2001) reviews traditional cueing hierarchy approaches as well as modified approaches (descending hierarchy only). Generalization to untrained items and tasks is inconsistent across studies. Nonetheless, this approach has great value in its stimulation and strengthening of the semantic and phonological connections to the lexicon.

The choice of using a semantic or phonological cueing hierarchy to stimulate word retrieval could be based on whether the word production disorder involves lexical–semantic or phonological–lexical connections. However, given the interactive nature of the semantic–lexical–phonological network and the likelihood that a person with aphasia will have some difficulty with both semantic and phonological connections to the lexicon, it may be a good strategy to use both hierarchy types. This approach has been used effectively by Wambaugh and colleagues (Wambaugh, Cameron, Kalinyak-Fliszar, Nessler, & Wright, 2004; Wambaugh, Doyle, Martinez, & Kalinyak-Fliszar, 2002; Wambaugh, Linebaugh, Doyle, Martinez, & Kalinyak-Fliszar, 2001) to improve retrieval of object and verb names. They examined the relative effectiveness of these treatments in relation to the locus of word retrieval impairment. For object naming, they found that both treatments were effective whether the retrieval disorder was more semantically based or more phonologically based (Wambaugh et al., 2001). In the case of verb retrieval, the effectiveness of phonological and semantic cueing treatments varied across the participants in that study (Wambaugh et al., 2004). Additional case studies

and case series studies are needed to determine which factors (e.g., type and severity of impairment) predict a benefit from cueing hierarchies.

Contextual Repetition and Production Priming

Contextual repetition and production priming, two related techniques, use massed repetition priming of a set of words that are semantically related, phonologically related, or unrelated (N. Martin, Fink, & Laine, 2004; N. Martin, Fink, Renvall, & Laine, 2006; Renvall, Laine, & Martin, 2007). They can be used to target semantic–lexical connections or lexical–phonological connections depending on the relationship among the words to be trained. The idea behind this approach is that if a set of words is primed repeatedly, and those words are also semantically related (for example), the repetition priming will increase the strength of the semantic–lexical connections, and the semantic relationships will enhance this priming further by virtue of the increased activation of shared features among the words in the set. This logic was applied also to the predictions about effects of training phonologically related words in a single set using the massed repetition priming.

The first studies using this technique used repetition priming only. This was found to be effective only when the impairment affecting word retrieval did not involve semantic–lexical connections. N. Martin et al. (2006) propose that the reduced effectiveness in this situation is because repetition can occur without the speaker ever accessing the connections beyond the lexical network, that is, the semantic–lexical connections. Thus, the pattern of short-term improvement (resulting from temporarily elevated activation of lexical entries from bottom-up phonological input) and no long-term carryover or generalization is typically observed when the semantic–lexical pathway is damaged. If that pathway is preserved, however, repetition priming is effective. In this situation, lexical entries that are primed by phonological input effectively spread their activation to semantic levels of representation, providing a deeper and more enduring encoding of the word–concept associations.

N. Martin et al. (2006) propose that modifications be made to the contextual repetition priming procedure to enhance stimulation of the semantic–lexical pathways. Renvall et al. (2007) add semantic and phonological tasks to the repetition priming procedure. These modifications resulted in improved naming in both participants of that study, one with semantic–lexical pathway anomia and the other with a phonological assembly disorder. Generalization to untrained words was not observed in either case.

Fink, Martin, and Berkowitz (2008) used contextual production priming to stimulate the semantic–lexical connections of a patient for whom this pathway was moderately impaired. Production priming is similar to repetition priming, but rather than just using repetition, a comprehension task (word-to-picture matching) and naming of multiple exemplars of an object are used to stimulate bottom-up and top-down use of the semantic–lexical pathway. Fink et al. (2008) postulate that direct priming of the production pathway between semantics and the lexicon strengthens this connection and improves word retrieval and is maintained. This hypothesis was confirmed. They found that short-term improvement and maintenance are strongest when the words being trained are unrelated to each other, *but* these gains were not evident at follow-up. In contrast, when words being trained were semantically related, there were modest short-term gains, but improvements in naming were maintained at 1-month follow-up. Thus, for the participant in this study, training in a context that directly stimulates the impairment underlying anomia (semantic–lexical connections) was most effective with respect to maintenance of improvement.

Phonological Priming

Massed repetition of a word or massed production of a word is one form of priming. Phonological priming can occur if only part of a word is repeated. Wilshire and Saffran (2005) examined effects of phonological priming on two people with fluent aphasia. They used two types of phonological prime: rhyme primes and prime words that shared the initial phoneme of the target word. Evaluation of the word retrieval impairments of the participants in this study, I.G. and G.L., indicated that I.G.'s deficit was at Step 1 of lexical retrieval (activating the word form in the lexical network), and G.L.'s impairment was at Step 2, phonological encoding. The authors found that I.G. benefited from phonological primes that shared initial phonemes, and G.L. benefited from rhyme primes. They interpreted these results within the IA model of word production (Dell et al., 1997). Although this is not a treatment study per se, it suggests the value of research that tries to understand the effectiveness of priming and cue types within a context of a word retrieval model. This study suggests that the choice of phonological prime type should depend on the locus of the word retrieval disorder, activating the word form (Step 1) or encoding the phonology (Step 2). The next section reviews three studies that focus on treatment of the phonological encoding step. Two of them capitalize on residual strengths in

word processing, and the other targets the phonological encoding deficit directly.

Treatment of Phonological Encoding Impairments

The lexical–phonological connections in Dell's model are active in two steps. First, they actively participate in selection of the word representation (Step 1). Activation from the lexicon spreads to the phonological network and primes the phonemes of the words that are active in the lexical network. This activation feeds back to the lexicon and primes the target word and other word nodes that are phonologically related to the target. Although the phoneme nodes are primed (activation levels are raised), they are not retrieved until Step 2, phonological encoding. When a word is selected from the lexicon, it sends activation again to those phonemes primed in the phonological network and selects the most highly active ones, which are processed further as articulatory motor plans and movements. When the breakdown in the production process occurs at this point, the resulting syndrome is reproduction conduction aphasia. Often, there is only minimal involvement of input processes, but some cases present with both input and output difficulties (Corsten, Mende, Cholewa, & Huber, 2007).

Indirect Treatments of Phonological Encoding

Some treatments for phonological encoding disorders use indirect approaches to stimulating accurate production. Two of these are described next.

1. *Oral reading.* Boyle (1989) used oral reading as a vehicle task to reduce the rates of phonemic paraphasias in the production pattern of a person with conduction aphasia, N.K. Treatment stimuli included three sets of word, phrase, and sentence lists. Syllable length of the words in the sets increased from one in the first set to three in the third set. N.K. read these stimuli aloud, and when a phonemic paraphasia occurred, he was provided with a cueing hierarchy. First, he was to read the word silently and think about how it should sound. He then read the target word aloud again. If the response was in error, a repetition cue was provided. The outcome of this experimental program was a reduction in N.K.'s phonemic paraphasias in connected speech and a reduction in his rate of speech. In her evaluation of these results, Boyle emphasizes the benefits of using a relatively intact ability (oral reading) as a vehicle to

improve a related but impaired ability, phonological encoding in production.

2. *Oral reading plus other tasks.* Peach (1996) also used an oral reading approach to treat what he called a phonological output-planning deficit. In conjunction with oral reading, he used tasks directed toward improving auditory comprehension, naming, and sentence formulation. His evaluation of his client's language abilities indicated impaired repetition and naming but relatively intact oral reading and writing. Peach hypothesized that in oral reading, his client was able to use a lexical strategy to structure phonological output planning. The first step of the therapy procedure was to attempt to read a word aloud. When an error occurred, the client would then write the word. This was intended to increase the salience of the word's phonological features. If the response was still incorrect, the incorrect phonemes were paired with the same phoneme in a key word that the client was able to read correctly. If the word was still not read correctly, a repetition cue was provided. This treatment resulted in improvements on trained and untrained words. Also, performance on the naming and repetition subtests of the Western Aphasia Battery (Kertesz, 1982) improved.

Direct Treatment of Phonological Encoding Disorders

Other approaches to treatment of phonological encoding disorders are more direct and often rely on tasks that make explicit those word and sound retrieval functions that are normally automatic. These approaches involve improving skills in editing one's own output and practice in producing words with increasingly complex phoneme sequences. Three of the more direct approaches to treatment are described next.

1. *Input and output tasks to improve phonological encoding.* Corsten et al. (2007) developed a treatment that uses both input and output phonological processing tasks. The authors tested the effectiveness of their treatment program for P.S., a person with both input and output phonological encoding difficulties. The primary task was to practice minimal phonemic contrasts. Stimuli were varied for the location of the contrast (onset or rhyme), lexicality (word and nonwords), and phonological complexity. Also, a series of input and output control tasks was used to monitor progress during treatment: auditory discrimination, matching a spoken pseudoword to one of four written pseudowords that were phonologically related, rhyme judgment for words and pseudowords, and repetition and oral reading of words and pseudowords. The gains made by P.S. were treatment specific. That is, improvements were observed on tasks that involved sublexical processing. These results indicate that treating an impairment directly can be effective.

2. *Phonological components analysis.* Leonard, Rochon, and Laird (2008) designed a phonological components treatment similar in format to the semantic feature analysis treatment discussed previously. A target picture (e.g., train) is placed in the center of a chart, and the client is asked to name the picture. Regardless of whether the client's response is accurate, he or she is then asked to respond to five questions pertaining to the phonological structure of the picture name. These questions ask for a rhyme, the first sound of the word, another word that starts with the same sound, the final sound, and the number of syllables. The chart is divided into areas around the pictured object for each of these components. If the client cannot answer these questions, he or she is given three possible responses written on a card. For example, for the target word train, three words are written on a card and one of them rhymes with train (e.g., lawn, cane, trade). The client is then asked to choose the word that rhymes with the name of the picture). The correct response (i.e., cane) is then written on the chart in the appropriate phonological components section. Following this procedure, the person is then asked to name the picture once more. If a correct response is given, the clinician provides positive feedback. If the response is still incorrect, the clinician asks the client to repeat the word.

This treatment was tested by Leonard et al. (2008) on 10 people with aphasia. Of these 10, 7 showed positive effects of treatment, and the treatment gains were maintained up to 4 weeks. In addition, some generalization to untreated items was observed.

3. Phonomotor treatment (Kendall, Pompon, Brookshire, Minkina, & Bislick, 2013; Kendall et al., 2008). This treatment is intended to directly target sound production and perception. The treatment is carried out over two stages. Stage 1 includes tasks that involve exploration of sounds, description of motor aspects of sounds, perception of sounds, and production of orthographic representations of sounds. In Stage 1, sounds are practiced in isolation. Stage 2 includes tasks similar to those used in Stage

1, but sounds are no longer practiced in isolation. The focus in Stage 2 is on sound sequences.

Kendall et al. (2008) tested the effectiveness of this treatment on 10 people with aphasia and, in particular, with impaired phonological processing. The primary outcome measure was accuracy of spoken word production in confrontation naming on the Object Action Naming Test (Druks & Masterson, 2000). Alternating between Lists A and B on this test, probes were administered at baseline, in treatment, and 1 week and 3 months following treatment. Secondary outcome measures included production of phonemes, nonword repetition, and discourse production using the Brookshire Discourse Production Test (Nicholas & Brookshire, 1993).

Participants received 96 hours of treatment over 10 weeks. Visual analysis of probe data and treatment effect sizes were used to evaluate the results. For most of these participants, there was evidence of positive effects of the treatment (increased accuracy in naming, nonword repetition, and phoneme production), and these effects were maintained up to 3 months after treatment ended. In addition, four of the participants showed generalization of improvement in the Brookshire Discourse Production Test (Nicholas & Brookshire, 1993).

In a second study (Kendall et al., 2013), the phonomotor treatment was tested on another 10 individuals with aphasia and phonological encoding impairment. The treatment stimuli were English phonemes in isolation, 72 nonwords and 39 real words that are low in phonotactic probability and high in neighborhood density. The choice of low phonotactic probability stimuli was motivated by the complexity hypothesis (Kiran & Thompson, 2003; Plaut, 1996), which claims that training of atypical exemplars of a category improve relearning (access to) both atypical and typical members of that category. The authors note also that they chose training stimuli with high neighborhood densities to maximize the number of word representations that linked with the trained phonemes and phoneme sequences. The primary prediction was that training on these stimuli would result in generalization to untrained stimuli.

Participants received 60 hours of treatment, scheduled as two 1-hour sessions per day, 5 days per week, for 6 weeks. The primary outcome measure was confrontation naming of the 39 pictured

nouns whose names were used in training and 37 pictured nouns that were untrained. The treatment resulted in a statistically significant improvement in naming of trained items, but not untrained items. These improvements were still evident 3 months following treatment. Regarding the minimal improvement in the untrained items, the authors note that this may have been due to the small number of participants.

Summary of Treatments for Word Retrieval Disorders

I have reviewed briefly some treatments of word retrieval disorders, some focusing on improving access to and retrieval of the word representation and others that target the phonological encoding step of word production. An evaluation of their effectiveness must take into account several considerations. It is relatively easy to effect short-term facilitation of the ability to retrieve a word. What is more difficult to achieve is (a) long-term maintenance of improved word and phoneme retrieval abilities and (b) generalization of improvements to untrained stimuli and to contexts other than the treatment setting. Some treatments fare better than others do with respect to maintenance and generalization. However, the treatment approaches I discussed *all* have value. Generalization, for example, seems most effectively achieved in the training protocols that include opportunities for self-generation of words (Boyle, 2004; Edmonds et al., 2009). Someone with a more severe anomia may not benefit from this protocol initially but may need to begin with a more direct facilitative treatment and progress to a treatment that includes self-generation of words. Thus, a clinician must consider severity when choosing from among these and other treatment approaches.

Another issue addressed in treatment research is whether to target an impairment directly or use residual strengths in the word-processing system to facilitate better function of the impaired component. Here again, it would seem that there is no single way to proceed. Both approaches have positive effects. A direct approach can lead to an errorful learning process but better maintenance of treatment gains (Fink, Berkowitz, & Martin, 2009). Less-direct treatment approaches that exploit use of more intact functions (e.g., oral reading for phonological encoding disorders; Boyle, 1989; Peach, 1996) may help the client develop strategies that promote endurance of treatment effects and generalization to other speaking contexts.

A final point to make concerns the need to make a connection between direct impairment-based treatments, such as have been described here, and the functional communication needs of the person with aphasia. As described in the case illustration for this chapter, the clinician must obtain and consider an assessment of the communication needs of the client when developing a treatment protocol. Also, it is important to determine what a client wants to gain from language treatment. Word retrieval disorders can have a tremendous impact on everyday communication activities. In many cases, direct treatment approaches *do* improve word retrieval. However, for most cases, word retrieval difficulties of some degree will be lifelong. Therefore, it is imperative that treatment protocols include strategies that will help the speaker cope with the word-finding difficulty in functional communication situations that are meaningful to the client.

FUTURE DIRECTIONS

In this chapter, I aimed to convince the reader of the value of using a model of word retrieval to guide the process of diagnosing and developing a treatment protocol for word production disorders in aphasia. Evaluation of a word retrieval disorder should yield information about its nature (word retrieval, phoneme assembly) and its severity. Traditional "box-and-arrow" language models provide a detailed framework within which the locus of language impairment can be identified. This kind of model informs the clinician about what components of the language system need to be addressed in treatment. For example, if there is evidence of difficulty in accessing words in the lexicon from semantics, treatment should focus on improving the link between words and their meanings. This is an important advance over earlier approaches to diagnosis and treatment that described impairments at the level of task (e.g., naming, reading comprehending).

However, there is still much to be learned about the dynamics of language processing and how to treat the processes that are impaired. We can say a naming impairment is due to a problem in accessing the words in the lexicon from semantics. This does not tell us the nature of the "access" impairment. Is the signal from semantics too slow? Is it fast enough to activate the word but does not endure long enough to keep that activation at a level needed to be retrieved in naming? The answers to these questions are important because treatment involves not only the content that is addressed but also the methods used to address it. How does the treatment method we use stimulate the language system? Priming treatments, for example, can facilitate or inhibit retrieval depending on the circumstances, such as type of prime and locus of language impairment (Fink et al., 2009). It is this kind of question that has motivated the direction of treatment research in recent years.

There is an increasing focus on achieving greater understanding of the dynamics of treatment methods and how these affect the impaired and spared language processes in aphasia. This line of research involves application of computational models of language processing that are capable of generating hypotheses about the dynamics of language and how damage to the language system will affect functions such as word retrieval or word recognition. This approach to understanding aphasia and its rehabilitation is timely as it will take us to a level of understanding the effects of brain damage on language processing that will be more directly translatable to the development of effective treatment methods that maximize generalization and maintenance of treatment results.

Case Illustration 9.1

You are a clinician working in a rehabilitation hospital setting. You have just received an outpatient referral requesting you to evaluate Mr. N. While looking over his medical records, you observe that he has had a left thalamus cerebrovascular accident with hemorrhage. Intake forms indicate that Mr. N. is 59 years old, African American. He is college educated with a bachelor of arts degree in theology. He is an ordained minister, and he is currently serving as pastor in a local church. Records also indicate no hemiparesis or visual difficulties. However, a mild aphasia was noted, in particular, an anomia.

Mr. N. was scheduled for evaluation. Although married, he came to the clinic on his own, using public transportation. Mr. N.'s conversational speech was fluent with no syntactic difficulties. The main problem, as reported in his medical records, was a severe word-finding difficulty. Mr. N. expressed some distress about his circumstances, saying he could not find the words for his sermons.

(continues)

Because naming difficulty is the most prominent symptom, you first administer the BNT (Kaplan et al., 2001). The BNT provides a direct measure of his ability to retrieve names of pictured objects. You also administer the Western Aphasia Battery–Revised (WAB-R; Kertesz, 2006), which provides an overall measure of language ability, including comprehension and production, and yields an aphasia quotient and estimate of aphasia type in the classical taxonomy of aphasia syndromes (e.g., Broca's, Wernicke's). Also, the WAB-R provides information about word retrieval in contexts other than picture naming, including responsive naming, word fluency, and sentence completion. This information will be useful as you develop a treatment protocol that will improve or facilitate naming ability.

To further assess the integrity of phonological, lexical, and semantic levels of processing, you administer several tests of single-word and nonword repetition and reading from the PALPA (Kay et al., 1992). You choose tests that vary characteristics of stimuli sensitive to each level of processing: imageability, frequency, lexicality (word or nonword), and word length. To assess repetition ability, you administer numbers 7 (Word repetition, syllable length varied); 8 (Nonword repetition, syllable length varied); and 9 (Word repetition, imageability and frequency varied). To assess reading ability, you administer 30 (Word reading, syllable length varied); 31 (Word reading, imageability and frequency varied); 32 (Word reading, grammatical class varied); and 36 (Nonword reading, syllable length varied). You also administer some verbal short-term memory (STM) span tasks that vary these same characteristics but for word sequences rather than single words. You recognize that Mr. N.'s aphasia is somewhat mild except for the anomia, and for this reason his performance on single-word processing tests might be unimpaired. In repetition of word sequences, however, effects of phonological, lexical, or semantic variables may become more apparent (e.g., N. Martin, 2001; N. Martin, Kohen, & Kalinyak-Fliszar, 2010; N. Martin & Saffran, 1990, 1997). Thus, you have created a short battery of span tasks that vary stimulus characteristics as an informal measure of phonological, lexical, and semantic processing beyond single-word verbal STM.

Finally, you want to know more about Mr. N.'s functional/social communication needs and the impact of his stroke on his general outlook and sense of well-being. To gain insight into this aspect of Mr. N.'s overall communication profile, you administer the Burden of Stroke Scale (Doyle et al., 2004), which assesses the physical, cognitive, and psychological burden of stroke.

The results of your evaluation show the following:

1. *BNT.* Mr. N. was able to name only 25 of 60 pictures but did produce another 20 when given phonemic cues. The types of errors that he made on this test were primarily omissions ("I can't say the name") or semantic descriptions (*canoe* → "it's some kind of boat"). There were no phonological errors in his naming or in any of his conversational speech.

2. *WAB-R.* Mr. N.'s Aphasia Quotient was 91.3, and his Aphasia Type was determined to be Anomic. The most relevant results of the WAB-R indicate good auditory comprehension, mild difficulty with repetition, impaired naming except in the context of responsive speech (0.80 correct) and sentence completion (1.00 correct).

3. *PALPA.* On the PALPA repetition and reading tests, Mr. N. made no errors in any variations of word and nonwords.

4. *Verbal span tasks.* On the verbal span tasks that you created, his span ranged from four to five items on most tasks but was reduced somewhat for nonword span and span for words of low frequency and low imageability. Word length did not affect his span, but nonword span (2.40) was less than word span (4.6). His errors in span task, as in picture naming, were primarily omissions. Mr. N. did not make phonological errors.

5. *Burden of Stroke Scale.* This evaluation revealed that Mr. N. was not experiencing physical limitations from his stroke but did feel that social needs were different from before the stroke, especially those involving communication with others.

The evaluation shows that the source of Mr. N.'s anomia is impaired semantic activation of word representations in the lexicon. The integrity of lexical and phonological representations is quite good because they are accessible via input phonological processes (as in word and nonword repetition). Input activation of the semantic representations is also quite good, as indicated by his good comprehension scores on the WAB-R. However, the spread of activation from a word's semantic representation to the word form in the lexicon is slow or weak.

(continues)

Mr. N.'s word retrieval does improve when a phonemic cue is provided. This along with his excellent repetition and reading skills are positive aspects of his profile that should help Mr. N. develop some self-cueing strategies to facilitate word retrieval. Thus, therapy should focus on helping Mr. N. to use written words to generate a phonemic cue that in turn will serve to cue a spoken word that he is having difficulty retrieving (see N. Martin, 2008, and L. Nickels, 1992, for examples of this treatment approach). A goal for improved functional communication is for Mr. N. to learn how to prepare his sermons with written key words that will enable him to retrieve them fluently in the context of his oral sermons.

Case Illustration 9.2

Ms. L. is a 41-year-old female who experienced a left cerebral artery infarct 18 months prior to her evaluation with you. She is college educated and worked as a writer for a local newspaper. Mrs. L. lives on her own and is close with her parents and two siblings, who live in the Philadelphia region. She hopes to return to her position at some point.

The results of your evaluation show the following:

1. *BNT.* Ms. L. was able to name only 27 of 60 pictures and was able to name another 10 when given phonemic cues. The types of errors that she made on this test were semantic substitutions (beaver → raccoon) and target-related phonological errors (e.g., octopus→ /a–ka-fEs/. Phonological errors were also present in her conversational speech, and she frequently tried to correct these.
2. *WAB-R.* Ms. L.'s Aphasia Quotient was 79.7, and her Aphasia classification according to the WAB-R was conduction aphasia. She demonstrated good auditory comprehension, moderate difficulty with repetition, impaired naming, with mostly semantic and phonological errors.
3. *PALPA* word repetition and reading tests. Ms. L. made errors on 0.44 of the words in the repetition test and .34 of the words in the reading test. On both tests, she made more errors on low-imageability words. On the PALPA nonword reading test, she was only able to repeat 0.15 of the nonwords correctly.
4. *Verbal span tasks.* Mrs. L's verbal span size varied depending on the items she had to recall: nonwords (1.0), low frequency-low imageability words (2.4), high frequency-high imageability words (3.8), and digits (4.0). It was lower for longer words as well. Her error responses were primarily phonological substitutions or omissions.
5. Ms. L. complained of reading and writing difficulties, and the written versions of lexical decision and oral reading tests on the PALPA indicated that she had phonological dyslexia and dysgraphia.
6. *Burden of Stroke Scale.* This evaluation revealed that Ms. L. was not affected by experiencing physical limitations from her stroke, and she was able to communicate her needs well with others. Her primacy concern was that she would not be able to return to work as a writer.

The evaluation shows that the source of Ms. L.'s naming difficulties is an impairment in encoding word phonology. Activation of the word forms from semantics is intact, but encoding of the phonology linked to that phonological form is impaired. Input activation of the semantic representations is also quite good, as indicated by her good comprehension scores on the WAB-R, but repetition of words and nonwords is impaired. Consistent with this phonological impairment, Ms. L. also demonstrates phonological dyslexia and dysgraphia. Goals in therapy should focus on improving auditory–verbal and visual–written phonological abilities. It would also be important to link direct impairment-based treatment of these skills with functional activities that relate to her goals to return to work as a news writer.

STUDY QUESTIONS

1. What are the three stages of word retrieval in the word production process?
2. How do speech errors made in everyday conversation inform about the cognitive organization of the language production system?
3. How do discrete-stage models of word production differ from IA models of word production? How are the two types of models similar?
4. One effect that has been observed in research on speech errors is the lexical bias effect. Describe what this effect is and what it tells us about the organization of the word production system.
5. What are the different types of word production disorders, and how do they reflect breakdown at different steps in models of word production?
6. What are some standard tasks that can be used to diagnose a word production disorder in a streamlined fashion?
7. How can the characteristics of test stimuli (words and nonwords) be manipulated to test the integrity of semantic, lexical, and phonological processing of words?
8. When someone cannot repeat nonwords and tends to produce word errors when trying to repeat a nonword, what does this tell us about a possible source of the person's word production difficulty?
9. Identifying methods that promote generalization of treatment gains from trained to untrained stimuli is an important objective in aphasia rehabilitation. Explain the reasons why this is important and how researchers have tried to achieve this goal.
10. Describe and critically evaluate one or more of the treatment approaches described in this chapter that aim to improve the function of Step 1 of word production (retrieving the word).
11. Describe and critically evaluate one or more of the treatment approaches described in this chapter that aim to improve the function of Step 2 of word production (phonological encoding).
12. Once you have identified an appropriate treatment approach that directly targets the source of the word production impairment, how would you integrate that direct treatment activity with the need to promote better functional communication abilities of your client?

ACKNOWLEDGMENTS

Preparation of this chapter was supported by grants from the National Institutes of Health (NIDCD), R01 DC 01924-14, R21 DC008782-02, R01 DC013196-01 to Temple University (PI: N. Martin). The ideas put forth in this chapter were fostered by many helpful discussions with my colleagues and friends, Matti Laine, Gary Dell, Myrna Schwartz, Ruth Fink, Francine Kohen, and Michelene Kalinyak-Fliszar; and my mentor and dear friend, the late Eleanor Saffran. I am grateful to them as well as the many people with aphasia and word production disorders whom I have had the privilege to know and to work with over the years.

REFERENCES

Abel, S., Wilmes, K., & Huber, W. (2007). Model-oriented naming therapy: Testing predictions of a connectionist model. *Aphasiology*, *21*(5), 411–447.

Baars, B. J., Motley, M. T., & MacKay, D. G. (1975). Output editing for lexical status in artificially elicited slips of the tongue. *Journal of Verbal Learning and Verbal Behavior*, *14*, 382–391.

Berndt, R. S. (1988). Category-specific deficits in aphasia. *Aphasiology*, *2*, 237–240.

Boyle, M. (1989). Reducing phonemic paraphasias in the connected speech of a conduction aphasic subject. *Proceedings: 18th Clinical Aphasiology Conference* (pp. 379–393). Cape Cod, MA: College-Hill Press.

Boyle, M. (2004). Semantic feature analysis treatment for anomia in two fluent aphasia syndromes. *American Journal of Speech-Language Pathology*, *13*, 236–249.

Boyle, M., & Coelho, C. A. (1995). Application of semantic feature analysis as a treatment for aphasic dysnomia. *American Journal of Speech-Language Pathology*, *4*, 94–98.

Bredart, S., & Valentine, T. (1992). From Monroe to Moreau: An analysis of face naming errors. *Cognition*, *45*, 187–223.

Brown, R., & McNeill, D. (1966). The "tip of the tongue" phenomenon. *Journal of Verbal Learning and Verbal Behavior*, *5*, 325–337.

Burke, D., MacKay, D. G., Worthley, J. S., & Wade, E. (1991). On the tip-of-the-tongue: What causes word finding failures in young and older adults? *Journal of Memory and Language*, *30*, 237–246.

Caramazza, A. (1997). How many levels of processing are there in lexical access? *Cognitive Neuropsychology, 14,* 177–208.

Coelho, C. A., McHugh, R., & Boyle, M. (2000). Semantic feature analysis as a treatment for aphasic dysnomia: A replication. *Aphasiology, 14,* 133–142.

Corsten, S., Mende, M., Cholewa, J., & Huber, W. (2007). Treatment of input and output phonology in aphasia: A single case study. *Aphasiology, 21*(6/7/8), 586–603.

Dell, G. S. (1986). A spreading activation theory of retrieval in language production. *Psychological Review, 93,* 283–321.

Dell, G. S., Martin, N., & Schwartz, M. F. (2007). A case-series test of the interactive two-step model of lexical access: Predicting word repetition from picture naming. *Journal of Memory and Language, 56,* 490–520.

Dell, G. S., & O'Seaghdha, P. G. (1992). Stages in lexical access in language production. *Cognition, 42,* 287–314.

Dell, G. S., & Reich, P. A. (1981). Stages in sentence production: An analysis of speech error data. *Journal of Verbal Learning and Verbal Behavior, 20,* 611–629.

Dell, G. S., Schwartz, M. F., Martin, N., Saffran, E. M., & Gagnon, D. A. (1997). Lexical access in aphasic and non-aphasic speakers. *Psychological Review, 104,* 801–838.

Doyle, P. J., McNeil, M. R., Mikolic, J. M., Prieto, L., Hula, W. D., Lustig, A. P., et al. (2004). The Burden of Stroke Scale (BOSS) provides valid and reliable score estimates of functioning and well-being in stroke survivors with and without communication disorders. *Journal of Clinical Epidemiology, 57*(10), 997–1007.

Druks, J., & Masterson, J. (2000). *An object and action naming battery.* East Sussex, UK: Psychology Press.

Edmonds, L. A., Nadeau, S. E., & Kiran, S. (2009). Effect of verb network strengthening treatment (VNeST) on lexical retrieval of content words in sentences in person with aphasia. *Aphasiology, 23*(3), 402–424.

Fink, R., Berkowitz, R., & Martin, N. (2009, May 26–May 31). *Interference and facilitation effects of semantic and phonological contextual priming: A treatment case study.* Paper presented at the Clinical Aphasiology Conference, Keystone, CO.

Fink, R. B., Martin, N., & Berkowitz, R. (2008, October 19–22). *Contextual priming revisited: Effects of a technique to maximize access to and from semantics.* Paper presented at the Academy of Aphasia, Turku, Finland.

Foygel, D., & Dell, G. S. (2000). Models of impaired lexical access in speech production. *Journal of Memory and Language, 43,* 182–216.

Francis, W. N., & Kucera, H. (1982). *Frequency analysis of English usage: Lexicon and grammar.* Boston: Houghton-Mifflin.

Fromkin, V. A. (1971). The non-anomalous nature of anomalous utterances. *Language, 47,* 27–52.

Gagnon, D. A., Schwartz, M. F., Martin, N., Dell, G. S., & Saffran, E. M. (1997). The origins of formal paraphasias in aphasics' picture naming. *Brain & Language, 59,* 450–472.

Garrett, M. F. (1975). The analysis of sentence production. In G. H. Bower (Ed.), *The psychology of learning and motivation* (Vol. 9, pp. 133–177). New York: Academic Press.

Garrett, M. F. (1976). Syntactic processes in sentence production. In R. J. Wales & E. Walker (Eds.), *New approaches to language mechanisms* (pp. 231–255). Amsterdam: North Holland.

Garrett, M. F. (1980). Levels of processing in sentence production. In R. J. Wales & E. C. T. Walker (Eds.), *New approaches to language mechanisms.* (pp. 231–255). Amsterdam: North Holland.

Garrett, M. F. (1982). Production of speech: Observations from normal and pathological language use. In A. Ellis (Ed.), *Normality and pathology in cognitive functions* (pp. 19–76). London: Academic Press.

Garrett, M. F. (1988). Processs in language production. In F. J. Newmeyer, *Linguistics: The Cambridge survey: Volume 3. Language: Psychological and biological aspects* (pp. 69–96). Cambridge, UK: Cambridge University Press.

Goodglass, H., Kaplan, E., & Barresi, B. (2000). *Boston Diagnostic Aphasia Examination-3.* Philadelphia: Taylor & Francis.

Greenwald, M. L., Raymer, A. M., Richardson, M. E., & Rothi, L. J. G. (1995). Contrasting treatments for severe impairments of picture naming. *Neuropsychological Rehabilitation, 5,* 17–49.

Haarbauer-Krupa, J., Moser, L., Smith, G., Sullivan, D. M., & Szekeres, S. F. (1985). Cognitive rehabilitation therapy: Middle stages of recovery. In M. Ylvisaker (Ed.), *Head injury rehabilitation: Children and adolescents* (pp. 287–310). San Diego, CA: College Hill Press.

Harley, T. A. (1984). A critique of top-down independent levels models of speech production: Evidence from non-plan internal speech errors. *Cognitive Science, 8,* 191–219.

Harley, T. A. (1990). Environmental contamination of normal speech. *Applied Psycholinguistics, 11,* 45–72.

Harley, T. A. (1995). Connectionist models of anomia: A reply to Nickels. *Language and Cognitive Processes, 10,* 47–58.

Harley, T. A. (2001). *The psychology of language: From data to theory* (2nd ed.). Hove, UK: Psychology Press.

Hillis, A. E. (1993). The role of models of language processing in rehabilitation of language impairments. *Aphasiology, 7,* 5–26.

Hillis, A. E. (1998). Treatment of naming disorders: New issues regarding old therapies. *Journal of International Neuropsychological Society, 4,* 648–660.

Jescheniak, J. D., & Levelt, W. J. M. (1994). Word frequency effects in speech production: Retrieval of syntactic information and of phonological form. *Journal of Experimental Psychology: Learning, Memory and Cognition, 20,* 824–843.

Jones, H. G. V., & Langford, S. (1987). Phonological blocking in the tip-of-the-tongue state. *Cognition, 26,* 115–122.

Kaplan, E., Goodglass, H., & Weintraub, S. (2001). *Boston Naming Test* (2nd ed.). Philadelphia: Lippincott Williams & Wilkins.

Kay, J., Lesser, R., & Coltheart, M. (1992). *PALPA: Psycholinguistic Assessments of Language Processing in Aphasia.* Hove, UK: Erlbaum.

Kendall, D. L., Pompon, R. H., Brookshire, C. E., Minkina, I., & Bislick, L. (2013). An analysis of aphasic naming errors as an indicator of improved linguistic processing following phonomotor treatment. *American Journal of Speech-Language Pathology, 22,* S240–S249.

Kendall, D. L., Rosenbek, J. C., Heilman, K. M., Conway, T., Klenberg, K., Gonzalez-Rothi, L., et al. (2008). Phoneme-based rehabilitation of anomia in aphasia. *Brain and Language, 105,* 1–17.

Kertesz, A. (1982). *Western Aphasia Battery.* San Antonio, TX: Pearson.

Kertesz, A. (2006). *Western Aphasia Battery—Revised.* San Antonio, TX: Pearson.

Kiran, S., & Thompson, C. K. (2003). The role of semantic complexity in treatment of naming deficits: Training semantic categories in fluent aphasia by controlling exemplar typicality. *Journal of Speech Language and Hearing Research, 46*(4), 773–787.

Kittredge, A. K., Dell, G. S., Verkuilen, J., & Schwartz, M. F. (2008). Where is the effect of lexical frequency in word production? Insights from aphasic picture naming errors. *Cognitive Neuropsychology, 25*(4), 463–492.

Laine, M., & Martin, N. (1996). Lexical retrieval deficit in picture naming: Implications for word production models. *Brain and Language, 53*, 283–314.

Lambon Ralph, M. A., Lowe, C., & Rogers, T. T. (2007). Neural basis of category-specific semantic deficits for living things: Evidence from semantic dementia, HSVE and a neural network model. *Brain, 130*, 1127–1137.

Laws, K. R., Adlington, R. L., Gale, T. M., Moreno-Martínez, F. J., & Sartori, G. (2007). A meta-analytic review of category naming in Alzheimer's disease. *Neuropsychologia, 45*(12), 2674–2682.

Leonard, C., Rochon, E., & Laird, L. (2008). Treating naming impairments in aphasia: Findings from a phonological components analysis treatment. *Aphasiology, 22*(9), 923–947.

Levelt, W. J. M. (1989). *Speaking: From intention to articulation.* Cambridge, MA: MIT Press.

Levelt, W. J. M., Roelofs, A., & Meyer, A. S. (1999). A theory of lexical access in speech production. *Behavioral and Brain Sciences, 22*, 1–38.

Levelt, W. J. M., Schriefers, H., Vorberg, D., Meyer, A. S., Pechmann, T., & Havinga, J. (1991). The time course of lexical access in speech production: A study of picture naming. *Psychological Review, 98*, 122–142.

Linebaugh, C. W. (1983). Treatment of anomic aphasia. In W. H. Perkins (Ed.), *Current therapy of communication disorders: Language handicaps in adults* (pp. 35–43). New York: Thieme-Stratton.

Linebaugh, C. W., & Lehrner, L. H. (1977). Cueing hierarchies and word retrieval: A therapy program. In R. H. Brookshire (Ed.), *Clinical aphasiology proceedings* (pp. 19–31). Minneapolis, MN: BRK.

Martin, N. (2001). Repetition in aphasia: Theoretical and clinical implications. In R. Berndt (Ed.), *Handbook of neuropsychology* (Vol. 3, 2nd ed., pp. 136–156). Amsterdam: Elsevier.

Martin, N. (2008). Intervention for anomic aphasia from a cognitive impairment-based perspective. In N. Martin, C. K. Thompson, & L. Worrall (Eds.), *Aphasia rehabilitation: The impairment and its consequences* (pp. 199–218). San Diego, CA: Plural.

Martin, N., Dell, G. S., Saffran, E. M., & Schwartz, M. F. (1994). Origins of paraphasias in deep dysphasia: Testing the consequences of a decay impairment in an interactive spreading activation model of language. *Brain and Language, 47*, 609–660.

Martin, N., Fink, R., & Laine, M. (2004). Treatment of word retrieval with contextual priming. *Aphasiology, 18*, 457–471.

Martin, N., Fink, R., Laine, M., & Ayala, J. (2004). Immediate and short-term effects of contextual priming on word retrieval. *Aphasiology, 18*, 867–898.

Martin, N., Fink, R., Renvall, K., & Laine, M. (2006). Effectiveness of contextual repetition priming treatments for anomia depends on intact access to semantics. *Journal of International Neuropsychological Society, 12*, 1–14.

Martin, N., Gagnon, D., Schwartz, M. F., Dell, G. S., & Saffran, E. M. (1996). Phonological facilitation of semantic errors in normal and aphasic speakers on a picture naming task. *Language and Cognitive Processes, 11*, 257–282.

Martin, N., Kohen, F. P., & Kalinyak-Fliszar, M. (2010, May 23–27). *A processing approach to the assessment of language and verbal short-term memory abilities in aphasia.* Paper presented at the Clinical Aphasiology Conference, Charleston, SC.

Martin, N., & Saffran, E. M. (1990). Repetition and verbal STM in transcortical sensory aphasia: A case study. *Brain and Language, 39*, 254–288.

Martin, N., & Saffran, E. M. (1997). Language and auditory-verbal short-term memory impairments: Evidence for common underlying processes. *Cognitive Neuropsychology, 14*(5), 641–682.

Martin, N., & Saffran, E. M. (2002). The relationship of input and output phonology in single word processing: Evidence from aphasia. *Aphasiology, 16*, 107–150.

Martin, N., Saffran, E. M., & Dell, G. S. (1996). Recovery in deep dysphasia: Evidence for a relation between auditory-verbal STM and lexical errors in repetition. *Brain and Language, 52*, 83–113.

Martin, N., Schwartz, M. F., & Kohen, F. P. (2005). Assessment of the ability to process semantic and phonological aspects of words in aphasia: A multi-measurement approach. *Aphasiology, 20*(2/3/4), 154–166.

Martin, N., Weisberg, R. W., & Saffran, E. M. (1989). Variables influencing the occurrence of naming errors: Implications for models of lexical retrieval. *Journal of Memory and Language, 28*, 462–485.

Martin, R., & Lesch, M. F. (1996). Associations and dissociations between language impairment and list recall: Implications for models of STM. In S. E. Gathercole (Ed.), *Models of short-term memory* (pp. 149–178). Hove, UK: Psychology Press.

Martin, R., Lesch, M., & Bartha, M. (1999). Independence of input and output phonology in word processing and short-term memory. *Journal of Memory and Language, 41*, 3–29.

Massaro, M. E., & Tompkins, C. A. (1992). Feature analysis for treatment of communication disorders in traumatically brain injured patients: An efficacy study. *Clinical Aphasiology, 22*, 245–256.

McClelland, J. L., & Rumelhart, D. E. (1988). *Explorations in parallel distributed processing.* Cambridge, MA: MIT Press.

Nicholas, L. E., & Brookshire, R. H. (1993). A system for quantifying the informativeness and efficiency of the connected speech of adults with aphasia. *Journal of Speech and Hearing Research, 36*, 338–350.

Nickels, L. (1992). The Autocue? Self-generated phonemic cues in the treatment of a disorder of reading and naming. *Cognitive Neuropsychology, 9*, 155–182.

Nickels, L. A., & Howard, D. (1995). Aphasic naming: What matters? *Neuropsychologia, 33*, 1281–1303.

Patterson, J. (2001). The effectiveness of cueing hierarchies as a treatment for word retrieval. ASHA Special Division 2. *Perspectives on Neurophysiological and Neurogenic Speech and Language Disorders, 11*, 11–18.

Peach, R. K. (1996). Treatment for aphasic phonological output planning deficits. *Clinical Aphasiology, 24*, 109–120.

Pease, K. M., & Goodglass, H. (1978). The effects of cuing on picture naming in aphasia. *Cortex, 14*, 178–189.

Plaut, D. C. (1996). Relearning after damage in connectionists networks: Toward a theory of rehabilitation. *Brain and Language, 52*(1), 25–82.

Plaut, D. C., & Shallice, T. (1991). Effects of word abstractness in a connectionist model of deep dyslexia. *Proceedings of the 13th Annual Conference of the Cognitive Science Society* (pp. 73–78). Hillsdale, NJ: Erlbaum.

Raymer, A. M., Thompson, C. K., Jacobs, B., & Le Grand, H. R. (1993). Phonological treatment of naming deficits in aphasia: Model-based generalization analysis. *Aphasiology, 7,* 27–54.

Renvall, K., Laine, M., & Martin, N. (2007). Treatment of anomia with contextual priming: Exploration of a modified procedure with additional semantic and phonological tasks. *Aphasiology, 21,* 499–527.

Schriefers, H., Meyer, A. S., & Levelt, W. J. M. (1990). Exploring the time course of lexical access in production: Picture-word interference studies. *Journal of Memory and Language, 29,* 86–102.

Schwartz, M. F., & Brecher, A. (2000). A model-driven analysis of severity, response characteristics, and partial recovery in aphasic's picture naming. *Brain and Language, 73,* 62–91.

Schwartz, M. F., Dell, G. S., Martin, N., Gahl, S., & Sobel, P. (2006). A case series test of the two-step interactive model of lexical access: Evidence from picture naming. *Journal of Memory and Language, 54,* 228–264.

Schwartz, M. F., Saffran, E. M., Bloch, D. E., & Dell, G. S. (1994). Disordered speech production in aphasic and normal speakers. *Brain and Language, 47,* 52–88.

Stemberger, J. P. (1982). *The lexicon in a model of language production.* Unpublished doctoral dissertation, University of California, San Diego.

Stemberger, J. P. (1985). An interactive model of language production. In A. W. Ellis (Ed.), *Progress in the psychology of language* (Vol. 1, pp. 143–186). Hillsdale, NJ: Erlbaum.

Walker, J. A., & Dell, G. S. (2006). Speech errors reflect newly learned phonotactic constraints. *Journal of Experimental Psychology: Learning, Memory and Cognition, 32*(2), 387–398.

Wambaugh, J. L., Cameron, R., Kalinyak-Fliszar, M., Nessler, C., & Wright, S. (2004). Retrieval of action names in aphasia: Effects of two cueing treatments. *Aphasiology, 18*(11), 979–1004.

Wambaugh, J. L., Doyle, P. J., Martinez, A. L., & Kalinyak-Fliszar, M. M. (2002). Effects of two lexical retrieval cueing treatments on action naming in aphasia. *Journal of Rehabilitation Research and Development, 39*(4), 455–466.

Wambaugh, J. L., Linebaugh, C. W., Doyle, P. J., Martinez, A. L., & Kalinyak-Fliszar, M. M. (2001). Effects of two cueing treatments on lexical retrieval in aphasic speakers with different levels of deficit. *Aphasiology, 15*(10/11), 933–950.

Wilshire, C., & Saffran, E. M. (2005). Contrasting effects of phonological priming in aphasic word production. *Cognition, 95,* 31–71.

OBJECTIVES

The reader will be able to:

1. **Distinguish between indirect and direct route reading processes, as outlined by the dual-route model.**

2. **Understand how the connectionist model explains nonword and real-word errors.**

3. **Describe alexia subtypes.**

4. **Understand the most appropriate diagnostic procedure to differentiate between alexia subtypes.**

5. **Apply effective treatment strategies for acquired alexias.**

The Acquired Disorders of Reading

Ellyn A. Riley, C. Elizabeth Brookshire, and Diane L. Kendall

INTRODUCTION

The process of reading has been debated much in psycholinguistic, neurolinguistic, and educational literature for many years. Much of this literature discusses the process of reading and proposes theoretical models to describe its components. Most of these models involve some variation of a process for perceiving a printed word, analyzing the components of a printed word, understanding the word the print represents, and in the case of reading aloud, orally producing the word. Some reading models specify the process of print analysis in more detail by defining separate processes for recognizing specific features of letters, recognizing letters from those features, and recognizing graphemes from the letters. Other models define separate processes for accessing the lexical entry of a word and accessing the word's meaning. For oral word reading, some theoretical models define separate processes for accessing the sounds composing the word and articulating those sounds to produce it.

DUAL-ROUTE MODELS

Although reading models are designed to represent the reading process in both typical and disordered readers, some of the first models of reading evolved from examining reading patterns in patients with acquired alexias. In 1973, Marshall and Newcombe described a model of oral reading that offered an interpretation for various types of acquired alexia. This model was a precursor to the current dual-route cascaded (DRC) model of reading, a model that conceptualizes oral reading as a serial process with two separate routes: one for lexical and one for nonlexical reading (see Figure 10.1) (Coltheart, Rastle, Perry, & Langdon, 2001). For each of these reading routes, the model conceptualizes the reading process as a series of modules, each specified for a particular task in the reading process.

The *visual feature analysis* module is involved in analyzing the individual visual parts of each letter (e.g., the letter P consists of a single vertical line attached to a single line curved to the right). The *letter analysis* module is involved in identifying the letter, identifying the letter's position in relation to other letters, and identifying the graphemes in the word (e.g., *bush* contains four letters, *b-u-s-h,* but only three graphemes, b-u-sh). The *orthographic input lexicon* contains a store of the visual forms of known, familiar words (e.g., the visual word form of *candle* would be accessed at this level, but the visual form of the pseudoword *tandle* would not be accessed here). The *semantic system* is involved in associating the visual form of the word to the meaning of the word (e.g., the visual form *cat* is associated with a small, furry animal

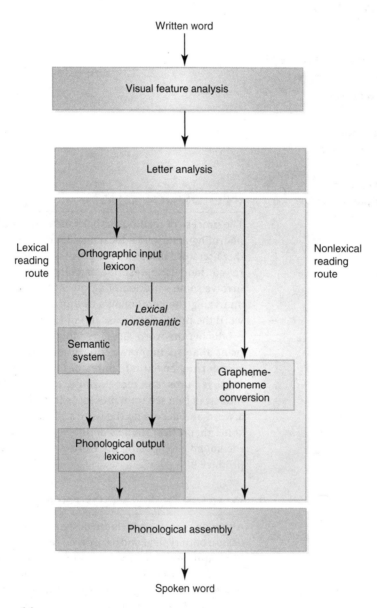

Figure 10.1 Dual-route model.

Modified from Coltheart, M., Rastle, K., Perry, C., & Langdon, R. (2001). DRC: A dual route cascaded model of visual word recognition and reading aloud. *Psychological Review, 108*(1), 204–256.

with four legs). The *grapheme–phoneme conversion* module involves translating the graphemes in a word to their corresponding phonemes (e.g., the graphemes t-i-p would be translated to the phonemes /t/, /ɪ/, /p/). The *phonological output lexicon* contains a store of the phonological forms of known, familiar words (e.g., the phonological form /tɪp/ would be accessed at this level, but the pseudoword /fɪp/ would not be accessed here). The *phonological assembly* module involves breaking down the phonological form into individual phonemes for speech production (e.g., the phonological form of /kɪp/ would be broken down to /k/, /ɪ/, /p/). In this model, the visual feature analysis, letter analysis, orthographic input lexicon, and grapheme–phoneme conversion modules are hypothesized to be involved only in the reading process, while the semantic system, phonological output lexicon, and phonological assembly modules are hypothesized to be involved in language processes other than reading, such as spontaneous speech production and repetition. Although this model's fundamental distinction lies between lexical and nonlexical reading, within lexical reading, two routes are proposed: a lexical–semantic route and a lexical–nonsemantic route. When reading a word via the lexical nonsemantic route, the features of a word's letters activate the word's letter units; then, letters activate the word's entry in the orthographic input lexicon, which activates the corresponding word entry in the phonological output lexicon, which activates the word's phonemes. This route could only possibly be used for oral reading and not reading comprehension because the meaning of the word is never accessed. In contrast, the lexical–semantic route could be used for oral reading as well as reading comprehension. The lexical–semantic route would operate similarly to the lexical–nonsemantic route except that the semantic system (i.e., word meaning) would be accessed between the orthographic input lexicon and the phonological output lexicon. According to this model, when reading a pseudoword or an unfamiliar word with regular spelling-to-sound rules, the nonlexical or sublexical route would be used. In this route, the letter string is converted into a phoneme string, assembled in a serial fashion with each grapheme converted to its corresponding phoneme (i.e., more commonly known as "sounding out the word").

CONNECTIONIST MODELS

In contrast to the serial processing of dual-route models, the connectionist triangle model explains oral reading as a single-route process involving bidirectional connections between orthography, meaning, and phonology units (Figure 10.2) (Harm & Seidenberg, 1999; Plaut,

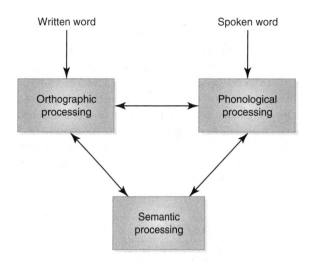

Figure 10.2 Connectionist triangle model.
Modified from Seidenberg, M., & McClelland, J. (1989). A distributed, developmental model of word recognition and naming. *Psychological Review, 96*(4), 523–568.

1999; Plaut, McClelland, Seidenberg, & Patterson, 1996; Seidenberg & McClelland, 1989). Proponents of this model argue that word reading is accomplished by the interaction of orthographic, semantic, and phonological information that is not specified only for the reading process, but is used for all types of language processing. Instead of postulating that the language system is made up of "rules" governing processing as the dual-route models do, connectionists argue that language knowledge is graded, and that learning language involves a process of statistical learning, or learning based on the probability of grapheme or phoneme patterns occurring in different contexts. This model would predict that in any language modality, processing occurs by comparing language input (via orthography or phonology) to information previously acquired, looking for consistency between the two.

In this model, a specific distinction is not made between lexical and nonlexical reading; however, because orthography, semantics, and phonology all interact in this model and processing can proceed bidirectionally, the model can still explain both types of reading. In the case of orally reading a word and processing the word's meaning (i.e., lexical–semantic reading), this model would predict that grapheme representations would be accessed first by searching for similarity among previously observed orthographic contexts, followed by access to the semantic information associated with the word, and finally ending with accessing the phoneme pattern previously associated with this grapheme pattern and using the phonological representation to produce the word.

In the case of orally reading a word without processing the word's meaning (i.e., lexical–nonsemantic reading), this model predicts that the grapheme representation would be accessed first, followed by directly accessing the word's corresponding phonological representation. A process similar to lexical–nonsemantic reading would be involved in pseudoword reading in the connectionist model, comparing grapheme patterns in the pseudoword to previously observed grapheme patterns, followed by accessing the phoneme pattern previously associated with this grapheme pattern.

ACQUIRED ALEXIA

Caused by an acquired disease of the central nervous system such as stroke or traumatic brain injury, acquired alexia results from damage to the mature reading system and manifests as an impairment in the comprehension of written language. Although several subtypes of acquired alexia have been discussed in the literature, acquired reading disorders can be divided into peripheral and central alexias, each category representing deficits in different stages of the reading process. Peripheral subtypes affect early stages of the reading process and involve difficulty perceiving the written word. Peripheral alexias include pure alexia, neglect alexia, attentional alexia, and visual alexia (Ellis & Young, 1988). Central subtypes affect later stages of the reading process and involve impairments in lexical or sublexical processing. Central alexias include surface alexia, deep alexia, and phonological alexia (Ellis & Young, 1988).

Peripheral Alexia Subtypes

Pure Alexia

Pure alexia involves an impairment in the way written words are perceived and analyzed during reading, specifically manifesting as an impairment in the simultaneous, parallel identification and processing of letters in a written word (Patterson & Kay, 1982; Warrington & Shallice, 1980). In an unimpaired system, the perception and processing of the letters in most words can be accomplished simultaneously (e.g., in the word *dog*, the initial letter *d* can be perceived and processed in relatively the same time frame as the final letter *g*). In pure alexia, however, letters are perceived and processed in a serial fashion (e.g., in the word *dog*, the initial letter *d* must be perceived, processed, and identified

before the second letter *o* can be processed, which is perceived, processed, and identified before the final letter *g*). This process, known as *letter-by-letter* reading, is extremely slow as a result of the patient having to identify each individual letter to slowly build the word. In other words, the patient essentially needs to spell out the entire word before being able to read it.

Pure alexia can be explained in dual-route reading models by an impairment at an early level of visual orthographic analysis, possibly occurring between the levels of *visual feature analysis* and *letter analysis*. Although most letters are perceived and identified correctly, the exchange of information between these processing levels is limited, with resources limited to processing a single letter at a time. Whereas dual-route models present a plausible explanation for pure alexia, connectionist models do not really present a specific explanation for this or other peripheral subtypes. Connectionist models combine all orthographic analysis into a single processing stage and do not differentiate between the analysis of single letters and overall orthographic patterns. Although the model contains an orthographic processing stage, it could be argued that pure alexia as well as other peripheral alexia subtypes occur because of impairment prior to the level of orthographic processing represented in the model and are therefore not relevant to discuss in the context of connectionist models.

Neglect Alexia

Neglect alexia involves an impairment in the way written words are perceived and analyzed during reading, specifically manifesting as an impairment in correctly identifying initial or final letters in words (Ellis, Flude, & Young, 1987). It is important to note that this impairment is specific to the perception of orthographic forms and is not the same as a general visual neglect. In neglect alexia, individuals produce spatially consistent errors at either end of a word. For example, if the person exhibits a left-sided neglect alexia, the person produces errors at the beginning of words in single-word oral reading tasks, while reading remains relatively unimpaired at the end of the word (e.g., *cat* produced as *bat*; *book* produced as *look*). In contrast, if an individual exhibits a right-sided neglect alexia, the individual produces the beginning of the word correctly but produces the end of the word incorrectly or omits it (e.g., *cat* produced as *car*; *book* produced as *boot*).

Neglect alexia can be explained in dual-route reading models by an impairment at the level of visual orthographic analysis, likely to occur specifically at the level of letter analysis. In this case, either before or after the point of neglect, the individual with alexia is unable to correctly identify the printed orthographic symbol (e.g., in a left-sided neglect alexia, the letter *c* in the word *cat* could be identified as *b*), resulting in activating an inaccurate target in the orthographic input lexicon (e.g., the orthographic form *bat* would be activated), semantic system (e.g., the semantic information for the word *bat* would be activated), and phonological output lexicon (e.g., the phonological form /bæt/ would be activated), leading to processing of inaccurate phonemes at the level of phonological assembly. Although the parts of the model following letter analysis are intact, because letter analysis processing is impaired, the inaccurate information is passed to all the following modules for processing, resulting in an inaccurate production. As with pure alexia, although dual-route models present a plausible explanation for neglect alexia, connectionist models do not really present a specific explanation for this alexia subtype.

Attentional Alexia

Attentional alexia involves an impairment in the way written words are perceived and analyzed during reading, specifically manifesting as incorrect productions of letters in a word as the result of interference from other letters in the word (Shallice & Warrington, 1977). Individuals exhibiting attentional alexia produce errors because of the influence of other letters occurring in the written context (e.g., *riverbank* produced as *biverbank*; *hot meal* produced as *hot heal*; *butterfly* produced as *flutterfly*; *bare* produced as *rare*).

Attentional alexia can be explained in dual-route reading models by an impairment at the level of visual orthographic analysis, likely to occur specifically at the level of letter analysis. In this case, the person is unable to correctly identify the spatial orientation of some letters in relation to others (e.g., for the word *bad*, the presence of the letter *d* could influence the perception of other letters, resulting in the person perceiving the word *dad*), resulting in activating an inaccurate target in the orthographic input lexicon (e.g., the orthographic form *dad* would be activated), semantic system (e.g., the semantic information for the word *dad* would be activated), and phonological output lexicon (e.g., the phonological form /dæd/ would be activated), leading to processing of inaccurate phonemes at the level of phonological assembly. As with pure and neglect alexia, although dual-route models present a plausible explanation for attentional

alexia, connectionist models do not really present a specific explanation for this alexia subtype.

Visual Alexia

Visual alexia involves an impairment in the way written words are perceived and analyzed during reading, specifically manifesting as production of a word that is visually similar to the target word (Marshall & Newcombe, 1973). The error patterns demonstrated in visual alexia are similar to those of neglect alexia except that the errors in visual alexia do not demonstrate a pattern of spatial consistency, and errors almost always represent real-word substitutions. The errors observed in visual alexia are also not specific to consonants or vowels but could occur at any point in the word on any type of letter and appear as letter or syllable substitutions, additions, or omissions (e.g., *butter* produced as *better*; *applause* produced as *applesauce*; *prince* produced as *price*).

Visual alexia can be explained in dual-route reading models by an impairment at the level of letter analysis or at the level of the orthographic input lexicon. If the impairment originates from letter analysis, the individual is unable to perceive correctly all the letters in the word (e.g., for the word *butter*, the misperception of the first vowel could result in perceiving the word *better*), resulting in activating an inaccurate target in the orthographic input lexicon (e.g., the orthographic form *better* would be activated), semantic system (e.g., the semantic information for the word *better* would be activated), and phonological output lexicon (e.g., the phonological form would be activated), leading to processing of inaccurate phonemes at the level of phonological assembly. If the impairment originates from the orthographic input lexicon, the person with alexia visually perceives the word correctly, but when similar words are activated in the orthographic input lexicon, selection of a visually similar word form occurs, resulting in inaccurate activation for the remaining parts of the process.

As with other peripheral alexias, although dual-route models present a plausible explanation for visual alexia, if it is considered a problem with perceiving the written form of the word, connectionist models do not really present a specific explanation for this alexia subtype. If visual alexia is conceptualized as an impairment in selecting an appropriate orthographic form, however, connectionist models could explain it as a reduced ability to activate correct forms or to inhibit incorrect forms at the level of orthographic processing.

Central Alexia Subtypes

Surface Alexia

Surface alexia involves an impairment in the way written words are processed during lexical reading, specifically manifesting as impaired reading of irregularly spelled words with relatively intact reading of regularly spelled real and pseudowords (Marshall & Newcombe, 1973). For example, the word *yacht* is considered an irregular word because it is pronounced /jat/ although it would be pronounced /jɔtʃt/ if regular spelling rules were applied; the word *bike* is considered a regular word because it is pronounced using a specific and predictable spelling rule (if a word ends in *e*, the preceding vowel is pronounced as a long vowel). In surface alexia, the person produces regular words such as *bike* more accurately than irregular words such as *yacht*. The errors produced by individuals with surface alexia can consist of visual errors (e.g., *blank* produced as *bank*), regularization errors (e.g., *pint* produced as /pɪnt/), and sometimes errors with visual and semantic overlap with the target (e.g., *car* produced as *cab*).

Surface alexia can be explained in dual-route reading models by an impairment at the level of the orthographic input lexicon, impairment in accessing the semantic system, or impairment in selection at the level of the phonological output lexicon. If errors are predominantly visual in nature, dual-route models explain them as occurring because of inappropriate selection at the level of the orthographic input lexicon, resulting in the subsequent activation of the semantic and phonological information for the visually similar word (e.g., for the word *blank*, other visually similar words are activated, and the incorrect word *bank* could be selected instead of the correct target, resulting in access to the semantic and phonological information for the word *bank*). If the lexical reading route is impaired, dual-route models predict that one possibility is to use the other unimpaired route for reading. Regularization errors can be explained by a dual-route model as an overreliance on the grapheme–phoneme conversion reading route caused by impairment in selection at the level of the phonological output lexicon (e.g., if the patient is unable to select the correct phonological form for the word *pint*, the grapheme–phoneme conversion route could be used to produce the word, resulting in the word pronounced using regular spelling rules—/pɪnt/). Dual-route models explain errors with both visual and semantic overlap with the target word as an impairment in accessing the semantic system from the orthographic input lexicon. In this case, a correct orthographic form could have been selected at the orthographic input lexicon, but incorrect selection occurs in the semantic system (e.g., the word *car* would be selected in the orthographic input lexicon along with other visually similar words like *cab* and *cat*; in the semantic system, other semantically related words would be activated like *cab* and *truck*; at this point, inaccurate selection could occur for *cab* because it was first active in the orthographic input lexicon and then active again in the semantic system).

In contrast to the dual-route approach of providing separate explanations for different types of reading errors, connectionist models explain surface dyslexia as a symptom of a general semantic impairment that is not specific to reading. Evidence for this explanation stems primarily from reports of individuals who demonstrate reading patterns consistent with surface alexia as well as co-occurring symptoms of semantic dementia, a type of dementia associated with the decline of semantic memory (Woollams, Ralph, Plaut, & Patterson, 2007). For connectionist models, all reading errors associated with surface alexia stem from weakened activations at the level of semantic processing.

Deep Alexia

Deep alexia involves an impairment in the way written words are processed during lexical and nonlexical reading, specifically manifesting as impaired pseudoword reading in conjunction with the production of semantic and visual errors in oral reading (Marshall & Newcombe, 1973; Patterson & Marcel, 1977; Shallice & Warrington, 1975). Although the literature offers various descriptions of deep alexia, individuals exhibit several hallmark symptoms, including (a) severely impaired pseudoword reading (e.g., inability to orally read *blik*); (b) semantic errors in oral reading (e.g., *apple* produced as *banana*; *window* produced as *door*); (c) visual errors in oral reading (e.g., *table* produced as *cable*; *goal* produced as *goat*); (d) morphological errors in oral reading (e.g., *baking* produced as *baked*; *drives* produced as *drive*); (e) an imageability effect in word reading, with greater success in reading concrete, imageable words (e.g., higher accuracy reading *horse* in comparison to *freedom*); and (f) a part-of-speech effect with more accurate word reading for content words compared to function words (e.g., higher accuracy reading *bee* compared to *be*).

Dual-route models have traditionally explained deep alexia as a dual impairment of nonlexical and lexical reading routes. In this explanation, errors in pseudoword reading can be explained as an impairment in grapheme–phoneme conversion, and lexical errors (especially semantic errors) can be explained as an impairment somewhere along the lexical route, in semantic access, semantic processing, or phonological processing. One recently proposed theory (failure of inhibition theory, FIT) suggests that symptoms of deep alexia (most specifically the production of semantic errors) result from a failure to inhibit selection of inappropriate targets at the level of the phonological output lexicon (Colangelo & Buchanan, 2006, 2007). However, other evidence indicates that individuals with deep alexia demonstrate differences in semantic processing that are not limited to reading, suggesting that semantic errors may be caused by impairment occurring prior to phonological processing (Riley & Thompson, 2010).

Although the FIT (Colangelo & Buchanan, 2006, 2007) and evidence from Riley and Thompson (2010) most directly address the question of lexical–semantic errors in deep alexia raised by dual-route model explanations, both are also compatible with connectionist model explanations of deep alexia. In a connectionist model, deep alexia can be explained either by a weakened phonological system (compatible with FIT) or by weakened connections between semantic and phonological processing (compatible with evidence from Riley & Thompson, 2010).

Phonological Alexia

Phonological alexia involves an impairment in the way written words are processed during nonlexical reading, specifically manifesting as impaired pseudoword reading in conjunction with the absence of semantic reading errors (Beauvois & Dérouesné, 1979; Dérouesné & Beauvois, 1979; Ellis & Young, 1988). In pseudoword oral reading, lexicalization errors (e.g., pseudoword, *blaf,* produced as real word *black*) are common in phonological alexia but are not always observed. In addition to this hallmark symptom of phonological alexia, in more recent years, studies have recognized that individuals with phonological alexia often demonstrate several overlapping symptoms with deep alexia, including visual errors and imageability effects, with semantic errors as the only consistent defining symptom between the two disorder subtypes (Crisp & Lambon Ralph, 2006; Friedman, 1996; Glosser & Friedman, 1990).

Dual-route models have traditionally explained phonological alexia as an impairment of the nonlexical reading route. More specifically, in this model, errors in pseudoword reading can be explained as an impairment in grapheme–phoneme conversion. Lexicalization and visual errors are explained in a dual-route model as an overreliance on lexical route reading (e.g., as a result of nonlexical route impairment, pseudoword *tavder* is

processed using the lexical route and read as real word *ladder,* which is both a lexicalization error and visually similar to the pseudoword target). However, imageability effects are more difficult to explain using a dual-route model because imageability effects are generally associated with semantic processing, and dual-route models do not explicitly conceptualize an interaction between semantic processing and nonlexical reading. Connectionist models explain phonological alexia primarily as a general weakening of phonological processing. Although some evidence suggested that individuals with phonological alexia do not demonstrate a general phonological impairment (Coltheart, 1996; Tree & Kay, 2006), others argued that growing evidence suggests that phonological impairment in these patients exists beyond the realm of reading and overlaps in spelling as well as other tasks not involving orthographic processing (Patterson & Lambon Ralph, 1999; Rapcsak et al., 2009; Welbourne & Lambon Ralph, 2007).

Deep and Phonological Alexia: Two Sides of the Same Coin?

Most existing literature treats phonological and deep alexia as separate subtypes of acquired alexia. However, some researchers suggest that phonological and deep alexia are not really separate disorders, but simply lie along a continuum of reading deficit, with phonological alexia representing the mild end and deep alexia representing the severe end of the continuum (Crisp & Lambon Ralph, 2006; Friedman, 1996; Glosser & Friedman, 1990). This view is based on evidence of significant symptom overlap between individuals with diagnoses of phonological or deep alexia as well as recovery patterns (Crisp & Lambon Ralph, 2006). Friedman (1996) reports five individuals whose reading deficits appeared to change over their recovery period, with symptoms of deep alexia eventually evolving into symptoms of phonological alexia. For all the individuals with alexia reviewed in this study, the first sign of recovery was a significant decrease and eventual disappearance of semantic reading errors. The last symptom affected was pseudoword reading, which significantly improved but did not fully recover in any of the individuals, suggesting that deep and phonological alexia are not independent disorders but represent differing levels of severity (Friedman, 1996). Proponents of the continuum theory provide some rather convincing supporting evidence. One possible explanation why previous studies did not adopt a spectral view of alexia may be that published research studies present a disproportionate number of cases from opposite ends of the continuum (i.e., more intermediary cases exist, but go unreported).

Associations Between Alexia and Aphasia

Typically, individuals with peripheral alexia do not have a co-occurring aphasia; however, the two language disorders are not mutually exclusive. In pure alexia, the most studied peripheral alexia subtypes, writing and spelling, are usually intact and language is fairly unimpaired with occasional cases of anomia (Friedman & Hadley, 1992). Typically, central alexias tend to co-occur with aphasia; however, the presence and subtype of aphasia vary greatly across individuals, and more evidence is necessary to draw accurate conclusions about these associations. Although the current evidence is not conclusive, cases of surface alexia have often reported fluent aphasia (Friedman & Hadley, 1992), cases of deep alexia have often reported nonfluent (often Broca's) aphasia (Coltheart, Patterson, & Marshall, 1980), and cases of phonological dyslexia have reported either no aphasia or mild aphasia (Coltheart, 1996). A recent retrospective study of oral reading abilities in a mixed group of 100 individuals with aphasia reported that the majority (68%) of the group presented with alexia, with sublexical alexia (phonological or deep) the most common subtype of alexia (Brookshire, Wilson, Nadeau, Gonzalez-Rothi, & Kendall, 2014).

Associations Between Alexia and Lesion Site

For the peripheral alexias, most lesions have been identified in areas of the brain associated with visual processing; however, lesion site varies greatly across individuals, and more research is necessary before definitive correlations can be made. The one exception is for pure alexia, which seems to be consistently associated with lesions in the left occipital lobe and the splenium of the corpus callosum (Friedman & Glosser, 1998; Friedman & Hadley, 1992). In the central alexias, lesion site varies greatly across subtypes and individuals. However, several studies report trends, including left temporal or temporoparietal lesions in surface alexia (Friedman & Hadley, 1992), extensive left hemisphere lesions in deep alexia (Coltheart et al., 1980; Friedman & Glosser, 1998), and left perisylvian or left superior temporal lesions in phonological alexia (Beeson, Rising, Kim, & Rapcsak, 2010; Friedman & Glosser, 1998).

ASSESSMENT

To determine the type of alexia, severity, and underlying psycholinguistic mechanisms contributing to the reading disorder, the clinician must conduct a sensitive and specific assessment. Screening tests of reading that are embedded as subtests of classic aphasia testing are included in the Boston Diagnostic Aphasia Examination (BDAE-3; Goodglass, Kaplan, & Barresi, 2001) and the Western Aphasia Battery—Revised (WAB-R; Kertesz, 2006). A detailed assessment can also be conducted using standardized research experimental assessments, or unstandardized stimuli.

Standardized Assessments

The following standardized assessments are commonly used to assess the nature, severity, and type of reading impairments in individuals with aphasia and non–brain-damaged adults or children.

- The Psycholinguistic Assessments of Language Processing in Aphasia (PALPA; Kay, Lesser, & Coltheart, 1992) is intended to be used for clinical and research purposes. The PALPA is modeled within current cognitive models of language and includes a set of resource materials enabling the user to select language tasks that can be tailored to the investigation of an individual patient's impaired and intact abilities. The PALPA consists of 60 tests of components of language structure, such as orthography and phonology, word and picture semantics, and morphology and syntax. Many of the subtests have normative data, and many are devoted to written language. Although the PALPA is one of the most comprehensive assessments of reading function, there are drawbacks, such as original norms are only for British English and the brevity of the stimulus word lists.
- The Reading Comprehension Battery for Aphasia, second edition (RCBA; LaPointe & Horner, 1998) provides a systematic evaluation of the nature and degree of reading impairment in adults with aphasia, including oral reading comprehension. The RCBA can be individually administered in 30 minutes with 20 subtests covering single-word comprehension for visual confusions, auditory confusions, and semantic confusions; functional reading; synonyms; sentence comprehension; short paragraph comprehension; paragraphs; and morphosyntactic reading with lexical controls.
- The Gray Oral Reading Test—4 (Wiederholt & Bryant, 2001) is intended for use for individuals 6 to 18 years of age to assess oral reading rate, fluency,

and comprehension. The test stimuli include 13 passages that are controlled for a variety of features of words and sentences.

- The Gates–MacGinitie Reading Test (GMRT; Gates & MacGinitie, 1978) is intended for use for individuals age 6 to 18 years to measure reading achievement. The GMRT is a timed multiple-choice test administered in groups. It provides scores in four areas: literacy concepts, oral language concepts, and letters and letter-sound correspondences.
- The Woodcock–Johnson III Diagnostic Reading Battery (WJ-III DRB; Woodcock, Mather, & Schrank, 2004) incorporates several subtests, including word identification, passage comprehension, nonword reading, reading fluency, and sound awareness. This battery provides normative values for individuals from age 2 to 90 years.

Research experimental assessments include the Battery of Adult Reading Function (Rothi, Coslett, & Heilman, 1984), the Maryland Reading Battery (Berndt, Haendiges, Mitchum, & Wayland, 1996), and the Johns Hopkins University Dyslexia Battery (Goodman & Caramazza, 1986).

Unstandardized Assessment

The following unstandardized assessments are commonly used to assess the nature, severity, and type of reading impairments in individuals with aphasia.

- *Peripheral assessment:* To ascertain that the reading deficit is not the result of early visual perception or peripheral mechanisms, an assessment of shape/letter matching and abstract letter identification can be used. For shape/letter matching, the clinician asks the individual with alexia to select two identical shapes from an array of nonsense shapes or to match letters of the same case and font. Abstract letter identities can be assessed with a task of letter matching across case or font and with a letter recognition task such as a forced-choice task in which the individual must distinguish correct letters from mirror-reversed letters.
- *Central assessment:*
  1. *Visual word recognition:* To assess whether the person with alexia has activation of the lexeme from orthography, a visual lexical decision task can be used. In this task, equal numbers of real words and nonwords are used as stimuli. A real word or nonword is presented randomly, and the individual is asked to respond whether the stimulus is a real word. Depending on the severity

level of the alexia, stimuli may be manipulated to include nonwords composed of legal and illegal phonotactic orthographic structure, high- and low-frequency real words, and irregularly spelled real words.

  2. *Semantic processing:* To assess access to semantics from visual orthography, several tasks can be conducted. A *category sorting task*, for example, includes written words belonging to a particular semantic category (e.g., tools, fruits, vegetables, transportation). The person with alexia is given these written words on index cards randomly ordered across various semantic categories and is asked to sort the cards into an appropriate category. Another semantic processing task is *cross-modality matching*, by which a single written word is matched with a corresponding picture or object. A *semantic associate matching task* can be used to assess semantic activation: A picture is shown, and the individual is asked to match the picture correctly to one picture in a field of three semantically related written words (e.g., picture of a tree is presented and written word stimuli are *branch, leaf, tree*). A final task that can be used to detect the integrity of the orthographic-to-semantic network is to *match a written word with a written definition*.
  3. *Nonlexical processing:* An evaluation of the aspects of the reading process that do not involve the lexical–semantic system includes an assessment of *graphemic parsing, graphemic blending,* and *grapheme-to-phoneme letter conversion*. To assess graphemic parsing, real-word and nonword stimuli can be visually presented, and the person with alexia must segment the word into smaller units, such as syllables or phonemes. For example, the real word *boxcar* is segmented into two real words, *box + car*. A nonword such as "drislee" would be segmented into *dris + lee*. Graphemic blending could be elicited for individual graphemes (b + e + d = bed) and syllables (ba + by = baby). Grapheme-to-phoneme letter conversion tasks assess the activation of orthographic and phonological representations and can be assessed by presenting individual written letters and asking the patient to produce the corresponding sound. *Pseudohomophone* pairs may also be used. They are pairs of phonetically identical letter strings where one string is a word and the other is a nonword (e.g., *groan/grone* and *crane/crain*).

INTERVENTION

Application of the International Classification of Functioning, Disability, and Health Model to Acquired Disorders of Reading

The International Classification of Functioning, Disability and Health, known more commonly as ICF, is a classification of health and health-related domains (World Health Organization, 2001). These domains are classified from body, individual, and societal perspectives by means of body functions, body structures, activities and participation, and environmental factors. The American Speech-Language-Hearing Association (ASHA, 2002) recommends using the WHO ICF as a framework for the assessment and treatment of individuals with neurogenic language disorders so that assessment and treatment address the spectrum of difficulty that individuals with communication disorders may encounter.

Communication and, in particular, reading are included in several aspects of the ICF. For example, the "Body Functions" section contains information related to voice and speech functions (b3) and mental functions (receptive and expressive aspects of language) that include silent reading comprehension and reading aloud. Three chapters in the "Activities and Participation" section describe behaviors for which reading is a necessary element. Chapter 1 (d1), "Learning and Applying Knowledge," includes information about learning, applying the knowledge that is learned, thinking, solving problems, and making decisions. Chapter 3 (d3), "Communication," includes general and specific features of communicating by language, signs, and symbols, including receiving and producing messages, carrying on conversations, and using communication devices and techniques. Chapter 8 (d8), "Major Life Areas," is about carrying out the tasks and actions required to engage in education, work, and employment and to conduct economic transactions.

Impairment-Based Approaches and Strategies

The Academy of Neurologic Communication Disorders and Sciences (ANCDS) and Special Interest Group 2 of ASHA (Neurophysiology and Neurogenic Speech and Language Disorders) developed evidence-based practice guidelines for the management of communication disorders in neurologically impaired individuals (Golper et al., 2001). The goal of the project "is to improve quality of services to individuals with neurologic communication disorders by assisting clinicians in decision-making about the management of specific populations through guidelines based on research evidence" (p. 1). To that end, an exhaustive, balanced, and inclusive literature review was conducted to encompass the available research evidence and expert opinion. The aphasia treatment studies were reviewed, and within that body of literature, 70 alexia treatment studies completed between 1964 and 2010 were evaluated (http://aphasiatx.arizona.edu/written_reading). Studies were coded for type of design (between group, within group, single subject, and case study); class of study (strongest, intermediate, weakest); and phase of treatment research (1–5) (Robey & Schultz, 1998).

To determine the most appropriate treatment approach for an individual with acquired alexia, it is essential for the clinician to link the behaviors observed in the standardized or unstandardized assessment with the underlying mechanism of impairment as theoretically described previously in this chapter. At that point, the clinician can evaluate the treatment programs described in the following sections, as well as others in the literature, for appropriateness to match the level of severity and stimulability of the individual with alexia. To that end, it is not the purpose of this chapter to present details for each treatment program; instead, the goal is to highlight the most recent and effective programs for each alexia type. However, four selected treatments for each alexia type and four text-level treatments are described in Tables 10.1 to 10.4 to provide more information regarding typical treatment stimuli, procedures, and outcomes used for reading interventions.

Pure Alexia

Eight studies published between 1991 and 2010 for rehabilitation of pure alexia were evaluated for the evidence-based practice guidelines, of which five were phase I (Arguin & Bub, 1994; Behrmann & McLeod, 1995; Lott & Friedman, 1999; Maher, Clayton, Barrett, Schober-Peterson, & Rothi, 1998; Seki, Yajima, & Sugishita, 1995) and four were phase II (Lott, Carney, Glezer, & Friedman, 2010; Sage, Hesketh, & Lambon Ralph, 2005; Tuomainen & Laine, 1991; Viswanathan & Kiran, 2005). The studies ranged in sample size from 1 to 3, and all employed a multiple-baseline, single-subject design. These eight studies employed the following treatment strategies to rehabilitate the underlying mechanisms of pure alexia:

multiple oral rereading (Tuomainen & Laine, 1991); speeded letter-matching tasks (Arguin & Bub, 1994); parallel processing of letters (Behrmann & McLeod, 1995); tactile–kinesthetic (Lott & Friedman, 1999; Lott et al., 2010; Seki et al., 1995); exploration of residual abilities through lexical treatment (Maher et al., 1998); letter-by-letter reading (Viswanathan & Kiran, 2005); and combination of whole-word, tactile–kinesthetic, and letter-by-letter reading (Sage et al., 2005). All treatment strategies were judged to be Class 3 (weakest strength).

More recently, Ablinger and Domahs (2009) successfully applied a whole-word reading approach to a single individual with pure alexia. In this study, they aimed to stimulate, via brief whole-word presentations, parallel grapheme processing. In the whole-word recognition task, words were repeatedly presented with limited exposure duration. The individual with alexia was asked to read the words aloud. Results showed improvement in word-reading performance for trained and control words. See Table 10.1 for a detailed description of selected pure alexia treatment studies.

Surface Alexia

Seven studies for rehabilitation of surface alexia published between 1989 and 2000 were evaluated for the evidence-based practice guidelines, of which six were phase I (Coltheart & Byng, 1989; De Partz, Seron, & Van der Linden, 1992; Ellis, Lambon Ralph, Morris, & Hunter, 2000; Friedman & Robinson, 1991; Moss, Gonzalez Rothi, & Fennell, 1991; Scott & Byng, 1989) and one was phase II (Weekes & Coltheart, 1996). The studies all were $n = 1$ and employed a single-subject baseline design or case study approach. Treatment strategies employed for surface alexia included lexical reading treatment (Coltheart & Byng, 1989; Scott & Byng, 1989); training grapheme-to-phoneme correspondence rules (Friedman & Robinson, 1991); speeded presentation (Moss et al., 1991); visual imagery (De Partz et al., 1992), mixed lexical reading and homophone spelling (Weekes & Coltheart, 1996); and naming and single-word reading (Ellis et al., 2000). All treatment strategies were judged to be Class 3 (weakest strength). See Table 10.2 for a detailed description of selected surface alexia treatment studies.

Phonological and Deep Alexia

Sixteen studies for rehabilitation of phonological and deep alexia published between 1986 and 2010 were evaluated for the evidence-based practice guidelines, of which 13 were phase I (De Partz, 1986; Friedman & Lott, 2002; Kendall, Conway, Rosenbek, & Gonzalez-Rothi, 2003; Kendall, McNeil, & Small, 1998; Laine & Nieme, 1990; Lott, Sample, Oliver, Lacey, & Friedman, 2008; Lott, Sperling, Watson, & Friedman, 2009; Mitchum & Berndt, 1991; Peach, 2002; Ska, Garneau-Beaumont, Chesneau, & Damien, 2003; Sperling, Lott, Snider, & Friedman, 2005; Stadie & Rilling, 2006; Yampolsky & Waters, 2002) and 3 were phase II (Beeson et al., 2010; Bowes & Martin, 2007; Lacey, Lott, Snider, Sperling, & Friedman, 2010). The most common treatment strategy employed to rehabilitate deep and phonological alexia is the retraining of grapheme-to-phoneme or bigraph–biphone correspondences (Bowes & Martin, 2007; De Partz, 1986; Friedman & Lott, 2002; Kendall et al., 1998; Laine & Nieme, 1990; Mitchum & Berndt, 1991; Peach, 2002; Yampolsky & Waters, 2002). Kendall et al. (2003) employed a purely phonological treatment using individual phonemes in the context of nonwords. Stadie and Rilling (2006) used phonological and semantic cueing, while Lott et al. (2008) employed phonological self-cueing. Beeson et al. (2010) implemented a two-stage interactive treatment involving reading and spelling components. Two other treatment approaches used with various amounts of success were priming (Ska et al., 2003) and speeded functor reading (Sperling et al., 2005).

More recently, Brookshire, Conway, Pompon, Oelke, and Kendall (2014) looked at effects of phonomotor treatment on the reading abilities of eight individuals with phonological alexia, and Riley and Thompson (2015) investigated effects of phonological complexity (sonority) during grapheme-to-phoneme training in five individuals with phonological alexia. See Table 10.3 for a detailed description of selected phonological–deep alexia treatment studies.

Text-Based Reading Treatment Approaches

Although improving text-level reading and comprehension is the ultimate goal of reading treatment, research in alexia has primarily been focused on training reading at the single-word level, as is evident in the studies mentioned previously. In these treatment studies, text-level reading is typically only mentioned as it relates to generalization effects across other reading contexts, which tend to be limited. Specific treatments focusing on text-level reading and comprehension are not frequently encountered in the alexia literature, and the motivations for these approaches are quite varied.

Table 10.1 Description of Pure Alexia Treatment Studies

Reference	Design	Site of Lesion(s)	Treatment Type	Target Behavior	Stimuli	Procedure	Intensity and Frequency	Outcome
Ablinger & Domahs (2009)	Case study (n = 1)	L MCA/PCA CVA	Whole word (limited exposure)	Word reading and letter ID	160 real words (80 trained, 80 control) between 1 and 3 syllables; words contained "difficult" letters the pt had difficulty naming	Training began with auditory–visual verification tasks (pt decided if written word matched spoken word) to familiarize pt with stimuli. Then, whole-word recognition training began. Pt briefly (1,000 ms) saw target word on screen and was asked to read it. Each word was randomly seen 4 times each session. Feedback was provided if pt was unable to correctly read target.	2 sessions/d, 5 days/wk for 4 weeks	Improved speed and accuracy of cross-case matching and reading of words and text
Lott et al. (2010)	Case series (n = 3)	L CVA; L parietal-occipital hemorrhage; L occipital CVA	Tactile–kinesthetic at letter level	Reading of untrained words in "free vision"	Phase 1: 26 alphabetic letters; Phase 2: 450 nonpronounceable letter strings and 450 words 4 to 8 letters in length matched for orthographic similarity; Untrained list: 40, six-letter, two-syllable low-frequency regularly spelled words	Phase 1 (letter naming): (1) trace each letter with and then without pen strokes provided, (2) copy each letter onto palm, (3) copy on palm and name it Phase 2a (rapid letter naming): (1) name letters in isolation and then in letter strings as fast as possible Phase 2b (rapid letter-by-letter word reading): name each letter in the word and then read the word as fast as possible; 3 blocks of 25 letter strings or words presented each session	1 h/day, 3x/wk, plus home practice 3x/d during Phase 1 only	Phase 1 did not improve reading; continued practice (Phase 2) improved reading speed and accuracy of untrained words without overt use of trained strategy

Study	Design	Lesion	Treatment approach	Target	Stimuli	Treatment steps	Dosage	Outcomes
Sage et al. (2005)	Case study (n = 1)	L parietal-temporal CVA followed 2 months later by L occipital hemorrhage	Tactile–kinesthetic at whole-word and letter levels	Word reading	Three 30-word lists matched for length, frequency, imageability, and AOA; lists consisted of triads (first 3 letters identical), words related to ADLs, and words of personal interest to the pt	Family was trained to deliver txt and therapist visited once/week. Treatment 1 (word therapy): Pt (1) traces around the shape of the word focusing on visual features, (2) looks at final 3 letters (in red font), (3) looks and listens to word read aloud by family member, (4) looks, listens, and then repeats 5 times Treatment 2 (letter therapy): (1) Family member reads aloud each target word one letter at a time and traces the letter onto pt's palm. Pt repeats word. (2) Same as Step 1 except pt reads aloud word after letters are traced. (3) Cards are shuffled, and Step 2 is repeated. (4) Pt reads aloud each letter and says word. Errorless learning feedback was provided.	Word therapy: 10 words/wk for 7 weeks; letter therapy: 30-item word list trained over 7 weeks	improved accuracy and speed on treated items; attempted use of whole-word reading instead of letter-by-letter strategy; decreased omissions and increased semantic and visual errors; letter ID remained impaired
Viswanathan & Kiran (2005)	Case study (n = 1)	L occipito-temporal-parietal CVA	Sublexical conversion and semantic feature analysis	Word reading	22 regularly spelled words matched for frequency, familiarity, and number of letters and syllables divided into trained and untrained lists; each word in one list was semantically related to a word in the other list	11 regular words trained using the following steps: (1) oral reading of target word, (2) written spelling, (3) identification of letters of the word from phonological and orthographic distracters, (4) identification of randomly presented letters of target word, (5) oral reading of letter names of target word, (6) description of semantic features of the target word, and (7) oral reading of the target word	2 baseline sessions and 20 probe sessions.	Improved oral reading accuracy for trained and untrained words; generalization to spelling of untrained words.

Note: ADLs, activities of daily living; AOA, age of acquisition; CVA, cerebrovascular accident; ID, identification; L, left; MCA, middle cerebral artery; PCA, posterior cerebral artery; pt, participant; txt, treatment.

Table 10.2 Description of Surface Alexia Treatment Studies

Reference	Design	Site of Lesion(s)	Treatment Type	Target Behavior	Stimuli	Procedure	Intensity and Frequency	Outcome
Coltheart & Byng (1989)	Case study (n = 1)	R temporal and L temporal-parietal s/p skull fx	Whole word with mnemonic support	Txt 1: Irregular word reading Txt 2 and 3: high-frequency words	Txt 1: 24 irregular words containing "-ough" (e.g., cough) Txt 2: 54 high-frequency words Txt 3: 101 high-frequency words	Txt 1: Each word was printed on a card alongside a picture representing the word. Pt read aloud each word and recorded progress in daily log. Txt 2 and 3: Words were accompanied by symbols selected by pt and therapist. Pt used mnemonic to assist in reading aloud each word.	Txt 1: 15 minutes/d at home for 5 weeks Txt 2: 15 minutes/d at home for 1 week Txt 3: not specified	Txt 1: 100% oral reading accuracy of all 24 words and maintained 1 year later Txt 2 and 3: Improved reading of trained words with some generalization to untrained words
R. B. Friedman & Robinson (1991)	Case study (n = 1)	L temporal-occipital CVA	Whole word	Reading of words with ambiguous vowels	16 vowel groups with inconsistent vowels (e.g., ow- as in cow, row) and words with and without the "rule of e" (e.g., rate, rat) represented in 253 words; words divided into treatment and control groups	Each vowel group (e.g., -ow) was represented on a card with the top half representing words with one pronunciation (e.g., cow) and the lower half another pronunciation (e.g., row). One to three vowel groups were trained each session. The pt read aloud each word independently or following verbal model when necessary.	7 sessions over 13 weeks plus daily home practice 15 to 30 minutes	improved reading of trained words, with poor generalization to untrained words with the same ambiguous vowels

Study	Design	Etiology	Treatment Approach	Target	Stimuli	Treatment	Dosage	Outcome
Moss et al. (1991)	Case study (n = 1)	R frontal craniotomy and L frontotemporal contusion s/p CHI	Whole word	Oral reading and reading comprehension	Task 1: 100 words, 10 per session; Task 2: 10 irregularly spelled words; Task 3: 5-sentence paragraphs containing homographic pairs	Treatment consisted of 3 tasks: Task 1: Forced semantic analysis (pt saw a word for 1 second and named semantic category). Task 2: Rapid reading aloud of irregular words. Task 3: Homophone selection (pt read paragraph silently and selected appropriate homophone based on context, e.g., flower/flour).	10, one-hour sessions over 2-week period	Increased reading rate while maintaining or improving accuracy
Weekes & Coltheart (1996)	Case study (n = 1)	R frontal contusion, L occipital fx, L postparietal extradural hematoma s/p car accident	2 treatments: whole-word reading and spelling with mnemonic support	Txt 1: Reading "exception" words; Txt 2: homophone spelling	Txt 1: 80 exception words (e.g., choir) divided into trained and untrained groups matched for word length and frequency; Txt 2: 62 homophones divided into trained and untrained groups	Txt 1: Each target word was presented on a card with a corresponding picture and the "conventional letter-sound rule pronunciation" printed below. Pt read aloud treated words with feedback from clinician. Txt 2: Each target word (e.g., peak) was shown with a picture and the correct spelling. On a separate card, the corresponding homophone (e.g., peek) was presented for pt to make comparison between the spellings and associate the mnemonics with the word.	Txt 1: 15 minutes/d for 7 days; Txt 2: 3 h/d for 3 days	Txt 1: Improved reading accuracy of trained and some untrained words; spelling of trained words did not improve. Txt 2: improved spelling of trained words; no generalization to spelling of untrained words

Note: CHI, closed head injury; CVA, cerebrovascular accident; fx, fracture; L, left; pt, participant; R, right; s/p, status post; txt, treatment.

Table 10.3 Description of Phonological/Deep Alexia Treatment Studies

Reference	Design	Site of Lesion(s)	Treatment Type	Target Behavior	Stimuli	Procedure	Intensity and Frequency	Outcome
Beeson et al. (2010)	Single-subject design (n = 2)	L CVA in perisylvian cortical regions	2 stages: phonological and then interactive (sublexical and lexical)	Sound-letter correspondences; nonword spelling	Stage 1: 20 consonants, 12 vowels, and corresponding "key" words (e.g., pie for /p/) Stage 2: regular and irregular words	Stage 1: Cueing hierarchy was used to train phoneme-grapheme correspondence: (1) write the letter that goes with the target phoneme; (2) think of "key" word paired to target phoneme and try to write it; (3) show picture of key word, write the word, and underline target phoneme; (4) copy key word. Phonological tasks (e.g., segmentation) using RWs and NWs were also trained. Stage 2: Trained a spelling problem-solving strategy: (1) attempt plausible spelling using phoneme-grapheme knowledge; (2) check spelling using lexical knowledge; (3) use electronic device to check and correct spelling errors	1 h/d, 3 d/wk for 12 to 14 weeks; homework 45 min/d, 5 d/wk	Improved phonological processing; improved reading and spelling of untrained RVs and NWs; improved spelling with use of electronic spelling aid.
Bowes & Martin (2007)	Longitudinal case study (n = 1)	L CVA involving frontal and parietal lobes and insular cortex	Bigraph-biphone segment blending	Reading and writing of nonwords, words, and phrases	Txt 1: 30, one-syllable NWs; with CVC, CCVC, CVCC structure Txt 2: 80, two-syllable RWs with CVCVC, CVVCVC, CVCCVC structure Txt 3: 48 noun/ verb and verb/noun phrases	Txt 1: 1-syllable reading: read bigraphs and then blend together into whole word; 1-syllable writing: repeat and write spoken biphones and then write each bigraph to spell whole word Txt 2: 2-syllable-reading: progress from reading bigraphs to syllables to whole word (e.g., CA-ME-EL CA-MEL, CAMEL); 2-syllable writing: write spoken bigraphs, then spoken syllable, and then whole word Txt 3: Reading phrases: Nouns and verbs read syllable by syllable and then as a phrase; writing phrases: each word spelled by emphasizing syllable-by-syllable strategy	1 h/d, 2 to 3 d/wk over 3 years	Pt improved from impaired 1-syllable word reading to accurate reading and writing at phrase level.

Study	Design	Participants	Treatment	Outcome measure	Stimuli	Treatment description	Dosage	Results
Brookshire et al. (2014)	Single-group pre-/post-txt (n = 8)	all pts had L CVAs	Phonomotor treatment (multimodal txt of phonology)	Oral reading of untrained real words and nonwords; comprehension of single words and text	English phonemes; 42, one- or two-syllable RWs and 72 one- or two-syllable NWs with low phonotactic probability and high neighborhood density	Stage 1 (about 20 hours): Train all English phonemes in isolation via multimodal tasks, including motor description, perception, production, and sound-to-letter correspondences Stage 2 (about 40 hours): Train phonologic sequence knowledge in NWs and then RWs via tasks, such as repetition, minimal pair discrimination, phoneme parsing and blending, reading, and spelling	2 h/d, 5 d/wk for 6 weeks	Improved NW repetition of trained and untrained items and improved reading accuracy of untrained regular and irregular RWs and NWs for all 8 pts with maintenance at 3-month follow-up; only 1 pt showed improved single-word and text comprehension.
Riley & Thompson (2015)	Single subject, multiple baseline (n = 5)	All pts had L CVAs	Phonological complexity (sonority) training	Oral reading of initial consonant clusters in real and nonwords	Initial consonant clusters with large (pl) and small (gl) sonority differences; for each cluster, a list of 20 RVs and 20 NWs created	Two consonant clusters (one simple, one complex) were selected for each pt. Three pts were trained on the complex cluster, and 2 pts were trained on the simple cluster. Pt was asked to read aloud a target word and then complete 3 phonological tasks: (1) phoneme segmentation, (2) grapheme-phoneme matching, and (3) phoneme blending	Maximum of 10 weeks (20 sessions) per consonant cluster	All pts improved on trained clusters; 2 of 3 pts in the "complex" (e.g., "gl-") training showed generalization to the untrained "simple" cluster ("kl-"); pts in "simple" condition (e.g., "pl-") did not show generalization to "complex" cluster ("gl-").

Note: CVA, cerebrovascular accident; L, = left; NW, nonword; pt, participant; RW, real word; txt, treatment.

Among the specific text-level reading treatments available, some focus on training the phonological aspects of reading in an attempt to increase reading fluency at the text level (Multiple Oral Re-Reading, MOR; Lacey et al., 2010; Moyer, 1979) or to boost phonological skills and reading fluency to divert more resources to reading comprehension (Oral Reading for Language in Aphasia, ORLA; Cherney, 2010a; Cherney, Merbitz, & Grip, 1986). Several studies have investigated the use of MOR as a treatment for alexia and, in general, have shown an increase in reading fluency on trained and untrained text (reviewed in Kim & Russo, 2010; Lacey et al., 2010). A few studies have used ORLA to improve reading comprehension in persons with alexia (Cherney, 2004; Cherney et al., 1986) and have shown improvements in reading fluency, but evidence for improved reading comprehension is limited and varies across individuals. In a series of case studies by Webster and colleagues (2013), a participant who received ORLA training did not demonstrate any change in reading comprehension from pre- to posttreatment. A computerized version of the treatment has also been tested (Cherney, 2010b), and similar outcomes have been reported. In terms of phonological text-based approaches, both MOR and ORLA improve reading fluency at the text level; however, evidence of positive effects on reading comprehension is much weaker.

In contrast, other approaches focus on training strategies for summarizing information (Attentive Reading and Constrained Summarization [ARCS]; Rogalski & Edmonds, 2008; Webster et al., 2013) and strategies for identifying key words and main ideas from text (Proposition Identification and Constrained Summarization [PICS]; Webster et al., 2013). ARCS involves reading a passage of text aloud, followed by focused silent reading and concluding in an oral summary delivered by the participant. ARCS was originally developed to improve discourse, but using the same protocol, Webster and colleagues (2013) reported improvements in reading comprehension from pre- to posttreatment and from posttreatment to follow-up. This preliminary evidence suggests that ARCS treatment may have some potential as a treatment for alexia, but improvements demonstrated were not statistically significant and have only been shown for reading comprehension in a single case. PICS is similar to ARCS in terms of providing opportunities for focused reading and oral summarization, but PICS differs from ARCS in that it requires the participant to explicitly identify key words and main ideas from the passage before providing an oral summary. In the case study reported by Webster and colleagues (2013), the participant undergoing PICS treatment did not improve her ability to identify main ideas in the trained passages and showed minimal (and statistically insignificant) improvements on standardized reading comprehension measures. Overall, strategy-based text reading treatments offer little evidence to support their use as reading comprehension treatments for alexia. However, research investigating these strategy-based approaches is still in the preliminary stages, and it is too early to draw meaningful conclusions. See Table 10.4 for a detailed description of selected text-level reading treatments.

FUTURE DIRECTIONS

Directions for future research in acquired disorders of reading are needed in the areas of assessment, treatment, and elucidating neural substrates.

Assessment: While few standardized assessments exist to assess acquired reading disorders, most lack support of essential standardization criteria, such as content validity, construct validity, specificity, and sensitivity. Further, assessment to understand reading abilities as related to the ICF model (WHO, 2001) is essential. As it stands, most available tools that assess reading are directed at the level of impairment, and items/stimuli need to be created to assess reading performance for societal participation.

Treatment: When conducting clinical research in the field of alexia rehabilitation, a clear foundation must be set to develop foundational knowledge that can later support inferences of causality as well as conclusions that can be generalized to the larger population being sampled. To date, essentially all published rehabilitation studies for the acquired alexias have focused on phases I and II (Robey, 2004). Future research is needed to extend existing knowledge of phase II treatment protocols into phase III.

Neural Substrates: Although it is widely agreed that reading entails multiple cognitive processes, there is little evidence for localization of these processes. Research combining functional and structural neuroimaging with behavioral performance is needed to determine the precise mechanisms that account for the acquired alexias.

Table 10.4 Description of Text-Level Reading Treatments

Reference	Design	Site of Lesion(s)	Treatment Type	Target Behavior	Stimuli	Procedure	Intensity and Frequency	Outcome
Lacey et al. (2010)	Case series (n = 6; four phonological and two pure alexia pts)	5 pts with L CVA; 1 pt with skull fx with L hemorrhage	Multiple Oral Re-Reading (MOR)	Oral text reading	300- word text passages that were trained, untrained with 60–80% overlap with trained passages, or control with minimal overlap with trained passages.	Each session trained a different passage. Pt read aloud the passage as fast and accurately as possible. Clinician pointed to incorrect word(s) and prompted pt to reread and if necessary provided repetition. Pt read passage 3 times during session and then 5 times/d at home and called in once per week to read aloud over the phone so clinician could provide feedback.	2 h/d, 1 d/wk for 8 weeks, plus homework	MOR improved reading accuracy and rate of untrained passages that contained overlap with the trained passages. No generalization to untrained passages that did not have overlap of words with trained passages. Reading comprehension of passages was not measured.
Cherney (2010a)	Pre-/post-txt (n = 25 individuals with nonfluent aphasia)	Single L CVA	Oral Reading for Language in Aphasia (ORLA)	Oral text reading and general language measures	Sentences of various lengths (Level 1: 3–5 words; Level 2: 8–12 words; Level 3: 15–30 words; Level 4: 50–100 words). Sentences contained various vocabulary items and grammatical structures.	(1) Pt listened to and looked at written sentence twice; (2) pt read aloud sentence twice with therapist; (3) pt identified two or three words and read them aloud; (4) pt read sentence aloud again in unison with therapist. About 30 sentences practiced each session.	24 sessions, two to three times/week	The severe pt group showed improved WAB-AQ, WAB reading, and RCBA scores. Moderate pt group showed improved WAB-AQ and WAB discourse scores. Mild group showed improved WAB-AQ, WAB writing, and WAB discourse scores.

(continued)

Table 10.4 Description of Text-Level Reading Treatments (*continued*)

Reference	Design	Site of Lesion(s)	Treatment Type	Target Behavior	Stimuli	Procedure	Intensity and Frequency	Outcome
Webster et al. (2013)	Single subject, multiple baseline (n = 1)	Single L CVA	Attentive Reading and Constrained Summarization (ARCS)	Paragraph-level reading comprehension	Articles from local newspapers or news websites.	(1) Pt read a whole passage aloud; (2) pt read passage again silently in 2- or 3-sentence chunks; (3) pt provided a short oral summary.	Twelve 45-minute to 1-hour sessions over 6 weeks	Nonsignificant increase in reading comprehension on DCT and nonsignificant increase in reading speed. Pt reported feeling more confident about reading.
Webster et al. (2013)	Single subject, multiple baseline (n = 1)	L MCA CVA	Proposition Identification and Constrained Summarization (PICS)	Paragraph-level reading comprehension	Articles from local newspapers or news websites.	Pt read passage as many times as necessary and then identified "key messages," wrote down key words, and provided an oral summary.	1-hour sessions, twice per week over 4 weeks	Nonsignificant increase in reading comprehension on DCT and RCBA and nonsignificant decrease in reading speed. Pt reported enjoying reading again.

Note: CVA, cerebrovascular accident; DCT, Discourse Comprehension Test (Brookshire & Nicholas, 1993); fx, fracture; L, left; MCA, middle cerebral artery; pt, participant; RCBA, Reading Comprehension Battery for Aphasia (La Pointe & Horner, 1998); txt, treatment; WAB, Western Aphasia Battery (Kertesz, 1982).

Case Illustration 10.1

As a clinician working in a private practice, you are conducting an evaluation of a 53-year-old man. At the initial session, you review his medical records and obtain background demographic information. You learn your patient is a right-handed male with a doctoral degree in psychology who was employed as a hospital administrator prior to onset of a left middle cerebral artery cerebral vascular accident 2 years prior. Reports from the speech–language clinician at the outpatient rehabilitation unit state that "his language is indicative of a severe nonfluent aphasia with alexia, agraphia, and apraxia of speech." Based on this background information, you determine which formal measures you need to administer during your first evaluation session.

To quantify the nature and severity of aphasia and suspected word retrieval impairments, you administer the WAB (Kertesz, 1982) and the Boston Naming Test (BNT; Kaplan, Goodglass, & Weintraub, 1983). To determine involvement of the speech motor articulatory system, you administer the Apraxia Battery for Adults (ABA-2; Dabul, 2000). To evaluate reading performance, you administer the RCBA (LaPointe & Horner, 1998). Finally, at this initial evaluation, you ask your patient to take home and complete the ASHA Functional Assessment of Communication Skills for Adults (FACS) (Frattali, Thompson, Holland, Wohl, & Ferketic, 1995) to identify and quantify the communication strengths and weaknesses at the Activity and Participation levels of the ICF model.

Based on data collected from these formal tests, you determine that your patient presents with severe nonfluent aphasia (WAB aphasia quotient: 31/100). His speech production is nonfluent and characterized by struggling, groping, inability to repeat phonemes or words; you noted fewer errors in automatic speech (e.g., counting) compared to volitional speech. These behaviors are consistent with apraxia of speech. In addition, he shows poor comprehension for yes/no questions, object/picture identification, and commands. Performance on the BNT shows 13/60 spontaneously correct, indicating difficulty with lexical retrieval or speech motor programming difficulties. In terms of reading, on the RCBA (LaPointe & Horner, 1998) your patient had an overall performance of 6.5/10. These results, however, do not reveal the type of alexia, but instead indicate global difficulty in reading performance.

To delineate the underlying mechanisms involved in the reading process, and thus determine the type of alexia, you administer a variety of orthographic stimuli. Through this unstandardized reading evaluation, you find that your patient is unable to read aloud letters, single-syllable real words, and consonant–vowel (CV) nonwords. He can point to nonwords with 73% accuracy and real words with 83% accuracy in a field of three and match homophones to pictures with 61% accuracy. The discrepancy between his poorer performance on nonword and homophone reading compared to real-word reading indicates an indirect reading route impairment. Finally, to assess integrity of phonological processing, the Lindamood Auditory Conceptualization (LAC; Lindamood & Lindamood, 1998) test and the Comprehensive Test of Phonological Processing (CTOPP; Wagner, Torgesen, & Rashotte, 1998) reveal significant impairment in the ability to discriminate, blend, and segment phonemes.

Based on your reading evaluation, you determine your patient has a phonological alexia. In the presence of his aphasia, you determine that your therapy will focus on the following four areas: (a) rebuilding an underlying impairment in phonology (e.g., Kendall et al., 2003); (b) in the face of a co-occurring aphasia, considering an intensive program that has been shown to generalize to language function (Kendall et al., 2008); (c) educating family members regarding the nature of his alexia and aphasia; and (d) encouraging social networking to stimulate language recovery.

STUDY QUESTIONS

1. How is the process of lexical–semantic reading conceptualized differently in dual-route and connectionist models?
2. What are the four subtypes of peripheral alexia and the three subtypes of central alexia?
3. What is the primary difference between deep and phonological alexias?
4. How do connectionist models explain nonword reading errors in deep and phonological alexias?

5. How does the dual-route model explain lexicalization errors in surface alexia?

6. List formal and informal assessments of alexia.

7. What is the difference between central versus peripheral mechanisms in reading?

8. Describe three nonlexical assessment procedures.

9. How does the ICF incorporate reading?

10. Describe how treatment for surface alexia might differ from treatment for phonological or deep alexia.

REFERENCES

Ablinger, I., & Domahs, F. (2009). Improved single-letter identification after whole-word training in pure alexia. *Neuropsychological Rehabilitation, 19*(3), 340–363.

American Speech-Language-Hearing Association. (2002). Scope of practice in speech-language pathology. *Communication Disorders Quarterly, 23*(2), 77–83.

Arguin, M., & Bub, D. N. (1994). Pure alexia: Attempted rehabilitation and its implications for interpretation of the deficit. *Brain and Language, 47*, 233–268.

Beauvois, M. F., & Dérouesné, J. (1979). Phonologic alexia: Three dissociations. *Journal of Neurology, Neurosurgery and Psychiatry, 42*(12), 1115–1124.

Beeson, P., Rising, K., Kim, E. S., & Rapcsak, S. Z. (2010). A treatment sequence for phonologic alexia/agrapha. *Journal of Speech, Language and Hearing Research, 53*, 450–468.

Behrmann, M., & McLeod, J. (1995). Rehabilitation for pure alexia: Efficacy of therapy and implications for models of normal word recognition. *Neuropsychological Rehabilitation, 5*(1–2), 149–180.

Berndt, R. S., Haendiges, A. N., Mitchum, C. C., & Wayland, S. C. (1996). An investigation of non-lexical reading impairments. *Cognitive Neuropsychology, 13*, 763–801.

Bowes, K., & Martin, N. (2007). Longitudinal study of reading and writing rehabilitation using a bigraph-biphone correspondence approach. *Aphasiology, 21*(6), 687–701.

Brookshire, C. E., Conway, T., Pompon, R., Oelke, M., & Kendall, D. (2014). Effects of intensive phonomotor treatment on reading in eight individuals with aphasia and phonological alexia. *American Journal of Speech-Language Pathology, 23*, S300–S311.

Brookshire, C. E., Wilson, J., Nadeau, S., Gonzalez-Rothi, L. J., & Kendall, D. (2014). Frequency, nature, and predictors of alexia in a convenience sample of individuals with chronic aphasia. *Aphasiology, 28*(2), 1464–1480.

Brookshire, R. H., & Nicholas, L. E. (1993). *Discourse comprehension test*. Tucson, AZ: Communication Skill Builders.

Cherney, L. R. (2004). Aphasia, alexia and oral reading. *Topics in Stroke Rehabilitation, 11*, 22–36.

Cherney, L. R. (2010a). Oral reading for language in aphasia: Impact of aphasia severity on cross-modal outcomes in chronic nonfluent aphasia. *Seminars in Speech and Language, 31*, 42–51.

Cherney, L. R. (2010b). Oral reading for language in aphasia (ORLA): Evaluating the efficacy of computer-delivered therapy in chronic nonfluent aphasia. *Topics in Stroke Rehabilitation, 17*(6), 423–431.

Cherney, L. R., Merbitz, C., & Grip, J. (1986). Efficacy of oral reading in aphasia treatment outcome. *Rehabilitation Literature, 47*, 112–119.

Colangelo, A., & Buchanan, L. (2006). Implicit and explicit processing in deep dyslexia: Semantic blocking as a test for failure of inhibition in the phonological output lexicon. *Brain and Language, 99*, 258–271.

Colangelo, A., & Buchanan, L. (2007). Localizing damage in the functional architecture: The distinction between implicit and explicit processing in deep dyslexia. *Journal of Neurolinguistics, 20*(2), 111–144.

Coltheart, M. (1996). Phonological dyslexia: Past and future issues. *Cognitive Neuropsychology, 13*(6), 749–762.

Coltheart, M., & Byng, S. (1989). A treatment for surface dyslexia. In X. Seron & G. Deloche (Eds.), *Cognitive approaches in neuropsychological rehabilitation* (pp. 159–174). London: Erlbaum.

Coltheart, M., Patterson, K., & Marshall, J. (1980). *Deep dyslexia*. London: Routledge & Kegan Paul.

Coltheart, M., Rastle, K., Perry, C., & Langdon, R. (2001). DRC: A dual route cascaded model of visual word recognition and reading aloud. *Psychological Review, 108*(1), 204–256.

Crisp, J., & Lambon Ralph, M. (2006). Unlocking the nature of the phonological-deep dyslexia continuum: The keys to reading aloud are in phonology and semantics. *Journal of Cognitive Neuroscience, 18*(3), 348–362.

Dabul, B. (2000). *Apraxia Battery for Adults* (2nd ed.). Austin, TX: Pro-Ed.

De Partz, M. (1986). Re-education of a deep dyslexic patient: Rationale of the method and results. *Cognitive Neuropsychology, 3*, 149–177.

De Partz, M. P., Seron, X., & Van der Linden, M. V. (1992). Re-education of surface dysgraphia with a visual imagery strategy. *Cognitive Neuropsychology, 9*, 369–401.

Dérouesné, J., & Beauvois, M. F. (1979). Phonological processing in reading: Data from alexia. *Journal of Neurology, Neurosurgery and Psychiatry, 42*(12), 1125–1132.

Ellis, A. W., Flude, B. M., & Young, A. W. (1987). "Neglect dyslexia" and the early visual processing of letters in words. *Cognitive Neuropsychology, 4*, 439–464.

Ellis, A. W., Lambon Ralph, M. A., Morris, J., & Hunter, A. (2000). Surface dyslexia: Description, treatment, and interpretation. In E. Funnell (Ed.), *Case studies in the neuropsychology of reading* (pp. 85–122). Hove, UK: Psychology Press.

Ellis, A. W., & Young, A. W. (1988). *Human cognitive neuropsychology*. Hove, UK: Erlbaum.

Frattali, C. M., Thompson, C. M., Holland, A. L., Wohl, C. B., & Ferketic, M. M. (1995). The FACS of life ASHA facs— A functional outcome measure for adults. *ASHA, 37*(4), 40–46.

Friedman, R. (1996). Recovery from deep alexia to phonological alexia: Points on a continuum. *Brain and Language, 52*, 114–128.

Friedman, R., & Glosser, G. (1998). Aphasia, alexia, and agraphia. In H. S. Friedman (Ed.), *Encyclopedia of mental health* (pp. 137–148). San Diego, CA: Academic Press.

Friedman, R., & Hadley, J. (1992). Letter-by-letter surface alexia. *Cognitive Neuropsychology, 9*(3), 185–208.

Friedman, R., & Lott, S. N. (2002). Successful blending in a phonological reading treatment for deep alexia. *Aphasiology, 16*, 355–372.

Friedman, R. B., & Robinson, S. R. (1991). Whole-word training therapy in a stable surface alexic patient: It works. *Aphasiology, 5*, 521–527.

Gates, A., & MacGinitie, W. (1978). *Gates–MacGinitie Reading Tests*. New York: Teachers College Press.

Glosser, G., & Friedman, R. (1990). The continuum of deep/phonological alexia. *Cortex, 26*(3), 343–359.

Golper, L., Wertz, R., Frattali, C., Yorkston, K., Myers, P., Katz, R., et al. (2001). *Evidence-based practice guidelines for the management of communication disorders in neurologically impaired individuals: Project introduction*. Retrieved from http://www.ancds.org/assets/docs/EBP/practiceguidelines.pdf

Goodglass, H., Kaplan, E., & Barresi, B. (2001). *Boston Diagnostic Aphasia Examination* (3rd ed.). New York: Lippincott Williams & Wilkins.

Goodman, R., & Caramazza, A. (1986). *Johns Hopkins University Dyslexia Battery*. Baltimore: Johns Hopkins University Press.

Harm, M., & Seidenberg, M. (1999). Phonology, reading acquisition, and dyslexia: Insights from connectionist models. *Psychological Review, 106*(3), 491–528.

Kaplan, E., Goodglass, H., & Weintraub, S. (1983). *The Boston Naming Test*. Philadelphia: Lea & Febiger.

Kay, J., Lesser, R., & Coltheart, M. (1992). *Psycholinguistic Assessments of Language Processing in Aphasia (PALPA)*. Hove, UK: Erlbaum.

Kendall, D., Conway, T., Rosenbek, J., & Gonzalez-Rothi, L. (2003). Phonological rehabilitation of acquired phonological alexia. *Aphasiology, 17*(11), 1073–1095.

Kendall, D., Rosenbek, J., Heilman, K., Conway, T., Klenberg, K., Gonzalez Rothi, L., et al. (2008). Phoneme-based rehabilitation of anomia in aphasia. *Brain and Language, 105*(1), 1–17.

Kendall, D. L., McNeil, M. R., & Small, S. L. (1998). Rule-based treatment for acquired phonological dyslexia. *Aphasiology, 12*, 587–600.

Kertesz, A. (1982). *Western Aphasia Battery*. New York: Grune & Stratton.

Kertesz, A. (2006). *Western Aphasia Battery–Revised*. San Antonio, TX: Pearson.

Kim, M., & Russo, S. (2010). Multiple Oral Rereading (MOR) treatment: Who is it for? *Contemporary Issues in Communication Science and Disorders, 37*, 58–68.

Lacey, E., Lott, S., Snider, S., Sperling, A., & Friedman, R. (2010). Multiple oral re-reading treatment for alexia: The parts may be greater than the whole. *Neuropsychological Rehabilitation, 20*(4), 601–623.

Laine, M., & Nieme, J. (1990). Can the oral reading skills be rehabilitated in deep dyslexia? In M. Hietanan, J. Vilkki, M.-L. Niemi, & M. Korkman (Eds.), *Clinical neuropsychology: Excursions into the field in Finland* (pp. 80–85). Rauma, Finland: Suomen Psykologinen Seura.

LaPointe, L. L., & Horner, J. (1998). *Reading Comprehension Battery for Aphasia* (2nd ed.). Tigard, OR: C.C. Publications.

Lindamood, P. C., & Lindamood, P. D. (1998). *The Lindamood Phoneme Sequencing Program for Reading, Spelling and Speech*. Austin, TX: Pro-Ed.

Lott, S., Carney, A., Glezer, L., & Friedman, R. (2010). Overt use of a tactile/kinaesthetic strategy shifts to covert processing in rehabilitation of letter-by-letter reading. *Aphasiology, 24*(11), 1424–1442.

Lott, S., Sample, D., Oliver, R., Lacey, E., & Friedman, R. (2008). A patient with phonological alexia can learn to read "much" from "mud pies." *Neuropsychologia, 46*, 2515–2523.

Lott, S. N., & Friedman, R. B. (1999). Can treatment for pure alexia improve letter-by-letter reading speed without sacrificing accuracy? *Brain and Language, 67*, 188–201.

Lott, S. N., Sperling, A. J., Watson, N. L., & Friedman, R. B. (2009). Repetition priming in oral text reading: A therapeutic strategy for phonologic text alexia. *Aphasiology, 23*(6), 659–675.

Maher, L., Clayton, M., Barrett, A., Schober-Peterson, D., & Rothi, L. (1998). Rehabilitation of a case of pure alexia: Exploiting residual abilities. *Journal of the International Neuropsychological Society, 4*(6), 636–647.

Marshall, J., & Newcombe, F. (1973). Patterns of paralexia: A psycholinguistic approach. *Journal of Psycholinguistic Research, 2*(3), 175–199.

Mitchum, C. C., & Berndt, R. S. (1991). Diagnosis and treatment of the non-lexical route in acquired dyslexia: An illustration of the cognitive neuropsychological approach. *Journal of Neurolinguistics, 6*, 103–137.

Moss, S. E., Gonzalez Rothi, L. J., & Fennell, E. B. (1991). Treating a case of surface dyslexia after closed head injury. *Archives of Clinical Neuropsychology, 6*, 35–47.

Moyer, S. (1979). Rehabilitation of alexia: A case study. *Cortex, 15*, 139–144.

Patterson, K., & Lambon Ralph, M. (1999). Selective disorders of reading? *Current Opinion in Neurobiology, 9*, 235–239.

Patterson, K. E., & Kay, J. (1982). Letter-by-letter reading: Psychological descriptions of a neurological syndrome. *Quarterly Journal of Experimental Psychology, 34A*, 411–441.

Patterson, K. E., & Marcel, A. J. (1977). Aphasia, dyslexia and the phonological coding of written words. *Quarterly Journal of Experimental Psychology, 29*, 307–318.

Peach, R. K. (2002). Treatment for phonological dyslexia targeting regularity effects. *Aphasiology, 16*(8), 779–789.

Plaut, D. (1999). A connectionist approach to word reading and acquired dyslexia: Extension to sequential processing. *Cognitive Science, 23*(4), 543–568.

Plaut, D., McClelland, J. L., Seidenberg, M. S., & Patterson, K. (1996). Understanding normal and impaired word reading: Computational principles in quasi-regular domains. *Psychological Review, 103*(1), 56–115.

Rapcsak, S., Beeson, P., Henry, M., Leyden, A., Kim, E., Rising, et al. (2009). Phonological dyslexia and dysgraphia: Cognitive mechanisms and neural substrates. *Cortex, 45*(5), 575–591.

Riley, E. A., & Thompson, C. K. (2010). Semantic typicality effects in acquired dyslexia: Evidence for semantic impairment in deep dyslexia. *Aphasiology, 24*, 802–813.

Riley, E. A., & Thompson, C. K. (2015). Training pseudoword reading in acquired dyslexia: A phonological complexity approach. *Aphasiology, 29*(2), 129–150.

Robey, R. (2004). A five-phase model for clinical-outcome research. *Journal of Communication Disorders, 37*, 401–411.

Robey, R. R., & Schultz, M. C. (1998). A model for conducting clinical-outcome research: An adaptation of the standard protocol for use in aphasiology. *Aphasiology, 12*, 787–810.

Rogalski, Y., & Edmonds, L. A. (2008). Attentive reading and constrained summarisation (ARCS) treatment in primary progressive aphasia: A case study. *Aphasiology, 22*(7–8), 763–775.

Rothi, L. J., Coslett, H. B., & Heilman, K. M. (1984). *Battery of Adult Reading Function, Experimental Edition*. Unpublished test.

Sage, K., Hesketh, A., & Lambon Ralph, M. (2005). Using errorless learning to treat letter-by-letter reading: Contrasting word versus letter-based therapy. *Neuropsychological Rehabilitation, 15*, 619–642.

Scott, C., & Byng, S. (1989). Computer assisted remediation of a homophone comprehension disorder in surface dyslexia. *Aphasiology, 3*, 301–320.

Seidenberg, M., & McClelland, J. (1989). A distributed, developmental model of word recognition and naming. *Psychological Review, 96*(4), 523–568.

Seki, K., Yajima, M., & Sugishita, M. (1995). The efficacy of kinesthetic reading treatment for pure alexia. *Neuropsychologia, 33*, 595–609.

Shallice, T., & Warrington, E. (1975). Word recognition in a phonemic dyslexic patient. *Quarterly Journal of Experimental Psychology, 27*, 187–199.

Shallice, T., & Warrington, E. (1977). The possible role of selective attention in acquired dyslexia. *Neuropsychologia, 15*, 31–41.

Ska, B., Garneau-Beaumont, D., Chesneau, S., & Damien, B. (2003). Diagnosis and rehabilitation attempt of a patient with acquired deep dyslexia. *Brain & Language, 53*, 359–363.

Sperling, A. J., Lott, S. N., Snider, F. S., & Friedman, R. B. (2005). Speeded functor reading: A new treatment program for phonological text alexia. *Brain & Language, 95*, 209–210.

Stadie, N., & Rilling, E. (2006). Evaluation of lexically and nonlexically based reading treatment in a deep dyslexic. *Cognitive Neuropsychology, 23*(4), 643–672.

Tree, J., & Kay, J. (2006). Phonological dyslexia and phonological impairment: An exception to the rule? *Neuropsychologia, 44*(14), 2861–2873.

Tuomainen, J., & Laine, M. (1991). Multiple oral rereading technique in rehabilitation of pure alexia. *Aphasiology, 5*, 401–409.

Viswanathan, M., & Kiran, S. (2005). Treatment for pure alexia using a model based approach: Evidence from one acute aphasic individual. *Brain & Language, 95*, 204–206.

Wagner, R. K., Torgesen, J. K., & Rashotte, C. A. (1998). *Comprehensive Test of Phonological Processing (CTOPP)*. Austin, TX: Pro-Ed.

Warrington, E., & Shallice, T. (1980). Word-form dyslexia. *Brain, 30*, 99–112.

Webster, J., Morris, J., Connor, C., Horner, R., McCormac, C., & Potts, A. (2013). Text Level reading comprehension in aphasia: What do we know about therapy and what do we need to know? *Aphasiology, 27*(11), 1362–1380.

Weekes, B., & Coltheart, M. (1996). Surface dyslexia and surface dysgraphia: Treatment studies and their theoretical implications. *Cognitive Neurophysiology, 13*, 277–315.

Welbourne, S. R., & Lambon Ralph, M. A. (2007). Using parallel distributed processing models to simulate phonological dyslexia: The key role of plasticity-related recovery. *Journal of Cognitive Neuroscience, 19*, 1125–1139.

Wiederholt, J. L., & Bryant, B. R. (2001). *GORT 4: Gray Oral Reading Tests examiner's manual*. Austin, TX: Pro-Ed.

Woodcock, R. W., Mather, N., & Schrank, F. A. (2004). *The Woodcock–Johnson III Diagnostic Reading Battery*. Rolling Meadows, IL: Riverside.

Woollams, A., Ralph, M., Plaut, D., & Patterson, K. (2007). SD-squared: On the association between semantic dementia and surface dyslexia. *Psychological Review, 114*(2), 316–339.

World Health Organization. (2001). *International classification of functioning, disability, and health*. Geneva, Switzerland: Author.

Yampolsky, S., & Waters, G. (2002). Treatment of single word oral reading in an individual with deep dyslexia. *Aphasiology, 16*, 455–471.

OBJECTIVES

The reader will be able to:

1. **Discriminate between the neurological and the neuropsychological approach in the description of writing disorders.**

2. **Define key terms used in relation to writing deficits in aphasia.**

3. **Demonstrate knowledge of the normal processes involved in writing and how these might break down in aphasia.**

4. **Plan an appropriate assessment protocol leading to the diagnosis and treatment of writing.**

5. **Interpret data in light of models of writing.**

6. **Hypothesize about the underlying nature of a writing deficit in a client with aphasia.**

7. **Choose an appropriate client-specific treatment for writing deficits.**

8. **Make evidence-based assessment and treatment decisions for writing disorders.**

Written Language and Its Impairments

Ilias Papathanasiou and Zsolt Cséfalvay

INTRODUCTION

Written language is a major communication channel that is parallel, rather than subordinate, to spoken language (McNeil & Tseng, 1990). Disorders of written language invariably reflect the dysfunction of a complex cognitive system. They are defined as the family of written language disorders resulting from central or peripheral neurological damage and are described under the collective term *agraphia* (Roeltgen, 1994). Within aphasia rehabilitation, disorders of writing have received less attention compared to other modalities of language. According to McNeil and Tseng (1990), this is mainly because speech is recognized as the major channel of communication, and writing is considered secondary to speech because of its later acquisition and its later neural development. Moreover, the investigations of normal writing have received little scientific attention. Consequently, compared to other aspects of communication, our scientific knowledge of the recovery of writing is restricted.

WHAT IS WRITTEN LANGUAGE?

The production of written language is a rather complicated process. For writing to take place, the integration of four main different elements, which are supported by a variety of functional systems, is necessary (Tseng & McNeil, 1997). The first element is the linguistic content of the message, which includes lexical selection, inflection, and word order in accordance with the semantic and grammatical rules of the language. The second element is the spelling of individual words, which includes letter selection, order, and grapheme-to-phoneme conversion rules, all important for word-level production. The third element is the visuospatial organization and sequencing of graphic symbols, which includes the individual characteristics and strokes of the letters, spacing, and so forth. The final element is the motoric organization of the orthographic output, which includes body posture, handgrip, eye–hand coordination, and direction and speed of writing.

Neuropsychological models of single-word production classify the preceding elements into two major functional systems: linguistic and motor (Rapcsak & Beeson, 2000). The linguistic component is responsible for selecting the appropriate words for written output and for providing information about the correct spelling. In addition, linguistic procedures are used to retrieve the orthographic forms of familiar words from lexical memory and to assemble plausible spelling for unfamiliar words and pronounceable nonwords. The motor component contains an independent set of procedures that convert graphemic information into movements of the pen. Graphemic information is generated from the linguistic spelling systems and is not specific to any particular modality of output because it is externalized via oral spelling, typing, or spelling with anagrams (Tainturier & Rapp, 2001). Rapcsak and Beeson (2000) suggest that written language results from the integration and interaction of processes involving more than one functional system, which makes writing one of the most variable aspects of cognitive performance in neurologically intact adults.

Orthographic variability affects the psycholinguistic and neuropsychological processing of the writing act; consequently, the identification and description of writing impairments are not always easy. Because of its complexity, written language impairment has various clinical manifestations. Orthographies are notoriously diverse. Alphabetical systems in which graphemes are mostly linearly mapped from the phonemes of the spoken language are not universal. For example, the orthographies used by many Asian languages emphasize the importance of the syllabic unit as their own spelling principle. To understand these mechanisms, several neuroanatomically and neuropsychologically based models have been proposed.

CLASSIFICATION OF WRITTEN LANGUAGE DISORDERS AND THEIR NEUROANATOMIC SUBSTRATES

Writing, because of its complexity, is easily affected following brain lesions. Such disorders of writing are called agraphia or dysgraphia. Usually, in the neurological classification the term *agraphia* is used,

while in the neuropsychological classification the term *dysgraphia* is used. The term *agraphia* was first used by Benedick in 1865, but Ogle (1867) was one of the first to describe the issues of lesion localization for agraphia based on his observation that aphasia and agraphia usually co-occur. The first classification of the agraphias was by Nielsen (1946), who also proposed that agraphia can present in isolation without any other associated signs. However, such a "pure" agraphia is rare (Roeltgen, 1994).

In the last decades, two different approaches to classification of written language disorders have been proposed, the neurological and the neuropsychological. The neurological classification views agraphia as a syndrome with a cluster of symptoms, whereas in the neuropsychological classification, written language disorders are considered an impairment of one or more of the components of cognitive processes of the model. The proponents of a neuropsychological taxonomy hypothesize that each element within the processing model is also neurologically distinct and can therefore be selectively impaired by focal brain lesion. There are a lot of similarities between the two approaches.

The Neurological Classification of Disorders of Writing

The neurological classification, as described by Roeltgen (1994), proposes five types of agraphia: pure agraphia, agraphia with alexia, aphasic agraphia, apraxic agraphia, and spatial agraphia. *Pure agraphia* is the disorder in which patients present with a selective agraphia in the absence of any other language disturbance (Rosati & de Bastiani, 1981). The lesion sites associated with pure agraphia are variable and include Exner's area in the second left frontal gyrus (Aimard, Devick, Lebel, Trouila, & Boisson, 1975; Vernea & Merory, 1975); the posterior perisylvian region (Rosati & de Bastiani, 1981); the superior parietal lobe (Basso, Taborielli, & Vignolo, 1978); the left occipital lobe (Kapar & Lawton, 1983); the posterior insula and posterior putamen (Roeltgen, 1985, 1991); and the basal ganglia (Laine & Marttila, 1981). This variability in localization of selective writing impairment indicates that a single center for writing is unlikely to exist. Writing itself is a complex task that requires the dynamic participation of multiple brain regions.

Agraphia with alexia is also called parietal agraphia because the two symptoms occur together in the absence of aphasia, usually in patients with parietal lobe lesions (Kaplan & Goodglass, 1981). This type of agraphia is similar to that seen in patients with fluent aphasia, and frequently these patients present with mild anomic aphasia (Benson & Cummings, 1985) and produce poorly formed graphemes (Roeltgen, 1993).

Aphasic agraphia is the type of agraphia associated with a specific aphasic syndrome, and its pattern in general has been reported to be similar to the disorder of oral output (Benson & Cummings, 1985), although discrepancies have been reported (Roeltgen, 1993). The neurological lesion in patients with this type of agraphia is thought to match the lesion site of their aphasic syndrome. For example, the lesions in an individual with agraphia and Broca's aphasia are similar to those found in individuals with Broca's aphasia (Roeltgen, 1994). In Broca's aphasia, two distinct subtypes of agraphia have been described; one is characterized by difficulty in grapheme production, and the other is associated with agrammatism (Kaplan & Goodglass, 1981). In conduction aphasia, agraphia is characterized by poor word spelling, with real words spelled better than nonwords (Marcie & Hecaen, 1979). In Wernicke's aphasia, agraphia is characterized by having normal output with well-formed graphemes and a decreased production of substantive words and incorrect spelling (Benson & Cummings, 1985). In transcortical motor aphasia and in transcortical sensory aphasia, the agraphia is similar to the one presented in Broca's and Wernicke's aphasia, respectively, while in mixed transcortical aphasia, patients present with non-fluent writing that improves with copying (Roeltgen, 1994).

Apraxic agraphia is characterized by difficulty in forming graphemes when writing to dictation (Roeltgen, 1993). Alexander, Fisher, and Friedman (1992) suggest that apraxic agraphia is a specific disorder of learned movements and is associated with lesions of the superior parietal lobe. Also, unilateral apraxic agraphia has been observed in patients with corpus callosum lesions (Watson & Heilman, 1983).

Spatial agraphia is characterized by production of duplicate strokes during grapheme formation, trouble with writing in a horizontal line, and intrusions of blank irregular spaces between graphemes (Roeltgen, 1994). This type of agraphia is associated with lesions of the nondominant parietal lobe (Ellis, Young, & Flude, 1987).

Although the types of agraphias just described, as classified by the neurological approach, attempt to explain the behavioral and clinical–pathological aspects of agraphias, inconsistencies and controversies do exist. For example, two different subtypes of agraphia may present with similar disturbances. Furthermore, in the last decade, the focus of research has shifted to the neuropsychological processing models, and the neuropsychological classification has dominated the recent agraphia literature. Therefore, the concept of agraphia syndrome has been criticized and has received progressively less attention. Consequently, the terminology described previously has limited application in current clinical practice (Basso & Maragnolo, 2000).

Lurian Approach to Writing Disorders

When reading Luria's seminal writings, published more than 50 years ago, where he describes the assessment of spoken and written language, we cannot ignore the similarities between his view and the current descriptions of the writing process and the agraphias (i.e., from a cognitive neuropsychological view). His work can be seen as a link between the neurological symptom-based description of writing disorders and the current cognitive models of writing.

Luria (1963) viewed writing as a complex function (a *dynamic functional system*) that consists of integrated basic components. Even if the functional system appears unitary on the surface, its inner structure is composed of a complex integration of multiple independent components. The impairment of any one of these components can lead to the impairment of the whole functional system or of specific systems containing this component. Using Luria's example and his terminology, the process of writing can be affected differently when different parts of the brain are damaged. That is, in the case of a lesion in the acoustic processing centers (left superior temporal lobe), copying and writing of highly automatized words would be preserved because they do not require any acoustic analysis of words, but writing to dictation would be strongly affected because, in this process, the acoustic analysis of phonemes plays an important role. The nature of the deficit is different when the left inferior premotor area is involved. Perseverations in writing occur because of the problem in sequencing elements (impaired kinetic melody), such as graphemes or syllables, but writing of isolated letters is preserved (see also Cséfalvay, 2003). Therefore, Luria's approach was the first attempt at a molecular analysis of the cognitive architecture underlying written language.

The Neuropsychological Classification of Disorders of Writing

From a neuropsychological perspective, the classification of the dysgraphia is based on the theoretical model of the writing process. The value of the model can be judged by its ability to account for patterns of abnormal performance often observed in clinical situations. Therefore, before we describe the various agraphia types, it is important to have an understanding of the written language-processing models.

Models of Written Language

Since the early 1980s, the description of written language production and its errors in individuals with acquired dysgraphia has been predominantly based on the information-processing model of normal language. As part of this approach, researchers have attempted to create comprehensive functional models of the writing process (Ellis, 1982; Ellis & Young, 1988; Goodman & Caramazza, 1986a; Margolin, 1984; Patterson & Shewell, 1987). The majority of the current models of written language have their roots in the notion of cognitive architecture. According to Rapp and Gotsch (2001), the term *cognitive architecture* refers to the various mental operations that are involved in a function such as writing. A description of the cognitive architecture of a task does not specify only the functions of the various cognitive processes, but also the relationship between them. A distinction is made between cognitive functions and behavioral tasks because the former include processes that are essential in more than one behavioral task.

Most of the current models of writing are based on the single-word processing logogen model introduced by Morton in 1980. Following Morton's model, a number of efforts have been made to construct comprehensive functional models of the writing process (Ellis, 1982, 1988; Goodman & Caramazza, 1986a; Margolin, 1984; Rapcsak, 1997; Rapcsak & Beeson, 2000; Rapp & Gotsch, 2001; Roeltgen, 1985, 1993; Shallice, 1988; Van Galen, 1991). All of these models share the same concepts of processing as originally described by Morton (1980), but they have evolved through the years based on evidence provided from experimental and clinical studies (see Rapcsak & Beeson, 2000, for review).

The current version of this model for writing to dictation is presented in Figure 11.1, and written picture naming is presented in Figure 11.2. This model distinguishes between central linguistic processes that generate spelling for words and nonwords and peripheral processes, which convert graphemes into motor commands for writing. This distinction is based on the view of the writing process as having two components—linguistic and motor, as described by the cognitive neuropsychological approach.

Rapcsak and Beeson (2000) suggest that during writing to dictation, the central spelling processes described

by this model follow one of three central routes for processing writing. These routes are *lexical–semantic*, *lexical–nonsemantic*, and *nonlexical* (see Figure 11.1). The proposed routes differ in the kinds of linguistic operations they perform and the types of spelling tasks they support. In all routes, there are processing components that are shared. These components are at a prelexical level that involves the processing of the auditory stimulus and at a postlexical level known as the "graphemic buffer," where spelling is represented as temporally ordered strings of graphemes. The *graphemic buffer* is a working memory system that temporarily stores abstract graphemic representations while they are being converted into codes appropriate for various output modalities (Caramazza, Miceli, Villa, & Romani, 1987; Miceli, Silveri, & Caramazza, 1985).

The *nonlexical route* (Route 3 in Figure 11.1) is used to process stimuli not represented in the individual's spelling vocabulary (i.e., unknown words or nonwords). This processing is based on at least two steps: First, the auditory stimulus is segmented into its component phonemes, following which each phoneme is converted to a corresponding grapheme. The *lexical routes* (Routes 1 and 2 in Figure 11.1) are used to generate spelling for familiar words. Lexical spelling is achieved by retrieving the orthographic word representations from the orthographic output lexicon, the memory store of learned spellings of familiar words or written word forms. Access to stored words (i.e., specific orthography) plays an important role in spelling by both lexical routes. However, there are critical differences in the way orthographic representations are retrieved in the two routes. In spelling via the *lexical–semantic route* (Route 1 in Figure 11.1), a semantic code activates the appropriate orthographic word form. The semantic input to orthography can be direct (via Route 1 in Figure 11.1) or indirect via the phonological representation of the word (from the semantic system to phonological output lexicon and then to the orthographic output lexicon). However, the role of this phonological representation is still controversial and debatable (Tainturier & Rapp, 2001).

On the contrary, spelling via the *lexical–nonsemantic route* (Route 2 in Figure 11.1) relies on the transcoding between the spoken and written forms of the same words using connections that bypass the semantic system. So, the heard word first activates its representation in the auditory input lexicon (a storage of the auditory form of the words), which leads to retrieval of the corresponding representation from the phonological output lexicon (a storage of the phonological form of the word), which in turns activates the appropriate orthographic word form in the orthographic output lexicon.

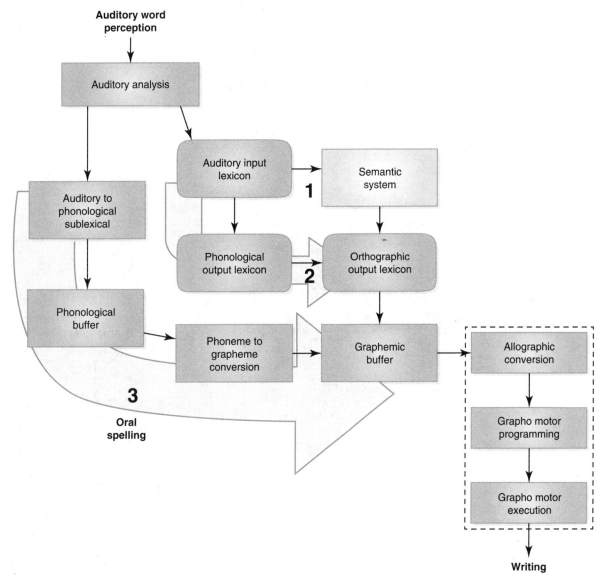

Figure 11.1 The neuropsychological model showing the three routes used during writing to dictation tasks. Route 1 is lexical–semantic, Route 2 is lexical–nonsemantic, and Route 3 is nonlexical. The dotted shape indicates peripheral processes.

Although the existence of these different spelling processes involved in these routes has been assumed in most written language research, there is little consensus concerning the specific nature of these processes and the relation and interaction between them (Tainturier & Rapp, 2001). Campbell (1983) has shown that the spelling of unfamiliar words and nonwords is based on lexical analogies to real words. On the other hand, the influence of the nonlexical route is revealed by the presence of plausible phonological errors in normal subjects during spelling of real words (Ellis, 1982), suggesting the presence of a nonlexical strategy to generate spelling when the word-specific spelling information is unavailable.

So, the independence of these spelling routes is still controversial.

However, during a written picture-naming task, the proposed routes differ in their linguistic operations compared to a task of writing to dictation (see Figure 11.2). In written picture naming, the visual analysis of the picture triggers the visual distinctive characteristics of the item, which in turn activate the appropriate concept within the semantic system. Then, the writing of the corresponding label can be performed by three routes: *the direct semantic route*, where the semantic system accesses the orthography of the word directly in the orthographic output lexicon (Route 1 in Figure 11.2); *the indirect semantic*

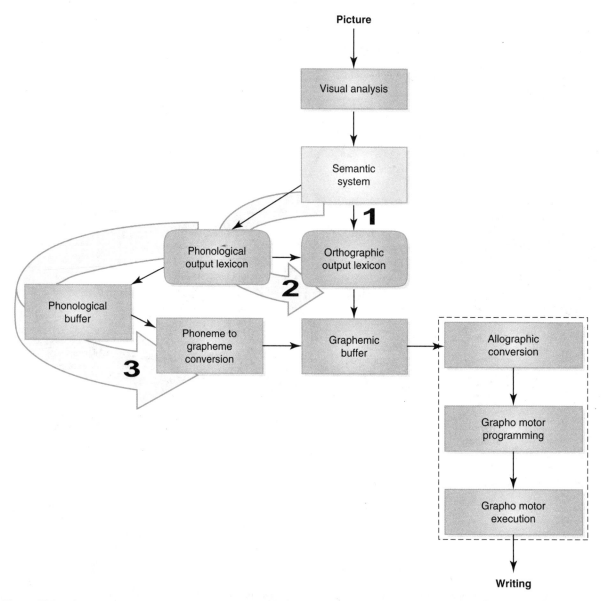

Figure 11.2 The neuropsychological model showing the three routes used during a written confrontation naming task. Route 1 is lexical–semantic, Route 2 is indirect lexical–semantic, and Route 3 is phoneme mediated. The dotted shape indicates peripheral processes.

route, where the retrieval of the orthographic word form is mediated by its phonological form via the phonological output lexicon (Route 2 in Figure 11.2); and finally *the phoneme-mediated route*, where each word is transformed into its individual phonemic components, a phoneme-to-grapheme conversion process is performed, and the information is relayed to the graphemic buffer for eventual execution (Route 3 in Figure 11.2). This last route is commonly used by individuals who tend to sound out each word before writing it. This strategy is particularly prevalent in languages with a more transparent writing

system (i.e., a high level of phoneme-to-grapheme correspondence).

The peripheral components of the model describe the motor elements of writing that come into focus below the level of the graphemic buffer, where the abstract graphemic representations are converted into letter codes. At the peripheral level, the graphemic information is externalized into movements of the pen through sequential processes (Rapcsak & Beeson, 2000; Schomaker & Van Galen, 1996). The first of these processes is known as *allographic conversion*: The selection of the appropriate letter shapes takes place based on the strings of graphemes held in the graphemic buffer. The remaining processing components are concerned with the programming and execution of writing movements required to produce the letter shapes identified by the allographic conversion. This process is known as *graphic motor programming* and includes visual kinesthetic engrams that contain abstract spatiotemporal codes. The graphic motor programs specify the sequence, direction, task space geometry, and joint space geometry that are necessary for the creation of the allographs.

Rapcsak and Beeson (2000) suggest that although the graphic motor programs are letter specific, they are effector independent in the sense that they do not determine which muscle groups are to be recruited for movement execution. Typically, the distal muscles of the hand and the wrist perform writing when using a pen, but writing on a blackboard is accomplished with the proximal muscles of the shoulder and the elbow (Mack, Gonzalez Rothi, & Heilman, 1993). Individuals can also write by using different limbs or even the mouth. However, the overall letter shape remains remarkably constant when produced by muscle effector systems with different biomechanic properties, which suggests the existence of effector independent abstract motor programs for writing (Wright, 1990).

The final step of the writing process involves the translation of the information of the graphic motor programs into *graphic motor execution*, containing sequences of motor commands to specific muscle effector systems. At this stage, the appropriate synergies of agonist and antagonist muscles are recruited, and concrete movement patterns specifying the details of stroke size, duration, and force of writing occur. Because the motor context of writing is not always the same, actual movement parameters must be recruited by the given biophysical context to produce the appropriate letter as a sequence of rapid movements. The production of the letters continuously provides visual and kinesthetic feedback, which plays an important role in updating graphic motor programs regarding which strokes have already been executed (Margolin, 1984). Also, it is essential to maintain the correct spacing of letters, the straight line of writing, and the proper orientation on the page (Smyth & Silvers, 1987).

Neuropsychological Disorders of Writing

Different forms of dysgraphia in neurologically impaired individuals should be directly interpretable with reference to specific functional components of the model described previously (Rapcsak & Beeson, 2000). Based on these models, the evaluation and interpretation of errors observed in patients with dysgraphia should be directly interpretable in reference to specific components of the model. Rapcsak and Beeson (2000) suggest that the validity of this approach is based on the assumption that in addition to having psychological reality, the hypothesized processing modules are neurologically distinct and therefore can be selectively impaired by focal brain damage. Also, it is assumed that the "damaged" processing component is identifiable through the careful analysis of impaired and preserved abilities, and that its putative neural substrate can be inferred from anatomic lesion localization studies. Therefore, in "pure" cases only a single processing component is implicated.

Roeltgen (1994) describes the same processing model and attempts to make clinical pathologic connections between lesion and behavior. However, he suggests that because of the complexity of writing and its sensitivity to cerebral dysfunction, no single site can be considered a "center for writing," but that certain patterns of agraphic performance and types of agraphia are associated with particular lesions. In everyday clinical practice, brain damage does not necessarily respect the functional distinctions of cognitive models, and clinicians frequently come across patients with various degrees of damage to multiple processing components showing great variability in response to treatment. According to these models, disorders of writing are classified as central or peripheral dysgraphia. In central dysgraphias, the locus of deficit is located in the central spelling routes (i.e., lexical–semantic, lexical–nonsemantic, or nonlexical), resulting in lexical (or surface), phonological, deep, semantic, and graphemic buffer dysgraphia (Rapcsak & Beeson, 2000). In peripheral dysgraphia, the main difficulties involve the selection or production of letters in handwriting and are labeled as allographic, apraxic, motor nonapraxic, and spatial (afferent) dysgraphia.

Central Dysgraphia *Lexical*, or *surface*, *dysgraphia* is characterized by a particular difficulty spelling irregular and ambiguous words as a result of damage to the orthographic output lexicon (Goodman & Caramazza, 1986a). In such individuals, the orthographic representations of words are lost or degraded so that they only show partial knowledge of known words. Patients have difficulty spelling familiar words, especially words that contain ambiguous or irregular phoneme–grapheme mappings. In contrast, spelling of regular words is relatively preserved, as is the ability to spell unfamiliar words or nonwords. Errors in spelling ambiguous or irregular words are usually phonologically plausible (e.g., "oshen" for *ocean*). In addition to the strong effect of orthographic regularity, spelling is influenced by word frequency, with an advantage of high-frequency words over low-frequency ones. However, spelling performance is typically unaffected by other lexical–semantic variables such as imageability (i.e., high-imageability or concrete words such as *apple* versus low-imageability or abstract words such as *pride*) and grammatical word class (i.e., content words, including nouns, verbs, and adjectives versus functors such as prepositions, pronouns, articles, and auxiliaries). In cases with this type of dysgraphia, the loss or unavailability of stored word-specific orthographic information forces patients to generate spellings by relying on the preserved nonlexical route. As indicated previously, this route is primarily used to compute plausible spellings for unfamiliar words and nonwords, but it can also handle regular words that strictly obey phoneme–grapheme conversion rules. However, attempts to spell ambiguous or irregular words by the nonlexical route result in phonologically plausible errors.

This type of dysgraphia is most commonly associated with posterior temporal lesions (Goodman & Caramazza, 1986a). In contrast, Roeltgen and Heilman (1984) propose that the critical lesion site is located between the junction of the posterior angular gyrus and the parietal lobule. Reduced metabolic activity in the left angular gyrus has also been revealed in patients with Alzheimer's disease with impairment of lexical spelling (Peniello et al., 1995), making this region a possible neural substrate for the orthographic output lexicon. However, recently Rapcsak and Beeson (2004) reported behavioral and neuroanatomic observations in patients with lexical dysgraphia that are consistent with functional imaging studies of writing in neurologically intact individuals and that provide converging evidence for the role of the left posterior inferior temporal cortex in spelling. Together, these findings implicate the left posterior inferior temporal cortex as a possible neural substrate of the orthographic output lexicon that contains stored memory representations for the written forms of familiar words.

In *phonological dysgraphia*, there is marked impairment of nonword spelling with selectively preserved real-word spelling resulting from a dysfunction of the nonlexical spelling route (Shallice, 1981). The spelling impairment may be attributable to at least two qualitatively different types of processing deficits. Some patients seem to have lost their knowledge of phoneme–grapheme correspondence rules, as suggested by their inability to write even single letters correctly when given their characteristic sounds. Others can translate single phonemes into the appropriate graphemes, and in these cases the nonlexical spelling deficit may reflect an inability to segment novel auditory stimuli into their constituent sounds. However, it is important to keep in mind that defective phoneme–grapheme transcoding may also be caused by perception of the stimuli (i.e., phoneme discrimination deficit) or reduced phonological short-term memory.

In pure cases of phonological dysgraphia, spelling of familiar words (including ambiguous and irregular words) can be performed at a fairly high level, consistent with preserved access to representations in the orthographic output lexicon via the lexical-semantic route. The fact that spelling in phonological dysgraphia relies on a lexical–semantic strategy is also suggested by the observation that some patients cannot write words to dictation unless they have access to their meaning. Furthermore, spelling performance may be influenced by lexical–semantic variables such as imageability, grammatical word class, and frequency. Specifically, some patients spell high-imageability words better than low-imageability words, and content words may have an advantage over functors. In addition, high-frequency words may be spelled more accurately than low-frequency words are. Orthographic regularity, however, does not have a significant effect on spelling. Spelling errors in phonological dysgraphia are usually phonologically implausible, although they may have visual similarity to the target (e.g., "towen" for *tower*). Morphological errors (e.g., "works"–"working") and functor substitutions (e.g., "over"–"here") are also observed occasionally.

In most individuals with nonlexical route impairment, spelling has also some degree of concomitant lexical–semantic spelling impairment, suggesting the importance of phonological processes for both nonword and word spelling (Henry, Beeson, Stark, & Rapcsak, 2007). Phonological dysgraphia is typically seen following left perisylvian lesions (Roeltgen, Sevush, & Heilman, 1983). Roeltgen (1985) suggested that lesions in patients with this type of dysgraphia overlap in the region of the anterior supramarginal gyrus, concluding that this perisylvian cortical area is important for spelling via the nonlexical route.

Deep dysgraphia has several linguistic characteristics in common with phonological dysgraphia, but it is distinguishable from phonological dysgraphia by the presence of prominent semantic errors in writing because semantic representations are damaged or the process of retrieving the correct orthographic representation is difficult (Hatfield, 1985). The types of errors observed in this form of agraphia are similar to those in phonological dysgraphia plus semantic errors. Semantic errors in writing indicate dysfunction of the lexical–semantic spelling route and may reflect several different processing impairments. Possible mechanisms include damage to the semantic system or faulty transmission of information between the semantic system and the orthographic output lexicon (Figure 11.1). In writing to dictation, semantic errors may also result from damaged connections between the auditory input lexicon and the semantic system (Figure 11.1). However, dysfunction of the lexical–semantic route alone is not sufficient to explain semantic errors in writing to dictation because the correct spelling of the target word could potentially be generated by spelling routes that normally bypass the semantic system and are therefore not susceptible to errors based on word meaning. Specifically, potential semantic errors could be blocked by phonology-to-orthography transcoding via either the lexical–nonsemantic or the nonlexical spelling routes. For instance, although the damaged lexical–semantic route may activate the entry *banana* in the orthographic output lexicon in response to the dictated word *apple*, the overt semantic error could be avoided if the phonological code / æpəl / was simultaneously released from the phonological output lexicon and provided a second source of input to orthography via the lexical–nonsemantic spelling route (Figure 11.1, Pathways 2 and 3) or if the correct spelling was computed by phoneme–grapheme conversion via the nonlexical route. Therefore, the appropriate conditions for semantic errors arise when the output of the dysfunctional lexical–semantic spelling route remains completely unconstrained by orthographic information generated by the lexical–nonsemantic and nonlexical routes.

An adequate linguistic explanation of deep dysgraphia requires that we postulate multiple processing impairments affecting all three central spelling routes. Rapcsak and Beeson (2000) suggest that these patients use the damaged lexical–semantic route for spelling. As in phonological dysgraphia, the spelling impairment in deep dysgraphia is influenced by lexical features such as concreteness/imageability, word class, and frequency, which might suggest that these two types of dysgraphia are not two distinct syndromes but belong to the same continuum of writing impairments (Rapcsak & Beeson, 2000). Patients with deep dysgraphia have large left hemisphere lesions that typically involve most of the perisylvian language zone. However, there is an intriguing possibility that, in deep dysgraphia, writing is no longer controlled by the damaged left hemisphere and that its characteristic features reflect the limitations of the intact right hemisphere (Rapcsak, Beeson, & Rubens, 1991).

Semantic dysgraphia is characterized by impairment in conceptually mediated writing tasks such as spontaneous writing and written naming, while writing to dictation is spared, although word meaning cannot be accessed (Patterson, 1986). Semantic dysgraphia is caused by damage to the lexical–semantic route, and individuals with this type of dysgraphia have particular difficulty with homophone words because they use the lexical–nonsemantic and the nonlexical routes for spelling (e.g., they would write *pear* and *pair* randomly because they cannot rely on semantic context to disambiguate). However, writing to dictation is relatively preserved because this task can be accomplished without semantic mediation by relying on the lexical–nonsemantic or nonlexical spelling routes. By using spelling routes that bypass the semantic system, patients with semantic agraphia can write familiar words to dictation even when the words' meanings are not understood (either because of damage to the semantic system or because of a disconnection of the semantic system from the auditory input lexicon).

Accurate spelling of ambiguous and irregular words without comprehension of their meaning in semantic agraphia provides the best available evidence for the existence of a lexical–nonsemantic spelling route (i.e., direct transcoding between phonological and orthographic lexical representations via Route 2 in 11.1) because these words could not be spelled correctly by relying on a nonlexical strategy. Patients with semantic dysgraphia do not constitute a homogeneous group with respect to lesion localization. Among the reported sites are various extraperisylvian lesions (Roeltgen, Rothi, & Heilman, 1986) and posterior temporoparietal areas because homophone errors have also been observed in patients with lexical dysgraphia (Hatfield & Patterson, 1983). At the present time, there is no conclusive evidence of the precise neuroanatomic substrate of this type of dysgraphia.

Individuals with dysgraphia caused by *graphemic buffer impairment* present with errors of grapheme identity and order in all spelling tasks regardless of word status, with all written output modalities affected (Caramazza et al., 1987; Miceli et al., 1985). A dysfunction of the graphemic buffer involves defective short-term storage of graphemic information. Writing is impaired in all tasks, including spontaneous writing, delayed copying, written naming, and writing to dictation and is not affected by lexical variables such as frequency, imageability, or word class. In contrast, word length has a significant effect on performance, with shorter words more accurate than longer words because of increased demand on short-term storage capacity. Because the graphemic buffer is a central processing component that supports all possible modalities of output, qualitatively similar errors are observed in writing, oral spelling, typing, and spelling with anagram letters.

Dysfunction of the buffer interferes with the short-term retention of information concerning the identity and serial ordering of stored graphemes. Spelling errors take the form of letter substitutions, deletions, additions, and transpositions, and their frequency increases as a function of word length. The distribution of errors may also be influenced by letter position. In some cases, more errors were produced on letters at the end of the word, consistent with the hypothesized serial left-to-right read-out process from the buffer (i.e., items retrieved last are more vulnerable to degradation because they have to be retained in memory longer). Errors on terminal letters may decrease in frequency if patients are asked to spell backward, suggesting that it is the order of retrieval rather than the spatial position of the letter within the word that is the critical factor. In other patients, spelling errors primarily involved letters in the middle of the word. The usual explanation offered for this phenomenon is that letters in internal positions are more susceptible to interference by neighboring items than are letters located at either end. Lesion sites in individuals with this type of dysgraphia have been variable. Involvement of left hemisphere frontoparietal cortical systems in working memory and spatial attention is common, but more specific localization is not possible at this time (Rapcsak & Beeson, 2000).

Peripheral Dysgraphia *Allographic dysgraphia* is characterized by an inability to generate or select the correct letter shapes in handwriting, while oral spelling remains spared (Patterson & Wing, 1989). Individuals with this type of dysgraphia present with writing impairment specific to case (upper versus lower) or style (print versus cursive). They display case-mixing errors and substitution of similar letter forms as a result of defective assignment of letter shapes to abstract graphemic representation held in the graphemic buffer. This can be caused either by a production deficit (e.g., failure to create the appropriate letter because of a failure to remember letter shapes; Kartsounis, 1992) or by a selection deficit (e.g., mixing upper- and lowercase letters; De Bastiani & Barry, 1989). In the majority of cases with this type of dysgraphia, the lesion has involved the left parieto-occipital region (Rapcsak & Beeson, 2000).

Apraxic dysgraphia is characterized by poor letter formation that cannot be attributed to impaired letter shape knowledge or to sensorimotor, extrapyramidal, or cerebellar dysfunction affecting the writing limb. These individuals are unable to execute the sequences of strokes necessary to produce the letter from the specified allographic code while oral spelling, typing, and spelling with anagrams are spared and letter imagery is preserved (Baxter & Warrington, 1986). These individuals make gross errors of letter morphology, including spatial

distortions, stroke insertions, and deletions, which sometimes make writing completely illegible. This is the result of destruction or disconnection of the graphic motor programs or damage to the systems responsible for translating these programs into accurate movement planning. In apraxic dysgraphia, lesions are generally located in the hemisphere contralateral to the dominant hand. However, the exact lesion site remains unspecified and has variously been reported as the parietal lobe at the junction of the angular gyrus and the superior parietal lobule (Alexander et al., 1992), the premotor cortical areas near the foot of the second frontal convolution (also known as Exner's writing center; Hodges, 1991), or the supplementary motor area (Watson, Fleet, Rothi, & Heilman, 1986).

Rapcsak and Beeson (2000) suggest that the motor programming of writing is mediated by a distributed neural network, which includes both posterior and anterior cortical components with distinct functional roles. More specifically, they suggest that the parietal lobe is the area where graphic motor programs are stored, and that the frontal premotor areas are involved in translating these programs into graphic innervation patterns. The critical role of these areas is supported by functional neuroimaging studies in normal subjects (Seitz et al., 1997).

Motor nonapraxic dysgraphia are characterized by defective regulation of movement force, speed, and amplitude in handwriting (Rapcsak & Beeson, 2000). A typical nonapraxic dysgraphia is the micrographia observed in cases of Parkinson's disease and the disjointed and irregular writing movements observed in cerebellar disorders. These dysgraphia are the result of dysfunction of motor systems involved in controlling the kinematic parameters of writing. Brooks (1986) suggests that basal-ganglia-thalamo-cortical and corticocerebellar motor loops are the possible neural substrates of a distributed system that generates and modulates innervation patterns for skilled limb movements, including innervation patterns for writing movements. This has been supported by regional blood flow and positron emission tomographic (PET) studies (Seitz et al., 1997).

Spatial or *afferent dysgraphia* arise from lesions that interfere with the ability to utilize sensory feedback for the control and execution of writing movements (Ellis, 1982; Lebrun, 1985). Errors in this type of dysgraphia include duplications or omissions of letters or strokes especially when writing sequences of similar items, difficulty keeping the line of writing straight, and difficulty maintaining proper spacing between letters and words. This type of dysgraphia is usually seen following nondominant parietal lesions (Ellis, 1982; Lebrun, 1985) but also has been observed in association with cerebellar dysfunction (Silveri, Misciagna, Leggio, & Molinari, 1997).

ASSESSMENT OF WRITING DISORDERS

Evaluation of acquired agraphia in individuals with neurological diseases is a complex endeavor because the task is not only to describe deficits in spelling and writing but also, if possible, to identify the underlying mechanism of the deficit in relation to the theoretical framework of writing processes. The goal is to go beyond the verification that symptoms exist.

A comprehensive assessment of agraphia must therefore include many different tasks allowing the analysis of both *central* and *peripheral* spelling processes. In the first case, *linguistic* components of writing and spelling are assessed, while in the second case, *motor* components of the writing process are evaluated. Obviously, this is a rather complex procedure, so many available diagnostic tools used in research and clinical practice focus only on some aspects of the evaluation of spelling and writing. Most of the existing assessment procedures contain a number of "artificial" tasks (such as copying, writing words and nonwords to dictation, etc.), activities that are rarely used in everyday life. To our knowledge, there is no formalized "functional evaluation of writing" published yet; however, in some tests, writing is included in the evaluation of functional communication (e.g., in the Communication Activities of Daily Living [CADL-2]; Holland, Frattali, & Fromm, 1999). Furthermore, from a functional perspective, while writing is part of the daily activities of normal adults (e.g., signing prescriptions, writing checks), the range of everyday writing practices of normal adults cannot be predicted from the existing functional assessments, so a questionnaire to establish the premorbid writing activities might be needed (Parr, 1992). Overall, a comprehensive writing assessment battery is still lacking in the aphasia literature.

Most comprehensive aphasia batteries, such as the Boston Diagnostic Aphasia Examination (BDAE-3; Goodglass, Kaplan, & Barresi, 2000) and the Western Aphasia Battery—Revised (WAB-R; Kertesz, 2007), contain subtests on writing, but these tasks should be used for *screening* acquired writing disorders. A comprehensive analysis of writing abilities must include a *spontaneous writing* sample (e.g., picture description or written narrative on a specific topic) and an analysis of *writing at the single-word level*. Furthermore, before assessing

writing, deficits of visual acuity, visual neglect, motor apraxia, and so forth must be excluded.

The process of spontaneous writing is a result of the integration of many different aspects of cognitive, linguistic, perceptual, and motor abilities (Beeson & Henry, 2008). The ability to write complex sentences or even paragraphs is for many patients with neurological disease limited, so the assessment is often focused primarily on single-word writing. For a detailed analysis of the spelling of single words, linguistically controlled agraphia batteries are needed, with test items (words and nonwords) selected according to certain lexical features, such as grammatical word class, word frequency, word length, word concreteness, regularity of spelling, and so on. Writing single words is most often evaluated in three types of tasks: *written picture naming, writing to dictation,* and *copying.* Obviously, different components of the cognitive architecture of writing are activated in these tasks. In all of the previously mentioned tasks, central and peripheral components of writing should also be investigated.

In the evaluation of spontaneous writing, we must keep in mind that the frequency of premorbid functional writing, as well as the level of automatization of this ability, varies. For people who use writing extensively, some tasks are highly automatized, and therefore the writing process could be affected differently from how it is affected in individuals who use writing only occasionally. Moreover, the clinician must consider the level of education, the age of the person, as well as the profession of the individual. Neither should the influence of computers on written communication be neglected. For many people, writing is now restricted almost exclusively to typing on a keyboard, so patterns of motor programs for handwriting are activated much less often than they were some years ago. Premorbid spelling and writing abilities and frequency of use should be investigated before any assessment starts, or at least before the qualitative analysis of writing begins.

Assessing Spontaneous Writing

Self-generated written communication is a useful task to determine the functional status of the lexical–semantic route that supports all conceptually driven writing tasks (Rapcsak & Beeson, 2000). This can be done by asking the patient to describe in writing his or her last vacation or to comment on some other topic. Using standard stimuli from aphasia batteries, such as the picture of a family having a picnic from the WAB-R (Kertesz, 2007) or a description of a well-known fairy tale, could help determine the access to main semantic concepts and words. The advantage of this complex task is that the clinician has the opportunity to go beyond the single-word level of writing and examine the grammatical aspects of written language. Some deficits in morphology (mainly in languages with rich and overtly realized morphology, e.g., Slovak or Hungarian) and syntactic complexity of written sentences can be elicited mostly in spontaneous writing. Hypotheses on the level of the impairment of central processes of writing can be formulated at this stage of assessment and verified further on the basis of single-word writing.

Assessing Single-Word Writing

Carefully selected and structured word lists, as well as pictures of objects and actions, are used in the assessment of single-word writing. Lexical properties such as word frequency, word length, imageability, regularity, lexicality, and word grammatical categories of test items can influence naming ability (Whitworth, Webster, & Howard, 2005). These features of the test items were taken into account when formalized agraphia test batteries were constructed. The following two published agraphia assessment tools are employed in research and clinical practice:

- Psycholinguistic Assessments of Language Processing in Aphasia (PALPA; Kay, Lesser, & Coltheart, 1992)
- Johns Hopkins University Dylexia and Dysgraphia Batteries (JHU Battery; Goodman & Caramazza, 1986b, published in Beeson & Henry, 2008)

There are several tasks in each of these agraphia assessment protocols: (a) written naming, (b) writing to dictation, and (c) copying. In these cases, the clinician has control over the items, so the target word is known, which makes the analysis of errors easier. In the JHU Dysgraphia Battery, comprehensive lists of words are selected to capture various linguistic variables: grammatical word class (nouns, adjectives, verbs, and functors); word concreteness (concrete versus abstract words); word frequency (high- and low-frequency words); nonwords (nonhomophone nonwords such as "berk," "foys," "sortain"); regularity of spelling (words with high and low probability of spelling, based on the transparency of phoneme–grapheme conversion); word length balanced for frequency, The JHU Dysgraphia Battery also contains oral spelling tasks, copy tasks (including the task to change words from uppercase to lowercase); and written naming (words balanced for frequency and number of letters).

Apart from these well-known test batteries, several formal and informal agraphia assessments exist in different countries, for example, the writing subtest of the Slovak Aphasia, Alexia and Agraphia Battery compiled by Cséfalvay, Egryová, and Wiedermann (2007). In addition to linguistically controlled word lists, this test contains subtests for sentence production and spontaneous writing (picture description). One important aspect of these "non-English" aphasia–alexia–agraphia test batteries is that, for languages with transparent orthography (e.g., Italian or Slovak), the evaluation of sublexical levels plays an important role. As Luzzatti, Colombo, Frustaci, and Vitolo (2000) point out, few studies have dealt with the nature of nonlexical routes and their disruption, which may be explained by the relatively reduced impact these routes have on the reading and writing of educated English-speaking adults. In fact, whereas in English these routes seem to be relevant only when writing new words, they appear to be more important in languages such as Italian, for which orthography is much more regular and predictable.

The administration of the test is followed by a detailed qualitative analysis of errors made in written production. The goal of this analysis is to formulate a hypothesis about the functional impairment of the components involved in the realization of a certain process. A characteristic pattern of acquired agraphia may result when certain component processes are disturbed (Beeson & Henry, 2008). Whitworth et al. (2005) list the following categories of errors in the written production of patients with neurological disease: additions, deletions, substitutions, transposition of letters, incomplete letters, the fusion of two letters, morphological errors, semantic errors, and regularization/phonologically plausible errors (for more detail, see Whitworth et al., 2005, pp. 86–96).

The classification of writing errors can also be helpful in the detection of salient features of a particular agraphia syndrome. As stated previously, there are three proposed routes in the model of writing (Figures 11.1 and 11.2): lexical–semantic, lexical–nonsemantic, and nonlexical (sublexical). Some components are involved in processing all routes (e.g., processing auditory stimuli, graphemic buffer), which implies that the impairment of the shared component will have an impact on many different writing tasks. As Basso (2003) states, a given component can operate normally only if it receives normal input, that is, if all the connected upstream components are undamaged. For instance, the integrity of the auditory input lexicon can be investigated only if the acoustic analysis is not disturbed.

In line with this idea, it is therefore important that the analysis of all the processes involved in the assessment tasks can be correctly performed only if all input and output components are taken into consideration. For example, difficulty in writing nonwords to dictation can be attributed exclusively to phoneme-to-grapheme conversion impairments only if nonword repetition and acoustic analysis skills are intact.

Central processes of writing are assessed during writing to dictation and written picture-naming tasks. Dictation of nonwords versus words assesses the ability of a person to write via the nonlexical versus the lexical routes of writing (regularization of nonwords to words indicates an impaired nonlexical route). Words controlled for imageability or grammatical class and homophones are used to assess impairment of the semantic system or access to the orthographic output lexicon, while the use of words controlled for frequency or regularity assesses the intactness of the orthographic output lexicon (reduced performance when spelling irregular words relative to regular words implies orthographic output lexicon impairment with spared phoneme–grapheme conversion). Finally, words controlled for word length assess the function of the graphemic buffer.

Peripheral processes for handwriting, for example, components such as allographic conversion, graphic motor programs, and graphic innervation patterns (see Figure 11.1), can be evaluated during all tasks, but specifically in copying words, copying nonwords, and transcoding letters. Beeson and Rapcsak (2002) state that immediate copying tasks provide an examination of writing without demands on central spelling processes, as well as a means to examine the motor aspects of writing. Careful observation of writing during copying tasks is therefore important. The comparison of performance in oral and written spelling can help differentiate between peripheral or central problems in writing. For example, significantly better oral than written spelling confirms deficits in the peripheral components of writing.

INTERVENTION APPROACHES TO WRITING DISORDERS

Traditional aphasia rehabilitation has focused on oral rather than on written language. Within written language, writing has received even less attention than reading has. Clinical priorities, resource constraints, and possibly even lack of expertise may be some of the reasons for this relative neglect (Whitworth et al., 2005). Nevertheless, recent studies have shown that therapy for writing can help individuals with agraphia improve their writing skills (as described further in this chapter). However, virtually none of these studies describe therapy approaches using the International Classification of Functioning, Disability, and Health framework (body functions, activity restrictions, and participation limitations), known more commonly as ICF (World Health Organization [WHO], 2001).

Still, writing is a functional activity in many settings, and agraphia has the potential to limit participation significantly, both as a specific communicative activity and as a compensatory mechanism for aphasia. For some people with aphasia, spoken communication impairments may be resistant to treatment, and writing may become a more realistic therapy goal (Beeson & Rapcsak, 2002). Writing has many uses in everyday communicative situations (shopping lists, telephone messages, greeting cards, etc.). In recent years, with the development of novel technology and social media, writing has become a required communicative function for texting, composing e-mails, and writing in Facebook, Twitter, blogs, and so on. According to a survey of participants with acquired brain injury, e-mail is often preferred to the telephone as a mode of communication for brain injury survivors for several reasons: They can write an e-mail at a time convenient to them; they can take as long as they need to read, write, and edit it; and there is less chance for breakdown in communication, so any embarrassing or intimidating situations can be avoided (Todis, Sohlberg, Hood, & Fickas, 2005). Moreover, with the increasing acceptability of spelling errors and abbreviations within social media and text messages, there is less pressure for written output to be fully "correct" in terms of spelling and grammar (Thiel, Sage, & Conroy, 2015). Fotiadou, Northcott, Chatzidaki, and Hilari (2014) suggest that the use of social media by people with aphasia should be further explored, both as a therapeutic outlet and as a way for people with aphasia to feel connected to a wider community. As a result, functional writing, that is, writing for real-life purposes, may become increasingly a more realistic rehabilitation goal for people with aphasia, and improving writing skills could provide greater opportunity for involvement in community life, which will enhance social participation.

Understanding the models of written language and gathering detailed information about writing impairments can lead to the development of appropriate clinical goals and maximize the recovery of writing skills in a person with aphasia and agraphia. So far, in the literature on written language impairment, studies are often limited to single cases or small groups of people with aphasia; yet, the authors have attempted to dovetail specific therapy approaches with a theoretical model of writing. As Hillis and Caramazza (1994) suggest, studies of writing should take into account the fact that treatment outcomes for similar patients may vary for numerous reasons, including individual variation in brain organization, motivation, and residual cognitive functioning. This in turn suggests a range of outcomes. The authors argue that (a) individuals with the same loci of impairment may require different treatment approaches; (b) different treatment approaches may be equally appropriate for different impairments; and (c) a given treatment strategy may affect several levels of processing impairment. Furthermore, the process of therapy might yield additional information about the nature of the impairment. This underlines the complexity of writing therapy and that therapy outcomes are subject to many variables related not only to the person with aphasia but also to the cognitive architecture and neural organization of writing.

Disorders of writing are considered a dysfunction of communication resulting from an organic neurological lesion (Roeltgen, 1994). This dysfunction typically results in impairment in linguistic or motor behaviors involved in writing. The cognitive neuropsychological model of writing described previously can guide the therapist in identifying the impaired processes and preserved functions that might be exploited to achieve improvement (Shallice, 2000). In addition, a writing impairment that results from damage to multiple processing components may never fit a specific agraphia profile, so a treatment approach that is designed to strengthen impaired processes and maximize the use of preserved abilities might be a valid approach, whether the patient has pure or complex agraphia (Rapcsak & Beeson, 2000). Decisions regarding which therapy approach to select are based on the relative sparing/impairment of each route, related intact abilities, and the impact that remediation of a route might have on the person's spelling.

During the acute stage of recovery, writing ability may progress rapidly as the effects of treatment coincide with physiologic recovery mechanisms (Rapcsak & Beeson, 2000). During this period, therapy goals should aim to enhance this recovery and reactivate the temporarily impaired written language function. So, therapy should focus on those parts of the functional system that are temporarily suppressed or inefficient. Techniques such as direct stimulation, indirect stimulation, and deblocking, which involve structured methods of response elicitation and selective reinforcement of correct responses within controlled levels of difficulty, are used (Rosenbek, LaPointe, & Wertz, 1989) within a specific cueing hierarchy that facilitates correct responses (Hillis & Caramazza, 1989). Also at this stage, writing therapy can provide persons with minimal speech output with an alternative means of communication.

During the more chronic stages, the recovery of writing is based on the principles of the cognitive neuropsychological model described previously. Therapy for central agraphias comprises three main approaches: Therapy can focus on strengthening the lexical routes, strengthening the nonlexical route, or using a combination of these approaches (Carlomagno, Iavarone, & Colombo, 1994; Hillis, 1992). Some approaches target writing skills in an item-specific manner (i.e., word by word), whereas other procedures focus on the processes that influence spelling of more than one lexical item. However, even in treatments described as process specific, there is a dynamic interplay among damaged and preserved functional components, and that performance reflects the summation of available visual, semantic, phonological, and motor graphemic information (Hillis, 1991). Beeson, Hirsch, and Rewega (2002) describe a problem-solving approach to agraphia treatment by which two patients interactively use the partially damaged lexical and nonlexical spelling routes to resolve spelling errors. They argue that a problem-solving approach is less limiting in terms of treatment generalization than is an item-specific approach. Still, the decision to use strategic interactive or item-specific treatment depends on the available intact cognitive mechanisms for a given individual at a given time in his or her rehabilitation process.

Thiel et al. (2015) evaluated the writing therapy literature in terms of its efficacy in adults with acquired dysgraphia. The studies reviewed were categorized according to type of treatment (impairment-based or assistive technology training) and outcome measures (single words or sentences). Subsequently, the studies fell in three distinct categories: impairment-based (i.e., relearning-based) writing therapies targeting single words; impairment-based writing therapies targeting sentences; and training in the use of assistive technologies. In the following sections, we review each of these categories through description of sample studies, which are intended to be representative rather than exhaustive. Furthermore, we discuss potential generalization to functional writing and subsequently to functional communication, which are necessary elements to reduce activity limitations and enhance social participation according to the ICF framework.

Impairment-Based Writing Therapies: Targeting Single Words

Therapy Strengthening the Lexical Routes

Studies suggest that it is possible to improve writing by strengthening the lexical–semantic route by focusing the intervention on specific loci of writing impairment within this route. Thus, for individuals whose orthographic representations are damaged or unavailable and for whom a nonlexical strategy is not feasible (as in phonological or deep dysgraphia), treatment may be administered with the goal of rebuilding specific representations in the orthographic output lexicon. Because many of these individuals also have significant aphasia, an item-specific lexical spelling treatment may be used to develop a functional written vocabulary that can augment, or substitute for, spoken language (Beeson, 1999; Clausen & Beeson, 2003; Robson, Marshall, Chiat, & Pring, 2001).

Treatment of Impaired Semantics Hillis (1991) reports that in some cases the underlying semantic deficits observed in writing may reflect an impairment within the semantic system so that lexical errors are evident in all modalities, while in other cases the semantic representations seem to be intact. In the former cases, teaching distinctions between semantically related items brought about improvement across all modalities, but in the latter cases writing improvement was achieved by improving the links between the semantic system and the orthographic output lexicon (i.e., by facilitating the restoration of degraded orthographic representations). Another treatment approach uses a visual and semantic cueing hierarchy (Carlomagno et al., 1994; Hillis, 1991). When Carlomagno et al. (1994) used this approach, they reported improvement in three subjects by strengthening the residual links between the semantic system and the orthographic output lexicon, while Hillis (1991) found that this approach also generalized to oral naming in one person with semantic deficits and improved writing in another individual with graphemic buffer damage.

Lexical Spelling Treatment Aliminosa, McCloskey, Goodman-Schulman, and Sokol (1993) used a delayed copying strategy with a patient who presented with impairments to the orthographic output lexicon, to phoneme–grapheme conversion, and possibly to the graphemic buffer. They reported improvement in the trained items, but no generalization was observed, suggesting improvement in the availability of specific stored orthographic representations. Rapp and Kane (2002) studied two individuals with agraphia presenting with selective deficits: One individual had a deficit of the orthographic output lexicon, and the other had a deficit of the graphemic buffer. The authors found that both individuals exhibited long-lasting word-specific benefits from the treatment. However, the individual with the graphemic buffer deficit exhibited generalization to untreated words, whereas the person with an impaired orthographic output lexicon did not. The authors suggest that generalization is determined by the specific cognitive component(s) that underlie the deficit.

Seron, Deloche, Moulard, and Rousselle (1980), who used a computer program to train five individuals with agraphia resulting from multiple processing deficits, describe a similar item-specific approach. The computer program prompted the typing of target words by presenting a series of blank spaces, one for each letter of the word. This approach strengthened the orthographic representations of the trained items, but retesting indicated that the improvement was not maintained. Therefore, additional training or concomitant semantic stimulation may be required to strengthen the lexical–semantic route adequately. As mentioned, many individuals with damage to nonlexical spelling procedures also have a concomitant impairment of the lexical–semantic spelling route. Several effective treatment protocols that include the task of arranging anagram letters to spell target words have been reported (Beeson, 1999; Beeson et al., 2002; Hillis, 1989), such as the lexical approach called Anagram and Copy Treatment (ACT). The treatment procedure uses a task hierarchy to elicit the correct spelling of the target words through the arrangement of anagram letters, followed by repeated copying of the word. The goal is to strengthen the orthographic representations of specific words. After correct anagram arrangement and copying of the word, recall trials require repeated correct spelling from memory. The ACT approach relies heavily on home practice (at least 30 minutes per day) that involves repeated copying of target words elicited with drawings or photographs. Another lexical spelling treatment relying heavily on home practice is Copy and Recall Treatment (CART; Beeson, 1999; Beeson et al., 2002; Beeson, Rising, & Volk, 2003; Clausen & Beeson, 2003). In this treatment, individuals repeatedly copy target words and then test their memory by covering up the written example and attempting to recall the spelling. During the treatment sessions, patients are trained to appropriately implement CART home practice and check the accuracy of their responses. Typically, five words are targeted for treatment at one time, with additional sets of words added sequentially as a criterion is met. For individuals who can repeat spoken words, CART can also be implemented with verbal repetition of target words to improve both written and spoken naming (Beeson & Egnor, 2006). The model for spoken repetition can be provided by any voice-recording device (tape, voice output augmentative device, etc.). Patients are trained to produce both spoken and written responses for each target during their daily homework. This "CART-plus-repetition" treatment resulted in positive gains in both written and spoken modalities for two individuals with moderate aphasia and severe agraphia (Beeson & Egnor, 2006).

Improvements made using ACT and CART tend to be item specific but can be highly functional when target words are individually selected and personally relevant. For example, written targets may be proper names, including those of family, friends, and favorite restaurants, allowing for specific, meaningful exchange of information. When applying this strategy within the WHO ICF framework, we can consider CART as a therapy protocol targeting the activity limitation level in addition to the function level. CART has proven beneficial in individuals with severe aphasia, even those with minimal pretreatment spelling skills (Beeson et al., 2003). Words practiced using the CART protocol may also be trained in the context of group treatment sessions, where each individual is given opportunities to communicate using practiced written words (Clausen & Beeson, 2003). This type of treatment has resulted in increased use of written targets in structured group settings and also in the context of conversation with unfamiliar partners. Other strategies used to strengthen the lexical–semantic route are the reestablishment of the correct spelling of homophone words by matching homophone words with respective pictures (Behram, 1987; Weekes & Coltheart, 1996); a visual imagery strategy for misspelling of irregular or ambiguous words (de Partz, Seron, & Van der Linden, 1992); the use of preserved spelling abilities for specific words as a self-cue mechanism to evoke lexical items starting with the same grapheme or phoneme (Hatfield, 1983); and the segmentation of long words into meaningful subsegments (de Partz, 1995).

Therapy Strengthening the Nonlexical Route

In cases where the lexical–semantic route is not available or too impoverished, spelling may be achieved through the nonlexical route by means of phoneme–grapheme correspondences, especially when the person is able to say the word (Cardell & Chenery, 1999; Hillis & Caramazza, 1994; Hillis Trupe, 1986). Carlomagno et al. (1994) report significantly improved spelling in six

cases when a nonlexical strategy was used in combination with a visual semantic approach. This strategy aimed for the reestablishment of sound-to-letter correspondences for selected consonants and consonant–vowel syllables.

Hillis and Caramazza (1994) described a treatment approach used in a case with orthographic output lexicon impairment. The patient had good access to the phonological output lexicon, and she was taught, by using a cueing hierarchy, the graphemic representations of the initial letters of 30 "key words," which in turn were used to self-cue correct orthographic representations and to self-monitor for semantic paragraphias. Pound (1996) also describes improvement in written spelling in a case with relatively intact oral spelling, where remediation was focused on the use of phoneme–grapheme correspondences to spell and then self-correct graphemic representations. In this study, the person was trained on the following steps during treatment: orally spell each target word before attempting to write it; self-dictate each letter while writing one letter at a time; examine the written word one letter at a time while orally spelling the word again; self-correct any noted errors; use an alphabet card if a model is needed; and finally inspect the entire word to check it against the orthographic representation for the word. Although spelling accuracy was not perfect posttreatment, this procedure proved successful in improving the patient's written spelling to a level commensurate with performance in oral spelling.

Furthermore, Beeson, Rising, Kim, and Rapcsak (2010) explored the application of interactive treatment as a complement to phonological treatment in two individuals with phonological alexia and dysgraphia. In this study, they examined the therapeutic effects of a two-stage treatment: phonological treatment followed by interactive treatment. The treatment sequence was intended to strengthen phonological processing abilities and the links between sounds and letters and then promote interactive use of nonlexical and residual lexical knowledge to resolve spelling errors. Phonological treatment was directed toward improving sound–letter correspondences for consonants and vowels and retraining nonlexical skills in the context of spelling nonwords. The interactive treatment guided participants to use phonological skills and residual orthographic knowledge to generate plausible spellings and to detect and correct spelling errors. Treatment emphasized spelling rather than reading, but naturally the writing tasks inherently stimulated reading as well. Following therapy, both participants improved phonological processing abilities and reading/spelling via the nonlexical route. They also improved spelling of real words and were able to detect and correct most residual errors using an electronic spelling aid. This suggests that behavioral treatment served to strengthen phonological skills supporting reading and spelling and provided a functional compensatory strategy to overcome residual weaknesses.

Finally, in individuals with deep dysgraphia, strengthening sound-to-letter conversion skills may provide access to initial graphemes, serving to prevent semantic errors and support activation of the orthographic output lexicon (Bub & Kertesz, 1982). In other words, semantic errors in writing might be avoided or self-corrected if a patient has at least some ability to translate the initial sounds of a word into corresponding graphemes.

Therapy for Graphemic Buffer Impairment

In cases of selective impairment to the graphemic buffer, the spared cognitive processes for spelling may provide a means to compensate (or self-correct) for spelling errors. For instance, individuals with some degree of preservation of nonlexical and lexical–semantic spelling processes may be trained to use strategies for self-correction of spellings (Hillis & Caramazza, 1987). Such strategies may include examining spellings to evaluate their accuracy (i.e., comparing to representations in the orthographic lexicon) and sounding out each word as it is written (to call attention to phonologically implausible misspellings). Spelling treatments targeting impaired lexical spelling procedures have resulted in improvement for individuals with deficits at the level of the orthographic output lexicon as well as the graphemic buffer, indicating that a single treatment approach may prove beneficial for more than one component of the spelling process. Raymer, Cudworth, and Haley (2003) used a modified version of CART to address a spelling impairment involving both the orthographic output lexicon and the graphemic buffer, and they documented improvements at both levels of processing in a single patient.

On the other hand, Panton and Marshall (2008) described a therapy study of a person with graphemic buffer impairment in whom thinking about language processing contributed to successful functional therapy and allowed an examination of the relationship between decreased function and participation restriction as defined by the ICF. This study is the only one using the principles of the WHO ICF framework in writing impairment. In this case, therapy had a double focus: spelling therapy (function level) and functional application of this skill, more specifically, taking a message in a work environment (activity limitation level). Following therapy, the individual with agraphia showed increased buffer capacity, as demonstrated by improvement in word spelling, a shift in the position of errors (errors occurred later in words after therapy), and an increase in number of words recorded during the functional task of taking down a message (i.e., representing generalization to untreated words).

Therapy for Peripheral Dysgraphia

Contrary to central dysgraphia, little attention has been given to peripheral dysgraphia treatment (Rapcsak & Beeson, 2000). In general, treatment of individuals with peripheral dysgraphia aims to reestablish letters and word production; however, slow, deliberate, and feedback dependent it may be. When graphic motor control is regained, treatment can be directed toward improving the automaticity of the motor programs. Strategies using a hierarchy of visual feedback or verbal reminders have been found to be effective (Oliveira, Gurd, Nixon, Marshall, & Passingham, 1997). Also, self-dictation procedures have proven beneficial in improving spelling in individuals with preserved oral relative to written spelling (Pound, 1996; Ramage, Beeson, & Rapcsak, 1998).

Evaluation of the Impairment-Based Writing Therapies Targeting Single Words

Thiel et al. (2015), in their review of agraphia therapies, evaluated 49 studies of impairment-based writing therapies. Twenty-two were single-case studies, 24 multiple-case studies, and 3 group studies. The participants were described to have a range of aphasia and dysgraphia types and severities. Therapy approaches used were informed by extensive assessments of the participants' spelling and language skills guided by the cognitive neuropsychological model. Outcomes were usually measured using either spelling to dictation or written picture description tasks. All of these studies reported positive outcomes for treated or untreated items or on oral discourse tasks.

Thiel et al. (2015) also reviewed these studies in terms of generalization. From the reviewed studies, four studies have provided a therapy targeting single words but have also assessed generalization to spontaneous writing (Carlomagno & Parlato, 1989; Hillis & Caramazza, 1994; Pound, 1996; Raymer et al., 2003). Seven studies evaluated the effects of a spelling therapy with an additional phase to encourage generalization to functional use of words learned in therapy for face-to-face conversations

(Beeson, 1999; Beeson et al., 2002, 2003; Clausen & Beeson, 2003; Jackson-Waite, Robson, & Pring, 2003; Robson et al., 2001; Robson, Pring, Marshall, Morrison, & Chiat, 1998). Four of the seven studies targeting conversational writing supported their results with statistical analyses (Clausen & Beeson, 2003; Jackson-Waite et al., 2003; Robson et al., 1998, 2001), and all of these found significant changes to functional writing. However, Robson et al. (2001) only found significant gains in a message assessment (measuring communicative use of writing) for one of three participants. Six studies encouraged participants to generalize therapy gains (often involving the use of a strategy such as oral spelling or phoneme-to-grapheme conversion) to more natural writing contexts, such as letters, e-mails, and essays (Beeson, Rewega, Vall, & Rapcsak, 2000; de Partz et al., 1992; Greenwald, 2004; Hillis & Caramazza, 1987; Mortley, Enderby, & Petheram, 2001; Panton & Marshall, 2008). Although all of the studies reported improvements, only one (Panton & Marshall, 2008) subjected their data to statistical analysis and found significant changes to note-taking ability.

In conclusion, people with acquired dysgraphia can relearn a list of single words targeted in therapy and in some cases can improve their writing of words that were not practiced in therapy. Furthermore, there has been some limited evidence that these therapies can have practical benefits: Participants can be trained to use learned words or spelling strategies to communicate functionally.

Impairment-Based Writing Therapies: Targeting Sentences

People with aphasia and writing impairment present with difficulties not only in single-word written production but also in production of sentences or text. Salis and Edwards (2010) treated the written production of transitive and intransitive verbs as well as subject–verb (SV) and subject–verb–object (SVO) sentences in a participant with moderate-to-severe aphasia and apraxia of speech. The aim was to improve the participant's ability to convey information; therefore, as the participant found it difficult to produce function words (e.g., the), she was discouraged from using them. The progressive (-ing) form of the verb was trained for each sentence. Verbs and sentences were targeted simultaneously within sessions with a "cue-and-copy" approach to treatment. In each session, the participant was first asked to write the verb depicted in a picture and was provided with orthographic cues on failed attempts. The same procedure was then followed for the nouns

(for subjects and objects). She was encouraged to use names of friends and family members as the subject of sentences instead of pronouns. The treatment resulted in significantly improved verb and sentence production, although the participant found transitive verbs more difficult than intransitive verbs. Generalization occurred to some untreated verbs and sentences; however, no generalization to everyday writing contexts was observed.

Four other studies aimed to improve writing syntax (Jacobs & Thompson, 2000; Mitchum, Haendiges, & Berndt, 1993; Murray & Karcher, 2000; Murray, Timberlake, & Eberle, 2007). The syntactic structures targeted included SVO (Mitchum et al., 1993; Murray & Karcher, 2000); object cleft (Jacobs & Thompson, 2000, p. 6); passive sentences (Jacobs & Thompson, 2000); and object- and subject-extracted embedded who-question sentences (Murray et al., 2007). All of the written sentence therapy studies reported improvements to trained sentences, with two reporting gains to trained verbs (Mitchum et al., 1993; Murray & Karcher, 2000). Two showed improvements to untrained sentences (Jacobs & Thompson, 2000; Murray et al., 2007). Only one study used statistical analyses to demonstrate significant improvements on their measures (Mitchum et al., 1993)

Evaluation of the Impairment-Based Writing Therapies: Targeting Sentences

As Thiel et al. (2015) described, three of these studies have included measures of spontaneous writing (Mitchum et al., 1993; Murray & Karcher, 2000; Murray et al., 2007). Using assessments such as picture description and narrative and procedural discourse tasks (e.g., describing how to carry out an everyday task such as making scrambled eggs), they have found that written sentence therapies have led to such changes as significant improvements to syntax; number of lexical verbs and content (Mitchum et al., 1993); a higher number of function words; longer, more grammatical sentences; more substantive verbs and fewer unsuccessful sentences (Murray & Karcher, 2000); and an increase in number of words, correct information units (CIUs), words per minute, CIUs per minute, percentage of CIUs, ratio of open to closed class words, and number of substantive verbs (Murray et al., 2007).

In summary, written sentence therapy studies have provided some evidence that people with aphasia and acquired dysgraphia not only can relearn the spelling of single words but also can learn how to construct sentences with them. Furthermore, this type of therapy has had positive effects on spontaneous writing. However, this evidence has been limited by the relative dearth of studies and number of participants.

Training in the Use of Assistive Technologies

As described, the development of novel technologies has increased the need for writing to be a functional goal in the rehabilitation process. Furthermore, these technologies can be used as a tool to facilitate learning to spell new words or as an aid to help the person with aphasia compensate for his or her writing impairments. Fluhardy (1993) reported that the use of partial lexical knowledge or preserved phonological knowledge in a patient with aphasia was sufficient to allow the use of an electronic dictionary to facilitate a self-correction strategy. Beeson et al. (2000) investigated a spelling treatment designed to promote interactive use of residual lexical and nonlexical abilities in two individuals with acquired spelling impairment using a problem-solving approach to spelling. Prior to the initiation of the interactive treatment, the participants demonstrated the ability to generate phonologically plausible spellings for many of the words that they could not spell. Training focused first on detection and self-correction of spelling errors. Then, the participants were trained to use an electronic spelling device to resolve spelling difficulties in a problem-solving manner so that they would become able to check spelling independently. For example, an individual might use a sublexical strategy to generate an initial spelling (e.g., "sepost" for *supposed*) and then evaluate this spelling relative to residual lexical knowledge for the target through the use of the electronic device (resulting in a closer approximation, such as "suposed"). Both participants improved not only their spelling abilities when using the device but also spelling of untrained words without the device. Some of the spelling attempts provided evidence of interactive use of lexical and nonlexical information because they contained phonologically plausible segments combined with low-frequency phoneme–grapheme mappings that were correct for the target word. Improvements following treatment appeared to reflect an increase in the detection and self-correction of such errors, suggesting a therapeutic effect of the relatively explicit training to use information from both lexical and nonlexical processing to resolve spelling errors.

This study used an assistive device to augment the effects of impairment-based therapy. However, several studies have reported the use of computer technologies to directly compensate for writing difficulties, rather than as an adjuvant to traditional therapy for agraphia (Armstrong & Macdonald, 2000; Behrns, Hartelius, & Wengelin, 2009; Bruce, Edmundson, & Coleman, 2003; Estes & Bloom, 2011; King & Hux, 1995; Manasse, Hux, & Rankin-Erickson, 2000; Nicholas, Sinotte, & Helm-Estabrooks, 2005, 2011). Five of these had single-case designs, and three were multiple case studies. Five technologies were used in these studies: voice recognition software (VRS), speech synthesizer software, predictive writing software, spell-checker software, and C-Speak Aphasia (CSA). Voice recognition software generates text as the user speaks into a microphone attached to a computer (Bruce et al., 2003; Estes & Bloom, 2011; Manasse et al., 2000). It has been tested in three studies on participants with mild-to-moderate fluent aphasia, reasonably good reading skills, and more severely impaired written language (Bruce et al., 2003; Estes & Bloom, 2011; Manasse et al., 2000), as the aim is to compensate for poor writing skills by using the more intact spoken language. As well as measuring improvements to the speech recognition accuracy of the software, these studies measured changes to written production, through either composite picture description tasks (Bruce et al., 2003; Estes & Bloom, 2011) or an essay about a chosen topic (Manasse et al., 2000). With the software, all participants demonstrated improvements, such as increased vocabulary and syntax (Estes & Bloom, 2011; Manasse et al., 2000), more content (Bruce et al., 2003; Estes & Bloom, 2011), and longer and more complex texts (Bruce et al., 2003) compared to writing with no support. Bruce et al. (2003) also found that texts were produced more quickly with the software. However, the participant in the study by Manasse et al. (2000) produced less text with the VRS than by typing, which the authors hypothesized may be due to the software's misperception of her words and the extra time needed to correct the spellings.

In contrast to VRS, speech synthesizer software, word prediction (or word prompt) software, and spell-check software are used to facilitate the writing process (rather than being an alternative to writing). Speech synthesizer software provides speech output for any part of a text that the user chooses to highlight (Armstrong & Macdonald, 2000; King & Hux, 1995). This can be a letter, word, sentence, or paragraph. Although this was developed to aid reading, it also functions as an editing tool for writing. Predictive writing software provides a list of possible words as letters are typed into the word processor (Armstrong & Macdonald, 2000; Behrns et al., 2009; Mortley et al., 2001; Murray

& Karcher, 2000). This list narrows as more letters of the word are typed. The user can select the required word from the list without having to type the entire word. Spell-checker software alerts the user to a word that has been incorrectly spelled or to a sentence or phrase that is ungrammatical and suggests alternatives (Behrns et al., 2009). These technologies have been used successfully in three studies to compensate for writing or editing difficulties in participants with mild, moderate, and severe nonfluent aphasia (Armstrong & Macdonald, 2000; Behrns et al., 2009; King & Hux, 1995). C-Speak Aphasia is a picture-based, alternative communication computer program (Nicholas & Elliott, 1998). The user selects icons from semantic categories and creates messages with them that are then spoken by the computer or converted into written words sent by e-mail (Nicholas et al., 2011). In two studies, Nicholas and colleagues evaluated the effects of this program on the functional spoken and written communication of participants with severe nonfluent aphasia and a range of auditory comprehension and nonverbal cognitive abilities (Nicholas et al., 2005, 2011). Five participants in the first study (Nicholas et al., 2005) and 10 in the second study (Nicholas et al., 2011) were trained to use the program over at least 6 months. The training consisted of three modules in which participants learned how to use CSA for generative language (i.e., producing statements, questions, and commands), communicating by telephone, and communicating via writing or e-mail. Within the writing module, participants learned to combine preprogrammed phrases and novel vocabulary via picture selections. These messages could then be converted into text and sent as e-mails. Outcomes were measured through repeated probing of five communication tasks. The writing task comprised writing a birthday card and a grocery list. Nicholas et al. (2005) found that three of five participants communicated more information using CSA than without. However, none of the participants communicated more information on the writing tasks with CSA. In the Nicholas et al. (2011) study, four participants communicated substantially more information in the CSA condition than in their "off-computer" condition. One participant performed better using CSA for the writing task.

Finally, Beeson, Higginson, and Rising (2013) reported a patient with Broca's aphasia, severe apraxia of speech and global dysgraphia, who was trained to use the typing feature of his cellular phone, with the ultimate goal of using text messaging for communication. A multiple baseline design was used. Relearning and maintenance of single-word spelling of targeted items was examined in response to the traditional CART treatment program for handwriting. A new paradigm using one-handed typing on a cell phone keyboard (texting version of CART) was used in writing text messages. The results showed marked improvement in spelling and spoken naming, with stronger maintenance of handwriting than cell phone typing. However, training resulted in functional use of texting that continued 2 years after treatment.

In summary, the results of this small group of studies evaluating assistive technologies suggested that these devices can be useful for some people with aphasia and dysgraphia to compensate for impairments in written word retrieval, spelling, monitoring, and editing and allow for more complex and meaningful messages to be conveyed.

CONCLUSIONS AND FUTURE DIRECTIONS

In this chapter, we described the different written language impairments and a framework for assessment and treatment of these impairments. Writing impairments can result from damage to one or more of the critical components of the cognitive processes that support written spelling. Treatment studies demonstrated that therapy directed toward lexical–semantic and nonlexical spelling processes can improve spelling abilities of individuals with acquired writing impairments or can be used efficiently to compensate for the impaired components. However, while most of the studies so far have focused at the body function level, we see an increased attempt to integrate functional writing, which will reduce the activity limitation and enhance social participation as rehabilitation goals. This may also represent an increased need for functional writing due to the development of social media and the novel technologies. So, in the future, we expect to see more therapy approaches focusing on the everyday functional writing needs of these patients in accordance with the ICF framework.

We expect that advances in our understanding of the cognitive processes and neural substrates that support writing will continue to influence treatment approaches for acquired disorders of writing. We expect that the knowledge gained from functional neuroimaging and computational modeling of normal and disordered language process research will be complemented by behavioral research. Advances in these areas may provide insights that improve our understanding of the nature of reading and spelling impairments, as well as maximize the efficacy, effectiveness, and efficiency of behavioral treatments. Finally, the increased attention to evidence-based practice in speech–language pathology has promoted increased rigor in the experimental designs used to examine treatment outcomes. Ideally, treatment research should serve to clarify candidacy for particular treatment approaches, which in turn can serve to guide clinicians as they select treatments for particular individuals according to their needs in their everyday environments.

Case Illustration 11.1

Ray suffered a left cerebrovascular accident at the age of 55 years following a middle cerebral artery occlusion. He presents with aphasia and right hemiparesis. Previously, he worked as a college professor and political counselor. He attended the university clinic 1 year poststroke. At that time, he had resumed his role as counselor, and he was receiving outpatient services twice weekly. Regarding his communication skills, he was coping with auditory comprehension and expressive language because he was able to follow everyday conversation and contribute to debates. He was also coping with reading because he was understanding lengthy work documents, but he was not coping with writing. Premorbidly, he wrote extensively and was an excellent speller, but now he shows marked spelling difficulties in all writing. He wants to develop better handwritten skills for taking messages and taking simple notes in meetings.

Assessment

During the assessment of his writing abilities, the clinician raised the following questions to form a hypothesis for Ray's level of impairment and functioning:

- What are Ray's current single-word writing skills?
- Which processing impairments got in the way of single-word writing?
- Which strategies was he using?

The clinician used the following assessment tasks:

- Informal written picture naming/description
- Writing words to dictation controlled for frequency, imageability, length, and regularity
- Writing nonwords to dictation
- Written message task (taking notes from a recorded message)

The assessment findings of Ray's writing skills revealed that, on the written naming/description task he was able to access target words and to compose sentences, but he presented with frequent spelling difficulties, for which he showed awareness and attempted corrections unsuccessfully. However, his performance in writing to dictation was influenced only by word length and not by word frequency, imageability, and regularity. Similarly, word length influenced his writing of nonwords. His errors were letter deletions (SOF for "soaf"), letter additions (BURDL for "birl"), letter substitutions, and letter transpositions. These observations indicated a deficit at the level of the graphemic buffer because (a) there is a problem with spelling, not with word access; (b) there is a word length effect but no frequency or imageability effect; and (c) there are errors at the grapheme level but not at the word level.

To assess Ray's writing strategies, the clinician used a written message task. During this task, Ray was asked to write down as much as he could about two recorded phone messages and one recorded news story, which were played three times each. He was instructed to use any resources at his disposal (abbreviations, symbols, drawings). Ray attempted a key word strategy with some success and attempted to use some abbreviations, but he omitted many key words or makes errors, and it was difficult to derive information from his notes.

In sum, the assessment revealed that his strengths included his word access abilities, his ability to detect his errors, and his ability to use some spontaneous compensatory strategies. His weaknesses were his impaired graphemic buffer storage (particularly for longer words), his frequent errors that he was unable to correct even if he could detect them, and his limited success in using compensatory strategies.

(continues)

Therapy

The therapy goals were set with Ray to enable him to take short written notes and messages by focusing on the following strategies:

- Improving spelling performance in a functional set of lexical items
- Improving note-taking strategies
- Improving the capacity of the graphemic buffer
- Using the notes to compose an e-mail

Ray received 12 hours of therapy over 6 weeks using the lexical spelling therapy (Beeson et al., 2002; Rapp & Kane, 2002). Sixty words related to his counseling role were used (30 used in therapy and 30 used as control probes). In each therapy session, Ray practiced 10 words during the following activities:

- Written spelling of each word to dictation
- Written spelling of each word from letter-by-letter dictation
- Copying each word
- Delayed recall of written word (elicited with partially obscured written stimuli)
- Repeating each word in syllables during spelling
- Completing worksheets for home practice (copying, anagram sorting, word completion)

Furthermore, during therapy, Ray was taught a strategy to improve his note-taking skills. The task used is for Ray to listen to a recorded message and then take notes using the following strategies:

- Write down key points.
- Do not: record verbatim, concentrate on spelling.
- Do: Use abbreviations, symbols, relevant punctuation.
- Read back notes.
- Discuss skills used and their effectiveness.

Therapy Outcome

Following therapy, the written message task was readministered. Ray's notes were given to "blind" judges, who were asked to write down the content of the original message. Ray's performance was evaluated by the following criteria:

- The number of message components detected by the judges pre- versus posttherapy (each judge sees only one version of each message)
- The percentage of message components detected by the judges from Ray's notes
- A qualitative analysis of the written messages

Posttherapy, Ray wrote more key words and more sentences/linked words, increased his use of symbols and punctuation, and increased his use of compensatory strategies. Regarding his written word-processing skills, there was some evidence of increased graphemic buffer capacity because a generalized improvement in word spelling was observed, as well as a shift in the position of errors (errors occur later in words after therapy). Finally, the increase in words in his messages included untreated as well as treated items. Furthermore, he was able to compose an e-mail with his notes and send it to his clinician.

Conclusions

This is an example of a therapy approach in which using a language-processing perspective contributes to a positive functional outcome. By relying on the ICF framework, it became clear that Ray's improvement in writing can be interpreted as a decrease in activity restriction and an increase in activity participation.

Source: Adapted from Panton & Marshall (2008). Improving spelling and everyday writing after a CVA: A single case therapy study. *Aphasiology, 22*(2), 164–183.

STUDY QUESTIONS

1. Compare and contrast the terms *agraphia* and *dysgraphia.*
2. Describe the two theoretical models associated with the writing process.
3. Cite and define the central processes of writing. Give an example of a frequent error you might observe in each of the central dysgraphia.
4. Cite and define the peripheral processes of writing.
5. What type of dysgraphia is characterized by a word length effect and why?
6. Based on the theoretical model, what can you conclude after each of the following assessment tasks: writing nonwords to dictation, writing words to dictation, writing homophones to dictation, written picture naming, word copying?
7. Describe a type of lexical treatment for writing.
8. What is meant by an interactive, problem-solving approach to writing treatment?
9. Describe an example of treatment for graphemic buffer impairment.
10. Describe strategies that will aim to improve functional writing in a person with aphasia and dysgraphia.

REFERENCES

Aimard, G., Devick, M., Lebel, M., Trouila, M., & Boisson, D. (1975). Agraphie pure (dynamique) d'origine frontale. *Revue Neurologique, 7,* 505–512.

Alexander, M. P., Fisher, R. S., & Friedman, R. (1992). Lesion localization in apraxic agraphia. *Archives of Neurology, 49,* 246–251.

Aliminosa, D., McCloskey, M., Goodman-Schulman, R., & Sokol, S. M. (1993). Remediation of acquired dysgraphia as a technique of testing interpretations of deficits. *Aphasiology, 7(1),* 55–69.

Armstrong, I., & Macdonald, A. (2000). Aiding chronic written language expression difficulties: A case study. *Aphasiology, 14,* 93–108

Basso, A. (2003). *Aphasia and its therapy.* Oxford, UK: Oxford University Press.

Basso, A., & Maragnolo, P. (2000). Cognitive neuropsychological rehabilitation: The emperor's new clothes? *Neuropsychological Rehabilitation, 10(3),* 219–230.

Basso, A., Taborielli, A., & Vignolo, L. A. (1978). Dissociated disorders of speaking and writing in aphasia. *Journal of Neurology, Neurosurgery and Psychiatry, 41,* 556–563.

Baxter, D. M., & Warrington, E. K. (1986). Ideational agraphia: A single case study. *Journal of Neurology, Neurosurgery and Psychiatry, 49,* 369–374.

Beeson, P. M. (1999). Treating acquired writing impairment: Strengthening graphemic representations. *Aphasiology, 13,* 767–785.

Beeson, P. M., & Egnor, H. (2006). Combining treatment for written and spoken naming. *Journal of the International Neuropsychological Society, 12,* 816–827.

Beeson, P. M., & Henry, M. (2008). Comprehension and production of written words. In R. Chapey (Ed.), *Language intervention strategies in aphasia and related neurogenic communication disorders* (5th ed., pp. 654–688). Baltimore: Lippincott Williams & Wilkins.

Beeson, P. M., Higginson, K., & Rising, K. (2013). Writing treatment for aphasia: A texting approach. *Journal of Speech, Language, and Hearing Research, 56,* 945–955.

Beeson, P. M., Hirsch, F. M., & Rewega, M. A. (2002). Successful single word writing treatment: Experimental analysis of four cases. *Aphasiology, 16(4/5/6),* 473–491.

Beeson, P. M., & Rapcsak, S. Z. (2002). Clinical diagnosis and treatment of spelling disorders. In A. E. Hillis (Ed.), *The handbook of adult language disorders: Integrating cognitive neuropsychology, neurology, and rehabilitation* (pp. 101–121). Philadelphia: Psychology Press.

Beeson, P. M., Rewega, M. A., Vall, S., & Rapcsak, S. Z. (2000). Problem solving approach to agraphia treatment: Interactive use of lexical and sublexical routes. *Aphasiology, 14(5/6),* 551–565.

Beeson, P. M., Rising, K., Kim, E. S., & Rapcsak, S. Z. (2010). A treatment sequence for phonological alexia/agraphia. *Journal of Speech, Language, and Hearing Research, 53(2),* 450–468.

Beeson, P. M., Rising, K., & Volk, J. (2003). Writing treatment for severe aphasia: Who benefits? *Journal of Speech and Hearing Research, 46,* 1038–1060.

Behram, M. (1987). The rites of righting writing: Homophone remediation in acquired dysgraphia. *Cognitive Neuropsychology, 4,* 365–384.

Behrns, I., Hartelius, L., & Wengelin, Å. (2009). Aphasia and computerised writing aid supported treatment. *Aphasiology, 23,* 1276–1294.

Benedick, M. (1865). *Uber Aphasie, Agraphie und verwandte pathologische Zustande.* Wiener medizinishe Presse Pr 6.

Benson, D. F., & Cummings, J. L. (1985). Agraphia. In P. J. Vinken, G. W. Bruyn, H. L. Klawns, & J. A. M. Fredericks (Eds.), *Handbook of clinical neurology* (Vol. 45, pp. 457–472). Amsterdam: Elsevier.

Brooks, V. B. (1986). *The neural basis of motor control.* New York: Oxford University Press.

Bruce, C., Edmundson, A., & Coleman, M. (2003). Writing with voice: An investigation of the use of a voice recognition system as a writing aid for a man with aphasia. *International Journal of Language & Communication Disorders, 38,* 131–148.

Bub, D., & Kertesz, A. (1982). Deep agraphia. *Brain and Language, 17,* 146–165.

Campbell, R. (1983). Writing nonwords to dictation. *Brain and Language, 19,* 153–178.

Caramazza, A., Miceli, G., Villa, G., & Romani, C. (1987). The role of the graphemic buffer in spelling: Evidence from a case of acquired dysgraphia. *Cognition, 26,* 59–85.

Cardell, E. A., & Chenery, H. J. (1999). A cognitive neuropsychological approach to the assessment and remediation of acquired dysgraphia. *Language Testing, 16*, 353–388.

Carlomagno, S., Iavarone, A., & Colombo, A. (1994). Cognitive approaches to writing rehabilitation: From single case to group studies. In M. J. Riddoch & G. W. Humphreys (Eds.), *Cognitive neuropsychology and cognitive rehabilitation* (pp. 485–502). Hillsdale, NJ: Erlbaum.

Carlomagno, S., & Parlato, V. (1989). Writing rehabilitation in brain damaged adult patients: A cognitive approach. In X. Seron & S. Deloche (Eds.), *Cognitive approaches in neuropsychological rehabilitation* (pp. 179–209). Hillsdale, NJ: Erlbaum.

Clausen, N. S., & Beeson, P. M. (2003). Conversational use of writing in severe aphasia: A group treatment approach. *Aphasiology, 17*, 625–644.

Cséfalvay, Zs. (2003). Lurian approach to aphasia therapy—a review. In I. Papathanasiou & R. Blesser (Eds.), *The sciences of aphasia: From therapy to theory* (pp. 111–120). Oxford, UK: Elsevier.

Cséfalvay, Zs., Egryová, M., & Wiedermann, I. (2007). *Diagnostika a terapia afázie, alexie a agrafie* [Diagnostics and therapy of aphasia, alexia and agraphia]. Bratislava, Slovakia: Kaminský.

De Bastiani, P., & Barry, C. (1989). A cognitive analysis of an acquired dysgraphic patient with an allographic writing disorder. *Cognitive Neuropsychology, 6*, 25–41.

de Partz, M. P. (1995). Deficits of the graphemic buffer: Effects of a written lexical segmentation strategy. *Neuropsychological Rehabilitation, 5*(1/2), 129–147.

de Partz, M. P., Seron, X., & Van der Linden, M. V. (1992). Re-education of surface dysgraphia with a visual imagery strategy. *Cognitive Neuropsychology, 9*, 369–401.

Ellis, A. W. (1982). Spelling and writing (and reading and speaking). In A. W. Ellis (Ed.), *Normality and pathology in cognitive functions* (pp. 113–146). London: Academic Press.

Ellis, A. W. (1988). Normal writing processes and peripheral acquired dysgraphias. *Language and Cognitive Processes, 3*, 99–127.

Ellis, A. W., & Young, A. W. (1988). *Human cognitive neuropsychology.* Hillsdale, NJ: Erlbaum.

Ellis, A. W., Young, A. W., & Flude, B. M. (1987). "Afferent dysgraphia" in a patient and in normal subjects. *Cognitive Neuropsychology, 4*, 465–486.

Estes, C., & Bloom, R. L. (2011). Using voice recognition software to treat dysgraphia in a patient with conduction aphasia. *Aphasiology, 25*, 366–385.

Fluhardy, G. (1993). Use of an electronic dictionary to compensate for surface dysgraphia. *Journal of Cognitive Rehabilitation, 11*, 28–30.

Fotiadou, D., Northcott, S., Chatzidaki, A., & Hilari, K. (2014). Aphasia blog talk: How does stroke and aphasia affect a person's social relationships? *Aphasiology, 28*(11), 1281–1300.

Goodglass, H., Kaplan, E., & Barresi, B. (2000). *Boston Diagnostic Aphasia Examination* (3rd ed.). New York: Psychological Assessment Resources.

Goodman, R. A., & Caramazza, A. (1986a). Aspects of spelling process: Evidence from a case of acquired dysgraphia. *Language and Cognitive Processes, 1*, 263–296.

Goodman, R. A., & Caramazza, A. (1986b). *The Johns Hopkins University Dyslexia and Dysgraphia Batteries.* Unpublished report.

Greenwald, M. (2004). "Blocking" lexical competitors in severe global agraphia: A treatment of reading and spelling. *Neurocase, 77*, 156–174.

Hatfield, F. M. (1983). Aspects of acquired dysgraphia and implication for re-education. In C. Code & D. J. Muller (Eds.), *Aphasia therapy* (pp. 157–169). London: Whurr.

Hatfield, F. M. (1985). Visual and phonological factors in acquired dysgraphia. *Neuropsychologia, 23*, 13–29.

Hatfield, F. M., & Patterson, K. (1983). Phonological spelling. *Quarterly Journal of Experimental Psychology, 35A*, 451–468.

Henry, M. L., Beeson, P. M., Stark, A. J., & Rapcsak, S. Z. (2007). The role of left perisylvian cortical regions in spelling. *Brain and Language, 100*(1), 44–52.

Hillis, A. E. (1989). Efficacy and generalization of treatment for aphasic naming errors. *Archives of Physical Medicine and Rehabilitation, 70*, 632–636.

Hillis, A. E. (1991). Effects of separate treatments for distinct impairments within the naming process. *Clinical Aphasiology, 19*, 255–265.

Hillis, A. E. (1992). Facilitating written production. *Clinics in Communication Disorders, 2*, 19–33.

Hillis, A. E., & Caramazza, A. (1987). Model-driven treatment of dysgraphia. In R. H. Brookshire (Ed.), *Clinical aphasiology* (pp. 84–105). Minneapolis, MN: BRK.

Hillis, A. E., & Caramazza, A. (1989). The graphemic buffer and attentional mechanisms. *Brain and Language, 36*, 208–235.

Hillis, A. E., & Caramazza, A. (1994). Theories of lexical processing and rehabilitation of lexical deficits. In M. J. Riddoch & G. W. Humphreys (Eds.), *Cognitive neuropsychology and cognitive rehabilitation* (pp. 449–484). Hillsdale, NJ: Erlbaum.

Hillis Trupe, A. E. (1986). Effectiveness of retraining phoneme to grapheme conversion. In R. H. Brookshire (Ed.), *Clinical aphasiology* (pp. 163–171). Minneapolis, MN: BRK.

Hodges, J. R. (1991). Pure apraxic agraphia with recovery after drainage of a left frontal cyst. *Cortex, 27*, 469–473.

Holland, A. L., Frattali, C., & Fromm, D. (1999). *Communicative Activities in Daily Living (CADL-2).* Austin, TX: Pro-Ed.

Jackson-Waite, K., Robson, J., & Pring, T. (2003). Written communication using a Lightwriter in undifferentiated jargon aphasia: A single case study. *Aphasiology, 17*, 767–780.

Jacobs, B. J., & Thompson, C. K. (2000). Cross-modal generalization effects of training noncanonical sentence comprehension and production in agrammatic aphasia. *Journal of Speech, Language, and Hearing Research, 43*, 5–20.

Kapar, N., & Lawton, N. F. (1983). Dysgraphia for letters: A form of motor memory deficit? *Journal of Neurology, Neurosurgery and Psychiatry, 50*, 1125–1129.

Kaplan, E., & Goodglass, H. (1981). Aphasia-related disorders. In M. T. Sarno (Ed.), *Acquired aphasia* (pp. 303–359). New York: Academic Press.

Kartsounis, L. D. (1992). Selective lower case letter ideational dysgraphia. *Cortex, 28*, 145–150.

Kay, J., Lesser, R., & Coltheart, M. (1992). *PALPA: Psycholinguistic Assessments of Language Processing in Aphasia.* Hove, UK: Erlbaum.

Kertesz, A. (2007). *Western Aphasia Battery—Revised.* New York: Grune & Stratton.

King, J., & Hux, K. (1995). Intervention using talking word processing software: An aphasia case study. *Augmentative and Alternative Communication, 11*, 187–192.

Laine, T. N., & Marttila, R. J. (1981). Pure agraphia: A case study. *Neuropsychologia, 19*, 311–316.

Lebrun, Y. (1985). Disturbances of written language and associated abilities following damage to the right hemisphere. *Applied Psycholinguistics, 6*, 231–260.

Luria, A. R. (1963). *Restoration of function after brain injury.* London, UK: Pergamon Press.

Luzzatti, C., Colombo, C., Frustaci, M., & Vitolo, F. (2000). Rehabilitation of spelling along the sub-word level routine. *Neuropsychological Rehabilitation, 10*(3), 249–278.

Mack, L., Gonzalez Rothi, L. J., & Heilman, K. M. (1993). Hemispheric specialization for handwriting in right handers. *Brain and Cognition, 21*, 80–86.

Manasse, N. J., Hux, K., & Rankin-Erickson, J. L. (2000). Speech recognition training for enhancing written language generation by a traumatic brain injury survivor. *Brain Injury, 14*, 1015–1034.

Marcie, P., & Hecaen, H. (1979). Agraphia: Writing disorders associated with unilateral cortical lesions. In K. M. Heilman & E. Valenstein (Eds.), *Clinical neuropsychology* (pp. 92–127). New York: Oxford University Press.

Margolin, D. I. (1984). The neuropsychology of writing and spelling: Semantic, phonological, motor and perceptual processes. *Quarterly Journal of Experimental Psychology, 36A*, 459–489.

McNeil, M. R., & Tseng, C. H. (1990). Acquired neurogenic dysgraphias. In L. L. LaPointe (Ed.), *Aphasia and related neurogenic language disorders* (pp. 147–176). New York: Thieme Medical.

Miceli, G., Silveri, M. C., & Caramazza, A. (1985). Cognitive analysis of a case of pure dysgraphia. *Brain and Language, 25*, 187–212.

Mitchum, C. C., Haendiges, A. N., & Berndt, R. S. (1993). Model-guided treatment to improve written sentence production: A case study. *Aphasiology, 7*, 71–109.

Mortley, J., Enderby, P., & Petheram, B. (2001). Using a computer to improve functional writing in a patient with severe dysgraphia. *Aphasiology, 15*, 443–461.

Morton, J. (1980). The logogen model and orthographic structure. In U. Frith (Ed.), *Cognitive approaches in spelling* (pp. 117–133). London: Academic Press.

Murray, L. L., & Karcher, L. (2000). A treatment for written verb retrieval and sentence construction skills. *Aphasiology, 14*, 585–602.

Murray, L. L., Timberlake, A., & Eberle, R. (2007). Treatment of underlying forms in a discourse context. *Aphasiology, 21*, 139–163.

Nicholas, M., & Elliott, S. (1998). *C-Speak aphasia: A communication system for adults with aphasia.* Solana Beach, CA: Mayer-Johnson.

Nicholas, M., Sinotte, M. P., & Helm-Estabrooks, N. (2005). Using a computer to communicate: Effect of executive function impairments in people with severe aphasia. *Aphasiology, 19*, 1052–1065.

Nicholas, M., Sinotte, M. P., & Helm-Estabrooks, N. (2011). C-Speak aphasia alternative communication program for people with severe aphasia: Importance of executive functioning and semantic knowledge. *Neuropsychological Rehabilitation, 21*, 322–366.

Nielsen, J. M. (1946). *Agnosia, apraxia, aphasia: Their value in cerebral localization.* New York: Hoeber.

Ogle, J. W. (1867). Aphasia and agraphia. *Report of Medical Research Council of St. George's Hospital (London), 2*, 83–122.

Oliveira, R. M., Gurd, J. M., Nixon, P., Marshall, J. C., & Passingham, R. E. (1997). Micrographia in Parkinson's disease: The

effect of providing external cues. *Journal of Neurology, Neurosurgery and Psychiatry, 63*, 429–433.

Panton, A., & Marshall, J. (2008). Improving spelling and everyday writing after a CVA: A single-case therapy study. *Aphasiology, 22*(2), 164–183.

Parr, S. (1992). Everyday reading and writing practices of normal adults: Implications for aphasia assessment. *Aphasiology, 6*(3), 273–283.

Patterson, K. (1986). Lexical but nonsemantic spelling? *Cognitive Neuropsychology, 3*(3), 341–367.

Patterson, K., & Shewell, C. (1987). Speak and spell: Dissociations and word class effects. In M. Coltheart, G. Santori, & R. Job (Eds.), *The cognitive neuropsychology of language* (pp. 273–294). Hillsdale, NJ: Erlbaum.

Patterson, K., & Wing, A. M. (1989). Processes in handwriting: A case for case. *Cognitive Neuropsychology, 6*, 1–23.

Peniello, M. J., Lambert, J., Eustache, F., Petit-Taboue, M. C., Barre, L., Viader, F., et al. (1995). A PET study of the functional neuroanatomy of writing impairment in Alzheimer's disease: The role of the left supramarginal and angular gyri. *Brain, 118*, 697–707.

Pound, C. (1996). Writing remediation using preserved oral spelling: A case for separate output buffers. *Aphasiology, 10*(3), 283–296.

Ramage, A., Beeson, P. M., & Rapcsak, S. Z. (1998, June). *Dissociation between oral and written spelling: Clinical characteristics and possible mechanisms.* Paper presented at the Clinical Aphasiology Conference, Asheville, NC.

Rapcsak, S. Z. (1997). Disorders of writing. In L. J. Gonzalez Rothi & K. M. Heilman (Eds.), *Apraxia: The neuropsychology of action* (pp. 149–172). Hove, UK: Psychology Press.

Rapcsak, S. Z., & Beeson, P. M. (2000). Agraphia. In S. E. Nadeau, L. J. Gonzalez Rothi, & B. Crosson (Eds.), *Aphasia and language: Theory to practice* (pp. 184–220). New York: Guildford Press.

Rapcsak, S. Z., & Beeson, P. M. (2004). The role of left posterior inferior temporal cortex in spelling. *Neurology, 62*, 2221–2229.

Rapcsak, S. Z., Beeson, P. M., & Rubens, A. B. (1991). Writing with the right hemisphere. *Brain and Language, 41*, 510–530.

Rapp, B., & Gotsch, D. (2001). Spelling disorders: Cognitive theory in clinical practice. In R. S. Bernt (Ed.), *Language and aphasia. Volume 3. Handbook of neuropsychology* (2nd ed., pp. 221–238). Amsterdam: Elsevier.

Rapp, B., & Kane, A. (2002). Remediation of deficits affecting different components of the spelling process. *Aphasiology, 16*(4/5/6), 439–454.

Raymer, A. M., Cudworth, C., & Haley, M. A. (2003). Spelling treatment for an individual with dysgraphia: Analysis of generalization to untrained words. *Aphasiology, 17*, 607–624.

Robson, J., Marshall, J., Chiat, S., & Pring, T. (2001). Enhancing communication in jargon aphasia: A small group study of writing therapy. *International Journal of Communication Disorders, 36*, 471–488.

Robson, J., Pring, T., Marshall, J., Morrison, S., & Chiat, S. (1998). Written communication in undifferentiated jargon aphasia: A therapy study. *International Journal of Language & Communication Disorders, 33*, 305–328.

Roeltgen, D. P. (1985). Agraphia. In K. M. Heilman & E. Valenstein (Eds.), *Clinical neuropsychology* (2nd ed., pp. 75–96). New York: Oxford University Press.

Roeltgen, D. P. (1991). Prospective analysis of writing and spelling. Part II: Results not related to localization. *Journal of Clinical and Experimental Neuropsychology, 13*(1), 48–62.

Roeltgen, D. P. (1993). Agraphia. In K. M. Heilman & E. Valenstein (Eds.), *Clinical neuropsychology* (3rd ed., pp. 63–89). New York: Oxford University Press.

Roeltgen, D. P. (1994). Localization of lesions in agraphia. In A. Kertesz (Ed.), *Localization and neuroimaging in neuropsychology* (pp. 377–406). London: Academic Press.

Roeltgen, D. P., & Heilman, K. M. (1984). Lexical agraphia: Further support for the two system hypothesis of linguistic agraphia. *Brain, 107*, 811–827.

Roeltgen, D. P., Rothi, L. G., & Heilman, K. M. (1986). Linguistic semantic agraphia: A dissociation of the lexical spelling system from semantics. *Brain and Language, 27*, 257–280.

Roeltgen, D. P., Sevush, S., & Heilman, K. M. (1983). Phonological agraphia: Writing by the lexical semantic route. *Neurology, 33*, 755–765.

Rosati, G., & de Bastiani, P. (1981). Pure agraphia: A discreet form of aphasia. *Journal of Neurology, Neurosurgery and Psychiatry, 44*, 266–269.

Rosenbek, J. C., LaPointe, L. L., & Wertz, R. T. (1989). *Aphasia: A clinical approach.* Austin, TX: Pro-Ed.

Salis, C., & Edwards, S. (2010). Treatment of written verb and written sentence production in an individual with aphasia: A clinical study. *Aphasiology, 24*, 1051–1063.

Schomaker, L. R. B., & Van Galen, G. P. (1996). Computer models of handwriting. In T. Dijkstra & K. de Smedt (Eds.), *Computational psycholinguistics* (pp. 386–420). Exeter, UK: Taylor & Francis.

Seitz, R., Canavan, A. G., Yaguez, L., Herzog, H., Tellman, L., Knorr, U., et al. (1997). Representations of graphomotor trajectories in the human parietal cortex: Evidence for control processing and automatic performance. *European Journal of Neurosciences, 9*, 378–389.

Seron, X., Deloche, G., Moulard, G., & Rousselle, M. (1980). A computer based therapy for the treatment of aphasic subjects with writing disorders. *Journal of Speech and Hearing Disorders, 45*, 45–58.

Shallice, T. (1981). Phonological agraphia and the lexical route in writing. *Brain, 104*, 413–429.

Shallice, T. (1988). *From neuropsychology to mental structure.* Cambridge, UK: Cambridge University Press.

Shallice, T. (2000). Cognitive neuropsychology and rehabilitation: Is pessimism justified? *Neuropsychological Rehabilitation, 3*(10), 209–217.

Silveri, M. C., Misciagna, S., Leggio, M. G., & Molinari, M. (1997). Spatial agraphia and cerebellar lesion: A case report. *Neurology, 48*, 1529–1532.

Smyth, M. M., & Silvers, G. (1987). Functions of vision in the control of handwriting. *Acta Psychologica, 65*, 47–64.

Tainturier, M.-J., & Rapp, B. (2001). The spelling process. In B. Rapp (Ed.), *The handbook of cognitive neuropsychology* (pp. 263–290). Philadelphia: Psychology Press.

Thiel, L., Sage, K., & Conroy, P. (2015). Retraining writing for functional purposes: A review of the writing therapy literature. *Aphasiology, 29*(4), 423–441.

Todis, B., Sohlberg, M., Hood, D., & Fickas, S. (2005). Making electronic mail accessible: Perspectives of people with acquired cognitive impairments, caregivers and professionals. *Brain Injury, 19*, 389–401.

Tseng, C. H., & McNeil, M. R. (1997). Nature and management of acquired neurogenic dysgraphias. In L. L. LaPointe (Ed.), *Aphasia and related neurogenic language disorders* (pp. 172–200). New York: Thieme Medical.

Van Galen, G. P. (1991). Handwriting: Issues for a psychomotor theory. *Human Movement Science, 10*, 165–192.

Vernea, J. J., & Merory, J. (1975). Frontal agraphia (including a case report). *Proceedings of the Australian Association of Neurologists, 12*, 93–99.

Watson, R. T., Fleet, W. S., Rothi, L. J., & Heilman, K. M. (1986). Apraxia and the supplementary motor area. *Archives of Neurology, 43*, 787–792.

Watson, R. T., & Heilman, K. M. (1983). Callosal apraxia. *Brain, 106*, 391–404.

Weekes, B., & Coltheart, M. (1996). Surface dyslexia and surface dysgraphia: Treatment studies and their theoretical implications. *Cognitive Neuropsychology, 13*(2), 277–315.

Whitworth, A., Webster, J., & Howard, D. (2005). *A cognitive neuropsychological approach to assessment and intervention in aphasia: A clinician's guide.* Hove, UK: Psychology Press.

World Health Organization (WHO). (2001). *International classification of functioning, disability and health: ICF.* Geneva, Switzerland: Author.

Wright, C. E. (1990). Generalised motor programs: Re-evaluating claims of effector independence in writing. In M. Jeannerod (Ed.), *Attention and performance XXIII* (pp. 294–320). Hillsdale, NJ: Erlbaum.

Disorders of Sentence Processing in Aphasia

Jane Marshall

INTRODUCTION

Fans of Chelsea football club will recall the 2009 match in which Barcelona knocked them out of the Champion's League. The aggrieved London side was convinced that they were victims of several poor decisions by the referee. Here is a quotation from their captain, John Terry:

> People are saying we shouldn't have reacted the way we did but the fact is that six decisions went against us. For the ref not to give one of them is unusual. (Fifield & Lawrence, 2009)

I include this quotation not because I am a Chelsea fan (far from it), but to show how everyone calls on the grammatical devices of their language to convey meaning. Terry builds complex structures and manipulates tense, aspect, and negative morphology to make his points, and all with far less effort than it takes to clear a ball off the line. If these devices were not available to him because of aphasia, there is no doubt that he could get some of his meaning across, particularly his outrage, but the details of his case would be lost.

Let us now turn to Ron, an individual who is in this situation. He is attempting to describe a clip from a Laurel and Hardy film:

> Two men . . . straight [gestures tall person] and then . . . [gestures fat person asleep] then river . . . river and then . . . asleep . . . and then snoozing. And then one . . . bye! [waves] and then . . . [gestures splashing] Oy! and then obviously wet, dripping wet and Ollie [gestures drying] and rip rip [gestures wringing handkerchief] and all right? [gestures thumbs up] . . . all right [gestures moving on] and then river . . . [gestures falling under water] . . . dripping wet and then . . . oh hang on . . . horse or donkey . . . then sit down. (from Cairns, Marshall, Cairns, & Dipper, 2007, p. 126)

Ron conveys a number of the entities involved in the clip (men, river, Ollie, and donkey), mainly by using his relative strength with nouns. He also makes it clear that an outbreak of slapstick has taken place, partly from his adjective phrases (*dripping wet*) and partly from his gestures. Yet, beyond this, it is difficult to determine what has happened. This is partly because of the dearth of verbs, with just two correct verbs contributing to the narrative (*snoozing* and *sit*). Even more critically, his speech lacks structure. So, we are not sure who has fallen into the river, who is doing the drying, or who is sitting down (in fact, Ollie falls in, Stan attempts to dry him with his handkerchief, which he periodically wrings out, and the donkey sits down).

Ron's speech contains few verbs, no word order structure, and practically no grammatical morphology. In other people with aphasia, problems are more selective. So, P.B. in the following quotation uses an impressive array of word and grammatical markers, but has substantial difficulties in composing word order:

> PB: *One woman and a cat is buying the man and paying the money the till.*
> Target: *A woman sells a cat to a man.* (Marshall, Chiat, & Pring, 1997, p. 859)

Such dissociations suggest that aphasia can impair some aspects of sentence processing more than others. They also call for tailored therapies that address the person's specific area of difficulty. This chapter considers three such areas: structure, verb processing, and grammatical morphology. Within each area, different theoretical accounts of the deficit are considered and different therapeutic responses described. The chapter then discusses whether grammatical competence outstrips performance in some people with aphasia and the degree to which this should influence clinical practice. Finally, it describes an approach to therapy that places the focus on conversation.

First, some terms and concepts are introduced.

AGRAMMATISM AND PARAGRAMMATISM

Sentence-level problems in aphasia are often associated with agrammatism. This term is used to describe a constellation of speech symptoms, including omissions of grammatical morphology, simplified syntactic structures, and reduced verb production (see Mitchum & Berndt, 2008). Agrammatism typically occurs in Broca's aphasia, so it is often associated with halting or

speech dyspraxia. Ron in the previous example displays agrammatism.

The problems of agrammatism are rarely confined to production. Many individuals also exhibit difficulties with sentence comprehension, at least when tests require syntactic processing (Caramazza & Zurif, 1976). So, when hearing the sentence "The boy is pushed by the girl," a speaker with agrammatism may be unable to choose between the target picture and its semantic reversal (a boy pushing a girl).

Theories of agrammatism abound. For example, some argue that there is a central syntactic disorder (e.g., Grodzinsky, 2000). Others use differences between speakers to argue that problems arise from various points of failure in a sentence-processing system (Mitchum & Berndt, 2008). A further proposal suggests that syntax is intact but slow to activate in agrammatism, and that many of the observed symptoms are therefore a strategic response to the problem (Kolk, 2006). As discussed in this chapter, all of these theories have influenced therapeutic practice.

The patterns of agrammatism contrast sharply with those of paragrammatism (see Butterworth & Howard, 1987). Here, grammatical elements are present but anomalous. Thus, a key symptom is the substitution, rather than omission, of grammatical morphology. There are also structural errors, some of which seem to reflect the blending of alternative structures, or anomalies arising from lexical errors (see the examples that follow). Paragrammatism typically occurs in cases of fluent aphasia, particularly Wernicke's aphasia. Here are examples of paragrammatic errors (Edwards, 2005, pp. 52 & 48, respectively):

> "I'm very want it" (possibly a blend of "I want it" and "I'm very keen on it")
> "I know it but I just can't sentence it" (possibly a lexical substitution of sentence for say)

There are competing views about the origins of paragrammatism. Butterworth and Howard (1987) argue that syntax is present but poorly controlled. One consequence of this is the generation of multiple syntactic options for each utterance, leading to blend errors. An alternative view states that patterns in agrammatism and paragrammatism are often more similar than different, and that speakers with paragrammatism have impaired access to syntactic processes (Edwards, 2005). This suggests that, as with the nonfluent speakers, we need to understand the individual processing difficulties of people with paragrammatism to arrive at a therapeutic response.

SENTENCE COMPLEXITY

It is reasonable to assume that sentence difficulties in aphasia will be affected by complexity. However, what constitutes complexity is not obvious. Take the following sentences:

1. The enormous snarling dog bit the harmless little cat.
2. The cat was bitten.

Sentence 1 is obviously longer and more elaborate than 2. Yet, is it more complex? First, the elaboration may support comprehension ("snarling" animals are much more likely to bite than "harmless" ones). Second, sentence 2 is a passive, that is, the object noun phrase has been moved from its canonical position after the verb to the start of the sentence. There is good evidence that people with aphasia pay a heavy price for argument movement of this kind, even with sentences that look deceptively simple (Bastiaanse & van Zonneveld, 2005; McAllister, Bachrach, Waters, Michaud, & Caplan, 2009). Indeed, some theories of agrammatism argue that difficulties with phrase movement are a critical symptom of the disorder (Grodzinsky, 2000). As described further in this chapter, specific therapy approaches have been developed to address the problem.

A SENTENCE-PROCESSING MODEL

The production model of Garrett (1988) has provided a framework for many sentence-level therapies in aphasia (and see Levelt, 1999, for a similar model). This model assumes that sentence production entails a number of processing levels or stages (Figure 12.1). The first generates the message or conceptual form of the sentence. Here, the speaker decides what to say. Garrett considered this level of processing to be nonlinguistic, although this view is not shared by Levelt (1989; also see arguments that follow).

The functional level creates the predicate argument structure. Here, the speaker must select a verb that maps onto the message content together with its argument structure. So, for example, the verb *give* specifies a three-place argument structure, allowing the roles of agent (the giver), theme (the object that changes hands), and goal (the recipient of the transaction) to be expressed. The noun representations are also accessed and assigned to the verb argument slots. Note that at this stage the spoken (or written) forms of words are not specified. Thus, the model assumes two stages of lexical access, with semantic/syntactic processing preceding phonological processing.

With the predicate argument structure in place, the speaker is ready to construct the surface form of the sentence. This occurs at the positional level. Here, the phrase structure of the sentence is specified and the phonologies of words retrieved. With the phrase structure comes the grammatical morphology, such as noun determiners and verb endings. Finally, phonetic encoding prepares the sentence for articulation.

This sentence-processing model encouraged clinicians to look below the surface symptoms displayed by speakers with aphasia and to consider the underlying reason for those symptoms. They particularly stimulated the view that early stages of processing may be breaking down and so need assistance in therapy.

STRUCTURAL IMPAIRMENTS

Conceptual Processing

A number of clinicians and researchers have suggested that aphasic problems in building structure may arise in the early conceptual processes of message generation (Dipper, Black, & Bryan, 2005; Marshall, 2009; Marshall

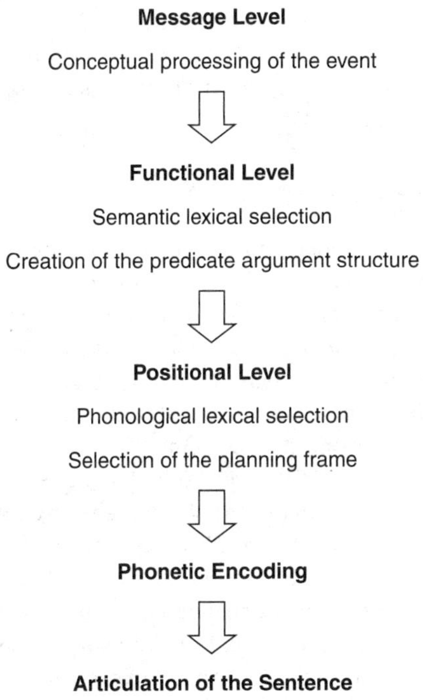

Message Level

Conceptual processing of the event

Functional Level

Semantic lexical selection

Creation of the predicate argument structure

Positional Level

Phonological lexical selection

Selection of the planning frame

Phonetic Encoding

Articulation of the Sentence

Figure 12.1 A model of sentence production.

Modified from Garrett, 1988. Processes in language production. In F. J. Newmeyer (Ed.), *Linguistics: The Cambridge survey: 111. Language: Psychological and biological aspects.* Cambridge, UK: Cambridge University Press.

& Cairns, 2005; Marshall, Pring, & Chiat, 1993). Part of their argument rests with the complexity of these processes. For example, when describing an event, the speaker has to determine the main entities involved and their respective roles. A number of perspective decisions also have to be made, for example, about which aspects of the event are to be given prominence in the description and which left out. Time and aspect are also marked in terms of whether the event is past, current, or ongoing.

Such decisions must be linguistically sensitive. In other words, the speaker has to construct a message that can be mapped onto the language that he or she plans to use. Time information is a good example here, in that this has to be specified if the speaker's language employs tense, but can be omitted if not. We can further illustrate the point by considering cross-linguistic differences in verb meanings. Take the English and British Sign Language (BSL) verbs for cutting events. English verbs typically focus on effect, as in *cleave*, *slice*, and *trim*. In contrast, BSL verbs place greater emphasis on manner, particularly on the instrument used. So, BSL employs a different verb to describe cutting with a knife as opposed to cutting with scissors. We can assume, therefore, that users of English and BSL have to construct rather different conceptual messages to access their "cutting" verbs. The English user will foreground the consequence of the event, while the BSL user must focus more on how it was carried out (for further arguments, see Dipper et al., 2005, and Marshall, 2009).

Assessing the Problem

If verb and sentence production depend on specialized, linguistically sensitive cognition, this could be a source of difficulty in aphasia. To investigate this possibility, there are a number of nonverbal tasks that require the person to make judgments about events, examples being the Event Perception Test (Marshall, Chiat, & Pring, 1999), the Kissing and Dancing Test (Bak & Hodges, 2003), and the Role Video (Marshall et al., 1993). In the last task, the person tested sees a video clip of an action and has to select a photo illustrating the outcome. For example, one film shows a woman setting fire to a box, and the photos show a burned box, a burned newspaper, and a torn-up box. Half the items in the test entail events with two people, with the hypothesis that these place a greater demand on role processing. So, one such item involves a man splashing a woman, with the photos showing the woman soaking wet (target), the woman with a black eye (event distractor), and the man soaking wet (role distractor). To succeed with these items, the person tested has to be clear not only about the nature of the event, but also about who played which role. If the person is not, he or she is in danger of selecting the role distractor. This was exactly the pattern shown by M.M., the person investigated by Marshall et al. (1993, and see Case Illustration 12.1).

Patterns of naming can offer further insights. The clinician might ask the client to describe action pictures and note which items are named and in what order. A tendency to name items that are peripheral to the main event might be a signal that message-level processing is breaking down. This was the pattern shown by M.M. (Marshall et al., 1993). For example, she mentioned items of clothing worn by the people in the picture and component parts of objects, rather than the main argument nouns. She also produced more of these augmentative nouns than unimpaired controls on the same task.

The study by Cairns et al. (2007) suggests that naming order is also informative. Cairns et al. worked with Ron, introduced at the start of this chapter. He and a group of healthy controls were shown action pictures involving people and objects. For example, one picture showed a cowboy cutting a cake with a sword. The nouns in the pictures were carefully matched for frequency and familiarity, and their images were balanced for size and page position. So, in half the items the person in the role of agent appeared on the left of the picture, and in half he or she appeared on the right. The task in this experiment was not to describe the picture. Rather participants were simply asked to name what they could see. The researchers were interested in the number of entities named and their order, with the supposition that this would illuminate participants' perspective on the event.

Controls behaved in a consistent manner. They typically named only the three key entities in the event and in a preferred order. Most controls started with the agent, then named the theme, and finally the instrument. So, a typical response to our example picture was *cowboy*, *cake*, and *sword*. Ron differed from the controls in two ways. First, he named more items, with a mean score of 4.93 nouns per picture, compared to 3.01 for the controls. Second, his order of naming was much less consistent. Like the controls, he tended to start with the agent noun but was much more likely to name the instrument or a peripheral noun ahead of the theme.

In interpreting these findings, the authors suggest that patterns of naming in the controls reflected their organized perspective on the event. They were clearly homing in on the main entities and had uncovered their roles, given that these determined the order of naming. Although

Ron was clearly still perceiving agency, in other respects his naming seemed less driven by a structured representation of the event. He was not isolating the key argument nouns from more peripheral entities and was less focused on role dynamics than the controls.

Therapy at the Level of the Event

It seemed that both M.M. and Ron struggled to generate focused and organized conceptual representations. Helping them to do so should therefore provide a platform for improved linguistic structure in their output.

Cairns (2006) provided this help by using perspective cues. A small group of people with aphasia, including Ron, was asked to access verbs in response to video clips of reverse role events. These were selected to pose a perspective dilemma. For example, one video showed a woman chasing a man, which can either be described from the woman's point of view (using verbs like *chase* and *pursue*) or the man's (using verbs like *flee* or *run away*).

Two types of cue were provided. One was a pure perspective cue. Here, the events were filmed in such a way that one participant was clearly highlighted more than the other. So, the chasing event might be shown with a strong focus on the woman. The other type of cue was "perspective plus language." The perspective films here were re-presented together with a sentence completion cue. For example, the person saw the film in which the woman chaser is strongly focused and heard "Sharon (bleep) Paul." These cued conditions were compared to a neutral condition, in which the event was shown without highlighting one or other of the participants and without a language cue.

Cairns (2006) hypothesized that verb production would increase when perspective cues were available. This was indeed the case. The effect, however, was small and only significant when the filming manipulation was combined with a language cue. It seemed that participants needed maximal help to organize their focus and so access the verb lexicon.

In the Cairns study, participants were provided only once with a perspective and language cues. It seems reasonable to suppose that more marked effects would emerge from a therapy program targeting event processing. Marshall et al. (1993) attempted such a program with M.M.; it is described in Case Illustration 12.1. Encouragingly, this did improve verb argument structure in her output and in ways that made a difference to observers. However, gains were only evident in picture description tasks and not in more spontaneous conditions, such as narrative and conversation.

Case Illustration 12.1: Therapy at the Level of the Event

M.M. had chronic aphasia following a left hemisphere stroke in her 50s. She had severely agrammatic speech, with no word order structure and barely any verbs. Here are some examples:

"Mother's day . . . er Nicola . . . meals . . . flowers . . . chocolates" (describing her weekend)
"Woman . . . books . . . duster . . . blue . . . shoes" (describing a picture of a woman dusting books)

M.M. had good comprehension of concrete nouns but poor understanding of verbs and sentences. She also made errors on two nonverbal tests of event conceptualization, the Event Perception Test and the Role Video. The researchers concluded that M.M. had a verb impairment that was underpinned by difficulty in processing events. It seemed that M.M. was unable to make the crucial focus and role decisions required for verb selection and the expression of verb argument relationships.

Therapy aimed to help M.M. make decisions about events, such as what is the main event, who or what is involved, and what role they are playing in the event. It was hypothesized that improved event processing would stimulate the production of verbs and verb argument structure. Twelve hours of therapy were delivered over 4 weeks.

The therapy stimuli consised of 18 video-recorded events. These were presented in a hierarchy:

Level 1: people acting on objects (e.g., a man ironing a shirt)
Level 2: instruments acting on objects (e.g., a hammer breaking a cup)
Level 3: interactive events involving two people (e.g., a woman punching a man)

(continues)

M.M. watched each event and was asked to make a series of decisions about them. These were to identify the agent (e.g., she was asked: "Who is in charge of the action?"); to identify the theme/patient ("Which object was changed by the event?"); and to identify the nature of the action. Associated photographs helped M.M. signal her decisions. For example, she indicated the nature of the action by selecting an appropriate outcome photo (e.g., an ironed rather than a torn shirt). Following these stages, M.M. was asked to access a verb that could describe the event. If necessary, she was provided written verb options for selection.

After therapy, M.M. scored at ceiling on the Event Perception Test and Role Video. A picture description task also showed improved verb access, more word order structure, and a greater tendency to name argument rather than peripheral nouns. These changes made M.M.'s production more comprehensible to observers. Less optimistically, M.M.'s production only improved when describing two-argument events, such as a woman driving a car (this was the type of event worked on in therapy). She was no better with three-argument events, such as a man giving flowers to a woman. There were also no changes in an open narrative task.

Adapted from Marshall, J., Pring, T., & Chiat, S. (1993). Sentence processing therapy: Working at the level of the event. *Aphasiology, 7*, 177–199.

Building the Predicate Argument Structure

The examples of aphasic speech at the start of this chapter showed that sentence disorders often compromise word order. In Ron's speech, word order is almost completely lacking, while in P.B.'s it is anomalous.

Two seminal papers in the 1980s explored the word-order problem in agrammatic aphasia. One showed that whether or not sentence word order could be produced depended critically on who or what was involved (Saffran, Schwartz, & Marin, 1980). When describing events in which people acted on objects, the participants with agrammatism achieved a high level of success. However, when the event involved two people or an object acting on a person, production disintegrated. The parallel study showed that there were equivalent problems in understanding word order (Schwartz, Saffran, & Marin, 1980). This showed that comprehension of even simple reversible sentences, which contain two nouns that could plausibly act as agent, was poor. So, when hearing the sentence "The man kisses the woman," participants might point to a picture in which a woman kisses a man.

Why was word order breaking down? The researchers were able to dismiss conceptual-level difficulties because the participants were able to act out their understanding of the events. Rather, they suggested that the problem lay with computing the first level of linguistic structure, which specifies the meaning relations of the sentence. In terms of Garrett's model (see Figure 12.1), these speakers were failing to generate the predicate argument structure at the functional level and therefore were not mapping this onto the surface form of the sentence. As a result, they had no principle mechanism for composing (or understanding) word order. Their few successes, for example, in describing events in which people acted on things, probably arose from the normal tendency to mention people first.

Assessing the Problem

Problems with predicate argument structure are signaled by reduced or anomalous word order in output. This can be examined by using picture description tasks. Useful examples are the Test of Thematic Role Production in Aphasia (Whitworth, 1996), the Sentence Production Test for Aphasia (Wilshire, Lukkien, & Burmester, 2014) and the Verb and Sentence Test (VAST; Bastiaanse, Edwards, & Rispens, 2002). The last includes a sentence anagram task, which investigates whether the client can order sentence fragments to describe a picture. The client can also be asked to retell a familiar story so that phrase structure can be analyzed (see protocol in Berndt, Wayland, Rochon, Saffran, & Schwartz, 2000).

Sentence-to-picture matching tasks can be used to explore the understanding of word order. These must include semantically reversible sentences, which demand syntactic processing, and should probe a range of syntactic structures. Examples are available in the Psycholinguistic Assessments of Language Processing in Aphasia (PALPA; Kay, Lesser, & Coltheart, 1992) and the VAST (Bastiaanse et al., 2002).

Therapy for Problems With Word Order

Sentence generation might be addressed using the Sentence Production Program for Aphasia (SPPA;

Helm-Estabrooks & Nicholas, 2000). This practices eight different sentence structures in a hierarchy of difficulty. Target sentences are embedded in a brief narrative context. This context is read to the participant, and the target sentence is modeled. The participant is then invited to repeat the target in response to a question. At the next level of difficulty, the target is not modeled. Rather, it has to be produced purely from the context and the question. SPPA is based on the Helm Elicited Language Program for Syntax Stimulation (HELPSS). Evaluations of HELLPS have shown successful training of target sentence structures, with generalization to untrained exemplars (e.g., Doyle, Goldstein, & Bourgeois, 1987; Fink et al., 1995; Helm-Estabrooks & Ramsberger, 1986). Gains on measures of connected speech, however, are not always achieved (see Doyle et al., 1987).

An alternative approach to sentence building is mapping therapy. This helps clients to delineate the meaning relationships of sentences and express those relationships through the surface form, particularly in terms of word order. Thus, the therapy requires the person to think about the roles in any event being described and where these roles are positioned in the sentence.

There are several variants of mapping therapy. Some use mainly comprehension tasks, such as matching spoken reversible sentences to pictures (Berndt & Mitchum 1998; Mitchum, Haendiges, & Berndt, 1995). Another variant involves unpicking the meaning relations of given written sentences (Jones, 1986; Schwartz, Saffran, Fink, Myers, & Martin, 1994). Here, the person has to mark the constituents in sentences and point to those constituents in response to questions from the therapist. For example, with the sentence, "The man next door is washing his car," the client may be asked to mark and point to the subject noun phrase in response to the question: "Who is washing the car?"

Other therapies place greater emphasis on production by helping the person to compose word order to describe pictured events (Carragher, Sage, & Conroy, 2015; Harris, Olson, & Humphreys, 2012; Marshall et al., 1997; Nickels, Byng, & Black, 1991; Rochon, Laird, Bose, & Scofield, 2005). Case Illustration 12.2 describes one of these approaches.

Perhaps the most novel account of mapping therapy used the participant's intact mathematical abilities to scaffold his understanding of language (Byrne & Varley, 2011). A series of therapy steps encouraged the participant, S.O., to draw analogies between mathematical and verbal expressions. For example, one stage aimed to underscore the importance of the verb by likening it to the operator in a mathematical expression. In this stage, S.O. was presented with mathematical problems that were missing the operator, such as: $3\_4 = 7$ and $3\_4 = -1$. The missing operators were associated with verbs with positive (e.g., *drinks* for +) or negative connotations (e.g., *spills* for –). The complete mathematical expressions were then associated with complete sentences. So, $3 + 4 = 7$ was associated with "The lady drinks the wine," while $3 - 4 = -1$ was associated with "The woman spills the wine." A later stage employed reversed mathematical expressions (such as $10 - 2 = \_$; $2 - 10 = \_$) to illustrate how word order expresses reversible linguistic relations.

There is a reasonable evidence base for mapping therapy, drawn from both single-case (Berndt & Mitchum 1998; Byng, 1988; Byng, Nickels, & Black, 1994; Harris et al., 2012; Jones, 1986; Le Dorze, Jacob, & Coderre, 1991; Marshall et al., 1997; Mitchum, Greenwald, & Berndt, 1997; Nickels et al., 1991) and small-group studies (Carragher et al., 2015; Fink, Schwartz, & Myers, 1998; Rochon et al., 2005; Schwartz et al., 1994; see also reviews in Marshall, 1995, and Mitchum, Greenwald, & Berndt, 2000). All studies show good posttherapy acquisition of treated sentence types, even when tested with novel exemplars. For example, after therapy A.E.R. (see Case Illustration 12.2) demonstrated improved production and comprehension of two argument sentences, which was the type worked on in the treatment, and Rochon et al. (2005) brought about improvements with passives.

The case for more widespread effects from mapping therapy is less clear cut. For example, in most studies generalization into untreated sentence types is either absent (e.g., Fink et al., 1998) or inconsistent (e.g., Rochon et al., 2005; Schwartz et al., 1994). This point is illustrated by comparing outcomes with P.B. (Marshall et al., 1997) and A.E.R. (Nickels et al., 1991). P.B. worked on three-argument verbs that express change of possession (such as lend/borrow) and communication (such as teach/learn). After therapy, his descriptions of these event types improved (as measured in a picture description task), despite no changes with two-argument structures. A.E.R., in contrast, did improve with two-argument structures having addressed these in therapy, while remaining completely unable to combine three arguments with a verb.

A further question is whether there are cross-modality benefits, for example, where comprehension therapy improves production. Early mapping papers (Byng, 1988; Jones, 1986) suggested that there might be. However, these findings were not consistently replicated in later studies. For example, Berndt and Mitchum (1998) and Rochon et al. (2005) did not achieve generalization, although Harris et al. (2012) did.

Finally, and critically, is the question of whether the benefits of mapping therapy extend beyond clinical tests into everyday language. A number of studies demonstrate change on spoken narratives following therapy, for example, with respect to structural complexity or the realization of grammatical morphology(e.g., Byng, 1988; Nickels et al., 1991; Rochon et al., 2005; Schwartz et al., 1994). Carragher and colleagues (Carragher et al., 2015) also examined the realization of verbs in conversational speech. Disappointingly, there were no changes across the group ($N = 9$) following therapy, although three participants demonstrated individual improvements.

Case Illustration 12.2: Mapping Therapy With A.E.R.

A.E.R. had chronic aphasia following a left hemisphere stroke. His speech was severely agrammatic, with few verbs, virtually no structure, and limited grammatical morphology. This fragment from his retelling of Cinderella is typical:

"the aunties is ball … and (10 seconds) the maid is (7 seconds) … no"

Although lexical comprehension was good, A.E.R.'s understanding of even simple sentences was poor. When tested, his errors typically involved selecting the reversal distractor. With "the queen splashes the nun," he might point to the picture of the nun splashing the queen. Nickels and colleagues concluded that A.E.R. could not relate sentence word order to meaning; that is, he had a mapping problem.

The first stage of their mapping therapy used a comprehension task. A.E.R. was shown two related action pictures. For example, one pair showed a robber writing a letter and a monk writing a letter. He was provided with four sentence fragments, written on separate cards: "the robber," "the monk," "the letter," "writes." These were initially color coded, with nouns in red and the verb in green. He was also given a sentence frame, consisting of two horizontal red lines separated by a horizontal green line. A.E.R.'s task was to select a picture and then construct a sentence to describe it using the given sentence fragments and cue frame. Once this was achieved, he was asked to change the sentence to describe the other picture. Feedback emphasized how the sentence word order related to meaning. For the example, the therapist would point out that the pictures had different agents, so required different first sentence nouns. Therapy progressed through several stages; for example, different parts of the sentences were contrasted, and reversible sentences were introduced.

The next stage moved into production. Here, A.E.R. was asked to describe the pictures verbally, using the color-coded sentence frame as a cue. Typically, he would produce the sentence nouns first, in which case the therapist would ask him to indicate where in the sentence frame these should be located. The verb was then either provided for him or elicited via phonological cues. As in the previous example, feedback emphasized the implications of word order, and therapy progressed through different sentence types. In a final stage, A.E.R. was encouraged to generate sentences to describe personally relevant materials, such as family photographs, and to describe events in his own life.

Production was evaluated by asking A.E.R. to tell a story before and after therapy and via an action picture description task. After therapy, A.E.R. produced more verb argument structure and fewer isolated noun phrases on these tasks. He also showed improvement on a sentence-to-picture matching test, but only with the type of sentence (agentive subject-verb-object [SVO]) worked on in therapy.

Sources: Adapted from Nickels, L., Byng, S., & Black, M. (1991). Sentence processing deficits: A replication of treatment. *British Journal of Disorders of Communication, 26,* 175–199; and Byng, S., Nickels, L., & Black, M. (1994). Replicating therapy for mapping deficits in agrammatism: Re-mapping the deficit? *Aphasiology, 8*(4), 315–341.

Dealing With Complex Structures

Mapping between the predicate argument structure and surface form of the sentence varies in complexity. Canonical SVO sentences are relatively straightforward because they obey simple correspondence rules, such as "name the agent first." However, as described at the start of this chapter, this is not the case for more complex forms, like passives, which entail argument movement.

Assessing the Problem

A number of tasks can be used to explore the impact of sentence complexity. Clinicians can analyze production elicited through picture description and narrative to determine the range of structures in the person's output. If moved argument structures are not used spontaneously, attempts can be made to elicit them. For example, the clinician can present an action picture and ask the client to start a description with the theme rather than the agent. The picture might show a boy kicking a ball, and the clinician asks the client to describe it starting with "the ball." The VAST (Bastiaanse et al., 2002) has sentence anagram tasks that can be used to explore skills with passive and question forms.

The Northwestern Assessment of Verbs and Sentences (NAVS; Thompson, 2011; Cho-Reyes & Thompson, 2012) includes a Sentence Production Priming Test. This elicits three canonical and three noncanonical sentence types, ranging in complexity from simple actives ("The dog is chasing the cat") to object relative clauses ("Pete saw the dog who the cat is chasing"). The test employs black-and-white drawings of paired reversible events. For example, one plate shows a drawing of a cat chasing a dog and one of a dog chasing a cat. The examiner describes one drawing with a sentence prime ("The dog is chased by the cat"). The person being tested is then required to describe the other drawing using the same sentence structure.

Turning to input, sentence comprehension tests can be used to compare understanding of simple and moved argument forms. Examples are available in the PALPA (Kay et al., 1992) and VAST (Bastiaanse et al., 2002). The NAVS (Thompson, 2011) includes a sentence-to-picture matching task, which assesses the same range of sentence types that are explored in production.

Therapy for Complex Structures

Clients who can manage simple, but not complex, forms may benefit from the Treatment of Underlying Forms (TUF) (Thompson, 2008). This has been applied to a range of structures, including wh- questions, clefts, and passives (see example sentences that follow). The therapy starts with an active sentence that, through a series of stages, is transformed into the target structure. The client is then invited to repeat the transformation independently and practice producing the spoken form following a prime from the therapist (see Case Illustration 12.3 for a fuller account).

Example Sentences:

1. The boy pinched the teacher. (Active)
2. Who did the boy pinch? (Object question, involves wh- movement)
3. It was the teacher who the boy pinched. (Object cleft, involves wh- movement)
4. The teacher was pinched by the boy. (Passive, involves NP- movement)
5. The parent saw the teacher who the boy pinched. (Object relative clause structure with wh- movement)

The effectiveness of TUF has been explored in a number of single-case and small-group studies (Ballard & Thompson, 1999; Jacobs & Thompson, 2000; Thompson, Shapiro, et al., 1997; Thompson, Shapiro, & Roberts, 1993; Thompson, Shapiro, Tait, Jacobs, & Schneider, 1996). All achieved good outcomes for treated structures and some generalization to untreated ones. Generalization only occurred to structures that were linguistically similar to the treated forms. For example, treatment using object cleft structures improved production of object wh- questions because these involve similar syntactic operations, but not passives, which involve a different type of movement (Thompson, Shapiro, et al., 1997). Generalization was also most likely from complex-to-simple forms (Thompson & Shapiro, 2007; Thompson, Shapiro, Kiran, & Sobecks, 2003). So, treating complex sentences like Sentence 5 has been shown to benefit simpler related structures like Sentences 2 and 3, but not the other way round. One study showed that computerized delivery of TUF is as effective as clinician-delivered therapy and elicits similar patterns of generalization (Thompson, Choy, Holland, & Cole, 2010).

The complex structures treated in TUF may not seem obvious targets for aphasia therapy, especially if the person is struggling to express basic verb argument relationships. Is there any evidence, therefore, that TUF improves everyday language? In several of the studies, pre- and posttherapy discourse samples were collected and analyzed, with some encouraging changes (see Thompson & Shapiro, 2007). For example, Thompson et al. (1996) found more verbs and better use of verb argument structure in the posttherapy samples. Participants also became more ambitious, in that they produced more complex sentence forms and more verbs combined with sentence complements. Ballard and Thompson (1999) explored the communicative value of such changes. They found that discourse became more informative and coherent after therapy, although not for all participants.

Finally, it is important to know whether TUF benefits both production and comprehension. Jacobs and Thompson (2000) examined this and found that both modalities could be trained. There was also some cross-modal generalization in that therapy working on comprehension helped production. Comprehension gains are not only of theoretical interest but also are functionally desirable because people with aphasia can choose to edit complex forms from their own output but cannot necessarily edit them from the language of others.

Case Illustration 12.3: TUF Treatment Protocol for Training Object wh- Questions

Step 1: Thematic role training

The person with aphasia is shown a picture of a semantically reversible event, such as a boy kissing a girl. The corresponding sentence is also presented, on separate cards, for example:

[THE BOY] [IS] [KISSING] [THE GIRL]
Additional cards [WHO] and [?] are put next to the picture.

The therapist identifies the roles of the sentence constituents in the following manner: "This is kissing [*pointing to the verb*]; it is the action of the sentence. This is the boy [*pointing to the subject*]; he is the person doing the kissing. And this is the girl [*pointing to the object*]; she is the person being kissed." The client is then asked to identify the sentence roles in response to questions from the therapist and to read or repeat the sentence again.

Step 2: Sentence building

The therapist explains that they are going to turn the original sentence into a question. The object noun phrase [THE GIRL] is replaced by [WHO]. The therapist explains that this is done because the girl is *who* is kissed. The question mark is put at the end of the sentence, and the therapist explains that this is necessary to show that the new sentence is a question. The person with aphasia now sees:

[THE BOY] [IS] [KISSING] [WHO] [?]

Finally, the therapist demonstrates subject auxiliary verb inversion and shows that the [WHO] card has to be moved to the start of the sentence, resulting in the final question form. The person with aphasia reads or repeats the question.

Step 3: Thematic role training

The therapist explains that the roles in the sentence are the same as in the old one. The client is asked to point to and name each constituent, for example: "Show me the action."

Step 4: Practice

The cards are arranged back into the original active sentence. The client is asked to transform it into a question, with support as required from the therapist.

Source: Adapted from Thompson, C. (2008). Treatment of syntactic and morphological deficits in agrammatic aphasia. Treatment of underlying forms. In R. Chapey (Ed.), *Language intervention strategies in aphasia and related neurogenic communication disorders* (5th ed., pp. 735–754). Baltimore: Lippincott Williams and Wilkins.

VERB IMPAIRMENTS

Models like those of Garrett and Levelt place a heavy burden of responsibility on the verb. Once the verb is selected, its syntactic properties become available. These specify the phrase structures that can be combined with it and indicates where, in the structures, the message roles should be located. To exemplify, *give* specifies a three-place argument structure (agent/theme/goal) with the following phrase options:

> NP (agent) V NP (theme) PP (goal) as in:
> The man gives the money to the boy.
> NP (agent) V NP (goal) NP (theme) as in:
> The man gives the boy the money.

Failure to access verbs will therefore, deprive the speaker of many of the resources that he or she needs to build sentences.

There is good evidence that many people with aphasia are particularly poor at retrieving verbs. For example, they omit verbs from their spontaneous speech and name object pictures significantly better than action pictures (see reviews in Conroy, Sage, & Lambon Ralph, 2006; Druks, 2002; Marshall, 2003). Such problems are often (although not always) associated with nonfluent and agrammatic forms of aphasia (Luzzatti et al., 2001).

Difficulties with verbs may be selective. Verbs that combine with several arguments are often particularly hard to produce (e.g., Cho-Reyes & Thompson, 2012; Dragoy & Bastiaanse, 2010). Thus, *give* (a three-argument verb) may be more problematic than *laugh* (a one-argument verb). Whether or not a verb has optional argument structures may also be important. For example, the verb *deliver* can be produced with two arguments ("The postman delivered the letter") or with three ("The postman delivered the letter to the house"). Such multiple structural options may add to the complexity of verb processing (Thompson, Lange, Schneider, & Shapiro, 1997), although not in all cases (Kim & Thompson, 2000). Unaccusative verbs, such as *bloom* can also be particularly difficult for speakers with agrammatism (Thompson, 2003; Thompson & Lee, 2009). It is thought that this is because the theme (rather than the agent) of these verbs is mapped onto the subject noun phrase ("The flower [THEME] bloomed").

Reasons for verb impairments are probably various. In some cases, they may be due to syntactic problems, which inhibit processing of syntactically elaborated lexical representations. In line with this, Kemmerer (2000) shows that the grammatical properties of verbs may be particularly inaccessible in cases of verb impairment.

In other cases, problems may relate more to meaning. Put most simply, verb impairments may reflect impaired access to action knowledge, a view that is supported by the observed overlap between the neural regions involved in action and verb processing (Kemmerer, Gonzalez Castillo, Talavage, Patterson, & Wiley, 2008; Pulvermuller, 2005). We also know that verbs as a class are less imageable than nouns, which may account for their vulnerability (Bird, Howard, & Franklin, 2003). More subtly, verbs package meaning differently from nouns. Concrete nouns typically refer to unitary, stand-alone objects, examples being *table, car,* and *anaconda*. Verbs, in contrast, express a particular focus on an action. So (i) in Figure 12.2 could be described as *lifting, carrying,* or *holding*, depending on the speaker's perspective.

The dilemma becomes even greater when more information enters the scene. Thus, the introduction of the truck in image (ii) (Figure 12.2) licenses numerous other

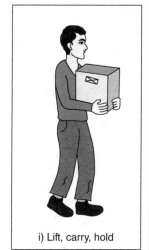

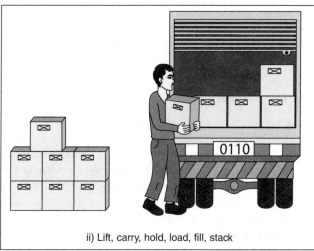

i) Lift, carry, hold

ii) Lift, carry, hold, load, fill, stack

Figure 12.2

contenders, such as *load*, *fill*, and *stack*. For reasons such as these, Black and Chiat (2000, 2003) argue that the "tightness of fit" between verbs and their referents is low, much lower than for nouns. Of course, this is particularly true for verbs that take multiple arguments.

The lack of one-to-one mapping between verbs and their referents suggests that their production entails considerable cognitive mediation. If semantic or event processing are impaired, such mediation will be compromised. It may also be impaired by executive problems, which affect cognitive organization and planning. Indeed, it has been shown that verb impairments can arise in cases of frontotemporal dementia associated with executive disorders (Silveri, Salvigni, Cappa, Della Vedova, & Puopolo, 2003). Furthermore, easing the executive demands of the task (e.g., by changing the stimuli) can facilitate verb production in these cases (D'Honincthun & Pillon 2005).

Assessing the Problem

An obvious sign of a verb impairment is the omission of verbs in spontaneous or elicited speech (see Ron's sample at the start of this chapter). Comparing the number of nouns and verbs in a conversational or narrative sample is therefore a good place to start (Berndt et al., 2000, give control data). Picture description and naming tasks can be used to elicit verbs. The Object and Action Naming Battery (Druks & Masterson, 2000) provides matched sets of nouns and verbs, so that naming can be compared across classes. The VAST (Bastiaanse et al., 2002) contains a verb-naming task and a sentence completion task eliciting inflected and uninflected verbs. The NAVS (Thompson, 2011) includes a verb-naming test that contrasts production of one, two, and three argument verbs. Verb comprehension can be tested in isolation by asking the person to match a spoken verb to an action picture. Tasks are available in the VAST (Bastiaanse et al., 2002) and the NAVS (Thompson, 2011).

Therapy for Verb Impairments

If verbs are impaired, they are a worthy target for intervention. A lack of verbs debars expression of a range of events and situations. It also severely limits sentence construction, not only because all sentences have to have a verb, but also because verbs provide much of the material needed for sentence generation.

A number of studies have attempted to improve verb retrieval using naming therapy approaches, similar to those developed for nouns (e.g., Carragher, Sage, &

Conroy, 2013; Edwards & Tucker, 2006; Edwards, Tucker, & McCann, 2004; Marshall, Pring, & Chiat, 1998; McCann & Doleman, 2011; Mitchum & Berndt, 1994; Raymer & Ellsworth, 2002; Wambaugh, Doyle, Martinez, & Kalinyak-Fliszar, 2002; Wambaugh & Ferguson, 2007). Tasks included word-to-picture matching, forming semantic associations with target verbs, semantic feature analysis, picture naming in response to semantic or phonological cues, naming to definition, repetition, and sentence completion. In a fairly recent addition to the literature, such tasks were delivered in an errorless paradigm (Conroy, Sage, & Lambon Ralph, 2009a), whereby maximal cues ensured a high degree of success during therapy.

Outcomes from these studies typically show that naming of treated verbs improved posttherapy, but with limited or no generalization to untreated verbs (see review in Webster & Whitworth, 2012). Associated gains in sentence production and spontaneous speech vary both within and across studies (and are not always assessed). For example, one of the three people treated by Edwards and Tucker (2006) improved significantly on sentence production, while the two others did not. Carragher and colleagues (2013) examined the effect of therapy on spontaneous speech by calculating the proportion of verbs produced in samples of conversation. This measure identified positive change in only three of the nine participants. Studies comparing different tasks and approaches reported no clear advantage for one over the other. For example, Raymer and Ellsworth (2002) found that semantic cueing, phonological cueing, and simple repetition were equally effective in improving verb naming and the use of treated verbs in sentences. Similarly, Conroy et al. (2009a) found that outcomes from errorful and errorless approaches were equivalent.

Several studies incorporated gesture tasks in therapy (Boo & Rose, 2011; Carragher et al., 2013; Pashek, 1998; Rodriguez, Raymer, & Gonzalez Rothi, 2006; Rose & Sussmilch, 2008). For example, the "gesture-only" treatment used by Boo and Rose (2011) provided the participant with a model gesture for a target verb alongside the spoken word. He was then invited to repeat the word and gesture three times. Those who employed gesture therapy hypothesized that gestures facilitate access to the semantic features of verbs, possibly by recruiting the neural networks involved in actions. In line with this view, Pashek (1998) found that verb naming was indeed helped by a therapy combining verbal and gestural cues, more so than when verbal cues were used alone. However, subsequent studies did not demonstrate a clear advantage for gesture therapy over other approaches. For example, both participants in the study of Boo and Rose

(2011) benefited from a combined gesture and semantic therapy but were equally helped by the contrastive therapies that omitted gesture.

Further verb therapy approaches place greater emphasis on the role of the verb in a sentence. Such programs either avoid naming tasks altogether (Bastiaanse, Hurkmans, & Links, 2006; Links, Hurkmans, & Bastiaanse, 2010) or extend them into sentence production (Webster, Morris, & Franklin, 2005). The Bastiaanse et al. (2006) study required participants to carry out sentence completion tasks with either an infinitive or finite (inflected) verb,[1] and then produce full sentences in response to pictures. Outcomes were measured with a sentence completion task like that used in therapy, although with different verbs. Both participants showed improved production of finite verbs on this task. Encouragingly, they also performed better on a test of everyday language, suggesting that treatment gains had generalized beyond the clinical setting. Webster et al. (2005) used three components to therapy: semantically based naming tasks, identifying arguments in action pictures, and building sentences from provided verbs. The authors argue that therapy improved verb naming and sentence production. Gains were evident not only on constrained tests, but also on a narrative discourse task.

Conroy and colleagues (Conroy, Sage, & Lambon Ralph, 2009b) compared the treatment of verbs in a sentence context with a single-word condition. Therapy used decreasing cues, which minimized errors during the therapy task, while maintaining effort. In the word condition, these progressed from repeating verbs to naming them in response to decreasing phonological cues. Verb production was also required in the sentence condition, but the cues were embedded within a sentence. Seven people received therapy, with broadly similar results. Production of treated verbs improved, while untreated controls remained virtually unchanged. There was no advantage for sentence over word therapy. Indeed, word therapy achieved marginally greater gains.

Verb network strengthening treatment (VNeST) targets the retrieval of verbs within sentences, specifically by focusing on their thematic roles (Edmonds, Nadeau, & Kiran, 2009). In the first two steps of therapy, participants are given a written verb and asked to generate at least three agents and three patients that can combine with that verb. For example, for the verb *measure,* they might offer *chef, carpenter*, and *mechanic* as agents and *sugar, lumber*, and *bumper* as corresponding patients. In these stages, participants are cued with "who" and "what" cards. They are also provided with written options for selection if they are unable to generate nouns themselves. The third step uses questions to extend the verb associations. For example, the participant might be asked "When does a chef measure sugar?" or "Why?" The fourth step offers written sentences for semantic judgment, half of which contain inappropriate arguments ("The snake carries the papers"). Finally, participants are asked to generate agents and patients again, but without the cue cards.

Evaluations of VNeST (Edmonds & Babb, 2011; Edmonds et al., 2009) have demonstrated improved production of nouns and verbs in sentences, with generalizations to untreated stimuli. Gains in connected speech (e.g., elicited via complex picture description) were also evident, although not in all participants. Recent studies have reported the successful combination of VNeST with group therapy (Hoover, Caplan, Waters, & Budson, 2015) and computer administration of the protocol (Furnas & Edmonds, 2014).

The reviewed studies indicate that practicing verbs in therapy will typically improve their retrieval. Some studies also report generalization to untreated verbs. However, this is by no means the case for all, making the selection of useful and relevant therapy stimuli essential. Improved verb access is often accompanied by improved sentence production. But, this does not always occur and is not measured in all studies. As yet, it is not possible to determine the most effective verb therapy technique. Gains have been reported from a range of approaches, and when therapies have been compared, no clear winner has emerged. Of course, it is likely that different treatment approaches will benefit different individuals, depending on the nature of their problem. However, the basis on which to make such selections remains unclear. Further comparisons between treatment approaches, particularly exploring issues of candidacy, are needed. Thompson and Shapiro (2007) have also argued that therapy working on complex verbs should be explored, as this may promote generalization beyond the treatment targets.

IMPAIRMENTS WITH GRAMMATICAL MORPHOLOGY

Many speakers with aphasia make errors with both free-standing and bound grammatical morphology. So, they often omit "little words," like auxiliaries, and strip content words of their inflections. In some cases, speech is totally devoid of syntactic markers. In others, the problems are selective, with the common finding that verb morphology is more impaired than noun (e.g., Faroqi-Shah & Thompson 2004). Within the category of verb inflections, tense is often particularly vulnerable (Arabatzi & Edwards 2002; Stavrakaki & Kouvava 2003), resulting in substitutions of verb forms or (in English) overuse of the progressive –ing. These patterns are illustrated by the following examples:

> *"this guy … he sleep."*
> *"And then … asleep . . . and then snoozing."*
> *(Both extracts from Cairns, 2006)*

The origin of tense impairments is disputed. One debate centers on the issue of regularity. Ullman and colleagues (1997, 2005) found that irregular inflections, such as *bought*, were more likely to be realized in agrammatism than regular ones, such as walk*ed*. This was interpreted within the dual-route theory of morphology. Under this account, regular inflections are attached to the stem by rule-based operations, whereas irregular forms are encoded, as a whole, within the lexicon. The dissociation reflects damage to the affixing operations, with relatively intact lexical access.

One problem for this view is that not all studies find the regular/irregular dissociation (Bird, Lambon Ralph, Seidenberg, McCleland, & Patterson, 2003; Faroqi-Shah & Thompson, 2007). Indeed, in the preceding samples, *sleep* is not inflected for past tense, despite being an irregular verb. Some authors (Bird, Lambon Ralph, et al., 2003; Braber, Patterson, Ellis, & Lambon Ralph, 2005) also made the point that regular tense forms are typically more phonologically complex than irregular ones; for example, they often entail an additional syllable or final consonant cluster. So, when regular forms *are* impaired, it could be their phonology that causes the problem.

An alternative proposal, put forward by Faroqi-Shah and Thompson (2007), suggests that speakers with agrammatism are unable to map the semantic specification of tense, developed during conceptual processing, onto the required verb form. Their evidence is derived from sentence completion tasks, showing that participants with aphasia struggled to select verb forms that were compatible with a given temporal marker. Here is an example:

> Yesterday I _____ a suitcase
> (Response options: *will carry, was carrying, is carried*)

Strikingly, the same participants coped much better when completion simply required compliance with local syntactic constraints. Here is an example of this type of task:

> The man was _____ the Canadian border.
> (Response options: *cross, crosses, crossing*)

It seems that these participants still knew the grammatical well-formedness rules for tense. But, integrating this knowledge with meaning was a step too far (Faroqi-Shah & Thompson, 2007).

Whatever the theory, an obvious question is the degree to which morphological impairments affect communication. Take the following extracts from D.O.R., a speaker with aphasia studied by Druks and Carroll (2005):

> *"Maybe two or three weeks time go abroad."*
> *"Tuesday is hoovering and dusting."*

Despite being unable to manipulate tense, D.O.R. conveyed time information successfully in these samples by using temporal words and phrases. It is clear that the first utterance relates to a future event and the second to habitual, and hence, present tense activities. On the face of it, this speaker is not paying a high price for his tense impairment. However, this may be understating the case. D.O.R. produced few verbs in connected speech, far fewer than nouns and other word classes. Interestingly, this discrepancy was much less evident in single-word tasks, where he was required simply to name objects and actions. Taking this evidence, the authors argued that D.O.R.'s tense impairment lay at the heart of his verb deficit. Stripped of tense, verbs had lost their grammatical status. Thus, they could still be employed to some extent in naming, but not in connected speech. It seemed, therefore, that a relatively "pure" problem with tense had far-reaching ramifications for D.O.R.'s entire verb system.

Assessing the Problem

Analyses of conversation, narrative, and picture description samples may point to a problem with grammatical morphology. For example, the therapist might find that few verbs are correctly inflected (see procedure in Berndt et al., 2000).

Tense can be explored through informal sentence completion tasks, by which the person has to select a correctly inflected verb to complete a sentence (see previous examples). Time sequence action pictures can also be used to elicit tensed verbs. For example, one set might show a man entering a shop, buying a newspaper, and leaving the shop ("He is going to buy a paper"; "He is buying a paper"; "He bought a paper"). Judgment tasks, in which the client has to detect morphological anomalies in given sentences, can explore skills on input.

Assessment should consider the degree to which any morphological problem impairs communication and, therefore, whether this is a priority for therapy. Following Druks and Carroll (2005), the therapist may hypothesize that restoration of tense could lead to improved verb use and verb argument structure, with consequent benefits for communication. Tense may also be a target for a client with high-level language abilities who needs grammatically correct language to resume work or education.

Therapy for Tense

Mitchum and Berndt (1994) present an early example of therapy for tense. M.L. had disordered sentence production with frequent verb omissions. An initial program of verb therapy brought about naming gains with verbs, but no benefits for connected speech or sentence production. The authors hypothesized that M.L. could not exploit his improved verb access because of an additional problem in accessing the grammatical elements of the verb phrase. The second therapy program aimed to remediate this problem, specifically by working on tense.

The therapy task involved ordering triads of time-sequenced pictures, showing events that were about to happen, happening, and just completed. M.L. was then asked to describe each picture using tensed sentences. Consistent time cues were provided. So, for the future events, the therapist might say, "The man is *about to* do something," and for past events, "He has *already* done this." Other cues involved reminding M.L. to use tense morphology and chaining progressive parts of the target sentence, such as "The man has … " or "The man is … ."

After therapy, M.L. was more able to use tensed sentences in picture description. This improvement generalized to verbs that had not featured in therapy, including irregular ones. There were also more widespread benefits for sentence production in terms of semantic and syntactic integrity.

Faroqi-Shah (2008) tested two therapy approaches for tense deficits. One, termed *morphophonological treatment*, involved repeated input and output practice with inflected forms, but with minimal emphasis on meaning. The input tasks included auditory discrimination of inflected verbs ("Do these words sound the same: *washes, washed*?") and lexical decision with legal and illegal verb forms (*washed* versus *digged*). Output tasks included being asked to generate as many inflected forms as possible from a given verb and transformation tasks, for example, where a given present tense verb had to be changed to past tense.

This therapy was contrasted with morphosemantic treatment, which placed a far greater emphasis on meaning. Example input tasks included judging sentence anomalies, such as "Yesterday the boy will wash his hands," and comprehension tasks in which a given sentence had to be matched to one of three pictures on the basis of tense. Production tasks entailed completing or ordering appropriately tensed sentences to describe a given picture.

Four participants were randomly assigned to the two treatment conditions. Results for the morphophonological treatment were disappointing, in that participants were no better at using tense morphology after therapy than before. Furthermore, when affixes were produced, they were often anomalous, as illustrated by the following example:

> Target: The lady will peel the potatoes.
> "Tomorrow … the … he peeled. She is peeling."

Results from the morphosemantic treatment were much more encouraging, with gains both in the number and the accuracy of inflections used. Two participants also showed generalization to both regular and irregular verbs, regardless of which type was treated.

A recent study again used morphosemantic therapy to promote tense marking in six people with agrammatic aphasia (Faroqi-Shah, 2013). Three participants received training on regular verbs, such as rake (*rake → raked*), and three were trained on irregular verbs, such as drink (*drink → drank*). Theory suggests that tense processing with irregular verbs entails default affixation with the regular ending (-ed), which is then blocked in favor of the correct, lexically specified form. The author therefore hypothesized that training with irregular forms might promote generalization to regularly tensed verbs, whereas the reverse was not anticipated. Results were broadly in line with this hypothesis. All participants improved on trained verbs. There was also encouraging generalization to untrained regular verbs, regardless of whether regular or irregular verbs were treated in therapy. Generalization to untrained irregular verbs, however, was poor, even in the participants who were trained on irregular stimuli.

The final study reviewed in this section incorporated tense exercises into a mapping therapy program (Harris et al., 2012). The participant had to describe reversible pictures, such as "a boy following a dog," using both active and passive sentences. He also had to answer questions about the thematic roles in the pictures. Tense practice was elicited by asking him to describe the events as if they happened yesterday. Following therapy, there were improvements in both sentence and tense production. There was also generalization of tense marking to untreated regular and irregular verbs. Interestingly, the latter was confined to verbs that came from the same quasi-regular cluster. So, training on *catch-caught* and *fight-fought* stimulated generalization to *think-thought* and *bring-brought*.

The studies reviewed in this section suggest that therapy can improve tense marking in people with agrammatic aphasia, with some generalization to untrained verbs. It is also clear that therapy should emphasize the meaning of tense markers as well as their form. The results offer some pointers with respect to therapy stimuli. It seems that irregular tense marking needs to be specifically addressed in therapy. Indeed, work with irregular verbs may bring about generalized skills, even with regular affixation. Treating verbs from quasi-regular clusters (*keep-kept*; *sleep-slept*; *creep-crept*) is also advocated.

COMPETENCE VERSUS PERFORMANCE

There is evidence that many speakers with agrammatism are less impaired than they seem. In other words, they possess grammatical competences that are only revealed by certain tests. An early indication of this was the finding that people with agrammatism could carry out sentence judgment tasks, which required them to detect grammatical violations in spoken sentences (Linebarger, Schwartz, & Saffran, 1983). Further evidence came from the results of priming. Hartsuiker and Kolk (1998) tested 12 people with agrammatism in three conditions: spontaneous speech, picture description, and picture description with priming. In the last condition, participants were first asked to repeat a sentence and then describe a picture. So, they might be asked to repeat, "The speaker is interrupted by the noise,"[2] and then describe a picture in which a golfer is struck by lightning. Normal language users typically show priming effects in this task: They describe the picture with a sentence that is syntactically similar to the prime. This was also true of the speakers with agrammatism. Most strikingly, the priming condition elicited complex forms that were rarely, if ever, observed in their spontaneous output. So, for example, seven of those tested produced passives. It seemed that the assistance provided by the prime exposed skills that would otherwise never see the light of day.

Such findings have generated the view that there is not a syntactic deficit in agrammatism after all (see Kolk, 2006, 2008). Rather, these speakers are wrestling with a timing problem, whereby their syntactic knowledge is slow to activate and subject to abnormal levels of decay. Their observed symptoms, such as the use of simplified structures and omissions of grammatical morphology, are adaptive responses to this problem; that is, these speakers are using elliptical forms that can be handled within a short temporal window.

Implications for Assessment

The hypothesis that competence may outstrip performance in agrammatic aphasia has important implications for assessment. It suggests that we need to employ testing that can expose latent skills, judgment and priming tasks being obvious candidates. For example, the therapist may ask the client to repeat a given sentence before attempting a picture description task to see if this primes production. It is also important to note the degree to which clients can be cued. For example, the clinician may note that sentence production improves if the client is cued with the first word or provided with the verb. Both these findings may point to important latent skills.

The VAST (Bastiaanse et al., 2002) contains a useful array of tasks to explore sentence production, including sentence anagrams. These may reveal word order skills that are masked in more demanding tasks, like picture description.

Implications for Therapy

If agrammatic symptoms are strategic adaptations to a problem, we need to be cautious about attacking those symptoms in therapy. In other words, the investment required to improve one aspect of sentence production may be so great that another is bound to suffer. Springer, Huber, Schlenck, and Schlenck (2000) adopt this view. Like Kolk, they saw the telegrammatic utterances of agrammatism as a strategic response to a deficit. Their Reduced Syntax Therapy (REST) therefore aimed to maximize rather than eliminate this strategy. In this approach, patients were encouraged to produce word order structures of increasing length, while being discouraged from producing morphosyntactic elements, such as verb endings and noun determiners. Minimalism and economy of effort were actively promoted, as this dialogue from the therapy exemplifies:

> *Therapist: Imagine there was an accident and you want to send a telegram, but you do not have the money to pay for a long message. You can only choose three words. What has happened? Listen to the story: On a skiing holiday, your friend Monica has broken her leg, and her mother must be informed as soon as possible. You have only enough money for three words. What three words would you use? . . . Can you tell me the three words? (Springer et al., 2000, p. 295).*

Eleven people with long-standing agrammatism were provided with 30 hours of REST, with positive outcomes for nine. After therapy, these individuals displayed expanded word order structures and increased verb use in their spontaneous speech. Surprisingly, four also showed an increase in the number of closed-class words (such as auxiliaries and determiners) despite the fact that these were discouraged by the treatment. Four of the improving patients were assessed again at least 10 months after the end of therapy; encouragingly, three were still showing significant benefits. A subsequent study involving Dutch speakers (Ruiter, Kolk, & Rietveld, 2010) reported similarly positive results from REST.

Linebarger and colleagues also believe that competence outstrips performance in people with aphasia and have developed a computer therapy aid that aims to expose their latent skills (e.g., Linebarger, Schwartz, Romania, Kohn, & Stephens, 2000). This aid, termed the *SentenceShaper*, removes all time pressure over production and allows the person to generate and elaborate on output through processes of experimentation, trial, and error. The aid has a number of key features:

- It records and stores fragments of speech produced by the person with aphasia and replays these when an icon is clicked.
- It allows the person to assemble passages of connected speech by ordering the recorded fragments (ordering is accomplished by dragging the icons into slots in a given frame).
- It provides lexical support through side buttons; by clicking on these, the person with aphasia can access a number of prerecorded high-frequency verbs and prepositions, with the selection customized by the clinician.
- Above all, the system offers a medium for self-directed and independent practice.

A series of studies has shown that SentenceShaper improves the grammatical integrity (Linebarger et al., 2000; Linebarger, McCall, & Berndt, 2004) and informativeness (Bartlett, Fink, Schwartz, & Linebarger, 2007) of aided production in speakers with aphasia. Importantly, gains have also been observed in unaided production (Linebarger, McCall, Virata, & Berndt, 2007), suggesting that practice with SentenceShaper brings about durable changes in sentence performance. There is also evidence that the aid can be combined with therapist input to target specific structures and so improve the quality and complexity of output (McCall, Virata, Linebarger, & Berndt, 2009).

The developers of SentenceShaper have produced a handheld version of the device, called *SentenceShaper To Go*. This can be preprogrammed with spoken messages that have been composed using the SentenceShaper software, which can be played during communicative interactions. There is preliminary evidence that dialogues supported by SentenceShaper To Go are more informative than unaided production (Linebarger, Romania, Fink, Bartlett, & Schwartz, 2008). Users also responded positively to the device and could perceive applications for it

in their everyday lives (True, Bartlett, Fink, Linebarger, & Schwartz, 2010).

AGRAMMATISM AND CONVERSATION

The therapy approaches described in this chapter are all supported by some evidence of clinical effectiveness, albeit often from single-case or small-group studies. Therapy benefits are typically revealed by clinical language tests, such as picture description or sentence-to-picture matching tasks. Generalization to more functional uses of language is varyingly assessed and less often demonstrated. In particular, few studies have explored the impact of therapy on conversation (see arguments in Beeke, Maxim, Best, & Cooper, 2011, and Carragher et al., 2015).

Investigations based on conversation analysis have suggested that the utterances produced in conversation by speakers with agrammatism are qualitatively different from the utterances produced in formal assessment tasks (Beeke, Maxim, & Wilkinson, 2007; Beeke, Wilkinson, & Maxim, 2003). It is argued that some speakers employ a "conversational grammar." This consists of systematic combinations of content words, time markers, reported speech, and gesture to communicate key concepts. Beeke et al. (2011, p. 223) cited the following example: "June, three-tier wedding cake, I make it." Here, a temporal marker ("June") is combined with a noun phrase ("three-tier wedding cake") and a comment ("I make it") to convey a planned future event. The authors suggest that such topic comment structures are typically employed in agrammatic conversation to signal a change of subject, whereas, an alternative form (adjective + because + reason) is preferred for the communication of an opinion.

A number of therapy proposals flow from these observations. If agrammatic conversation has its own conventions for building structure, therapy working on formal sentence skills may not readily generalize to that context. Rather, Beeke et al. (2011) suggest that therapy should directly target the "grammar of conversation" (p. 224). This approach takes naturally occurring and unconstrained conversational data as its starting point. Videos of conversation are viewed and discussed by the therapist, client, and conversational partner. Together, they identify strategies that are employed by the person with aphasia to convey meaning and consider additional strategies that could be employed. The behaviors of the conversational partner are also analyzed to reveal those that do (and do not) facilitate successful turns. Such analyses generate a number of therapy objectives, for both the client and the conversation partner. For example, the client might aim to make more use of alternative communication modalities, such as writing and drawing, or target increased use of key words. The partner might aim to check more often whether a turn is complete or use additional methods to seek clarification. Barrier behaviors, which obstruct conversation, are also identified for reduction. Therapy sessions then practice conversations, using the target strategies, with feedback from the therapist. This approach exemplifies the psychosocial therapy focus on environmental factors according to the International Classification of Functioning, Disability, and Health (World Health Organization, 2001).

A recent project attempted this therapy with 10 couples (Beeke et al., 2011). Rather than seeking change on formal language tests, the researchers examined change in conversation. In particular, they hoped that therapy would reduce the number of incomplete turns on the part of the person with aphasia and lessen the need for repair from the partner. Quantifiable data were also collected with respect to the number of facilitative and nonfacilitative (barrier) behaviors observed before and after therapy. Outcomes varied; however, reports from some of the participants showed that both conversational partners were able to adopt at least some of the strategies targeted in therapy, with benefits for the construction of turns in conversation (Beeke et al., 2014, 2015).

CONCLUSIONS AND FUTURE DIRECTIONS

This review considered a range of approaches to sentence therapy in aphasia. These target several aspects of production, including the conceptual preparations for language, building the predicate argument structure, generating complex forms, verb access, and morphology. It has also considered the proposal that there are concealed grammatical competences in aphasia that can be revealed through therapeutic aids, such as Sentence Shaper.

For the clinical practitioner, selecting between the various treatment approaches is not easy and is not helped by the obvious contradictions in the literature. Take the very different views of Springer et al. (2000) and Thompson and Shapiro (2007). According to Springer et al., the syntactic omissions in agrammatism reflect a strategic response to the deficit, one that should be harnessed in therapy. Thus, treatment aims to reduce complexity in output by eliminating grammatical morphology, in the hope that this would release resources for word order. Thompson and Shapiro (2007), in contrast,

specifically champion complexity, with the argument that therapy targeting complex forms is most likely to achieve generalization.

How can the seeming contradictions be reconciled? In the lexical domain, there have been similar debates about therapy content, with numerous approaches evaluated (e.g., see Nickels, 2002). It has been argued, however, that some of the differences between these approaches are more apparent than real, and that all essentially target the mapping of meaning onto form (Howard, 2000).

Problems in mapping between meaning and form may also lie at the heart of sentence impairments in aphasia. However, here the challenges are far greater than in single-word production. The meanings that are mapped onto verbs and sentences are complex and relational. They also have to be shaped into a form that is compatible with language. The target words and structures are similarly demanding. Verbs have more multidimensional representations than nouns and have to be combined with word order and morphology to construct sentences. Elaborated language, for example, with moved arguments or embedded clauses, raises the bar further, not only because the forms themselves are more complex but also because the mappings between those forms and meaning are more opaque.

Following this line, it could be argued that all the reviewed sentence therapies essentially help with this core problem of mapping meaning onto form. Progressing through the production stages, some help the person to package meaning appropriately for language by working at the conceptual level. Others help the person relate that meaning to a target verb or word order structure. In the case of the treatment devised by Faroqi-Shah (2008), therapy pays attention to the features of meaning that are mapped onto morphological aspects. Therapy has also exploited strategic devices that assist mapping, SentenceShaper being an excellent example. Finally, conversation analysis has been used to explore the transmission of meaning during interaction.

A proposed route into therapy, therefore, starts with the following question: What meaning(s) does the person want to express, and what happens when he or she attempts to map those meanings onto form? Put differently, to what extent can he or she convey the target meanings during communication exchanges? Observation and assessment attempt to pin down the problem. The person may, for example, show problems of conceptual focus, with disorganized naming and poor event judgments. He or she may be unable to access the verbs needed or combine those verbs with structure. The individual may be unable to convey time or aspect, with morphological omissions or substitutions. A further issue is whether the person, or people in the environment, could make better use of strategies to overcome the problems. For example, partners could ask homing-in questions that scaffold structure or help the person focus on the meanings that he or she wants to express (see Worrall, 2008, for strategic approaches). Therapy selection is then driven by the principle of semantic dividend. In effect, the therapist targets skills that will make the greatest difference to communication. Given the interconnectedness of sentences, this may involve work at multiple levels of processing.

This proposal by no means solves the therapy dilemma. It does, however, place the focus squarely on meaning. As proposed by Beeke et al. (2011), it also pays attention to the person's use of language, not only as a desired generalization from therapy but also as its starting point. Finally, it clarifies the therapy goal, which is to expand the meanings that the person can convey. To date, most therapy studies have aimed to show an increased use of the target forms, be they verbs, verb argument structures, or morphology. Ideally, such an increase is shown not only in clinical elicitation tasks, but also in more naturalistic language. Just as crucially, however, we need to explore the communicative consequences of these gains. This requires a different approach to outcome measurement, for example, by using conversational and interactive tasks. Although such measures were featured in some studies (e.g., Ballard & Thompson, 1999; Carragher et al., 2015; Hoover et al., 2015), they need to become the norm.

STUDY QUESTIONS

1. A man with aphasia produces almost no verbs in spontaneous speech and names objects much more successfully than actions. Consider all the reasons why this may be so.

2. On hearing the sentence "The man is chasing the woman," a man with aphasia points to a picture of a woman chasing a man. Why might he make this error? How would you explore the different possibilities?

3. A therapist notices that almost all the verbs produced by a client with aphasia are uninflected.

How could she explore this pattern further? What factors should she take into account when deciding whether to treat the morphological impairment?

4. How could you explore whether a client has latent or concealed grammatical skills?

5. A client with agrammatic aphasia reports feeling excluded in conversation (e.g., because he cannot ask questions or get his ideas across). What strategies could a therapist promote to improve his participation in conversation?

NOTES

1. Therapy exploited two structural options in Dutch: verb final constructs using infinite verbs or verb medial constructs with finite verbs.

2. This is an English translation of the Dutch sentence used in the experiment.

REFERENCES

Arabatzi, M., & Edwards, S. (2002). Tense and syntactic processes in agrammatic aphasia. *Brain and Language, 80,* 314–327.

Bak, T., & Hodges, J. (2003). Kissing and dancing—a test to distinguish lexical and conceptual contributions to noun/verb and action/object dissociation: Preliminary results in patients with frontotemporal dementia. *Journal of Neurolinguistics, 16,* 169–181.

Ballard, K., & Thompson, C. (1999). Treatment and generalisation of complex sentence production in agrammatism. *Journal of Speech, Language and Hearing Research, 42,* 690–707.

Bartlett, M., Fink, R., Schwartz, M., & Linebarger, M. (2007). Informativeness ratings of messages created on an AAC processing prosthesis. *Aphasiology, 21*(5), 475–498.

Bastiaanse, R., Edwards, S., & Rispens, J. (2002). *The Verb and Sentence Test.* Bury St Edmunds, UK: Thames Valley Test.

Bastiaanse, R., Hurkmans, J., & Links, P. (2006). The training of verb production in Broca's aphasia: A multiple baseline across behaviours study. *Aphasiology, 20*(2/3/4), 298–311.

Bastiaanse, R., & van Zonneveld, R. (2005). Sentence production with verbs of alternating transitivity in agrammatic Broca's aphasia. *Journal of Neurolinguistics, 18,* 57–66.

Beeke, S., Beckley, F., Johnson, F., Heilemann, C., Edwards, S., Maxim, J., et al. (2015). Conversation focused aphasia therapy: Investigating the adoption of strategies by people with agrammatism. *Aphasiology, 29*(3), 355–377.

Beeke, S., Johnson, F., Beckley, F., Heilemann, C., Edwards, S., Maxim, J., et al. (2014). Enabling better conversations between a man with aphasia and his conversation partner: Incorporating writing into turn taking. *Research on Language and Social Interaction, 47*(3), 292–305.

Beeke, S., Maxim, J., Best, W., & Cooper, F. (2011). Redesigning therapy for agrammatism: Initial findings from the ongoing evaluation of a conversation based intervention study. *Journal of Neurolinguistics, 24*, 222–236.

Beeke, S., Maxim, J., & Wilkinson, R. (2007). Using conversation analysis to assess and treat people with aphasia. *Seminars in Speech and Language, 28*(2)136–147.

Beeke, S., Wilkinson, R., & Maxim, J. (2003). Exploring aphasic grammar 2: Do language testing and conversation tell a similar story? *Clinical Linguistics and Phonetics, 17*, 109–134.

Berndt, R., & Mitchum, C. (1998). An experimental treatment of sentence comprehension. In N. Helm-Estabrooks & A. Holland (Eds.), *Approaches to the treatment of aphasia* (pp. 91–112). San Diego, CA: Singular.

Berndt, R., Wayland, S., Rochon, E., Saffran, E., & Schwartz, M. (2000). *Quantitative production analysis.* Hove, UK: Psychology Press.

Bird, H., Howard, D., & Franklin, S. (2003). Verbs and nouns: The importance of being imageable. *Journal of Neurolinguistics, 16*, 113–149.

Bird, H., Lambon Ralph, M., Seidenberg, M., McCleland, J., & Patterson, K. (2003). Deficits in phonology and past tense morphology: What's the connection? *Journal of Memory and Language, 48*(3), 502–526.

Black, M., & Chiat, S. (2000). Putting thoughts into verbs: Developmental and acquired impairments. In W. Best, K. Bryan, and J. Maxim (Eds.), *Semantic processing: Theory and practice* (pp. 52–79). London: Whurr.

Black, M., & Chiat, S. (2003). Noun-verb dissociations: A multifaceted phenomenon. *Journal of Neurolinguistics, 16*, 231–250.

Boo, M., & Rose, M. (2011). The efficacy of repetition, semantic, and gesture treatments for verb retrieval and use in Broca's aphasia. *Aphasiology, 25*(2), 154–175.

Braber, N., Patterson, K., Ellis, A., & Lambon Ralph, M. (2005). The relationship between phonological and morphological deficits in Broca's aphasia: Further evidence from errors in verb inflection. *Brain and Language, 92*, 278–287.

Butterworth, B., & Howard, D. (1987). Paragrammatism. *Cognition, 26*, 1–37.

Byng, S. (1988). Sentence processing deficits: Theory and therapy. *Cognitive Neuropsychology, 5*(6), 629–676.

Byng, S., Nickels, L., & Black, M. (1994). Replicating therapy for mapping deficits in agrammatism: Re-mapping the deficit? *Aphasiology, 8*(4), 315–341.

Byrne, C., & Varley, R. (2011). From mathematics to language: A novel intervention for sentence comprehension difficulties in aphasia. *Journal of Neurolinguistics, 24*, 173–182.

Cairns, D. (2006). *Processing events: Investigating event conceptualisation in aphasia.* Unpublished doctoral dissertation, City University, London.

Cairns, D., Marshall, J., Cairns, P., & Dipper, L. (2007). Event processing through naming: Investigating event processing in people with aphasia. *Language and Cognitive Processes, 22*, 210–233.

Caramazza, A., & Zurif, E. (1976). Dissociation of algorithmic and heuristic processes in language comprehension: Evidence from aphasia. *Brain and Language, 3*, 572–582.

Carragher, M., Sage, K., & Conroy, P. (2013). The effects of verb retrieval therapy for people with non-fluent aphasia: Evidence from assessment tasks and conversation. *Neuropsychological Rehabilitation, 23*(6), 846–887.

Carragher, M., Sage, K., & Conroy, P. (2015). Outcomes of treatment targeting syntax production in people with Broca's type aphasia: Evidence from psycholinguistic therapy tasks and everyday conversation. *International Journal of Language and Communication Disorders, 50*(3), 322–336

Cho-Reyes, S., & Thompson, C. (2012). Verb and sentence production and comprehension in aphasia: Northwestern Assessment of Verbs and Sentences (NAVS). *Aphasiology, 26*(10), 1250–1277.

Conroy, P., Sage, K., & Lambon Ralph, M. (2006). Towards theory driven therapies for aphasic verb impairments: A review of current theory and practice. *Aphasiology, 20*(12), 1159–1185.

Conroy, P., Sage, K., & Lambon Ralph, M. (2009a). The effects of decreasing and increasing cue therapy on improving naming speed and accuracy for verbs and nouns in aphasia. *Aphasiology, 23*(6), 707–730.

Conroy, P., Sage, K., & Lambon Ralph, M. (2009b). A comparison of word versus sentence cues as therapy for verb naming in aphasia. *Aphasiology, 23*(4) 462–482.

D'Honincthun, P., & Pillon, A. (2005). Why verbs could be more demanding of executive resources than nouns: Insight from a case study of a fv-FTV patient. *Brain and Language, 95*, 36–37

Dipper, L. T., Black, M., & Bryan, K. L. (2005). Thinking for speaking and thinking for listening: The interaction of thought and language in typical and non-fluent comprehension and production. *Language and Cognitive Processes, 20*(3), 417–441.

Doyle, P. J., Goldstein, H., & Bourgeois, M. S. (1987). Experimental analysis of acquisition and generalization of syntax in Broca's aphasia: A generalization and social validation study. *Journal of Speech and Hearing Disorders, 52*, 143–155.

Dragoy, O., & Bastiaanse, R. (2010). Verb production and word order in Russian agrammatic speakers. *Aphasiology, 24*, 28–55.

Druks, J. (2002). Verbs and nouns–A review of the literature. *Journal of Neurolinguistics, 15*(3–5), 289–315.

Druks, J., & Carroll, E. (2005). The crucial role of tense for verb production. *Brain and Language, 94*, 1–18.

Druks, J., & Masterson, J. (2000). *An object and action naming battery.* Hove, UK: Psychology Press.

Edmonds, L., & Babb, M. (2011). Effect of verb network strengthening treatment in moderate-to-severe aphasia. *American Journal of Speech Language Pathology, 20*, 131–145.

Edmonds, L., Nadeau, S., & Kiran, S. (2009). Effect of Verb Network Strengthening Treatment (VNeST) on lexical retrieval of content words in sentences in persons with aphasia. *Aphasiology, 23*, 402–424.

Edwards, S. (2005). *Fluent aphasia.* Cambridge, UK: Cambridge University Press.

Edwards, S., & Tucker, K. (2006). Verb retrieval in fluent aphasia: A clinical study. *Aphasiology, 20*(7), 644–675.

Edwards, S., Tucker, K., & McCann, C. (2004). The contribution of verb retrieval to sentence construction: A clinical study. *Brain and Language, 91*, 78–79.

Faroqi-Shah, Y. (2008). A comparison of two theoretically driven treatments for verb inflection deficits in aphasia. *Neuropsychologia, 46*, 3088–3100.

Faroqi-Shah, Y. (2013). Selective treatment of regular versus irregular verbs in agrammatic aphasia: Efficacy data. *Aphasiology, 27*(6), 678–705.

Faroqi-Shah, Y., & Thompson, C. (2004). Semantic, lexical and phonological influences on the production of verb inflections in agrammatic aphasia. *Brain and Language, 89*, 484–498

Faroqi-Shah, Y., & Thompson, C. (2007). Verb inflections in agrammatic aphasia: Encoding of tense features. *Journal of Memory and Language, 56*, 129–151.

Fifield, D., & Lawrence, A. (2009, May 7). Chelsea rage at referee for not giving them four penalties. *The Guardian*, Sport, p. 1.

Fink, R. B., Schwartz, M., & Myers, J. (1998). Investigations of the sentence query approach to mapping therapy. *Brain and Language, 65*, 203–207.

Fink, R. B., Schwartz, M. F., Rochon, E., Myers, J. L., Socolof, G. S., & Bluestone, R. (1995). Syntax stimulation revisited: An analysis of generalization of treatment effect. *American Journal of Speech Language Pathology, 4*, 99–104.

Furnas, D., & Edmonds, L. (2014). The effect of computerised Verb Network Strengthening Treatment on lexical retrieval in aphasia. *Aphasiology, 28*(4), 401–420.

Garrett, M. (1988). Processes in language production. In F. J. Newmeyer (Ed.), *Linguistics: The Cambridge Survey: 111. Language psychological and biological aspects.* (pp 69–98) Cambridge, UK: Cambridge University Press.

Grodzinsky, Y. (2000). The neurology of syntax: Language use without Broca's area. *Behavioural and Brain Sciences, 23*, 1–21.

Harris, L., Olson, A., & Humphreys, G. (2012). Rehabilitation of past tense verb production and non-canonical sentence production in left inferior frontal non-fluent aphasia. *Aphasiology, 26*(2), 143–161.

Hartsuiker, R., & Kolk, H. (1998). Syntactic facilitation in agrammatic sentence production. *Brain and Language, 62*, 221–254.

Helm-Estabrooks, N., & Nicholas, M. (2000). *Sentence production program for aphasia.* Austin, TX: Pro-Ed.

Helm-Estabrooks, N., & Ramsberger, G. (1986). Treatment of agrammatism in long-term Broca's aphasia. *British Journal of Disorders of Communication, 21*, 39–45.

Hoover, E., Caplan, D., Waters, G., & Budson, A. (2015). Effects of impairment-based individual and socially oriented group therapies on verb production in aphasia. *Aphasiology, 29*(7), 781–798

Howard, D. (2000). Cognitive neuropsychology and aphasia therapy: The case of word retrieval. In I. Papathanasiou (Ed.), *Acquired neurogenic communication disorders* (pp. 76–99). London: Whurr.

Jacobs, B., & Thompson, C. (2000). Cross-modal generalization effects of training noncanonical sentence comprehension and production in agrammatic aphasia. *Journal of Speech, Language and Hearing Research, 43*, 5–20.

Jones, E. (1986). Building the foundations of sentence production in a non-fluent aphasic. *British Journal of Disorders of Communication, 21*, 63–82.

Kay, J., Lesser, R., & Coltheart, M. (1992). *Psycholinguistic Assessments of Language Processing in Aphasia (PALPA).* Hove, UK: Erlbaum.

Kemmerer, D. (2000). Grammatically relevant and grammatically irrelevant features of verb meaning can be independently impaired. *Aphasiology, 14*(10), 997–1020.

Kemmerer, D., Gonzalez Castillo, J., Talavage, T., Patterson, S., & Wiley, C. (2008). Neuroanatomical distribution of five semantic components of verbs: Evidence from fMRI. *Brain and Language, 107*, 16–43.

Kim, M., & Thompson, C. (2000). Patterns of comprehension and production of nouns and verbs in agrammatism, Implications for lexical organisation. *Brain and Language, 74*, 1–25.

Kolk, H. H. J. (2006). How language adapts to the brain. In L. Progovac, K. Paesani, E. Casielles, & E. Barton (Eds.), *The syntax of nonsententials: Multi-disciplinary perspectives* (pp. 229–258). Philidelphia: Benjamins.

Kolk, H. H. J. (2008). Time in agrammatic aphasia. Commentary on Wearden. *Language and Learning, 58*(Suppl. 1), 173–177.

Le Dorze, G., Jacob, A., & Coderre, L. (1991). Aphasia rehabilitation with a case of agrammatism: A partial replication. *Aphasiology, 5*, 63–85.

Levelt, W. (1989). *Speaking: From intention to articulation.* Cambridge, MA: MIT Press.

Levelt, W. (1999). Producing spoken language: A blueprint of the speaker. In C. Brown & P. Hagoort (Eds.), *The neurocognition of language* (pp. 83–114). Oxford, UK: Oxford University Press.

Linebarger, M., McCall, D., & Berndt, R. (2004). The role of processing support in the remediation of aphasic language production disorders. *Cognitive Neuropsychology, 21*, 267–282.

Linebarger, M., McCall, D., Virata, T., & Berndt, R. (2007). Widening the temporal window: Processing support in the treatment of aphasic language production. *Brain and Language, 100*, 53–68.

Linebarger, M., Romania, J., Fink, R., Bartlett, M., & Schwartz, M. (2008). Building on residual speech: A portable processing prosthesis for aphasia. *Journal of Rehabilititon Research and Development, 45*(9), 1401–1414.

Linebarger, M., Schwartz, M., Romania, J., Kohn, S., & Stephens, S. (2000). Grammatical encoding in aphasia: Evidence from a processing prosthesis. *Brain and Language, 75*, 416–427.

Linebarger, M., Schwartz, M., & Saffran, E. (1983). Sensitivity to grammatical structure in so-called agrammatic aphasics. *Cognition, 13*, 361–392.

Links, P., Hurkmans, J., & Bastiaanse, R. (2010). Training verb and sentence production in agrammatic Broca's aphasia. *Aphasiology, 24*, 1303–1325.

Luzzatti, C., Raggi, R., Zonca, G., Pistarini, C., Contardi, A., & Pinna, G. (2001). On the nature of the selective impairment of verb and noun retrieval. *Cortex, 37*, 724–726.

Marshall, J. (1995). The mapping hypothesis and aphasia therapy. *Aphasiology, 9*, 517–539.

Marshall, J. (2003). Noun-verb dissociations: Evidence from acquisition and developmental and acquired disorders. *Journal of Neurolinguistics, 16*, 67–84.

Marshall, J. (2009). Framing ideas in aphasia: The need for thinking therapy. *The International Journal of Language and Communication Disorders, 44*(1), 1–14.

Marshall, J., & Cairns, D. (2005). Therapy for sentence processing problems in aphasia: Working on thinking for speaking. *Aphasiology, 19*, 1009–1020.

Marshall, J., Chiat, S., & Pring, T. (1997). An impairment in processing verbs' thematic roles: A therapy study. *Aphasiology, 11*, 855–876.

Marshall, J., Chiat, S., & Pring, T. (1999). *The Event Perception Test.* Bicester, UK: Winslow Press.

Marshall, J., Pring, T., & Chiat, S. (1993). Sentence processing therapy: Working at the level of the event. *Aphasiology, 7,* 177–199.

Marshall, J., Pring, T., & Chiat, S. (1998). Verb retrieval and sentence production in aphasia. *Brain and Language, 63,* 159–183.

McAllister, T., Bachrach, A., Waters, G., Michaud, J., & Caplan, D. (2009). Production and comprehension of unaccusatives in aphasia. *Aphasiology, 23*(7–8), 989–1004.

McCall, D., Virata, T., Linebarger, M., & Berndt, R. (2009). Integrating technology and targeted treatment to improve narrative production in aphasia: A case study. *Aphasiology, 23*(4) 438–502.

McCann, C., & Doleman, J. (2011). Verb retrieval in nonfluent aphasia: A replication of Edwards & Tucker, 2006. *Journal of Neurolinguistics, 24,* 237–248.

Mitchum, C., & Berndt, R. (1994). Verb retrieval and sentence construction: Effects of targeted intervention. In G. Humphreys & M. Riddoch (Eds.), *Cognitive neuropsychology and cognitive rehabilitation* (pp. 317–348). Hove, UK: Erlbaum.

Mitchum, C., & Berndt, R. (2008). Comprehension and production of sentences. In R. Chapey (Ed.), *Language intervention strategies in aphasia and related neurogenic disorders* (5th ed., pp. 632–653). Baltimore: Lippincott Williams & Wilkins.

Mitchum, C., Greenwald, M., & Berndt, R. (1997). Production-specific thematic mapping impairment: A treatment study. *Brain and Language, 60,* 121–123.

Mitchum, C., Greenwald, M., & Berndt, R. (2000). Cognitive treatments of sentence processing disorders: What have we learned? *Neuropsychological Rehabilitation, 10*(3), 311–336.

Mitchum, C., Haendiges, A., & Berndt, R. (1995). Treatment of thematic mapping in sentence comprehension: Implications for normal processing. *Cognitive Neuropsychology, 12,* 503–547.

Nickels, L. (2002). Therapy for naming disorders: Revisiting, revising and reviewing. *Aphasiology, 16,* 935–980.

Nickels, L., Byng, S., & Black, M. (1991). Sentence processing deficits: A replication of treatment. *British Journal of Disorders of Communication, 26,* 175–199.

Pashek, G. (1998). Gestural facilitation of noun and verb retrieval in aphasia: A case study. *Brain and Language, 65,* 177–180.

Pulvermuller, F. (2005). Brain mechanisms linking language and action. *Nature Reviews Neuroscience, 6,* 576–582.

Raymer, A., & Ellsworth, T. (2002). Response to contrasting verb retrieval treatments: A case study. *Aphasiology, 16*(10/11), 1031–1045.

Rochon, E., Laird, L., Bose, A., & Scofield, J. (2005). Mapping therapy for sentence production impairments in non fluent aphasia. *Neuropsychological Rehabilitation, 15*(1), 1–36.

Rodriguez, A., Raymer, A., & Gonzalez Rothi, L. (2006). Effects of gesture + verbal and semantic-phonologic treatments for verb retrieval in aphasia. *Aphasiology, 20*(2/3/4), 286–297.

Rose, M., & Sussmilch, G. (2008). The effects of semantic and gesture treatments on verb retrieval and verb use in aphasia. *Aphasiology, 22*(7/8), 691–706.

Ruiter, M., Kolk, H., & Rietveld, T. (2010). Speaking in elipses: The effect of a compensatory style of speech on functional communication in chronic agrammatism. *Neuropsychological Rehabilitation, 20,* 423–458.

Saffran, E., Schwartz, M., & Marin, O. (1980). The word order problem in agrammatism, II Production. *Brain and Language, 10,* 263–280.

Schwartz, M., Saffran, E., Fink, R., Myers, J., & Martin, N. (1994). Mapping therapy: A treatment programme for agrammatism. *Aphasiology, 8,* 19–54.

Schwartz, M., Saffran, E., & Marin, O. (1980). The word order problem in agrammatism 1. Comprehension. *Brain and Language, 10,* 249–262.

Silveri, M., Salvigni, B., Cappa, A, Della Vedova, C., & Puopolo, M. (2003). Impairment of verb processing in frontal variant-frontotemporal dementia. A dysexecutive symptom. *Dementia and Geriatric Cognitive Disorders, 16,* 296–300.

Springer, L., Huber, W., Scnhlenck, K-J., & Schlenck, C. (2000). Agrammatism: Deficit or compensation? Consequences for aphasia therapy. *Neuropsychological Rehabilitation, 10*(3), 279–309.

Stavrakaki, S., & Kouvava, S. (2003). Functional categories in agrammatism: Evidence from Greek. *Brain and Language, 86,* 129–141.

Thompson, C. (2003). Unaccusative verb production in agrammatic aphasia: The argument structure complexity hypothesis. *Journal of Neurolinguistics, 16,* 151–161.

Thompson, C. (2008). Treatment of syntactic and morphological deficits in agrammatic aphasia: Treatment of underlying forms. In R. Chapey (Ed.), *Language intervention strategies in aphasia and related neurogenic communication disorders* (5th ed., pp. 735–754). Baltimore: Lippincott Williams and Wilkins.

Thompson, C. (2011). *Northwestern assessment of verbs and sentences.* Evanston, IL: Northwestern University.

Thompson, C., Choy, J., Holland, A., & Cole, R. (2010). Sentactics® computer-automated treatment of underlying forms. *Aphasiology, 24*(10), 1242–1266.

Thompson, C., Lange, K., Schneider, S., & Shapiro, L. (1997). Agrammatic and non brain damaged subjects' verb and verb argument structure production. *Aphasiology, 11,* 473–490.

Thompson, C., & Lee, M. (2009). Psych verb production in agrammatic Broca's aphasia. *Journal of Neurolinguistics, 22,* 354–369.

Thompson, C., & Shapiro, L. (2007). Complexity in treatment of syntactic deficits. *American Journal of Speech-Language Pathology, 16,* 30–42.

Thompson, C., Shapiro, L., Ballard, J., Jacobs, K., Schneider, S., & Tait, M. (1997). Training and generalized production of wh- and NP- movement structures in agrammatic aphasia. *Journal of Speech and Hearing Research, 40,* 228–244.

Thompson, C., Shapiro, L., Kiran, S., & Sobecks, J. (2003). The role of syntactic complexity in treatment of sentence deficits in agrammatic aphasia: The complexity account of treatment efficacy (CATE). *Journal of Speech, Language and Hearing Research, 42,* 690–707.

Thompson, C., Shapiro, L., & Roberts, M. (1993). Treatment of sentence production deficits in aphasia: A linguistic specific approach to wh-interrogative training and generalization. *Aphasiology, 7,* 111–133.

Thompson, C., Shapiro, L., Tait, M., Jacobs, B., & Schneider, S. (1996). Training wh-question production in agrammatic aphasia: Analysis of argument and adjunct movement. *Brain and Language, 52,* 175–228.

True, G., Bartlett, M., Fink, R., Linebarger, M., & Schwartz, M. (2010). Perspectives of persons with aphasia towards SentenceShaper To Go: A qualitative study. *Aphasiology, 24*(9), 1032–1050.

Ullman, M., Corkin, S., Coppola, M., Hickok, G., Growdon, J., Koroshetz, W., et al. (1997). A neural dissociation within language: Evidence that the mental dictionary is part of declarative memory, and that grammatical rules are processed by the procedural system. *Journal of Cognitive Neuroscience,9*(2) 266–276.

Ullman, M., Pancheva, R., Love, T., Yee, E., Swinney, D., & Hickok, G. (2005). Neural correlates of lexicon and grammar: Evidence from the production, reading and judgement of inflection in aphasia. *Brain and Language, 93*, 185–238.

Wambaugh, J., Doyle, P., Martinez, A., & Kalinyak-Fliszar, M. (2002). Effects of two lexical retrieval cueing treatments on action naming in aphasia. *Journal of Rehabilitation Research and Development, 39*(4), 455–466.

Wambaugh, J., & Ferguson, M. (2007). Application of semantic feature analysis to retrieval of action names in aphasia. *Journal of Rehabilitation Research and Development, 44*, 381–394.

Webster, J., Morris, J., & Franklin, S. (2005). Effects of therapy targeted at verb retrieval and the realisation of the predicate argument structure: A case study. *Aphasiology, 19*(8), 748–764.

Webster, J., & Whitworth, A. (2012). Treating verbs in aphasia: Exploring the impact of therapy at the single word and sentence levels. *International Journal of Language and Communication Disorders, 47*(6), 619–636.

Whitworth, A. (1996). *Thematic Roles in Production (TRIP).* London: Whurr.

Wilshire, C., Lukkien, C., & Burmester, B. (2014). The Sentence Production Test for Aphasia. *Aphasiology, 28*(6), 658–691.

World Health Organization. (2001). *International classification of functioning, disability and health.* Geneva, Switzerland: Author.

Worrall, L. (2008). Interventions for agrammatism from a consequences perspective. In N. Martin, C. Thompson, & L. Worrall (Eds.), *Aphasia rehabilitation: The impairment and its consequences* (pp. 155–170). San Diego, CA: Plural.

OBJECTIVES

The reader will be able to:

1. Identify the main principles and distinctions among approaches to assessment of everyday talk, including a discourse perspective, conversation analysis, and a narrative approach.

2. Recognize the potential for integration of selected aspects of the assessment approaches with clinical practice.

3. Recognize the application of selected aspects of these approaches within holistic intervention planning in clinical practice.

4. Critically evaluate the theoretical and evidence base for these perspectives as applied within aphasia clinical research.

Approaches to Assessment and Treatment of Everyday Talk in Aphasia

Elizabeth Armstrong, Lucy Bryant, Alison Ferguson, and Nina Simmons-Mackie

INTRODUCTION

Everyday talk involves an exchange of information between conversational partners, but talk also presents and shapes the identity and social relationship of the interactants. We define *talk* broadly as the communicative elements involved in face-to-face interaction, including spoken language, gesture, body language, facial expression, prosody, gaze, and vocalizations. Everyday talk is often equated with the term *functional communication*. Functional communication refers to everyday communicative activities and situations.

Although many early studies of aphasia focus on the word or sentence level of language, more recently researchers and clinicians have been interested in functional communication and the discourse level of aphasic communication—that is, communication beyond the single-sentence level. Many diverse realms of research have assisted in the understanding of how aphasia affects everyday talk and functional communication, including behavioral, psycholinguistic, and sociolinguistic perspectives on communication in aphasia.

The talk of people with aphasia has long been investigated, and early functional approaches to the observation of everyday talk made use of behavioral observation tools for analysis (Holland, Frattali, & Fromm, 1999). Brady, Kelly, Godwin, and Enderby (2012) suggest that these tools remain the primary means of investigating functional communication in aphasia within clinical settings by acting as an efficient conduit to interpreting communicative ability. For example, Sarno's Functional Communication Profile (1969) involves rating functional tasks such as indicating yes or no or reading newspaper headlines. Informal behavioral assessments involve observation of daily functional activities, such as talking on the phone or purchasing an item. Such functional approaches provide important insights into the aspects of function described as activity and social participation within frameworks such as the International Classification of Functioning, Disability, and Health (ICF; World Health Organization [WHO], 2001, p. 325). For example, through observing simulated interaction using a doctor–patient scenario, assessment can be made of a client's ability to handle an interview situation—his or her ability to ask questions, answer questions, or comprehend what is said within a specific context. Intervention from a functional approach is similarly influenced by behavioral paradigms, focusing on identification of specified target behaviors and the scaffolding of performances related to activity or social participation. In other words, the clinician identifies key communicative behaviors that limit or enhance the client's participation in a functional activity and then designs interventions that specifically address performance of the activity.

Psycholinguistic methods focus on highly controlled sampling of language, primarily at the word and sentence levels. These approaches draw from a variety of psycholinguistic and neurolinguistic theories of language processing (e.g., Riddoch & Humphreys, 1994). The clinician or researcher in this situation systematically presents carefully selected stimuli to the person with aphasia, noting patterns of responses. Such approaches shed light on potential associations between language behaviors and neurological impairment. For example, explorations of performance on repetition of real words and nonwords provide the platform for hypotheses regarding differential diagnosis with both the Geschwind/Boston model and more recently developed information-processing models of aphasia. Intervention from such frameworks tends to be based on assumptions of recovery in line with stimulation of neurological pathways, and intervention is primarily focused on the impairment aspects of the ICF—problems with language processing and underlying neurological pathways.

Developments in the theoretical frameworks and methodological advances associated with sociology, sociolinguistics, and other social sciences have provided additional ways to understand the nature and impact of aphasia (e.g., Goodwin, 2003). These developments serve as the basis for the approaches discussed in this chapter, including discourse, conversation, and narrative analysis of aphasic communication. A *discourse perspective* focuses on the language use of people with aphasia in natural contexts, paying particular attention to how language is used for different purposes and in different ways. For example, this perspective can illuminate how a person with severe word-finding difficulty makes use of other language resources to provide cohesion in describing events. Such a perspective has variously been argued to provide insights into impairment (e.g., through comparison with slips-of-the-tongue evidence); activity (e.g., through providing detailed empirical description of performance on specified speaking tasks); and social participation (e.g., through consideration of the social roles enacted within natural discourse settings). This perspective has similarly influenced a range of interventions, providing both a context and a focus for therapy. The approach known as *conversation analysis* similarly focuses on real-life interactions and provides a well-developed and highly specified framework for understanding the interactive structure within which the person with aphasia is communicating and to date has been applied primarily with a focus on social participation. Interventions that make use of conversation analysis have integrated aspects of counseling (e.g., through engaging people with aphasia and their family members in active reflection on their interaction), behavioral scaffolding and shaping, as well as opportunities for use of learned therapeutic strategies in real-world settings. Most recently, research has also acknowledged the role of *personal narratives* in shaping a person's adjustment to life with aphasia. This research has been centrally concerned with understanding the impact of aphasia on the person's sense of self and his or her place within the social environment, and as such relates closely with what is described within the ICF framework as Personal Factors as well as social participation. Personal Factors within the ICF are not currently coded specifically because of issues concerning cultural variability (Threats, 2007) but go beyond such factors as age, race, gender, and education to include "coping styles . . . overall behavior pattern and character style, individual psychological assets" (WHO, 2001, p. 17). A focus on narratives from an identity perspective is a relatively new innovation in aphasiology and provides clinicians with a window into personal characteristics that may influence the rehabilitation and adjustment process, for example, resilience.

RATIONALE FOR DISCOURSE, CONVERSATION ANALYTIC, AND NARRATIVE APPROACHES

An understanding of everyday talk of people with aphasia provides significant insights into multiple domains of the ICF, including impairment/language processing, social participation, and psychosocial adjustment. Although impairment has long been a focus of aphasia assessment and intervention, the domains of activity, social participation, and personal/psychosocial factors have only relatively recently become prevalent topics in research and clinical literature. Activity and social participation are key aspects of living life with aphasia. In fact, research suggests that people's overall well-being and quality of life are strongly influenced by their level of social participation and quality of social relationships (e.g., Cruice, Worrall, Hickson, & Murison, 2003; Hilari, Needle, & Harrison, 2012). Furthermore, psychosocial adjustment, including factors such as confidence, self-esteem, and identity, are critical elements of living successfully with a communication disorder. Intervention restricted to the impairment of aphasia might fail to address important issues that influence real-life communication. Thus, assessment and intervention targeting functional communication and life participation are imperative in ensuring meaningful outcomes in aphasia. A focus on discourse, conversation, or narrative potentially provides the clinician with information across the ICF domains of impairment (e.g., language processing), activities and participation, and psychosocial factors (i.e., personal factors).

In the following sections, we provide a snapshot of these three analytic approaches to understanding functional communication in aphasia. Readers should note that the terms used to describe each approach are labels of convenience and draw together diverse approaches and paradigms. Many of these are explored in more depth elsewhere, and of course, still more warrant far more attention than can be provided within this chapter.

DIFFICULTIES WITH EVERYDAY TALK: SYMPTOMS OF DISCOURSE BREAKDOWN

Lexical–Syntactic Breakdown

Studies of aphasic discourse are plentiful and have raised a number of issues related to language use—originally in monologues and more recently in dialogues as well. Monologic studies are typically concerned with aspects such as amount of information conveyed by the aphasic speaker, variety of word types used, grammatical accuracy and complexity, cohesion, and overall coherence of a text, as well as issues related to specific meanings, such as the conveying of emotions. Although word-finding difficulties have been identified at the single-word level, and syntactic problems at the sentence level in tests that are decontextualized from everyday language, discourse studies have explored how such difficulties manifest in connected speech.

In terms of amount of information conveyed during discourse, it is unsurprising and well acknowledged that people with aphasia produce less information than speakers without aphasia on a variety of discourse tasks (e.g., Doyle et al., 2000; Marini, Andreetta, del Tin, & Carlomagno, 2011). Nicholas and Brookshire (1993) examine the relevance and information accuracy of individual words in the discourse of the speaker with aphasia, defining the notion of *correct information unit* (CIU) as a measure of the relevance of lexical items to the discourse in which they occurred. They found that subjects without brain damage produced more words overall, more CIUs, and a higher percentage of CIUs than subjects with aphasia did, as they expected. In an effort to quantify informativeness further, Nicholas and Brookshire also looked at words and CIUs produced per minute and found higher scores for the subjects without aphasia than for the subjects with aphasia.

Studies also document significant problems in the discourse of speakers with aphasia in terms of incidence of paraphasias and neologisms and increased frequency of usage of deictics and nonspecific lexical items such as *something, somewhere* (e.g., Boyle, 2014; Falconer & Antonucci, 2012). Studies have also explored the levels of cohesion and coherence of a text (e.g., Wright & Capilouto, 2012). Speakers with aphasia have been found to have reduced global coherence at the macrostructural level, associated with disruptions across the microstructure, including at the lexical, syntactic, and semantic levels.

In terms of syntactic breakdown, errors documented have included a range of omissions of various grammatical structures typical of errors seen at the sentence level alone, such as the subject of a sentence, its main verb, required functors, inflections, and content/function words (e.g., Milman, Dickey, & Thompson, 2008). In many of the studies, syntactic complexity has been measured in terms of amount of embedding or subordination present (e.g., Gordon, 2008) or number of arguments attached to the verb (e.g., Barbieri, Basso, Frustaci, & Luzzatti, 2010; Thompson, Riley, den Ouden,

Meltzer-Asscher, & Lukic, 2013; Webster, Franklin, & Howard, 2001). Overall, speakers with aphasia have been found to have less grammatically complex language than normal speakers do.

Although the majority of grammatical errors have been demonstrated in the speech of speakers with Broca's aphasia or agrammatism (e.g., Grodzinsky, 1990), speakers with fluent aphasia have also been noted to demonstrate grammatical errors (e.g., Bastiaanse, Edwards, & Kiss, 1996). However, the basis for such errors may differ from that of speakers with agrammatic aphasia in that the apparent syntactic errors may be accounted for in lexical semantic terms (for discussion, see Edwards & Bastiaanse, 1998).

More recently, semantic aspects of discourse have been further investigated using concepts such as "evaluative language" (e.g., E. Armstrong, Mortensen, Ciccone, & Godecke, 2012; E. Armstrong & Ulatowska, 2007; Olness & Englebretson, 2011; Ulatowska, Reyes, Santos, & Worle, 2010). *Evaluative language* refers to the language of emotion or opinion giving and involves the use of emotive words and phrases as well as such phenomena as repetition (for emphasis), reported speech (to convey immediacy of emotion), and metaphor. Studies found that speakers with aphasia often retain the ability to use evaluative or emotive words in a coherent manner even when referential narrative content is compromised, and that they can provide reflections and comments about their feelings and the events occurring throughout a text; however, they are restricted in these resources as with other lexical resources. Hence, their abilities to convey feelings and express their opinions are restricted.

Conversation Breakdown

The difficulties speakers with aphasia face in terms of their actual lexical–syntactic resources inevitably interfere with the flow of conversation in terms of aspects such as turn taking and breakdown repair (Schegloff, Jefferson, & Sacks, 1977). Conversation analysis has enabled researchers and clinicians to observe the dynamic nature of interactions between people with aphasia and their conversation partners.

Conversation analysis demonstrates both the challenges and strategic successes of individuals with aphasia and their conversation partners (e.g., Beeke, Wilkinson, & Maxim, 2007; Wilkinson, 2015). The person with aphasia and conversation partners are known to adapt numerous collaborative strategies, such as joint production, repetition, guessing, and completion, to overcome trouble or breakdown in conversation.

However, both also use behaviors that can be potentially disruptive to the conversation flow. For example, when asked for clarification of something said, a person with aphasia may simply repeat what he or she said in the first place rather than rephrase or try to elaborate. Some conversation partners use "test questions" to ask for known information, or they ask the person with aphasia to say a particular word when the partner already knows the meaning the person is attempting to convey (e.g., Simmons-Mackie & Kagan, 1999). Such behaviors potentially delay the conversation and cause frustration for the communicative partner.

The difference between aphasic language structure in structured monologue (picture description, elicited storytelling such as *Cinderella*) and natural dialogue has also been highlighted (E. Armstrong, Ciccone, Godecke, & Kok, 2011; Beeke, Wilkinson, & Maxim, 2003; Herbert, Gregory, & Best, 2014). For example, Beeke and colleagues report on a speaker with aphasia who demonstrates subject–verb–object structures commonly in monologue, although slowly, but rarely in dialogue, where more unconventional forms were used to convey meaning, and with less effort, presumably to facilitate the flow of conversation.

In addition, the phenomenon of conversation partners speaking for people with aphasia has also been noted, with numerous purposes and outcomes of this behavior identified (e.g., Croteau, Le Dorze, & Morin, 2008). One person speaking for another can certainly have negative consequences in one situation. For example, Croteau and Le Dorze (2006) discuss this behavior in terms of overprotection of the aphasic conversation partner and minimizing that person's conversational participation. However, it may also be perceived as an opportunity for the person with aphasia to communicate through another supportive person and be an active participant in the conveying of meanings (Simmons-Mackie, Kingston, & Schultz, 2004).

Psychosocial Breakdown

Researchers have identified a variety of psychosocial consequences of aphasia that, although attributable to the communication disability, affect nonlinguistic aspects of the self, such as communicative confidence, self-esteem, and identity. For example, Shadden (2005) describes aphasia as "identity theft" in which the person with aphasia loses key aspects of the preonset self-image. Simmons-Mackie (2001) argues that psychosocial issues and communication are inseparable, and communication intervention must include attention to the psychosocial consequences of aphasia. Simmons-Mackie and Damico (2010) demonstrate how discourse and conversational interaction can be used as a "window" into identity and social roles and how narrative approaches to clinical management of aphasia can help to target these indirect consequences.

ASSESSMENT ISSUES

A Discourse Perspective

As demonstrated, language does not occur in a vacuum. It occurs in a context or variety of contexts covering a variety of purposes that require different linguistic outputs. Although some authors dismiss context as occurring outside language, hence not directly relevant to the way language is organized, others argue that language and context are inextricably interwoven (e.g., Labov, 1977/2006). Language is seen as a resource that is learned in a variety of contexts so that language patterns occur systematically linked with situational variables. Conversely, the context of a situation is also defined by the language used. For example, language used in a casual conversation differs from that of a formal letter in terms of grammar and vocabulary, and it is through the observation of these forms that a certain text can be identified as either a casual or formal interaction. This interwoven view of language and context makes their analysis inseparable, as opposed to more formal views of language that encourage analysis of vocabulary and syntactic skills outside functional contexts, as is the case with many standardized tests.

Aphasiologists have been aware for many years that the expressive and receptive skills of people with aphasia can vary across contexts, yet there has been relatively little systematic analysis of the sources of this variability. Factors such as listener familiarity, topic, and emotionality have been identified as affecting such aspects as vocabulary, cohesion, and coherence (Borod et al., 2000). Studies have examined speakers with aphasia talking across many different genres, ranging from spontaneous narratives about such events as their stroke, both happy and frightening events (Ulatowska & Olness, 2001), and daily activities (e.g., Bastiaanse et al., 1996), to structured narratives based on picture descriptions, story retelling (McNeil, Doyle, Fossett, & Park, 2001), and set interactive tasks such as barrier games (e.g., Hengst, 2003). Although conclusions have often been drawn about aphasic discourse by collapsing the results of divergent discourse samples and genres, we now know that different contexts and elicitation techniques have an effect on the discourse produced, and results across such contexts should not be equated. For example, it has been found that stories elicited from stimuli such as "Talk about what is going on in the picture(s)" were impoverished in terms of story structure compared with those elicited with prompts such as "I want you to look at the picture(s) and tell me a story that has a beginning, middle, and end" (e.g., Wright & Capilouto, 2009). This suggests that stories elicited by the latter sentence tend to prompt the temporal sequential aspect of a narrative and improve overall coherence, whereas the former statement prompts description only rather than true narrative. Hence, it is important for clinicians to ensure a representative sample of a speaker's discourse before inferring ability level.

It is also important to emphasize that where psycholinguistic/cognitive neuropsychological approaches to aphasia focus primarily on the impairment, studies of everyday discourse examine the ways people with aphasia actually convey meanings successfully as well as their limitations in this regard. Hence, an assessment should provide a speaker with aphasia with as many opportunities to convey strengths as possible (e.g., across different genres) to gain as full a picture as possible of the person's skills in everyday situations.

Although different types of discourse are noted in some of the preceding studies, a systematic theory of context is rarely used (e.g., a categorization of genres predicting different types of discourse according to different variables). Variables such as listener familiarity, topic, and elicitation technique are often described or manipulated in some way, but theoretical frameworks regarding what could be expected under certain conditions are rarely used. Theories of context addressing such issues have been written about for many years (e.g., Hymes, 1974) and have enabled analysts to systematically examine contextual variables and their relationship to a variety of behaviors, including language behaviors. Such frameworks allow us to make predictions about and to gain insights in terms of not only the form of behaviors but also their functions. One such theory that appears to be clearly accessible for clinical purposes, having already been used on a limited basis (see E. Armstrong, 2005b), is that of Halliday (Halliday & Matthiessen, 2004)—systemic functional linguistics. Halliday sees discourse as a semantic unit rather than a grammatical one. He identifies three functions of language that interact systematically with extralinguistic variables to form context (see Table 13.1).

The experiential (informational or transactional) nature of aphasic discourse has been the focus of aphasia researchers for many years. For example, considerable research has addressed the information expressed

Table 13.1 Context and Language Use

Aspect of Context	Metafunction of Language Use	Examples of Influences	Examples of Linguistic Resources
Field	Experiential	Purpose of talk, topic	Transitivity (who is doing what to whom): Actor, Sayer, Recipient, Goal, Attribute, Process; Processes (verb types): material (e.g., walk, swim); relational (e.g., be, have); mental (e.g., think, believe); verbal (e.g., say, talk); behavioral (e.g., sneeze, breathe)
Tenor	Interpersonal	Role relationships between interactants (e.g., familiarity, power)	Mood (subject, finite, signaling declarative, imperative); modality (e.g., must, should, could, might)
Mode	Textual	With/without visual contact (e.g., written text versus phone contact vs. face-to-face contact)	Cohesion : coreference ellipsis lexical relationships (e.g., synonymy, antonymy, collocation)

Data from Halliday, M. A. K., and Matthiessen, C.(2004). *An introduction to functional grammar* (3rd ed.). New York: Arnold.

in narratives produced by people with aphasia, using measures that operationally define content or information units (as previously discussed). Less attention has been paid to the interactional or interpersonal aspects of aphasic discourse (Ferguson, 1992). However, when considering discourse from within a contextual framework, some interesting patterns emerge. For example, although a clinician might discover that a person with aphasia can produce only a certain number of content units per minute and may work with the person to increase this through various word-finding strategies, there may be a pattern to the kinds of content units or meanings that the person finds easier or more difficult. Further exploration of the semantic resources used in discourse might reveal that the person is able to relate events relatively well (e.g., using verbal processes such as *walking, writing, eating*) but provides limited attitudes or feelings in the recount (e.g., through the use of verbal processes such as *think, feel, believe, love*). This might limit the person's ability to tell an interesting story or to convey aspects of identity related to his or her attitudes and may be significant to the ability to engage others in conversations (E. Armstrong, 2005a). From an interpersonal language perspective, a person with aphasia may be restricted in the range of modality resources that assist in conveying politeness, for example, "*Could* you . . . ?" or "I *might* go now." From a textual perspective, one of the problems encountered commonly by individuals with aphasia is ensuring that the person or thing to which they are referring is clear. For example, word-finding difficulty might result in the use of pronouns without

clear referents rather than specific nouns (Ulatowska, Weiss-Doyell, Freedman-Stern, & Macaluso-Haynes, 1983). On the other hand, some resources for creating coherence may be retained, for example, the ability to form cohesive ties through lexical relationships such as synonymy, antonymy, or the ability to use conjunctions appropriately (Lock & Armstrong, 1997).

Hence, when assessing the communication skills of a person with aphasia, the three-function framework described previously can be used as the basis of observation (Ferguson, 2000), with a view to providing directions for intervention. We suggest that a discourse perspective provides for the systematic analysis of context, combined with that of corresponding linguistic features, and that such an analysis can create a framework that is clinically relevant for both the assessment and treatment purposes of aphasia. In combining the two, the framework addresses the patterns of lexicogrammatical deficit/usage in aphasia, as well as the social impacts of aphasia and ways in which interpersonal relationships via verbal interactions are affected by aphasia.

Conversation Analysis

Conversation analysis is a qualitative approach to analyzing discourse that seeks to discover social order within the structure of talk-in-interaction and build an understanding of the resources employed by speakers to accomplish their interactive goals. Conversation analysis focuses on the collaborative construction of meaning by participants. Whereas a discourse perspective may look particularly at moments in interaction where the speaker alone is talking (e.g., telling a story), conversation analysis looks at such a moment of talking within its conversational context of preceding and subsequent turns of talk. This focus on two-way (or multiparty) interaction drives the sampling for conversation analysis to more natural contexts than is strictly necessary for those working from a discourse perspective, although discourse analysis has also increasingly focused on interactions in more recent years (e.g., Matthiessen, Lukin, Butt, Cleirigh, & Nesbitt, 2005). In the use of conversation analytic approaches, it is important to involve additional conversation partners and ideally real-world contexts. Some assessments emanate from structured or manipulated conversations, such as that of Ramsberger and Rende (2002), who propose an assessment based on the person with aphasia retelling the story of an episode from a well-known television show to someone who had not seen the episode. Other studies argue for more natural conversations and encourage data being gathered in the person's home as well as within the clinic setting (e.g., Davidson, Worrall, & Hickson, 2008). An accessible clinical tool based on a conversation analytic perspective is the Conversation Analysis Profile for People With Aphasia (CAPPA; Whitworth, Perkins, & Lesser, 1997). Studies highlight the idiosyncratic nature of conversations and relationships; hence, careful analysis of specific couples' patterns and their attitudes toward these patterns is recommended (Lock et al., 2001).

Narrative Perspective

A narrative perspective involves listening for and to the life experiences and personal perspectives of those who are affected by aphasia (Hinckley, 2007). For example, Frank (1995) describes the "quest narrative" as one of several possible narratives that result after illness. When clients are immersed in the quest narrative, they typically expect a cure effected by an expert therapist and may not realize their own power and responsibility as therapy partners in effecting carryover. Outcomes of therapy with such a passive therapy partner might be less successful than for a person with aphasia whose narrative regarding aphasia involves a confident and action-oriented perspective.

Narrative approaches require that clinicians attempt to learn about the individual's life before onset and the person's current cultural perspectives, values, hopes, and expectations for the future. Such information is typically gleaned from interviews and conversations; thus, approaches that incorporate discourse sampling into

telling aspects of the individual's life story provide an efficient method of gathering both discourse and narrative data.

In addition, a narrative approach involves looking for "tells" (something the person does or says that conveys their perspective regarding what is going on) in everyday conversation (Simmons-Mackie & Damico, 2010). For example, consider the client who was asked to construct a sentence with the word *nothing* and who responded, "I am aphasia, I am nothing"; she was clearly providing a personal perspective on her life with aphasia.

Finally, in interpreting the findings from discourse, conversation, and narrative assessments, personal style and personality should always be considered. Asking family members and friends for their feedback in relation to specific findings from samples of discourse can be helpful because this provides them with a greater opportunity to comment constructively rather than simply being asked if the person's talk is different from before the stroke. Furthermore, others can provide information about helpful discourse strategies and barriers to participation in interactions and elaborate on their experience in conversing with the person with aphasia.

PRACTICAL ANALYSIS ISSUES

Practical issues exist when implementing any form of assessment using connected language samples, whether discourse, conversation, or narrative analysis. The volume of language required for an adequate analysis of language ability and the skills necessary to collect and analyze such samples pose barriers to clinical implementation of language analysis. Multiple studies recognize and discuss the clinical limitations of discourse analysis, with particular reference to the time required (e.g., Togher, 2001). Boles and Bombard (1998) investigate the length of sample needed to accurately represent language ability in four people with aphasia. They suggest a 5- to 10-minute sample of discourse is necessary to reliably estimate language ability. When coupled with estimates that full transcription of language samples, multilevel analysis, and interpretation of results take up to 60 minutes for every minute of language sampled, analysis appears impractical even on a single-case basis (L. Armstrong, Brady, Mackenzie, & Norrie, 2007).

Developments in computer technology present a potential means to overcome this barrier of inefficiency. While the process of manual analysis requires transcription and separate coding and analysis of multiple linguistic behaviors, computer software has the potential to assist and therefore hasten the transcription process and to calculate multiple discourse measures simultaneously (e.g., Systematic Analysis of Language Transcripts [SALT 2012] Clinical Version; Miller, Andriacchi, & Nockerts, 2012). The speed of such software is not the only advantage of computer-assisted language analysis. By determining multiple measures using a single tool, the clinician requires training in the use of only one piece of software. Using alternative manual calculations, training is required for each analysis procedure that is to be completed. A further benefit of automated analysis is seen in the application of complex functions to linguistic data to calculate the distribution of a behavior throughout discourse. These complex measures account for a greater amount of the variation that arises due to differences inherent in text, including length and style (Fergadiotis, Wright, & West, 2013). While this may be ideal in research, the complexity of the mathematical functions applied to calculate distributions complicates clinical interpretation of language outcomes.

This interpretation of language analysis can act as a further practical barrier to the use of functional language as a clinical tool. Discourse and other functional approaches to aphasia often provide a descriptive analysis of linguistic and communicative behaviors. While language behaviors are qualitatively identified, analysis often transforms these data into numerical output. This numeric information represents the ability to utilize specific behaviors. While explicit instruction is not available for interpretation of results, as is used to determine performance in standardized testing, these data permit simple comparisons between individuals or within individuals over time and complex statistical analyses for research purposes. Some knowledge of linguistics, language structure, and aphasic impairment is necessary for accurate interpretation of results from manual or computerized analysis, although this is provided through professional training (Jaecks, Hielscher-Fastabend, & Stenneken, 2012).

Other alternatives to automated analyses include both online ratings (e.g., L. Armstrong et al., 2007) or models enabling prioritization of the focus of assessment. Olness, Gyger, and Thomas (2012) provide a model of discourse assessment known as narrative functionality, which addresses the factors noted and suggests ways of tailoring focus to a client's stage postonset of aphasia. Olness et al. suggest that in the inpatient rehabilitation setting, cohesive referencing abilities associated with word-finding difficulties could be monitored. In the outpatient stages where more adaptive strategies are the focus, alternative strategies of referencing could be monitored, for example, use of alternative words

(related through synonymy, collocation) or even substitution or ellipsis. In the final stages, "overall referential and evaluative functionality" (p. 63) can be monitored, including the use of such devices as repetition and use of modality where the interpersonal function is of ultimate interest as the person attempts to maximize social participation.

INTERVENTION

The ways in which discourse and conversation are used in intervention cover a wide range of therapy goals (see Table 13.2). For some interventions, the focus of therapy is on discourse-level features, while for other approaches, the discourse provides the context of therapy in which specific aspects of language can be practiced. Regardless of the focus of therapy, all approaches to intervention aim for improvements to be observable in the everyday interactions of clients, so discourse offers the opportunity to evaluate the outcome of therapies. However, aphasia affects more than language, with clients trying to adjust to living with the consequences of aphasia on their ability to interact with family, friends, and others. The psychosocial consequences of aphasia have long been recognized in the field, and counseling can occur through the medium of discourse (Ireland & Wotton, 1996). This section discusses each of these ways of using discourse in intervention.

Focus ON Discourse

Clinicians who work with people who have cognitive communication disability associated with traumatic brain injury or right hemisphere damage will be familiar with therapy approaches that focus on particular aspects of the discourse or conversation structure itself because these disorders frequently disrupt discourse-level aspects of language use, such as turn taking and cohesion. Penn, Jones, and Joffe (1997) outline an approach called *hierarchical discourse therapy* that explicitly links levels of cognitive demand with discourse to provide a structure for this kind of therapy. However, people with specific aphasia also have disrupted discourse because of their specific language difficulties at the word and sentence levels, so therapy targeting discourse is also appropriate for this population. For example, Armstrong (1991) presents an outline of how cohesion might be targeted in therapy. For example, the notion of cohesive chains (words that relate to each other in a particular discourse) contribute to discourse continuity; working with a client on cohesive relationships such as synonymy (e.g., good,

Table 13.2 Discourse and Intervention

Relationship Between Discourse and Therapy	Explanation	Examples of Therapy Goals
The **focus** of therapy is ON discourse-level features.	Therapy goals aim to improve an aspect of discourse or conversation (i.e., language above the level of word or sentence).	To improve cohesion, coherence in discourse To improve turn taking in conversation
Discourse provides the **context** of therapy IN which specific aspects of language can be practiced.	Therapy goals aim to improve an aspect of word- or sentence-level processing, using interactions involving discourse or conversation.	To promote lexical retrieval (using self-cues) in a storytelling task To improve lexical retrieval in role-play of service encounter
Specific aspects of language are being targeted FOR the **outcome** of eventual use in discourse.	Therapy goals aim to improve an aspect of cognitive–linguistic processing, using word- or sentence-level tasks and evaluating generalization through discourse or conversation measures.	To promote word retrieval in single-word picture-naming task, measuring generalization in test–retest story retell procedure
Discourse provides the **medium** THROUGH which psychosocial consequences of language impairment can be managed.	Therapy goals aim to improve an aspect of psychosocial recovery, using therapeutic interaction involving discourse or conversation.	To promote self-esteem, in a group activity using the development of personal portfolios or life stories

fantastic), antonymy (e.g., happy, sad), and collocation (e.g., weather, bad, wet, humid) within the context of a particular topic could enhance this. Penn and Beecham (1992) present a case study of a multilingual speaker for whom the discourse targets include circumlocution. In a review of the literature on conversation therapy, Simmons-Mackie, Savage, and Worrall (2014) describe multiple approaches to working on conversation within a discourse context. Many of these studies demonstrate the positive impact of focusing intervention directly on improving conversation between people with aphasia and their regular communication partners (e.g., Beckley et al., 2013; Beeke et al., 2014; Wilkinson & Wielaert, 2012). In fact, substantial empirical evidence is available from the research into intervention with conversation partners, which has focused on conversation-level strategies to improve communication effectiveness and ease (Simmons-Mackie, Raymer, Armstrong, Holland, & Cherney, 2010). For example, therapy based on conversation analysis appears to show promise when directed toward a range of conversation partners of people with aphasia (e.g., Cunningham & Ward, 2003; Hickey, Bourgeois, & Olswang, 2004; Kagan, Black, Duchan, Simmons-Mackie, & Square, 2001).

Therapy IN Discourse Context

Most clinicians include in their therapy planning opportunities for the person with aphasia to use the targets of language therapy within a discourse context, for example, within role-plays (Hinckley & Carr, 2005); scripts (see computer-based innovations for script-based therapy; Cherney, Halper, Holland, & Cole, 2008); or through conversational coaching (Hopper, Holland, & Rewega, 2002). Whitney and Goldstein (1989) provide a good example of this way of using discourse in their study involving three people with aphasia who worked on self-monitoring of revisions, repetitions, and pauses in discourse, resulting in a significant reduction of these behaviors and an associated improvement in listener perceptions. More recently, researchers have recognized that the kind of language targets that would have traditionally been treated in word or sentence tasks can be treated within the discourse context (e.g., Murray, Timberlake, & Eberle, 2007). Within group therapy in particular, conversation provides the major context for all therapy targets (Simmons-Mackie, Elman, Holland, & Damico, 2007). One of the challenges for clinicians when using discourse/conversation contexts in therapy is to preserve authenticity and naturalness (Holland, 1998). As Togher (2003) discusses, many interactions within the clinical setting are highly unnatural and contrived, and even when role-plays and orchestrated group interactions approximate typical interactions, the therapeutic agenda necessarily affects the nature of the interaction.

Discourse as Outcome for Therapy

Numerous studies acknowledge the importance of discourse measures as functional outcomes for impairment-based treatments (e.g., del Toro et al., 2008). For example, Hickin, Best, Herbert, Howard, and Osborne (2001) discuss the importance of ascertaining whether treatment gains in picture naming generalize to conversation, and Coelho (2007) argues for the recognition of discourse measures (e.g., productivity, efficiency, content accuracy and organization, story grammar and coherence, and topic management) as ideally suitable and indeed necessary for measuring outcomes from treatment for traumatic brain injury. There have been mixed findings to date in terms of generalization of skills learned in treatment to nonclinical situations and everyday discourse. These findings emanate from a variety of treatment types, including word-based therapies and conversational therapies. Conroy, Sage, and Lambon Ralph (2009) studied seven people with aphasia of various severities and type and demonstrated that gains made through naming therapy did generalize to connected speech. Conversely, Wallace and Kimelman (2013) report a case series in which three people with aphasia demonstrated improvement in naming following intervention, but these gains did not generalize to discourse.

Although most clinicians recognize the role of discourse as an outcome measure for mild aphasia, the work of Weinrich, McCall, Boser, and Virata (2002) identifies the importance of discourse outcomes for people with severe aphasia. In their study on treatment of five people with severe aphasia using the Computerized Visual Iconographic Communication (C-VIC) system, the therapy focused on single-word and sentence tasks, while outcome measures also included narrative and procedural discourse tasks (e.g., describing how to make an omelet). They reported changes at the word and sentence levels but not on the discourse tasks, again highlighting the need to measure all levels of language usage before claiming efficacy of treatments.

Some conversational therapies, such as those mentioned in the previous two sections, have demonstrated generalization from treatment contexts to spontaneous conversations (e.g., Cunningham & Ward, 2003; Hickey et al., 2004; Sorin-Peters & Patterson, 2014). Hence, although findings about generalization have been varied, researchers and clinicians are increasingly looking to discourse measures as a way of tapping whether clinical treatment gains have an effect on the person's everyday talking. The extent to which clinical treatment gains generalize to everyday discourse outside the clinical environment is a constant challenge of every type of treatment with every type of client. Discourse measures provide an avenue for exploring this vital issue.

Discourse as Medium for Management of Psychosocial Consequences of Aphasia

Clinicians routinely listen to the stories of their clients and use counseling principles to deal with psychosocial issues (Holland, 2007). One approach with close links to discourse theory is often characterized as a narrative approach, and it offers a systematic way of interpreting the stories and a framework for addressing their significance (Corsten, Konradi, Schimpf, Hardering, & Keilmann, 2014; Greenhalgh & Hurwitz, 1998). Because perceived loss of identity has been highlighted as a major problem for people with aphasia (Shadden, 2007), such stories are not merely incidental to the therapy process. Thus, a narrative approach to therapy involves expanding the therapy session from focusing only on language to focusing on the lived experience of aphasia. Rather than usurping the role of trained counselors, the speech–language clinician assists the recovery process by really listening to clients, understanding who they are, and "co-constructing clinical interactions in such a way as to create authentic relationships aimed at effecting relevant change" (Simmons-Mackie & Damico, 2010, p. 52).

Clearly, discourse is a key medium in such an approach. In addition, specific activities such as journaling and portfolio development provide ways for people with aphasia to tell their stories and gain insight into living with aphasia (Pound, Parr, Lindsay, & Woolf, 2000). Discourse within group aphasia therapy is also an excellent medium for addressing psychosocial issues. As Wilkinson and colleagues (1998) point out, there is a close relationship between language and psychosocial issues, so clinicians need to recognize that working with conversational interaction necessarily involves working with interpersonal relationships. This recognition is evident in the work of Boles, who has applied the principles of counseling and discourse analysis to intervention for couples when one has aphasia (Boles & Lewis, 2003).

CONCLUSIONS AND FUTURE DIRECTIONS

This chapter examined key perspectives in everyday talk in aphasia and provided an overview of how these can be used in clinical assessment and treatment frameworks. Because everyday talk is the ultimate focus of both the person with aphasia and his or her family, it is increasingly acknowledged in clinical fields as a valid focus of intervention and as an important source of communication information and client profiling not available from standardized tests. Conveying meanings to each other is the fundamental function of communication, and addressing the variety of meanings conveyed across a variety of contexts is essential if we are to capture a holistic picture of a person's communicative life. The three perspectives presented here represent a potential coalescence of frameworks drawn from linguistics, sociology, and psychology, each complementing the other.

To further explore everyday talk in aphasia and implications for treatment, numerous directions are possible. Continuing a focus on discourse occurring in natural situations is essential. Where early studies examined contrived discourse, often with the researcher acting as listener/conversation partner, future studies must continue to search out authentic contexts with real-life conversation partners of the person with aphasia. With technology moving forward continually and becoming increasingly portable and accessible, recording interactions in a variety of situations will be even more easily possible, with less technological intrusion, for example, through the use of personal technologies such as mobile phones, iPods, and MP3 players, which all have a recording capacity and to which many people have access. Of course, ethical issues related to anonymity, consent of conversation partners, and confidentiality must be considered; however, new avenues for recording interactions widen the scope of possible access to natural everyday discourse.

Technological development will also support the analysis of language samples once collected. Future investigation will determine the effectiveness of computerized applications to assist functional language analysis. Research supports the use of these assessment methods, although practical issues impede clinical implementation. Supporting the clinical use of discourse measurement may generate the necessary efficiency to increase the use of language structures beyond the sentence in assessment and intervention.

Factors related to gender, personality, premorbid discourse style, and the effects of emotion are also areas for future investigation that will shed light on language variety rather than assuming a normative approach to discourse phenomena. The most recent work examining the effects of different conversation partners on the discourse of people with aphasia will also continue, with further contextually driven analyses of these effects. Acknowledging the complexity of discourse and influencing factors, integration of multifunctional perspectives in assessment and treatment should provide a new lens on the impairment and provide a link to the individual's activity and participation levels referred to in the ICF model. Once discourse meanings are considered beyond the referential meanings often investigated in studies of single words, a closer link is obvious between language and interpersonal interactions.

With increased understanding of the dynamics of discourse, additional discourse treatments will emerge, utilizing natural conditions as well as the largely controlled conditions used to date. Although the challenge of discourse treatments is to provide a natural context and at the same time sufficiently control the data to be manageable, newer qualitative and descriptive frameworks may supply the answer to trying to fit a square peg into the round hole of experimental design applied to psycholinguistic and sociolinguistic studies.

Another important consideration for the future is the cultural context of discourse. Across-language comparisons in single-case studies are emerging and are highlighting areas where theoretical concepts in aphasia may be challenged (e.g., Abuom & Bastiaanse, 2012). Many aphasic discourse investigations to date have examined predominantly English language/Western cultural discourse contexts. Future research into discourse should expand on existing investigations that identify the cultural variations that differentiate aspects such as discourse structure, conversational rules, and narrative principles. In an area often focused on normal versus pathological phenomena, it is crucial to highlight cultural factors affecting language use to minimize clinical judgments of pathology and to broaden the notion of language and communication norms to include the variety of discourse phenomena that occur across languages.

Reports of conversation and discourse frameworks being incorporated into aphasia treatments are increasing in frequency in the research literature, providing a growing and promising evidence base for the clinical usefulness of such frameworks. Further research will provide greater insights into such aspects as those discourse components most amenable to change, the most significant components of partner training, and the relative stability of different discourse types of measures.

Case Illustration 13.1

In the preceding discussion of approaches to therapy, we identified four ways in which discourse and conversation might play a role in intervention. We illustrate these ways of using discourse and conversation in therapy in one case: Jan (pseudonym). Although we discuss these interventions separately, readers should note that in everyday clinical practice, these roles overlap and may differ in their priority for the client at different stages of recovery.

Jan is a 65-year-old woman who experienced aphasia following a stroke. Jan lives with her husband, Joe. She describes herself as very sociable and has lots of friends with whom she mixes frequently. Interests included genealogy as well as other historical matters, reading, and travel. During her working life, she worked as a typist, bookkeeper, and courier.

Computed tomographic (CT) scanning performed 4 to 5 days after the stroke showed no abnormality, and no further CT scans were performed. Immediately after the stroke, Jan's clinical signs consisted of fluent aphasia, right-sided hemiparesis, some upper limb dyspraxia, and right-sided hemianopia. Her hemiparesis, dyspraxia, and hemianopia resolved within a month after onset, but the aphasia persisted. At 12 months postonset, Jan's rating on the Boston Diagnostic Aphasia Examination (BDAE; Goodglass, Kaplan, & Barresi, 2000) Severity Rating Scale is 3, indicating a moderate degree of aphasia, with significant anomia. She has been categorized as having a fluent aphasia. The following discourse sample is one of a series of recounts obtained at this time, this particular one being a response to "Tell me about a happy experience."

Discourse sample: Jan's Wedding Recount at 12 Months Postonset

Key: Processes (verb types): Relational—*italics*; mental—UPPERCASE; material—**bold**; verbal—underlined.

1. Yes I got **married** at uh Saint Vincent's at Ashfield.
2. And that's where I told you my reception was at um . . . called the was called the Amery the Amery.
3. And uh that's been **pulled down** now.
4. And of course that's where I had to **go** and **get** whatever it *was* I had to **do** up there.
5. It *was* funny.
6. And uh um we *had* a very nice wedding.
7. And it *was* uh.
8. I THINK.
9. We *had* about 60 70 guests.
10. And it *was* about 8 no . . . in the af the morning the morning at about half past 12.
11. And uh what else would you LIKE to . . .

Clinician: What about the reception?

12. What *was* it like?
13. It *was* exciting naturally.
14. Because you're nervous.
15. But I *had* uh my naseral.
16. My little bridesmaid *was* only a small little person.
17. And uh I LOVED my reception.
18. It *was* beautiful you know.
19. And everything *was* uh.
20. It *was* a beautiful old place.
21. It *was* . . . lovely.
22. And everything was **looked after**.
23. And it *was* beautiful.
24. **Going** up to your.
25. To **take** your nice to your clothes.

(continues)

26. To **take off** your wedding frock.
27. And it *was* really very nice.
28. I LOVED it.
29. It *was* beautiful.
30. Then I **came** to Canberra for my honeymoon.

Jan's husband, Joe, has discussed with the treating clinician his distress when he sees her struggling, particularly in front of others, and his uncertainty about supplying the words for Jan. Thus, for Jan, an important part of her intervention will need to include ensuring that her husband, Joe, feels comfortable in conversation with her. Joe will be her major conversation partner because their adult children have left the family home, and he will accompany her as she attends her medical appointments and as they take up their former social activities of bowling and attending Rotary Club functions.

In terms of focusing ON discourse-level features, in this text, Jan produced numerous evaluations and descriptions of the day (e.g., *it was exciting, it was beautiful, it was really very nice, you were nervous, it was a lovely old place*). She predominantly uses the verb *to be*—classified as a relational process—to describe attitudes (*it was really very nice, it was beautiful, it was exciting*) or to describe entities (*it was a beautiful old place, my little bridesmaid was only a small little person*), but she can provide few details of actual events in the day. In all, she used 19 relational (in italics) and 4 mental verbs (in capitals) to convey feelings and attitudes, 10 material verbs (in bold) to describe actions, and 2 verbal processes (underlined), *told* and *call*.

Because this sample is a recount, it is appropriate that Jan uses mainly statements, so this sample does not provide an opportunity to look at her use of mood resources (i.e., to modulate meaning). However, Jan did use some interpersonal resources to add shades of meaning in terms of her evaluations. For example, the adjuncts *naturally* and *of course*, the projected mental phrase *I think* indicating uncertainty, the intensifier *very*, and the choice of evaluative lexical items *beautiful, lovely, exciting, nice,* all add to Jan's presentation of her perspective on events. From a textual perspective, the restrictions on Jan's lexical repertoire are obvious. Nevertheless, she obtains a degree of lexical cohesion through repetition of lexical items. Interestingly, this might be considered pathological or compensatory. For example, Jan emphasizes the pleasantness of the day through repetition of *nice, beautiful*. However, as well as repetition, she was able to create connections throughout the text through collocation of words related to the topic (e.g., *wedding, reception, wedding frock, bridesmaid*). In addition, continuity of the chains in which Jan is the agent is present (e.g., *I loved my reception/I loved it*), and she demonstrates intact use of pronouns. Overall, then, in Jan's discourse, we see limited experiential information but relatively strong interpersonal resources and some textual resources. Further sampling would be essential to gauge the representativeness of the findings discussed for Jan's discourse. However, it is important to note the discourse approach provides information about strengths and problematic usage that occurs across contexts and in specific contexts—so therapy is designed to elicit and facilitate language use for both particular situations and for general use.

For Jan, treatment directed toward problematic usage could focus on increasing her access to widen the variety of other verb types to broaden the meanings she could convey throughout the text, for example, incorporating traditional therapy structure (e.g., Rodriguez, Raymer, & Rothi, 2006) within discourse contexts such as personal recounts. Also, from a strength perspective, Jan's strong use of relational processes and interpersonal resources could form the basis for communication activities designed to maximize effectiveness, that is, to form the basis for conversational scripts and coaching (Hopper et al., 2002). Thus, a discourse perspective informs both the selection of linguistic items for therapy as well as the types of contextual situations in which the therapy would most usefully be embedded.

From a conversational perspective, but still focusing on discourse-level phenomena, analysis of their conversation together indicates that Joe tends to provide prompts and cues (e.g., first letter of the word) that are less effective than those identified by the clinician (e.g., semantic cues). In discussion with Joe and Jan, the clinician also identifies that Jan would like to set up an agreed signal (eye gaze) to Joe to indicate when she would appreciate his *speaking* on her behalf in the company of others. Therapy tasks are planned to work through a hierarchy, from short scripted role-plays through to role-plays of anticipated social encounters, and finally using reflection on free-flowing conversation.

(continues)

In terms of focusing on therapy IN a discourse context, Jan also has significant anomia, and when she describes what she wants out of therapy, she says she would "just like to get the words out." Naming therapy will make use of the approach of semantic feature analysis (Boyle, 2011; Boyle & Coehlo, 1995), and although the naming strategies involved in this approach will initially be introduced to Jan through explanation at word and sentence levels, therapy tasks will be provided within a sustained thematically unified discourse context, for example, procedural discourse tasks.

In terms of discourse as a medium for management of psychosocial issues, Jan and Joe may well benefit from the opportunity to explore their communication issues within a broader spectrum of life issues. The use of journaling and portfolio development in particular could be explored as a way for them to tell their stories as part of living with aphasia (Pound et al., 2000). Explicit work on narrative that makes use of the person's reflections on his or her story and its meaning for their personal identity and adaptation may also be of benefit (Hinckley, 2007).

In deciding on the most salient measures of outcome, the clinician will select discourse measures that meet the following criteria: relevant to targets of treatment, replicable, and time efficient to collect. For the preceding therapy plans, the clinician must measure the number of different categories of verb types as a percentage of total verbs to see potential changes in access to verbs for different genres. To evaluate the effect of training interactive partner strategies, the clinician can use observations taken "online" during a natural conversation among Jan, Joe, and an unfamiliar clinician, using the categories developed to describe *speaking-for* behaviors by Croteau and others (Croteau, Le Dorze, & Baril, 2007). In addition, the clinician can use measures of participation in conversation developed by Kagan and colleagues that provide two observational measures that allow him or her to rate each person, Jan and Joe, as they engage in conversation. The measures are both reliable and sensitive to change over time (Kagan et al., 2004). Lexical access for nouns in discourse will be observed through a transcription of a short personal recount elicited by the unfamiliar clinician in the context of the conversation ("What happened when you had your stroke?") and analyzed using the measures noted by Hickin and colleagues (2001): nouns as a proportion of content words in the sample, nouns per clause (per turns in Hickin's conversational sample), and measures such as hesitation phenomena (pauses and filled pauses), circumlocutions and semantic paraphasias, phonological errors, neologisms, overuse of pronouns, and comments on word retrieval such as "oh, what's it called?" to demonstrate difficulties experienced by the speaker in actual word retrieval.

STUDY QUESTIONS

1. What are the differences and similarities between discourse, conversation analysis, and narrative perspectives as discussed in this chapter?
2. How might these approaches be complementary?
3. How might contextual factors affect discourse output?
4. Would severity of aphasia influence the choice of a certain approach? If so, how? If not, why not?
5. Would type of aphasia influence the choice of a certain approach? If so, how? If not, why not?
6. What is the difference between experiential meanings and interpersonal meanings?
7. What might the discourse of a speaker be like when focusing on one type of meaning versus another, that is, either mainly experiential or mainly interpersonal?
8. How do the notions of *deficit* and *strength* apply to these approaches in terms of treatment directions?
9. What are the potential benefits of undertaking a narrative approach with a person with aphasia?
10. Can relatives/significant others participate in any/all of these approaches to assessment and treatment?

REFERENCES

Abuom, T. O., & Bastiaanse, R. (2012). Characteristics of Swahili-English bilingual agrammatic spontaneous speech and consequences for understanding agrammatic aphasia. *Journal of Neurolinguistics, 25*(4), 276–293.

Armstrong, E. (1991). The potential of cohesion analysis in the analysis and treatment of aphasic discourse. *Clinical Linguistics & Phonetics, 5*(1), 39–51.

Armstrong, E. (2005a). Expressing opinions and feelings in aphasia: Linguistic options. *Aphasiology, 19*(3/5), 285–296.

Armstrong, E. (2005b). Language disorder: A functional linguistic perspective. *Clinical Linguistics & Phonetics, 19*(3), 137–153.

Armstrong, E., Ciccone, N., Godecke, E., & Kok, B. (2011). Monologues and dialogues in aphasia: Some initial comparisons. *Aphasiology, 25*(11), 1347–1371.

Armstrong, E., Mortensen, L., Ciccone, N., & Godecke, E. (2012). Expressing opinions and feelings in an aphasia group setting. *Seminars in Speech & Language, 33*(1), 16–26.

Armstrong, E., & Ulatowska, H. K. (2007). Making stories: Evaluative language and the aphasia experience. *Aphasiology, 21*(6), 763–774.

Armstrong, L., Brady, M., Mackenzie, C., & Norrie, J. (2007). Transcription-less analysis of aphasic discourse: A clinicians dream or a possibility? *Aphasiology, 21*(3–4), 355–374.

Barbieri, E., Basso, A., Frustaci, M., & Luzzatti, C. (2010). Argument structure deficits in aphasia: New perspective on models of lexical production. *Aphasiology, 24*(11), 1400–1423.

Bastiaanse, R., Edwards, S., & Kiss, K. (1996). Fluent aphasia in three languages: Aspects of spontaneous speech. *Aphasiology, 10*(6), 561–575.

Beckley, F., Best, W., Johnson, F., Edwards, S., Maxim, J., & Beeke, S. (2013). Conversation therapy for agrammatism: Exploring the therapeutic process of engagement and learning by a person with aphasia. *International Journal of Language and Communication Disorders, 48*(2), 220–239.

Beeke, S., Johnson, F., Beckley, F., Heilemann, C., Edwards, S., Maxim, J., et al. (2014). Enabling better conversations between a man with aphasia and his conversation partner: Incorporating writing into turn taking. *Research on Language and Social Interaction, 47*(3), 292–305.

Beeke, S., Wilkinson, R., & Maxim, J. (2003). Exploring aphasic grammar 2: Do language testing and conversation tell a similar story? *Clinical Linguistics & Phonetics, 17*(2), 109–134.

Beeke, S., Wilkinson, R., & Maxim, J. (2007). Grammar without sentence structure: A conversation analytic investigation of agrammatism. *Aphasiology, 21*(3/4), 256–282.

Boles, L., & Bombard, T. (1998). Conversational discourse analysis: Appropriate and useful sample sizes. *Aphasiology, 12*(7–8), 547–560.

Boles, L., & Lewis, M. (2003). Working with couples: Solution focused aphasia therapy. *Asia Pacific Journal of Speech, Language and Hearing, 8*, 153–159.

Borod, J. C., Rorie, K. D., Pick, L. H., Bloom, R. L., Andelman, F., Campbell, A. L., et al. (2000). Verbal pragmatics following unilateral stroke: Emotional content and valence. *Neuropsychology, 14*(1), 112–124.

Boyle, M. (2011). Discourse treatment for word retrieval impairment in aphasia: The story so far. *Aphasiology, 25*(11), 1308–1326.

Boyle, M. (2014). Test–retest stability of word retrieval in aphasic discourse. *Journal of Speech, Language & Hearing Research, 57*(3), 966–978.

Boyle, M., & Coehlo, C. (1995). Application of semantic feature analysis as a treatment for aphasic dysnomia. *American Journal of Speech Language Pathology, 4*(4), 94–98.

Brady, M., Kelly, H., Godwin, J., & Enderby, P. (2012). Speech and language therapy for aphasia following stroke. *Cochrane Database of Systematic Reviews, 16*(5), CD000425. doi:10.1002/14651858.CD000425.pub3

Cherney, L. R., Halper, A. S., Holland, A., & Cole, R. (2008). Computerized script train ing for aphasia: Preliminary results. *American Journal of Speech-Language Pathology, 17*(1), 19–34.

Coelho, C. (2007). Management of discourse deficits following traumatic brain injury: Progress, caveats and needs. *Seminars in Speech & Language, 28*(2), 122–131.

Conroy, P., Sage, K., & Lambon Ralph, M. (2009). Improved vocabulary production after naming therapy in aphasia: Can gains in picture naming generalise to connected speech? *International Journal of Language & Communication Disorders, 44*(6), 1036–1062.

Corsten, S., Konradi, J., Schimpf, E., Hardering, F., & Keilmann, A. (2014). Improving quality of life in aphasia—evidence for the effectiveness of the biographic-narrative approach. *Aphasiology, 28*(4), 440–452.

Croteau, C., & Le Dorze, G. (2006). Overprotection, "speaking for," and conversational participation: A study of couples with aphasia. *Aphasiology, 20*(2–4), 327–336.

Croteau, C., Le Dorze, G., & Baril, G. (2007). Development of a procedure to evaluate the contributions of persons with aphasia and their spouses in an interview situation. *Aphasiology, 21*(6/7/8), 791–801.

Croteau, C., Le Dorze, G., & Morin, C. (2008). The influence of aphasia severity on how both members of a couple participate in an interview situation. *Aphasiology, 22*, 802–812.

Cruice, M., Worrall, L., Hickson, L., & Murison, R. (2003). Finding a focus for quality of life with aphasia: Social and emotional health, and psychological well-being. *Aphasiology, 17*(4), 333–353.

Cunningham, R., & Ward, C. D. (2003). Evaluation of a training programme to facilitate conversation between people with aphasia and their partners. *Aphasiology, 17*(8), 687–707.

Davidson, B., Worrall, L., & Hickson, L. (2008). Exploring the interactional dimension of social communication: A collective case study of older people with aphasia. *Aphasiology, 22*(3), 235–257.

del Toro, C. M., Altmann, L. P., Raymer, A. M., Leon, S., Blonder, L. X., & Gonzalez Rothi, L. J. (2008). Changes in aphasic discourse after contrasting treatments for anomia. *Aphasiology, 22*(7/8), 881–892.

Doyle, P. J., McNeil, M. R., Park, G., Goda, A., Rubenstein, E., Spencer, K., et al. (2000). Linguistic validation of four parallel forms of a story retelling procedure. *Aphasiology, 14*, 537–549.

Edwards, S., & Bastiaanse, R. (1998). Diversity in the lexical and syntactic abilities of fluent aphasic speakers. *Aphasiology, 12*(2), 99–117.

Falconer, C., & Antonucci, S. M. (2012). Use of semantic feature analysis in group discourse treatment for aphasia: Extension and expansion. *Aphasiology, 26*(1), 64–82.

Fergadiotis, G., Wright, H. H., & West, T. M. (2013). Measuring lexical diversity in narrative discourse of people with aphasia. *American Journal of Speech-Language Pathology, 22*(2), S397–S408.

Ferguson, A. (1992). Interpersonal aspects of aphasic communication. *Journal of Neurolinguistics, 7*(4), 277–294.

Ferguson, A. (2000). Maximising communicative effectiveness. In N. Muller (Ed.), *Pragmatic approaches to aphasia* (pp. 53–88). Amsterdam: Benjamins.

Frank, A. W. (1995). *The wounded storyteller: Body, illness, and ethics.* Chicago: University of Chicago Press.

Goodglass, H., Kaplan, E., & Barresi, B. (2000). *BDAE-3: Boston Diagnostic Aphasia Examination* (3rd ed.). Austin, TX: Pro-Ed.

Goodwin, C. (Ed.). (2003). *Conversation and brain damage.* Oxford, UK: Oxford University Press.

Gordon, J. K. (2008). Measuring the lexical semantics of picture description in aphasia. *Aphasiology, 22*(7–8), 839–852.

Greenhalgh, T., & Hurwitz, B. (Eds.). (1998). *Narrative based medicine: Dialogue and discourse in clinical practice.* London: BMJ Books.

Grodzinsky, Y. (1990). *Theoretical perspectives on language deficits.* Cambridge, MA: MIT Press.

Halliday, M. A. K., & Matthiessen, C. (2004). *An introduction to functional grammar* (3rd ed.). New York: Arnold.

Hengst, J. (2003). Collaborative referencing between individuals with aphasia and routine communication partners. *Journal of Speech, Language, and Hearing Research, 46*(4), 831–848.

Herbert, R., Gregory, E., & Best, W. (2014). Syntactic versus lexical therapy for anomia in acquired aphasia: differential effects on narrative and conversation. *International Journal of Language & Communication Disorders, 49*(2), 162–173.

Hickey, E., Bourgeois, M., & Olswang, L. (2004). Effects of training volunteers to converse with nursing home residents with aphasia. *Aphasiology, 18*(5/6/7), 625–637.

Hickin, J., Best, W., Herbert, R., Howard, D., & Osborne, F. (2001). Treatment of word-retrieval in aphasia: Generalisation to conversational speech. *International Journal of Language & Communication Disorders, 36*(Suppl. 1), 13–18.

Hilari, K., Needle, J., & Harrison, K. (2012). What are the important factors in health-related quality of life for people with aphasia? A systematic review. *Archives of Physical Medicine and Rehabilitation, 12*(93), S86–S95.

Hinckley, J., & Carr, T. (2005). Comparing the outcomes of intensive and non-intensive context-based aphasia treatment. *Aphasiology, 19*(10–11), 965–974.

Hinckley, J. J. (2007). *Narrative-based practice in speech-language pathology.* San Diego, CA: Plural.

Holland, A. (1998). Why can't clinicians talk to aphasic adults? Comments on supported conversation for adults with aphasia: Methods and resources for training conversational partners. *Aphasiology, 12*(9), 844–847.

Holland, A. (2007). *Counseling in communication disorders: A wellness perspective.* San Diego, CA: Plural.

Holland, A., Frattali, C., & Fromm, D. (1999). *Communication Activities of Daily Living (CADL-2)* (2nd ed.). Austin, TX: Pro-Ed.

Hopper, T., Holland, A., & Rewega, M. (2002). Conversational coaching: Treatment outcomes and future directions. *Aphasiology, 16*(7), 745–761.

Hymes, D. (1974). *Foundations in sociolinguistics: An ethnographic approach.* Philadelphia: University of Pennsylvania Press.

Ireland, C., & Wotton, C. (1996). Time to talk: Counselling for people with dysphasia. *Disability and Rehabilitation, 18*(11), 585–591.

Jaecks, P., Hielscher-Fastabend, M., & Stenneken, P. (2012). Diagnosing residual aphasia using spontaneous speech analysis. *Aphasiology, 26*(7), 953–970.

Kagan, A., Black, S. E., Duchan, F. J., Simmons-Mackie, N., & Square, P. (2001). Training volunteers as conversation partners using "Supported conversation for adults with aphasia." *Journal of Speech, Language and Hearing Research, 44*(3), 624–638.

Kagan, A., Winckel, J., Black, S., Duchan, J. F., Simmons-Mackie, N., & Square, P. (2004). A set of observational measures for rating support and participation in conversation between adults with aphasia and their conversation partners. *Topics in Stroke Rehabilitation, 11*(1), 67–83.

Labov, W. (2006). The transformation of experience in narrative. In A. Jaworski & N. Coupland (Eds.), *The discourse reader* (2nd ed., pp. 214–226). London: Routledge. (Original work published 1977)

Lock, S., & Armstrong, L. (1997). Cohesion analysis of the expository discourse of normal, fluent aphasic and demented adults: A role in differential diagnosis? *Clinical Linguistics & Phonetics, 11*(4), 299–317.

Lock, S., Wilkinson, R., Bryant, K., Maxim, J., Edmundson, A., Bruce, C., et al. (2001). Supporting Partners of People With Aphasia in Relationships and Conversation (SPPARC). *International Journal of Language & Communication Disorders, 36*(Suppl.), 25–30.

Marini, A., Andreetta, S., del Tin, S., & Carlomagno, S. (2011). A multi-level approach to the analysis of narrative language in aphasia. *Aphasiology, 25*(11), 1372–1392.

Matthiessen, C., Lukin, A., Butt, D., Cleirigh, C., & Nesbitt, C. (2005). A case study of multi-stratal analysis. *Australian Review of Applied Linguistics, 19*, 123–150.

McNeil, M. R., Doyle, P. J., Fossett, T. R. D., & Park, G. H. (2001). Reliability and concurrent validity of the information unit scoring metric for the story retelling procedure. *Aphasiology, 15*(10/11), 991–1006.

Miller, J. F., Andriacchi, K., & Nockerts, A. (2012). Systematic Analysis of Language Transcripts—SALT (Version SALT 2012 Clinical Version). Middleton, WI: SALT Software.

Milman, L. H., Dickey, M. W., & Thompson, C. K. (2008). A psychometric analysis of functional category production in English agrammatic narratives. *Brain & Language, 150*(1), 18–31.

Murray, L., Timberlake, A., & Eberle, R. (2007). Treatment of underlying forms in a discourse context. *Aphasiology, 21*(2), 139–163.

Nicholas, L. E., & Brookshire, R. H. (1993). A system for quantifying the informativeness and efficiency of the connected speech of adults with aphasia. *Journal of Speech & Hearing Research, 36*, 338–350.

Olness, G. S., & Englebretson, E. F. (2011). On the coherence of information highlighted by narrators with aphasia. *Aphasiology, 25*(6–7), 713–726,

Olness, G., Gyger, J., & Thomas, K. (2012). Analysis of narrative functionality: Toward evidence-based approaches in managed care settings. *Seminars in Speech and Language, 33*(1), 55–67.

Penn, C., & Beecham, R. (1992). Discourse therapy in multilingual aphasia: A case study. *Clinical Linguistics & Phonetics, 6*(1–2), 11–25.

Penn, C., Jones, D., & Joffe, V. (1997). Hierarchical discourse therapy: A method for the mild patient. *Aphasiology, 11*(6), 601–613.

Pound, C., Parr, S., Lindsay, J., & Woolf, C. (2000). *Beyond aphasia: Therapies for living with communication disability.* Bicester, UK: Speechmark.

Ramsberger, G., & Rende, B. (2002). Measuring transactional success in the conversation of people with aphasia. *Aphasiology, 16*(3), 337–353.

Riddoch, M. J., & Humphreys, G. W. (1994). *Cognitive neuro-psychology and cognitive rehabilitation*. London: Erlbaum.

Rodriguez, A. D., Raymer, A. M., & Rothi, L. J. G. (2006). Effects of gesture + verbal and semantic-phonological treatments for verb retrieval in aphasia. *Aphasiology, 20*(2–4), 286–297.

Sarno, M. T. (1969). *The Functional Communication Profile: Manual of directions*. New York: Institute of Rehabilitation Medicine.

Schegloff, E. A., Jefferson, G., & Sacks, H. (1977). The preference for self-correction in the organization of repair in conversation. *Language, 53*, 361–382.

Shadden, B. (2005). Aphasia as identity theft: Theory and practice. *Aphasiology, 19*(3/4/5), 211–223.

Shadden, B. (2007). Rebuilding identity through stroke support groups: Embracing the person with aphasia and significant others. In R. Elman (Ed.), *Group treatment of neurogenic communication disorders* (2nd ed., pp. 111–126). San Diego, CA: Plural.

Simmons-Mackie, N. (2001). Social approaches to aphasia intervention. In R. Chapey (Ed.), *Language intervention strategies in aphasia and related neurogenic communication disorders* (pp. 246–268). Philadelphia: Lippincott Williams & Wilkins.

Simmons-Mackie, N., & Damico, J. (2010). Exploring clinical interaction in speech-language therapy: Narrative, discourse and relationships. In R. Fourie (Ed.), *Therapeutic processes for communication disorders: A guide for clinicians and students*. London: Psychology Press.

Simmons-Mackie, N., Elman, R., Holland, A., & Damico, J. S. (2007). Management of discourse in group therapy for aphasia. *Topics in Language Disorders, 27*(1), 5–23.

Simmons-Mackie, N., & Kagan, A. (1999). Communication strategies used by "good" versus "poor" speaking partners of individuals with aphasia. *Aphasiology, 13*, 807–820.

Simmons-Mackie, N., Kingston, D., & Schultz, M. (2004). Speaking for another: The management of participant frames in aphasia. *American Journal of Speech Language Pathology, 13*(2), 114–127.

Simmons-Mackie, N., Raymer, S., Armstrong, E., Holland, A., & Cherney, L. (2010). Partner training in aphasia: A systematic review. *Archives of Physical Medicine and Rehabilitation. 91*(12), 1814–1837.

Simmons-Mackie, N., Savage, M., & Worrall, L. (2014). Conversation therapy for aphasia: A qualitative review of the literature. *International Journal of Language & Communication Disorders, 49*(5), 511–526.

Sorin-Peters, R., & Patterson, R. (2014). The implementation of a learner-centred conversation training programme for spouses of adults with aphasia in a community setting. *Aphasiology, 28*(6), 731–749.

Thompson, C., Riley, R., den Ouden, D., Meltzer-Asscher, A., & Lukic, S. (2013). Training verb argument structure production in agrammatic aphasia: Behavioral and neural recovery patterns. *Cortex, 49*(9), 2358–2376.

Threats, T. T. (2007). Access for persons with neurogenic communication disorders: Influences of personal and environmental factors of the ICF. *Aphasiology, 21*, 67–80.

Togher, L. (2001). Discourse sampling in the 21st century. *Journal of Communication Disorders, 34*(1–2), 131–150.

Togher, L. (2003). Do I have green hair? "Conversations" in aphasia therapy. In S. Parr, J. Duchan, & C. Pound (Eds.), *Aphasia inside out: Reflections on communication disability* (pp. 65–79). Maidenhead, UK: Open University Press.

Ulatowska, H. K., & Olness, G. (2001). Dialectal variants of verbs in narratives of African Americans with aphasia: Some methodological considerations. *Journal of Neurolinguistics, 14*(2), 93–110.

Ulatowska, H. K., Reyes, B., Santos, T., & Worle, C. (2010). Stroke narratives in aphasia: The role of reported speech. *Aphasiology, 25*(1), 93–105

Ulatowska, H. K., Weiss-Doyell, A., Freedman-Stern, R., & Macaluso-Haynes, S. (1983). Production of narrative discourse in aphasia. *Brain and Language, 19*, 317–334.

Wallace, S. E., & Kimelman, M. D. Z. (2013). Generalization of word retrieval following semantic feature treatment. *NeuroRehabilitation, 32*(4), 899–913.

Webster, J., Franklin, S., & Howard, D. (2001). An investigation of the interaction between thematic and phrasal structure in nonfluent agrammatic subjects. *Brain & Language, 78*(2), 197–211.

Weinrich, M., McCall, D., Boser, K. I., & Virata, T. (2002). Narrative and procedural discourse production by severely aphasic patients. *Neurorehabilitation & Neural Repair, 16*(3), 249–274.

Whitney, J. L., & Goldstein, H. (1989). Using self-monitoring to reduce disfluencies in speakers with mild aphasia. *Journal of Speech & Hearing Disorders, 54*(4), 576–586.

Whitworth, A., Perkins, L., & Lesser, R. (1997). *Conversation Analysis Profile for People with Aphasia (CAPPA)*. London: Whurr.

Wilkinson, R. (2015). Conversation and aphasia: Advances in analysis and intervention. *Aphasiology, 29*(3), 257–268.

Wilkinson, R., Bryan, K., Lock, S., Bayley, K., Maxim, J., Bruce, C., et al. (1998). Therapy using conversation analysis: Helping couples adapt to aphasia in conversation. *International Journal of Language & Communication Disorders, 33*, 144–149.

Wilkinson, R., & Wielaert, S. (2012). Rehabilitation targeted at everyday communication: Can we change the talk of people with aphasia and their significant others within conversation? *Archives of Physical Medicine & Rehabilitation, 93*(2, Suppl.), S70–S76.

World Health Organization. (2001). *ICF: International Classification of Functioning, Disability and Health*. Geneva, Switzerland: Author.

Wright, H. H., & Capilouto, G. J. (2009). Manipulating task instructions to change narrative discourse performance. *Aphasiology, 23*(10), 1295–1308.

Wright, H. H., & Capilouto, G. J. (2012). Considering a multi-level approach to understanding maintenance of global coherence in adults with aphasia. *Aphasiology, 26*(5), 656–672.

OBJECTIVES

The reader will be able to:

1. Understand what the quality-of-life approach in aphasia means.

2. Develop understanding and awareness of key concepts and definitions associated with quality of life.

3. Develop awareness of quality-of-life tools available for use with people with aphasia and their families.

4. Appreciate how the quality-of-life approach underpins the whole of intervention.

Quality-of-Life Approach to Aphasia

Katerina Hilari and Madeline Cruice

INTRODUCTION

As a profession, we have been moving toward a better understanding of how communication and communication disability affect quality of life (QOL), how intervention influences QOL, as well as effecting communicative improvements. Our growing evidence base has thus far considered how to predict, describe, change, and measure QOL in aphasia, and how family members or other communication partners are involved in QOL evaluations. This chapter defines QOL and related concepts and references relevant research.

A substantial proportion addresses measurement issues, approaches, and tools that can be used in the management of individuals with aphasia. We also present clinical applications of a QOL approach in clinical management across different stages of service delivery using case illustrations and how we anticipate QOL moving forward in the next decade.

QUALITY OF LIFE AND RELATED CONCEPTS

Following are several reasons why it is essential to address people with aphasia within the context of their QOL:

- *A drive to contextualize all rehabilitation for the client and family:* Using a QOL approach allows us to better understand and measure the impact of disease on the client's life as a whole (Patrick & Erickson, 1993) and to incorporate the client's perspective in clinical decision making (Mayou & Bryant, 1993).
- *A client focus and consumer inclusion in decision making in health care in the 21st century:* For example, in the United Kingdom,

service delivery and organization should be informed by clients' and caregivers' views (Department of Health, 2007; NHS Executive, 1999). Similarly, in the United States, the Food and Drug Administration (FDA) encourages the use of patient-reported outcomes, such as QOL outcomes, in the evaluation of the effectiveness of interventions (US Department of Health and Human Services FDA Center for Drug Evaluation and Research, Center for Biologics Evaluation and Research, Center for Devices and Radiological Health, 2006).

- *Guidelines by professional bodies:* In the United States, the American Speech-Language-Hearing Association (ASHA) scope of practice document identifies as the overall objective of speech–language pathology services optimizing individuals' ability to communicate and swallow, thereby improving QOL (ASHA, 2007). Similarly, the Speech Pathology Australia Association (SPAA) scope of practice statement describes that one of the many possible outcomes to be achieved through the provision of speech pathology services is the improvement in general health, well-being, and QOL (Speech Pathology Australia, 2015). Finally, in the United Kingdom, professional guidelines identify as key aims of stroke and aphasia rehabilitation to maximize the patients' social rehabilitation and their sense of well-being/QOL and to minimize the distress and stress of the family (Intercollegiate Stroke Working Party, 2012; Royal College of Speech and Language Therapists, 2006).

- *Stakeholder priorities:* In Scotland, consensus-focused research conducted in partnership with stroke survivors, caregivers, and health professionals revealed 10 top priorities for life with stroke, including best ways for recovery from aphasia, coping with speech problems, coming to terms with the long-term consequences of stroke, and improving confidence after stroke (Pollock, St George, Fenton, & Firkins, 2012). Internationally, people with aphasia and family members have agreed on desired outcomes after stroke and aphasia and focused on communication; life participation; attitudes, awareness and education; emotional (and physical) well-being; health (and support) services; and recovery (Wallace et al., submitted). Both studies demonstrate that the consequences of stroke and aphasia are far reaching with implications for practitioner assessment and intervention.

Before looking at how we can measure and explore QOL in people with aphasia, we explain what QOL and related concepts, that is, emotional state, social participation, social support, well-being, and life satisfaction, actually mean. We also look at what we know about these areas in relation to people with aphasia and their families. We refer to key findings from the growing evidence base in each section.

Quality of Life and Health-Related Quality of Life

In 1975, Medline introduced QOL as a heading, and it was accepted as a concept by Index Medicus in 1977 (Bowling, 1995). Since then, there has been an explosion of interest in the area, with more than 20,000 new papers indexed under "quality of life" published in the decade from 2000 to 2009; and more than 81,000 from 2005 to 2014. Bowling (1995) points out that QOL is "an amorphous concept that has a usage across many disciplines … and theoretically incorporates all aspects of an individual's life" (p. 2).

The World Health Organization (WHO) defines QOL as follows:

> An individual's perception of their position in life in the context of the culture and value systems in which they live and in relation to their goals, expectations, standards and concerns. It is a broad ranging concept affected in complex ways by the person's physical health, psychological state, level of independence, social relationships, and their relationships to salient features of their environment. (WHOQOL Group, 1995, p. 1405)

Health-related quality of life (HR-QOL) is a related but narrower term. HR-QOL is concerned with the impact of a health state on a person's ability to lead a fulfilling life (Bullinger, Anderson, Cella, & Aaronson, 1993). It incorporates the individual's subjective evaluation of his or her physical, mental/emotional, family, and social functioning (Berzon, Hays, & Shumaker, 1993; de Haan, Aaronson, Limburg, Langton Hewer, & van Crevel, 1993; Hays, Anderson, & Revicki, 1993). Within adult neurogenic communication disorders, it is fair to say that the majority of the evidence in QOL lies in aphasic populations.[1] This evidence base has grown steadily in the last decade, with research from Australia, England, and North America the main contributors. Key findings include these:

- Aphasia has a profoundly negative impact on QOL both personally and socially, as identified by participants in a metasynthesis of qualitative studies of QOL with stroke (Moeller & Carpenter, 2013).

- The QOL of people with aphasia is distinguished from that of people without stroke and aphasia on independence, social relationships, and access to aspects of the environment (K. Ross & Wertz, 2003).
- People with aphasia have poorer HR-QOL and report fewer social and leisure activities than people with stroke without aphasia, even when their physical abilities, emotional well-being, and social support are comparable (Hilari, 2011).
- Communication ability, and to a lesser degree the individual's level of linguistic ability, predicts an aphasic person's HR-QOL and well-being (Cruice, Worrall, Hickson, & Murison, 2003; Hilari, Wiggins, Roy, Byng, & Smith, 2003).
- Individuals with severe aphasia have significantly lower HR-QOL compared to their general aphasic peers (Hilari & Byng, 2009). Using generic measures of HR-QOL and well-being, family members acting as proxy respondents for their aphasic partners rate the aphasic person's QOL (on global or physical-specific questions) predictably and significantly lower than the aphasic person would him- or herself (Cruice, Worrall, Hickson, & Murison, 2005). Conversely, using a stroke- and aphasia-specific measure of HR-QOL, family members were better judges of their partner's QOL (Hilari, Owen, & Farrelly, 2007).
- Activities, verbal communication, people, body functioning, stroke, mobility, personal outlook, independence, home, and health are important to the QOL of individuals with aphasia. Discussions with family members reveal that emotional consequences, ability to socialize, psychological impact, financial issues, and a need for purpose were also important (Cruice, Hill, Worrall, & Hickson, 2010).
- Summarizing factors that affect HR-QOL postaphasia, a recent systematic review synthesized the evidence of 14 studies: HR-QOL was negatively affected by emotional distress/depression, severity of aphasia and communication disability, other medical problems, activity limitations, and aspects of social network and support (Hilari, Needle, & Harrison, 2012). Themes drawn from qualitative studies add to these findings. A meta-analysis of qualitative studies identified seven overarching themes related to living successfully with aphasia: participation, meaningful relationships, support, communication, positivity, independence and autonomy, and seeing living successfully with aphasia as a journey over time (Brown, Worrall, Davidson, & Howe, 2012).

With respect to the broad and emerging evidence base on impact of aphasia on families, the following key findings are known:

- Families experience a broad range of consequences (many negative) with aphasia, including having to handle stress, changes in own self-care, more responsibilities in domestic life, changes to social life of family and friends specifically decreased time for leisure and withdrawal from social situations, and changes in employment, education, and volunteering (Grawburg, Howe, Worrall, & Scarinci, 2013; Winkler, Bedford, Northcott, & Hilari, 2014).
- Living successfully with aphasia for family members is influenced by seven elements: getting involved in life, support for the person with aphasia, communication, family members' own needs, putting life in perspective, focusing on and celebrating strengths and improvements, and experiences with services (Brown, Worrall, Davidson, & Howe, 2011). These findings were echoed by Winkler et al. (2014), who identified positive reframing, allocating time to oneself, and seeking support from family and friends as helpful strategies for family members to adjust to their new roles.
- Finally, family members' reflections on the rehabilitation goals they had for themselves included a specific goal around caring for one's own well-being, which was especially important given the emotional and mental impact and fatigue that family members experienced (Howe et al., 2012).

Emotional State and Depression

Emotional state can be described as emotional health or emotional distress, mood, depression, and anxiety. Emotional state is difficult to define: Within the WHO's framework, emotional state is considered through the domain of psychological health, which includes negative and positive feelings (WHOQOL Group, 1993). Others consider it as depression and define it as a universal condition that exists on a continuum from normal mood swings to a pathological state (Zung, cited in McDowell & Newell, 1996). Although *emotional health* is a more neutral term, *depression* is more widely and easily understood.

Given that poststroke depression can be present in as many as 62–70% of people with aphasia (Kauhanen et al., 2000), and it is one of three major issues in poststroke QOL (Bays, 2001), depression is an essential consideration in adult clinical practice. Emotional distress or mood also strongly predicts HR-QOL and well-being in chronic aphasia (Cruice et al., 2003; Hilari, Wiggins, et al., 2003; Hilari et al., 2012): The higher the degree of distress, the lower the person's QOL. Emotional responses to aphasia change over time. The work of Parr, Byng, and Gilpin (1997) with 50 individuals with aphasia illustrates a range of responses to aphasia, such as fear, anxiety, bewilderment, despair, fury, amusement, frustration, isolation, shock, embarrassment, depression, and as time goes by, resignation or increasing confidence. There is a sense that emotional responses related to aphasia gradually become more stable and predictable. Although this may be true, it should not mask the swings of feeling that can still occur years after the stroke or the intensity of the distress that can be experienced over years.

Addressing depression in people with aphasia poststroke is an important consideration. There is promising evidence for psychological interventions: A multicenter randomized controlled trial (n = 105) of behavior activation therapy (BAT) delivered by assistant psychologists to stroke patients with aphasia found that mood was significantly better at the 6-month follow-up in those who received BAT compared to usual care (Communication and Low Mood [CALM] trial; Thomas, Walker, Macniven, Haworth, & Lincoln, 2013).

Arguably, speech and language clinicians may have a key role to play in supporting people with aphasia's emotional well-being. The Royal College of Speech and Language Therapists guidelines state that speech and language clinicians working with people with aphasia should aim to "address emotional health and enable participation" (p. 98) (Royal College of Speech and Language Therapists, 2005); an Australian survey found that the majority of aphasia-specialist speech and language clinicians provided counseling either frequently (27%) or very frequently (39%) (Rose, Ferguson, Power, Togher, & Worrall, 2014). Yet, evidence on the impact of speech and language pathology therapeutic intervention on depression and well-being is mixed. For example, Ross, Winslow, Marchant, and Brumfitt (2006) found no significant group change using the Hospital Anxiety and Depression Scale (HADS; Zigmond & Snaith, 1983) for seven individuals with aphasia after completing an 11-week program of disability awareness and advocacy sessions. The researchers note that some individuals reported more favorable outcomes posttreatment, whereas, others within the group had less favorable outcomes, affecting the overall group analysis. A similar nonsignificant finding, using the Affect Balance Scale (Bradburn, 1969), was noted in Lyon et al.'s (1997) study of 10 individuals with aphasia completing a 20-week communication partners training program. Still, more recently a small proof-of-concept study (Northcott, Burns, Simpson, & Hilari, in press) explored a novel psychosocial therapy approach, *solution-focused brief therapy* (SFBT), for people with chronic aphasia (n = 5). Both qualitative and quantitative results described improvements in participants' communicative participation and mood, with large effect sizes (Cohen's d = 0.79–0.81) (using the Communicative Participation Item Bank, Baylor et al., 2013, and the General Health Questionnaire, Goldberg, 1972). Further research with larger samples and with attention to individual and not only group change will move the field forward in this crucial area of addressing depression in poststroke aphasia.

Thus, identifying which factors predict emotional distress poststroke is important to detect those at risk for depression and target intervention appropriately. In a recent systematic review (Kutlubaev & Hackett, 2014), depression after stroke was associated with prestroke depression, more severe neurological deficit, and physical disability both in the acute phase and at later stages poststroke. People with aphasia were excluded in most of the studies included in this review. However, people with aphasia were included in one recent study that explored predictors of emotional distress at 1 and 6 months poststroke (Thomas & Lincoln, 2008). Expressive aphasia and dependence in personal activities of daily living (ADL) predicted distress at 1 month poststroke. Stroke severity, expressive aphasia, and distress at 1 month poststroke predicted distress at 6 months. A further study also explored distress in a sample of stroke survivors that included people with aphasia (Hilari et al., 2010). People were seen soon after their stroke and 3 and 6 months later. The study found that the strongest predictors of emotional distress were stroke severity at baseline, low social support at 3 months, and loneliness and low satisfaction with social network at 6 months poststroke. In this study, although aphasia was not a predictor of distress at any time point, still, at 3 months poststroke, people with aphasia were significantly more likely to suffer from emotional distress (93%) than were people without aphasia (50%) (Hilari et al., 2010).

Caregivers of individuals with stroke often have elevated levels of depression in both the acute and chronic stages poststroke (Han & Haley, 1999). Frequent or common concerns for caregivers in stroke or aphasia are lack of information generally or specifically about aphasia; need for psychosocial support and hopefulness; and poor follow-up procedures for initiating rehabilitation in the home (Avent et al., 2005; Ski & O'Connell, 2007). Family members are often worried about the person with aphasia, report changed relationships and loss of spare time, and feeling lonely and resentful (Winkler et al., 2014). Understanding how clinicians and therapy services can support the caregiver and determining what contributes to caregiver burden, distress, and lack of coping are areas that deserve more attention in both research and clinical practice.

Well-Being and Life Satisfaction

Well-being is a concept related to QOL. Definitions of subjective well-being (the overarching more common concept) all center on an individual's cognitive and emotional judgment of his or her life experience, which may range on a continuum from positive to negative and reflect the individual's implicit standards (Fuhrer, 1994). Subjective well-being usually comprises three different constructs: life satisfaction, positive affect, and negative affect. Life satisfaction is a cognitive evaluation of where one is in life now compared to one's aspirations. Positive affect is the experience of positive feelings and is more dependent on external stimulation than internal control. Finally, negative affect is the experience of negative feelings such as anxiety or sadness, and the reverse is true, that is, it is more dependent on internal control.

There seems to be a link between language, communication, and psychological well-being in people with chronic aphasia (Cruice et al., 2003). Psychological well-being is thought to comprise the three constructs of subjective well-being described previously and mental health. The research found that participants with better language and better functional communication abilities had significantly higher psychological well-being in three specific areas: "personal growth" (being open to new experiences), "positive relations with others" (having satisfying high-quality relationships), and "self-acceptance" (a positive attitude toward oneself and one's past life). There is limited evidence for improved well-being from therapy, with a single study by Lyon and colleagues (1997), who found that their 10 participants had higher scores on the Psychological Well-Being Index (instrument developed by the authors) after their 20-week communication partners intervention program.

Interviews with 50 people with aphasia reveal various factors that contributed to life satisfaction (Parr, cited in Jordan & Kaiser, 1996). Decreased life satisfaction was attributed to physical (tiredness, volatility, irritability, life dominated by physiotherapy exercises); material (loss of work, loss of car, loss of income, drop in standards); social (restriction of social life, loss of contacts, boredom); and emotional (loss of confidence, fear of another stroke) factors. Increased life satisfaction in life with aphasia included freedom from previous restrictions (more time, more relaxed, life is slower, more laid back, free from work, reduced drinking); family and social life (family seems closer, partner closer, partnership closer, relationship improved, people more friendly, people helping); and enhanced sense of the value of life (Parr, cited in Jordan & Kaiser, 1996).

Social Participation and Social Support

Within the WHO International Classification of Functioning, Disability, and Health (ICF) framework (WHO, 2002), *participation* is defined as involvement in a life situation. Thus, social participation can be seen as involvement in social life situations. Older individuals with aphasia report a range of activities as important in QOL, some of which are specific social activities (such as dining or going out with friends), and others involve other people in a social sense (such as learning a foreign language or playing golf; Cruice, Hill, et al., 2010). Research shows that in general, individuals with aphasia have fewer regular social activities compared to their peers without aphasia and would generally value doing more social activities (Cruice, Worrall, & Hickson, 2006). Moreover, research with people with severe aphasia shows that they are particularly prone to social isolation and exclusion (Parr, 2007).

Social participation is linked to social networks and social support. We know that people are influenced by the quality and quantity of their social relationships. For example, people with strong social relations have lower morbidity and mortality (House, Robbins, & Metzner, 1982), better possibility of recovery or survival after illness (Glass & Maddox, 1992), and better psychological health, well-being, and QOL (Aneshensel & Frerichs, 1982; Billings & Moos, 1982; Turner, 1981).

A social network can be seen as "the web of identified social relationships that surround an individual and the characteristics of those linkages" (Bowling, 1997, p. 90). Cohen and Wills (1985) suggest the role of a social network is to provide a sense of social integration. Functional social support, on the other hand, comprises a person's subjective experience of support and the degree to which interpersonal relationships serve particular needs (Hilari & Northcott, 2006). Social networks can be seen as the structure through which social support is provided (Lin, Dean, & Ensel, 1981). Individuals with aphasia have been found to have smaller social networks, that is, fewer social contacts in their network and specifically fewer friend relationships, than their nonaphasic peers (Cruice et al., 2006; Hilari & Northcott, 2006; Northcott & Hilari, 2011). There is, however, considerable range in social networks; for example, in one study, one individual named only 5 social contacts who were important in the individual's life, and another individual named 51 people (see Cruice et al., 2006). Thus, it is not possible to assume that persons with aphasia have homogeneous social participation patterns.

The evidence base clearly suggests the need to consider social participation with respect to QOL: Social relationships are a key discriminator between aphasic and nonaphasic QOL (K. Ross & Wertz, 2003); loneliness and low satisfaction with one's social network contribute to long-term emotional distress after stroke and aphasia (Hilari et al., 2010); individuals with aphasia who are involved in more activities have more favorable HR-QOL (Hilari, Wiggins, et al., 2003); and social interaction and activities outside the home have been shown to improve following yearlong rehabilitation programs (Sarno, 1997).

ASSESSING QOL AND HR-QOL

Before looking at assessing QOL and related concepts in people with aphasia, we highlight general information on the purposes of QOL assessment. This section also lists types of measures and approaches that a clinician can use, depending on the aim of the assessment.

There are several purposes for using QOL instruments. An authority body, the Scientific Advisory Committee of the Medical Outcomes Trust (2002), described these as follows:

- Assessing general or specific populations
- Screening
- Diagnosing
- Evaluating impact of (community) interventions/policies
- Evaluating efficacy and effectiveness of (health-care) interventions
- Conducting economic evaluations of interventions
- Using quality improvement and assurance programs in health care
- Monitoring general or specific populations over time

Note that a clinician's typical purpose for assessing QOL, monitoring *individuals* over time ideally to determine change from intervention, is absent from this list. It is fair to say that organizations (such as the Medical Outcomes Trust) interested in QOL on a grand scale have group, financial, and resource interests in mind, which are at odds with the individualized approach implicit for clinicians. In our profession so far, QOL is typically considered an additional outcome for measurement to identify the impact that speech–language therapy intervention has had on an individual's situation (e.g., A. Ross et al., 2006; Sarno, 1997; Van der Gaag et al., 2005).

The purpose for assessing QOL also depends on time postonset. It is likely that at acute and inpatient time periods, the clinician is foremost interested in screening to identify and address depression. In the rehabilitation (hospital or community) phase, the clinician might use tools to determine client interests and priorities to contextualize goals and therapy and tools to capture social participation changes. Different tools are needed

for each of these stages and to justify the cost of the rehabilitation services. Research from different countries suggests that QOL measures are variably used in clinical practice, for example, only 3 of 70 Australian aphasia clinicians surveyed (Verna, Davidson, & Rose, 2009) reported using a QOL measure, and all reported the Visual Analogue Self-Esteem Scale (VASES, Brumfitt & Sheeran, 1999), and similarly in the United Kingdom, the VASES was the most common QOL tool (Brumfitt, 2006; ten Kate, 2014). More recently, an international survey of aphasia clinicians from 16 countries ($N = 579$), involving substantial samples from Europe ($n = 179$), the United Kingdom ($n = 171$), United States ($n = 62$), and Australia ($n = 51$) found that 128 clinicians used QOL measures; the most common measure used was the Stroke and Aphasia Quality of Life scale (SAQOL-39: Hilari, Byng, Lamping, & Smith, 2003; Hilari et al., 2009; Hilari et al., in press). Generally, a most sensible use of QOL instruments is in gathering information for therapy planning so that intervention is focused on the individual's needs and desires and takes into consideration his or her interests. This is often conducted in clinical practice but has yet to be researched and evaluated to determine whether QOL-driven approaches to therapy result in similar or greater outcomes for the client than do clinician-led approaches to therapy planning.

Types of Measures and Approaches

There are many different ways of measuring QOL and HR-QOL, and the choice of what measure to use depends primarily on the purpose of the assessment.[2]

Generic and Condition-Specific Scales

In health-related research, the most commonly used measures are multi-item scales. Early measures were developed and rated by clinicians and were mostly limited to functional abilities (e.g., Karnofsky, Abelmann, & Craver, 1948). Following this, a number of ADL scales were developed, and gradually in the 1970s and 1980s, measures of health status started emerging. Such measures included the Sickness Impact Profile (SIP; Bergner, Bobbitt, Carter, & Gilson, 1981) and the Nottingham Health Profile (NHP; Hunt, McKenna, McEwen, Williams, & Papp, 1981). Since then, numerous HR-QOL scales have been developed. In 1992, the Short-Form 36 Health Survey (SF-36) was developed (J. E. Ware, Snow, & Kosinski, 1993), which is today the most commonly used health status measure. Unlike many other scales, the SF-36 has been extensively tested for its psychometric properties and evaluated in many populations. It is a generic measure that covers the domains of physical functioning, role limitations caused by physical health problems, bodily pain, social functioning, mental health, role limitations caused by emotional problems, vitality/energy/fatigue, and general health perceptions. The SF-36 reflects the challenges inherent in any general health measurement: An instrument should be broad in scope but not unwieldy, and a trade-off has to be made between covering many topics superficially and achieving detailed coverage of a few, that is, comprehensiveness versus precision (McDowell & Newell, 1996). The main advantage of generic measures is that they allow comparisons between different disease groups (Patrick & Erickson, 1993). Moreover, interventions can affect outcomes that are not condition specific, and generic measures may pick up QOL changes that were not anticipated and thus, not included in condition-specific measures.

Apart from generic measures of health status or HR-QOL, such as the SF-36, which have not been designed with a specific population in mind, there are also disease- or condition-specific measures. These are developed with specific populations in mind, for example, stroke, and they are not intended for general application (see the section "Stroke- and Aphasia-Specific HR-QOL Scales" in this chapter for further examples).

The main advantage of condition-specific measures is their increased validity and sensitivity (Bech, 1993). They are more likely than generic measures to detect small but clinically significant changes in health status (Patrick & Deyo, 1989). Moreover, they can reduce respondent burden by, including only relevant questions. Ideally, both types of measures should be used with clients because they complement one another in the information they provide. Moreover, the clients we see often have more than one underlying problem (e.g., a client may have both aphasia and dyspraxia or a client with Parkinson's disease may also have a stroke and aphasia).

Utility Measures

Another type of HR-QOL measure developed by health economists is utility assessments that are designed specifically for use in economic evaluations. The cost-effectiveness of interventions can be evaluated by calculating quality-adjusted life years (QALYs) (e.g., Weinstein & Stason, 1976). In QALYs, improvements in length of life and HR-QOL are amalgamated into one single index. Each life year is quality adjusted with a utility value, where 1 equals full health. Utility measures, such as the EuroQol/EQ-5D (European Quality of Life – 5 Dimensions; EuroQol Group, 1990), are increasingly used in clinical trials to evaluate the cost-effectiveness of interventions. In the field of aphasia, studies

exploring the costs of delivering a service are emerging (e.g., Van der Gaag & Brooks, 2008).

Individualized Measures

Another approach in the measurement of QOL and HR-QOL attempts to take individuals' own conceptualizations into account. In one technique (O'Boyle, McGee, Hickey, O'Malley, & Joyce, 1992), human judgment analysis is used. The respondents were not given a set questionnaire but were asked to nominate the five most important areas of their lives and rate their function in these areas. This technique is known as the Schedule for the Evaluation of Individual Quality of Life (SEIQOL). In a similar approach, respondents were asked to rate the most important areas of their lives affected by their condition and rate how badly affected each one was (Patient Generated Index; Ruta, Garratt, Leng, Russell, & MacDonald, 1994). These measures represent advances in developing more patient-centered HR-QOL outcomes (Bowling, 1995; Staniszewska, 1999), but more work is needed on their acceptability with different condition groups (Bowling, 1995).

Qualitative Approaches

Qualitative approaches have also been used in the assessment of QOL/HR-QOL and have been effectively conducted with individuals with mild-to-moderate aphasia. These include interviewing techniques, such as semistructured and structured interviewing, and ethnographic approaches, such as participant or nonparticipant observation, and analysis of artifacts, for example, diaries. Such qualitative methods are frequently employed to examine the impact of aphasia on family members' lives (Grawburg et al., 2013). Advocates of ethnographic approaches highlight their suitability for people with severely compromised language. Still, QOL is generally defined as a subjective phenomenon. This makes it hard to observe without making value judgments that link the observed behavior to the assumed subjective perception.

In short, a variety of different measures exists for the assessment of HR-QOL. The decision on what measure to use depends primarily on the purpose of the assessment and also on practical considerations (e.g., respondent burden, respondent communication skills, time constraints, resources). For example, if a service provider wants to compare the cost-effectiveness of two interventions, then a utility measure would be the most likely choice. On the other hand, if a clinician wants to collate HR-QOL data of groups of patients to measure the effectiveness of a therapy program, then a scale would be a more likely choice. If a clinician wants to find out about a specific client's QOL to guide goal setting and therapy, then a semistructured interview perhaps in combination with a scale may be a more appropriate approach.

Issues in Assessing QOL and Related Concepts With People With Aphasia

The very nature of aphasia, as a language and communication impairment, poses a serious challenge in assessing HR-QOL in an optimal way, that is, through participant self-report. People with aphasia are likely to have difficulty understanding some of the items in HR-QOL scales or questions asked and expressing their responses. This necessitates special attention on the selection and presentation of the materials to be used and the skills of the interviewer. For people with very severe aphasia, proxy respondents may have to be used. We discuss these issues in turn.

Selection and Presentation of Materials

In selecting a measure to assess QOL/HR-QOL or related areas in people with aphasia, the clinician should check measures for their linguistic and reading complexity and length and choose those that may be easier for people with aphasia. The chosen scale's presentation should then be modified to make it more accessible to people with aphasia. Previous studies suggest and test various methods (Hilari & Byng, 2001; Townend, Brady, & McLaughlan, 2007; Worrall et al., 2005). Scales can be reproduced and printed in an aphasia-friendly format, using large font (minimum point size 14), printing keywords in bold, presenting few items per page, and where appropriate using preprepared images. Moreover, practice items can be introduced to ensure that participants understand the format of each questionnaire and its response options. Last, lead-in sentences can be added to focus respondent attention, for example, "The next set of questions asks about your feelings."

Interviewer Skills

Speech and language clinicians have a special role to play in facilitating the communication of people with aphasia. Studies exploring the QOL of people with aphasia have typically employed speech and language clinicians as interviewers because of their special skills. They can read aloud the items and provide cues to facilitate understanding, check that the respondent has understood, and provide options to facilitate responding (Cruice, Hirsch, Worrall, Holland, & Hickson, 2000;

Hilari & Byng, 2001). Moreover, they need to monitor the respondents for signs of fatigue or distress and address these as necessary.

Use of Proxies

When people have such severe aphasia that they are unable to report for themselves on their QOL, then a person who knows them well, most commonly their significant other, can be asked to report for them. Typically, the proxy respondent is not asked for his or her own opinion but rather for what he or she thinks the person with aphasia would say if the person with aphasia could report for him- or herself. During assessment of the QOL of people with severe aphasia using proxies, it is important to remind the proxies frequently that they should be reporting as the person with aphasia would. For example, "What would Joan say to this question?" can be helpful in focusing the proxy appropriately.

If we are to use proxy respondents to obtain information on the QOL of people with severe aphasia, then we need to know how well proxies agree with the patients' self-evaluations. In the general medical literature, a systematic review of studies using proxy respondents with various population groups (not including people with aphasia) concludes that (a) agreement between proxy and self-report is better for more concrete, observable domains (e.g., physical) than for less-observable domains (e.g., psychosocial); and (b) proxies tend to score the patients as more severely affected than the patients score themselves (Sneeuw, Sprangers, & Aaronson, 2002).

Two studies have looked at proxy and self-report agreement with people with aphasia. One used generic QOL scales (Cruice et al., 2005) and the other the SAQOL-39 item (Hilari et al., 2007). As previously, they found that agreement was higher for objective rather than subjective domains and that proxies rated people with aphasia as more severely affected than people with aphasia rated themselves. However, the differences in the Hilari et al. (2007) study were small to moderate (effect sizes 0.2–0.5), suggesting that they may not be clinically significant. Readers are encouraged to read these sources because much detailed information is available within each.

In short, proxy evaluations of QOL for people with aphasia cannot be used interchangeably with self-reports. For some measures, for example, aphasia-friendly measures such as the SAQOL-39, proxy ratings may be more accurate than for generic measures. Clinicians need to be aware of the negative bias of proxy ratings, particularly on subjective domains, to be able to interpret proxy evaluations.

Assessment Tools for People With Aphasia and Their Families

In this section, we present a range of scales that can be used to assess QOL, HR-QOL, social participation, social support, and emotional distress in people with aphasia and their families. We present in more detail measures that have been extensively tested or successfully used with people with aphasia and their families.

Generic Health Status and QOL Scales

This section describes three generic health status or QOL instruments. The first has already been introduced in this chapter. Measuring HR-QOL, the SF-36 (J. J. Ware & Sherbourne, 1992; J. E. Ware et al., 1993) assesses eight health concepts, as described previously. It is the most widely used health status scale and has well-evidenced psychometric properties. It yields eight subscale scores across physical and mental health that give rise to two composite scores. Scoring and interpreting these are complex, and the results are not transparent to the clinician or client. The instrument contains yes/no questions, true/false questions, and frequency questions, and the average time for self-completion is reportedly 10 minutes (Bell & Kahn, 1996; Hayes, Morris, Wolfe, & Morgan, 1995), although it takes much longer with respondents with aphasia (on average, 23 minutes for people with mild-moderate aphasia; Cruice, 2001). The SF-36 has various instructions, question formats, and response formats as well as a high linguistic complexity that makes it difficult for respondents with aphasia. Subsequently, many of the items require a lot of cueing, particularly for those respondents with more severe linguistic impairment (Cruice, 2001). It is important to note that using the SF-36 in aphasiology warrants further attention, as research conducted with 30 individuals with chronic aphasia revealed that it did not adequately assess social HR-QOL functioning (Cruice, Worrall, & Hickson, 2010).

The Dartmouth Primary Care Cooperative Information Project COOP Charts Nelson et al., 1987) measure functional status through overall assessment of biological, physical, emotional and social well-being, and QOL. Designed to screen patients in primary care, the illustrated response options suggest their potential use with people with aphasia. They include nine charts, each of which poses a single question and has an illustrated five-point response scale, which includes written description, picture presentation, and numbers (see Figure 14.1). The charts take less than 5 minutes to complete with normal populations (on average, 12 minutes with respondents with aphasia; Cruice, 2001), and their reliability and validity are proven (Nelson, Landgraf, Hays, Wasson, & Kirk, 1990). Compared to the SF-36, the COOP Charts are accessible, relatively easy to complete, and transparent in scoring. Although there is no psychometric data for individuals with aphasia, the instrument is suggested for further research and clinical use and has been used in research exploring social participation of Dutch individuals with aphasia (Dalemans, De Witte, Beurskens, Van Den Heuvel, & Wade, 2010).

The EQ-5D is a self-report popular measure of health outcome and is used across a range of health conditions. Designed by EuroQol, the EQ-5D is a brief measure comprising two pages: a descriptive evaluation of five dimensions (mobility, self-care, usual activities, pain/discomfort, and anxiety/depression) and a visual analogue scale of best-to-worst imaginable health state. The tool exists in two versions: three levels (no problems, some or moderate problems, extreme problems) and five levels (no problems, slight problems, moderate problems, severe problems, and extreme problems). Two scores are generated and compared to existing values available from the EuroQol website. As a utility index (as well as health status tool), the EQ-5D has been used to explore cost-effectiveness of community services for living with aphasia (Van der Gaag & Brooks, 2008) and is being increasingly preferred and used in stroke units and community services, although full evidence for its application is still needed.

A final generic QOL/HR-QOL measure to consider is the World Health Organization QOL-100 (WHOQOL-100) instrument and the smaller WHOQOL BREF (26 items only), which were designed by the WHOQOL Group (1995). The content for the WHOQOL-100 was drawn both from scientific experts and from the lay field, from a number of different international collaborating centers, and has passed through substantial rigorous pilot testing. The measure has at its core the definition of QOL described at the beginning of this chapter and measures functioning and satisfaction from the respondent's point of view. The WHOQOL-100 has six domains: physical health, psychological, level of independence, social relations, environment, and spirituality/religion/personal beliefs. The WHOQOL BREF contains only the physical, psychological, social relationships, and environment domains. It is somewhat disappointing that in the BREF version, the number of items pertaining to social relationships (highly relevant for adults with acquired neurological conditions generally) is substantially reduced compared to the 100-item version. The WHOQOL-100 is complex both linguistically and cognitively and would require substantial facilitation for individuals with aphasia.

Social Activities

During the past 4 weeks . . .
Has your physical and emotional health limited
your social activities with family, friends, neighbors, or groups?

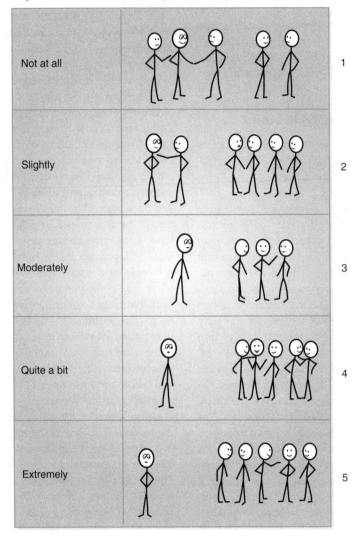

Figure 14.1 Social activities chart.
© Trustees of Dartmouth College/CO-OP Project, 2010.

However, K. Ross and Wertz (2003) used the BREF version successfully in their study and show that it is a useful tool that can discriminate between adults with and without chronic aphasia. It requires respondents to think over the past 4 weeks and keep their standards, hopes, pleasures, and concerns in mind when answering. Although the response format stays consistent with a 5-point scale, the scale descriptors change several times through the instrument, which may be a challenge for individuals with comprehension difficulties. The WHOQOL BREF is available through the WHO website and can be downloaded in PDF format.

Stroke- and Aphasia-Specific HR-QOL Scales

A number of scales have been developed to assess HR-QOL in people with stroke. These are as follows, in publication order:

1. The Stroke-Adapted Sickness Impact Profile (SA-SIP30; Van Straten et al., 1997)
2. The Stroke-Specific Quality of Life Scale (SS-QOL; Williams, Weinberger, Harris, Clark, & Biller, 1999)
3. The Stroke Impact Scale (SIS; Duncan et al., 1999)
4. The Newcastle Stroke-Specific Quality of Life Scale (NEWSQOL; Buck, Jacoby, & Ford, 2001)

5. The Burden of Stroke Scale (BOSS; Doyle, McNeil, Hula, & Mikolic, 2003)
6. The SAQOL-39 (Hilari, Byng, et al., 2003; Hilari et al., 2009)

The first of these scales, the SA-SIP30, was not developed in consultation with people with stroke and aphasia, but rather was adapted from the generic SIP. Scales 2 and 3 (SS-QOL and SIS) are commonly used scales, especially in the United States, for the assessment of HR-QOL in people with stroke. However, people with aphasia were excluded from the psychometric testing. People with aphasia were involved in the development of the NEWSQOL, but as in the previous scales, they were excluded from psychometric testing. The BOSS was designed to measure patient-reported difficulty in multiple domains of functioning, psychological distress associated with specific functional limitations, and general well-being in stroke survivors. The 12 subscales address mobility, self-care, swallowing, communication, cognition, social relations; energy and sleep; and positive mood, negative mood, domain mood, domain satisfaction, and domain restriction. Aspects of the BOSS have been well tested with people with aphasia (Doyle et al., 2003), and psychometric testing with 178 stroke survivors (one third with aphasia) confirmed internal consistency, test–retest reliability, construct validity, and responsiveness to change in the first year poststroke (Doyle, McNeil, Bost, Ross, Wambaugh, Hula, & Mikolic, 2007). The BOSS also provides three composite scores of physical limitations, cognitive limitations, and psychological distress, the last of which may be particularly helpful for aphasia clinicians.

The SAQOL-39 was developed through adapting the SS-QOL for use with people with aphasia (Hilari & Byng, 2001). It taps the people's subjective evaluation of functioning in four domains: physical (e.g., "How much trouble did you have walking?"), psychosocial (e.g., "Did you feel that you were a burden to your family?"), communication (e.g., "How much trouble did you have finding the word you wanted to say?"), and energy (e.g., "Did you feel too tired to do what you wanted to do?"). The SAQOL-39 contains 39 items, each of which is scored on a 5-point scale (two response formats: 1 = could not do it at all, 5 = no trouble at all; 1 = definitely yes, 5 = definitely no) and provides an overall score and four domain scores (score range 1 to 5). High scores indicate better HR-QOL. Figure 14.2 shows one of the pages of the SAQOL-39, with items from the psychosocial domain.

The SAQOL-39 was tested for its psychometric properties in a group of 83 people with chronic aphasia in the United Kingdom and demonstrated good accessibility, reliability, and validity (Hilari, Byng, et al., 2003). It has been translated and adapted for use in several languages and cultures, including Chinese, Dutch, Finnish, Flemish, German, Greek, Hindu, Italian, Japanese, Korean, Norwegian, Portuguese (for Brazil and Portugal), Spanish (for Mexico and Spain), Swedish, and Turkish (contact Hilari for references).

More recently, the SAQOL-39 was tested in people with stroke with and without aphasia and the SAQOL-39generic (SAQOL-39g) emerged. The SAQOL-39g has the same items as the SAQOL-39 but has three domains: physical, psychosocial, and communication. The SAQOL-39g shows good reliability and validity and differentiates people by stroke severity and Visual Analogue Scale–defined QOL. Moderate changes from 2 weeks to 6 months supported the SAQOL-39g's responsiveness to change (Hilari et al., 2009). An additional advantage of the SAQOL-39, is its stability when administered over the

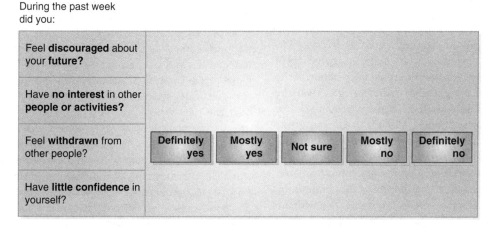

Figure 14.2 One page of the SAQOL-39, comprising four questions from the psychosocial domain.
Courtesy of Katerina Hilari.

phone or as a postal survey (Caute, Northcott, Clarkson, Pring, & Hilari, 2012).

Qualitative QOL Assessments

Qualitative QOL assessment, such as in-depth interviewing (Parr et al., 1997), semistructured interviewing (Le Dorze & Brassard, 1995; Zemva, 1999), and structured interviewing (Cruice, Hill, et al., 2010), have been used with people with aphasia. Research carried out with older individuals with aphasia illustrates that activities, verbal communication, people, and body functioning were core factors influencing their current and future QOL (Cruice, Hill, et al., 2010). Additional factors included stroke, mobility, positive personal outlook, dependence/independence, home, and health. These factors were identified from the analysis of participants' responses to six questions (see Farquhar, 1995, and Cruice, Hill, et al., 2010). A trained speech–language clinician facilitated a supported and structured interview to allow individuals with aphasia to express their views. There was, however, a noticeable impact on participants' capacity to express their views, and clinicians and individuals need to employ all means of expression and communication to support this exchange.

Emotional Distress

Many scales can be used to evaluate emotional distress, so we report two of the most commonly used ones here: the General Health Questionnaire (GHQ) and the Geriatric Depression Scale (GDS). Before addressing these, two scales specifically developed for people with aphasia are worth a mention. The Visual Analogue Mood Scales (VAMS; Stern, 1997) were developed specifically for post-stroke patients with aphasia to address the barriers of other measures: length and linguistic, cognitive, memory, and attention demands (Stern, 1999). With two positive mood scales (energetic, happy) and six negative mood scales (afraid, confused, sad, angry, tired, and tense), it has an obvious bent toward a negative state. Relatively recent research has identified that reversing the position of the positive mood state images (happy and energetic) with the other anchor (neutral) resulted in better psychometrics for people with aphasia (Kontou, Thomas, & Lincoln, 2012). The Stroke Aphasic Depression Questionnaire (Sutcliffe & Lincoln, 1998) is a 10-item questionnaire completed by a caregiver or observer to identify depression in stroke patients with aphasia. It was designed for community-living individuals and is increasingly being used with different populations (e.g., nursing home residents without major communication and cognitive difficulties; Sackley, Hoppitt, & Cardoso, 2006).

The GHQ (Goldberg, 1972) is a measure of distress that has been extensively used as a screening tool for psychiatric disorders. It was designed to identify two main types of problems: the inability to carry out normal functions and the appearance of new distressing symptoms (Goldberg & Hillier, 1979). The original 60-item version covers four elements of distress: depression, anxiety, social impairment, and hypochondriasis. The shortened versions (30-, 28-, 20-, and 12-item) do not include 12 items on somatic symptoms that were answered positively by physically ill people (Goldberg, 1972; Goldberg & Hillier, 1979). This reduces the number of false-positive responses. Its psychometric properties have been extensively tested with very good results (for reviews, see Goldberg & Williams, 1988; Vieweg & Hedlund, 1983). The GHQ has been used with people with stroke (e.g., Dennis, O'Rourke, Lewis, Sharpe, & Warlow, 2000; Dennis, O'Rourke, Slattery, Staniforth, & Warlow, 1997) and people with aphasia (e.g., the GHQ-12 in Hilari, Byng, et al., 2003; Hilari et al., 2010). Johnson et al. (1995) compared the GHQ-28 with the HADS in terms of screening for depression and anxiety after stroke. The patients were diagnosed using the *Diagnostic and Statistical Manual of Mental Disorders*, third edition (DSM-III; American Psychiatric Association, 1980) criteria. They found that the GHQ was superior to the HADS, and it had the best overall performance for specificity, sensitivity, and predictive validity. The GHQ-12 and the GHQ-28 are more appropriate for use with people with aphasia than are the longer versions of the instrument because they have comparable psychometric properties and yet are considerably shorter, reducing respondent burden. The GHQ is frequently used with family members in studies investigating changes and impact of aphasia (Grawburg et al., 2013).

The GDS (Brink et al., 1982) has been used with individuals with and without aphasia to determine the presence of depressive symptoms or normal/low mood (Cruice, 2001; Cruice et al., 2003). It was originally developed as a screening test for depression in older adults and exists as a 30-item tool and an abbreviated 15-item version. Respondents indicate "yes" or "no" to the questions depending on how they have felt over the past week. Questions are counterbalanced, alternating positive and negative responses, and one point is counted for each depressive answer. In the 15-item version, a score of 0–4 indicates normal emotional health status, 5–9 indicates mild depression, and 10–15 moderate-to-severe depression. The GDS has good reliability, validity, sensitivity, and specificity for healthy older people (McDowell & Newell, 1996); however, aphasia-specific information is not available for this tool.

Social Participation and Social Support

The Social Support Survey (SSS; Sherbourne & Stewart, 1991) assesses the perceived availability of four types of support (tangible, emotional/informational, social companionship, and affectionate support). It consists of 19 items, which means it is brief enough to minimize respondent burden. The response format is a 5-point scale going from "none of the time" to "all of the time." Average scores are calculated ranging from 1 to 5, with high scores indicative of higher social support. It has a sound basis guided by theory on the most important dimensions of support (e.g., Cohen & Wills, 1985). Its items were designed specifically to be short, simple, and easy to understand, restricted to one idea in each item. It has good psychometric properties (Sherbourne & Stewart, 1991), which were tested on a group of chronically ill outpatients. It is, therefore, applicable to patient populations who may have greater-than-average needs for various forms of social support (Sherbourne & Stewart, 1991). All this makes it suitable for use with people with aphasia.

The Community Integration Questionnaire (CIQ; Willer, Rosenthal, Kreutzer, Gordon, & Rempel, 1993) was developed for traumatic brain injury and comprises 15 items in three areas of home integration, social integration, and productive activities. Scoring is based on the frequency with which the individual performs the item. The CIQ includes some complex language, and an adapted picture-supported version has been developed by Dutch researchers (Dalemans et al., 2010) for use with people with aphasia.

A different approach to measuring social participation is social network analysis (Antonucci & Akiyama, 1987), which involves interviewing respondents about their important regular social contacts and recording the relationship and type and frequency of each social contact. Set categories exist for relationship, type, and frequency so that each contact is coded in a consistent manner and data can be compared across individuals or groups. Prompt cards with pictorial support help the respondent to stay on track during the interview and are especially helpful for aphasic respondents. Although this approach originates in the nonaphasic literature, it has been used effectively with aphasic individuals (see Cruice et al., 2006). Although it is a time- and language-intensive exercise, it is extremely informative and can be greatly facilitated by interviewing respondents in their own home where they have easy access to photographs or a family member to assist the process. More recently, a measure has been developed to assess social networks, including components of social networks, frequency and type of contact, and satisfaction with network, specifically for people with stroke and aphasia (Northcott & Hilari, 2013). Although it does not yield the wealth of information social network analysis does, clinicians and researchers may still use the Stroke Social Network Scale (SSNS), for example, to understand better what happens to social networks after stroke; which aspects are more vulnerable (e.g., friends); and how social networks relate to other variables, such as psychological well-being.

Because there were few measures available to evaluate social activity participation in the late 1990s, a new tool was developed, the Social Activities Checklist (SOCACT; Cruice, 2001). This tool quantifies participants' range and frequency of involvement in social activities. Based on research and questionnaires within stroke, gerontology, and mental health, the 20-item SOCACT measures social, informal, and formal social activities checked for regular or average participation across frequencies of weekly, biweekly, monthly, rarely, not at all, and not applicable. No immediate time frame is imposed. Preliminary psychometric analysis of this instrument indicates that while there is questionable internal consistency, there is known group validity (i.e., the tool discriminates performance for individuals with and without aphasia), and it may be used clinically to explore individuals' views about their social participation for goal planning (Aujla, Botting, Worrall, Hickson, & Cruice, 2015).

Measures Specific for People With Aphasia

The VASES was specifically developed to measure self-esteem in people with aphasia (Brumfitt & Sheeran, 1999). It is a 10-item scale, each item consisting of two pictures presented horizontally with a verbal label (e.g., "optimistic" and "not optimistic") and a 5-point response scale. It places limited linguistic demands on the respondent and has a simple, straightforward response format. Because of its pictorial format, the VASES has also been used as a measure of emotional distress in people with aphasia (Thomas & Lincoln, 2008). The internal consistency, test–retest reliability, and construct validity of the VASES have been tested on controls (university students) and people with aphasia with good results. The VASES is a popular tool and is used in small-scale evaluation studies in England (e.g., A. Ross et al., 2006) and large-scale correlational and descriptive studies in North America (e.g., Vickery, 2006, for inpatient rehabilitation study).

The Communication Disability Profile (CDP) is a measure of the impact of living with aphasia (Swinburn & Byng, 2006). It comprises four sections: activity (covering talking, expression, understanding, reading, and writing); social participation (in terms of "things they have to do," "things they want to do," and "how things are at home"); external influences (barriers and facilitators of communication); and emotional consequences (both positive and negative). People receive scores expressed as a percentage in activities, participation, and emotions. The CDP contains pictures to facilitate the comprehension of people with aphasia. It is completed in discussion with a clinician. The psychometric properties of the CDP require full testing; the Activities and Participation sections have high and acceptable test–retest reliability, but the Emotions section does not demonstrate adequate reliability (Chue, Rose, & Swinburn, 2010).

Inspired by CDP item content, the Aphasia Impact Questionnaire (AIQ-19) was developed by Connect, the communication disability network in the United Kingdom (http://www.ukconnect.org). The AIQ is a 19-item, patient-reported outcome measure designed to evaluate communication, participation, and well-being, particularly in relation to community service for people with aphasia. Preliminary evidence suggests that Connect services (befriending, conversation groups, counseling, conversation partners, and drop-in) improve individuals' scores on all AIQ domains: communication, social participation, and well-being (Swinburn, McVicker, & Cruice, 2012). Good preliminary psychometrics has been found for internal consistency and some aspects of validity for the AIQ-19.

The Quality of Communication Life Scale (Paul et al., 2004), published by ASHA, assesses the impact of an individual's communication disability on a number of areas of his or her life: relationships; communication interactions; participation in social, leisure, work, and education activities; and overall QOL. The scale is presented as one item per page, with a vertical 10-cm scale anchored by pictures and keywords at each end. Although the tool has been available some years now, little to no research about it has been published internationally.

Finally, the Assessment for Living With Aphasia (ALA; Kagan et al., 2010), was developed at the Aphasia Institute in Toronto, Canada. The purpose of this scale is to capture real-life outcomes of interventions for people living with aphasia. The ALA addresses language impairment, participation, personal and environmental factors, and a dynamic interconnecting aspect referred to as "living with aphasia." More information about the background research and pictorially represented example items of the ALA can be found in the work of Kagan et al. (2007). Psychometric evaluation showed acceptable reliability and validity, and the tool is considered accessible by people with aphasia (Simmons-Mackie et al., 2014).

In summary, a number of tools are available to measure QOL and HR-QOL, emotional distress, social participation, and social support in people with stroke and aphasia. Scales that are accessible to people with aphasia and with good psychometric properties are recommended for use (e.g., SAQOL-39, COOP Charts). Readers are advised to look for future publications reporting further on the development of newer scales (e.g., AIQ, ALA).

CLINICAL APPLICATIONS

To date there is limited knowledge in terms of which specific interventions improve QOL in people with aphasia. There is promising evidence for intensive comprehensive aphasia programs (Rodriguez et al., 2013) and for models of community service provision (e.g., Legg, Stott, Ellis, & Sellars, 2007; Mumby & Whitworth, 2012; van der Gaag et al., 2005). Yet, further research in these areas with larger sample sizes and appropriate control groups will increase our confidence in these findings. Encouragingly, a number of randomized controlled trials of intensive aphasia therapy are currently under way around the world, incorporating generic (Nouwens et al., 2013) and stroke- and aphasia-specific HR-QOL outcome measures (Baumgaertner et al., 2013; Godecke et al., 2014), and they can begin to shed some light on which interventions improve QOL.

Clinicians can pursue a QOL approach in intervention for adults with neurological conditions in different ways. These relate to assessments used to measure change and outcome of intervention, methods or assessments used to gather information about the client and set therapy goals, and different degrees of involving the client in management. We discuss two different ways here. The first is an extension of the traditional approach to practice, which is to start with the client's core impairment (in speech, or language, or mixed, however it presents) and expand the scope outward to include communication activities, social participation, and QOL. The clinician may select a range of methods, including interview, instruments, and tests, to profile the individual's strengths, weaknesses, interests, and priorities. If the clinician actively takes into account the client's priorities and concerns and goals in therapy are set collaboratively with the client and relevant others, then additional outcomes around improved QOL can be anticipated, although they are not often explicitly targeted. An example of this follows in the case of T.E. (Best, Greenwood, Grassly, & Hickin, 2008; Greenwood, Grassly, Hickin, & Best, 2010).

A second way is to start, continue, and finish with QOL in mind, structuring assessment and therapy from the client's perspective after having determined the client's desire for therapy, priorities, standards, and personal aspirations in initial QOL interviews and selecting areas for further assessment based on that. Such an approach is not an alternative or addition to typical approaches to aphasia therapy, for example, neuropsychological or functional communication approaches. It is more of an overarching philosophy that can encompass different approaches and methods depending on what works best for each client at different stages of recovery and life after stroke and aphasia.

A QOL approach to intervention is not only what is done in therapy (i.e., which program is followed, which assessment is used as a baseline) but also the how of therapy and practice. By this we mean that the attitude, philosophy of professional practice, communication skills, and interpersonal skills of the clinician matter as much as the quality and skill that underpin the therapy program. Clinicians who share the decision making collaboratively with clients, seek to build the client's confidence at all times, encourage clients to pursue goals of their choice, and support and facilitate the client without creating dependency support a QOL approach to practice. Case vignettes illustrating these two approaches are described in the case illustrations in this chapter.

CONCLUSIONS AND FUTURE DIRECTIONS

Throughout this chapter, we considered areas of focus for future research, for example, which factors relate to depression in people with aphasia poststroke, which factors contribute to carer burden, and how clinicians and services can best support people with aphasia and their caregivers. This section presents some further suggestions.

We have demonstrated that the evidence on how aphasia affects people's QOL is accumulating. Yet, little is known about the QOL of people with severe aphasia (Hilari & Byng, 2009; Parr, 2007). An accumulation of research evidence from different paradigms, such as proxy data, ethnographic explorations, and social indicators research, can begin to unravel what the big picture is for them. It will help us understand what life is like with severe aphasia, what the main issues are in relation to QOL, and what we can do about them.

Moreover, routine clinical practice needs to make more use of assessment tools tapping into QOL and related concepts, such as emotional well-being and social participation, and devote more time to goal planning in intervention. Some measures currently exist, such as the AIQ, the ALA, and the SAQOL-39, that have been specifically developed for people with stroke and aphasia. Furthermore, researchers in the

field have successfully adapted and used a range of other measures with people with aphasia. Still, more research is needed on making assessment tools accessible to people with aphasia, and clinicians need to be more aware of available tools (e.g., see McDowell, 2006) and use them in their practice. A recent survey of the Aphasia Committee of the International Association of Logopedics and Phoniatrics, involving more than 500 participants from 16 countries, looked at speech and language clinicians' perspectives and practices on QOL. Clinicians were well informed on what constitutes QOL, considered QOL important, used informal approaches to explore it, and aimed to address QOL goals in their practice; yet, the majority did not evaluate QOL in a systematic way (Hilari et al., in press).

Furthermore, we need to know more about what it is in intervention that has positive effects on people with aphasia's QOL—is it the what or the how or a combination of both or more than either of these? We advocate taking a QOL approach to clinical practice with individuals with aphasia, which means structuring assessment and therapy from the client's perspective; taking into account the client's priorities, standards, and concerns; and selecting areas for further assessment and goals of therapy based on that, across all the stages of service provision. More systematic, experimental research is needed in this area.

We are entering a new phase of interest and exploration in QOL in speech pathology generally and are continuing to deepen our understanding of QOL in aphasia for individuals and their families. In the near future, we are likely to see (a) increased use of emotional distress and mood measures with patients and clients, either in the speech pathology profession alone or in conjunction with clinical psychologists; (b) increased use (pilots and trials) of existing, modified, and new QOL measures in aphasia, including research into methods and tools to effectively and reliably explore and assess QOL with clients with severe linguistic impairments; and (c) increased use of QOL as an outcome of both speech pathology–specific interventions and broader rehabilitation interventions.

In the more distant future, we will head toward (a) understanding what constitutes a *better* QOL across the different stages of service provision or recovery and living with aphasia; (b) understanding how client and family QOL affect each other; (c) using QOL measures for information gathering, goal setting, and therapy planning on a more routine basis; and (d) developing an advanced knowledge and skills base in aphasia integrating our ranges of approaches (whether they be neuropsychological, functional, life participation, or social model) for the end goal, which is the best service provision possible for people with aphasia, their families, and their communities.

Case Illustration 14.1: Exploring Broader Outcomes

Intervention does not have to be directly targeted on improving QOL to produce changes that have a positive effect on people's lives. T.E. is a published example of how impairment-based therapy can lead to psychosocial benefits (Best et al., 2008; Greenwood et al., 2010).

T.E. is 67 years old and has suffered a left hemisphere stroke resulting in anomic aphasia. He lives with his wife and has two children and four grandchildren. Prior to his stroke, he ran his own building company, and his wife reports that he was a strong, outgoing character. His assessment focused on his language skills and is summarized in Table 14.1. The results suggested that T.E. had good auditory comprehension and semantic processing (e.g., spoken word and sentence-to-picture matching: 100%) but had difficulties in mapping semantics to phonology (e.g., word reading: 88%) and later-stage phonological processing (e.g., nonword reading: 27%).

Therapy aimed to improve T.E.'s word finding in isolation and in connected speech and to see whether this would have any impact on activity, participation, and emotional well-being. T.E. received therapy in two phases: in Phase 1, T.E. had eight weekly sessions of therapy, which used a hierarchy of phonological and orthographic cues to improve his word retrieval (see also Hickin, Best, Herbert, Howard, & Osborne, 2002). In Phase 2, T.E. had another eight sessions working on word retrieval in connected speech, in a hierarchy of functional tasks, based on a therapy program described by Herbert, Best, Hickin, Howard, and Osborne (2003). Some of the words targeted in therapy were personally relevant. The team used impairment-based measures (e.g., picture naming, retelling of the Cinderella story) to check improvements in word finding and the CDP, (described previously in this chapter) to explore changes in T.E.'s activities, participation, and emotions.

The outcomes of this therapy program were very positive:

- T.E.'s word finding in isolation significantly improved posttherapy.
- He also produced more content words in conversation following therapy.
- T.E. achieved significantly higher scores on the CDP Activity, Participation, and Emotions sections posttherapy. These changes seem to represent real gains in day-to-day life and confidence. For example, the authors stated

Table 14.1 T.E.'s Assessment Scores

Area	Test	Score
Cognition	Pyramids and Palm Trees (n = 52)	100%
	Raven's Coloured Progressive Matrices (n = 12)	83%
Comprehension	Spoken word–picture matching (n = 30)	100%
	Written word–picture matching (n = 30)	100%
	Spoken sentence–picture matching (n = 16)	100%
	Written sentence–picture matching (n = 16)	91%
Expression	Picture naming (n = 200)	74%[a]
	Written naming (n = 40)	65%
	Repetition (n = 182)	87%
	Word reading (n = 182)	88%
	Nonword reading (n = 26)	27%

[a] Errors: Semantic = 16%; phonological = 50%.

(continues)

that he would answer the phone and go out independently and that he felt more positive about himself with aphasia.

- Last, there was a significant positive relationship between changes in word finding (naming 200 items) and changes in CDP scores (activity ratings) across the course of the study.

These results are important. They highlight the fact that impairment-based therapy, when carefully targeted to an individual's interests, can produce changes not only in the therapy room but also in what people do in real life and how they feel about it.

Case Illustration 14.2: Using QOL Measures in Therapy Planning

In this case, 30 people with aphasia participated in a doctoral research project investigating the relationship between variables of communication (linguistic and sensory functioning, functional communication, social participation) and variables of QOL, HR-QOL, and well-being (Cruice, 2001; Cruice et al., 2003). One of these participants, Jane, was a single woman of 64 years who was retired from her job as a TAB (betting agency) supervisor. She lived independently in her own villa in a retirement village complex. She had had a stroke 65 months prior to participating in the study and was no longer involved with any speech pathology services. Through the research project, Jane completed 15 assessments/questionnaires (standardized and author developed), and her scores/responses on a selection of these are reported in Table 14.2. To aid interpretation of her information, where appropriate, her scores are reported in the context of the mean of the overall sample that took part in the research.

In terms of her profile (Table 14.2), Jane had a mild aphasic linguistic impairment, was a particularly effective communicator, was quite involved in communicative and social activities, and had many social contacts in her life. Although Jane participated in a high number of social activities, she reported wanting to do more socially.

Table 14.2 Jane's Profile

Area	Test	Score
Language functioning	Western Aphasia Battery	78
Functional communication	Communication Activities of Daily Living Revised (CADL-2)	84
	Communicative Activities Checklist	35 activities (average = 29)
Social participation	Social Activities Checklist	15 activities (average = 13)
	Social Network Analysis	23 social contacts (average = 21)
Emotional health	Geriatric Depression Scale	1 (average = 3.6)
Quality of life	Global 5-Point Rating	3 or "average" (average = 4 or "good")
	How I Feel About Myself (psychological well-being scale)	75 (range 24–120; average = 88.1)

Jane reported a normal emotional state and average global life quality, and her psychological well-being score was lower than the average for the sample (Table 14.2). She also answered questions about her HR-QOL. Her

(continues)

responses to the Dartmouth COOP Charts are interpreted as follows: moderate physical fitness (able to walk at a medium pace), slightly bothered by emotional problems, no difficulty with daily activities, slightly limited social activities, no pain, no change in health, very good overall health, as much social support as she wanted, and in terms of QOL, good and bad parts about equal. Finally, Jane's responses to the structured QOL questions were as follows:

How would you describe the quality of your life? And why do you say that?

Oh … I'd say it's in three-quarters, well, it's not very, it's not very good but it's in between, yeah yeah. Well because I can't read, I can't write, I can't write anything, different things they an annoy me because I can't do them, and ah … I can't drive the car anymore so that drives me … [*laugh*] it's different things that I can't do these days, yeah.

What things give your life quality?

Oh … I think … I spose when I go out with the girls and, um … we laugh and everything, that's probably good yeah. And ah … yeah I … um … quality um … when I go swim, usually when we go swimming I like, we, usually go with three girls, and I like to go with them and I'll have a laugh with them even, yeah, but ah … what else? … is that alright?

What things take quality away from your life?

I can't read it's driving me mad [*laugh*], and I can't even write very good, I can do a couple of little things, I can't read er. Write like that, so it's not very good, yeah … I think that's about it. Um. No that's about it I think.

What would make the quality of your life better?

Um … just being able to read I spose and write and do different things I used to, these days I just can't do it. But then I can, I can um ah can go out and do things so I'm lucky in that way I'm not as though I have to stay here all the time.

What would make the quality of your life worse?

Worse? … If I couldn't read, if I couldn't do anything, I'd be worse yeah yeah yes it would be hard it would be awful if you couldn't read or write or do anything you wanted to. I spose I shouldn't I shouldn't really say all the time what's wrong with me, because really there isn't that much wrong with me when you think of it, I can read and I can I know what I can do I can watch the television I can go out so I really shouldn't complain.

Does communication have an impact on the quality of your life? If yes, then how?

Communication, what with friends? … Does it have anything to do? … oh yeah yeah yeah yes has to be.

The first step the clinician can take toward determining goals for intervention is to look across the range of assessments and questionnaires and integrate the information. The clinician must consider the following:

- Jane's strengths (effective verbal and functional communicator, able to articulate and reflect, healthy emotional state, good physical fitness)
- What her priorities might be (reading, writing, more social activities, possibly getting out more; note also that although Jane has relatively *mild impairment in language functioning*, her responses suggest she does not talk the way she used to and there is a sense of loss when she describes her speech)
- Whether improving areas of relative weakness will be of importance to her (sense of well-being, reading, and writing)
- What is important to maintain (socialization and friendship, swimming)

The clinician needs to find out more information about Jane's current and desired level of reading[3] and writing and probe further her desire for more social activities—Are these more activities in general, or going to them more frequently, or finding new activities? The clinician also needs to determine what prevents Jane from currently doing this (she has hinted that independent transport may be an issue because she no longer drives). Her responses also suggest a need to explore what Jane's self-perception of her communication is, what she would desire overall,

(continues)

and also what contact with others with aphasia after stroke she has had (people's attitudes are often influenced by participating in aphasia groups).

In terms of service provision, therapy with a social frame of reference would support her desires, for example, community-based therapy in a library or local venue with others (possibly her friends) based around meaningful activities (possibly a book club or local reading group). This would be one way of taking forward a QOL approach based on Jane's presentation in the original research study, and it does not preclude other goals and directions that readers may identify from her case.

A paper by Ylvisaker and Feeney (2000) provides further reading on an approach to intervention that is more likely to sit within the QOL approach. These two researchers and clinicians invite readers to reflect on the sequence and progression of assessment and intervention activities. In particular, they propose clinicians *reverse* the "traditional impairment-disability-handicap hierarchy" (p. 411) beginning with participation in everyday life routines and thereafter focusing on reducing social handicap, reducing disability, and reducing impairment. The relationships between the client's general and specific goals and the sequence of intervention were clearly discussed, using the case of Jason. Although Jason is a young man with an acquired brain injury and significant life issues, the paper is relevant for clinicians working with individuals with aphasia. In Jane's case, the paper might encourage us to reflect on how long- and short-term goals might relate to one another, based on the broad assessment information that has been gathered. Further guided reading is recommended with the case of G.J., whose clinical management is contrasted from a functional–social perspective (Simmons-Mackie, 2008) and an impairment perspective (Howard, 2008). Although the nature of the impairment between cases differs (G.J. has severe apraxia of speech and aphasia, compared to Jane's mild aphasia), the case comparison illustrates features relevant to Jane: participation-oriented assessment, emphasis on well-being and identity, assessment and outcome measurement across multiple domains, capitalization on strengths, and gaining a proper understanding of the nature or cause of the difficulty. Integrating approaches (e.g., Garcia, 2008) are the way forward for contemporary practice and are well adopted by the current profession (Rose et al., 2014; Verna et al., 2009).

STUDY QUESTIONS

1. How is HR-QOL distinguished from QOL?
2. What are the key factors that affect HR-QOL in people with chronic aphasia?
3. What are the key factors contributing to high emotional distress after stroke?
4. How does aphasia affect people's social participation and social support systems?
5. Why is it important to assess QOL/HR-QOL in intervention with people with aphasia?
6. What are the main challenges in measuring QOL/HR-QOL in people with aphasia?
7. What scales could a clinician working with people with aphasia use to measure the following items:
   a. HR-QOL
   b. Emotional distress
   c. Social support
   d. Social activities
8. How would the QOL approach to aphasia influence your intervention?

NOTES

1. An excellent grounding in this area can be gained from reading special issues: *Folia Phoniatrica et Logopedica* has a special issue on QOL in press; and *Aphasiology* published the "Quality of Life in Aphasia" special issue in 2003. It contains seminal papers and example approaches to interventions supporting QOL with aphasia.

2. For the reader interested in the details of different measurement tools that are available on the market, the text *Measuring Health: A Guide to Rating Scales and Questionnaires* by Professor Ian McDowell is the book of choice. The third edition was published in 2006 and reviews more than 100 instruments; however, the second edition in 1996 (by McDowell and Newell) is equally useful, with approximately 80 instruments covered. This text is attractive for its inclusion of the instruments, enabling clinicians to make judgments about the appropriateness for clients; for its excellent reviews of the psychometric properties for each instrument; and for its breadth, covering physical, social, and psychological health, pain, mental status, depression, and general health.

3. As well as discussing this with Jane, the clinician can also return to the detailed information already collected, for example, look at each of her responses to the 45-item communicative activities checklist, identify what communicative activities she did not check off, and use this as the basis for further discussion (also looking for overlap with reading and writing as mentioned in the QOL interview).

REFERENCES

American Psychiatric Association (1980). *DSM-III: Diagnostic and Statistical Manual of Mental Disorders* (3rd ed.). Washington DC: Author.

American Speech-Language-Hearing Association. (2007). *Scope of practice in speech-language pathology* [Scope of Practice]. Retrieved from http://www.asha.org/policy

Aneshensel, C. S., & Frerichs, R. R. (1982). Stress, support, and depression: A longitudinal causal model. *Journal of Community Psychology, 10*, 363–376.

Antonucci, T. C., & Akiyama, H. (1987). Social networks in adult life and a preliminary examination of the convoy model. *Journal of Gerontology, 42*(5), 519–527.

Aujla, S., Botting, N., Worrall, L., Hickson, L., & Cruice, M. (2015). Preliminary psychometric analyses of two assessment measures quantifying communicative and social activities: The COMACT and SOCACT. *Aphasiology.* doi: 10.1080/02687038.2015.1074655

Avent, J., Glista, S., Wallace, S., Jackson, J., Nishioka, J., & Yip, W. (2005). Family information needs about aphasia. *Aphasiology, 19*(3–5), 365–375.

Baumgaertner, A., Grewe, T., Ziegler, W., Floel, A., Springer, L., Martus, P., et al. (2013). FCET2EC (From controlled experimental trial to = 2 everyday communication): How effective is intensive integrative therapy for stroke-induced chronic aphasia under routine clinical conditions? A study protocol for a randomized controlled trial. *Trials, 14*, 308.

Baylor, C., Yorkston, K., Eadie, T., Kim, J., Chung, H., & Amtmann, D. (2013). The Communicative Participation Item Bank (CPIB): Item bank calibration and development of a disorder-generic short form. *Journal of Speech, Language, and Hearing Research, 56*(4), 1190–1208.

Bays, C. (2001). Quality of life of stroke survivors: A research synthesis. *Journal of Neuroscience Nursing, 33*(6), 310–316.

Bech, P. (1993). Quality of life measurement in chronic disorders. *Psychotherapy and Psychosomatics, 59*, 1–10.

Bell, D., & Kahn, C. (1996). Assessing health status via the World Wide Web. In J. C. Cimino (Ed.), *Proceedings of the AMIA annual fall symposium* (pp. 338–342). Philadelphia: Hanley & Belfus.

Bergner, M., Bobbitt, R., Carter, W., & Gilson, B. (1981). The Sickness Impact Profile. *Medical Care, 19*, 787–805.

Berzon, R., Hays, R. D., & Shumaker, S. A. (1993). International use, application and performance of health-related quality of life instruments. *Quality of Life Research, 2*, 367–368.

Best, W., Greenwood, A., Grassly, J., & Hickin, J. (2008). Bridging the gap: Can impairment-based therapy for anomia have an impact at the psycho-social level? *International Journal of Language and Communication Disorders, 43*(4), 390–407.

Billings, A. G., & Moos, R. H. (1982). Stressful life events and symptoms: A longitudinal model. *Health Psychology, 1*, 99–117.

Bowling, A. (1995). *Measuring disease.* Buckingham, UK: Open University Press.

Bowling, A. (1997). *Measuring health. A review of quality of life measurement scales.* Buckingham, UK: Open University Press.

Bradburn, N. (1969). *The structure of psychological well-being.* Chicago: Aldine.

Brink, T. L., Yesavage, J. A., Lum, O., Heersema, P., Adey, M. B., & Rose, T. L. (1982). Screening tests for geriatric depression. *Clinical Gerontology, 1*, 37–43.

Brown, K., Worrall, L. E., Davidson, B., & Howe, T. (2012). Living successfully with aphasia: A qualitative meta-analysis of the perspectives of individuals with aphasia, family members, and speech-language pathologists. *International Journal of Speech-Language Pathology, 14*, 141–155.

Brown, K., Worrall, L., Davidson, B., & Howe, T. (2011). Living successfully with aphasia: Family members share their views. *Topics in Stroke Rehabilitation, 18*(5), 5376–548.

Brumfitt, S. (2006). Psychosocial aspects of aphasia: Speech and language therapists' views on professional practice. *Disability & Rehabilitation, 28*(8), 523–534.

Brumfitt, S., & Sheeran, P. (1999). *VASES: Visual Analogue Self-Esteem Scale.* Bicester, UK: Winslow Press.

Buck, D., Jacoby, A., & Ford, G. (2001). Reliability and validity of "NEWSQOL": The Newcastle Stroke-specific Quality of Life Measure. *Quality of Life Research, 10*, 258.

Bullinger, M., Anderson, R., Cella, D., & Aaronson, N. K. (1993). Developing and evaluating cross cultural instruments: From minimum requirements to optimal models. *Quality of Life Research, 2*, 451–459.

Caute, A., Northcott, S., Clarkson, L., Pring, T., & Hilari, K. (2012). Does mode of administration affect health-related quality of life outcomes after stroke? *International Journal of Speech-Language Pathology, 14*(4), 329–337.

Chue, W., Rose, M., & Swinburn, K. (2010). The reliability of the communication disability profile: A patient-reported outcome measure for aphasia. *Aphasiology, 24*(6–8), 940–956.

Cohen, S., & Wills, A. B. (1985). Stress, social support, and the buffering hypothesis. *Psychological Bulletin, 98*(2), 310–357.

Cruice, M. (2001). *Communication and quality of life in older people with aphasia and healthy older people.* Unpublished doctoral dissertation, Department of Speech Pathology and Audiology, University of Queensland, Brisbane, Australia.

Cruice, M., Hill, R., Worrall, L., & Hickson, L. (2010). Conceptualising quality of life for older people with aphasia. *Aphasiology, 24*(3), 327–347.

Cruice, M., Hirsch, F., Worrall, L., Holland, A., & Hickson, L. (2000). Quality of life for people with aphasia: Performance on and usability of quality of life assessments. *Asia Pacific Journal of Speech, Language and Hearing, 5*, 85–91.

Cruice, M., Worrall, L., & Hickson, L. (2006). Quantifying aphasic people's social lives in the context of their non-aphasic peers. *Aphasiology, 20*(12), 1210–1225.

Cruice, M., Worrall, L., & Hickson, L. (2010). Health-related quality of life in people with aphasia: Implications for fluency disorders quality of life research. *Journal of Fluency Disorders*, *35*, 173–189.

Cruice, M., Worrall, L., Hickson, L., & Murison, R. (2003). Finding a focus for quality of life with aphasia: Social and emotional health, and psychological well-being. *Aphasiology*, *17*(4), 333–353.

Cruice, M., Worrall, L., Hickson, L., & Murison, R. (2005). Measuring quality of life: Comparing family members' and friends' ratings with those of their aphasic partners. *Aphasiology*, *19*(2), 111–129.

Dalemans, R. J., De Witte, L. P., Beurskens, A. J., Van Den Heuvel, W. J. A., & Wade, D. T. (2010). An investigation into the social participation of stroke survivors with aphasia. *Disability and Rehabilitation*, *32*(20), 1678–1685.

de Haan, R., Aaronson, N., Limburg, M., Langton Hewer, R., & van Crevel, H. (1993). Measuring quality of life in stroke. *Stroke*, *24*, 320–327.

Dennis, M., O'Rourke, S., Lewis, S., Sharpe, M., & Warlow, C. (2000). Emotional outcomes after stroke: Factors associated with poor outcome. *Journal of Neurology, Neurosurgery and Psychiatry*, *68*, 47–52.

Dennis, M., O'Rourke, S., Slattery, J., Staniforth, T., & Warlow, C. (1997). Evaluation of a stroke family care worker: Results of a randomised controlled trial. *British Medical Journal*, *314*, 1071.

Department of Health. (2007). *House of Commons Health Committee Patient and Public Involvement in the NHS: Third Report of Session 2006-07 Volume I Report, HC 278-I*. Retrieved November 10, 2015, from http://webarchive.nationalarchives.gov.uk/20080814090418/dh.gov.uk/en/Publicationsandstatistics/Publications/PublicationsPolicyAndGuidance/DH_076380

Doyle, P., McNeil, M., Bost, J., Ross, K., Wambaugh, J., Hula, W., et al. (2007). The Burden of Stroke Scale (BOSS) provided valid, reliable, and responsive score estimates of functioning and well-being during the first year of recovery from stroke. *Quality of Life Research*, *16*, 1389–1398.

Doyle, P., McNeil, M., Hula, W., & Mikolic, J. (2003). The Burden of Stroke Scale (BOSS): Validating patient-reported communication difficulty and associated psychological distress in stroke survivors. *Aphasiology*, *17*(3), 291–304.

Duncan, P. W., Wallace, D., Lai, S.-M., Johnson, D., Embretson, S., & Jacobs Laster, L. (1999). The Stroke Impact Scale Version 2.0. Evaluation of reliability, validity, and sensitivity to change. *Stroke*, *30*, 2131–2140.

EuroQol Group. (1990). EuroQol: A new facility for the measurement of health related quality of life. *Health Policy*, *16*, 199–208.

Farquhar, M. (1995). Elderly people's definitions of quality of life. *Social Science and Medicine*, *41*(10), 1439–1446.

Fuhrer, M. (1994). Subjective well-being: Implications for medical rehabilitation outcomes and models of disablement. *American Journal of Physical Medicine and Rehabilitation*, *73*(5), 358–364.

Garcia, L. (2008). Chapter 19: A treatment plan for a letter-by-letter reader: Intervention from an integrated perspective. In N. Martin, C. Thompson, & L. Worrall (Eds.), *Aphasia rehabilitation: The impairment and its consequences* (pp. 231–258). San Diego, CA: Plural.

Glass, A. T., & Maddox, G. L. (1992). The quality and quantity of social support: Stroke recovery as a psycho-social transition. *Social Science and Medicine*, *34*, 1249–1261.

Godecke, E., Ciccone, N. A., Granger, A. S., Rai, T., West, D., Cream, A., et al. (2014). A comparison of aphasia therapy outcomes before and after a Very Early Rehabilitation programme following stroke. *International Journal of Language & Communication Disorders*, *49*, 149–161.

Goldberg, D. P. (1972). *The detection of psychiatric illness by questionnaire*. London: Oxford University Press.

Goldberg, D. P., & Hillier, V. F. (1979). A scaled version of the General Health Questionnaire. *Psychological Medicine*, *9*, 139–145.

Goldberg, D. P., & Williams, P. (1988). *A user's guide to the General Health Questionnaire (GHQ)*. Oxford, UK: NFER-Nelson.

Grawburg, M., Howe, T., Worrall, L., & Scarinci, N. (2013). Third party disability in family members of people with aphasia: A systematic review. *Disability & Rehabilitation*, *35*(16), 1324–1341.

Greenwood, A., Grassly, J., Hickin, J., & Best, W. (2010). Phonological and orthographic cueing therapy: A case of generalised improvement. *Aphasiology*, *24*(9), 991–1016.

Han, B., & Haley, W. E. (1999). Family caregiving for patients with stroke. Review and analysis. *Stroke*, *30*(7), 1478–1485.

Hayes, V., Morris, J., Wolfe, C., & Morgan, M. (1995). The SF-36 Health Survey Questionnaire: Is it suitable for use with older adults? *Age and Aging*, *24*, 120–125.

Hays, R. D., Anderson, R., & Revicki, D. (1993). Psychometric considerations in evaluating health-related quality of life measures. *Quality of Life Research*, *2*, 441–449.

Herbert, R., Best, W., Hickin, J., Howard, D., & Osborne, F. (2003). Combining lexical and interactional approaches to the treatment of word-finding deficits in aphasia. *Aphasiology*, *17*, 1163–1189.

Hickin, J., Best, W., Herbert, R., Howard, D., & Osborne, F. (2002). Phonological therapy for word finding difficulties: A re-evaluation. *Aphasiology*, *16*(Special Issue), 981–999.

Hilari, K. (2011). The impact of stroke: Are people with aphasia different to those without? *Disability and Rehabilitation*, *33*(3), 211–218.

Hilari, K., & Byng, S. (2001). Measuring quality of life in aphasia: The Stroke-Specific Quality of Life Scale. *International Journal of Language and Communication Disorders*, *36*(Suppl.), 86–91.

Hilari, K., & Byng, S. (2009). Health-related quality of life in people with severe aphasia. *International Journal of Language and Communication Disorders*, *44*(2), 193–205.

Hilari, K., Byng, S., Lamping, D. L., & Smith, S. C. (2003). Stroke and Aphasia Quality of Life Scale–39 (SAQOL-39): Evaluation of acceptability, reliability and validity. *Stroke*, *34*(8), 1944–1950.

Hilari, K., Klippi, A., Constantinidou, F., Horton, S., Penn, C., Raymer, S., et al. (2015). Quality of life in aphasia: An international perspective. A survey of clinician views and practices from 16 countries. *Folia Phoniatrica et Logopedica*. *67*(3)

Hilari, K., Lamping, D. L., Smith, S. C., Northcott, S., Lamb, A., & Marshall, J. (2009). Psychometric properties of the Stroke and Aphasia Quality of Life scale (SAQOL-39) in a generic stroke population. *Clinical Rehabilitation*, *23*(6), 544–557.

Hilari, K., Needle, J. J., & Harrison, K. L. (2012). What are the important factors in health-related quality of life for people with aphasia? A systematic review. *Archives of Physical Medicine and Rehabilitation, 93*, S86–S95.

Hilari, K., & Northcott, S. (2006). Social support in people with chronic aphasia. *Aphasiology, 20*(1), 17–36.

Hilari, K., Northcott, S., Roy, P., Marshall, J., Wiggins, R. D., Chataway, J., et al. (2010). Psychological distress after stroke and aphasia: The first six months. *Clinical Rehabilitation, 24*(2), 181–190.

Hilari, K., Owen, S., & Farrelly, S. J. (2007). Proxy and self-report agreement on the Stroke and Aphasia Quality of Life scale (SAQOL-39). *Journal of Neurology, Neurosurgery and Psychiatry, 78*, 1072–1075.

Hilari, K., Wiggins, R. D., Roy, P., Byng, S., & Smith, S. C. (2003). Predictors of health-related quality of life (HRQL) in people with chronic aphasia. *Aphasiology, 17*(4), 365–381.

House, J. S., Robbins, C., & Metzner, H. L. (1982). The association of social relationships and activities with mortality: Prospective evidence from the Tecumseh Community Health Study. *American Journal of Epidemiology, 116*, 123–140.

Howard, D. (2008). Chapter 8: Treatment for a case of severe apraxia of speech and aphasia: An impairment-based perspective. In N. Martin, C. Thompson, & L. Worrall (Eds.), *Aphasia rehabilitation: The impairment and its consequences* (pp. 109–123). San Diego, CA: Plural.

Howe, T., Davidson, B., Worrall, L., Hersh, D., Ferguson, A., Sherratt, S., et al. (2012). "You needed to rehab … families as well": Family members' own goals for aphasia rehabilitation. *International Journal of Language and Communication Disorders, 47*(5), 511–521.

Hunt, S. M., McKenna, S. P., McEwen, J., Williams, J., & Papp, E. (1981). The Nottingham Health Profile: Subjective health status and medical consultations. *Social Science and Medicine, 15*, 221–229.

Intercollegiate Stroke Working Party. (2012). *National clinical guideline for stroke* (4th ed.). London: Royal College of Physicians.

Johnson, G., Burvill, P. W., Anderson, C. S., Jamrozik, K., Stewart-Wynne, E. G., & Chakera, T. M. (1995). Screening instruments for depression and anxiety following stroke: Experience in the Perth community stroke study. *Acta Psychiatrica Scandinavica, 91*, 252–257.

Jordan, L., & Kaiser, W. (1996). *Aphasia: A social approach.* Cheltenham, UK: Thornes.

Kagan, A., Simmons-Mackie, N., Rowland, A., Huijbregts, M., Shumway, E., McEwen, S., et al. (2007). Counting what counts: A framework for capturing real-life outcomes of aphasia intervention. *Aphasiology, 22*(3), 258–280.

Kagan, A., Simmons-Mackie, N., Victor, J. C., Carling-Rowland, A., Hoch, J., Huijbregts, M., et al. (2010). *Assessment for Living With Aphasia (ALA).* Toronto: Aphasia Institute.

Karnofsky, D. A., Abelmann, W. H., & Craver, L. F. (1948). The use of nitrogen mustards in the palliative treatment of carcinoma. *Cancer, 1*, 634–656.

Kauhanen, M. L., Korpelainen, J. T., Hiltunen, P., Maatta, R., Mononen, H., Brusin, E., et al. (2000). Aphasia, depression, and non-verbal cognitive impairment ischaemic stroke. *Cerebrovascular Disease, 10*, 455–461.

Kontou, E., Thomas, S., & Lincoln, N. (2012). Psychometric properties of a revised version of the Visual Analog Mood Scales. *Clinical Rehabilitation, 26*(12), 1133–1140.

Kutlubaev, M. A., & Hackett, M. L. (2014). Part II: Predictors of depression after stroke and impact of depression on stroke outcome: An updated systematic review of observational studies. *International Journal of Stroke, 9*(8), 1026–1036.

Le Dorze, G., & Brassard, C. (1995). A description of the consequences of aphasia on aphasic persons and their relatives and friends based on the WHO model of chronic diseases. *Aphasiology, 9*(3), 239–255.

Legg, L., Stott, D., Ellis, G., Sellars, C. (2007). Volunteer stroke service (VSS) groups for patients with communication difficulties after stroke: A qualitative analysis of the value of groups to their users. *Clinical Rehabilitation, 21*(9), 794–804.

Lin, N., Dean, A., & Ensel, W. M. (1981). Social support scales: A methodological note. *Schizophrenic Bulletin, 7*, 73–89.

Lyon, J. G., Cariski, D., Keisler, L., Rosenbek, J., Levine, R., Kumpula, J., et al. (1997). Communication partners: Enhancing participation in life and communication for adults with aphasia in natural settings. *Aphasiology, 11*(7), 693–708.

Mayou, R., & Bryant, B. (1993). Quality of life in cardiovascular disease. *British Medical Journal, 69*, 460–466.

McDowell, I. (2006). *Measuring health: A guide to rating scales and questionnaires.* New York: Oxford University Press.

McDowell, I., & Newell, C. (1996). *Measuring health: A guide to rating scales and questionnaires.* New York: Oxford University Press.

Moeller, D., & Carpenter, C. (2013). Factors affecting quality of life for people who have experienced a stroke. *International Journal of Therapy and Rehabilitation, 20*(4), 207–216.

Mumby, K., & Whitworth, A. (2012). Evaluating the effectiveness of intervention in long-term aphasia post-stroke: The experience from CHANT (Communication Hub for Aphasia in North Tyneside). *International Journal of Language & Communication Disorders, 47*, 398–412.

Nelson, E., Landgraf, J., Hays, R., Wasson, J., & Kirk, J. (1990). The functional status of patients: How can it be measured in physicians' offices? *Medical Care, 28*(12), 1111–1126.

Nelson, E., Wasson, J., Kirk, J., Keller, A., Clark, D., Dietrich, A., et al. (1987). Assessment of function in routine clinical practice: Description of the COOP Chart method and preliminary findings. *Journal of Chronic Disease, 40*(1), 55S–63S.

NHS Executive. (1999). *Clinical governance in the new NHS.* London: NHS Executive Quality Management Branch.

Northcott, S., Burns, K., Simpson, A., & Hilari, K. (2015). "Living with aphasia the best way I can": A feasibility study exploring solution focused brief therapy for people with aphasia. *Folia Phoniatrica et Logopedica. 67* (3)

Northcott, S., & Hilari, K. (2011). Why do people lose their friends after a stroke? *International Journal of Language & Communication Disorders, 46*(5), 524–534.

Northcott, S., & Hilari, K. (2013). Stroke Social Network Scale: Development and psychometric evaluation of a new patient-reported measure. *Clinical Rehabilitation, 27*(9), 823–833.

Nouwens, F., Dippel, D. W., de Jong-Hagelstein, M., Visch-Brink, E. G., Koudstaal, P. J., & de Lau, L. M. (2013). Rotterdam Aphasia Therapy Study (RATS)–3: The efficacy of intensive cognitive-linguistic therapy in the acute stage of aphasia: design of a randomised controlled trial. *Trials, 14*, 24.

O'Boyle, C. A., McGee, H., Hickey, A., O'Malley, K., & Joyce, C. R. (1992). Individual quality of life in patients undergoing hip replacement. *Lancet, 339*, 1088–1091.

Parr, S. (2007). Living with severe aphasia: Tracking social exclusion. *Aphasiology, 21*(1), 98–123.

Parr, S., Byng, S., & Gilpin, S. (1997). *Talking about aphasia.* Philadelphia: Open University Press.

Patrick, D. L., & Deyo, R. A. (1989). Generic and disease-specific measures in assessing health status and quality of life. *Medical Care, 27,* S217–S232.

Patrick, D. L., & Erickson, P. (1993). Assessing health-related quality of life for clinical decision making. In S. R. Walker (Ed.), *Quality of life assessment: Key issues in the 1990s* (pp. 11–63). Dordrecht, Netherlands: Kluwer Academic.

Paul, D., Holland, A., Frattali, C., Thompson, C., Caperton, C., & Slater, S. (2004). *Quality of Communication Life Scale (ASHA QCL).* Rockville, MD: American Speech-Language-Hearing Association.

Pollock, A., St George, B., Fenton, M., & Firkins, L. (2012). Top ten research priorities relating to life after stroke—Consensus from stroke survivors, caregivers, and health professionals. *International Journal of Stroke, 9*(3), 313–320.

Rodriguez, A. D., Worrall, L., Brown, K., Grohn, B., McKinnon, E., Pearson, C., et al. (2013). Aphasia LIFT: Exploratory investigation of an intensive comprehensive aphasia programme. *Aphasiology, 27,* 1339–1361.

Rose, M., Ferguson, A., Power, E., Togher, L., & Worrall, L. (2014). Aphasia rehabilitation in Australia: Current practices, challenges and future directions. *International Journal of Speech-Language Pathology, 16,* 169–180.

Ross, A., Winslow, I., Marchant, P., & Brumfitt, S. (2006). Evaluation of communication, life participation and psychological well-being in chronic aphasia: The influence of group intervention. *Aphasiology, 20*(5), 427–448.

Ross, K., & Wertz, R. (2003). Quality of life with and without aphasia. *Aphasiology, 17*(4), 355–364.

Royal College of Speech and Language Therapists. (2005). *Clinical guidelines.* Oxon, UK: Speechmark.

Royal College of Speech and Language Therapists. (2006). *Communicating Quality 3: The RCSLT's guidance on best practice in service organisation and provision.* London: Author.

Ruta, D. A., Garratt, A. M., Leng, M., Russell, I., & MacDonald, L. (1994). A new approach to the measurement of quality of life: The Patient Generated Index (PGI). *Medical Care, 32,* 1109–1126.

Sackley, C., Hoppitt, T., & Cardoso, K. (2006). An investigation into the utility of the Stroke Aphasic Depression Questionnaire (SADQ) in care home settings. *Clinical Rehabilitation, 20,* 598–602.

Sarno, M. (1997). Quality of life in aphasia in the first post-stroke year. *Aphasiology, 11*(7), 665–679.

Scientific Advisory Committee of the Medical Outcomes Trust. (2002). Assessing health status and quality-of-life instruments: Attributes and review criteria. *Quality of Life Research, 11,* 193–205.

Sherbourne, C. D., & Stewart, A. L. (1991). The MOS Social Support Survey. *Social Science and Medicine, 32,* 705–714.

Simmons-Mackie, N. (2008). Chapter 7: Intervention for a case of severe apraxia of speech and aphasia: A functional-social perspective. In N. Martin, C. Thompson, & L. Worrall (Eds.), *Aphasia rehabilitation: The impairment and its consequences* (pp. 75–108). San Diego, CA: Plural.

Simmons-Mackie, N., Kagan, A., Victor, J. C., Carling-Rowland, A., Mok, A., Hoch, J., et al. (2014). The assessment for living with aphasia: Reliability and construct validity. *International Journal of Speech-Language Pathology, 16*(1), 82–94.

Ski, C., & O'Connell, B. (2007). Stroke: The increasing complexity of carer needs. *Journal of Neuroscience Nursing, 39*(3), 172–179.

Sneeuw, K. C., Sprangers, M. A., & Aaronson, N. K. (2002). The role of health care providers and significant others in evaluating the quality of life of patients with chronic disease. *Journal of Clinical Epidemiology, 55*(11), 1130–1143.

Speech Pathology Australia. (2015). Scope of practice in speech pathology. Retrieved November 5, 2015, from http://www.speechpathologyaustralia.org.au/library/20150720%20-%20Scope%20of%20Practice%20-%20FINAL.pdf

Staniszewska, S. (1999). Patient expectations and health related quality of life. *Health Expectations, 2,* 93–104.

Stern, R. (1997). *Visual analog mood scales manual.* Lutz, FL: Psychological Assessment Resources.

Stern, R. (1999). Assessment of mood states in aphasia. *Seminars in Speech and Language, 20*(1), 33–50.

Sutcliffe, L. M., & Lincoln, N. B. (1998). The assessment of depression in aphasic stroke patients: The development of the Stroke Aphasic Depression Questionnaire. *Clinical Rehabilitation, 12,* 506–513.

Swinburn, K., & Byng, S. (2006). *The Communication Disability Profile.* London: Connect.

Swinburn, K., McVicker, S., & Cruice, M. (2012). Measuring outcomes in community services: Patient reported outcome measurement for people with aphasia. *International Journal of Stroke, 7*(Suppl. 2), 30.

ten Kate, O. (2014). *Increasing everyday use of wellbeing and health-related quality of life measures.* Unpublished MSc in speech and language therapy dissertation, Division of Language and Communication Sciences, City University London.

Thomas, S. A., & Lincoln, N. B. (2008). Predictors of emotional distress after stroke. *Stroke, 39*(4), 1240–1245.

Thomas, S. A., Walker, M. F., Macniven, J. A., Haworth, H., & Lincoln, N. B. (2013). Communication and Low Mood (CALM): A randomized controlled trial of behavioural therapy for stroke patients with aphasia. *Clinical Rehabilitation, 27*(5), 398–408.

Townend, E., Brady, M., & McLaughlan, K. (2007). A systematic evaluation of the adaptation of depression diagnostic methods for stroke survivors who have aphasia. *Stroke, 38,* 3076–3083.

Turner, R. J. (1981). Social support as a contingency in psychological well-being. *Journal of Health and Social Behavior, 22,* 357–367.

US Department of Health and Human Services FDA Center for Drug Evaluation and Research, US Department of Health and Human Services FDA Center for Biologics Evaluation and Research, & US Department of Health and Human Services FDA Center for Devices and Radiological Health. (2006). Guidance for industry: Patient reported outcome measures: Use in medical product development to support labelling claims: Draft guidance. *Health and Quality of Life Outcomes, 4*(79). doi:10.1186/1477-7525-4-79

Van der Gaag, A., & Brooks, R. (2008). Economic aspects of a therapy and support service for people with long-term stroke and aphasia. *International Journal of Language and Communication Disorders, 43*(3), 233–244.

Van der Gaag, A., Smith, L., Davis, S., Moss, B., Cornelius, V., Laing, S., et al. (2005). Therapy and support services for people with long-term stroke and aphasia and their relatives: A six-month follow-up study. *Clinical Rehabilitation, 19*(4), 372–380.

Van Straten, A., de Haan, R. J., Limburg, M., Schuling, J., Bossuyt, P. M., & van den Bos, G. A. M. (1997). A stroke-adapted

30-item version of the Sickness Impact Profile to assess quality of life (SA-SIP30). *Stroke, 28,* 2155–2161.

Verna, A., Davidson, B., & Rose, T. (2009). Speech-language pathology services for people with aphasia: A survey of current practice in Australia. *International Journal of Speech-Language Pathology, 11*(3), 191–205.

Vickery, C. (2006). Assessment and correlates of self-esteem following stroke using a pictorial measure. *Clinical Rehabilitation, 20,* 1075–1084.

Vieweg, B. W., & Hedlund, J. L. (1983). The General Health Questionnaire (GHQ): A comprehensive review. *Journal of Operational Psychiatry, 14,* 74–81.

Wallace, S., Worrall, L., Rose, T., Le Dorze, G., Cruice, M., Isaksen, J., et al. (submitted). Which outcomes are most important to people living with aphasia? An international nominal group technique study framed within the ICF. *Disability and Rehabilitation.*

Ware, J. E., Jr., Snow, K. K., & Kosinski, M. (1993). *SF-36 Health Survey: Manual and interpretation guide.* Boston: Health Institute, New England Medical Center.

Ware, J. J., & Sherbourne, C. D. (1992). The MOS 36-item short-form survey (SF-36): I. Conceptual framework and item selection. *Medical Care, 30,* 473–483.

Weinstein, M. C., & Stason, W. B. (1976). *Hypertension: A policy perspective.* Cambridge, MA: Harvard University Press.

WHOQOL Group. (1993). Study protocol for the World Health Organization project to develop a quality of life assessment instrument (WHOQOL). *Quality of Life Research, 2,* 153–159.

WHOQOL Group. (1995). The World Health Organization Quality of Life Assessment (WHOQOL): Position paper from the World Health Organization. *Social Science and Medicine, 41,* 1403–1409.

Willer, B., Rosenthal, M., Kreutzer, J. S, Gordon, W. A., & Rempel, R. (1993). Assessment of community integration following rehabilitation for traumatic brain injury. *Journal of Head Trauma Rehabilitation, 8,* 75–87.

Williams, L. S., Weinberger, M., Harris, L. E., Clark, D. O., & Biller, H. (1999). Development of a stroke-specific quality of life scale. *Stroke, 30,* 1362–1369.

Winkler, M., Bedford, V., Northcott, S., & Hilari, K. (2014). Aphasia Blog Talk: How does stroke and aphasia affect the carer and their relationship with the person with aphasia? *Aphasiology, 28,* 1301–1319.

World Health Organization. (2002). *Towards a common language for functioning, disability and health. ICF.* Geneva, Switzerland: Author.

Worrall, L., Rose, T., Howe, T., Brennan, A., Egan, J., Oxenham, D., et al. (2005). Access to written information for people with aphasia. *Aphasiology, 19,* 923–929.

Ylvisaker, M., & Feeney, T. (2000). Reflections on Dobermans, poodles, and social rehabilitation for difficult-to-serve individuals with traumatic brain injury. *Aphasiology, 14*(4), 407–431.

Zemva, N. (1999). Aphasic patients and their families: Wishes and limits. *Aphasiology, 13*(3), 219–234.

Zigmond, A. S., & Snaith, R. P. (1983). The Hospital Anxiety and Depression Scale. *Acta Psychiatrica Scandinavica, 67,* 361–370.

OBJECTIVES

The reader will be able to:

1. Understand how to be an effective client-centered therapist.

2. Know the psychological and social factors that often accompany life with aphasia.

3. Identify assessment approaches and interventions that are inclusive of the psychosocial impact of aphasia.

4. Understand the skills and strategies necessary to support people as they learn to live with aphasia.

Living With Aphasia: A Client-Centered Approach

Bronwyn Davidson and Linda Worrall

INTRODUCTION

A client-centered approach to aphasia intervention underpins therapy that is responsive to the priorities and needs of people with aphasia and their families. This approach is congruent with intervention framed within the International Classification of Functioning, Disability, and Health (ICF) of the World Health Organization (WHO) (2001) in that it is holistic and inclusive of therapy that addresses neurolinguistic changes as well as the personal and social communication factors that often accompany aphasia. Thus, this chapter has a dual focus: first, to discuss core features of "client-centered" intervention and, second, to examine the psychosocial impact of aphasia as well as assessment and therapy that are inclusive of this dimension of life with aphasia.

For people with aphasia and others in their world, life with aphasia is accompanied by psychosocial adjustments. In the past decade in particular, there has been a call for health professionals to learn from the insider perspective, to listen to the stories of people with aphasia and their families. Increasingly, services are challenged to respond to the ongoing social, psychological, and medical impact of neurological changes to a person's language-processing and communicative abilities. Social approaches to aphasia rehabilitation have heralded interventions that give attention to communicative participation throughout the clients' journey following the onset of aphasia, the reduction of barriers to effective communication for people with aphasia, and the education of both members of a communication dyad and the community at large.

This chapter aims to provide the clinician with an understanding of the factors inherent in being a client-centered therapist. The chapter addresses how to learn from the lived experiences of people with aphasia and their family and friends. Understanding the impact of aphasia on a person's identity, mood, and social relationships is central to the provision of holistic and client-centered speech–language pathology services. This chapter addresses the professional skills and strategies required to engage in client-centered therapy. It includes a case study that illuminates approaches to assessment and intervention that address life participation and psychosocial adjustment in aphasia. In conclusion, factors that enable successful living with aphasia are discussed.

A FOCUS ON CLIENT-CENTEREDNESS

According to Hughes, Bamford, and May (2008), client-centeredness encompasses three necessary conditions of a therapeutic relationship: empathetic understanding, unconditional positive regard, and therapeutic genuineness. Within the health professions, its meaning has been extended to broader aspects of communication, including the provision of information to enable clients to make informed decisions (Grenness, Hickson, Laplante-Levesque, & Davidson, 2014; Law, Baptiste, & Mills, 1995; Sumsion & Law, 2006).

In 2008, Hughes and associates published results of a literature search and their analysis of identified reviews and articles on types of "centeredness" in health care; these included client-centeredness, family-centeredness, patient-centeredness, person-centeredness, and relationship-centeredness. Although Hughes et al. (2008) recognized that different types of centeredness may be required in different contexts (e.g., family-centeredness in working with pediatric oncology patients), they found 10 themes that were featured in all types of centeredness, as summarized in Table 15.1. In the context of this chapter, these 10 themes are described in relation to client-centered approaches to aphasia intervention. The 10 themes are discussed in terms of their relevance to the speech–language clinician's role in the provision of client-centered services for people with aphasia and their families.

Respect for Individuality and Values

The foundation of a respectful relationship is the value placed on a person's individuality, privacy, and dignity. Health and community services are continually challenged to both recognize and respond to differences of culture, age, gender, socioeconomic position, and personal factors. Respect for individuality is essential if health and community workers are to provide optimal and equitable services to all members of a society. In everyday practice, clinicians are likely to encounter people whose values and attitudes differ markedly from their own. As discussed by Holland (2007b), a way to approach differences in values is to develop the ability to take another's perspective. The demonstration of empathy demands the ability to shift perspective from your own to "walk in another's shoes." Therefore, it is imperative that health professionals are aware of their own personal values and how these may affect their relationships with clients and colleagues and the therapy services in which they engage. In addition, respect of individuality and values comes through getting to know the person with aphasia and his or her context, and this can simply be accomplished by asking the person to tell you about him- or herself. Of equal importance is the need for health professionals to understand and adhere to the ethical standards and values of their profession.

Meaning

An understanding of *meaning* has two different, though related, prongs. First, a client-centered therapist seeks to understand the meaning of aphasia as experienced by his or her clients and their families. The second prong relates to the need for therapy to address those communication functions and activities that hold meaning for that individual. Since the seminal work of Parr, Byng, Gilpin, and Ireland (1997), there has been an increasing interest in research that explores the phenomenological experience of aphasia. Whereas a number of studies have examined the meaning of living with aphasia for the person with aphasia (K. Brown, Worrall, Davidson, & Howe, 2010; Davidson, Worrall, & Hickson, 2008; Parr et al., 1997), the perspective and experiences of family, friends, and speech–language clinicians are increasingly being investigated (Avent et al., 2005; Croteau & Le Dorze, 2001; Michallet, Le Dorze, & Tétreault, 2001; Michallet, Tétreault, & Le Dorze, 2003; Worrall et al., 2010; Zemva, 1999).

Listening to the stories and metaphors used by people with aphasia and their families provides a window into their unique world, their understanding, experiences, and needs (Davidson, Worrall, & Hickson, 2003; Ferguson et al., 2010). As described by Barrow (2008), listening to how people talk about the consequences of acquired aphasia helps health professionals gain insight into how people construe disability and communication

Table 15.1 Summary of Factors Related to Client-Centeredness in Aphasia Intervention

Themes	Relevance to Client-Centered Aphasia Services and Speech–Language Pathology Practice
Respect for individuality and values	The speech–language clinician values and respects individual differences and the diverse ways in which aphasia may be experienced. The speech–language clinician is sensitive to cultural values and differences.
Meaning	The speech–language clinician seeks the insider perspective and listens and observes to better understand the client's experience of illness, change, and aphasic language.
Therapeutic alliance	The therapeutic relationship is a partnership of respect, trust, and confidentiality. The speech–language clinician demonstrates empathy and seeks to convey realistic hope.
Social context and relationships	The speech–language clinician takes the person's living situation and vocational, social, and leisure activities into account. The speech–language clinician works together with the family, friends, and work associates of the person with aphasia to facilitate understanding of aphasia and to enable optimal communication with the person.
Inclusive model of health and well-being	An integrated holistic approach to disability is valued. A biopsychosocial approach (e.g., ICF framework) is adopted. Assessment and intervention outcomes are inclusive of measures of impairment, activity, and participation as well as personal and environmental factors. A focus on quality of life is maintained.
Expert lay knowledge	The client as expert is recognized. Learning from the client is valued. The person with aphasia and family may contribute to service delivery and evaluation of services.
Shared responsibility	Shared decision making and goal setting are encouraged. The speech–language clinician seeks user involvement in services and is aware of service users' rights and responsibilities.
Communication	The speech–language clinician is committed to aphasia-accessible communication. Written information is modified to enable comprehension of health information. Supported communication is provided.
Autonomy	The speech–language clinician respects the rights of the person with aphasia and family members to make choices about care in accordance with principles of self-determination.
Professional as person	The speech–language clinician commits to ongoing professional and personal development. The speech–language clinician is a reflective practitioner who seeks professional support and mentoring.

Data from Hughes, J. C., Bamford, C., & May, C. (2008). Types of centeredness in health care: Themes and concepts. *Medicine Health Care and Philosophy, 11*(4), 455–463.

disability in particular. Seeking meaning is also to be understood through the lens of culture and cultural differences. Recent research provides a poignant reminder of cultural experiences of aphasia and aphasia services as recorded in Maori and indigenous Australian stories (Armstrong, Hersh, Hayward, Fraser, & Brown, 2012; McLellan, McCann, Worrall, & Harwood, 2014). For example, in a study about Maori experiences of aphasia, a family member emphasized how language is central to their cultural lives and that the loss of language affects the communication of culture through storytelling and singing: "For Maori, language is precious. And without it, we're, well we are a bit lost I think. It is just the way the whole world ticks, through language and singing" (McLellan et al., 2013, p. 9).

The highly individualized experiences of living with aphasia need to be taken into account if professionals are to come to terms with the meaning of having aphasia for each of their clients. The following quotations from two people with aphasia serve to illustrate different ways in which people discuss the meaning of aphasia. Ram Dass (2000), in his struggle to understand his experience of being aphasic, wrote the following:

From the inside, the aphasia doesn't seem like a breakdown of concepts, but like an undressing of the concepts. It's as if there's a dressing room where concepts get clothed in words, and that's the part of my brain that was affected by the stroke. It took me a while after I'd had the stroke to figure out what was going on. I had to sort out that distinction between words and concepts. (p. 190)

Chris Ireland, a poet who has aphasia, described it as follows:

> *My language has changed but not how I use it. Like before, I use it to match my feelings, to analyse. I go for meanings and understanding. Language like tools. . . . Reading is still hard and less pleasure than before. . . . So frustrating: means me cut off to learn knowledge. Being in my own private word . . . world. Miss reading novels. Catch expression and inner feelings, more like poetry. (Ireland & Pound, 2003, p. 146)*

Engaging in therapy that holds meaning for the person with aphasia is to achieve personalized client-centered therapy. Simmons-Mackie (2008), in describing social approaches to aphasia intervention, refers to therapy that increases the person's successful participation in authentic communication events. Lyon (2004) describes treatment that makes a difference in the everyday life of the person that fits with the life schemas and life agendas of those affected by aphasia. A first step is to discover the communicative activities and interactions that are relevant and important for the person. This can be conceptualized as a focus on the person's everyday functioning and the social and emotional factors of significance for that person. Worrall's Functional Communication Therapy Planner (1999) provides a structure for clinicians to plan and deliver therapy that takes into account the client's interests, focuses on activities relevant to the client, and allows the client to drive the decision-making process.

Therapeutic Alliance

The importance of the relationship between therapist and client cannot be overemphasized. Holland (2007b) describes that although speech–language clinicians bring to the therapeutic relationship expertise in specific clinical areas (e.g., knowledge and skills in the assessment and treatment of specific disorders of communication such as aphasia), an important skill is effective counseling of clients and family members to support behaviors that optimize quality of life. In this respect, the aphasia clinician can be viewed as a resource, a person who through the development of a positive therapeutic alliance affords his or her clients a relationship of care, trust, and hope. Client and clinician develop a relationship to work together on areas such as the following:

- Social communication
- Language processes
- Conversation skills
- Feelings of loss and recovery
- Confidence and identity

- Life participation
- Diminished barriers to effective communication
- Facilitation of social connectedness

Further evidence of a positive therapeutic alliance is the process of collaborative goal setting in which client and therapist work together to identify goals and to determine an intervention program. It is through collaborative planning that clinicians share their knowledge and skills and commit to accompany the person with aphasia on the path to rehabilitation. Increasingly, in the field of aphasiology, a therapeutic alliance develops not only with the person with aphasia, but also with family and other communication partners, including friends, employers, and hospital and residential care staff.

Social Context and Relationships

Communication is the currency of relationships, and individuals' sense of self is defined by their communicative style. It is not surprising that the sudden and distinctive changes to language and interactional communication that accompany aphasia affect a person's sense of identity, mood, and social adjustment. Understanding how people experience the impact of aphasia in their social communication and social relationships is important in client-centered care and integral to interventions that address the ICF domains of Activities and Participation while taking into account Personal and Environmental Factors.

Simmons-Mackie (2008), in discussing social approaches to aphasia intervention, wrote, "The goal of a social approach is to promote membership in a communicating society and participation in personally relevant activities for those affected by aphasia" (p. 290). Tuning in to the natural and stimulating flow of everyday communication and the range of social relationships engaged in by their clients can provide health professionals with tangible evidence of ways to enhance social communication for those with aphasia. One way for clinicians to become conversant with the social context of their clients is to conduct home visits and to observe the person with aphasia within his or her usual social world. Another is to work with the person to complete a social network analysis (see Simmons-Mackie, 2008), detailing family and friendship relationships and identifying regular communication partners.

The onset of aphasia affects family communication and may result in changes in family roles and relationships. Respect, education, and care for family members are required. Le Dorze, Tremblay, and Croteau (2009), in reporting a qualitative longitudinal case study of a daughter's adaptation process, draw attention to the need for speech–language clinicians to be aware of the impact of aphasia on a daughter's relationship with her father and of the uniqueness of parent–child relationships. A central element in this daughter's experience was how her relationship with her father changed because they could not have real conversations anymore. To date, the majority of literature concerning how families are affected by aphasia refers to spouses. Although authors have suggested that family members be included in therapy programs and receive information, support, and counseling (Chapey et al., 2008; Le Dorze, Croteau, Brassard, & Michallet, 1999; Pound, Parr, & Duchan, 2001), it is suggested that increased attention be given to the inclusion of relevant family members (including children and siblings) in rehabilitation care. Further, this research illuminates adaptation as an evolving process involving both negative and more positive consequences. The possibility of third-party disability in which family may exhibit stress and social isolation, and possibly depression, as the result of their family member's aphasia is not to be overlooked.

Friends are another important component of a person's social life and relationships. To date, intervention communication partner training programs have focused on work with spouses or other family members. Davidson, Howe, Worrall, Hickson, and Togher (2008) describe the potential benefits of friendship to a person's social communication, to the maintenance of identity and positive relationships, and to connecting or reconnecting with life. Clinicians are challenged to be creative in designing programs that are inclusive of work with friends of people with aphasia to facilitate the maintenance of friendships and the person's engagement in enjoyable, supportive, and satisfying social relationships.

Inclusive Model of Health and Well-Being

Within this text, several references have been made to the World Health Organization ICF model (WHO, 2001). This international classification with its biopsychosocial approach to disability provides the framework for an inclusive approach to understanding an acquired communication disorder such as aphasia. The ICF framework illustrates the interacting factors that contribute to a health condition and the lived experience of aphasia. Inclusive approaches to aphasia rehabilitation demand an understanding by speech–language clinicians of the person's language impairment and its consequences (Martin, Thompson, & Worrall, 2008). Worrall (2008) discusses how the ICF framework may inform a "consequences approach"

to aphasia treatment, which recognizes that aphasia has a significant impact on people's lives and the lives of their family, friends, and colleagues. The consequences of living with aphasia may include both negative and positive changes. For some, this is manifest in changes in identity, relationships, and life roles or changes in quality of life, depression, and social isolation. For others, the joy of survival and discovering different meaning in life and relationships are described as positive gains. Therapy informed by a consequences approach may target interventions with an emphasis on the Participation component of the ICF framework through attention to communication activities and contextual factors (both environmental factors and personal factors).

Attention to the well-being of clients is paramount in client-centered care. As described by Pound (2004), for an individual to reconstrue his or her sense of identity to incorporate the physical, emotional, and lifestyle changes associated with a new state of being (living with aphasia) is not an easy transition. Wider concepts of health and well-being are discussed by Pound (2011). Coordinated services that address a person's health, psychological, and social factors across the continuum of care are required.

Assessment and outcome measures need to reflect an inclusive model of health and well-being for people with aphasia. A recent initiative in this regard has been the development of the Living With Aphasia Framework for Outcome Measurement (A-FROM; Kagan et al., 2008). A related assessment is the Assessment for Living With Aphasia (ALA; Kagan et al., 2010), a tool designed to measure the domains represented in the A-FROM. A-FROM is an adaptation of WHO's ICF. The ALA questions target all A-FROM domains, including language impairment, life participation, environmental support, and personal/psychosocial factors that affect quality of life with aphasia.

Expert Lay Knowledge

It is consistent with the social model that people with disabilities are recognized as experts in their own conditions (Byng & Duchan, 2005). People who have aphasia are truly expert in conveying what life with aphasia involves and in educating others. This role of the person with aphasia as expert contrasts with traditional treatments in which the person with aphasia is the novice who is trying to learn from the speech–language clinician as expert. Pound (2004) raises awareness that all too often people with aphasia feel disengaged from life, excluded from involvement in decision making and participation in organizations and training. One way of actively valuing the expertise of people with aphasia is to engage them as trainers in education and awareness-raising initiatives.

Avent, Patterson, Lu, and Small (2009) report on a project in which a man with aphasia taught student clinicians how to communicate with people with aphasia in conversational group treatment sessions. A further example of people with aphasia as experts is provided in a chapter by Worrall, Davidson, Howe, and Rose (2007), "Clients as Teachers: Two Aphasia Groups at the University of Queensland." In both groups, one a "transition group" and the other an "Internet group," clients with aphasia contributed to the training of speech–language pathology students. In the transition group, clients who have lived with aphasia for several years assisted people with recently acquired aphasia as they transited from hospital-based rehabilitation to community living. In the Internet trainers group, clients with aphasia learned to train other people with aphasia to use the Internet. The training conversation partners program developed by Aura Kagan (Kagan, 1995, 1998; Kagan, Black, Duchan, Simmons-Mackie, & Square, 2001) usefully highlights the notion of communicative competence and ways to teach nonaphasic communication partners to acknowledge the competence of the person with aphasia. Furthermore, the work of Connect, the Communication Disability Network in the United Kingdom, bears witness to the expert knowledge and work of employees and volunteers with aphasia (e.g., Byng, Cairns, & Duchan, 2002; Parr, Pound, & Hewitt, 2006; Pound, Duchan, Penman, Hewitt, & Parr, 2007).

Shared Responsibility

In client-centered services, shared decision making and goal setting are encouraged. The importance of understanding similarities and differences in the identified rehabilitation goals of people with aphasia, family members, and clinicians has been highlighted in recent research (Sherratt, Worrall, Hersh, Howe, & Davidson, 2015). The speech–language clinician seeks to collaborate with clients and families and other health-care workers in setting goals for rehabilitation and is aware of the person's rights and responsibilities. In a study that investigated goal setting in the subacute rehabilitation setting, Leach, Cornwell, Fleming, and Haines (2010) identify a number of barriers and fewer facilitators to patient-centered goal setting. The most commonly reported advantage of a patient-centered approach was its effects on increased patient motivation. Rehabilitation therapists perceived expressive language as a barrier, thus highlighting the need

to attend to ways in which people with aphasia may participate fully in joint goal setting. Discrepancies between therapists' and patients' goals and limitations on therapists' time were also identified as barriers. Strategies required to overcome these problems included the need for education to overcome differences in knowledge and understanding of the goal-setting process and allocation of time to build a positive relationship between therapist and client. A practical example of ways to achieve shared goal setting with people with aphasia is the work of Bornman and Murphy (2006), who have used Talking Mats, a low-tech communication framework based on the ICF, to enable people with aphasia to be empowered to participate in shared goal setting. The Talking Mat addresses holistic issues (impairment, activities and participation, and contextual factors for each individual) and helps people with aphasia see their lives in perspective and identify the areas of strength and success as well as prioritize areas of difficulty.

Alan Hewitt and Sally Byng (2003) describe how they worked together to find ways of involving people with aphasia in the running of a voluntary sector organization. They suggest that engagement in services involves "being and feeling valued." They challenge service providers to broaden their understanding of what therapy services might offer and how services are established and monitored. Their suggestion is for people with aphasia to be involved in consultation, planning about services to be provided, and the delivery of services. Their work represents an example of people with aphasia and professionals sharing responsibility in ways that enable people to reconnect with life.

Communication

Communication in the context of living with aphasia can be seen as a two-way street. Speech–language clinicians learn from communicating openly with their clients, and clients learn from clear and accessible communication with health professionals. The speech–language clinician is committed to providing and enabling aphasia-accessible communication. Written information is modified to facilitate comprehension of information on health conditions and intervention choices (Rose, Worrall, & McKenna, 2003).

Enabling optimal communication between the person with aphasia and his or her communication partners is a major focus of therapy and educational programs. "Supported communication" is provided (Kagan, 1995, 1998; Kagan et al., 2001). A recommended therapeutic intervention with a focus on training communication partners is Supporting Partners of People With Aphasia in Relationships and Conversation (SPPARC; Lock, Bryan, & Wilkinson, 2001). The therapist analyzes conversations between the person with aphasia and his or her spouse to identify and teach strategies that facilitate optimal communication.

One of the identified barriers to achieving optimal communication for people living with aphasia is time. Not only may the person with aphasia require time to process language, but also participation in a fast-paced social world may require services and people to accommodate different time frames (Parr, Paterson, & Pound, 2003). People with aphasia and their families reiterate that they want information about aphasia and stroke (and other health conditions) early, and they want ongoing information about rehabilitation, community options, and services throughout their lives.

In this context, it is timely to consider that the functions of communication are both transactional (information transfer) and interactional (relationship building) (G. Brown & Yule, 1983; Simmons-Mackie, 2008). Effective communication in client-centered care requires attention to both the quality of rapport established between client and clinician and the clarity and accessibility of the information shared.

In specific situations, the concept of communication may extend to being an advocate for the person with aphasia.

Autonomy

A shift to conceptualize intervention programs in terms of adult learning, rather than clinical care, is in keeping with the aim of achieving personal autonomy for the person with aphasia and a client-centered and person-driven approach to adjusting to life with aphasia. Examples include the work of Sorin-Peters (2003), who reported on an approach to intervention for couples living with chronic aphasia that is based on an adult learning model and includes education, communication skill training, and counseling. Also, Avent and Austermann (2003) and Avent et al. (2009) describe the use of reciprocal scaffolding (i.e., an apprenticeship or reciprocal model of learning) as a potentially beneficial life participation approach for aphasia. One example of the use of reciprocal scaffolding is when an older man with aphasia, a former physicist, took up the role of science teacher with 4- to 5-year-old children and demonstrated how reapplication of prestroke vocational skills could enhance quality of life, improve language performance, and enable him to find new purpose in his life (Avent & Austermann, 2003).

Professional as Person

A professional attends to his or her own personal development. To be effective client-centered therapists, professionals must know themselves, their strengths, and their limitations. Self-respect, self-esteem, and self-knowledge are core attributes of a self-aware professional. Holland (2007b), in describing characteristics of good communication counselors, suggests self-examination as an ongoing and rewarding process whereby self-acceptance can be achieved. Holland suggests that clinicians can ask questions such as "Why does a session with this family make me happy?" or "Why do I leave my session with this client feeling sad?" or "Where does my anger with this client come from?" to shed light on their self-knowledge. Becoming a reflective practitioner who is able to learn from experience is fundamental to ongoing professional development (Schon, 1987). Maintaining clinical competence and a commitment to ongoing professional development are hallmarks of professional behavior.

THE SOCIAL AND EMOTIONAL IMPACT OF APHASIA

People with aphasia and their families frequently describe the experience of living life with aphasia as a journey. Common elements are the trauma and distress of finding oneself in unchartered waters and treading the unpredictable and personal road of loss, recovery, and adaptation. Sue Boazman (2003), a counselor and a person with aphasia, says that her recovery did not go up in a straight line, but went up and down. She describes the variations in her life after stroke as closely related to feelings of control and confidence. It has been suggested that an individual's emotional state affects motivation, language processing, and cognitive and physical performance (Herrmann & Wallesch, 1993).

Depression is a frequent sequela of life with aphasia for both the person and those close to him or her (Code & Herrmann, 2003). Reactions of grief, loss, fear, sadness, withdrawal, and reduced self-esteem can have a marked negative impact on a person's ability to engage in life and participate in rehabilitation programs. Psychosocial adjustment to life with aphasia is both complex and highly personal (Hemsley & Code, 1996). Work with people with aphasia and their families alerts clinicians to the role of personal factors, such as the attitude of the person to his or her aphasia, and psychological factors such as determination, coping skills, and personality as relevant to the person's adjustment to life with aphasia and level of participation in life. Identification and elaboration of the psychosocial and personal factors that bear on everyday communication performance are indicated if clients and clinicians are to engage in meaningful dialogue about priorities in therapy and life goals. As described by Code and Herrmann (2003), normally the best way to find out how someone is feeling is to ask him or her, even though it is recognized that communication impairments may affect a person's ability to verbally express emotions and explain concerns.

Although it is important to be cognizant of the negative impact that aphasia may have on a person's well-being, clinicians have much to learn from people with aphasia who enjoy and embrace life in the midst of change. Chris Ireland and Carole Pound (2003) describe how they celebrate the language of aphasia by making poetry with aphasia spellings, words, and ideas. Increasingly, the role of humor in dealing with stress, coping with illness, mitigating embarrassment, and building enjoyable social interactions and relationships is highlighted and promoted (Davidson, Worrall, et al., 2008; Simmons-Mackie, 2004; Simmons-Mackie & Schultz, 2003).

INTERVENTION APPROACHES THAT ADDRESS THE PSYCHOSOCIAL DIMENSION

The past decade has seen an increased emphasis in addressing in rehabilitation the psychosocial dimension of life with aphasia. Because communication is inherently a social act, it functions to allow people to share and convey information and plays a major role in social affiliation and in establishing social and emotional connectedness between people. These dual functions of communication are often referred to as transactional and interactional (Simmons-Mackie, 2008; Simmons-Mackie & Damico, 1995). A focus on the social and emotional dimensions of life with aphasia entails assessment and therapy that address social participation, communication between communication partners, environmental factors, and self-esteem and self-identity.

Assessment Inclusive of Psychosocial Factors

A client-centered approach demands that assessment be a collaborative process in which the clinician tunes in to persons with aphasia first and then works with them to assess the impact of aphasia on their language processing, everyday communication, and sense of self. Assessment of the person's language impairment

is not enough. Understanding of psychosocial factors is needed and may include assessment of social networks, psychological factors, and natural communication, including conversational skills.

Assessment of Social Networks

Code (2003) developed the Social Network of Aphasia Profile (SNAP), which asks people with aphasia and family members to keep a brief, structured, daily record of a person's social communication over a 7-day period. Each person with aphasia and his or her significant other record the identity of the person with whom they interacted, where the communication took place, the purpose of the contact, and the nature of the relationship.

Another means of collecting social network information is to use an adaptation of the Social Network Convoy Model, originally developed by Antonucci and Akiyama (1987) and explored further by Cruice, Worrall, and Hickson (2006). The model comprises concentric circles. Cruice et al. (2006) describe the layers of this model as representing social relationships of different levels of closeness. Thus, the central circle represents the person whose social network is being investigated. The next circle represents the person's closest relationships, often, including close family and close friends. The next, more outward circle represents family, friends, and colleagues with whom the person is less close but still closer than an acquaintance relationship. The most outward circle represents peripheral relationships. A Social Network Analysis allows the person with aphasia and the therapist to prepare a record of the person's social associations (family, friends, and acquaintances). Identification of people within the person's social network can inform and expand therapy and inform communication partner training.

Simmons-Mackie and Damico (1996, 2001) also describe the use of social networks and embed it as part of their Communication Profiling System (CPS). The CPS is a qualitative assessment that collects data using a contextual profile, a social network profile, a behavioral profile, and an affective profile. Data collection methods include interview, observation, and self-report.

Assessment of Psychological Factors

A number of options are available to clinicians and counselors wanting to gain insight into a person's psychosocial adjustment. These include observation of the person's mood and emotional state, the use of aphasia-accessible questionnaires and interviews, or the use of scales such as the Visual Analogue Mood Scales (VAMS; Arruda et al., 1996; Stern, Arruda, Hooper, Wolfner, & Morey, 1997) and Visual Analogue Self-Esteem Scale (VASES; Brumfitt & Sheeran, 1999). If it seems that the person is depressed, it is important that referral to an appropriate health professional or counselor occurs.

Assessment of Natural Communication, Including Conversational Skills

Building on the CPS of Simmons-Mackie and Damico (1996, 2001) and the research of Davidson, Worrall, and Hickson (Davidson, 2004; Davidson, Worrall, et al., 2008), an assessment process that provides a Social Communication Summary (SCS) is proposed. A personalized SCS provides a means for evaluating the everyday communication of the person with aphasia, including information relating to that person's regular conversation partners and conversational communication with family and friends. Assessment data for an SCS is collected from five sources: (a) aphasia-friendly social network analysis (which records details of the person with aphasia's family and friends); (b) qualitative interviews with the person with aphasia and family members; (c) communication details from a 7-day diary, kept by the person with aphasia or a significant other; (d) the video recording of conversations between the person with aphasia and two regular communication partners; and (e) rating scales completed by people with aphasia, family, and therapists for use in pre- and postintervention evaluations. An SCS provides a lens to understanding the person's communication abilities and challenges on a daily basis. Table 15.2 provides a summary of naturalistic assessment methods that therapists can usefully apply in clinical practice to address the client's social communication and psychosocial adjustment.

Therapy That Addresses Social Communication and Psychosocial Factors

This section addresses what the therapist can do in everyday clinical practice to facilitate a person's optimal communication and positive adaptation to life with aphasia. Collaborative goal setting and relationship-centered practice are the foundation of intervention that is responsive to the personal needs and desires of the person with aphasia and his or her family. The therapist together with the client sets goals and a therapy program, based on best available evidence of efficacious treatment methods and in accordance with

the client's priorities. The therapist must continually monitor the client's response to therapy, review goals, and be sensitive to the person's mood and psychological state. The following principles are core to a client-centered approach: Whether working directly on word finding, sentence production, or discourse, ensure that vocabulary, therapy resources, and conversation topics are relevant to the person and his or her everyday life; include therapy on conversation and storytelling; videotape conversations or other social communication for use in therapy; provide the option of individual or group therapy; include family in the intervention program; consider working on communication between the person with aphasia and his or her family or friends; link the client to rehabilitation and community services; and refer the person for counseling, if indicated. Following are a number of examples of intervention approaches with a focus on social participation and connectedness.

Life Participation Approach

Chapey et al. (2008) described the five core values of the Life Participation Approach to Aphasia (LPPA). The explicit goal of the LPPA approach is enhancement in life participation. All those affected by aphasia are entitled to service. The measures of success include documented life enhancement changes, and both personal and environmental factors are targets of intervention. This approach emphasizes the availability of services as needed at all stages of life with aphasia.

Group Therapy

Group therapy with people with aphasia has a long tradition but has been underutilized in service delivery. As described by Elman (2007b), group treatment approaches and goals are consistent with WHO's conceptual framework of disability, the ICF (WHO, 2001). Through participating with others affected by aphasia in group therapy, clients may learn together in an aphasia-accessible therapy setting. Group therapy may have as goals enhancing social participation and engagement in community living (Penman & Pound, 2007) and rebuilding personal identity (Shadden, 2007).

In group settings, people with aphasia have the opportunity to converse and to enjoy social interaction with others who understand the changes in social communication that accompany aphasia. Beeson and Holland (2007) remind us that one of the greatest losses experienced by people with aphasia is the reduced opportunities for everyday conversation. The psychosocial benefits

Table 15.2 Assessment Methods in Clinical Practice That Address Social Communication and Psychosocial Adjustment

Assessment Methods	Rationale for Clinical Application
Participant observation and recording of naturalistic communication (e.g., in the hospital, at home, in community settings)	Investigation of real-life communication situations ensures a focus on authentic communication for the person with aphasia.
Social network analysis	This identifies close and more distant members of the person's social network (family, friends, and acquaintances) to inform social communication approaches and include in therapy.
Use of structured diaries	Diaries kept by people with aphasia or significant others provide information on • The insider perspective • Social contacts • Places of communication • Everyday literacy • Leisure, education, and business activities
Complementary use of direct observation and qualitative interviewing	This provides information on a person's performance in everyday communication and personal accounts of life with aphasia.
Stimulated recall of videotaped communication events, especially conversations	Recall provides a medium for the person's description of experiences and feelings and their perceptions about different communication partners and events.
Conversation or discourse analysis	A detailed analysis is provided of interactional communication, including use of nonverbal resources (e.g., gesture), turn-taking, repair, structural exchange analysis.
Use of rating scales related to dimensions of everyday communication and mood or self-esteem identified as important by people with aphasia (e.g., satisfaction with and enjoyment of conversation)	These scales provide measures for pre- and postprogram evaluation and therapy outcome measurement.

of group participation are notable. Groups provide people with aphasia the opportunities to

• Enjoy social interaction
• Share frustrations and concerns
• Learn about aphasia and community support
• Develop a sense of self (with aphasia)
• Tell one's story
• Learn from others
• Offer support and encouragement to others
• Practice conversational skills using a total communication approach
• Engage in humorous interchanges
• Make friends

Indeed, Audrey Holland (2007c) reports on Roger Ross, a man who had aphasia, who wrote: "I have a sense that, after my stroke, I did not get better until I met with other people with the same problem."

Readers are directed to texts and articles on group therapy (Elman, 2007a; Lanyon, Rose, & Worrall, 2013; Marshall, 1999; Pound, Parr, Lindsay, & Woolf, 2000) to expand their understanding of group processes and different types of groups. Depending on the goals of therapy, clinician's workplace, and the time postonset of aphasia for the person and significant others, groups may take on different forms and focus. Examples of groups that may address psychosocial factors are discussed in the text edited by Elman (2007a) and may include learning about aphasia groups, personal portfolio groups, family education groups, conversation groups, transition groups, and Internet groups. Group therapy has the potential to address principles of aphasia therapy congruent with a social model philosophy (Byng & Duchan, 2005): equalizing social relations, creating authentic involvement, creating engaging experiences, establishing user control, and becoming accountable to users.

Conversation Therapy

Conversation therapy programs, including people with aphasia and their communication partners, are increasingly being reported (Fox, Armstrong, & Boles, 2009; Kagan et al., 2001; Wilkinson, 2015;Wilkinson, Bryan, Lock, & Sage, 2010). Indeed, ways of supporting the communication of people with aphasia across the continuum of care have been emphasized by Simmons-Mackie, King, and Beukelman (2013). While the majority of conversational partner training programs in aphasia have focused on family members, health workers, or volunteers, increasingly there is a call to also consider, including friends in conversation therapy. The underlying premise is that conversation dyads can learn to improve their social interaction. Thus, the inclusion of conversation therapy reflects an increased awareness of the relationship between psychosocial functioning of people with aphasia and interaction with their communication partners (Turner & Whitworth, 2006). Davidson et al. (2003) find that conversations were the most frequent communication activities of older people. Increasingly, clinicians address conversational skills in intervention programs through working with the person with aphasia and with conversational dyads (Cunningham & Ward, 2003; Lock et al., 2001; Oelschlaeger & Damico, 1998; Simmons-Mackie & Damico, 2007).

Working With Family, Friends, and Caregivers

Holland (2007a) asserts that aphasia is a family issue. It is also an issue for the long-standing friends of the person with aphasia, and it will also be an issue for any new friends. Aphasia is also a significant factor in the relationship between any caregivers involved with the person with aphasia. All of the people in the social network of the person with aphasia may be thought of as conversational partners.

There are many reasons why family, friends, and caregivers should be included in the rehabilitation process and should also be considered clients. The primary reason is that the family may be struggling with the impact aphasia has had on family relationships. Another important reason is that a facilitative conversational partner can reveal the competence of a person with aphasia (Kagan, 1995, 1998; Kagan et al., 2001), and finally, family, friends, and caregivers may be powerful partners in the rehabilitation process.

To be client-centered with family, friends, and caregivers is to recognize their needs and, if needed, provide intervention to meet those needs. Le Dorze and Signori (2010) highlight the fact that clinicians could benefit from the experience of caregivers to organize pertinent services. Hence, a client-centered approach begins with asking the conversational partners about the impact the aphasia has had on them and to describe their needs. Interventions such as referrals to counselors or caregiver groups may occur, but the speech–language clinician may also provide aphasia-specific interventions. These may include facilitating a family group of people with aphasia, coordinating a group for conversation partner training so that they can communicate effectively with the person with aphasia, or ensuring that friends are included in any information or education about aphasia.

Community Engagement Approaches

A client-centered approach recognizes that the person with aphasia lives within a community. People with aphasia face barriers and facilitators as they go about their everyday lives (see Howe, Worrall, & Hickson, 2008a, 2008b). This ultimately affects their degree of community participation and reintegration. The speech–language clinician's role is to work with the person with aphasia and the family to identify solutions. For example, if a client finds it difficult to use the automatic teller machine to withdraw money from the bank, the clinician can discuss aphasia and the special limitations of people with aphasia with the bank, and this discussion may result in solutions that can help many people with aphasia, not just that one client.

In many countries, active aphasia support organizations advocate on behalf of their members. Raising the awareness of aphasia in the community is often a major role of aphasia support organizations and speech–language clinicians, and people with aphasia can play a vital role in assisting organizations to get their message across. The Access to Life Toolkit (Parr, Hewitt, Wimborne, & Pound, 2008) from UK Connect provides resources on ways to improve communication access in interactions, documents, and environments.

In addition, support organizations can help people with aphasia make the transition from rehabilitation to living a full life in the community. As described by Shadden, Hagstrom, and Koski (2008), a sense of community is important in the social grounding of the experience of aphasia. Support organizations can help the person with aphasia make new friends, help others with aphasia in their community, or advocate on behalf of the aphasia community. Speech–language clinicians need to recognize the importance of support organizations by ensuring every client with aphasia has the opportunity to be involved with a support organization.

Counseling

An important skill for both students and practicing clinicians is the ability to offer effective communication counseling to clients and their families to support decisions and behaviors that optimize quality of life and adaptation to life with communication disability. Harry Clarke, a counselor and a person who has aphasia, describes his philosophy as "doing less, being more" (Clarke, 2003). He writes, "Whether I am just being with a client early on, or offering a more practical view later on, I believe that the art of listening to another person is a real gift that is of immeasurable value to the healing process" (p. 81). Whereas it is recognized that speech–language clinicians bring to their professional practice specific knowledge and skills in relation to the assessment and treatment of disorders of communication and swallowing, Ireland and Wotton (1996) and Holland (2007a, 2007b) emphasize the role of counseling in clinical practice.

In preparing to be an effective communication counselor, clinicians can ask the following questions raised by Holland in her book *Counseling in Communication Disorders* (2007b):

> "Am I a good listener?"
> "Do I demonstrate active, nonjudgmental listening?"
> "Am I a good communicator?"
> "Can I relate to clients and family members on their terms and at their level of understanding?"
> "Can I explain myself and convey information in lay terms?"

The very nature of aphasia and language breakdown presents special challenges to clinicians seeking to understand the emotional impact of language loss on a person's life. Thus, other questions to ask are "Can I listen comfortably to people who have trouble talking?" and "Can I listen to emotions?" Having a family focus in counseling can assist people with aphasia and family members in adjusting to life changes and communication changes within the family (Boles & Lewis, 2000; Sorin-Peters, 2004).

A commitment to developing counseling skills affords the clinician opportunities for self-growth and increased self-awareness. It is suggested that attributes to be valued in clinicians who are engaging in communication counseling are those of personal optimism, empathetic listening, enthusiasm, a keen sense of humor, flexibility, perceptiveness, a positive attitude, and the abilities to reflect and learn from experience.

As described by Holland (2007b), the intent of counseling with people with communication disability and their families is to help them achieve the following:

- To grieve what has been lost
- To understand what has happened as fully as possible
- To develop coping strategies and to increase resilience
- To make peace with the disorder
- To make sensible adaptations to the disorder
- To capitalize on strengths to minimize weaknesses
- To live as fully as possible, despite impairment (Holland, 2007b, p. 12)

Understanding the boundaries of communication counseling and counseling for other psychological or emotional problems is important. Referral of clients or family members to psychologists, psychiatrists, or social workers may be indicated.

Holland (2007a) also describes life coaching as a type of counseling in which the professional establishes empathy and provides information and support about stroke and aphasia throughout the recovery process. Life coaching involves an active listening process and can also guide individuals as they develop their own goals and problem solve their life issues. In discussing the assumptions that underpin this approach, Worrall et al. (2010) draw on their research studies and expand on the principles as described by Holland (2007a) as follows:

1. Learning to live successfully with aphasia does not occur immediately, rapidly, or spontaneously following stroke. It takes time and is different for every person.
2. Aphasia is a family concern and requires family involvement.
3. Given its chronicity, people do not "get over" aphasia. Rather, they learn to fit it and their new lifestyle into their lives (Worrall et al., 2010, p. 512).

Within the rehabilitation team, speech–language clinicians are well positioned to work alongside and with people with aphasia and their families. Through listening to individuals' stories, concerns, needs, and aspirations and being a resource to those seeking to navigate their way through life with aphasia, speech–language clinicians develop valuable communication counseling skills. Learning to be an empathetic listener and learning how to enable people with aphasia and families to express their emotions, clarify their needs, and face the necessary changes that accompany life with aphasia are rewarding attributes of client-centered therapists.

SKILLS AND STRATEGIES FOR THE CLIENT-CENTERED APHASIA THERAPIST

The following points illuminate ways in which speech–language clinicians may become client centered as they work with people with aphasia and their families throughout the continuum of care:

- Be a participant observer.
- Listen to the personal stories of people with aphasia (both life before aphasia and present).
- Learn from others: people with aphasia, family, friends, other staff, other aphasiologists.
- Make your expert knowledge accessible to people with aphasia, their families, and the community in which you work.
- Engage with the person with aphasia and his or her significant others (family, friends, community workers).
- Collaborate with the person with aphasia and his or her family in discussing goals and deciding on therapy approaches.
- Be flexible and resourceful.
- Recognize that the aphasia therapist's role encompasses a focus on "living life with aphasia" as well as "language intervention."
- Celebrate successes with your clients.

CONCLUSIONS AND FUTURE DIRECTIONS

Continued medicalization of aphasia may be counterproductive to responding to the everyday communication experiences and challenges of people who will live with chronic aphasia. We suggest that a client-centered approach provides a means for thinking creatively about how a person may negotiate the challenges of life with aphasia. Changes in practice are required while the person is in the acute stages and may begin while the person is in the hospital with a focus on social communication rather than just on illness. Examples include the following: Instead of commencing an interview with the question, "How long has it been since you had the stroke?" clinicians may ask, "Who did you talk with today?" Clinicians can check if the person can read the menu, and friends may be encouraged to bring photographs and invite the person to their home

after discharge from the hospital. A focus on client-centeredness, throughout the continuum of rehabilitation and community services for people with aphasia, ensures that the social, emotional, and communication needs of each individual are identified, monitored, and addressed.

A client-centered approach demands that family members and health professionals are educated in practices that enable shared decision making and collaborative problem solving. Thus, the goal is to ensure continued involvement of the person with aphasia in decisions that relate to his or her health care as well as participation in family, social, and business activities. As described by Lubinski (2008) in discussing the impact of stroke on individuals, on family systems, and within extended social systems, the communication life of the person with aphasia is enhanced when clinicians go beyond words to the function of communication and from function to context.

In considering future directions in client-centered therapy services for people with aphasia, the role of storytelling requires further attention in clinical intervention. As described by Wallace (1994), life stories allow clinicians and researchers to study how people ascribe meaning and communicate about life experiences within the framework of the present. Intervention programs that both enable storytelling by those with aphasia and attend to the content of specific stories told by people with aphasia and their families are indicated (Schroots & Birren, 2002; Shadden et al., 2008). Life stories have the potential to be important clinical tools for understanding the lived experience of life with aphasia.

K. Brown et al. (2010), in a qualitative interview study of 25 adults with aphasia, found the concept of living successfully with aphasia from the insider perspective to be complex and highly individualized. Core themes relating to living successfully with aphasia, as expressed by people with aphasia, were doing things, having meaningful relationships, striving for a positive way of life, and communicating. The challenge for health professionals is to be open to learn from clients, to seek to build the evidence base of practice in aphasiology across the continuum of care, and to recognize that the experience of living with aphasia is a deeply personal and individual one, one that involves the person and his or her relationships with family and friends. A commitment to a client-centered approach is a commitment to practice that is evidenced-based and values the priorities and life experiences of the person with aphasia.

Case Illustration 15.1

The case of J.B. draws on participant data from a doctoral research project that investigated the impact of aphasia on the everyday communication of older people (Davidson, 2004; Davidson, Worrall, & Hickson, 2006, 2008). The case includes excerpts from Davidson et al. (2006, pp. 5–8).

Case: Male J.B.

J.B. was a polite, reserved, yet sociable man with a keen interest in current affairs, sports, and reading history. When he was 60 years of age, he had a left cerebrovascular stroke that left him with a right hemiparesis, his arm and hand being affected most markedly. At 9 years poststroke, he walked independently, enjoyed participating in social activities with friends, and was an active member of an aphasia support group. His residual aphasia fits the description of an anomic-type aphasia (Western Aphasia Battery [WAB; Kertesz, 1982] Aphasia Quotient = 88.9) with associated moderate dysgraphia. He experienced a mild–moderate degree of nonfluency when discussing issues in depth and expressing abstract ideas. His Boston Naming Test (BNT; Kaplan, Goodglass, & Weintraub, 2001) score was 41 out of a possible 60. He was 69 years old at the time these case data were collected. J.B.'s results on the ASHA Functional Assessment of Communication Skills for Adults (ASHA FACS; Frattali, Thompson, Holland, Wohl, & Ferketic, 1995) were as follows:

Overall Communication Independence Score: 6.46 (scale 1 to 7)

Domain mean scores:

- Social Communication 6.24
- Communication of Basic Needs 6.71
- Reading, Writing, and Number Concepts 6.3
- Daily Planning 6.6

Prior to his stroke, J.B. worked and lived on his own, maintained his own apartment, and enjoyed socializing with friends, going to libraries and book shops, reading, sailing, gardening, and cooking. He described the experience of having a stroke as: "Terrible, yeah, awful. Still, it's life." Speech–language pathology reports from hospital therapists 1 month after his stroke recorded that J.B. had moderately severe nonfluent-type aphasia. In the first 4 months poststroke, J.B. received inpatient and then outpatient rehabilitation. Following hospitalization and early rehabilitation, J.B. moved to live with friends and attended outpatient rehabilitation twice weekly. Gradual improvement in language-processing skills and functional communication were noted, though J.B. was often withdrawn and rarely participated in group conversations. At 26 months postonset, he was referred to a community-based aphasia clinic, where he attended individual and group therapy. J.B. had a strong commitment to improving his own communication abilities. He also became involved in groups that promoted increased community awareness of aphasia and learning from each other. J.B. had a strong interest in reading and in sports, especially golf and sailing, and was a regular visitor at a sports club near his home.

The following case data exemplify the positive use of a communication diary in recording everyday social communication, the rich understanding gained from qualitative interviewing, and the practical insights obtained from videotaped naturalistic conversations.

J.B.'s Communication Diary

J.B. completed a 7-day diary using the Social Network of Aphasia Profile (Code, 2003), recording his social communication by printing with his left hand. J.B. presented with moderate acquired dysgraphia. He sought assistance from friends and the use of a dictionary when he experienced spelling difficulties. Written sentences were often agrammatic, and J.B. asked for help if extended writing was required. With some assistance, J.B. completed the brief 7-day structured diary himself. The diary recorded daily greetings and conversations with the friends he lived with; conversations with staff, friends, and acquaintances at the sports club that he visited on 5 of the 7 days; greetings and brief conversations with people in his neighborhood (including staff at the local

(continues)

school); a luncheon outing with a friend; and two visits to shops, one of which involved him taking a taxi. In the diary, J.B. described the purpose of the social contacts as *plans for the day, conversation, good morning and goodnight, chat have coffee, shopping, purchased an old painting, bought a new TV, met a few friends, had lunch, "Good day, How are you? Well, I hope."* The diary records indicated that during that week, J.B. spent around 27 hours in social activities away from home.

Qualitative Interviewing With J.B.

The interview was conducted at the home of J.B. He and two dogs were at home, and the interview took place at the kitchen table. J.B. demonstrated an interest in exploring the topic of the impact of aphasia on social communication, yet had marked difficulty explaining details. J.B. focused on talking about his current activities and friends. For example, the interviewer probed if some people were easier to have conversations with than others. The following is an excerpt from this recorded interview:

> Interviewer: Can you tell me about conversations with friends?
> J.B.: Ah, I, I reckon I can. Mark is a . . . He's a reporter . . . a reporter. He works for radio.
> Interviewer: He's a presenter.
> J.B.: Announcer yes, yes. He's a jolly well-founded fellow he knows what my stroke has been like.
> Interviewer: Yes.
> J.B.: Yeah.
> Interviewer: So, does it make a difference if people know what your stroke has been like?
> J.B.: Yes, yes . . . [and further in the interview]
> Interviewer: He's a good person to talk with, to converse with.
> J.B.: Yes, yes. He's . . . he's a good person. And . . . he takes the time. He takes the time um . . . [*pause*] the time he takes. . . .

The preceding exchanges were typical of the way J.B. described his social communication. J.B. became engaged in the interview and animated as he described his enjoyable social activities and time with friends. During the social communication interview, J.B. raised a number of other issues, including the following:

- Life is different after a stroke:

  I had great plans for before my stroke [pause] and it's all gone now.
  J.B.'s descriptions of aphasia:
  It is famous, ah . . . infamous thing . . . aphasia.
  It's complex, very complex. [Long pause]

- Factors that affect social interaction, including responses of communication partners. The interviewer asked if aphasia affected getting on with people.

  J. B.'s response: [*Pause*] Um, it does . . . yeah . . . um. It might be harder but manageable. Yeah. It's not right, but they tend to give it away. They cut you off. Not everyone, but some do. The . . . got aphasia, people, pushed to one side.

- Factors that support social communication, including rapport and empathy.

  He's understanding. We have lots of interests, driving, going down to . . . [coffee], sport...

- The impact of aphasia on specific communication activities.

  I never tell jokes. Stories, no you don't. . . . Stories, jokes will come anathema. The detail about the stories. It's er . . . It's difficult.
  I read quite a lot and . . . Stories . . . um . . . I find that . . . with stories . . . The won't the . . . the detail as much as the story I'm reading.

- Communication with different communication partners.

  Before my stroke, I talk to shopkeeper, tradespeople. It's easy. But aphasia . . . it's difficult. I think ah . . . if they were strangers, they don't know what aphasia is and um they can tell you . . . you can tell them you've got aphasia.
  When describing attendance at a community-based aphasia group:
  Fun, it's fun. And I meet friends, made lots of friends through that.

(continues)

Listening to J.B. highlighted the following three aspects of his lived experience of aphasia: the importance of his current regular social outings and contacts with people in his community and with others with aphasia; his perception that aphasia is very complex; and his difficulty telling the detail of stories.

Videotaped Conversations With Regular Communication Partners

Two conversations were videotaped. J.B. and the speech–language clinician viewed the recorded conversations to gain insight into J.B.'s perceptions of the effectiveness of the conversations with his friends. This video-stimulated recall process (Gass & Mackey, 2000) allows the person with aphasia to explain aspects of importance in everyday conversations and allows for goal setting for future therapy. The first conversation took place at the local sports club and involved a conversation over coffee and the daily newspaper with his friend, Mark, whom J.B. met on a regular basis. The second video segment was of communication with his friend Jill. The video segment with Jill was of a conversation around a table at their home. On viewing the video segments, J.B. became animated and spontaneously offered comparisons on the two interchanges. J.B. described the first video interchange as, "I think it's marvelous," and "um . . . two of us together, yeah, is enjoyable."

When commenting on the conversation with Jill, J.B. described some lack of symmetry in the communication:

I don't think I was equal with Jill. I'm . . . with Jill . . . I don't spend the time talking. . . . Jill was not as much interested, um interested in my . . . conversation with Jill.

The video-mediated recall activity provided a focus for J.B.'s comments about the impact of aphasia within a particular interchange:

There is a time when much I'm, I'm going to skay . . . say . . . is um . . . I can't get it out. . . . It slackens off a bit. More silences, yeah . . . because I went from there, I suddenly . . . couldn't answer anything.

J.B. indicated that meaningful interactions occurred when he was able to share about his life and his interests. Expressions of enjoyment and satisfaction occurred when J.B. felt connected with the other person and shared conversation on topics of mutual interest. Understandings gained from reviewing these videos allowed J.B. and his therapist to identify areas to be addressed in therapy.

Interventions to Address J.B.'s Social Communication and Life With Aphasia

This case study highlights a number of areas that are important in client-centered intervention for J.B. and that address his everyday communication with aphasia. First, we focus on conversation. Conversation analysis of the videotaped conversations of J.B. and his regular communication partner, Jill, provided insights into their patterns of turn-taking, episodes of breakdown in conversational flow, the repair strategies they used, and their verbal and nonverbal behaviors. J.B. and Jill were committed to working to improve their communicative effectiveness and benefited from therapy that included conversational partner training (as described by Lock et al., 2001).

Second, we examine the value of aphasia groups (see Elman, 2007a; Pound et al., 2000). J.B. reported the sense of affiliation he experienced through attending group therapy with others with aphasia and being an active member of an aphasia support group. In retrospect, J.B. and his friends would have benefited from a transition group that specifically addressed moving between hospital and community-based services. Such a group could provide timely information on services available and support groups and provide a forum for revisiting goals for intervention and life with aphasia. J.B. attended modules of group therapy at a community-based clinic.

Third, therapy addressed the psychosocial dimensions of adjusting to life with aphasia and the interactional nature of communication. In therapy with J.B., it was important to attend to the affective nature of communication and not focus solely on the accuracy of information transfer. Davidson, Worrall, et al. (2008) discuss factors inherent in positive social interaction:

- The concept of connectedness with communication partners
- The positive value of humor
- The role of phatic communication (including social chat, greetings)
- The ability to share stories and feelings

(continues)

Group interactions were an important component of J.B.'s intervention, evident by the fact that his confidence in communicating in social situations grew. J.B. experienced the safe, satisfying, and enjoyable social communication that accompanied being with others who shared the experience of having aphasia. In individual and group therapy, J.B. worked on his ability to relate stories of his travels, express his opinion, and share in lighthearted and humorous social conversations.

Ultimately, a client-centered approach with J.B. is one that tunes in to his story and his unique and dynamic experience of coming to terms with life with aphasia. For J.B., this journey is one of self-discovery involving personal and social challenges and changes. The challenge for speech–language clinicians is to be a resource to J.B. on that journey, to share their knowledge of aphasia and evidenced-based interventions, and to work collaboratively with J.B. and others to achieve J.B.'s goal of effective communication and a satisfying and enjoyable life.

STUDY QUESTIONS

1. Describe core elements of a client-centered approach to aphasia intervention.
2. Why is WHO's ICF a useful framework for describing a holistic approach to living with aphasia?
3. What is the intent of counseling people living with communication disability?
4. Describe skills and strategies of a client-centered therapist.
5. Identify assessment methods and outcome measures that may be useful in recording the psychosocial aspects of life with aphasia.
6. Describe core steps in preparing a social communication summary.
7. Describe how group therapy can address social communication for a person with aphasia.
8. Why is it important to include family and friends in intervention programs?

REFERENCES

Antonucci, T. C., & Akiyama, H. (1987). Social networks in adult life and a preliminary examination of the convoy model. *Journal of Gerontology*, 42(5), 519–527.

Armstrong, E., Hersh, D., Hayward, C., Fraser, J., & Brown, M. (2012). Living with aphasia: Three indigenous Australian stories. *International Journal of Speech-Language Pathology*, 14, 271–280.

Arruda, J. E., Stern, R. A., Hooper, C. R., Wolfner, G. D., Somerville, J. A., & Bishop, D. S. (1996). Visual analogue mood scales to measure internal mood state in aphasic patients: Description and initial validity evidence with normal and neurologically impaired subjects. *Archives of Clinical Neuropsychology*, 11(5), 364.

Avent, J., & Austermann, S. (2003). Reciprocal scaffolding: A context for communication treatment in aphasia. *Aphasiology*, 17(4), 397–404.

Avent, J., Glista, S., Wallace, S., Jackson, J., Nishioka, J., & Yip, W. (2005). Family information needs about aphasia. *Aphasiology*, 19(3–5), 365–375.

Avent, J., Patterson, J., Lu, A., & Small, K. (2009). Reciprocal scaffolding treatment: A person with aphasia as clinical teacher. *Aphasiology*, 23(1), 110–119.

Barrow, R. (2008). Listening to the voice of living life with aphasia: Anne's story. *International Journal of Language & Communication Disorders*, 43, 30–46.

Beeson, P. M., & Holland, A. (2007). Aphasia groups in a university setting. In R. Elman (Ed.), *Group treatment of neurogenic communication disorders: The expert clinician's approach* (2nd ed.). (pp 145-158) San Diego, CA: Plural.

Boazman, S. (2003). A time of transition: A matter of control and confidence. In S. Parr, J. Duchan, & C. Pound (Eds.), *Aphasia inside out: Reflections on communication disability*. (pp 32-40) Maidenhead, UK: Open University Press.

Boles, L., & Lewis, M. (2000). Solution-focused co-therapy for a couple with aphasia. *Asia Pacific Journal of Speech, Language, and Hearing*, 5(2), 73–78.

Bornman, J., & Murphy, J. (2006). Using the ICF in goal setting: Clinical applications using Talking Mats. *Disability and Rehabilitation: Assistive Technology*, 1(3), 145–154.

Brown, G., & Yule, G. (1983). *Discourse analysis*. Cambridge, UK: Cambridge University Press.

Brown, K., Worrall, L., Davidson, B., & Howe, T. (2010). Snapshots of success: An insider perspective on living successfully with aphasia. *Aphasiology*, 24(10), 1267–1295.

Brumfitt, S. M., & Sheeran, P. (1999). The development and validation of the Visual Analogue Self-Esteem Scale (VASES). *British Journal of Clinical Psychology*, 38, 387–400.

Byng, S., Cairns, D., & Duchan, J. (2002). Values in practice and practising values. *Journal of Communication Disorders*, 35, 89–106.

Byng, S., & Duchan, J. F. (2005). Social model philosophies and principles: Their applications to therapies for aphasia. *Aphasiology*, *19*(10–11), 906–922.

Chapey, R., Duchan, J., Elman, R., Garcia, L., Kagan, A., Lyon, J., et al. (2008). Life-participation approach to aphasia: A statement of values for the future. In R. Chapey (Ed.), *Language intervention strategies in aphasia and related neurogenic communication disorders.* (pp 279-289) Philadelphia: Lippincott Williams & Wilkins.

Clarke, H. (2003). Doing less, being more. In S. Parr, J. Duchan, & C. Pound (Eds.), *Aphasia inside out: Reflections on communication disability.* (80-90) Maidenhead, UK: Open University Press.

Code, C. (2003). The quantity of life for people with chronic aphasia. *Neuropsychological Rehabilitation*, *13*, 379–390.

Code, C., & Herrmann, M. (2003). The relevance of emotional and psychosocial factors in aphasia to rehabilitation. *Neuropsychological Rehabilitation*, *13*(1–2), 109–132.

Croteau, C., & Le Dorze, G. (2001). Spouses' perceptions of persons with aphasia. *Aphasiology*, *15*(9), 811–825.

Cruice, M., Worrall, L., & Hickson, L. (2006). Quantifying aphasic people's social lives in the context of non-aphasic peers. *Aphasiology*, *20*(12), 1210–1225.

Cunningham, R., & Ward, C. D. (2003). Evaluation of a training programme to facilitate conversation between people with aphasia and their partners. *Aphasiology*, *17*(8), 687–707.

Dass, R. (2000). *Still here: Embracing aging, changing and dying.* New York: Riverhead Books.

Davidson, B. (2004). *The impact of aphasia on the everyday communication of older people.* Unpublished doctoral dissertation, University of Queensland, Brisbane, Australia.

Davidson, B., Howe, T., Worrall, L., Hickson, L., & Togher, L. (2008). Social participation for older people with aphasia: The impact of communication disability on friendships. *Topics in Stroke Rehabilitation*, *15*(4), 325–340.

Davidson, B., Worrall, L., & Hickson, L. (2003). Identifying the communication activities of older people with aphasia: Evidence from naturalistic observation. *Aphasiology*, *17*(3), 243–264.

Davidson, B., Worrall, L., & Hickson, L. (2006). Social communication in older age: Lessons from people with aphasia. *Topics in Stroke Rehabilitation*, *13*(1), 1–13.

Davidson, B., Worrall, L., & Hickson, L. (2008). Exploring the interactional dimension of social communication: A collective case study of older people with aphasia. *Aphasiology*, *22*(3), 235–257.

Elman, R. (Ed.). (2007a). *Group treatment of neurogenic communication disorders: The expert clinician's approach* (2nd ed.). San Diego, CA: Plural.

Elman, R. (2007b). Introduction to group treatment of neurogenic communication disorders. In R. Elman (Ed.), *Group treatment of neurogenic communication disorders: The expert clinician's approach* (2nd ed., pp. 1–10). San Diego, CA: Plural.

Ferguson, A., Worrall, L., Davidson, B., Hersh, D., Howe, T., & Sherratt, S. (2010). Describing the experience of aphasia rehabilitation through metaphor. *Aphasiology*, *24*(6–8), 685–696.

Fox, S., Armstrong, E., & Boles, L. (2009). Conversational treatment in mild aphasia: A case study. *Aphasiology*, *23*(7), 951–964.

Frattali, C., Thompson, C. K., Holland, A., Wohl, C. B., & Ferketic, M. M. (1995). *American Speech-Language-Hearing Association Functional Assessment of Communication Skills for Adults (ASHA FACS).* Rockville, MD: American Speech-Language-Hearing Association.

Gass, S. M., & Mackey, A. (2000). *Stimulated recall methodology in second language research.* Mahwah, NJ: Erlbaum.

Grenness, C., Hickson, L., Laplante-Levesque, A., & Davidson, B. (2014). Patient-centred care: A review for rehabilitative audiologists. *International Journal of Audiology*, *53*, S60–S67.

Hemsley, G., & Code, C. (1996). Interactions between recovery in aphasia, emotional and psychosocial factors in subjects with aphasia, their significant others and speech pathologists. *Disability and Rehabilitation*, *18*(11), 567–584.

Herrmann, M., & Wallesch, C. W. (1993). Depressive changes in stroke patients. *Disability and Rehabilitation*, *15*(2), 55–66.

Hewitt, A., & Byng, S. (2003). From doing to being: From participation to engagement. In S. Parr, J. Duchan, & C. Pound (Eds.), *Aphasia inside out: Reflections on communication disability.* (pp 51-64) Maidenhead, UK: Open University Press.

Holland, A. (2007a). Counseling/coaching in chronic aphasia: Getting on with life. *Topics in Language Disorders*, *27*(4), 339–350.

Holland, A. (2007b). *Counseling in communication disorders: A wellness perspective.* San Diego, CA: Plural.

Holland, A. (2007c). The power of aphasia groups: Celebrating Roger Ross. In R. Elman (Ed.), *Group treatment of neurogenic communication disorders: The expert clinician's approach* (2nd ed.). (pp 249-256) San Diego, CA: Plural.

Howe, T. J., Worrall, L. E., & Hickson, L. M. H. (2008a). Interviews with people with aphasia: Environmental factors that influence their community participation. *Aphasiology*, *22*(10), 1–29.

Howe, T. J., Worrall, L. E., & Hickson, L. M. H. (2008b). Observing people with aphasia: Environmental factors that influence their community participation. *Aphasiology*, *22*(6), 618–643.

Hughes, J. C., Bamford, C., & May, C. (2008). Types of centredness in health care: Themes and concepts. *Medicine Health Care and Philosophy*, *11*(4), 455–463.

Ireland, C., & Pound, C. (2003). Celebrating aphasia poetry power. In S. Parr, J. Duchan, & C. Pound (Eds.), *Aphasia inside out: Reflections on communication disability.* (pp 144-162) Maidenhead, UK: Open University Press.

Ireland, C., & Wotton, G. (1996). Time to talk: Counselling for people with dysphasia. *Disability and Rehabilitation*, *11*, 585–589.

Kagan, A. (1995). Revealing the competence of aphasic adults through conversation: A challenge to health professionals. *Topics in Stroke Rehabilitation*, *2*, 15–28.

Kagan, A. (1998). Supported conversation for adults with aphasia: Methods and resources for training communication partners. *Aphasiology*, *11*, 693–703.

Kagan, A., Black, S. E., Duchan, J. F., Simmons-Mackie, N., & Square, P. (2001). Training volunteers as conversation partners using "Supported Conversation for Adults With Aphasia" (SCA): A controlled trial. *Journal of Speech Language and Hearing Research*, *44*(3), 624–638.

Kagan, A., Simmons-Mackie, N., Rowland, A., Huijbregts, M., Shumway, E., McEwen, S., et al. (2008). Counting what counts: A framework for capturing real-life outcomes of aphasia intervention. *Aphasiology*, *22*(3), 258–280.

Kagan, A., Simmons-Mackie, N., Rowland, A., Huijbregts, M., Shumway, E., McEwen, S., et al. (2010). *Assessment for Living With Aphasia.* Toronto: Aphasia Institute

Kaplan, E., Goodglass, H., & Weintraub, S. (2001). *Boston Naming Test* (2nd ed.). Baltimore: Lippincott Williams & Wilkins.

Kertesz, A. (1982). The Western Aphasia Battery. San Antonio, TX: Psychological Corporation, Harcourt Brace Jovanovich.

Lanyon, L. E., Rose, M. L., & Worrall, L. (2013). The efficacy of outpatient and community-based aphasia group interventions: A systematic review. *International Journal of Speech-Language Pathology, 15*, 359–374.

Law, M., Baptiste, S., & Mills, J. (1995). Client-centred practice: What does it mean and does it make a difference? *Canadian Journal of Occupational Therapy, 62*(5), 250–257.

Le Dorze, G., Croteau, C., Brassard, C., & Michallet, B. (1999). Research considerations guiding interventions for families affected by aphasia. *Aphasiology, 13*, 922–927.

Le Dorze, G., & Signori, F.-H. (2010). Needs, barriers and facilitators experienced by spouses of people with aphasia. *Disability and Rehabilitation, 32*(13), 1073–1087.

Le Dorze, G., Tremblay, V., & Croteau, C. (2009). A qualitative longitudinal case study of a daughter's adaptation process to her father's aphasia and stroke. *Aphasiology, 23*(4), 483–502.

Leach, E., Cornwell, P., Fleming, J., & Haines, T. (2010). Patient centered goal-setting in a subacute rehabilitation setting. *Disability and Rehabilitation, 32*(2), 159–172.

Lock, S., Bryan, K., & Wilkinson, R. (2001). *SPPARC: Supporting Partners of People With Aphasia in Relationships and Conversations*. Bicester, UK: Speechmark.

Lubinski, R. (2008). Environmental approach to adult aphasia. In R. Chapey (Ed.), *Language intervention strategies in aphasia and related neurogenic communication disorders* (5th ed., pp. 290–318). Philadelphia: Lippincott Williams & Wilkins.

Lyon, J. (2004). Evolving treatment methods for coping with aphasia approaches that make a difference in everyday life. In J. Duchan & S. Byng (Eds.), *Challenging aphasia therapies: Broadening the discourse and extending the boundaries* (pp. 54–82). Hove, UK: Psychology Press.

Marshall, R. C. (1999). *Introduction to group treatment for aphasia: Design and management*. Boston: Butterworth-Heinemann.

Martin, N., Thompson, C. K., & Worrall, L. E. (2008). *Aphasia rehabilitation: The impairment and its consequences*. San Diego, CA: Plural.

McLellan, K. M., McCann, C. M., Worrall, L. E., & Harwood, M. L. N. (2014). "For Māori, language is precious. And without it we are a bit lost": Māori experiences of aphasia. *Aphasiology, 28*, 453–470.

Michallet, B., Le Dorze, G., & Tétreault, S. (2001). The needs of spouses caring for severely aphasic persons. *Aphasiology, 15*(8), 731–747.

Michallet, B., Tétreault, S., & Le Dorze, G. (2003). The consequences of severe aphasia on the spouses of aphasic people: A description of the adaptation process. *Aphasiology, 17*(9), 835–859.

Oelschlaeger, M. L., & Damico, J. S. (1998). Joint productions as a conversational strategy in aphasia. *Clinical Linguistics and Phonetics, 12*(6), 459–480.

Parr, S., Byng, S., Gilpin, S., & Ireland, C. (1997). *Talking about aphasia: Living with loss of language after stroke*. Buckingham, UK: Open University Press.

Parr, S., Hewitt, A., Wimborne, N., & Pound, C. (2008). *The communication access toolkit*. London: Connect Press.

Parr, S., Paterson, K., & Pound, C. (2003). Time please! Temporal barriers in aphasia. In S. Parr, J. Duchan, & C. Pound (Eds.), *Aphasia inside out: Reflections on communication disability* (pp. 127–144). Maidenhead, UK: Open University Press.

Parr, S., Pound, C., & Hewitt, A. (2006). Communication access to health and social services. *Topics in Language Disorders, 26*(3), 189–198.

Penman, T., & Pound, C. (2007). Making connections: Involving people with aphasia as group facilitators. In R. Elman (Ed.), *Group treatment of neurogenic communication disorders: The expert clinician's approach* (2nd ed., pp. 233–247). San Diego, CA: Plural.

Pound, C. (2004). Dare to be different: The person and the practice. In J. Duchan & S. Byng (Eds.), *Challenging aphasia therapies: Broadening the discourse and extending the boundaries* (pp. 32–53). Hove, UK: Psychology Press.

Pound, C. (2011). Reciprocity, resources, and relationships: New discourses in healthcare personal, and social relationships. *International Journal of Speech-Language Pathology, 13*(3), 197–206.

Pound, C., Duchan, J., Penman, T., Hewitt, A., & Parr, S. (2007). Communication access to organisations: Inclusionary practices for people with aphasia. *Aphasiology, 21*(1), 23–38.

Pound, C., Parr, S., & Duchan, J. (2001). Using partners' autobiographical reports to develop, deliver, and evaluate services in aphasia. *Aphasiology, 15*, 477–493.

Pound, C., Parr, S., Lindsay, J., & Woolf, C. (2000). *Beyond aphasia: Therapies for living with communication disability*. Bicester, UK: Winslow.

Rose, T. A., Worrall, L. E., & McKenna, K. T. (2003). The effectiveness of aphasia-friendly principles for printed health education materials for people with aphasia following stroke. *Aphasiology, 17*(10), 947–963.

Schon, D. A. (1987). *Educating the reflective practitioner*. San Francisco: Jossey-Bass.

Schroots, J. J. F., & Birren, J. E. (2002). The study of lives in progress: Approaches to research on life stories. In G. D. Rowles & N. E. Schoenberg (Eds.), *Qualitative gerontology: A contemporary perspective* (pp. 51–67). New York: Springer.

Shadden, B. (2007). Rebuilding identity through stroke support groups: Embracing the person with aphasia and significant others. In R. Elman (Ed.), *Group treatment of neurogenic communication disorders: The expert clinician's approach* (2nd ed., pp. 111–126). San Diego, CA: Plural.

Shadden, B., Hagstrom, F., & Koski, P. R. (2008). *Neurogenic communication disorders: Life stories and the narrative self*. San Diego, CA: Plural.

Sherratt, S., Worrall, L., Hersh, D., Howe, T. & Davidson, B. (2015). Goals and goal setting for people with aphasia, their family members and clinicians. In R. J. Siegert & W. M. M. Levack (Eds.), *Rehabilitation goal setting: Theory, practice and evidence* (pp. 325–344). Boca Raton, FL: CRC Press, Taylor & Francis Group.

Simmons-Mackie, N. (2004). Just kidding! Humour and therapy for aphasia. In J. Duchan & S. Byng (Eds.), *Challenging aphasia therapies: Broadening the discourse and extending the boundaries* (pp. 101–117). Hove, UK: Psychology Press.

Simmons-Mackie, N. (2008). Social approaches to aphasia intervention. In R. Chapey (Ed.), *Language intervention strategies in aphasia and related neurogenic communication disorders* (5th ed., pp. 290–318). Philadelphia: Lippincott Williams & Wilkins.

Simmons-Mackie, N., & Damico, J. S. (1995). Communicative competence in aphasia: Evidence from compensatory strategies. *Clinical Aphasiology, 23*, 95–105.

Simmons-Mackie, N., & Damico, J. S. (1996). Accounting for handicaps in aphasia: Communicative assessment from an authentic social perspective. *Disability and Rehabilitation, 18*, 540–549.

Simmons-Mackie, N., & Damico, J. S. (2001). Intervention outcomes: A clinical application of qualitative methods. *Topics in Language Disorders, 22*(1), 21–36.

Simmons-Mackie, N., & Damico, J. S. (2007). Access and social inclusion in aphasia: Interactional principles and applications. *Aphasiology, 21*(1), 81–97.

Simmons-Mackie, N., King, J. M., & Beukelman, D. R. (Eds.). (2013). *Supporting communication for adults with acute and chronic aphasia.* Baltimore: Brookes.

Simmons-Mackie, N., & Schultz, M. (2003). The role of humour in therapy for aphasia. *Aphasiology, 17*(8), 751–766.

Sorin-Peters, R. (2003). Viewing couples living with aphasia as adult learners: Implications for promoting quality of life. *Aphasiology, 17*(4), 405–416.

Sorin-Peters, R. (2004). The evaluation of a learner-centred training programme for spouses of adults with chronic aphasia using qualitative case study methodology. *Aphasiology, 18*(10), 951–975.

Stern, R. A., Arruda, J. E., Hooper, C. R., Wolfner, G. D., & Morey, C. E. (1997). Visual analogue mood scales to measure internal mood state in neurologically impaired patients: Description and initial validity evidence. *Aphasiology, 11*(1), 59–71.

Sumsion, T., & Law, M. (2006). A review of evidence on the conceptual elements informing client-centred practice. *Canadian Journal of Occupational Therapy, 73*(3), 153–162.

Turner, S., & Whitworth, A. (2006). Conversational partner training programmes in aphasia: A review of key themes and participants' roles. *Aphasiology, 20*(6), 483–510.

Wallace, J. B. (1994). Life stories. In J. Gubrium & A. Sankar (Eds.), *Qualitative methods in aging research.* (pp 137-154) Thousand Oaks, CA: Sage.

Wilkinson, R. (2015). Conversation and aphasia: Advances in analysis and intervention. *Aphasiology, 29*(3), 257–268.

Wilkinson, R., Bryan, K., Lock, S., & Sage, K. (2010). Implementing and evaluating aphasia therapy targeted at couples' conversations: A single case study. *Aphasiology, 24*(6–8), 869–886.

World Health Organization. (2001). *International classification of functioning, disability and health: ICF.* Geneva, Switzerland: Author.

Worrall, L. (1999). *FCTP: Functional Communication Therapy Planner.* Bicester, UK: Winslow.

Worrall, L. (2008). Intervention for agrammatism from a consequences perspective. In N. Martin, C. K. Thompson, & L. E. Worrall (Eds.), *Aphasia rehabilitation: The impairment and its consequences* (pp. 155–169). San Diego, CA: Plural.

Worrall, L., Brown, K., Cruice, M., Davidson, B., Hersh, D., Howe, T., et al. (2010). The evidence for a life-coaching approach to aphasia. *Aphasiology, 24*(4), 497–514.

Worrall, L., Davidson, B., Howe, T., & Rose, T. (2007). Clients as teachers: Two aphasia groups at the University of Queensland. In R. Elman (Ed.), *Group treatment of neurogenic communication disorders: The expert clinician's approach* (2nd ed., pp. 127–144). San Diego, CA: Plural.

Zemva, N. (1999). Aphasic patients and their families: Wishes and limits. *Aphasiology, 13*(3), 219–224.

OBJECTIVES

As a result of this activity, the reader will be able to:

1. Identify the various factors that have an impact on aphasic impairments in multilingual persons.

2. Differentiate among the different language recovery patterns in multilingual persons with aphasia.

3. Employ meaningful principles to implement valid testing procedures that would lead to culturally, linguistically, and cognitively plausible intervention with multilingual persons with aphasia.

Aphasia in Multilingual Populations

José G. Centeno, Ladan Ghazi-Saidi, and Ana I. Ansaldo

INTRODUCTION

Culturally and linguistically heterogeneous societies, consisting of multiple ethnic groups with their individual cultural norms and languages, are commonplace worldwide. These diverse environments frequently result in bilingualism and multilingualism as routine communication styles. Given that there are approximately 7,102 languages and 195 sovereign states in the world (Ethnologue, 2015; World Atlas, 2015), it is evident that several languages coexist in a large number of countries, and individuals in those communities must necessarily be bilingual (speakers of two languages) or multilingual, also known as polyglots (speakers of more than two languages). For example, a large number of Europeans (57%) report that they know from one to two foreign languages (European Commission, 2015). Further, some countries have two official languages, a fact that particularly favors extensive bilingualism. This is the case of Canada, where, in addition to official language policies, high immigration has resulted in a largely multiethnic and multilingual society. Presently, based on the 2011 census, the Canadian population includes 6.6 million residents (20% of the population) whose mother tongue is a language other than French or English, the official languages, an increase of 1,558,000 (23.6%) since the 2001 census; 5.8 million individuals (17.5% of the population) speak both official languages (Statistics Canada, 2015a). In Quebec, the second most populous Canadian province after Ontario and the largest French-speaking community in North America, over 50% of the young generation are French–English bilinguals (Statistics Canada, 2015b). Likewise, the United States has a rich multilingual scenario. Of the 21% (60 million) persons who reported to speak a language other than English at home, close to 78% (47 million) of these individuals consider themselves to speak English from well to very well (Ryan, 2013).

In multilingual societies, communicatively impaired bilingual or multilingual adults in neurorehabilitation, like their monolingual counterparts, may receive speech therapy for acquired speech, language, or cognition problems after a stroke or other neurological pathologies. Serving patients with aphasia generally is a complex process. Yet, for speech–language clinicians working with bilingual or multilingual individuals with aphasia, there are additional conceptual and clinical challenges that may have an impact on the quality of service delivery (Centeno, 2009, 2015). Conceptual challenges include understanding the multiple complexities in bilingualism and their influence on the clinical profile exhibited by bilingual speakers with aphasia (Ansaldo, Marcotte, Scherer, & Raboyeau, 2008). Clinical difficulties encompass the particularities of both diagnostic and therapeutic procedures as well as securing the pertinent research evidence that would guide the assessment and treatment of bilingual individuals with aphasia in culturally and linguistically diverse (CLD) rehabilitation contexts (Ansaldo et al., 2008; Centeno, 2015; Kiran & Roberts, 2012; Kohnert, 2008; Penn, 2012). In fact, speech–language clinicians serving bilingual persons with neurogenic cognitive–communicative impairments, including aphasia, routinely face challenges from limited training and pertinent clinical resources (Centeno, 2015).

Contemporary accounts of bilingualism suggest that a multidisciplinary approach is necessary to interpret communication disorders in individuals with a bilingual or multilingual history. Bilingualism, often viewed within solely linguistic confines in speech–language pathology practice, is a multidimensional phenomenon that goes far beyond the linguistic domain. Bilingualism comprises experientially based sociocultural, linguistic, cognitive, and neurological processes that interact in ways more complex than those typically seen in monocultural and monolingual environments (e.g., Ansaldo et al., 2008; Bialystok, 2001; Centeno, 2007c; Martinovic & Altarriba, 2013; Pavlenko, 2005; Penn, 2023; Walters, 2005). Hence, in the case of bilingual patients with aphasia, minimizing challenges in service delivery may necessitate the use of broad foundational knowledge (Byng, Parr, & Cairns, 2003; Centeno, 2007c, 2008; Kohnert, 2008). Broad multidisciplinary bases have been proposed to strengthen the understanding of aphasic symptoms in monolingual persons and, in turn, implement well-principled services for these patients (Code, 2001). For bilingual or multilingual persons with aphasia, holistic conceptual approaches would ultimately facilitate two main goals: first, the accurate differential diagnosis between genuine disorders (resulting from the neurological damage) and

experiential behaviors (resulting from life experiences, including bilingual/multilingual histories) and second the design of plausible intervention contexts that would provide the optimal stimulation to enhance linguistic recovery, minimize the extent of the disability, and promote social functioning (Centeno, 2007c, 2009; Life Participation Approach to Aphasia Project Group, 2008; World Health Organization, 2001).

This chapter discusses conceptual and evidential bases, grounded in contemporary interdisciplinary accounts of bilingualism, including pertinent neuroscience evidence, to formulate an integrated perspective for the diagnosis and therapy of bilingual and multilingual speakers who experience aphasia. Our approach is based on the notion that the experiential premorbid background of bilingual and multilingual language users needs to be systematically considered for the thorough diagnostic description of their aphasia profiles and the design of optimal, personalized intervention contexts that would stimulate the linguistic, cognitive, and neurobiological processes supporting recovery in bilingual or multilingual persons in CLD aphasia intervention programs. The first sections of this chapter provide an overview of the foundational knowledge and pertinent research that would facilitate the understanding of the social, linguistic, communicative, cognitive, and neurolinguistic profiles that bilingual and multilingual patients bring to their aphasia services. Next, our discussion moves on to the application of those principles and evidence to implement culturally and linguistically suitable diagnostic and therapeutic procedures with those patients. Finally, future directions for clinical research and training that would strengthen aphasia services with bilingual and multilingual clients are discussed. For the sake of length, the chapter focuses on the main arguments and findings reported in the literature. Readers are encouraged to pursue the presented information further in the works cited throughout this chapter.

Throughout the discussion, the terms *bilingual*, *multilingual*, or *polyglot* are used interchangeably for two reasons: First, both bilingual and multilingual individuals (polyglots) may receive aphasia services; and second, the principles addressed in this chapter apply to both patient cohorts. In addition, information on bilingual Spanish–English Hispanic individuals in the United States is often used to illustrate the discussion, given that a large body of the clinically relevant research has focused on this population. It is expected that the principles based on Spanish–English speakers and other bilingual adults proposed in this chapter will be assessed clinically and, when necessary, adapted to the particularities of other bilingual and multilingual language users with aphasia.

EXPERIENTIAL FACTORS IN APHASIA SERVICES FOR BILINGUAL SPEAKERS

The following sections discuss critical information on the life experiences of bilingual speakers to highlight a number of sociocultural, acquisitional, communicative, and cognitive variables that may have strong repercussions in the diagnostic interpretation of bilingual aphasic symptoms and the implementation of suitable intervention approaches with this population.

Sociocultural History

Culture may be broadly defined as the life contexts that determine the psychological (e.g., values, behaviors, attitudes, etc.) and physical (i.e., food, religious icons, language, etc.) realities of a group of individuals and each of its members (Brozgold & Centeno, 2007; Salas-Provance, Erickson, & Reed, 2002). Each cultural or ethnic group members are characterized by a core of shared cultural bonds, such as language, ancestry, values, and religion. Some ethnic groups are considered a minority due to their smaller demographic representations. For example, in the United States, Hispanic persons are the largest minority, comprising 17% (53.8 million) of the total population, followed by Blacks 13.2% (41.8 million), Asians 5% (15.8 million), American Indians and Alaska Natives 1.2% (3.7 million), and Native Hawaiians and other Pacific Islanders 0.2% (0.6 million). The White majority presently constitutes 63% (199.3 million) of the population (US Census Bureau, 2012, 2014). While ethnic groups differ culturally among each other, there is also internal diversity within each ethnic group due to regions of origin (e.g., in the United States, Blacks may be from Africa, the Caribbean, or the United States [African Americans]); tribes or native groups of ancestry (e.g., Native Americans may be Indians [Navajo, Sioux, etc.], Eskimos, and Aleuts); life experiences (e.g., socioeconomic status [SES] background, occupation, educational history, etc.); language use; and cultural identity with the group (Centeno, 2007c, 2007d). In many ethnic groups, individuals become bilingual or multilingual, as they learn the majority language while continuing to use the language(s) of their group.

Given that aphasia rehabilitation programs focus on restoring language and communication abilities, it is crucial to understand the role that internal sociocultural forces within each ethnic group play on language use, particularly to assess the effect that these forces may have on attitudes affecting language choice for therapy and the overall understanding of the clinical program. Ethnic pride and cultural identity play a critical role in the perceptions that individuals have on the dialects (varieties of a language reflecting region or country of origin, age, SES background, etc.) they use and, when individuals are bilingual, on each of the languages they speak. For example, Hispanics in the United States, originating from many countries (Cuba, Puerto Rico, Mexico, etc.), generally want to be associated with the dialectal forms of Spanish and English consistent with their Spanish-speaking countries of ancestry and the US region where they have been raised (Torres, 1997; Zentella, 1997). Further, they may associate each language with a different cultural value. A study of a Puerto Rican community in a New York suburb found that younger members of this bilingual Spanish–English community were more acculturated to American values than their older counterparts, as suggested by their language practices (Torres, 1997). While most residents (61% of adults and 81% of teenagers) used both Spanish and English rather than either language exclusively across communication contexts, the younger cohort did not identify Spanish "as the language or even a language of the United States" (p. 29). In addition, to these young bilingual communicators, English was important for educational reasons, whereas Spanish was not.

In the development of ethnic identity (or cultural affinity) through acculturation or assimilation, language pride is a key element. The distinction between race and ethnicity is important in this process. While race refers to physical features, ethnicity (or ethnic identity) is a psychological state or a sense of affiliation to an ethnic group (Brozgold & Centeno, 2007). Cultural or ethnic identity formation occurs gradually over time through acculturation as an individual experiences changes in cultural practices and symbols, including language, values, beliefs, and overall lifestyle. Language use is the most frequent measure of acculturation (Marín, Organista, & Chun, 2003). Acculturation differs from assimilation. While acculturation involves changes toward another culture without completely losing the original cultural traits, assimilation results in complete absorption into another culture (Brozgold & Centeno, 2007; Phinney, 2003).

Cultural identification is not a uniform phenomenon within members of an ethnic group; its development depends on multiple personal and societal elements. At the personal level, several variables are important determinants in acculturation, such as age, gender, generation, urban versus rural locations, socioeconomic circumstances, and length of residence in the new country (Brozgold & Centeno, 2007; Torres, 1997; Zentella, 1997).

At the societal level, the process of acculturation is also dependent on the positive or negative attitudinal disposition from the larger majority group toward individuals of minority ethnic communities (Centeno, 2007d; Zentella, 1997). Lack of support and pressure from the majority group has an impact on the minority group members' self-perceptions and adherence to their own culture and language. In fact, some members of the group will likely tend to shift to the majority language because the minority language is seen as lacking prestige and not associated with academic achievement and economic progress (Appel & Muysken, 1987; Grosjean, 1982).

Acquisitional and Communicative Experiences

Interpreting language skills in bilingual persons with aphasia without taking into consideration the developmental experiences in the first (L1) and second (L2) language in each dual-language user as well as the typical expressive features in bilingual communication may lead to incomplete, and thus, inappropriate, descriptions of these patients. Bilingual acquisition modes and ultimate linguistic proficiency are highly variable across bilingual individuals. Multiple terms have been proposed to describe the numerous bilingual acquisitional contexts and the considerable diversity in the linguistic abilities of bilingual language users (e.g., incipient, balanced, subtractive, etc.) (Centeno, 2007a). In general, bilingual communication environments and their learners may be classified as simultaneous or sequential (successive). The term *simultaneous bilingual speakers* refers to young language learners regularly exposed to two languages since a very early age, whereas *sequential bilingual speakers* are introduced to L2 from late childhood onward (Centeno, 2007a). In both acquisitional contexts, mastery in each language critically depends on individual communication circumstances and acquisitional age. Individual communication scenarios shape exposure and practice in L1 and L2 for each bilingual learner along the oral–literate–metalinguistic continuum of language experiences (Bialystok, 2001). Linguistic experiences in L1 and L2 generally contrast among dual-language users in terms of communication contexts (e.g., home, work, and school); the language modalities employed (auditory comprehension, reading, oral expression, and writing); and the particular purposes for which each language is used (informal [e.g., conversing with relatives at home] versus formal [e.g., writing an academic assignment]), all critically shaped by individual socioeconomic, educational, and occupational circumstances (Manuel-Dupont, Ardila, Rosselli, & Puente, 1992; Muñoz & Marquardt, 2008; Penn, 2012). Further, for each bilingual speaker, because both languages are not uniformly used across all communication environments, overall linguistic knowledge is summative in nature, with both languages complementing each other as a result of their context-specific use. In terms of age, younger bilingual learners tend to outperform bilingual adults in final linguistic gains. While adult L2 learners may bring more mature and experienced linguistic and cognitive skills and strategies to the learning process, research evidence irrefutably confirms that final L2 achievements in young L2 learners tend to be better (see Centeno, 2007a, for review).

Further, bilingual speakers' discourse is characterized by special expressive features reflecting individual acquisition history in each language and discourse routines typical of language-contact situations as they occur in communication environments involving two or more languages. Bilingual expressive features may include the presence of a foreign accent in L2 (L1 phonological/phonetic transfer), using L1 sentence structure when speaking in L2 (L1 syntactic transfer), mixing both languages in utterances (code-mixing/-switching), using foreign words (borrowings) in another language, or being halting and dysfluent in L1 due to nonpathological loss of L1 skills (language attrition). Also, each of the languages used by a bilingual speaker represents a dialectal variety on its own, as mentioned previously (Centeno, 2007a; Hamers & Blanc, 2000; Zentella, 1997).

Language mixing, either as code-mixing or as code-switching, is a special expressive feature of bilingual communicators that deserves further consideration for its pragmatic and linguistic requirements. Bilingual speakers are not expected to mix languages or switch to a language that their interlocutors may not understand. Moreover, language mixing and switching may also be motivated by pragmatic factors involving social roles, topics of discussion, addressee specification, and conveying meaning above and beyond the explicit message. In this regard, some of the sociocultural factors discussed previously may similarly motivate the pragmatic contexts to use language switching and mixing. Finally, in linguistic terms, the use of either language may depend as well on the relative lexical availability and proficiency attained in either language (Ansaldo et al., 2008).

Cognitive Strategies

The interaction of language and cognition in bilingual and multilingual language users may include complex interconnections involving acquisitional environments, language use routines, and language–emotion associations in each language. In terms of acquisitional scenarios, differences in acquisitional environments (e.g., informal [social interactions] versus formal [academic settings] contexts) result in different modes of language practices and cognitive strategies. Hence, when either L1 or L2 is more frequently used in either conversational or formal educational contexts, the bilingual speaker would have different processing approaches routinely associated to each language.

According to Bialystok (2001), language proficiency can be characterized along an oral–literate–metalinguistic hierarchy with corresponding differences in cognitive requirements. For Bialystok, language proficiency may be viewed in terms of three broad communication domains of increasing complexity: oral (auditory comprehension and speaking), literate (reading and writing), and metalinguistic levels (language analysis). These domains have progressively higher levels of linguistic and cognitive demands of analysis, attention, and control. For example, within the oral domain, a bilingual speaker experiences varying linguistic and cognitive demands when conversing compared to giving a lecture. Similarly, for literacy tasks, reading and writing at different levels of competence (e.g., beginning versus fluent reading), for different purposes (e.g., studying versus perusing), and in different genres (e.g., e-mail versus essay) require different levels of language proficiency and cognitive demands (i.e., text analysis, lexical and sentential elements, etc.) (Bialystok, 2001; Centeno, 2007a).

Similarly, Paradis (2004) posited a possible impact of acquisitional language dynamics (simultaneous versus sequential bilingualism) on cognitive strategies. To Paradis, the mode of second language acquisition determines the cognitive operations involved in second language processing. More specifically, a first language or two languages simultaneously learned since a young age mostly through conversational communication (informal environments) relies on implicit/procedural memory strategies, whereas languages learned later in life, often in structured instructional contexts (formal environments), rely on explicit/declarative memory strategies (emphasizing metalinguistic knowledge).

Variability in cognitive processing may similarly apply to expressive skills in bilingual speakers. In contrast to other expressive features in bilingual discourse (i.e., transfer patterns, borrowing, etc.), language mixing (either as switching or mixing) imposes control demands on bilingual speakers to be pragmatically appropriate and to use the correct language switch for each listener, environment, and topic without any communication breakdowns (Ansaldo et al., 2008; Ansaldo & Marcotte, 2007). In addition, language switching appears to rely on executive function, a supramodal cognitive ability that can be affected by age, rate of information processing, and task demands (i.e., language switching during a naming task versus a translation task) (see Ansaldo & Marcotte, 2007, for discussion) and by brain damage to

specific neural circuits in the frontal lobes (Abutalebi et al., 2007; Ansaldo et al., 2008; Ansaldo & Marcotte, 2007). We revisit the role of attention–control mechanisms and procedural–declarative relationships further in this chapter when we discuss neurolinguistic considerations in aphasia profiles of bilingual speakers.

Information processing in bilingual individuals may also involve culturally determined psychosocial variables. In addition to its strictly linguistic dimensions (e.g., vocabulary, grammatical structure, etc.), language represents a powerful psychosocial element through which individuals experience and internalize their culture (Brozgold & Centeno, 2007; Hamers & Blanc, 2000; Martinovic & Altarriba, 2013; Penn, 2012). Each language, including its conceptual representations and affective responses, becomes deeply linked to the sociocultural world and associative relationships represented by personal interactions, settings, and themes experienced in each language (Pavlenko, 2005, 2006). Schrauf and Rubin (2000) examined the extent long-term memory for personal past, or autobiographical memory (experienced events specific to each individual; Baddeley, Eysenck, & Anderson, 2009), was encoded in a language-specific manner in bilingual Spanish–English speakers. Findings showed that autobiographical memories were encoded in the language in which they were experienced; memories experienced in Spanish or English were retrieved in the language in which the event took place.

Further, Altarriba (2003) added an affective dimension to the way bilingual individuals process experienced episodes in their two languages. When assessing mental representations of words in Spanish–English speakers, Altarriba found that emotion words in Spanish (L1), unlike their English (L2) counterparts, were more easily associated with contexts or specific episodes in which the words were coded. Altarriba argued that contextual differences in the use of both languages may explain these findings. Spanish may be used in private, more intimate settings allowing more emotional expression compared to English, which may be used for occupational and educational purposes. In fact, sociolinguistic and psycholinguistic accounts of bilingualism consistently suggest that language use practices and contexts throughout bilingual speakers' lives have an impact on their individual emotional associations with each language (Pavlenko, 2005, 2006; Torres, 1997). However, emotionality, like linguistic skills, may change with acculturation. Schrauf and Rubin (2004) reported that, for some bilingual individuals with many years of residence in the L2 (US) culture, acculturative forces may have influenced their ability to rate their autobiographical memories in L2 as having more intense emotional accompaniment than those in L1.

To summarize, research evidence suggests that factors such as acquisitional environments, language use routines, and language–emotion connections in each language may have an impact on the cognitive mechanisms employed while bilingual speakers use each of their languages. These cognition–language interactions seem to be molded by fluctuations in individual communication environments, educational experiences, and acculturation, hence resulting in variable linguistic input and concomitant cognitive demands for each language for each bilingual person throughout life (Centeno, 2007c; Pavlenko, 2005, 2006).

APHASIA IN BILINGUAL SPEAKERS

In addition to premorbid sociocultural, linguistic, and cognitive factors, accurate analysis of aphasic profiles in bilingual speakers requires an awareness of how aphasia may manifest in monolingual individuals in the two target languages spoken by the bilingual patient and in bilingual persons in general (Centeno, 2008, 2009, 2012). Knowledge of poststroke language deficits in monolingual speakers of the two languages spoken by the bilingual patient with aphasia allows comparisons of the linguistic deficits across the two languages and any aphasic symptoms or strategies in the bilingual client that do not correspond to those in the monolingual aphasia profiles. In fact, aphasic symptoms may manifest differently across languages (Menn, O'Connor, Obler, & Holland, 1995; Paradis, 2001). For example, though verb errors prominently occur in patients with agrammatism (syntactically impoverished utterances in the context of nonfluent aphasia) in all languages, the range and nature of errors differ across languages (Menn et al., 1995; Menn & Obler, 1990; see also Centeno, 2007b, 2012; Centeno & Cairns, 2010; Centeno & Obler, 2001).

Regarding bilingual speakers with aphasia, the clinical literature often tends to report the unusual cases. Yet, reviews of unselected aphasia cases suggest that two main postmorbid recovery patterns and deficits may occur in bilingual language users: parallel and nonparallel (Fabbro, 1999; Paradis, 2004). Parallel recovery, the most frequent profile, involves the simultaneous recovery of both languages. Though aphasia symptoms are similar in both languages, the actual expressive profile in each language may differ in patients with parallel recovery. Ansaldo, Ghazi-Saidi, and Ruiz (2010) reported a Spanish–English bilingual individual with parallel aphasia symptoms who showed a noun advantage when naming in Spanish and a verb advantage when naming in English; performance on nouns and verbs varied across languages depending on the task performed, with opposite verb–noun patterns in naming and translation tasks. In contrast, nonparallel recovery, which may occur in various ways, refers to an unequal order in the restitution of the languages or differences in their use. For example, both languages may be affected, although one more than the other (differential recovery); both languages may be alternatively affected over periods of time (antagonistic recovery); or only one language may be available after the stroke (selective recovery) (Fabbro, 1999; Paradis, 2004). Most often, the languages known by a multilingual speaker premorbidly are recovered proportionally to their prestroke proficiency, consistent with reports of parallel recovery as the most frequent pattern. Interestingly, when nonparallel recovery occurs, the language most frequently used by the patient at the time of the stroke is the most likely to be restituted, which is consistent with Pitre's principle, discussed further in this section (Albert & Obler, 1978; Centeno, 2010a; Goral, Levy, & Obler, 2002).

Explaining the possible neurological substrates and cognitive–linguistic operations responsible for parallel and nonparallel recovery has been attempted using both clinical and experimental evidence. Researchers essentially have aimed to specify language lateralization (specific hemisphere) and localization (specific hemispheric site) for L1 and L2 in the bilingual brain, based on the symptomatology of aphasia cases and experimental results from laterality measures, electrocortical stimulation, and neuroimaging techniques. The main questions driving these investigations focus on answering whether the bilingual brain is organized differently from the monolingual brain; whether neural organization for L1 is similar to or contrasts with that for L2; whether some important factors in bilingual development, such as age of L2 acquisition and L2 proficiency, have an effect on neural distribution; and whether typical skills in unimpaired bilingual discourse, such as language selection and translation, have an impact on neural organization (Abutalebi, Cappa, & Perani, 2005; Centeno, 2010a; Fabbro, 1999; Goral et al., 2002; Hull & Vaid, 2005; Paradis, 2004; Vaid, 2008).

Based on clinical cases, early accounts to explain the stronger poststroke language included the language most familiar to the patient at the time of the stroke (Pitre's principle); the language first acquired because it involves the oldest memories, most resistant to impairment (Ribot's principle); the language associated with the strongest affective experiences (Minkowski's account); and the language most useful to the patient at the time of the cerebral insult (Goldstein's account) (Paradis, 2004). To account for language localization, early reports of a possible higher incidence of crossed aphasia in bilingual and multilingual individuals (aphasia resulting from damage in the right hemisphere in right-handed individuals, the typically nondominant hemisphere for language) encouraged the speculation of right-sided language processing in these speakers. This early clinical evidence, presumably reported due to a tendency to publish unusual aphasic profiles in bilingual speakers, was invalidated by the overwhelming occurrence of aphasia in bilingual individuals after left-sided lesions, which strongly supported the left hemisphere to be dominant for both languages (Goral et al., 2002).

Contemporary explanations of selective (nonparallel) language loss or recovery in polyglots with aphasia implicate language representations or neurocognitive operations. In representational terms, selective language impairments reflect damage to specialized neural networks for each language, which may be housed in the same or different areas of the left or right hemisphere (Vaid, 2008). In contrast, neurocognitive accounts suggest that procedural–declarative memory processes or control mechanisms are involved in nonparallel language restitution. As mentioned, Paradis (2004) viewed bilingual acquisition as a process in which the language-learning environment may call for different procedural–declarative processing. Paradis (2004) associated such variable cognitive operations with different neural substrates, which in turn may affect language recovery depending on the site of cerebral insult. Simultaneous bilingual acquisition involves implicit/procedural memory strategies housed in subcortical neural regions, whereas successive bilingual learning depends on explicit/declarative memory strategies localized in cortical areas. Thus, in this perspective, nonparallel recovery may reflect the neurofunctional modularity (separation) of the languages known by the multilingual speaker; the language recovered in a nonparallel pattern would reflect the interplay of acquisitional environments, procedural/declarative memory traces affected, and the extent of subcortical–cortical damage.

Further, in more cognitive terms, Green (2005) and Green and Abutalebi (2008) proposed that, rather than deficits being a direct result of the neuroanatomical cerebral regions affected by the stroke, language impairments may result from the temporary or permanent disruption of neurofunctional control mechanisms that regulate the activation and inhibition of the linguistic systems by a complex interplay of language-specific and supramodal cognitive mechanisms (i.e., executive function). Specifically, cognitive control abilities encompass inhibition, selection, and switching abilities that are necessary to select the target language, and to inhibit the nontarget one, depending on communicative demands (Buchweitz & Prat, 2013). Green and Abutalebi (2008) proposed a dynamic model of language recovery

in bilingual individuals with aphasia, a model that is similar to their 2007 account (Abutalebi & Green, 2007) in regard to second language processing in healthy bilingual speakers. Specifically, according to the model (2007), the same neural network supports L1 and L2 processing, but processing of the weaker language (usually L2) may also involve the left prefrontal cortex, the basal ganglia, and the anterior cingulate cortex, as a function of L2 proficiency level. These areas are part of the cognitive control network; therefore, the status of cognitive control abilities is considered to have a direct impact on the language profile in bilingual aphasia (Ansaldo et al., 2010; Kong, Abutalebi, Lam, & Weekes, 2014). A typical manifestation of disrupted control in bilingual aphasia comes from the observation of alternate language switching or language mixing in this population (Ansaldo et al., 2010).

Experimental data, particularly laterality measures and electrophysiological and neuroimaging research, have yielded critical data that complement the preceding findings and arguments based on clinical evidence. Particularly, experimental data have provided insights into the inter- and intrahemispheric processing sites and the possible variables having an impact on neural language distribution in bilingual speakers to account for postmorbid language recovery. While the evidence is far from conclusive, findings support the dominant role of the left hemisphere in bilingual individuals, particularly its perisylvian regions, just like in monolingual persons; the possible recruitment of the right hemisphere in early stages of bilingualism and in low L2 proficiency; and the possible impact of proficiency, rather than acquisition age and exposure, on bilingual representation (Abutalebi et al., 2005; Centeno, 2010a; Fabbro, 1999; Hull & Vaid, 2005; Goral et al., 2002; Paradis, 2004; Vaid, 2008; see also Raboyeau et al., 2008, for evidence on right hemispheric participation in language learning in non–brain-damaged monolingual persons).

Both clinical and experimental data seem to converge in pointing to a higher incidence of overlapping L1-L2 cerebral sites over separate sites, consistent with the larger number of parallel aphasia cases relative to nonparallel cases in bilingual persons. Evidence on typical bilingual expressive features, such as language switching and selection, despite being scant, further supports the strong role of left foci in language representation in dual-language users (Hernández, Dapretto, Mazziotta, & Bookheimer, 2001; Rodriguez-Fornells, Rotte, Heinze, Nösselt, & Münte, 2002), particularly the left frontal–subcortical circuits, sites involved in executive function, a nonlinguistic ability with an important role in controlling language switching (see Ansaldo et al., 2008, for a review of this issue).

Evidence is still emerging. Inconsistencies and inter-subject variability persist. Similarly, there are method-ological concerns. Studies largely do not acknowledge the complexities in bilingual acquisition and discourse and their cognitive consequences or possible cross-language processing differences. Chief concerns include minimal or no information on the bilingualism history of the participants, focus on naming and the spoken modality for experimental tasks, and a small number of contrasting language pairs (see Centeno, 2010a; Vaid, 2008, for discussion).

APHASIA REHABILITATION WITH THE BILINGUAL INDIVIDUAL

Our preceding discussion highlighted important socio-cultural, acquisitional, communicative, and cognitive processes in the life experiences of multilingual lan-guage users with repercussions in our understanding of the language, communication, and thought pro-cesses of clients with aphasia and with a multilingual background. Our discussion also provided evidential insights that explicate the possible role of experien-tial factors in multilingual persons (i.e., acquisitional age, premorbid language use, and proficiency) in lan-guage localization and representation with implica-tions in aphasic language recovery in these individuals. The foregoing factors, when combined with realistic understandings of the culturally shaped attitudes and motivations that clients with aphasia from CLD environ-ments bring to the clinical process may enhance the effectiveness in service delivery. Next, we discuss how the preceding principles may be useful to understand, assess, and treat aphasia in multiple-language users and provide an illustrative case that shows how some of the principles may be applied to implement a personalized management program with a Spanish–English bilingual individual with aphasia.

Multicultural Considerations

Cultural characteristics of bilingual and multilingual clients receiving aphasia services differ among the members of ethnic/racial groups in CLD communities due to acculturative forces, as described previously. Depending on the extent of cultural affinity to the mainstream culture, individuals from minority groups in diverse societies will have various levels of attitudes to the health-care process in general, including ser-vices, the organizations that deliver those services, the interactions with clinical practitioners, and the materi-als and tasks used for service delivery, such as tests and therapy tools (Holland & Penn, 1995; Penn, 2012;

Tonkovich, 2002). Thus, delivering culturally compe-tent services requires a system-wide approach in which both health-care administrators and providers work together with realistic understandings of the clients' cultural realities (US Department of Health and Human Services, 2015). Speech–language clinicians working with bilingual minority individuals must then be cogni-zant of the cultural background of each bilingual client with aphasia to implement the most effective clinical strategies for individual clinical management. In fact, speech–language clinicians working in neurorehabili-tation are interested in more professional development opportunities to learn about realistic approaches to improve their services with minority bilingual adults (Centeno, 2015).

Degree of acculturation may interact with other factors in minority groups to have an impact on the dispositions brought to therapy by bilingual members of the various ethnic groups. Salas-Provance et al. (2002) showed that less educated, low-income, or older Hispanic individuals in the United States were less acculturated to US norms; for example, they tended to hold folk beliefs regarding health practices, such as consulting *curanderos* (healers) and using home remedies, whereas the youngest gen-erations and individuals with more years of education or access to the mainstream majority culture tended to be unsupportive of folklore and more inclined to uti-lize mainstream resources. Similarly, in line with tradi-tional, less acculturated attitudes, individuals from some minority groups, such as Christian African Americans, may view an illness and its resulting disability as arising from God's reaction to a sinful act (Tonkovich, 2002). Interestingly, minimal acculturation may interact with other factors in immigrant and minority groups, includ-ing stringent socioeconomic conditions, educational lim-itations, and lack of awareness of health-care resources, to synergistically trigger stressful living environments that affect responses to therapy as well as the emotional and physical health of minority individuals (Institute of Medicine, 2002; Myers, Lewis, & Parker-Dominguez, 2003; Zunker & Cummins, 2004).

Similarly, interactions during service delivery are shaped by cultural backgrounds. For example, tradi-tional Asian individuals may not make direct eye contact with the therapist as this behavior is not typical in the culture. For Asian and Arab clients, polite and reassuring responses to the practitioner may signal respect rather than actual agreement. In some Arab cultures, touch-ing during conversational exchanges is only acceptable between members of the same gender, which may result in physical distance in a clinical setting (see Tonkovich, 2002, for comprehensive review). For Hispanics, strong loyalty and solidarity among members of the same family (*familism*) may combine with a traditional high respect paid to the elderly and translate into considerable assistance or exaggerated help to the elderly person with aphasia by multiple family members (Centeno & Gingerich, 2007).

Cultural life experiences may also have an impact on the methods and tools used for assessment and therapy, as discussed in the next sections and illustrated in the clinical case at the end of this chapter.

Assessment Considerations

Assessment of multilingual persons with aphasia requires adapting the intake procedures as well as informal and formal assessment steps typically employed with monolingual clients to the special circumstances of bilingual persons in language rehabilitation. Thus, in addition to the standard collection of background information, such as medical, educational, occupational, and social factors, crucial details on the bilingualism history of each individual patient are collected to enhance accuracy in the interpretation of informal and formal diagnostic observations and, in turn, plan the most optimal therapy program (Centeno, 2009).

Bilingualism History

Knowledge of developmental linguistic and communicative experiences in L1 and L2 is critical to gain insights on possible premorbid language practices and proficiency with repercussions on poststroke language abilities and possible cognitive strategies reflecting acquisitional experiences in each language. A bilingual individual's prestroke language status can never be known precisely. Bilingualism questionnaires, however, are valuable tools to estimate the extent of linguistic experiences and mastery in adults from dual-language backgrounds (Centeno, 2010b; Kiran & Roberts, 2012; Roberts, 2008). Although these interview protocols have been used for research purposes primarily (e.g., Marian, Blumenfeld, & Kaushanskaya, 2007; Muñoz & Marquardt, 2008; Muñoz, Marquardt, & Copeland, 1999), they can be clinically adapted to be administered to the family and, if possible, the patient herself/himself to explore premorbid language dominance and mastery as well as the extent of L1 and L2 use in all modalities (reading, aural comprehension, writing, and speaking) and communication contexts (home, school, community, work) throughout life (Centeno, 2010b; Kiran & Roberts, 2012; Paradis, 1987). Similarly, as the cultural and emotional associations of either language spoken may influence performance (Altarriba, 2003; Brozgold & Centeno, 2007; Martinovic & Altarriba, 2013), questions

on language preference and attitudes to each language are critical issues, in particular regarding language choice for intervention (Brozgold & Centeno, 2007; Centeno, 2010b; Penn, 2012).

Informal Conversational Sampling

As in monolingual individuals with aphasia, conversational interactions with bilingual speakers and polyglots with aphasia can provide valuable insights on the receptive and expressive communication skills and strategies employed during informal discourse. In particular, spoken narratives, elicited using topics familiar to the patient (i.e., work, family, hobbies, etc.) (Pietrosemoli, 2007), provide qualitative information on communication strategies used in either language and the integrity of the various linguistic levels across languages (i.e., naming, comprehension and production at the utterance and discourse levels, etc.) (Penn, 2012). Given that bilingual individuals with aphasia may use communicative resources in each language separately or in combination (Ansaldo & Marcotte, 2007; Centeno, 2012; Müller & Guendouzi, 2009), collecting information on possible dissociations across language performance at different levels may provide important cues to guide intervention. Thus, different degrees of impairment in utterance construction in either language depend on the aphasia type, whereas potential errors are constrained by the structural characteristics of each language (Centeno, 2012; Menn et al., 1995; Paradis, 2001, 2008). The patient, however, may also combine available resources from each language to communicate, an expressive strategy akin to code-switching or code-mixing, in typical bilingual discourse (Centeno, 2007a). However, descriptions of the aphasic signs observed in either language for comparative purposes in clinical practice are critically scant (Paradis, 2001).

Conversational samples from bilingual clients with aphasia can reveal the impact of the brain damage on the use of typical expressive features in the bilingual discourse (i.e., language mixing and switching, transfer patterns, etc.) (Centeno, 2012; Kiran & Roberts, 2012). Changes between pre- and postlesion use of such expressive skills can be determined by inquiring efforts on the patient's premorbid discourse profile. Research has focused on the impact of aphasia on language switching, a typical bilingual feature. Given the cognitive control and attentional mechanisms deployed to achieve this challenging expressive skill (e.g., Ansaldo & Marcotte, 2007; Muñoz et al., 1999), language switching is particularly sensitive to cerebral damage. Although bilingual and multilingual persons with aphasia may show language-switching patterns of their original speech community, they may also switch between language more frequently than their healthy counterparts to take advantage of the less impaired language or to cope with an episode of expressive stress (Muñoz et al., 1999). There are instances, however, when the lesion location (i.e., frontal lobe damage) may limit the ability to control language switching, thus hindering the bilingual person with aphasia from avoiding the use of the wrong language with a unilingual interlocutor (Ansaldo et al., 2010; Ansaldo & Marcotte, 2007).

Formal Testing

Language tests provide a systematic means to collect language data, assess the degree of language impairment and recovery, and explore the nature of the deficits in either language. Yet, assessment and comparative interpretation of language recovery in bilingual speakers with aphasia are a challenge due to variability in language acquisition, educational experiences, differences in proficiency and use across bilingual individuals, and structural differences between languages (Centeno, 2009; Muñoz & Marquardt, 2008). Administration of culturally and linguistically equivalent diagnostic batteries to bilingual persons with aphasia is necessary for valid cross-language comparison, based on similar linguistic tasks reflecting linguistic areas (e.g., vocabulary, sentences, metalinguistic areas) and typical life experiences (i.e., activities, topics, academic exposure) in each language being tested (Centeno 2007c, 2009; Paradis, 2004).

Specifically, rather than using literal test translations and assessment formats designed from a monocultural perspective, testing activities must represent typical linguistic and conceptual factors consistent with communication, social, and educational experiences and test-taking strategies familiar to the bilingual individual with aphasia (Centeno, 2009; Paradis, 2004). For example, some sentence structures commonly used in English sentence repetition, such as the passive voice *The cat was chased by the dog*, are infrequent in spoken Spanish. Therefore, such items should not be administered, and only use items, such as active sentences (e.g., *The dog chased the cat*), more typical in Spanish usage. A similar approach must be taken when the test to be used contains linguistic stimuli (e.g., expressions and vocabulary) that do not represent the dialectal form of the language spoken by the client. Finally, attentional demands required by a formal test may be unfamiliar to some clients, particularly illiterate individuals or individuals with minimal academic experiences, not often exposed to formal, structured language tasks. These tasks could be adapted by providing increased illustrative instructions and more practice trials to enhance individuals' attention and focus (Centeno, 2009).

Securing valid culturally and linguistically appropriate aphasia tests in many languages is not always possible. The limited number of available assessment tools in languages other than English often do not meet the expected psychometric requirements for these measures (i.e., construct validity, content validity, test–posttest reliability, etc.) (Kennedy & Chiou, 2005; Roberts, 2008). In this case, administering adapted versions of available tests (see Table 16.1) rather than translations and using an interpreter, if necessary, are advised. Helpful guidelines to facilitate interpreter-assisted interactions have been proposed (American Speech-Language-Hearing Association, 2015; Isaac, 2005). The evaluator will have to use his or her discretion for final diagnostic impressions because, when adapting a test, the normative data from the original test cannot be employed to assess the patient (Roberts, 2008).

The *Bilingual Aphasia Test* (BAT; Paradis, 1987, 2010) may be an optional assessment tool to obtain complementary results not typically collected through standard aphasia tests. Created to systematically assess aphasia patterns in different pairs of languages, the BAT, a criterion-based measure, may be useful to obtain multi-modality information not obtained from typical aphasia batteries on poststroke linguistic processing. The BAT, only available from its author at this time (Paradis, 2010), explores the bilingualism history of each patient through a questionnaire and examines all language modalities, employing various tasks (e.g., spoken commands, word reading, naming, sentence formulation, etc.), and translation skills.

Although the BAT is available in over 60 languages and numerous language pairs, there is limited normative data on nonimpaired bilingual individuals for most languages. Available reports on intact bilingual speakers tested with the BAT suggest that acquisitional background, educational experiences, and age are crucial determinants in the L1–L2 profile of the bilingual persons assessed (Juncos-Rabadán, 1994; Manuel-Dupont et al., 1992; Muñoz & Marquardt, 2008). Specifically, bilingual speakers do better in their dominant language; educated bilingual individuals score higher than their less educated counterparts; performance is stronger in the language used academically for academically based tasks (e.g., grammaticality judgment, spoken and written complex sentences, and mental arithmetics); older bilingual persons score lower than their younger counterparts; and language loss (attrition) may be responsible for the poorer performance in the nondominant language (Juncos-Rabadán, 1994; Manuel-Dupont et al., 1992; Muñoz & Marquardt, 2008). Interestingly, for

Table 16.1 Frequently Used Aphasia Tests in Various Languages

Versions in English and Spanish

1. Boston Diagnostic Aphasia Examination, 3rd ed. (BDAE)
   Goodglass, Kaplan, and Barresi (2001)
   Evaluación de la Afasia y Trastornos Relacionados, 3rd ed. (EATR)
   Goodglass and Kaplan (2005)
2. Multilingual Aphasia Examination–English (MAE-E)
   Benton, Hamsher, and Sivan (1994)
   Multilingual Aphasia Examination–Spanish (MAE-S)
   Rey, Sivan, and Benton (1991)
3. Psycholinguistic Assessment of Language Processing in Aphasia (PALPA)
   Kay, Lesser, and Coltheart (1992)
   Evaluación del Procesamiento Lingüístico en la Afasia (EPLA)
   Valle and Cuetos (1995)

Versions in Multiple Languages

1. The Bilingual Aphasia Test (BAT)
   Paradis (1987, 2010)
   Available online: http://www.mcgill.ca/linguistics/research/bat/
2. The Aachen Aphasia Test
   Huber, Poeck, and Willmes (1984)

a number of subtests, unimpaired bilingual speakers may exhibit substantially low response rates in either or both languages. Such performance limitations in cases of healthy bilingual speakers suggest that these subtests may not be valid to assess aphasic difficulties as poor scores in the patients with aphasia cannot be attributed to the disorder. Items of these subtests may be modified or eliminated (Muñoz & Marquardt, 2008).

Thus, administration of the BAT may require adaptations, as demonstrated when this test was employed with persons with limited education (i.e., illiterate individuals) (Juncos-Rabadán, 1994). Indeed, as in monolingual individuals with aphasia, educational experiences are an important factor to consider when testing bilingual patients because limited academic experiences can result in depressed cognitive skills (e.g., conceptual similarities, phoneme segmentation, and delayed verbal memory) (Ostrosky-Solís, Lozano, Ramírez, & Ardila, 2007) that may affect language areas in testing (i.e., metalinguistic skills, phonological awareness, latency of response, etc.) (Centeno & Gingerich, 2007; see also Muñoz & Marquardt, 2008, for additional discussion on the role of education in bilingual language testing).

Intervention Considerations

The preceding discussion underscores the importance of well-principled assessment procedures that would facilitate the collection of the formal and informal diagnostic data necessary to implement individualized intervention strategies consistent with each multilingual patient's premorbid linguistic, communicative, and cognitive experiences (Centeno, 2009, 2010b). Research exploring the role of such experiential factors in the rehabilitation of multilingual individuals with aphasia is in its infancy. Intervention studies with these patients essentially have aimed to examine whether therapy should be conducted monolingually or bilingually and, if monolingually, what factors should be considered for language choice; whether there is transfer of therapy gains between the treated and nontreated language(s); and what factors support cross-language generalization (Ansaldo et al., 2010; Faroqi-Shah, Frymark, Mullen, & Wang, 2010; Goral, Rosas, Conner, Maul, & Obler, 2012; Kohnert, 2009).

Current intervention data are far from conclusive. Answers to the preceding questions appear to be complex. Studies have shown that treatment can help both treated and untreated languages, that the treated language may improve more than the untreated language, that both languages may improve simultaneously, or that there might not be any generalization to the untreated language. Despite such variability in the intervention outcomes, an important emerging trend in the evidence is that treating in one language, be it L1 or L2, may similarly help the untreated language in both structurally similar and structurally different languages, as long as therapy targets cross-linguistic similarities (Fabbro, 1999; Gil & Goral, 2004; Kohnert, 2009; Paradis, 2008). Still, a large number of intervening factors exist, such as premorbid language proficiency, type of aphasia, and treatment approach, whose impact on intervention needs to be clarified (Faroqi-Shah et al., 2010). However, because cross-linguistic generalization appears to occur when either language is used in systematic intervention (Kohnert, 2009; Kohnert & Peterson, 2012), exploiting those factors that enhance cross-language transfer seems to be a viable treatment approach.

In a recent review, Ansaldo and Ghazi-Saidi (2014) examined the possible determinants that may operate on promoting transfer of therapy gains between the treated and nontreated language(s), particularly because a unilingual treatment approach may often be the only option, given that the person with aphasia speaks a language other than that of the speech–language clinician. Ansaldo and Ghazi-Saidi (2014) advance the possibility that a number of factors, including word type, language distance, status of cognitive control abilities, and premorbid and postmorbid language proficiency in each language spoken by the patient, determine the potential for cross-linguistic effects of therapy gains. For example, transfer is better when treatment (a) targets both cognitive skills (e.g., card sorting, single-digit computations) and cross-linguistically similar word types (e.g., cognates: rosa/rose) relative to no cross-linguistic similarities (e.g., noncognates: apple/manzana) (Kohnert, 2008); (b) involves two structurally similar languages (Goral, Levy, & Kastl, 2010); (c) takes into consideration cognitive control issues related to specific expressive skills in bilingual discourse (i.e., code-switching in naming relative to translation) (Ansaldo et al., 2010; Ansaldo & Marcotte, 2007); and (d) considers prestroke and poststroke language routines and proficiency levels (Edmonds & Kiran, 2006; Gil & Goral, 2004; Goral et al., 2012).

Aphasia intervention research with bilingual speakers requires considerable further exploration. When interpreting research data on intervention issues, there are a number of variables to consider. First, for some studies, it is difficult to distinguish the positive effects of therapy on language gains from spontaneous recovery because those studies were conducted during the acute period of the aphasia. Second, factors related to the bilingual patient with aphasia, such as premorbid proficiency in either language, premorbid and postmorbid patterns of language use, and order of acquisition, may interact on therapy outcomes. Third, language variables affecting cross-language generalization may include the particular linguistic aspect (e.g., lexical production versus narrative comprehension) and the typological features of the language (e.g., tonal versus nontonal). Fourth, the majority of these studies have focused on naming skills, thus providing no insights into the possible factors with an impact on treatment of morphological or syntactic comprehension or production. Finally, important variables shaping therapy outcomes in monolingual individuals with aphasia, including type and severity of aphasia, premorbid health status, educational levels, and family support, may similarly be critical when treating multilingual persons with aphasia (Faroqi-Shah et al., 2010; Goral et al., 2012; Kohnert, 2009; Kohnert & Peterson, 2012; Paradis, 2004).

In addition to specific factors with an impact on therapy, research similarly has provided evidence on plausible treatment approaches. For example, as mentioned, coupling cognitive training (i.e., attention, categorization, or problem solving through tasks such as card sorting and single-digit computations) and language similarities (e.g., cognates) may help naming recovery better than when there are no language similarities (Kohnert, 2008). Intensive multimodality stimulation (combined use of speaking, writing, reading, etc.) may activate not only the specific aspects targeted during therapy but also underlying language components and cognitive processes of information organization and retrieval (Gil & Goral, 2004). Intervention targeting cognitive operations involved in typical expressive features in bilingual communicators similarly has been useful to treat naming skills in the context of pathological language mixing and switching (Ansaldo et al., 2010; Ansaldo & Marcotte, 2007). Specifically, using translation, an ability that often is less impaired than other linguistic skills in bilingual persons with aphasia (Paradis, 2004), may enhance conscious control of language selection and word retrieval during those episodes of erroneous language choice while naming. In this approach, translating essentially becomes a self-cueing mechanism for the patient (Ansaldo et al., 2010).

Moreover, adopting a therapy approach that stimulates both languages (as in translation) may be more ecologically valid because such an approach, while supporting the client's premorbid communication routines, would capitalize on the spared cross-linguistic L1–L2 links and make optimal use of the bilingual language system as a whole (Ansaldo et al., 2010; Kohnert & Peterson, 2012). This perspective contrasts with traditional one-language intervention, based on the earlier notion that treating more than one language might inhibit global speech recovery (Chlenov, 1948) and delay the recovery of all languages (Wald, 1958, 1961). Current understanding of the characteristics of the bilingual language system shows that it involves a complex integration of the two languages into one language system (Ansaldo et al., 2008). Thus, even in situations when only one language is recovered, bilingual intervention would seem to be a plausible approach on theoretical and sociolinguistic grounds. Bilingual therapy would provide a dual-language strategy to maximally stimulate the cognitive–linguistic mechanisms participating in the bilingual language system of the speaker and enhance the dual language use (language switching and mixing) typically employed by bilingual speakers in daily discourse.

Interestingly, findings from treatment studies support the possible connection between cognitive operations and linguistic retrieval to facilitate language recovery. This approach is consistent with notions that aphasia, although primarily considered a language impairment, may involve certain cognitive dysfunctions (Harley, 2008; Hillis & Newhart, 2008), thus suggesting that addressing possible cognitive operations underlying aphasic symptoms may speed recovery (see Cuetos & Centeno, 2009; Rapp, 2005, for discussion of cognitively based treatment of acquired linguistic impairments).

Similarly, integrating psychocognitive factors into bilingual aphasia therapy, considering the emotional dimension of language processing, may similarly be useful for language rehabilitation. Motivation and affect may strengthen a memory trace physiologically inhibited in the bilingual speaker with aphasia by the cerebral insult (Paradis, 2004). Further, because emotion words appear to be encoded in L1 and L2 differently and emotional scripts associated with each language may change with acculturation (Altarriba, 2003; Schrauf & Rubin, 2004), knowledge of contexts of acquisition, acculturation, and emotional connections to each language seems necessary for appropriate language and topic selection and to enhance recall during intervention (Brozgold & Centeno, 2007; Centeno, 2007c, 2010b).

Hence, as illustrated in our clinical illustration, knowing about the sociocultural history, acquisitional and communicative experiences, and routine cognitive strategies as well as the possible interactions among these elements in each bilingual person with aphasia may be helpful for language and communication enhancement. Optimal, personalized intervention contexts for bilingual and multilingual individuals with aphasia might benefit from integrating premorbid life experiences, communication practices, cognitive–linguistic interactions, and cultural realities in ways that can promote communication maximally utilizing sociocultural, processing, and linguistic resources familiar to the individual client.

FUTURE DIRECTIONS

Based on contemporary accounts of bilingualism and emerging neuroscience evidence, this chapter highlighted some possible relationships involving experiential background in multiple-language users (i.e., sociocultural history, linguistic and communicative experiences, and cognitive strategies) with consequences in the valid diagnostic analysis of aphasia profiles and the design of optimal, culturally suitable intervention contexts. Our discussion has clinical and research implications. Regarding assessment, there is an imperative need to develop valid diagnostic tools based on both sound psychometric principles and realistic linguistic, communicative, and cognitive experiences of persons with multilingual histories, especially those individuals from minority environments. These assessment measures should be equivalent across languages to facilitate accurate cross-language comparison of test results. Also, descriptive studies of aphasic symptomatology in underresearched languages are mandated to obtain the evidence to allow the systematic comparative analysis of the nature and incidence of errors between languages.

In terms of intervention, research has provided important preliminary evidence. Numerous questions remain, especially the role of intervening variables in therapy (e.g., spontaneous recovery, overall patient health, acquisitional factors, language similarities, etc.). Yet, there is reason for optimism and for increased research with bilingual speakers, particularly encouraged by neuroplasticity investigations supporting posttherapy language gains accompanied by neurological reorganization in monolingual patients with aphasia (Gonzalez-Rothi & Barrett, 2006; Marcotte & Ansaldo, 2010; Thompson, 2000). Similar studies on dual-language users, albeit extremely limited, have yielded consistent findings suggesting treatment-induced enhancement of neuroplastic changes (e.g., recruitment of undamaged left hemispheric language regions and right hemispheric homologous areas) (Meinzer, Obleser, Flaisch, Eulitz, & Rockstroh, 2007; see also Ansaldo et al., 2008, for discussion). The combined effect of experiential and environmental variables in multilingual contexts discussed in this chapter and the principles of experience-dependent plasticity in aphasia rehabilitation (e.g., timing, intensity, and richness of training) on the processes of neurological reorganization (i.e., new neuronal connections [collateral sprouting] to denervated areas on stimulation, possible involvement of right-sided homologous areas) (Raymer et al., 2008) have not been examined in detail in aphasia intervention with multilingual individuals. Given that richness of stimulation (e.g., conversational treatment relative to unguided socialization) may play a critical facilitation role in aphasia therapy (Raymer et al., 2008), studying the possible impact of holistic conversationally based treatment relative to narrow skill-based training (i.e., naming) on neuronal reactivation and growth would be a possible research direction in bilingual clients receiving aphasia intervention. Indeed, holistic interactive therapy would bring together language (i.e., target linguistic stimuli and multimodality stimulation); cognitive strengths (e.g., attention, representational schemata, and memory); communication contexts (e.g., interlocutors, themes, and settings); and motivation (i.e., conversational engagement) into an integrated paradigm that may stimulate linguistic and psycholinguistic resources, consistent with the social, acquisitional, and communicative history of each bilingual client with aphasia, to possibly favor neuronal activation (Centeno, 2007c).

Additional lines of research warrant attention. Given the frequent use of interpreters and cultural brokers by speech–language clinicians in CLD neurorehabilitation programs, including aphasia services (Centeno, 2015; Faroqi-Shah et al., 2010; Penn, 2012), outcome investigations when these linguistic–cultural assistants participate in aphasia treatment would be valuable. Finally, consistent with model-driven approaches to aphasia therapy based on the cognitive operations underlying acquired linguistic deficits (Cuetos & Centeno, 2009), treating bilingual speakers with aphasia may strongly benefit from model-driven descriptions of bilingual clients' language profiles and the preserved and disrupted cognitive mechanisms in the bilingual language system in each bilingual patient with aphasia (Green, 2005; Green & Abutalebi, 2008). This approach would reinforce preserved processors and, in turn, overcome the effects of disrupted operations to help the restoration of language and communication faculties (Ansaldo et al., 2010).

Theoretical models can be verified using novel technology such as neuroimaging. Functional connectivity, particularly, is a promising tool that may prove useful to reveal best therapy options for patients who speak more than one language because it can provide information on the brain networks involved in a task and their interconnections. Presently, most studies using functional connectivity to address brain networks based on theoretical models include healthy participants (Dodel et al., 2005; Ghazi-Saidi et al., 2013) and rarely include bilingual patients with aphasia (Abutalebi, Della Rosa, Tettamanti, Green, & Cappa, 2009). Nevertheless, the results of these studies suggest that there is a close interaction between cognitive control and language networks, thus highlighting the possible use of this technique to investigate the role of cognitive–linguistic interactions in therapy, such as in patients with pathological language mixing and switching.

Ultimately, the principles discussed here may serve as foundational knowledge to enhance service delivery. Speech–language clinicians presently working with bilingual and multilingual persons with aphasia in CLD adult health care routinely face challenges in service delivery due to limitations in their professional preparation and clinical resources to realistically serve these clients. These clinicians have great interest in improving current professional preparation for future providers and securing resources for presently licensed practitioners (Centeno, 2015). Thus, for training clinicians, the information presented here would provide helpful content for their clinical preparation. Practicing speech–language clinicians may adapt this information to minimize their training limitations and better serve multilingual patients with aphasia consistent with the therapy context (e.g., clinical facility, patient's home, etc.) and individual patient background (e.g., language history, premorbid routines, educational level, etc.). They can use the presented principles to enhance accuracy in their diagnostic interpretation of aphasia profiles in multilingual speakers and to design optimal, individual intervention programs that would stimulate the possible linguistic, cognitive, and neurological operations supporting linguistic and communicative recovery in each multilingual client with aphasia.

Case Illustration 16.1

This case concerns a bilingual patient with parallel language recovery consistent with Broca's aphasia in both languages

Overall Patient Description

R.T., a 68-year-old right-handed woman, had suffered a left-sided frontoparietal cerebrovascular accident (CVA). R.T. exhibited characteristic symptoms of Broca's aphasia in both Spanish and English. She demonstrated nonfluent, agrammatic oral expression (syntactically limited utterances) and difficulty with naming and sentence repetition. Comprehension was adequate for informal conversation in both languages, although some comprehension deficits (e.g., complex ideational material) were observed during formal testing. Her recovery pattern and deficits were parallel as both languages were restituted simultaneously and showed similar Broca's aphasia symptoms. The individual in this clinical case, reported previously (Centeno, 2009), was seen by the first author as a home care patient.

Bilingualism History

A bilingualism questionnaire, structured to explore R.T.'s age of onset of L2 experiences as well as the communication environments (home, school, community) and modalities (speaking, writing, reading) in which

(continues)

both languages were used (Centeno, 2010b), was administered to R.T.'s husband and daughter. The information collected revealed that R.T. was born in Venezuela and arrived in the United States when she was 32. Prior to arriving in the United States, she only spoke Spanish and learned English as a school subject in Venezuela. She did not use English outside school. In terms of education, she completed high school in Venezuela. Once in the United States, she married a bilingual Spanish–English man. She communicated with her husband and four children in Spanish and English. Her social networks and community were bilingual, although Spanish was the most frequently used language. R.T. worked as a cafeteria manager in New York City. She wrote and read in Spanish more frequently than in English. Her reading and writing in English primarily involved work-related activities. She primarily watched TV in Spanish.

Informal Sample

The informal language sample that follows illustrates R.T.'s recovery profile in conversation after she was asked what she did for work before her CVA. Her oral expression consisted of agrammatic utterances involving simple verb forms (*hacia, trabaja, trabajando*), literal paraphasias (*cafesia*/cafeteria, *kisen*/kitchen), and some typical features of bilingual speech, particularly mixed-language utterances (code-switching), with automatized formulaic expressions (*I don't know, day and night*) and borrowed words (*cafeteria*). She did not generate any utterances that did not fit into either the aphasic profile or typical expressions of bilingual discourse (see Muñoz et al., 1999).

> R.T. *Hacia… trabaja… I don't know… la cafesia…*
>
> Translation: Used to make… [he/she] works… I don't know… the cafeteria
>
> R.T. *Gente… big, big… kisen… kitchen… comida…*
>
> Translation: People… big, big… kitchen… kitchen… food…
>
> R.T. *Day and night… trabajando… papel* ("writing" gesture)
>
> Translation: Day and night… working… Paper

Formal Assessment

Formal testing included the administration of available versions of the BDAE (Goodglass & Kaplan, 1974, 1983) in each language at the time. R.T. demonstrated an overall higher performance in comprehension tasks (Spanish [S]: 50–90%; English [E]: 30–70%) than in expression tasks (S: 40–70%; E: 30–50%) for both languages with a tendency to perform better in Spanish than in English. Similarly, for reading, she performed better in Spanish than in English (S: 50–90%; E: 40–60%). Writing was not assessed due to a right-sided hemiparesis. Test results are reported in percentages because BDAE norms for Venezuelan Spanish speakers were not available in the literature, and the BDAE, available in Argentinean Spanish (Goodglass & Kaplan, 1974), required dialectal adaptations into Venezuelan Spanish (e.g., bird: *gorrión* [Argentina]/*pájaro* [Venezuela]).

Treatment Procedures

R.T. was seen by the first author for speech therapy at her home 4 weeks after her cerebral damage. Sessions were administered twice a week for 3 months before the patient changed residence. Once the diagnostic profile was developed, this information and the treatment program were explained to the patient and her immediate family. Both parties were particularly keen in knowing about the nature and goals of therapy and what the prognosis was. Throughout the program, the family episodically required encouragement to patiently allow R.T. to communicate rather than "speaking for her." Overall, relatives at home were supportive of the therapy program, showing considerable willingness to help a family member.

Intervention specifically was designed based on the sociocultural and acquisitional factors, collected from the intake procedures, particularly the bilingualism questionnaire, as well as the informal and formal diagnostic results. The bilingualism history suggested a premorbid use of both Spanish and English with a tendency to use both languages at home and English at work. Informal and formal diagnostic results showed that this client had

(continues)

a parallel recovery pattern consisting of naming deficits and agrammatic utterances in both languages and the use of typical expressive features of bilingual discourse.

Hence, treatment, while acknowledging premorbid cultural and linguistic experiences, aimed to facilitate naming and utterance construction using a cognitive approach grounded in the client's routine language practices. Treatment was conducted in both languages using translation and language switching to both maintain the client's premorbid bilingual mode of communication at home and provide her with a self-help strategy that would allow her to switch languages when experiencing expressive difficulties in either language. Although sessions were alternatively conducted in either Spanish or English, R.T. was allowed to switch from one language to the other if she needed to do it, a strategy consistent with the facilitation of cognitive control in bilingual speakers with aphasia (Ansaldo & Marcotte, 2007). Target utterances (short sentences, including vocabulary and verbs from topics and stories familiar to R.T.: *My hija canta en la iglesia* "My daughter sings in church") were auditorily presented by the clinician in the language of the session accompanied by visual contexts (pictures or actual objects). R.T. was asked to repeat the sentence, and when experiencing difficulty, she could switch to the other language. In this manner, as mentioned, translation and switching, while similarly giving the patient a compensatory strategy to help herself during expressive blocks, stimulated the patient cognitively through control and attention to retrieve the target utterances (Ansaldo & Marcotte, 2007; Green, 2005; Green & Abutalebi, 2008).

The bilingual approach to therapy was supported by research evidence that cross-linguistic facilitation may occur between treated and untreated languages in bilingual aphasia therapy (Kohnert, 2009; Kohnert & Peterson, 2012). Thus, in this case, both languages were treated, which suggests greater cross-language reinforcement. Therapy similarly involved familiar experiential routines about home, family, and work associated with each language, as conceptual context for language stimuli (i.e., vocabulary and sentences) and conversation. This functional approach, often involving family members as interlocutors, is consistent with evidence on language-specific emotional–cognitive relationships (Altarriba, 2003; Marian & Kaushanskaya, 2004; Schrauf & Rubin, 2000, 2004) and motivation and affect being important facilitating factors in recall (Paradis, 2004).

The client showed improvement in both languages, although she relied on Spanish more frequently than English, consistent with her premorbid language dominance pattern. Her family reported that RT appeared to enjoy the sessions, as demonstrated by her eagerness to follow up on the home practice given to her by the clinician and to use the utterances targeted during the sessions with her friends and relatives. A systematic long-term follow-up of this client could unfortunately not be continued because she changed residence after 3 months of therapy. Informal observations collected during the sessions, including an increased ease to name items and produce short phrases in both languages, provided informal evidence supporting the therapeutic approach. It is possible that spontaneous recovery may have also contributed to the patient's progress because intervention occurred during the patient's acute aphasia stage (Gil & Goral, 2004; Kohnert, 2009). Similar informal approaches, however, involving weekly clinical observations during treatment, have been useful to speech–language clinicians working in neurorehabilitation to monitor language changes and progress in bilingual individuals receiving aphasia therapy (Holland & Penn, 1995).

STUDY QUESTIONS

1. Explain how individual acculturation, bilingual/multilingual acquisition, and cognitive strategies before the cerebral damage can have an impact on aphasia testing and therapy with each bilingual/multilingual client.

2. Discuss the possible language recovery patterns in bilingual speakers with aphasia and the possible neurological and neurocognitive reasons for their occurrence.

3. Describe the aphasia assessment protocol that you would implement with a 35-year-old trilingual patient who has been living in Montreal, Canada, a bilingual French–English environment, for 6 years. This person, who did not know French or English, came from Portugal, where she only spoke Portuguese.

4. Describe the intervention protocol that you would employ if the evaluation in question 3 resulted in a diagnosis of nonparallel language recovery with Portuguese as the recovered language and Broca's aphasia.

REFERENCES

Abutalebi, J., Annoni, J. M., Zimine, I., Pegna, A.J., Seghier, M.L., Lee-Jahnke, H., et al. (2007). Language control and lexical competition in bilinguals: An event-related FMRI study. *Cerebral Cortex, 18*, 1496–1505.

Abutalebi, J., Cappa, S. F., & Perani, D. (2005). What can functional neuroimaging tell us about the bilingual brain. In J. F. Kroll & A. M. B. de Groot (Eds.), *Handbook of bilingualism: Psycholinguistic approaches* (pp. 497–515). New York, NY: Oxford University Press.

Abutalebi, J., Della Rosa, P. A., Tettamanti, M., Green, D. W., & Cappa, S. F. (2009). Bilingual aphasia and language control: A follow-up FMRI and intrinsic connectivity study. *Brain and Language, 109*, 141–156.

Abutalebi, J., & Green, D. W. (2007). Bilingual language production: The neurocognition of language representation and control. *Journal of Neurolinguistics, 20*, 242–275.

Albert, M., & Obler, L. K. (1978). *The bilingual brain*. New York, NY: Academic Press.

Altarriba, J. (2003). Does *cariño* equal liking? A theoretical approach to conceptual nonequivalence between languages. *International Journal of Bilingualism, 3*, 305–322.

American Speech-Language-Hearing Association. (2015). Collaborating with interpreters. Retrieved May 5, 2015, from http://www.asha.org/Practice-Portal/Professional-Issues/Collaborating-With-Interpreters/#_ga = 1.196149612.1729696513.1430845945

Ansaldo, A. I., Ghazi-Saidi, L., & Ruiz, A. (2010). Model-driven intervention in bilingual aphasia: Evidence from a case of pathological language mixing. *Aphasiology, 24*, 309–324.

Ansaldo, A. I., & Marcotte, K. (2007). Language switching in the context of Spanish-English bilingual aphasia. In J. G. Centeno, R. T. Anderson, & L. K. Obler (Eds.), *Communication disorders in Spanish speakers: Theoretical, research, and clinical aspects* (pp. 214–230). Clevedon, UK: Multilingual Matters.

Ansaldo, A. I., Marcotte, K., Scherer, L., & Raboyeau, G. (2008). Language therapy and bilingual aphasia: Clinical implications of psycholinguistic and neuroimaging research. *Journal of Neurolinguistics, 21*, 539–557.

Ansaldo, A. I., & Ghazi-Saidi, L. G. (2014). Aphasia therapy in the age of globalization: Cross-linguistic therapy effects in bilingual aphasia. *Behavioural Neurology, 2014*, Article ID 603085. Retrieved from http://dx.doi.org/10.1155/2014/603085

Appel, R., & Muysken, P. (1987). *Language contact and bilingualism*. London, UK: Arnold.

Baddeley, A., Eysenck, M. W., & Anderson, M. C. (2009). *Memory*. New York, NY: Psychology Press.

Benton, A. L., Hamsher, K., & Sivan, A. B. (1994). *Multilingual aphasia examination* (3rd ed.). Lutz, FL: Psychological Assessment Resources.

Bialystok, E. (2001). *Bilingualism in development: Language, literacy, and cognition*. Cambridge, UK: Cambridge University Press.

Brozgold, A., & Centeno, J. G. (2007). Sociocultural, societal, and psychological aspects of bilingualism: Variables, interactions, and therapeutic implications in speech-language pathology. In J. G. Centeno, R. T. Anderson, & L. K. Obler (Eds.), *Communication disorders in Spanish speakers: Theoretical, research, and clinical aspects* (pp. 67–81). Clevedon, UK: Multilingual Matters.

Buchweitz, A., & Prat, C. (2013). The bilingual brain: Flexibility and control in the human cortex. *Physics of Life Reviews, 10*, 428–443.

Byng, S., Parr, S., & Cairns, D. (2003). The science or sciences of aphasia? In I. Papathanasiou & R. De Bleser (Eds.), *The sciences of aphasia: From therapy to theory* (pp. 201–224). Oxford, UK: Pergamon.

Centeno, J. G. (2007a). Bilingual development and communication: Dynamics and implications in clinical language studies. In J. G. Centeno, R. T. Anderson., & L.K. Obler (Eds.), *Communication disorders in Spanish speakers: Theoretical, research, and clinical aspects* (pp. 46–56). Clevedon, UK: Multilingual Matters.

Centeno, J. G. (2007b). Canonical features in the inflectional morphology of Spanish-speaking individuals with agrammatic speech. *International Journal of Speech-Language Pathology, 9*, 162–172.

Centeno, J. G. (2007c). Considerations for an ethnopsycholinguistic framework for aphasia intervention. In A. Ardila & E. Ramos (Eds.), *Speech and language disorders in bilinguals* (pp. 213–234). New York, NY: Nova Science.

Centeno, J. G. (2007d). From theory to realistic praxis: Service-learning as a teaching method to enhance speech-language pathology services with minority populations. In A. J. Wurr & J. Hellebrandt (Eds.), *Learning the language of global citizenship: Service-learning in applied linguistics* (pp. 190–217). Bolton, MA: Anker.

Centeno, J. G. (2008, October). Multidisciplinary evidence to treat bilingual individuals with aphasia. *Perspectives on Communication Disorders and Sciences in Culturally and Linguistically Diverse Populations, 15*, 66–72.

Centeno, J. G. (2009). Serving bilingual patients with aphasia: Challenges, foundations, and procedures. *Revista de Logopedia, Foniatria, y Audiologia, 29*, 30–36.

Centeno, J. G. (2010a). Neurolinguistic and neurocognitive considerations of language processing in adult bilinguals. In J. Guendozi, F. Loncke, & M. J. Williams (Eds.), *The handbook of psycholinguistic and cognitive processes: Perspectives in communication disorders* (pp. 645–662). Oxford, UK: Taylor and Francis.

Centeno, J. G. (October, 2010b). The relevance of bilingualism questionnaires in the personalized treatment of bilinguals with aphasia. *Perspectives on Communication Disorders and Sciences in Culturally and Linguistically Diverse Populations, 17*, 65–73.

Centeno, J. G. (2012). Morphosyntactic features in the spoken language of Spanish-English bilinguals with aphasia. In M. Gitterman, M. Goral, & L. K. Obler (Eds.), *Aspects of multilingual aphasia* (pp. 207–223). Clevedon, UK: Multilingual Matters.

Centeno, J. G. (2015). Assessing services with communicatively-impaired bilingual adults in culturally and linguistically diverse neurorehabilitation programs. *Journal of Communication Disorders, 58*, 58-73.

Centeno, J. G., & Cairns, H. S. (2010). Frequency effects on verb inflection use by Spanish-speaking agrammatic individuals: Theoretical and clinical implications. *International Journal of Speech-Language Pathology, 12*, 35–46.

Centeno, J. G., & Gingerich, W. (2007). Ethical and methodological considerations in clinical communication research with

Hispanic populations. In J. G. Centeno, R. T. Anderson, & L. K. Obler (Eds.), *Communication disorders in Spanish speakers: Theoretical, research, and clinical aspects* (pp. 99–112). Clevedon, UK: Multilingual Matters.

Centeno, J. G., & Obler, L. K. (2001). Agrammatic verb errors in Spanish speakers and their normal discourse correlates. *Journal of Neurolinguistics, 14*, 349–363.

Chlenov, L. G. (1948). On aphasia in polyglots. In M. Paradis (Ed), *Readings on aphasia in bilinguals and polyglots* (pp. 445–543). Montreal, Canada: Didier.

Code, C. (2001). Multifactorial processes in recovery from aphasia: Developing the foundations for a multilevel framework. *Brain and Language, 77*, 25–44.

Cuetos, F., & Centeno, J. G. (2009). Applying cognitive neuropsychological principles to the rehabilitation of Spanish readers with acquired dyslexia. *Seminars in Speech and Language, 30*, 187–198.

Dodel, S., Golestani, N., Pallier, C., ElKouby, V., Le Bihan, D., & Poline, J. B. (2005). Condition-dependent functional connectivity: Syntax networks in bilinguals. *Philosophical Transactions of the Royal Society B: Biological Sciences, 360*, 921–935.

Edmonds, L., & Kiran, S. (2006). Effect of semantic naming treatment on crosslinguistic generalization in bilingual aphasia. *Journal of Speech, Language, and Hearing Research, 49*, 729–748.

Ethnologue. (2015). *Statistical summaries.* Retrieved March 26, 2015, from https://www.ethnologue.com/statistics.

European Commission. (2015). *Number of foreign languages known (self-reported) by age 2014.* Retrieved March 26, 2015, from http://ec.europa.eu/eurostat/web/products-datasets/-/edat_aes_l22.

Fabbro, F. (1999). *The neurolinguistics of bilingualism: An introduction.* East Sussex, UK: Psychology Press.

Faroqi-Shah, Y., Frymark, T., Mullen, R., & Wang, B. (2010). Effect of treatment for bilingual individuals with aphasia: A systematic review of the evidence. *Journal of Neurolinguistics, 23*, 319–341.

Ghazi-Saidi, L., Perlbarg, V., Marrelec, G., Pélégrini-Issac, M., Benali, H., & Ansaldo, A. I. (2013). Functional connectivity changes in second language vocabulary learning. *Brain and language, 124*, 56–65.

Gil, M., & Goral, M. (2004). Nonparallel recovery in bilingual aphasia: Effects of language choice, language proficiency, and treatment. *International Journal of Bilingualism, 8*, 191–219.

Goodglass, H., & Kaplan, E. (1974). *Evaluación de la afasia y de trastornos similares.* Buenos Aires, Argentina: Editorial Médica Panamericana.

Goodglass, H., & Kaplan, E. (1983). *The assessment of aphasia and related disorders.* Philadelphia, PA: Lea and Fabiger.

Goodglass, H., & Kaplan, E. (2005). *Evaluación de la afasia y trastornos relacionados* (3rd ed.). Madrid, Spain: Médica Panamericana.

Goodglass, H., Kaplan, E., & Barresi, B. (2001). *Boston Diagnostic Aphasia Examination* (3rd ed.). Philadelphia, PA: Lippincott Williams and Wilkins.

Gonzalez-Rothi, L., & Barrett, A. M. (2006). The changing view of neurorehabilitation: A new era of optimism. *Journal of the International Neuropsychological Society, 12*, 812–815.

Goral, M., Levy, E. S., & Kastl, R. (2010). Cross-language treatment generalisation: A case of trilingual aphasia. *Aphasiology, 24*(2), 170-187.

Goral, M., Levy, E., & Obler, L. K. (2002). Neurolinguistic aspects of bilingualism. *International Journal of Bilingualism, 6*, 411–440.

Goral, M., Rosas, J., Conner, P. S., Maul, K. K., & Obler, L. K. (2012). Effects of language proficiency and language of the environment on aphasia therapy in a multilingual. *Journal of Neurolinguistics, 25*, 538–551.

Green, D. (2005). The neurocognition of recovery patterns in bilingual aphasics. In J. F. Kroll & A. M. B. de Groot (Eds.), *Handbook of bilingualism: Psycholinguistic approaches* (pp. 516–530). New York, NY: Oxford University Press.

Green, D., & Abutalebi, J. (2008). Understanding the link between bilingual aphasia and language control. *Journal of Neurolinguistics, 21*, 558–576.

Grosjean, F. (1982). *Life with two languages: An introduction to bilingualism.* Cambridge, MA: Harvard University.

Hamers, J. F., & Blanc, M. H. A. (2000). *Bilinguality and bilingualism* (2nd ed.). Cambridge, UK: Cambridge University.

Harley, T. A. (2008). *The psychology of language: From data to theory* (3rd ed.). East Sussex, UK: Psychology Press.

Hernández, A., Dapretto, M., Mazziotta, J., & Bookheimer, S. (2001). Language switching and language representation in Spanish-English bilinguals: An fMRI study. *Neuroimage, 14*, 510–520.

Hillis, A. E., & Newhart, M. (2008). Cognitive neuropsychological approaches to treatment of language disorders: Introduction. In R. Chapey (Ed.), *Language intervention strategies in aphasia and related neurogenic communication disorders* (5th ed., pp. 595–604). Philadelphia, PA: Lippincott Williams and Wilkins.

Holland, A., & Penn, C. (1995). Inventing therapy for aphasia. In L. Menn, M. O'Connor, L. K. Obler, & A. Holland (Eds.), *Non-fluent aphasia in a multilingual world* (pp. 144–155). Amsterdam, the Netherlands: Benjamins.

Huber, W., Poeck, K., & Willmes, K. (1984). The Aachen aphasia test. *Advances in Neurology, 42*, 291–303.

Hull, R., & Vaid, J. (2005). Clearing the cobwebs from the study of the bilingual brain: Converging evidence from laterality and electrophysiological research. In J. F. Kroll & A. M. B. de Groot (Eds.), *Handbook of bilingualism: Psycholinguistic approaches* (pp. 480–496). New York, NY: Oxford University Press.

Institute of Medicine. (2002). *What healthcare providers need to know about racial and ethnic disparities in healthcare.* Retrieved April 8, 2006, from http://www.iom.edu.

Isaac, K. M. (2005). Managing linguistic diversity in the clinic: Interpreters in speech-language pathology. In M. J. Ball (Ed.), *Clinical sociolinguistics* (pp. 265–280). Malden, MA: Blackwell.

Juncos-Rabadán, O. (1994). The assessment of bilingualism in normal aging with the Bilingual Aplasia Test. *Journal of Neurolinguistics, 8*, 67–73.

Kay, J., Lesser, R., & Coltheart, M. (1992). *PALPA: Psycholinguistic assessments of language processing in aphasia.* Hove, UK: Erlbaum.

Kennedy, M., & Chiou, H.-H. (2005, June). Assessment tools for adolescents and adults in languages other than English. *Perspectives on Neurophysiology and Neurogenic Speech and Language Disorders, 15*, 20–23.

Kiran, S., & Roberts, P. (2012). What do we know about assessing language impairment in bilingual aphasia? In M. Gitterman, M. Goral, & L. K. Obler (Eds.), *Aspects of multilingual aphasia* (pp. 35–50). Clevedon, UK: Multilingual Matters.

Kohnert, K. (2008). *Language disorders in bilingual children and adults.* San Diego, CA: Plural.

Kohnert, K. (2009). Cross-language generalization following treatment in bilingual speakers with aphasia: A review. *Seminars in Speech and Languag, 30*, 174–186.

Kohnert, K., & Peterson, M. (2012). Generalization in bilingual aphasia treatment. In M. Gitterman, M. Goral, & L. K. Obler, (Eds.), *Aspects of multilingual aphasia* (pp. 207–223). Clevedon, UK: Multilingual Matters.

Kong, A. P. H., Abutalebi, J., Lam, K. S. Y., & Weekes, B. (2014). Executive and language control in the multilingual brain. *Behavioural neurology, 2014*, Article ID 527951. Retrieved from http://dx.doi.org/10.1155/2014/527951

Life Participation Approach to Aphasia Project Group. (2008). Life participation approach to aphasia: A statement of values for the future. In R. Chapey (Ed.), *Language intervention strategies in adult aphasia* (5th ed., pp. 279–289). Baltimore, MD: Lippincott, Williams and Wilkins.

Manuel-Dupont, S., Ardila, A., Rosselli, M., & Puente, A. E. (1992). Bilingualism. In A. E. Puente & R. J. McCaffrey (Eds.), *Handbook of neuropsychological assessment: A biopsychosocial perspective* (pp. 193–210). New York, NY: Plenum Press.

Marcotte, K., & Ansaldo, A. I. (2010). The neural correlates of semantic feature analysis in chronic aphasia: Discordant patterns according to etiology. *Seminars in Speech and Language, 31*, 52–63.

Marian, V., Blumenfeld, H. K., & Kaushanskaya, M. (2007). The language experience and proficiency questionnaire (LEAP-Q): Assessing language profiles in bilinguals and multilinguals. *Journal of Speech, Language, and Hearing Research, 50*, 940–967.

Marian, V., & Kaushanskaya, M. (2004). Self-construal and emotion in bicultural bilinguals. *Journal of Memory and Language, 51*, 190–201.

Marín, G., Organista, P. B., & Chun, R. M. (2003). Acculturation research: current issues and findings. In G. Bernal, J. E. Trimble, A. K. Burlew, & F. T. L. Leong (Eds.), *Handbook of racial and ethnic minority psychology* (pp. 208–219). Thousand Oaks, CA: Sage.

Martinovic, I., & Altarriba, J. (2013). Bilingualism and emotion: Implications for mental health. In T. K. Bhatia & W. C. Ritchie (Eds.), *The handbook of bilingualism and multilingualism* (pp. 292–320). Malden, MA: Blackwell.

Meinzer, M., Obleser, J., Flaisch, T., Eulitz, T., & Rockstroh, B. (2007). Recovery from aphasia as a function of language therapy in an early bilingual patient demonstrated by fMRI. *Neuropsychologia, 45*, 1247–1256.

Menn, L., & Obler, L. K. (Eds.) (1990). *Agrammatic aphasia: A cross-language narrative sourcebook* (Vols. 1–3). Amsterdam, the Netherlands: Benjamins.

Menn, L., O'Connor, M., Obler, L. K., & Holland, A. (Eds.). (1995). *Non-fluent aphasia in a multilingual world*. Amsterdam, the Netherlands: Benjamins.

Müller, N., & Guendouzi, J. A. (2009). Discourses of dementia: A call for an ethnographic, action research approach to care in linguistically and culturally diverse environments. *Seminars in Speech and Language, 30*, 198–206.

Muñoz, M. L., & Marquardt, T. P. (2008). The performance of neurologically normal bilingual speakers of Spanish and English on the short version of the Bilingual Aphasia Test. *Aphasiology, 22*, 3–19.

Muñoz, M. L., Marquardt, T. P., & Copeland, G. (1999). A comparison of the codeswitching patterns of aphasic and neurologically normal bilingual speakers of English and Spanish. *Brain and Language, 66*, 249–274.

Myers, H. F., Lewis, T. T., & Parker-Dominguez, T. (2003). Stress, coping, and minority health. In G. Bernal, J. E. Trimble, A. K. Burlew, & F. T. L. Leong (Eds.), *Handbook of racial and ethnic minority psychology* (pp. 377–400). Thousand Oaks, CA: Sage.

Ostrosky-Solís, F., Lozano, A., Ramírez, M. J., & Ardila, A. (2007). Neuropsychological profiles of adult illiterates and the development and application of a neuropsychological program for learning to read. In J. G. Centeno, R. T. Anderson, & L. K. Obler (Eds.), *Communication disorders in Spanish speakers: Theoretical, research, and clinical aspects* (pp. 256–275). Clevedon, UK: Multilingual Matters.

Paradis, M. (1987). *The assessment of bilingual aphasia*. Hillsdale, NJ: Erlbaum.

Paradis, M. (2001). By the way of preface: The need for awareness of aphasia symptoms in different languages. In M. Paradis (Ed.), *Manifestations of aphasic symptoms in different languages* (pp. 1–7). Amsterdam, the Netherlands: Pergamon Press.

Paradis, M. (2004). *A neurolinguistic theory of bilingualism*. Amsterdam, the Netherlands: Benjamins.

Paradis, M. (2008). Language and communication disorders in multilinguals. In B. Stemmer & H. A. Whitaker (Eds.), *The handbook of the neuroscience of language* (pp. 341–349). Amsterdam, the Netherlands: Academic Press.

Paradis, M. (2010). *The bilingual aphasia test—Online resources*. Retrieved April 17, 2010, from http://www.mcgill.ca/linguistics/research/bat/

Pavlenko, A. (2005). Bilingualism and thought. In J. F. Kroll & A. M. B. de Groot (Eds.), *Handbook of bilingualism: Psycholinguistic approaches* (pp. 433–453). New York, NY: Oxford University Press.

Pavlenko, A. (2006). Bilingual selves. In A. Pavlenko (Ed.), *Bilingual minds: Emotional experience, expression, and representation* (pp. 1–33). Clevedon, UK: Multilingual Matters.

Penn, C. (2012). Towards cultural aphasiology: Contextual models of service delivery in aphasia. In M. Gitterman, M. Goral, & L. K. Obler (Eds.), *Aspects of multilingual aphasia* (pp. 292–306). Clevedon, UK: Multilingual Matters.

Phinney, J. S. (2003). Ethnic identity and acculturation. In K. M. Chun, P. B. Organista, and G. Marín (Eds.), *Acculturation: Advances in theory, measurement, and applied research* (pp. 63–82). Washington, DC: American Psychological Association.

Pietrosemoli, L. G. (2007). Cohesion in the conversational samples of the conversational samples of Broca's aphasic individuals: Theoretical and clinical implications. In J. G. Centeno, R. T. Anderson., & L. K. Obler (Eds.), *Communication disorders in Spanish speakers: Theoretical, research, and clinical aspects* (pp. 198–213). Clevedon, UK: Multilingual Matters.

Raboyeau, G., De Boissezon, X., Marie, N., Balduyck, S., Puel, M., Bézy, C., et al. (2008). Right hemisphere activation in recovery from aphasia: Lesion effect or function recruitment? *Neurology, 70*, 290–298.

Rapp, B. (2005). The relationship between treatment outcomes and the underlying cognitive deficit: Evidence from the remediation of acquired dysgraphia. In J. Stark, N. Martin, & R. B. Fink (Eds.), *Aphasia therapy workshop: Current approaches to aphasia therapy—Principles and applications* (pp. 994–1008). Hove, UK: Psychology Press.

Raymer, A. M., Beeson, P., Holland, A., Kendall, D., Maher, L., Martin, N., et al. (2008). Translational research in aphasia: From neuroscience to neurorehabilitation. *Journal of Speech, Language, and Hearing Research, 51*, S259–S275.

Rey, G. J., Sivan, A. B., & Benton, A. L. (1991). *Multilingual aphasia examination-Spanish*. Lutz, FL: Psychological Assessment Resources.

Roberts, P. M. (2008). Issues in assessment and treatment for bilingual and culturally diverse clients. In R. Chapey (Ed.), *Language intervention strategies in aphasia and related neurogenic communication disorders* (5th ed., pp. 245–275). Baltimore, MD: Lippincott, Williams and Wilkins.

Rodriguez-Fornells, A., Rotte, M., Heinze, H. J., Nösselt, T., & Münte, T. F. (2002). Brain potential and functional MRI evidence for how to handle two languages with one brain. *Nature, 415*, 1026–1029.

Ryan, C. (2013). Language use in the United States: 2011. *US American Community Survey Reports, ACS-22*. Washington, DC: US Census Bureau.

Ghazi-Saidi, L., Perlbarg, V., Marrelec, G., Pélégrini-Issac, M., Benali, H., & Ansaldo, A. I. (2013). Functional connectivity changes in second language vocabulary learning. *Brain and language, 124*, 56–65.

Salas-Provance, M. B., Erickson, J. G., & Reed, J. (2002). Disabilities as viewed by four generations of one Hispanic family. *American Journal of Speech-Language Pathology, 11*, 151–162.

Schrauf, R. W., & Rubin, D. C. (2000). Internal languages of retrieval: The bilingual encoding of memories for the personal past. *Memory and Cognition, 28*, 616–623.

Schrauf, R. W., & Rubin, D. C. (2004). The "language" and "feel" of bilingual memory: Mnemonic traces. *Estudios de Sociolingüística, 5*, 21–40.

Statistics Canada. (2015a). *2011 National Household Survey: Immigration, place of birth, citizenship, ethnic origin, visible minorities, language and religion*. Retrieved March 29, 2015, from http://www.statcan.gc.ca/daily-quotidien/130508/dq130508b-eng.htm

Statistics Canada. (2015b). *Study: The evolution of English-French bilingualism in Canada from 1961 to 2011*. Retrieved March 29, 2015, from http://www.statcan.gc.ca/daily-quotidien/130528/dq130528b-eng.htm

Thompson, C. K. (2000). Neuroplasticity: Evidence from aphasia. *Journal of Communication Disorders, 33*, 357–366.

Tonkovich, J. D. (2002). Multicultural issues in the management of neurogenic communication and swallowing disorders. In D. E. Battle (Ed.), *Communication disorders in multicultural populations* (3rd ed., pp. 233–265). Boston, MA: Butterworth-Heinemann

Torres, L. (1997). *Puerto Rican discourse: A sociolinguistic study of a New York suburb*. Mahwah, NJ: Erlbaum.

US Census Bureau. (2012). *US census projections show a slower growing, older, more diverse nation a half century from now* (US Census Bureau News, Report CB12-243). Washington, DC: Author.

US Census Bureau. (2014). *Annual estimates of the resident population by sex, race, and Hispanic origins for the United States, states, and counties: April 1, 2010 to July 1, 2013*. Washington, DC: Author.

US Department of Health and Human Services. (2015). *National standards for cultural and linguistically appropriate services (CLAS) in health and health care*. Retrieved March 24, 2015, from https://www.thinkculturalhealth.hhs.gov/index.asp

Vaid, J. (2008). The bilingual brain: What is right and what is left? In J. Altarriba & R. R. Heredia (Eds.), *An introduction to bilingualism: Principles and processes* (pp. 129–146). New York, NY: Erlbaum.

Valle, F., & Cuetos, F. (1995). *EPLA: Evaluación del procesamiento lingüístico en la afasia*. Hove, UK: Erlbaum.

Wald, I. (1958). Zagadnienie afazji poliglotow. *Postepy Neurologii, Neurochirurgii i Psychiatrii, 4*, 183–211.

Wald, I. (1961). Problema afazii poliglotov. *Voprosy Kliniki I Patofiziologii Afazi, Moskva*, 140–176

Walters, J. (2005). *Bilingualism: The sociopragmatic-psycholinguistic interface*. Mahwah, NJ: Erlbaum.

World Atlas. (2015). *Countries of the world*. Retrieved March 26, 2015, from http://www.worldatlas.com/aatlas/populations/ctypopls.htm

World Health Organization. (2001). *International classification of functioning, disability, and health, ICF*. Geneva, Switzerland: Author.

Zentella, A. C. (1997). Spanish in New York. In O. Garcia and J. Fishman (Eds.), *The multilingual apple: Languages in New York City*. Berlin, Germany: Mouton de Gruyter.

Zunker, C. L., & Cummins, J. L. (2004). Elderly health disparities on the US-Mexico border. *Journal of Cross-Cultural Gerontology, 19*, 13–25.

RELATED COMMUNICATION DISORDERS

OBJECTIVES

The reader will be able to:

1. Define coarse semantic coding and identify two communicative forms or functions it may underlie.

2. Define suppression and identify two communicative forms or functions it may underlie.

3. Compare and contrast the coarse coding and suppression deficit hypotheses of right hemisphere disorder (RHD) cognitive–communicative disorders.

4. List two pieces of evidence consistent with the cognitive resources hypothesis of RHD cognitive–communicative disorders.

5. Describe the social cognition hypothesis of RHD cognitive–communicative disorders.

6. Identify three communicative deficits and three cognitive deficits that may typify RHD as specifically as possible (e.g., not just "figurative language" or "reading" or "attention" without further differentiation).

7. Compare and contrast viewer-centered, stimulus-centered, and object-centered neglect.

8. Compare and contrast the medical model with the International Classification of Functioning, Disability, and Health (ICF) model and the applied cognitive rehabilitation model for assessment and treatment.

9. Define the discrepancy between *knowing* (or *saying*) and *doing* that may characterize performance by adults with RHD, relate this distinction to two memory systems, and illustrate the distinction with examples of performance.

Nature and Assessment of Right Hemisphere Disorders

Connie A. Tompkins, Ekaterini Klepousniotou, and April G. Scott

INTRODUCTION

The focus of this chapter is the cognitive–communicative consequences of relatively focal damage to the right cerebral hemisphere, typically resulting from unilateral stroke, and the assessment of resulting disorders. It is generally accepted that people who have these disorders do not have aphasia, but the research in this area is so new that no specific communicative label or definition has been accepted. Typically, it is agreed that these disorders are not caused by sensory or motor (e.g., dysarthria) deficits or by cognitively deteriorating conditions.

Space limitations preclude us from providing original citations for much of the evidence that underpins our descriptions, recommendations, and conclusions. As a result, we often direct the reader to relevant reviews or summary sources.

THEORETICAL ACCOUNTS OF COGNITIVE–COMMUNICATION DEFICITS IN RIGHT HEMISPHERE DISORDERS

This section briefly addresses four influential accounts of performance in right hemisphere disorders (RHDs) as they relate to facets of normal right hemisphere (RH) processing. Further sections allude to other accounts of specific RHD deficits, but for the most part, theorizing about RHD communication and cognition remains in its infancy.

The Coarse Coding Deficit Hypothesis

Evidence suggests that there are cerebral hemispheric differences in how semantic representations of words are automatically accessed and in how word meanings are selected and suppressed. According to the leading view (e.g., Beeman, 1998; Jung-Beeman, 2005), the left hemisphere (LH) engages in fine semantic coding by strongly activating a small semantic field for an encountered word and rapidly inhibiting all but a limited subset of features that are related to the dominant or contextually appropriate meaning of that word (e.g., *round, red* as features of the word *apple*). By contrast, the RH is proposed to coarsely code information conveyed by lexical items, diffusely activating large semantic fields and maintaining activation for more distant meanings and features, regardless of their congruity with the linguistic context (e.g., *rotten* as a feature of *apple*). This RH maintenance function is presumed to support a revision process when selected interpretation is incorrect. An updated view of the fine–coarse coding hypothesis, namely, the bilateral activation, inhibition, and selection (BAIS) model, proposes bilateral roles for semantic integration and selection as well (Jung-Beeman, 2005). Coarse and fine semantic coding, engaging the RH and LH, respectively, occur in parallel and interact at every stage of processing (Jung-Beeman, 2005).

Coarse semantic activation and maintenance are hypothesized to make the RH sensitive to semantic overlap between words. Although evidence is mixed, it suggests that the RH may be specialized for making novel semantic connections (e.g., Mashal, Faust, Hendler, & Jung-Beeman, 2007) that aid the processing of unfamiliar sentences or that the RH may support additional processing required to make sense of distant semantic relations. These processes are posited to be important for some kinds of inferencing and nonliteral language interpretation.

Adults with RHD have been proposed to have a deficit in coarse semantic activation (e.g., Beeman, 1998). This hypothesis has two rationales. The first is a common, yet simplified, assumption: Damage in one brain hemisphere eliminates that hemisphere's processing contributions and causes overreliance on processes associated with the other hemisphere. Second, adults with RHD can have difficulties in the aspects of normal language comprehension that coarse coding is posited to underpin.

Three studies investigating the processing of particularly distant meanings or features of words (Grindrod, 2012; Klepousniotou & Baum, 2005; Tompkins, Fassbinder, Scharp, & Meigh, 2008) have reported evidence consistent with coarse coding deficits in adults with RHD. One study found that comprehension of implied information in narratives was poorer for adults with RHD with the clearest coarse coding deficit than for other adults with RHD, even after controlling for vocabulary knowledge and working memory capacity for language (WMCL; Tompkins, Scharp, Meigh, & Fassbinder, 2008). These subgroups of adults with RHD did not differ in comprehension of explicitly stated information. It should be noted that group average findings of coarse coding deficit do not characterize all individuals with RHD; indeed, many do not have coarse coding deficits (Scharp, Tompkins, & Blake, 2014). A voxelwise analysis of lesions in adults with RHD diagnosed with coarse coding deficit (Yang, Tompkins, Meigh, & Prat, in review) implicated posterior middle temporal gyrus, dorsolateral prefontal cortex (DLPFC), and lenticular nuclei in impairment of coarse semantic activation. Deficits in the maintenance of coarsely activated representations were associated with lesions in the temporal pole and DLPFC more medially.

The Suppression Deficit Hypothesis

Communication is filled with ambiguity. People regularly use polite, indirect forms to make requests; humor and jokes often hinge on secondary or unexpected meanings or features of a word or phrase; listeners frequently have to revise an initial inference. In normal comprehension, it is common to mentally activate multiple meanings of words and phrases, often without awareness or intention. Influential models of comprehension include a mechanism to attenuate activation for such information when it becomes superfluous or misleading and when it is inconsistent with a final interpretation of what someone or something means (see summary in Tompkins, 2008). Gernsbacher (1990) dubs this the suppression mechanism. Both brain hemispheres appear to participate in the suppression of contextually incompatible forms of homophones, whereas the LH may be more involved in suppressing irrelevant meanings of homographs (Faust & Gernsbacher, 1996).

Tompkins and colleagues have proposed and documented the suppression deficit hypothesis (for review, see Tompkins, 2008). They find that some adults with RHD activate multiple interpretations for ambiguous words, sentences, and phrases and demonstrate that reconciliation of competing activations is hampered by ineffective suppression. Tompkins's group and others (e.g., Klepousniotou & Baum, 2005) have documented ineffective suppression in several contexts for adults with RHD, many of whom sustain for too long the mental activation of contextually inappropriate meanings. In addition, several studies by these investigators (e.g., Tompkins, Fassbinder, Lehman-Blake, Baumgaertner, & Jayaram,

2004) demonstrate that the degree of ineffective suppression predicts general narrative comprehension by adults with RHD, even after controlling for vocabulary knowledge, working memory capacity, and age. These investigators argue that suppression deficit could account for difficulties in many language and cognitive tasks that support or induce competing interpretations.

Again, a group average finding of suppression deficit does not mean that every adult with RHD will have it (e.g., Scharp et al., 2014). A voxelwise analysis of RH lesions associated with suppression deficit (Yang et al., in press) implicated the inferior frontal gyrus and connected subcortical regions, as well as RH temporal pole.

Coarse coding and suppression act as complementary facets of normal comprehension. In an initial phase of comprehension, coarse coding activates semantically distant word meanings and features that may be less likely in the broader context (e.g., *rotten* as a feature of *apple* in the sentence "The apples were perfect for eating"). Suppression occurs after the broader context is taken into account and prunes irrelevances to shape a final interpretation. Suppression acts on even semantically near features and meanings if they become inappropriate in the broader context.

Although the suppression deficit and coarse coding deficit hypotheses have often been cast as competitors, they are not mutually exclusive. In addition to being associated with different RH lesion complexes (Yang et al., in press), the two deficits can co-occur in adults with RHD (for a review, see Tompkins, Lei, & Zezinka, 2015). Results interpreted in light of a suppression deficit (e.g., Forgács et al., 2012; Lovseth & Atchley, 2010) can also be interpreted in light of the revised BAIS model of the coarse semantic coding hypothesis (Jung-Beeman, 2005). A suppression deficit can lead to prolonged activation of contextually incompatible word meanings or features at any point along the semantic distance continuum, while a coarse coding deficit may affect only the most distant aspects of meaning.

The Cognitive Resources Hypothesis

Prior to their research on suppression, Tompkins's group pinpointed attentional processing demands and limits on attentional capacity or its allocation as key factors in the comprehension difficulties of adults with RHD. A series of studies documents that deficits of adults with RHD are not absolute in comprehension domains that are typically considered problematic (e.g., lexical metaphor, phrasal idiom, affect, emotional prosody, inference, inference revision, and activating subordinate and alternative meanings of words, phrases, and prosodic contours). "Typical" RHD deficits

are evident when tasks place relatively high demands on attentional resources but are minimized or absent under less demanding test conditions (see summaries in Tompkins, 1995; Tompkins et al., 2015). Inference revision performance of adults with RHD in demanding discourse conditions also is predicted by their estimated WMCL (Tompkins, Bloise, Timko, & Baumgaertner, 1994). The WMCL is an index of the ability to perform simultaneous language processing and storage operations. A "cognitive resources" hypothesis has been further substantiated by Joanette's group (e.g., Joanette & Goulet, 1998; Monetta & Joanette, 2003). The imprecision of this type of account, however, led us to examine suppression as a more specific mechanism underlying RHD discourse comprehension deficits. Suppression consumes processing capacity for adults with RHD and without brain damage (Tompkins, Lehman-Blake, Baumgaertner, & Fassbinder, 2002).

A number of neuroimaging studies suggest that the RH assists the LH in language computations by providing additional cognitive resource capacity when that of the LH is exceeded (e.g., Just, Carpenter, Keller, Eddy, & Thulborn, 2006). Involvement of the RH in language processing seems to increase with the complexity of the linguistic stimuli, being least involved at the lexical level and maximally involved in narrative discourse (e.g., Kuperberg, Lakshmanan, Caplan, & Holcomb, 2006; Xu, Kemeny, Park, Frattali, & Braun, 2005).

The Social Cognition Deficits Hypothesis

One account of RHD cognitive–communication deficits invokes social cognition (e.g., Brownell & Martino, 1998), including the ability to use appropriate politeness conventions and information about interpersonal relationships and to reason using a mental mechanism termed *theory of mind* (ToM; e.g., Happé, Brownell, & Winner, 1999). ToM allows people to understand and interpret their own and other people's mental states and hence to predict and explain their behavior. The RH may be critical for social cognition, more broadly defined as the ability to perceive, interpret, and provide an adequate response to affective and other interpersonal cues. According to the social cognition account, RHD can reduce the ability to engage in competent social relations and understand social information, and patients may become indifferent. These changes lead to impaired social judgments, reduced affect and goal-directed behavior, and self-monitoring deficits that also influence language performance.

Reasoning based on ToM requires the mental activation of multiple perspectives that eventually have to be reconciled. Thus, Tompkins's group (e.g., Tompkins, Baumgaertner, Lehman, & Fassbinder, 2000) suggested that difficulties could result in part from suppression deficits. More recently, Tompkins, Scharp, Fassbinder, Meigh, and Armstrong (2008), after removing confounding variables from stimuli often used to assess ToM, concluded that these difficulties may reflect, at least in part, problems with complex inferencing rather than inferences about mental states per se (see Weed, McGregor, Nielsen, Roepstorff, & Frith, 2010, for a similar account). The broader view of social impacts, however, is unique among current accounts and deserves further investigation.

Evidence about the neural underpinnings of ToM processing is mixed. There is consensus, however, that it involves a network of cognitive areas in which right dorsomedial frontal and right temporal areas are often included (e.g., Mason & Just, 2009).

SYMPTOMATOLOGY OF COGNITIVE–COMMUNICATION DISORDERS IN RIGHT HEMISPHERE DISORDER

This section briefly outlines the potential influence of RHD on the communicative domains of prosody, pragmatics and discourse, lexical–semantic processing, and reading and writing. The following material also addresses cognitive difficulties that can arise after RHD, including anosognosia, and problems in the domains of attention (including neglect syndrome), visual processing (perceptual/spatial), memory, and executive functioning. We include cognitive factors because they may underlie some or all of the communication difficulties of a patient with RHD. Beyond this, cognitive skills and deficits clearly affect performance in assessment and treatment.

Before continuing this section, we emphasize that adults with RHD are a heterogeneous group, and no one patient will have all of the symptoms identified here. There is little information about what accounts for this heterogeneity, so clinicians must be cautious not to think too narrowly or stereotypically about this patient group.

Prosody

Patients with RHD may exhibit aprosodia (e.g., Blake, 2007), an inability (or reduced ability) to produce or comprehend linguistic or affective information communicated by fundamental frequency, intensity, or duration cues in speech. Pell (1999) reports that patients with RHD use fewer prosodic cues to communicate emphasis in emotional utterances, a difficulty related to prosodic

encoding rather than emotional processing. In addition, adults with RHD may not exploit prosody effectively to signal changes in discourse structure (Hird & Kirsner, 2003). Clinically, patients with expressive aprosodia may have monotonous voices or sound hypermelodic. As summarized by Rosenbek et al. (2004), two major theories of expressive aprosodia emphasize either a motor impairment or a deficit in a "modality-specific nonverbal affect lexicon" (p. 787). Patients with RHD also may be impaired at judging emotion from the speech of others (Pell, 2006; E. D. Ross & Monnot, 2011) or at interpreting linguistic information signaled by prosody (e.g., syntactic markers; Joanette, Goulet, & Hannequin, 1990). In many cases, difficulties are related to perceptual impairments in prosodic decoding rather than the emotional or linguistic nature of the utterance (see Tompkins, 1995).

Discourse and Pragmatics

Discourse Production

Discourse macrostructures reflect the overall meaning, gist, topic, theme, or moral of a narrative and are needed to establish the narrative's global coherence. Adults with RHD may have difficulty generating discourse macrostructures. This difficulty may result from a variety of impairments, including a problem perceiving key contextual information, selecting and integrating contextually relevant information, or using world knowledge and text microstructure to derive appropriate macrostructure inferences (see also Gouldthorp, 2014, for evidence of greater intact RH involvement in interpreting global targets). *Microstructural content*, which can also be affected by RHD, refers to local discourse entities such as words, propositions, clauses, or turns in conversation.

Discourse superstructures are stored cognitive representations of the conventional elements of different discourse genres, such as narratives, overlearned procedures, and conversations. Adults with RHD may be impaired at this level as well. For example, they may not supply an initial setting when telling a story, or they may attempt to continue a conversation with someone who is signaling the end of the exchange. The bases of these deficits are unknown, but they could be caused by problems in selective attention (going straight to the heart of a story without introduction; being diverted from the conversational script) or other cognitive impairments (e.g., not perceiving confusion in their listeners).

Overall, there is considerable variability in discourse production after RHD, as illustrated in Table 17.1. This is likely the result of inconsistencies among studies

Table 17.1 Some Contrasting Findings in Discourse Production After a Right Hemisphere Disorder

Diminished informational content (prepositions, t-units, episodes) versus propositional content and accuracy similar to comparable non–brain-damaged adult speakers

Fewer words than normal (paucity) versus same number of words versus more words or more words per turn (verbosity)

Wandering from the point versus topic maintenance skills similar to those of control speakers

Poor error monitoring in discourse versus as many successful repairs as control speakers

Productions based on scripts, which are common scenarios like ordering a meal in a restaurant, that include tangential associations versus those that terminate prematurely

Difficulty telling an integrated story versus producing a fully integrated story that is unrelated to the stimulus situation

Impaired organization on story recall versus impaired memory for story schema

Loss of connecting line (coherence errors) in narrative productions versus comparable proportions of propositions that are central to, supportive of, or distracting from the main story line

Most important, core propositions produced versus inaccurate/incomplete main concepts

Higher proportions of literal concepts reflecting a tendency to itemize, rather than interpret, in picture descriptions versus no differences from age peers in proportions of literal and inferential concepts produced

Excessive detail and overpersonalization versus "unnecessary" detail and personal comments similar in extent to those produced by normally aging speakers

Adapted from Tompkins, C.A. *Right hemisphere communication disorders: Theory and management.* San Diego, CA: Singular. © 1995 Delmar Learning, a part of Cengage Learning, Inc./ Cengage Learning/ Nelson Education. Reproduced by permission. www.cengage.com/permissions

in terms of discourse models, sampling contexts, and patient factors.

Our patient T.N. illustrated some of these discourse characteristics. Some adults with RHD are terse to the point of seeming rude, but T.N. fit the stereotypic view, being overly verbose, egocentric, and tangential. When asked to explain how to make a sandwich, T.N. made various asides (e.g., "and I break the lettuce because I hate those big arched veins that stick up") and strayed into a full "lunch schema," including microwaving water for tea and putting applesauce on the side. In addition, his conversation was replete with ambiguous, vague, or absent referents, as when he spontaneously said, "You look just like her, you know."

Discourse Comprehension

The difficulty for adults with RHD in processing discourse at the macrostructure level may be evidenced in problems abstracting overall meanings, themes, or gists. Several neuroimaging studies corroborate RH involvement that increases as the complexity of linguistic stimuli increases, being the least evident at word level and maximally involved in narrative discourse (e.g., Xu et al., 2005; see also Braun, Guillemin, Hosey, & Varga, 2001; Kuperberg et al., 2006). Impairment in the ability to coherently integrate, interpret, and infer from discourse may lead to disorganized responses that seem impulsive or poorly thought out (Chantraine, Joanette, & Ska, 1998; Myers, 2001). These problems are pronounced in difficult listening situations, such as when spoken input is rapid (Titone, Wingfield, Caplan, Waters, & Prentice, 2001).

Patients with RHD may have particular difficulties when discourse contains ambiguous or conflicting elements that make multiple interpretations possible, as in sarcasm, irony, and figurative expressions (Murteira & Santos, 2013; for review, see Tompkins, 2008; Tompkins et al., in press). When a text (or discourse) contains incongruity or requires a revision of an initial inference, adults with RHD may have trouble forming coherent mental models of what is happening. Adults with RHD may have difficulty suppressing contextually inappropriate meanings of ambiguous inferences (Tompkins, Lehman-Blake, Baumgaertner, & Fassbinder, 2001; Tompkins et al., 2004) or information from a prior narrative time frame that is subsequently inhibited in ongoing comprehension (Scharp & Tompkins, 2013). Investigators such as Beeman (1993, 1998) have argued that patients with RHD do not generate bridging inferences to link current information in discourse with that in prior text. However, when task demands are reduced, adults with RHD can draw the types of inferences studied by Beeman (Tompkins et al., 2004). In general, patients with RHD have more trouble interpreting texts with conflicting elements when attentional task demands are high, when working memory resources are low, or when they have a suppression or coarse coding deficit (see Tompkins, 2008; Tompkins et al., 2015).

Tompkins's group has further demonstrated that patients with RHD can perform well when discourse information is coherent and consistent (e.g., Tompkins et al., in press). Leonard and colleagues (e.g., Leonard & Baum, 2005) also found that these patients are often unimpaired in their use of available contextual information. Along similar lines, Blake and Lesniewicz (2005) report that adults with RHD are able to generate predictive inferences, such as those deemed to require an intact RH (Beeman, Bowden, & Gernsbacher, 2000), when those inferences are strongly or moderately supported by a discourse context. Findings like these underpin one component of Contextual Constraint Treatment (Tompkins, Blake, Scharp, Meigh, & Wambaugh, 2013; Tompkins, Scharp, Meigh, Blake, & Wambaugh, 2012), which improves the efficiency of basic coarse coding (Blake, Tompkins, Scharp, Meigh, & Wambaugh, 2015) or suppression (Tompkins et al., 2013) processes and generalizes to narrative comprehension.

The RHD population has other discourse-processing strengths that can be exploited in assessment and treatment (Tompkins et al., in press). These include better comprehension of main ideas than details and of explicit than implied information; typically retained knowledge of essential elements of common scripts; and in limited-demand conditions, ability to infer from and profit from context of various sorts (e.g., referential, semantic, emotional) and in various forms (e.g., explicit themes, redundancy, schema-related expectations) and to make some kinds of inference revisions.

Pragmatics

Pragmatics refers to the context-appropriate, social use of language and communicative functions and is often assessed in discourse and conversation. The RH seems to play an important role in pragmatic aspects of language and to be necessary for interpreting utterances in context. Pragmatic deficits are manifested in various forms or domains and have been suggested by some investigators to be central to the communication impairments associated with RHD (for reviews, see Blake, 2007; Johns, Tooley, & Traxler, 2008; Sherratt & Bryan, 2012). However, pragmatic deficits in RHD have often been demonstrated with tasks that require meta-linguistic/metacognitive association and judgment and that do not reflect natural situations (e.g., Tompkins & Baumgaertner, 1998). For example, assessments often supply an isolated figurative expression and require patients to define it or to choose a picture that represents its meaning. Another common task is to have patients judge the appropriateness of a story character's actions or comments. In metacognitive tasks, performance can dissociate in either direction. A patient may act appropriately in response to an indirect request without correctly identifying a picture or phrase that is intended to represent the most appropriate action or may recite the steps needed to maintain a safe living environment without applying them.

Cummings (2007) echoes this concern about contrived measures that do not tap the natural use of language in context. We concur with Cummings, who notes the largely ad hoc nature of pragmatic research in clinical populations and recommends that future work should be motivated by current pragmatic theories.

Emotion and Nonverbal Communication Verbal animation and coverbal behavior may be reduced after RHD, although some adults with RHD may be extremely animated (for summary, see Tompkins, 1995). Mackenzie, Begg, Lees, and Brady (1997) report that 75% of adults with RHD at 3 months poststroke were rated as deficient in conversational eye contact, facial expression, or intonation. Based on facial expression alone, adults with RHD have been rated less likable than those with LHD or without brain damage (but not so when rated on conversational transcripts; Langer, Pettigrew, & Blonder, 1998).

Regarding emotional communication, Heilman (2009) catalogues a range of deficits that can occur with RHD and notes that typically they involve both positive and negative emotions. Beyond affective prosody deficits, RHD also often results in receptive and expressive difficulties in processing emotional faces. Heilman cites evidence that the discrimination and comprehension of emotional faces may be linked to the posterior superior temporal gyrus. Frontal lesions can lead to emotional disinhibition or lower intensity expressions (see also Alves, Aznar-Casanova, & Fukusima, 2009, for the role of the RH in a divided visual field study).

Tompkins (1995) notes that some work on emotional interpretation points to a relatively intact appreciation of emotional content in RHD but identifies problems when participants have to match their emotional inferences with specific settings or pictures. Problems may be magnified by, or the result of, deficits in processing the visuoperceptual, visuospatial, or acoustic/prosodic features of stimuli that convey emotion.

Speech Acts Some adults with RHD may have difficulty comprehending indirect requests (e.g., "Can you pass the salt?"), either taking them literally or, more often, choosing an action response that is inappropriate to the given situation (for review, see Tompkins, 1995). Production of indirect requests also may be problematic in RHD, with indirect hints the most affected (e.g., saying, "I'm having difficulty concentrating" in hopes that the listener will turn down the radio). Zaidel et al. (2000) report that adults with RHD and LHD were equally deficient in comprehension and production of basic speech acts (assertions, questions, requests, and commands) and comprehension of Gricean conversational implicatures of quantity, quality, relevance, and manner. More recently, Ribeiro, Mansur, and Radanovic (2015) demonstrated that adults with RHD were impaired in comprehending logical and pragmatic visual inferences, with a subgroup of individuals with posterior lesions performing worse than most. However, such deficits, demonstrated with metalinguistic association and judgment tasks, may be less apparent in natural situations. For example, in a clinical context, adults with RHD responded accurately to indirect requests such as "Can you sign your name on this sheet?" and "Could you name, in 30 seconds, as many words as you can starting with the letter *F*?" (Vanhalle et al., 2000).

Figurative and Other Implied Meanings Adults with RHD may have difficulty selecting a picture, word, or phrase that corresponds to a target idiom, metaphor, sarcastic statement, or other connotative meaning (see summary in Tompkins, 1995). More commonly, patients with RHD choose related nonliteral interpretations rather than literal ones. Again, however, the metacognitive demands of common assessments may obscure retained abilities. Furthermore, assessments often rely on visuoperceptual/spatial skills that can confound performance. Finally, the familiarity or relevance of expressions is likely to be important. Adults with RHD may comprehend figurative expressions that they use in conversation better than other nonliteral expressions.

Sensitivity to Listener Needs and Situation Theory of mind is a key concept in relation to sensitivity to listener needs. It affects choices ranging from referential and lexical selection to conversational management, as speakers try to make their contributions appropriate to their partners. Also, ToM is important for determining a speaker's communicative intention: Cummings (2005) places ToM squarely at the center of pragmatic interpretation.

The expressive communication of some adults with RHD suggests a deficit in this realm. Some initiate topics without informing the listener, are excessively verbose or terse, attempt few conversational repairs, or have difficulty taking a listener's perspective. To interpret such behaviors, it is important to know something about premorbid style. On the receptive side, metacognitive tasks suggest that some adults with RHD are poor at attributing intentions from knowledge of interpersonal relationships (Cheang & Pell, 2006; Kaplan, Brownell, Jacobs, & Gardner, 1990).

Happé et al. (1999) also report an RHD ToM deficit. In their study, however, ToM stories contained the perspectives of multiple characters, whereas control stories primarily did not. After equating ToM and control conditions and modifying the task response to reduce metalinguistic demands, adults with RHD did not display the deficits reported by Happé and colleagues (Tompkins, Scharp, Fassbinder, et al., 2008; see also Tompkins et al., in press, for a recent review). Happé and colleagues' participants may have had more severe RHD than Tompkins et al.'s, but this could not be determined from the article. Thus, it remains in question the extent to which adults with RHD have a fundamental ToM deficit.

Humor Clinically, some adults with RHD, particularly those with frontal lobe damage, react to cartoons with unrestrained hilarity. Some adults with RHD also have other humor appreciation difficulties, which likely have multiple roots, including visuoperceptual/spatial impairments; deficits in processing or interpreting situational, facial, and prosodic cues that signal humor; difficulty with alternate word meanings; or trouble integrating content across parts of a story. Concerning this last possibility, some patients with RHD appear to detect, but to have difficulty resolving, the contradiction that is often required for a story to be considered humorous (e.g., Bihrle, Brownell, & Gardner, 1988). These findings were corroborated in a magnetoencephalography study (Marinkovic et al., 2011) that reported joke selective activity emerging in the right prefrontal cortex. Cheang and Pell (2006), however, found the ability of participants with RHD to interpret humor from jokes to be relatively unimpaired.

Humor production has not been well documented. Clinical observation suggests humor that is at times disinhibited, crude, suggestive, or otherwise inappropriate in some adults with RHD.

Lexical–Semantic Processing

One of the RH's most prominent contributions to language processing is in the appreciation of lexical–semantic relations (see Tompkins et al., in press, for a review). Early work with patients with RHD suggested that they had problems with lexical ambiguity, and metaphor in particular, and it was proposed that secondary or subordinate (i.e., nonliteral, connotative) meanings are less available when the RH is dysfunctional (e.g., Brownell, Simpson, Bihrle, Potter, & Gardner, 1990). Early neuroimaging investigations (e.g., Bottini et al., 1994) suggest that the RH is critical for processing metaphoric language, but the results of this work were confounded by other factors. More current neuroimaging experiments have investigated the neural systems underlying the processing of ambiguous words, and although some have shown increased activation in the RH (e.g., Bilenko, Grindrod, Myers, & Blumstein, 2008; Mason & Just, 2007; Zempleni, Renken, Hoeks,

Hoogduin, & Stowe, 2007), others have not (e.g., Bedny, McGill, & Thompson-Schill, 2008; Grindrod, Bilenko, Myers, & Blumstein, 2008; T. M. Lee & Dapretto, 2006), leading to unanswered questions regarding the role of the RH in the processing of lexical ambiguity.

Recently, Klepousniotou, Gracco, and Pike (2014) demonstrated primary involvement of the ventral operculum (Brodmann area 44) of the inferior frontal gyrus, bilaterally, in activating and manipulating linguistic information in semantic memory. In addition, significant coactivations occurred in the anatomically and functionally connected inferior parietal lobule (IPL) (Brodmann area 40) bilaterally. The authors suggested that area 40 is involved in the mental manipulation and computation of meaning. When demands increase, such as when manipulating multiple alternative interpretations, the right IPL area 40 is differentially recruited to ensure successful meaning computation.

Whether or how the RH preferentially maintains features or meanings of words remains controversial, as well. Some work suggests that the RH maintains activation only for targets that are both categorically and associatively related (Bouaffre & Faita-Ainseba, 2007, but cf. Harpaz, Lavidor, & Goldstein, 2013, who also found RH involvement for words related only via association). Meyer and Federmeier's (2008) event-related potential results, obtained in an eye-tracking study, suggest that the RH actually allows subordinate meanings to decay and then reactivates them more quickly than the LH in contextually incompatible contexts. In addition, in the absence of context, Klepousniotou, Pike, Steinhauer, and Gracco (2012) found N400 priming effects predominantly over the RH for subordinate senses of metaphorical polysemies (such as *arm-couch*), unlike subordinate meanings of polarized homonyms (such as *ball-dance*). These effects were sustained over a long interval for polysemous but not homonymous words (MacGregor, Bouwsema, & Klepousniotou, 2015). As noted, the RH may be specialized for making novel semantic connections or may support additional processing required to make sense of distant semantic relations. These processes may be necessary to understand metaphors but are not confined to figurative language.

Reading and Writing

Reading and writing difficulties in RHD may be attributable to impairments in several mechanisms that encode and process visual information, such as the premotor programming of ocular scanning, allocation of spatial attention, or creation of visual representations. More basic deficits may include difficulties scanning a line of print, tracking back to the margin to find the beginning of the next line, or looking up and down on a page to locate or place information. Visual field cuts must also be considered as contributing factors.

Assessed primarily with oral reading tasks, *neglect dyslexia* is typically associated with the attentional disruptions of neglect syndrome, although the two do not always co-occur. Table 17.2 describes some characteristics and subtypes of neglect syndrome that also apply to neglect dyslexia. Chechlacz et al. (2012) reported neural correlates of neglect in a large group of stroke patients. At both subacute and chronic stages, both egocentric and allocentric neglect were associated with lesions in the right temporoparietal junction and along the superior longitudinal fasciculus; subacutely, right frontal lesions were also related to both types of neglect. Persistent egocentric neglect was associated with superior temporal gyrus lesions, extending into supramarginal gyrus, basal ganglia, and insula, while persistent allocentric neglect was related to angular gyrus lesions. Figure 17.1 illustrates two neglect subtypes as evidenced in reading, drawing, and a gap detection task.

Common word-level symptoms of neglect dyslexia are initial letter substitutions (e.g., *pillow/yellow*) or deletions (*read/tread*). Performance tends to be worse with greater separation between letters or when words are written on the left side of a page and is likely better with vertically displayed or orally spelled words (unless the client has a rare form of neglect dyslexia). Text-level symptoms may include omitting whole words at the beginning of a line or even the entire left side of a page.

Hillis and colleagues (2005) studied neglect dyslexia in a large RHD sample within 48 hours of stroke. Patients whose reading and spelling errors occurred mostly on the contralateral (left) side of words were given other tasks to distinguish stimulus-centered neglect dyslexia (defined by side of the stimulus—thus, errors on the contralateral side of words in both hemifields) from object-centered neglect dyslexia (defined by the side of the abstract representation of the [stimulus] word, that is, its beginning—thus, errors in reading standard print, vertical print, recognizing orally spelled words, and spelling words). One-third of the patients demonstrated viewer-centered neglect dyslexia, 22% stimulus centered, and 18% a combination of the two. Few patients had the object-centered pattern, and 58% did not exhibit neglect.

Spatial agraphia (sometimes called neglect dysgraphia) is a frequent writing difficulty in RHD. According to Ardila and Rosselli (1993), posterior damage is usually linked with spatial deficits (e.g., superimposition of words or elements of words; misgroupings of elements within and between words), while frontal damage is generally associated with mechanical or motor deficits (e.g., repetitions of features and letters). Patients with concomitant neglect

Table 17.2 Neglect Characteristics and Subtypes

General Characteristics

- *More common/severe/long lasting* in RHD than LHD
- *Most common* with middle cerebral artery lesions
- *Most often visual* but can affect auditory and tactile modalities
- *Can affect various domains*, singly or in combination: spatial (attentional/sensory and action–intentional/motor); personal; representational

Spatial Neglect

Attentional/sensory: Difficulty disengaging attention from ipsilesional frame of reference or attraction bias. *Frames of reference* include right versus left (in contralateral or ipsilateral space); contra versus ipsilesional; up versus down; proximal (near extrapersonal) versus distal (far extrapersonal); viewer versus stimulus/object centered. Lower left quadrant often most impaired.

- *Viewer centered (also known as egocentric):* Reference is viewer midline (head, trunk, retina).
- *Stimulus centered (also known as allocentric):* Reference is an object itself (including a word), regardless of where it is in viewer space.
- *Object centered:* Reference is the usual mental representation of an object (including a word), regardless of where it is or what form presented in (e.g., written vertically, spoken).
- *Environment centered:* Reference is left side of a group of stimuli or of a set of spatial coordinates (e.g., left side of a book or a room).

Action–intentional/motor: Difficulty moving/using contralesional side of the body unless strongly directed to do so. Often coexists with hemiparesis; more difficult to diagnose. Involves basal ganglia and dopaminergic system; also prefrontal, limbic, and temporoparietal. Frontal lesions more likely yield this than attentional/sensory neglect.[a] May be worse when movement is directed toward or performed in contralesional space. Includes the following:

- *Hypo-/akinesia:* Delayed/absent initiation of movement of eyes, head, limb, and/or body.
- *Hemiakinesia or motor impersistence:* Poor at sustaining an action.

Personal Neglect

Affects tasks such as grooming, dressing, eating, recognizing own body parts.

Representational Neglect

Impairments related to mental images of objects and locations (e.g., drawn or described from memory).

Note: LHD, left hemisphere damage; RHD, right hemisphere damage.

Medina, J., Kannan, V., Pawlak, M., Kleinman, J., Newhart, M., Davis, C., et al. (2009). Neural substrates of visuospatial processing in distinct reference frames: Evidence from unilateral spatial neglect. *Journal of Cognitive Neuroscience, 21,* 2073–2084.

[†]Heilman (2009).

syndrome may crowd their productions into the right side of the space provided or leave larger margins on the left side of a page, increasing in size from top to bottom. This last feature may be hard to separate from the large normative variation in left margin width on writing tasks, variation that increases with age (Azouvi et al., 2006).

Other impairments that can contribute to reading or writing difficulty include many of the cognitive deficits reviewed in the next portion of this chapter. For example, distractibility may make it hard for patients to pick up where they left off in a writing task, or difficulty organizing thoughts may result in ambiguous or poorly coherent sentences and texts. Adults with RHD also may have *reading comprehension* and *written expression* deficits for materials that create the processing difficulties described elsewhere in this chapter.

Cognition

Anosognosia

Anosognosia is a general term for a complex family of related disorders that may occur after RHD. Anosognosia can be defined as impaired awareness of deficits—motor, sensory, cognitive, emotional—or reduced insight into how those deficits affect daily functioning. Clinical presentations of anosognosia vary considerably across patients with RHD (Besharati, Crucianelli, & Fotopoulou, 2014). Patients may exhibit an unawareness of cognitive, emotional, or physical changes, and awareness may vary across domains. Any of these problems can hinder motivation for treatment and reduce prognosis for functional recovery (Gialanella, Monguzzi, Santoro, & Rocchi, 2005). Various terms describe specific types

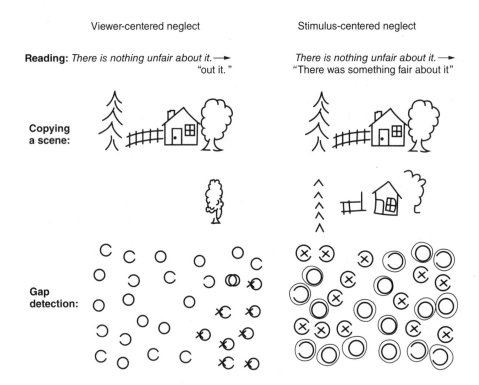

Figure 17.1 Viewer-centered and stimulus-centered neglect.

Taylor & Francis. Hillis, A. E., Newhart, M., Heidler, J., Marsh, E. B., Barker, P., & Degaonkar, M. (2005). The neglected role of the right hemisphere in spatial representation of words for reading. *Aphasiology, 19*(3/4/5), 225–238.

or facets of anosognosia, such as *asomatognosia* (lack of awareness of the existence of, or the condition of, some part[s] of the body) and *anosodiaphoria* (indifference to a deficit, most often paralysis).

Anosognosia tends to improve with time but can remain problematic in chronic patients. Although anosognosia is often categorized under executive function deficits, we emphasize it separately here because of its potentially important influence on treatment approach, treatment compliance, and functional recovery.

Attention

As previously noted, RHD appears to be linked with limitations of the capacity or allocation of attentional resources that are needed to perform cognitive–communicative processing. Other aspects of attention have been investigated as well. For example, the RH seems to subserve the bilateral *maintenance of arousal* (a physiological state of readiness), *alertness* to process an expected signal, and *sustained attention* (Keller, Schlenker, & Pigache, 1995). Although RHD results were not addressed separately, McDowd, Filion, Pohl, Richards, and Stiers (2003) report that patients have deficits in *dividing and switching attention*, and that

these deficits are related to self-reported physical and social outcomes, such as limitations in social activities and performance of family roles.

Posner (1994; Posner & Petersen, 1990), among others, distinguished the contributions of a posterior cerebral attention network from those of an anterior attention network. The posterior network, and particularly the posterior parietal cortex, is involved in maintaining alertness, orienting attention to particular locations in space, and reorienting attention to previously attended locations (see also Thiel, Zilles, & Fink, 2004). This network further disengages attention from a target, while the thalamus contributes to engaging attention on a target. In addition, the posterior system is thought to operate on the ventral ("what") pathway (Ungerleider & Haxby, 1994) when detailed processing of objects is necessary. The anterior attention network contributes primarily to selective attention and helps to filter, inhibit, and resolve attentional conflicts. This system includes medial and lateral prefrontal regions, anterior cingulate cortex, and basal ganglia connections.

More recently, it has been proposed that distinct forms of attentional orienting have distinct neural systems (e.g., Fox, Corbetta, Snyder, Vincent, & Raichle, 2006; Hutchinson, Uncapher, & Wagner, 2009). Automatic orienting (also called reflexive or exogenous attention) is subserved primarily by RH temporal, ventral posterior parietal (IPL and angular gyrus), and inferior/ventral frontal cortex. This network responds to abrupt changes in stimuli, filters irrelevant stimuli, and detects relevant input, particularly when salient or unexpected. Voluntary orienting (also called top-down or endogenous attention) is bilaterally mediated by parts of the dorsal posterior parietal and superior frontal cortex and is active when attention is purposely directed. Both types of attentional orienting can be disrupted in neglect syndrome.

Neglect syndrome, particularly spatial neglect, is likely the most clinically important attention deficit in adults with RHD because it is associated with poor functional outcomes (e.g., Jehkonen, Laihosalo, & Kettunen, 2006). Also called unilateral neglect, visual neglect, visuospatial neglect, hemispatial neglect, hemineglect, contralateral neglect, or (simply) neglect, neglect syndrome is a constellation of disorders of spatial exploration and selective attention that manifests primarily in a directional bias for perception, attention, or action and that cannot be explained by sensory or motor impairments. It is often characterized by difficulty disengaging attention from ipsilesional portions of space or stimuli and orienting to, acknowledging, responding to, or reporting stimuli located primarily in contralesional space (or contralesional portions of stimuli). Neglect often co-occurs with anosognosia, and nonlateralized components of attention (e.g., vigilance) can contribute to its functional impact. Table 17.2 provides further information about neglect and comparisons of performance in neglect subtypes (see also Figure 17.1).

The cognitive mechanisms, neural bases, and appropriate assessment and treatment of neglect all remain topics of debate. There is also controversy about the stability of neglect subtypes, particularly in the acute poststroke period (e.g., Hamilton, Coslett, Buxbaum, Whyte, & Ferraro, 2008; Marsh & Hillis, 2008). However, some neglect subtype classifications may be reliable (i.e., visuospatial, tactile, or combined; viewer centered versus object/stimulus centered), even in acute patients (Marsh & Hillis, 2008).

Visuoperceptual/Visuospatial Processing

Adults with RHD can have other visual processing problems that may depend on site of lesion. Separate streams exist in the central nervous system for identifying "what" something is and "where" in space it is located, with "what processing" involving the temporal association cortex and "where processing" relying on parietal regions.

Regarding what processing, adults with RHD typically have little difficulty identifying pictured objects (e.g.,

Myers & Brookshire, 1996) unless presented in unusual views (e.g., rotated, incomplete, fragmented) and devoid of context. Adults with RHD may be impaired in matching unfamiliar faces that are presented in different perspectives or lighting conditions. These bottom-up perceptual difficulties may not be apparent in more natural situations, where top-down knowledge and expectations can contribute to performance.

Regarding where processing, one common deficit is difficulty judging the slope and position of single line segments to match them to the same lines in a larger array. Adults with RHD also may produce drawings that are spatially incomplete or disorganized; the extent to which such impairments reflect problems with visual input processing, visual allocation of attention, or visuomotor output must be determined. Topographical difficulty, or confusion about location in space, can occur as well, affecting map reading, finding one's way in space, or describing how to get from one place to another.

Any such problems can be exacerbated by co-occurring, uncompensated visual field deficits or neglect.

Memory

A meta-analysis and review by Gillespie, Bowen, and Foster (2006) documents RHD deficits in nonverbal episodic memory, in both recall and recognition. These impairments are likely associated with early attentional or perceptual encoding problems. The RHD deficits are also evident in verbal episodic recall tasks such as story memory, word list learning, and paired-associate learning, which were linked with attentional deficits in several of the studies assessed. An imaging study of non–brain-damaged adults correlates episodic–autobiographical memory retrieval with RH frontotemporal and limbic regions (Markowitsch, 2008).

Many adults with RHD have deficits in estimated verbal WMCL (Tompkins et al., 1994). Good WMCL is associated with higher-level cognitive performance, such as resolving inconsistencies in narratives and revising inferences in tasks with relatively high processing demands. Marsh and Hillis (2008) indicate that impaired spatial working memory can co-occur with and complicate neglect syndrome.

Executive Functioning

Beyond problems with anosognosia, adults with RHD can have deficits in other aspects of executive functioning, including planning, organization, reasoning, and problem solving. Some component deficits may include problems in generating or appreciating alternative goals, organizational strategies, outcomes, or solutions to problems; in perceiving relevant properties or characteristics of a task or the task environment; or in various facets of information integration and inferencing. Difficulties have been documented in daily planning and organizational tasks involving, for example, record keeping, adhering to checklists, organizing schedules, keeping track of belongings, and managing time (Klonoff, Sheperd, O'Brien, Chiapello, & Hodak, 1990).

ASSESSMENT OF PATIENTS WITH RIGHT HEMISPHERE DISORDER

Historically, assessment for cognitive communication disorders has followed a medical model, in which the heart of the process is to identify a patient's *impairments*. The World Health Organization (WHO) International Classification of Functioning, Disability, and Health (ICF; WHO, 2001) reminds us to consider the patient's cognitive–communicative *activity limitations* and *participation restrictions* (which may or may not be directly predictable from a measured impairment; Tompkins, Lehman, Wyatt, & Schulz, 1998). *Contextual factors*, such as support, relationships, and attitudes, are also important to assess because they may be targets for treatment. McCue and colleagues (1994) describe an applied cognitive rehabilitation approach that emphasizes the *impact* of deficits and a focus on *obstacles*—which may include deficits and factors outside the patient—that interfere with patients achieving their goals. Note here that patients' goals are preeminent.

Assessment of adults with RHD is complicated by a number of factors (Tompkins, 1995), including the lack of normative data for many aspects of cognition and communication, a vast range of normal for many of these areas, a shortage of conceptually and psychometrically sound tests and measures, and a dearth of research to assist with the goals of assessment. In addition, there are few available psychometrically sound measures of activity limitations, participation restrictions, and obstacles to goal attainment beyond a patient's deficits.

With all this in mind, we turn next to the initial evaluation for patients with RHD. The purposes of assessment will change over time, of course, as when periodic measures are made to monitor the effects of treatment. As in other areas of language, communication, and cognition, a good evaluation relies on material from multiple sources, including past records, current case history, observations, interviews, questionnaires, simulations, and tests.

Initial Evaluation

Collecting Basic Information

Part of the initial appraisal involves collecting biographical information, including birth date; education; date of stroke onset; handedness; and preexisting language, cognitive, or learning deficits. Pertinent medical data include such things as the medical diagnosis and etiology, medications that could affect performance, and information on vision (acuity, fields, perception, neglect), hearing (acuity, discrimination), and mental status. Tompkins (1995) provides a complete list of such factors.

To supplement traditional case histories, clinicians should also gather information about (a) patients' and families' complaints and goals; (b) levels of distress or importance accorded to these complaints and goals; (c) patients' communicative contexts (e.g., work, leisure, social); (d) premorbid cognitive and communication abilities, styles, and needs in those contexts; (e) communicative strengths and strategies and general and specific coping styles and compensatory techniques; (f) sociocultural norms and expectations related to cognition and communication; (g) potential obstacles to goal attainment other than patients' deficits; and (h) resources available to assist recovery and facilitate life participation. Appendix 17A provides a sample case history supplement, and Appendix 17B provides a performance inventory for everyday tasks and environments. Both appendices address many of these issues and help point toward meaningful outcomes.

Because many patients with RHD lack full awareness of their strengths, weaknesses, and other obstacles to goal attainment, much of the interview or questionnaire information may have to come from family members, friends, or coworkers. As the Case Illustration further in this chapter highlights, it is important to interview more than one respondent.

Conducting Informal and Formal Assessments

Early informal assessment and observation can help identify behaviors that may signal impaired communication and cognition, as outlined in the previous section, "Symptomatology of Cognitive–Communication Disorders in Right Hemisphere Disorder." To focus and interpret assessment, it is also valuable to obtain samples of premorbid cognitive–communicative performances, such as work products, letters, or video interactions with family members.

Screening evaluations are also imperative, with formal screening detecting more problems than informal

Table 17.3 Examples of Potential Links Between Impairment and Activities Limitation for Adults With RHD

Impairment	Activities Limitation
Pragmatics; social comprehension, communication, and judgment	Difficulty participating in social interactions of all kinds (e.g., missing indirect "hints," emotional and nonverbal nuances; losing or alienating listeners through disinhibition and other unusual behavior; creating embarrassment for family that further limits opportunities)
Discourse and conversation; ambiguity and inference	Difficulty participating in social interactions (e.g., being misunderstood or misunderstanding others because of problems with cohesion, coherence, inference generation or revision, determination and designation of contextually relevant information, turn-taking, and topic control)
Reading and writing	Difficulty reading/writing for daily activities and interests (e.g., newspapers, recipes, instructions, phone books, schedules, messages/letters, checks, appointments, diary entries, lists)
Cognitive/perceptual, such as anosognosia, neglect and other facets of attention, visuoperceptual or spatial deficits, learning and memory deficits, executive function deficits	Difficulty participating in social interactions; increased risk for falls; difficulty with daily life activities such as dressing, grooming; loss of independence in daily activities because of family's concerns about awareness, planning, safety, and so forth (e.g., driving or other independent ambulation, cooking, handling money, shopping, keeping records, keeping track of belongings); diminished participation in hobbies involving visual perception or construction (e.g., woodworking; painting) or musical ability; diminished concentration or memory for various social, recreational, and vocational activities

Data from Tompkins, C. A., Lehman, M., Wyatt, A., Schulz, R. (1998). Functional outcome assessment of adults with right hemisphere brain damage. Seminars in *Speech and Language,* 19(3), 303–321.

screening (e.g., Hinckley, 2014). The Birmingham Cognitive Screen (BCoS; Humphreys, Bickerton, Samson, & Riddoch, 2012) is an option with relatively acceptable psychometric properties. A subset of tasks focused on spatial attention (neglect), controlled attention (executive functions), and memory is most relevant for adults with RHD. Its utility and predictive value were recently investigated in a large sample of individuals with stroke (Bickerton et al., 2014). Some clinicians use the Repeatable Battery for the Assessment of Neuropsychological Status Update (Randolph, 2012), but its validity evidence is incomplete, and its subtest reliability is insufficient to make decisions about individuals (French, Gotch, & Linck, 2014). Some clinicians like the Cognitive Linguistic Quick Test (Helm-Estabrooks, 2001), but caution is warranted in light of a small standardization sample, weak test–retest reliability estimates (with no data for clinical samples), and limited validity evidence. Recent research has documented some promising psychometric properties of BRAINscreen, a web-based, real-time system for cognitive screening (Zakzanis & Azarbehi, 2014); it will be interesting to watch for further validation evidence.

Structured informal assessment complements the formal assessment process to help determine reasons for patients' particular strengths and weaknesses (see Case Illustration 17.1 for an example). Structured informal assessment also helps to determine the effects of deficits on daily functioning. There are no data about the links between RHD cognitive–communicative impairments and activity limitations, but Table 17.3 presents some intuitions.

Tables 17.4 through 17.10 describe selected formal measures of cognitive–communicative disorders that have some psychometric foundations, although they vary widely in quality. Speech–language clinicians may not give all of these tests, but information about these measures is useful for evaluating the results of testing reported by rehabilitation specialists in other disciplines. Several other possible assessments are described in the accompanying text.

A note of caution is warranted about the metalinguistic (metacognitive) nature of typical clinical assessments for RHD. Most require patients to reflect on or make judgments about their language, cognition, or social communication, and their responses can be very different from their actual performances in daily life situations. As an example, think of how we may not be able to define a word (or a proverb or some other figurative phrase), but we can respond to it appropriately. Similarly, there may be big differences for patients between being able to describe how they would react in certain situations and their actual reactions. Metacognitive versus actual responses draw on different learning and memory systems (declarative versus procedural), and performance dissociations can go either direction (better at saying than doing; better at doing than saying). Clinicians can supplement metalinguistic responses with direct observations of relevant behavior and directed observations and reports by other members of the rehabilitation team, medical staff, or family and close friends of the patients.

Table 17.4 describes overall assessments of language, communication, or cognitive–communicative abilities in adults with RHD. These tests primarily assess the Impairment level of function, although some items target the Activity level (e.g., conversations in Right Hemisphere Language Battery–2 [RHLB-2], Protocole Montreal d'Evaluation de la Communication [MEC], and RIC Evaluation of Communication Problems in Right Hemisphere Dysfunction–Revised [RICE-R]; RICE-R writing tasks and Pragmatic communication skills rating). Caution is necessary in interpreting most of these tests, which share a number of limitations. For example, they tend to be normed on small samples of adults with RHD or only on adults without brain damage. Validity and reliability data are sparse and primarily based on very small samples. Also, formal tests often do not help identify underlying processes.

Although not intended for adults with RHD, various versions of the Ross Information Processing Assessment (e.g., RIPA-2; Ross-Swain, 1996) are commonly used clinically with these patients. Tompkins (1995) catalogues serious psychometric problems with the original (D. G. Ross, 1986), which are only somewhat improved in the RIPA-2. In one relevant study, all 94 non–brain-damaged adults were identified as having traumatic brain injury (TBI) based on RIPA-2 norms (Friehe & Schultz, 2003). Thus, we do not endorse this measure for clinical purposes.

Table 17.5 lists measures at the level of Activity and Participation that are appropriate for adults with RHD. Cautious interpretation is again warranted because of limitations in norms, psychometric properties, or a self-report format that may be invalidated by anosognosia or by patients' difficulty remembering limitations they have experienced.

The American Speech-Language-Hearing Association Functional Assessment of Communication Skills for Adults (ASHA FACS; Frattali, Thompson, Holland, Wohl, & Ferketic, 1995) may have some utility as an informal measure of communication activity in some adults with RHD (Tompkins et al., 1998), although it is not validated as a formal measure for this population. A number of other informal assessments have potential at the Activity

level. For example, Tompkins (1995) presents principles and proposed tasks to assess processes that underlie discourse processing, based on a useful model (Frederiksen, Bracewell, Breuleux, & Renaud, 1990), and summarizes some comprehensive analyses of narrative discourse production (such as Joanette and Goulet's [1990] approach for a picture description task). If faced with time constraints, clinicians could adopt part of this approach by, for example, applying the list of core propositions provided by Joanette and Goulet. These authors also advise tracking noncore propositions that may reflect tendencies to provide tangential or irrelevant responses.

Several other measures, not yet studied with adults with RHD, could be useful. These include Nicholas and Brookshire's main concept (1993b) and correct information unit (CIU; 1993a) metrics for quantifying the content of discourse in aphasia. The former indicates the accuracy and completeness of information determined to be central to a set of five elicitation tasks, while the latter indexes "informativeness" in terms of the number of relevant and intelligible words and can be calculated for any type of discourse. Measures of the percentage of words that are CIUs and CIUs per minute are more stable for adults with aphasia than are simple counts of CIUs.

Tompkins (1995) also recommends Promoting Aphasics' Communicative Effectiveness (PACE)-like "barrier tasks" as one way to structure an informal conversational evaluation and illustrates how such tasks can provide insights into communicative interactions. In barrier tasks, an individual tries to communicate some object, concept, picture sequence, and the like that is hidden behind a conversational barrier. Clients and clinicians take turns as message senders and receivers and can use any means possible to communicate. When patients are senders, clinicians may be able to observe strengths and weaknesses in areas such as presupposition and sensitivity to the partner (e.g., lexical selection, conciseness, relevance, formality, contingent responses, and feedback-based adaptations); speech act use (e.g., direct versus indirect commands); awareness of message adequacy (e.g., attempts to self-correct or clarify; nature and adequacy of those attempts); topic maintenance; and turn-taking. To see what patients will do to repair, clinicians can feign difficulty discerning a message, ask for clarification, do nothing, signal confusion nonverbally, or make an incorrect response. To observe patients' receptive abilities, clinicians acting as message senders can vary their utterances prosodically, facially, and so forth; use different types of speech acts; give vague information; or provide semantically or perceptually redundant information. The materials to be conveyed in such tasks can focus on potential problem areas, such as humor, emotion, or figurative meanings.

Table 17.4 General, Impairment-Based Measures of Language and Cognitive Communication in Adults With RHD

Measure	Description	Standardization Samples	Validity/Reliability	Other
Burns Brief Inventory of Communication and Cognition: Right Hemisphere Inventory (Burns, 1997)	Screens scanning and tracking, visuospatial skills, and prosody and abstract language. Criterion referenced; not intended for diagnosis. Designates "moderate impairment" to direct choice of functional treatment goals.	85 RHD	*Validity:* Content (limited), concurrent (limited), construct (incomplete/unconvincing). *Reliability:* Internal consistency, test–retest (small sample), interrater. Standard error for each task.	Qualitative scoring; gives possible reasons for poor performance; goal bank to help set functional goals, but goals based on deficits inferred from very small behavior samples; unknown effects of demographic variables.
Mini-Inventory of Right Brain Injury, 2nd edition (Pimental & Knight, 2000)	A screening in four processing domains: visuospatial/visuoperceptual and attentional; lexical knowledge; affective; behavioral. Also a right–left differentiation scale.	128 RHD 45 LHD 78 NBD	*Validity:* Content (overrepresentation of oral stimuli with spoken response), concurrent (small sample), construct identification (RHD versus LHD). *Reliability:* Internal consistency (acceptable). Lacks test–retest data.	Sensitivity/specificity not addressed. No data about effects of demographic variables. Some cutoff issues/overlap between RHD and LHD scores. Lacks norms/standard scores for the four domains and individual subtests.
Protocole Montreal d'Evaluation de la Communication (MEC; Joanette, Ska, & Côté, 2004)[a]	French language test. Targets linguistic and emotional prosody, verbal fluency, semantic judgment, conversational and narrative discourse, metaphor and indirect speech act interpretation, awareness of deficits. Focus on "verbal communication," not cognition.	180 (Quebec) French-speaking NBD to establish cut points	*Validity:* Content (limited). *Reliability:* Interrater (acceptable for most tasks). *Other:* Age, education effects on all tasks.	Cutoffs at 10th percentile for NBD controls, so some adults with NBD will be misidentified as having a deficit. Authors caution to consider premorbid ability when interpreting cutoffs.

(continues)

Table 17.4 General, Impairment-Based Measures of Language and Cognitive Communication in Adults With RHD (*continued*)

Measure	Description	Standardization Samples	Validity/Reliability	Other
Rehabilitation Institute of Chicago (RIC) Evaluation of Communication Problems in Right Hemisphere Dysfunction–Revised (RICE-R; Halper, Cherney, Burns, & Mogil, 1996)[b]	Targets five domains: visual scanning/tracking, writing, nonliteral language interpretation, behavioral observation profile, pragmatic communication skills rating.	40 RHD 36 NBD	*Validity:* Content (limited); construct (limited). *Reliability:* Internal consistency (acceptable for all but Writing); interrater (acceptable only for trained raters); mostly acceptable item and person separation reliability (per Rasch analysis).	This version provides administration guidelines. NBD sample biased toward females. Some cutoff issues (22% and 34% of NBDs classified as impaired on metaphorical language and completeness of narrative discourse, respectively).
Right Hemisphere Language Battery–2 (RHLB-2; Bryan, 1994)	Seven subtests: implied meaning comprehension, humor, lexical–semantic recognition, emphatic stress production, spoken metaphor appreciation, written metaphor appreciation, discourse production. Italian version (Zanini, Bryan, De Luca, & Bava, 2005).	40 RHD 40 LHD 30 NBD (444 NBD for Italian version)	*Validity:* Content (limited). *Reliability:* Test–retest; interrater (for discourse analysis).	Essentially the same items as original RHLB. See Tompkins (1995) for further comment.

Note: LHD, left hemisphere disorder; NBD, no brain damage; RHD, right hemisphere disorder.

[a]Brazilian version (Fonseca et al., 2008); developing Italian, European Spanish, German, English versions and brief versions for acute care screening.

[b]RICE-3 is essentially the same instrument as the RICE-R with the same standardization sample and psychometric data, but with some clarification of instructions and minor changes in format. Developed when RICE-R publisher stopped publishing the test (L. R. Cherney, 2015, personal communication). RICE-3 available from RIC: http://www.ricbookstore.org/detail.aspx?ID=76.

Table 17.5 Measures of Cognitive–Communicative Activity and Participation for Adults With RHD

Measure	Focus	Description, Standardization/Reliability/Validity	Other
Assessment of Language-Related Functional Activities (ALFA; Baines, Heeringa, & Martin, 1999)	Activity: Patient performs simulated language-related activities.	Ten subtests: Tell time, count money, address an envelope, solve daily math problems, write check/balance checkbook, understand medicine labels, use calendar, read instructions, use telephone, write phone message. Large standardization samples. Validity data limited/incomplete. Reliability data borderline-to-high for RHD sample, though none on test–retest reliability.	Addresses performances that are usually queried informally or not at all. No content in social communication/pragmatic areas that are especially important in RHD.
Burden of Stroke Scale (BOSS; Doyle et al., 2004, 2007; Doyle, McNeil, & Hula, 2003)	Activity and participation: Patient-reported assessment of physical and cognitive limitations and emotional distress.	Sixty-five items, 12 scales. Most relevant for this chapter are communication, cognition, social relations, and various mood and satisfaction scales. Also three composite scores: Physical Limitations, Cognitive Limitations, Emotional Distress. Test development and psychometrics are strong points.	Stroke patients with communication disorders have more difficulty and distress than those without communication disorders for Communication, Swallowing, and Social Relations scales and Cognitive composite score (Doyle et al., 2004).
Communication Activities of Daily Living–2 (CADL-2; Holland, Frattali, & Fromm, 1999)	Activity: Test of aspects of functional communication.	Ten communicative activities are sampled, including reading, writing, using numbers, social interaction, nonverbal communication, contextual communication, humor/metaphor/absurdity. Test development and psychometrics are strong points, though test–retest data obtained only for chronic aphasia.	Includes some qualitative scoring, for example, for both accuracy and adequacy. Norms combined for stroke patients with RHD and LHD. Also Spanish, Japanese versions.
Discourse Comprehension Test (DCT; Brookshire & Nicholas, 1993)[a]	Activity: Auditory (or silent reading) comprehension/retention of humorous narratives.	Two sets of five narratives. Yes/no questions assess stated and implied main ideas and details after each narrative. Some important factors considered in test development. Extensive evidence/arguments regarding validity and reliability but based on small samples, and some only for aphasia. Small standardization sample ($N = 20$ RHD); norms getting old.	Auditory version: Suppression function in adults with RHD predicts total DCT score (Tompkins et al., 2000, 2001, 2004); coarse coding in adults with RHD predicts comprehension of implied information (Tompkins, Scharp, Meigh, et al., 2008). Reading version: Norms only for NBD ($N = 20$); no cutoff score.
Pragmatic Protocol (Prutting & Kirchner, 1987)	Activity: General index of pragmatic abilities in unstructured conversation.	Thirty parameters represent three aspects of communication, rated based on 15-minute conversation: Verbal (speech acts, topic skills, turn-taking, lexical selection/use, stylistic variations); Paralinguistic (intelligibility, prosodics); Nonverbal (kinesics, proxemics).	Interscorer agreement high after 8–10 hours of training when 90% criterion reached during training. Scoring limited to "appropriate," "inappropriate," or "not observed."

Note: LHD, left hemisphere disorder; NBD, no brain damage; RHD, right hemisphere disorder.

[a]DCT, 2nd edition (1997); same instrument, published by PICA Programs (www.picaprograms.com)

Also potentially useful are (a) Hough and Pierce's (1994) Adult Social Communication Rating Scale, given to obtain communication partners' ratings of skills for initiating and maintaining conversations, dealing with feelings, generating alternatives to aggression, coping with stress, and advanced social conversation and planning skills; and (b) Gerber and Gurland's (1989) Assessment Protocol of Pragmatic Linguistic Skills, which focuses on social exchanges between familiar and unfamiliar partners. At the level of conversational turns, this profile addresses the nature and consequences of communication breakdowns, the resolution strategies used by speaker and conversation partner, and antecedent/consequent behaviors that contribute to successful and unsuccessful turn exchanges.

Solid measures at the level of Participation are as yet meager. The BOSS (Table 17.5) provides one good example, although the self-report format may be problematic for patients with RHD who have anosognosia. The ASHA's Quality of Communication Life Scale (Paul et al., 2004) is another patient self-rating that addresses social participation, well-being, and overall quality of life. The measure was standardized on a small sample of patients with speech, language, or cognitive deficits and provides a template for questions that could be asked informally of patients with adequate awareness.

The next five tables turn to cognitive measures. The relevant cognitive areas consist of multiple aspects and processes, so no single test will give a full picture of patients' strengths and weaknesses. In addition, some of the tasks are complex, requiring a variety of skills other than those a clinician wishes to assess. The entries in these tables were selected for one or more of the following reasons: The measures were developed for adults with RHD; developed for neurologically impaired patients, including some adults with RHD; sample a range of aspects of each domain; are better controlled for confounds than other similar measures; or have better psychometric properties than other similar measures. Again, such measures can be used to follow up on screening results and clinical hypotheses about what problems might underlie overt performance deficits.

Table 17.6 covers attention measures and Table 17.7 neglect measures. Because neglect tests vary in sensitivity, they should be used in combination. The varying sensitivity in part may be because studies of neglect tests have not routinely separated patients with different neglect subtypes (Marsh & Hillis, 2008). Some tests are starting to rectify this problem (e.g., the Apples cancellation task from the BCoS). In an investigation of neglect dyslexia within 48 hours of stroke, Hillis and colleagues (2005) reported that neglect patterns were consistent in reading and nonlanguage tasks, including scene copying

and gap detection (see Table 17.7), for example, viewer-centered neglect on both types of measures (see Figure 17.1 for an illustration). Dissociations have been reported in the literature, however.

Most of the available neglect measures address viewer-centered neglect in near extrapersonal space. Tasks that require reading, writing, and copying have the potential to detect object-/stimulus-centered neglect. Tasks of drawing from memory assess representational aspects of neglect. Neglect of far space has been examined with tasks such as projecting a slide of a scene from a lobby and asking the patient to identify all items in the scene. Virtual reality assessments, which will improve ecological validity, are beginning to be evaluated in the literature (e.g., Navarro, Lloréns, Noé, Ferri, & Alcañiz, 2013).

As noted in Table 17.7, the Catherine Bergego Scale (CBS; Azouvi et al., 1996, 2003) assesses various aspects of space and detects neglect in 76% of patients with RHD. Similar sensitivity is reported for four paper-and-pencil variables in a large patient sample (average 11 weeks postonset; Azouvi et al., 2006). The first two variables were the number of omissions and the starting point on the Bells cancellation test (Gauthier, Dehaut, & Joanette, 1989), with adults with RHD mainly starting on the right side of the page (although 20% of Azouvi et al.'s non–brain-damaged control subjects did not use a left-to-right pattern). A similar rightward bias has been reported as the only detectable residual deficit in patients whose neglect appears to have recovered (e.g., Mattingley, Bradshaw, Bradshaw, & Nettleton, 1994). The other key variables were performance on figure copying and clock-drawing tasks. Lindell et al. (2007) report that three paper-and-pencil tasks together detected 88% of neglect cases in a small group of patients (2–3 weeks postonset): Random Shape Cancellation (Weintraub & Mesulam, 1988), Complex Line Bisection (Butter, Mark, & Heilman, 1988), and Star Cancellation from the RBIT (Wilson, Cockburn, & Halligan, 1987; see Table 17.7). They did not include the CBS in their assessment.

Table 17.8 addresses selected measures of visual processing. Drawing a clock is a common task, despite its added demands for constructional, memory, and executive functions. With focal right parietal damage, severe spatial disorganization is common; frontal patients may have difficulty with the multiple demands of the task; and patients with right cortical or subcortical damage may reverse placement of numbers (Strauss et al., 2006). It can be difficult to determine why patients have trouble on this task, so follow-up probes are needed. Although the Hooper Visual Organization Test (Hooper, 1958) is also frequently given to assess visuospatial/perceptual performance, Strauss et al. (2006) note that the

Table 17.6 Selected Measures of Various Aspects of Attention

Measure	Focus	Description	Other[a]
Brief Test of Attention (Schretlen, 1997)	Impairment, Activity	Ten-minute screen of auditory divided attention. Reduces confounds (motor speed, visual scanning, long-term declarative memory).	Internal consistency, construct and ecological validity, low-to-adequate test–retest reliability, good parallel forms reliability, moderate sensitivity. Large adult normative sample (but 63% female).
Paced Auditory-Serial Addition Task (Gronwall, 1977; software package, Wingenfeld, Holdwick, Davis, & Hunter, 1999)[b]	Impairment, Activity	Fifteen- to 20-minute test of divided and sustained attention, working memory, information-processing speed. Requires arithmetic skills, rapid spoken response.	Internal consistency, ecological validity, adequate-to-high test–retest reliability. Reliability, validity data needed for 1999 computerized version. Various normative samples.
Ruff 2&7 Selective Attention Test (Ruff & Allen, 1992)	Impairment	Five-minute test of sustained and selective visual attention (automatic and controlled components).	Internal consistency, adequate-to-high test–retest reliability, good sensitivity. Provides standard error. Age, education effects. Large adult normative sample.
Symbol Digit Modalities Test (SDMT; Smith, 1991)[b]	Impairment, Activity	Five-minute test of divided visual attention, processing speed. Requires complex scanning/tracking. Oral, written formats. Incidental learning trial can be given.	Ecological validity, good sensitivity. Test–retest reliability data vary: good for original versions, less for incidental learning trial. Age, sex effects. Large adult normative samples.
Test of Everyday Attention (Robertson, Ward, Ridgeway, & Nimmo-Smith, 1994)[c]	Impairment, Activity	Forty-five- to 60-minute test with eight subtests that load on four factors: visual selective attention/speed, attentional switching, sustained attention, and auditory–verbal working memory.	Construct and ecological validity. No test–retest data for patients; mostly adequate-to-high for NBD sample (although compounded with alternate forms reliability). Standard error data in Crawford, Sommerville, and Robertson (1997). Limited norms (based on poorly described NBD sample) getting old. Moderate-to-good sensitivity. Age effects.

Note: NBD, no brain damage.

[a]Some of these comments are based on information compiled by Strauss, Sherman, and Spreen (2006) or entries in the Buros Mental Measurement Yearbooks (http://buros.unl.edu/buros/jsp/search.jsp).

[b]Many versions (see Strauss et al., 2006).

[c]Cantonese (Chan, Hoosain, & Lee, 2002) and Italian (Cantagallo & Zoccolotti, 1998) versions.

Table 17.7 Selected Measures of Neglect

Measure	Focus	Description	Other[a]
Balloons Test (Edgeworth, Robertson, & McMillan, 1998)	Impairment	Screens near extrapersonal space. Can rule out hemianopsia as cause of deficit.	Marginal-to-adequate test–retest reliability; acceptable construct (known groups) and convergent validity. Cutoffs based on 55 hospitalized controls (age about 64 years).
Catherine Bergego Scale (Azouvi et al., 1996, 2003)	Activity	Personal space, near and far extrapersonal space. Observe 10 daily activities. Detects neglect in 76% of patients with RHD. Most sensitive to neglect of left limbs, in dressing, and in collisions while moving.	Ecological, construct, criterion validity (Azouvi et al., 2006; Menon & Korner-Bitensky, 2004). Responsive to change in two cases, after visuo-spatio-motor cueing. Interrater reliability fair to high; no test–retest reliability data. Arbitrary cutoff points. Can be given as a self-report questionnaire to evaluate anosognosia.
Comb and Razor/Compact Test (Beschin & Robertson, 1997)	Activity	Screens personal space. Patient demonstrates use of common objects placed at midline.	Excellent test–retest reliability; construct validity (known groups).
Gap Detection (Ota, Fujii, Suzuki, Fukatsu, & Yamadori, 2001), modified by Marsh and Hillis (2008)[b]	Impairment	Near extrapersonal space; to detect egocentric and allocentric neglect. Patient identifies circles with/without a gap (on left/right side). Visual, tactile versions.	Experimental measure. No change in classification for small groups of acute patients (2- to 3-day interval between test and retest).
Line Bisection Test (Schenkenberg, Bradford, & Ajax, 1980)	Impairment	Screens near extrapersonal space. Mark the center of 18 horizontal lines.	Per Menon and Korner-Bitensky (2004): Acceptable construct, convergent, criterion validity; borderline-to-acceptable predictive. Strong test–retest reliability.
Rivermead Behavioral Inattention Test (RBIT; Wilson et al., 1987)	Impairment, Activity	Near and far extrapersonal space. Six conventional and nine behavioral subtests. A 10- to 15-minute short form: three conventional, five behavioral subtests (per Menon and Korner-Bitensky, 2004).	Per Menon and Korner-Bitensky (2004): Strong internal consistency, construct and ecological validity, test–retest and interrater reliability. Strong correlations between conventional and behavioral subtests (Hartman-Maeir & Katz, 1995).
Sunnybrook Neglect Assessment Procedure (Leibovitch, Vasquez, Ebert Beresford, & Black, 2012)	Impairment	Screens near extrapersonal space with five conventional tasks. Developed for quick bedside use in acute setting.	Adequate internal consistency, initial evidence of construct and concurrent validity, apparently good intra- and interscorer reliability.
Vest Test (Glocker, Bittl, & Kerkhoff, 2006)	Impairment, Activity	Screens personal space. Blindfolded patient manually scans front of vest to retrieve common objects from 24 pockets. Identifies personal neglect in 80% of patients with RHD with acute brain damage.	Low-to-adequate convergent validity, excellent internal consistency, good test–retest reliability. Cutoffs based on 50 healthy NBD controls, 92% of whom performed perfectly. No age effect when allowed 210 seconds to complete (but no participant above age 70 years).

Note: LHD, left hemisphere disorder; NBD, no brain damage; RHD, right hemisphere disorder.

[a]For more details on many of these and other measures, see Lindell et al. (2007) and Menon and Korner-Bitensky (2004). See Azouvi et al. (2006) for normative data on several neglect tests.

[b]The Apples cancellation task, from the better validated BCoS (Humphreys et al., 2012), is a similarly formatted visual task that uses large and small apples instead of circles.

Table 17.8 Selected Measures of Visual Perception and Visuospatial Processing

Measure	Focus	Description	Other[a]
Clock Drawing Test[b]	Impairment	Screens visuospatial (and other) skills	Construct validity (mostly for patients with dementia); ecological validity (healthy elders). Scorer reliability high for most scoring systems used with adults. Multiple quantitative and qualitative scoring systems for various versions (see Lezak, Howieson, & Loring, 2004; Strauss et al., 2006). Qualitative systems evaluate, for example, spatial/planning (e.g., neglect, gaps in number spacing, numbers outside clock face), clock size, omissions.
Facial Recognition Test (Benton & Van Allen, 1968; see Benton, Sivan, Hamsher, Varney, & Spreen, 1994)	Impairment	Ten to 15 minutes; recognition of unfamiliar faces. Also 7-minute Short Form	Construct validity. Internal consistency and test–retest reliability marginal for original; inadequate for Short Form. Sensitive to posterior RHD and RHD with neglect, but also impaired in patients with schizophrenia, multiple sclerosis, alcoholism, etc. Newer North American norms available. Interpretation note: Hairlines, eyebrows are not obscured, so normal scores can be obtained without intact face recognition.
Judgment of Line Orientation (Benton et al., 1994)	Impairment	Fifteen to 20 minutes; test of spatial perception and orientation. Also various short forms[c]	For original: Construct validity. Internal consistency high; test–retest reliability high (for small patient sample). Similar norms in United States and Europe. Extended norms for older African Americans (Lucas et al., 2005). In some studies, patients with RHD poorer than LHD, particularly with neglect, parietal damage.
Rivermead Perceptual Assessment Battery (Whiting, Lincoln, Bhavnani, & Cockburn, 1985)	Impairment, Activity	Sixteen tests for severe perceptual deficit. Intended for occupational therapists in United Kingdom.	Some construct validity; ecological validity. No internal consistency; widely varying test–retest stability data (for two small samples, one overwhelmingly male). Good interrater reliability. Limited normative sample. Does not discriminate between RHD and LHD. No evidence to support interpretations in the manual.
Visual Object and Space Perception Battery (Warrington & James, 1991)	Impairment	Eight brief tests of object/space perception. Intended to minimize confounds.	Some construct validity; better for object perception space perception tests. Reliability data from other sources; none in manual. Internal consistency adequate to low for a US sample. Test–retest reliability data available for only one test (identifying silhouettes of animals/objects in unusual views); high for healthy adults. Standardized in United Kingdom on hospitalized NBD. Norms not appropriate for older adults in the United States; Bonello, Rapport, and Millis (1997) gathered some norms from restricted region in the United States (see Strauss et al., 2006).

Note: LHD, left hemisphere disorder; NBD, no brain damage; RHD, right hemisphere disorder.

[a]Some of these comments are based on the information compiled by Strauss et al. (2006) or entries in the *Buros Mental Measurement Yearbooks* (http://buros.unl.edu/buros/jsp/search.jsp).

[b]Various versions; for example, in Boston Diagnostic Aphasia Examination (Goodglass, Kaplan, & Barresi, 2001) parietal lobe battery.

[c]Short forms correlate well with full test, but dissimilar severity categorization (Qualls, Bliwise, & Stringer, 2000) and limited test–retest reliability. Per Spencer et al. (2013), most are adequate only for screening, but one short form (Calamia, Markon, Denburg, & Tranel, 2011) has promise as a stand-alone instrument.

norms are quite outdated, and procedures for obtaining them were not sufficiently standardized. These authors conclude that a short version developed by Merten (2002), which includes improved administration and scoring procedures, may be more appropriate than the original test.

Table 17.9 includes selected memory measures. An experimental measure of auditory WMCL (Tompkins et al., 1994) has been used to assess the "central executive" component of working memory by engaging a patient in simultaneous processing and storage of sets of brief sentences (e.g., "You sit on a chair"). This task has good internal consistency and test–retest reliability and some evidence of construct validity, although from very small samples of adults with RHD or without brain damage (Lehman & Tompkins, 1998). In various studies, this measure has predicted auditory discourse comprehension for adults with RHD when task processing demands are presumed to exceed available working memory capacity. The Brief Assessment of Prospective Memory (Man, Fleming, Hohaus, & Shum, 2011), although developed for TBI, has promising psychometric properties, including acceptable test–retest reliability, and with appropriate cautions may be useful for adults with RHD. Several studies also report the development of intriguing virtual reality assessments of prospective memory as applied to individuals with TBI (Canty et al., 2014; Mioni, Rendell, Henry, Cantagallo, & Stablum, 2013).

Informal screening of memory function is also common. *Semantic memory* can be screened by asking patients about well-known facts (e.g., How many days are in a year?) and observing their adherence to common scripts. *Episodic memory* can be screened by asking about recent public events and autobiographical memories. *Working memory* is often screened by asking patients to spell the word *world* backward or with backward digit span tasks. Rough inferences about *metamemory* can be drawn by observing whether patients attempt to use any memory strategies or if they are aware of memory difficulties. And, as noted in Table 17.6, a measure of *incidental learning* can be obtained after administering the Symbol Digit Modalities Test (SDMT).

A few executive function assessments are described in Table 17.10. Many clinicians use the Wisconsin Card Sorting Test (Heaton, Chelune, Talley, Kay, & Curtiss, 1993, and other versions) as a measure of certain aspects of executive function. However, its reliability is quite low, and Strauss et al. (2006) recommend extreme caution in interpreting its results; Mueller and Dollaghan (2013) also demonstrate a lack of adequate diagnostic accuracy. Performance on such tests often varies with premorbid education or intellect. In addition, such measures may miss subtle difficulties because their structure obviates

the need for clients to generate their own complex plans, goals, and decisions (Lezak, 1983).

The Multiple Errands Test (MET; Shallice & Burgess, 1991) provides insight into higher functioning patients' planning, organizing, and rule following in a complex task with less structure and greater ecological validity. A simplified measure (Alderman, Burgess, Knight, & Henman, 2003) has also been adapted for use in the hospital (Knight, Alderman, & Burgess, 2002). Each of these has good sensitivity and specificity (based on small-sample studies) and some convincing evidence of construct validity; small-sample data for the hospital version also suggest adequate internal consistency and interrater reliability (Poulin & McDermott, 2013).

The Functional Assessment of Verbal Reasoning and Executive Strategies test (MacDonald, 2005) also offers a measure of some aspects of executive function, including planning, organization, prioritization with time constraints, and inhibition, in simulated everyday situations, such as planning an event or making a decision. Normed almost entirely on adults with TBI, the test is intended to detect subtle cognitive–communicative difficulties. MacDonald and Johnson (2005) provide evidence of good interrater reliability and initial sensitivity and specificity data, based on performance one standard deviation below that of a control group. Mueller and Dollaghan (2013), however, raise concerns about diagnostic accuracy.

Less complicated, but still potentially sensitive because of a lack of structure, is Boyd and Sautter's (1985) Executive Function Route Finding Task. Other ecologically oriented, virtual reality measures are being developed (e.g., Jovanovski, Zakzanis, Campbell, Erb, & Nussbaum, 2012; Rand, Rukan, Weiss, & Katz, 2009; Renison, Ponsford, Testa, Richardson, & Brownfield, 2012), and an emerging computerized measure addresses some executive skills in a social context (e.g., Kelly, McDonald, & Kellett, 2014).

There are a number of informal assessment options for anosognosia, though many involve a subjective report. Simple screening questions include "Why are you here?" and "What happened to you?" Awareness questionnaires (e.g., Fleming, Strong, & Ashton, 1996) include more in-depth items focused on the patient's awareness of changes in functioning, other people's concerns, and effects on everyday life. Forms such as those in Appendices 17A and 17B can be given to patients and other respondents to check for discrepancies. For more psychometrically sound options, the CBS (Azouvi et al., 1996, 2003), an activity-level measure of neglect described in Table 17.7, can be used as a self-report questionnaire and self-other ratings can be compared on the BRIEF-A (Table 17.10).

Table 17.9 Selected Measures of Various Aspects of Memory

Measure	Focus	Description	Other[a]
Benton Visual Retention Test (5th ed.; Sivan, 1992)	Impairment	Assesses immediate and (briefly) delayed visual memory recall, visual perception, visual construction	Adequate construct validity and reliability for scorers and alternate forms. Test–retest inconsistent for NBD adults. Lack of detail about normative samples; important variables not represented in norms (e.g., age, sex, SES, education). See Youngjohn, Larrabee, and Crook (1993) for adult age- and education-corrected norms.
Cambridge Prospective Memory Test (Wilson et al., 2005)	Activity	Assesses prospective memory, based on time cues and event cues	Reliability and validity data incomplete and from very small samples. Mixed group of patients performed worse than controls, except when patients took notes. Important variables not represented in patient norms (e.g., IQ, age).
Contextual Memory Test (Toglia, 1993)	Activity, Participation	Assesses metamemory: knowledge of memory limitations and strategy use	Reliability and validity adequate. Use norms cautiously: sample highly educated and homogeneous. Age, education affect performance; other potential reasons for poor performance not considered (e.g., depression).
Corsi Block-Tapping Task (Kessels, van Zandvoort, Postma, Kappelle, & de Haan, 2000)	Impairment	Assesses visuospatial memory span and memory for temporal information; visual working memory; correlates with visuospatial perception	Standardizes an otherwise highly variable task of tapping sequences of blocks after they are tapped by an examiner. No reliability and validity data for this version; construct validity inferred from extant literature. Limited normative data for healthy adults; somewhat better for small sample of adults with RHD (N = 22) without neglect. RHD worse than LHD. No sex differences. Corsi backward no more difficult than Corsi forward (Kessels, van den Berg, Ruis, & Brands, 2008).
Everyday Memory Questionnaire, Revised, Short Form (Short EMQ-R; Royle & Lincoln, 2008)	Activity, Participation	Assesses attitudes and beliefs about memory deficits	Strong correlations between short form and original long form. Strong internal consistency; some evidence of construct validity. Differentiates mixed group of stroke patients from NBD individuals (but NBD group much younger). Samples highly skewed female. No other demographic or cognitive information on samples.
Rey Complex Figure Test and Recognition Trial (Meyers & Meyers, 1995)	Impairment	Assesses immediate and delayed visual memory (recall and recognition), visual perception, visual construction	Standardizes an otherwise highly variable task of figure copying and reproduction. Provides a recognition trial, precise scoring criteria, information on older adults. Good construct, convergent, and discriminant validity; strong interrater reliability and temporal stability for brain-damaged patients and NBD adults. Strong correlation between immediate/delayed recalls for 100 patients suggests possibility of excluding delayed condition.

(continues)

Table 17.9 Selected Measures of Various Aspects of Memory *(continued)*

Measure	Focus	Description	Other[a]
Rivermead Behavioral Memory Test, 3rd edition (RBMT-3)[b] (Wilson et al., 2008)	Impairment, Activity	Screens and yields a General Memory Index for everyday memory (e.g., remembering a face, an appointment, a new route). Assesses immediate and delayed visual, verbal, and spatial recall and recognition. Also prospective memory, orientation, and new skill learning.	Reliability, validity mostly adequate. No standard error (and test–retest interval unknown); no sensitivity and specificity data. Updated norms (though not separated by sex). Alternate forms. Improvements in range of item difficulty, ethnic diversity in photos of people, control over verbal memory stories. Approximately 75 in clinical sample, with mixed etiologies.
Wechsler Memory Scale–Fourth Edition (Wechsler, 2009)	Impairment	Comprehensive assessment of immediate and delayed auditory verbal, visual, and spatial memory abilities, including working memory.	Substantial and impressive evidence of reliability and validity. Includes a briefer battery for older adults (ages 65–91).

Note: LHD, left hemisphere disorder; NBD, no brain damage; RHD, right hemisphere disorder.

[a]Some of these comments are based on the information compiled by Strauss et al. (2006) or entries in the *Buros Mental Measurement Yearbooks* (http://buros.unl.edu/buros/jsp/search.jsp).

[b]Original RBMT (Wilson, Cockburn, & Baddeley, 1985) available in various translations, including Dutch, German, Spanish, Chinese.

Table 17.10 Selected Measures of Various Aspects of Executive Functioning

Measure	Focus	Description	Other[a]
Behavior Rating Inventory of Executive Function–Adult Version (BRIEF-A; Roth, Isquith, & Gioia (2005)	Activity	Approximately 15-minute screen. Respondent and informant rate frequency of self-regulation behaviors in daily environment. Subscales: Inhibit, Shift, Emotional Control, Self-Monitor, Initiate, Working Memory, Plan/Organize, Task Monitor, Organization of Materials.	Strong norming procedure. Evidence of content, convergent, and discriminant validity (though often based on small samples). Moderate correlations self- and informant ratings. Extensive, strong evidence for internal consistency, test–retest, and interrater reliability.
Behavioral Assessment of the Dysexecutive Syndrome (BADS)[b] and Dysexecutive Questionnaire (DEX; Wilson, Alderman, Burgess, Emslie, & Evans, 1996)	Activity	Approximately 30-minute measure of organization, planning, self-monitoring, problem solving, impulsivity, inhibition, other executive functions. Aimed at predicting problems in everyday living. DEX comes with BADS. Twenty items assess changes in emotion, motivation, behavior, cognition. Two versions: Patient; Other rater.[c]	BADS: Construct, ecological, concurrent validity (with DEX). Poor internal consistency, good interrater reliability, low test–retest reliability (for small sample of NBD adults). Mixed patient sample; no severity information. Normative information incomplete. Some answers incorrect for North America; authors caution not to use Temporal Judgment task. DEX: Construct, concurrent validity (i.e., Other rater scores correlate with BADS total profile [but higher when for rehabilitation professionals than family]). No reliability data. No norms (problematic because NBD adults can present with "dysexecutive behavior"). Good internal consistency.
Hayling and Brixton Tests (Burgess & Shallice, 1997)	Impairment, Activity	Five-minute tests: Response inhibition (Hayling); Rule derivation and shifting (Brixton); Fluid ability (both). Brixton requires no verbal skill.	Hayling: Ecological, concurrent validity. Internal consistency variable for NBD, adequate for adults with frontal lesions. Adequate test–retest reliability for overall score and one response time score (but calculated for small NBD sample). No interrater reliability. Brixton: Concurrent validity. Internal consistency marginal (NBD adults). Adequate test–retest reliability (small NBD sample).
Naturalistic Action Test (Schwartz, Buxbaum, Ferraro, Veramonti, & Segal, 2003)	Activity	Observation of awareness and error correction in naturalistic action while patients perform tasks preparing buttered toast and coffee.	Normed on 100 stroke patients, 28 TBI patients, and 28 age-matched controls. Interrater reliability, internal consistency acceptable. Some evidence of test–retest reliability and of construct, concurrent criterion, and predictive validity. Results correlate with diminished attentional resource capacity, visuospatial impairments, and working memory.
Stroop Test[b] (e.g., Golden, 1978) or Victoria version (Regard, 1981)[d]	Impairment, Activity	Five-minute measure of goal maintenance, response inhibition.	Ecological, construct, concurrent, and predictive validity. Adequate test–retest reliability for interference score, though practice effects. Normative sample characteristics not clear for Golden version; better for Victoria version. Norms for older African Americans (Lucas et al., 2005). Low correlations among different versions of Stroop task.

Note: NBD, no brain damage.

[a]Some of these comments are based on the information compiled by Strauss et al. (2006) or entries in the *Buros Mental Measurement Yearbooks* (http://buros.unl.edu/jsp/search.jsp).

[b]Mueller and Dollaghan (2013) report inadequate diagnostic accuracy for this and many other executive function assessments.

[c]Patient versus other ratings may provide a measure of insight.

[d]Many other versions. Also, the Golden version has been translated into Spanish (Artiola i Fortuny, Romo, Heaton, & Pardee, 1999); the Victoria version to Cantonese (S. S. Lee, 2003).

A few final notes are in order about executive function screening. First, the potential contribution of neglect must be considered in interpreting commonly recommended indices of planning and execution, such as observing the use of space in construction, drawing, or copying tasks. Second, clinicians often screen for problem-solving deficits by presenting patients with hypothetical problems and asking how the patients would solve them. There are two main difficulties with such measures: They do not necessarily reflect patients' daily life problems, and they may yield a knowing versus doing dissociation. Such tasks may provide a window into a patient's suitability for treatments that involves metacognitive instruction. Whether or not patients can perform such tasks, assessment time should be spent identifying daily life problems that are causing difficulty or that may do so in the future and implementing behavioral observations to analyze these problems (e.g., their antecedents and consequents, other potential environmental contributions or obstacles, potential cognitive sources). The forms in Appendices 17A and 17B may provide useful information relative to everyday problems and needs.

Table 17.11 lists additional informal cognitive communication measures, including some potential simulations. The metalinguistic quality of many of these tasks should be kept in mind.

Making a Diagnosis

Diagnosis first involves determining whether patients' presentations are abnormal rather than premorbid, and, if so, how severely impaired. In the Case Illustration, for example, E.A.'s "vision problems" clearly were not premorbid, so the clinician documented them and provided a severity estimate (i.e., "moderate cognitive–communicative disorder characterized by moderate-severe viewer-centered spatial neglect and moderate neglect dyslexia"). Another issue in differential diagnosis for adults with RHD is to identify whether patients' profiles are more consistent with multiple or diffuse lesions commonly associated with certain neurologically deteriorating conditions. This distinction affects the determination of candidacy for treatment, the nature of prognostic statements and long-term goals, and most likely, the focus of treatment.

Formulating Initial Prognosis and Treatment Focus

Prognostic statements should address the question: "Prognosis for what?" Some possible answers are as follows: to be a rehabilitation candidate after discharge from acute care; to tolerate formal treatment; to make meaningful improvement on specified outcome measures after a period of treatment; or to function competently in the social environment.

There is little information to guide prognosis in RHD. The studies that associate neglect with poor outcome typically focus on physical outcomes or eventual placements. Poorer discourse comprehension has been linked to neglect in some of our studies, as well as to lower estimated attentional or working memory capacity in the absence of neglect. The presence (versus absence) of communicative disorders in RHD also seems to be associated with lower education, familial left-handedness, cortical (rather than subcortical) lesions, and anosognosia (Joanette et al., 1990). It is possible that some of the pragmatic/social interactional behaviors noted after RHD may interact with sex because women may be more attuned to social and emotional cues than men Cautious extrapolation from the aphasia literature suggests that initial severity of impairment may be an important predictor of eventual outcome in the impairment domain of functioning. Outcomes in the activity or participation domains may not be predicted very well by impairment-level measures (Tompkins et al., 1998).

FUTURE DIRECTIONS

Much remains to be done in this fascinating area of communication and cognition. Readers of this chapter will have noted several gaps, many of which are the result of the relatively recent attention given to RHD cognitive–communicative disorders. We identify three major future directions. First, we envision arriving at a good definition of these disorders, one that describes both exclusion and inclusion criteria, the potential bases of common deficits, and given this population's tremendous heterogeneity, factors that may affect the expression or nature of deficits in individual subsets of patients. Such a definition would lead to better impairment-level tests and measures, prognostic statements, and one hopes, treatment approaches. Second, we predict fuller information about cognitive–communicative abilities in RHD. For example, prospective memory, or remembering to do things in the future, has not yet been studied in RHD. Neither has acquisition of procedural memories, which may underlie the learning of new habits in treatment. Third, we foresee the development of better activity- and participation-level measures. A promising future approach involves selecting questions from a repository like the Communicative Participation Item Bank (Baylor, Yorkston, Eadie, Miller, & Amtmann, 2009) after it has been further validated for relevant populations and, someday, administering these questions via computer-adjusted testing, which will allow response-contingent follow-up.

Table 17.11 Other Potential Informal Measures for Cognitive–Communicative Deficits

---

Discourse and Pragmatics

Discourse Production

Sentential measures (e.g., average utterance length, number of incomplete utterances); semantic measures such as organization of content (e.g., includes elements appropriate to genre), quantity of content (e.g., sufficient, redundant), problems of content (accuracy of propositions, clarity of reference), inappropriate content (e.g., irrelevancies, personal/excessive).

Topic analysis (Hartley, 1995)—positive/negative conversational discourse/topic skills.

Discourse Comprehension (Many of these can also be assessed for Discourse Production.)

Number, accuracy, completeness of propositions recalled (explicit, inferred from text or general knowledge), including core or essential (state key elements underlying inferred propositions, e.g., relational cues needed to establish theme, plot, story resolution); optional; local (closely related to a specific proposition in the text); global (evaluate, summarize, or otherwise augment the text); self-generated (e.g., number of intrusions on story retell).

Contrast performance when text is internally consistent versus when it has inconsistencies; supplement recall with cues or choice recognition tasks; assess ease or difficulty of inference generation/revision using barrier tasks or, in any task, varying availability of inference-supporting information from text/general knowledge (via, e.g., manipulating prior themes, distance between inference-supporting elements, presence of intervening first-mention nouns/propositions between inference-supporting elements, provision/representation of key elements; perspective patient is asked to adopt when interpreting a text).

Ambiguity, Inference, and Metaphor

Test of Language Competence–Expanded Edition (Wiig & Secord, 1989): Comprehend lexical/syntactic ambiguity in sentences, alternative inferences, metaphors. Developed for adolescents; some data for NBD adults (Murray, 2002).

Emotion and Nonverbal Communication

Florida Affect Battery (Blonder, Bowers, & Heilman, 1991): Identify/discriminate five emotions conveyed via face and prosody.

New York Emotion Battery (Borod, Welkowitz, & Obler, 1992): Pose/spontaneously express, identify/discriminate eight emotions; has screening and nonemotional control tasks. Low test–retest reliability for RHD (Zgaljardic, Borod, & Sliwinski, 2002).

The Awareness of Social Inference Test (TASIT)[a]: Emotion Evaluation (McDonald, Flanagan, Rollins, & Kinch, 2003): Recognize specific emotions conveyed in audiovisual vignettes.

TASIT[a]: Social Inferences (McDonald et al., 2003): Interpret paralinguistic cues that indicate sincerity, sarcasm, or lying. Vignettes with or without added context.

Figurative Meanings

Familiar and Novel Language Comprehension Protocol (Kempler & Van Lancker, 1986): Identify pictures that represent familiar phrases (e.g., idioms, proverbs).

Sensitivity to Listener and Environment

Listening Behaviors Checklist (Hartley, 1995): Conversations, group activities rated for frequency of, for example, planning what to say rather than listening, providing nonverbal indications of understanding, responding appropriately to speaker's intent.

Discourse and Pragmatics

Social Comprehension and Judgment screening test (Sohlberg & Mateer, 1989): Explain reasons, actions, consequences, social appropriateness when asked open-ended questions about social situations.

TASIT[a]: Social Inferences, as above.

Other Pragmatics

Social Skills Checklist (Hartley, 1995): Addresses rituals, requesting/giving information, controlling (e.g., giving directions, inviting friends, offering something), sharing feelings.

(continues)

Table 17.11 Other Potential Informal Measures for Cognitive–Communicative Deficits

Discourse and Pragmatics

Lexical–Semantic Processing

The Word Test 2: Adolescent (Bowers, Huisingh, LoGiudice, & Orman, 2005): Generate synonyms, antonyms, definitions, multiple meanings.

Cookie Theft picture description: Literal and Interpretive concepts (Myers, 1979).

Variables That May Affect Performance

Single word: for example, word frequency, familiarity, concreteness

Sentence level: for example, semantic redundancy, inferential complexity, syntactic complexity

Discourse level: for example, salience (main idea versus detail); explicitness (directly versus indirectly stated); semantic redundancy; thematic consistency; clarity/ambiguity of picture stimuli; etc.

Simulations and Observations of Everyday Communicative Activities

Watch a video and ask patient to summarize for someone who comes in later (narrative production [macrostructure]; emotion; sustained attention; memory [encoding visual information]; executive function [EF]—planning, organization).

Feign misplacement of keys; ask patient where you might look (EF—identifying alternatives).

Feign strong concern/sadness; observe patient's response (social communication; interpretation of prosody/emotion).

Misstate name of patient's wife (social communication; EF—self-directing and initiating).

Hand patient a broken pencil to use; observe response (EF—self-directing and initiating).

Have someone new in the treatment room when patients arrive; see if patients introduce themselves (social discourse; EF—initiating).

Set up phone calls to schedule appointments or talk to grandchildren (discourse production scripts [genres]).

Have a conversation or treatment activity interrupted by a phone call (focused attention).

Play a card game such as blackjack or Go Fish, where patient has to initiate communication (EF—initiating, rule following).

Ask patient to get ticket or schedule information or to read a newspaper to find sports scores or information about sales, etc. (memory—for task goal, strategies to record the information; EF—organization, self-directing and initiating).

Observe initiation, style, appropriateness of communication during lunch, coffee break.

[a]Developed for, and initially validated with, traumatic brain injury (TBI); sensitive to severe impairment.

Case Illustration 17.1

E.A. was a 62-year-old man who ran his own landscaping business with his son-in-law. He was referred to us 10 days postonset of RH stroke, with a stated goal of returning to work as soon as possible. Before we met with E.A., we sent several forms and a questionnaire to his wife and daughter, requesting that they complete them as best they were able and bring them to our first meeting. A review of the forms (Case History Supplement, Appendix 17A; Performance Inventory, Appendix 17B) suggested some concerns for E.A.'s safety (crossing street and taking medications safely as a result of "vision problems," reported by daughter only) and potential problems with social communication or executive functioning (going off topic, lacking "manners" in some situations, losing track of mail). Responses to the Dysexecutive Questionnaire (Table 17.10) further suggested some impulsivity, lack of planning, disinhibition, and lack of concern. E.A. had not yet gone back to some of his premorbid activities, such as budgeting, doing outdoor chores, or playing poker with his buddies.

We engaged E.A. in conversation about his goals, his business, and what had happened to him and noted that social conventions and other aspects of pragmatics were mostly appropriate in this context. We recorded this conversation

(continues)

and rated it using the discourse analysis rating from the Right Hemisphere Language Battery–2 (see Table 17.4) and noted primarily a reduction in sentence stress and intonation. E.A. also exhibited a potential reduction in questioning; potentially overly long utterances and some wandering from the point that did not make an unfavorable impression; and occasional responses suggesting that he missed the point but usually with a logical digression.

To pinpoint the nature of the reported "vision problems," we did an informal screen for neglect that included asking E.A. to read aloud a sentence that remained semantically plausible when the first two words were removed. He omitted those two words. Performance was unchanged when another sentence was moved into his right visual field. Also, when asked to write his name, E.A. crowded it into the right half of the page. Accordingly, we assessed him more fully for neglect and for its implications for reading, writing, and drawing tasks that were important in his daily life. Testing suggested that E.A. had a moderate-severe viewer-centered extrapersonal spatial neglect and neglect dyslexia. The spatial neglect was evident in left-sided errors on the Gap Detection task (see Table 17.7); left-sided omissions on the Coin Sorting, Card Sorting, and Map Navigation subtests of the RBIT (Table 17.7) and in copying a sketch for a garden redesign project that we had asked his wife to bring; and impairments in determining which of two poker hands was a winner (two sets of five cards each were displayed on the table, one set above the other, and E.A. told us we were missing a card in the lower set). The neglect dyslexia was reflected in difficulty reading the left side of four-plus-digit numbers, single words, phrases, and sentences, singly and in discourse, as evidenced in informal testing (reading notations on the garden design sketch) and omissions on the Menu Reading, Article Reading, and Address and Sentence Copying subtests of the RBIT. The patient appeared to lack awareness of these difficulties: He did not express frustration or concern or attempt self-correction.

We assessed E.A.'s reading comprehension with the reading version of the Discourse Comprehension Test (DCT; Table 17.5). Performance was three standard deviations below the mean for non–brain-damaged individuals, incommensurate with his college degree and premorbid occupation. His neglect dyslexia seemed to account for much of this apparent deficit because his performance on auditory subtests was only one standard deviation below the mean. E.A.'s daughter wrote on her response forms that for her entire life, her father often "seems to have his head in the clouds," and he did not seem too different to her in that respect. We took this into account in interpreting E.A.'s occasionally distractible test performance and interactions with others, where he sometimes seemed to drift away, and indicated in E.A.'s chart the potential role of his premorbid function in such behaviors.

We aimed to untangle the nature of discourse comprehension deficits by attempting to improve the encoding of information in two ways. First, we used text material relevant to E.A.'s interests: a DCT-length paragraph we composed from material in the *Occupational Outlook Handbook* (Bureau of Labor Statistics, 2010) that described the training and education requirements and job prospects for a landscape architect, printed in the same font as the DCT passages. Second, we provided additional DCT passages in a larger, bold font to improve the perceptual salience of the information. E.A. did better on comprehension questions with the relevant material, but the font manipulation made no difference. This highlighted an important strength in E.A.'s access to and application of top-down knowledge in comprehension. It left unanswered the question of whether perceptual encoding affected his reading comprehension because perceptual encoding may not have been manipulated in the most beneficial way or the influence of perceptual factors may have been masked by E.A.'s neglect. E.A.'s clinician suspected other environmental contributions to his daily life comprehension, in that his wife spoke very rapidly and did not view him as having changed much.

In light of the daughter's concerns about reading and understanding medicine labels, we administered the appropriate subtest from the Assessment of Language-Related Functional Activities (Table 17.5). E.A.'s performance was indeed deficient on this task, and we counseled his wife to oversee his medication use.

STUDY QUESTIONS

1. What do you see as the two most significant unmet needs in the assessment of RHD cognitive–communicative disorders? What needs to be done first to address each of these? Could you begin to address them with your clients? Why or why not? And how?

2. Consider the initial evaluation process for RHD cognitive–communicative disorders. Which part(s) of the process have you had the most exposure to in your classes, readings, or clinical experience? Which part(s) have you had the least exposure to?

3. In what ways is assessment like a research project?

4. What are three ways in which assessment goes beyond "tests"?

5. Choose any three items from the appendices. For each item, what are two different ways you could use the information in the assessment process?

6. Choose three different individuals you communicate with on a regular basis (e.g., spouse, best friend, coworker, pastor). What are some of the ways you adjust your communication with these individuals? Consider the same question with relation to different environments or settings, rather than people, and again with relation to different purposes for communication.

7. Clinically, it is always important to think "What else could have caused this behavior/performance?" Choose three specific communicative or cognitive behaviors/performances and pose three potential reasons why a patient could exhibit each. Make two of these three reasons be potential underlying deficits and one be something outside the patient.

8. Choose any three of the objectives listed at the beginning of this chapter and read the chapter so that you can achieve them. To challenge yourself even further, read to achieve five or all of these outcomes.

REFERENCES

Alderman, N., Burgess, P. W., Knight, C., & Henman, C. (2003). Ecological validity of a simplified version of the Multiple Errands Shopping Test. *Journal of the International Neuropsychological Society, 9*(1), 31–44.

Alves, N. T., Aznar-Casanova, J. A., & Fukusima, S. S. (2009). Patterns of brain asymmetry in the perception of positive and negative facial expressions. *Laterality: Asymmetries of Body, Brain and Cognition, 14*(3), 256–272.

Ardila, A., & Rosselli, M. (1993). Spatial agraphia. *Brain and Cognition, 22*(2), 137–147.

Artiola i Fortuny, L., Romo, D. H., Heaton, R. K., & Pardee, R. E. (1999). *Manual de normas y procedimientos para la bateria neuropsicologica en espanol.* Lisse, the Netherlands: Swets & Zeitlinger.

Azouvi, P., Bartolomeo, P., Beis, J., Perennou, D., Pradat-Diehl, P., & Rousseaux, M. (2006). A battery of tests for the quantitative assessment of unilateral neglect. *Restorative Neurology and Neuroscience, 24*(4–6), 273–285.

Azouvi, P., Marchal, F., Samuel, C., Morin, L., Renard, C., Louis-Dreyfus, A., et al. (1996). Functional consequences and awareness of unilateral neglect: Study of an evaluation scale. *Neuropsychological Rehabilitation, 6*(2), 133–150.

Azouvi, P., Olivier, S., de Montety, G., Samuel, C., Louis-Dreyfus, A., & Tesio, L. (2003). Behavioral assessment of unilateral neglect: Study of the psychometric properties of the Catherine Bergego Scale. *Archives of Physical Medicine and Rehabilitation, 84*(1), 51–57.

Baines, K. A., Heeringa, H. M., & Martin, A. (1999). *Assessment of Language-Related Functional Activities.* Austin, TX: Pro-Ed.

Baylor, C. R., Yorkston, K. M., Eadie, T. L., Miller, R. M., & Amtmann, D. (2009). Developing the communicative participation item bank: Rasch analysis results from a spasmodic dysphonia sample. *Journal of Speech, Language and Hearing Research, 52*(5), 1302–1320.

Bedny, M., McGill, M., & Thompson-Schill, S. L. (2008). Semantic adaptation and competition during word comprehension. *Cerebral Cortex, 18*, 2574–2585.

Beeman, M. (1993). Semantic processing in the right hemisphere may contribute to drawing inferences from discourse. *Brain and Language, 44*(1), 80–120.

Beeman, M. (1998). Coarse semantic coding and discourse comprehension. In M. Beeman & C. Chiarello (Eds.), *Right hemisphere language comprehension: Perspectives from cognitive neuroscience* (pp. 255–284). Mahwah, NJ: Erlbaum.

Beeman, M. J., Bowden, E. M., & Gernsbacher, M. A. (2000). Right and left hemisphere cooperation for drawing predictive and coherence inferences during normal story comprehension. *Brain and Language, 71*(2), 310–336.

Benton, A. L., Sivan, A. B., Hamsher, K., Varney, N. R., & Spreen, O. (1994). Judgment of line orientation. In *Contributions to neuropsychological assessment: A clinical manual* (2nd ed., pp. 53–64). New York, NY: Oxford University Press.

Benton, A. L., & Van Allen, M. W. (1968). Impairment in facial recognition in patients with cerebral disease. *Transactions of the American Neurological Association, 93*, 38–42.

Beschin, N., & Robertson, I. (1997). Personal versus extrapersonal neglect: A group study of their dissociation using a reliable clinical test. *Cortex, 33*(2), 379–384.

Besharati, S., Crucianelli, L., & Fotopoulou, A. (2014). Restoring awareness: A review of rehabilitation in anosognosia for hemiplegia. *Revista Chilena de Neuropsicologia, 9*(1), 31–37.

Bickerton, W.-L., Demeyere, N., Francis, D., Kumar, V., Remoundou, M., Balani, et al. (2014). The BCoS cognitive profile screen: Utility and predictive value for stroke. *Neuropsychology.* http://dx.doi.org/10.1037/neu0000160

Bihrle, A. M., Brownell, H. H., & Gardner, H. (1988). Humor and the right hemisphere: A narrative perspective. In H. A. Whitaker (Ed.), *Contemporary reviews in neuropsychology* (pp. 109–126). New York, NY: Springer-Verlag.

Bilenko, N. Y., Grindrod, C. M., Myers, E. B., & Blumstein, S. E. (2008). Neural correlates of semantic competition during processing of ambiguous words. *Journal of Cognitive Neuroscience, 21*, 960–975.

Blake, M. L. (2007). Perspectives on treatment for communication deficits associated with right hemisphere brain damage. *American Journal of Speech-Language Pathology, 16*(4), 331–342.

Blake, M. L., & Lesniewicz, K. (2005). Contextual bias and predictive inferencing in adults with and without right hemisphere brain damage. *Aphasiology, 19*(3–5), 423–434.

Blake, M. L., Tompkins, C. A., Scharp, V. L., Meigh, K. M., & Wambaugh, J. L. (2015). Contextual Constraint Treatment for coarse coding deficit in adults with right hemisphere brain damage: Generalization to narrative discourse comprehension. *Neurpsychological Rehabilitation, 25*(1), 15–52.

Blonder, L. X., Bowers, D., & Heilman, K. M. (1991). The role of the right hemisphere in emotional communication. *Brain, 1149*(3), 1115–1127.

Bonello, P. J., Rapport, L. J., & Millis, S. R. (1997). Psychometric properties of the visual object and space perception battery in normal older adults. *Clinical Neuropsychologist, 11*(4), 436–442.

Borod, J. C., Welkowitz, J., & Obler, L. K. (1992). *The New York Emotion Battery.* Unpublished materials, Department of Neurology, Mount Sinai Medical Center, New York, NY.

Bottini, G., Corcoran, R., Sterzi, R., Paulesu, E., Schenone, P., Scarpa, P., et al. (1994). The role of the right hemisphere in the interpretation of figurative aspects of language: A positron emission tomography activation study. *Brain, 117*(6), 1241–1253.

Bouaffre, S., & Faita-Ainseba, F. (2007). Hemispheric differences in the time-course of semantic priming processes: Evidence from event-related potentials (ERPs). *Brain and Cognition, 63*(2), 123–135.

Bowers, L., Huisingh, R., LoGiudice, C., & Orman, J. (2005). *The WORD Test 2: Adolescent.* East Moline, IL: LinguiSystems.

Boyd, T. M., & Sautter, S. W. (1985). Route-finding: A measure of everyday executive functioning in the head-injured adult. *Applied Cognitive Psychology, 7*(2), 171–181.

Braun, A. R., Guillemin, A., Hosey, L., & Varga, M. (2001). The neural organization of discourse: An H215O-PET study of narrative discourse production in English and American sign language. *Brain, 124,* 2028–2044.

Brookshire, R. H., & Nicholas, L. E. (1993). *Discourse Comprehension Test (DCT).* Tucson, AZ: Communication Skill Builders.

Brookshire, R. H., & Nicholas, L. E. (1997). *Discourse Comprehension Test (2nd ed).* http://www.picaprograms.com/discourse_comprehension_test.htm.

Brownell, H., & Martino, G. (1998). Deficits in inference and social cognition: The effects of right hemisphere brain damage on discourse. In M. Beeman & C. Chiarello (Eds.), *Right hemisphere language comprehension: Perspectives from cognitive neuroscience* (pp. 309–328). Mahwah, NJ: Erlbaum.

Brownell, H. H., Simpson, T. L., Bihrle, A. M., Potter, H. H., & Gardner, H. (1990). Appreciation of metaphoric alternative word meanings by left and right brain-damaged patients. *Neuropsychologia, 28*(4), 375–383.

Bryan, K. L. (1994). *The Right Hemisphere Language Battery* (2nd ed.). London, UK: Whurr.

Bureau of Labor Statistics. (2010). *Occupational outlook handbook, 2010–11 edition.* Retrieved from http://www.bls.gov/OCO

Burgess, P. W., & Shallice, T. (1997). *The Hayling and Brixton tests.* Thurston, UK: Thames Valley Test Company.

Burns, M. S. (1997). *Burns Brief Inventory of Communication and Cognition.* San Antonio, TX: Psychological Corporation.

Buros Institute of Mental Measurements. (2101). *Buros mental measurements yearbooks.* Retrieved from https://www.ebscohost.com/academic/mental-measurements-yearbook

Butter, C. M., Mark, V. W., & Heilman, K. M. (1988). An experimental analysis of factors underlying neglect in line bisection. *Journal of Neurology, Neurosurgery, and Psychiatry, 51*(12), 1581–1583.

Calamia, M., Markon, K., Denburg, N. L., & Tranel, D. (2011). Developing a short form of Benton's Judgment of Line Orientation Test: An item response theory approach. *The Clinical Neuropsychologist, 25,* 670–684.

Cantagallo, A., & Zoccolotti, P. (1998). *Il Test dell'Attenzione nella vita Quotidiana (T.A.Q.): Il contributo alla standardizzazione italiana.* [A contribution on the Italian standardization of the Test of Everyday Attention.] *Rassegna di Psicologia, 15*(3), 137–157.

Canty, A. L., Fleming, J., Patterson, F., Green, H. J., Man, D., & Shum, D. H. (2014). Evaluation of a virtual reality prospective memory task for use with individuals with severe traumatic brain injury. *Neuropsychological Rehabilitation, 24,* 238–265.

Chan, R. C., Hoosain, R., & Lee, T. (2002). Reliability and validity of the Cantonese version of the test of everyday attention among normal Hong Kong Chinese: A preliminary report. *Clinical Rehabilitation, 16*(8), 900–909.

Chantraine, Y., Joanette, Y., & Ska, B. (1998). Conversational abilities in patients with right hemisphere damage. *Journal of Neurolinguistics, 11*(1–2), 21–32.

Cheang, H. S., & Pell, M. D. (2006). A study of humour and communicative intention following right hemisphere stroke. *Clinical Linguistics and Phonetics, 20*(6), 447–462.

Chechlacz, M., Rotshtein, P., Roberts, K. L., Bickerton W.-L., Lau, J. K. L., & Humphreys, G. W. (2012). The prognosis of allocentric and egocentric neglect: Evidence from clinical scans. *PLoS ONE, 7*(11): e47821. doi:10.1371/journal.pone.0047821

Crawford, J. R., Sommerville, J., & Robertson, I. H. (1997). Assessing the reliability and abnormality of subtest differences on the Test of Everyday Attention. *British Journal of Clinical Psychology, 36,* 609–617.

Cummings, L. (2005). *Pragmatics: A multidisciplinary perspective.* Edinburgh, Scotland: Edinburgh University Press.

Cummings, L. (2007). Pragmatics and adult language disorders: Past achievements and future directions. *Seminars in Speech and Language, 28*(2), 96–110.

Doyle, P. J., McNeil, M. R., Bost, J. E., Ross, K. B., Wambaugh, J. L., Hula, W. D., et al. (2007). The Burden of Stroke Scale (BOSS) provided valid, reliable, and responsive score estimates of functioning and well-being during the first year of recovery from stroke. *Quality of Life Research: An International Journal of Quality of Life Aspects of Treatment, Care and Rehabilitation, 16*(8), 1389–1398.

Doyle, P. J., McNeil, M. R., & Hula, W. D. (2003). The Burden of Stroke Scale (BOSS): Validating patient-reported communication difficulty and associated psychological distress in stroke survivors. *Aphasiology, 17*(3), 291–304.

Doyle, P. J., McNeil, M. R., Mikolic, J. M., Prieto, L., Hula, W. D., Lustig, A. P., et al. (2004). The Burden of Stroke Scale (BOSS) provides valid and reliable score estimates of functioning and well-being in stroke survivors with and without communication disorders. *Journal of Clinical Epidemiology, 57*(10), 997–1007.

Edgeworth, J. A., Robertson, I. H., & McMillan, T. M. (1998). *Balloons Test.* Bury St. Edmunds, UK: Thames Valley.

Faust, M. E., & Gernsbacher, M. A. (1996). Cerebral mechanisms for suppression of inappropriate information during sentence comprehension. *Brain and Language, 53*(2), 234–259.

Fleming, J. M., Strong, J., & Ashton, R. (1996). Self-awareness of deficits in adults with traumatic brain injury: How best to measure? *Brain Injury, 10*(1), 1–16.

Fonseca, R. P., Joanette, Y., Côté, H., Ska, B., Giroux, F., Fachel, J. M. G., et al. (2008). Brazilian version of the Protocole Montréal d'Evaluation de la Communication (Protocole MEC): Normative and reliability data. *Spanish Journal of Psychology, 11*(2), 678–688.

Forgács, B., Bohrn, I., Baudewig, J., Hofmann, M. J., Pléh, C., & Jacobs, A. M. (2012). Neural correlates of combinatorial semantic processing of literal and figurative noun noun compound words. *NeuroImage, 63*(3), 1432–1442.

Fox, M. D., Corbetta, M., Snyder, A. Z., Vincent, J. L., & Raichle, M. E. (2006). Spontaneous neuronal activity distinguishes human dorsal and ventral attention systems. *Proceedings of the National Academy of Sciences of the United States of America, 103*, 10046–10051.

Frattali, C. M., Thompson, C., Holland, A., Wohl, A., & Ferketic, M. (1995). *American Speech-Language-Hearing Association Functional Assessment of Communication Skills for Adults.* Rockville, MD: ASHA.

Frederiksen, C. H., Bracewell, R. J., Breuleux, A., & Renaud, A. (1990). The cognitive representation and processing of discourse: Function and dysfunction. In Y. Joanette & H. H. Brownell (Eds.), *Discourse ability and brain damage: Theoretical and empirical Perspectives* (pp. 19–44). New York, NY: Springer-Verlag.

French, B. F., Gotch, C. M., & Linck, J. (2014). Review of the Repeatable Battery for the Assessment of Neuropsychological Status update. Retrieved from Mental Measurements Yearbook, Volume 19..

Friehe, M., & Schultz, J. (2003). Performance of non-brain injured adults on the Ross Information Processing Assessment-2. *Journal of Medical Speech-Language Pathology, 11*(3), 147–156.

Gauthier, L., Dehaut, F., & Joanette, Y. (1989). The Bells Test: A quantitative and qualitative test for visual neglect. *International Journal of Clinical Neuropsychology, 11*(2), 49–54.

Gerber, S., & Gurland, G. (1989). Applied pragmatics in the assessment of aphasia. *Seminars in Speech and Language, 10,* 263–281.

Gernsbacher, M. A. (1990). *Language comprehension as structure building.* Hillsdale, NJ: Erlbaum.

Gialanella, B., Monguzzi, V., Santoro, R., & Rocchi, S. (2005). Functional recovery after hemiplegia in patients with neglect. *Stroke, 36,* 2687–2690.

Gillespie, D., Bowen, A., & Foster, J. (2006). Memory impairment following right hemisphere stroke: A comparative meta-analytic and narrative review. *Clinical Neuropsychologist; Neuropsychology, Development and Cognition, 20*(1), 59–75.

Glocker, D., Bittl, P., & Kerkhoff, G. (2006). Construction and psychometric properties of a novel test for body representational neglect (Vest Test). *Restorative Neurology and Neuroscience, 24*(4–6), 303–317.

Golden, C. J. (1978). *Stroop Color and Word Test: A manual for clinical and experimental uses.* Chicago, IL: Stoelting.

Goodglass, H., Kaplan, E., & Barresi, B. (2001). *Boston Diagnostic Aphasia Examination* (3rd ed.). Philadelphia, PA: Lippincott Williams & Wilkins.

Gouldthorp, B. (2014). Hemispheric differences in the processing of contextual information during language comprehension. *Laterality.* http://dx.doi.org/10.1080/13576 50X.2014.979194

Grindrod, C. M. (2012). Effects of left and right hemisphere damage on sensitivity to global context during lexical ambiguity resolution. *Aphasiology, 26*(7), 933–952.

Grindrod, C. M., Bilenko, N. Y., Myers, E. B., & Blumstein, S. E. (2008). The role of the left inferior frontal gyrus in implicit semantic competition and selection: An event-related fMRI study. *Brain Research, 1229,* 167–178.

Gronwall, D. M. A. (1977). Paced Auditory Serial Addition Task: A measure of recovery from concussion. *Perceptual and Motor Skills, 44,* 367–373.

Halper, A. S., Cherney, L. R., Burns, M. S., & Mogil, S. I. (1996). *Clinical management of right hemisphere dysfunction* (2nd ed.). Rockville, MD: Aspen.

Hamilton, R. H., Coslett, H. B., Buxbaum, J., Whyte, J., & Ferraro, M. K. (2008). Inconsistency of performance on neglect subtype tests following acute right hemisphere stroke. *Journal of the International Neuropsychological Society, 14*(1), 23–32.

Happé, F., Brownell, H., & Winner, E. (1999). Acquired "theory of mind" impairments following stroke. *Cognition, 3*(1), 211–240.

Harpaz, Y., Lavidor, M., & Goldstein, A. (2013). Right semantic modulation of early MEG components during ambiguity resolution. *NeuroImage, 82*(15), 107–114.

Hartley, L. L. (1995). *Cognitive-communicative abilities following brain injury: A functional approach.* San Diego, CA: Singular.

Hartman-Maier, A., & Katz, N. (1995). Validity of Behavioral Inattention Test (BIT): Relationships with functional tasks. *American Journal of Occupational Therapy, 49,* 507–516.

Heaton, R. K., Chelune, G. J., Talley, J. L., Kay, G. G., & Curtiss, G. (1993). *Wisconsin Card Sorting Test manual* (Rev. ed.). Los Angeles, CA: Western Psychological Services.

Heilman, K. H. (2009). Right hemispheric neurobehavioral syndromes. In J. Stein, R. L. Harvey, R. F. Macko, C. J. Winstein, & R. D. Zorowitz (Eds.), *Stroke recovery and rehabilitation* (pp. 201–212). New York, NY: Demos Medical.

Helm-Estabrooks, N. (2001). *Cognitive Linguistic Quick Test.* San Antonio, TX: Pearson.

Hillis, A. E., Newhart, M., Heidler, J., Marsh, E. B., Barker, P., & Degaonkar, M. (2005). The neglected role of the right hemisphere in spatial representation of words for reading. *Aphasiology, 19*(3/4/5), 225–238.

Hinckley, J. J. (2014). A case for implementation of cognitive-communication screenings in acute stroke. *American Journal of Speech-Language Pathology, 23,* 4–14.

Hird, K., & Kirsner, K. (2003). The effect of right cerebral hemisphere damage on collaborative planning in conversation: An analysis of intentional structure. *Clinical Linguistics & Phonetics, 17*(4&5), 309–315.

Holland, A. L., Frattali, C. M., & Fromm, D. (1999). *Communication activities of daily living* (2nd ed.). Austin, TX: Pro-Ed.

Hooper, H. E. (1958). *The Hooper Visual Organization Test manual.* Beverly Hills, CA: Western Psychological Services.

Hough, M. S., & Pierce, R. S. (1994). Pragmatics and treatment. In R. Chapey (Ed.), *Language intervention strategies in adult aphasia* (3rd ed., pp. 246–268). Baltimore, MD: Williams & Wilkins.

Humphreys, G. W., Bickerton, W.-L., Samson, D., & Riddoch, M. J. (2012). *Birmingham Cognitive Screen (BCoS).* Hove, UK: Psychology Press.

Hutchinson, J. B., Uncapher, M. R., & Wagner, A. D. (2009). Posterior parietal cortex and episodic retrieval: Convergent and divergent effects of attention and memory. *Learning & Memory, 16*(6), 343–356.

Jehkonen, M., Laihosalo, M., & Kettunen, J. (2006). Anosognosia after stroke: Assessment, occurrence, subtypes and impact on functional outcome reviewed. *Acta Neurologica Scandinavica, 114*(5), 293–306.

Joanette, Y., & Goulet, P. (1990). Narrative discourse in right-brain-damaged right-handers. In Y. Joanette & H. H. Brownell (Eds.), *Discourse ability and brain damage: Theoretical and empirical perspectives* (pp. 131–153). New York, NY: Springer-Verlag.

Joanette, Y., & Goulet, P. (1998). Right hemisphere and the semantic processing of words: Is the contribution specific or not? In E. Visch-Brink (Ed.), *Linguistic levels in aphasia* (pp. 19–34). San Diego, CA: Singular.

Joanette, Y., Goulet, P., & Hannequin, D. (1990). *Right hemisphere and verbal communication*. New York, NY: Springer-Verlag.

Joanette, Y., Ska, B., & Côté, H. (2004). *Protocole Montréal d' Évaluation de la Communication (Protocole MEC)*. Isbergues, France: Ortho-Edition.

Johns, C. L., Tooley, K., & Traxler, M. J. (2008). Discourse impairments following right hemisphere brain damage: A critical review. *Language and Linguistics Compass, 2*(6), 1038–1062.

Jovanovski, D., Zakzanis, K., Campbell, Z., Erb, S., & Nussbaum, D. (2012). Development of a novel, ecologically oriented virtual reality measure of executive function: The Multitasking in the City Test. *Applied Neuropsychology: Adult, 19*, 207–220.

Jung-Beeman, M. (2005). Bilateral brain processes for comprehending natural language. *Trends in Cognitive Sciences, 9*(11), 512–518.

Just, M. A., Carpenter, P. A., Keller, T. A., Eddy, W. F., & Thulborn, K. R. (2006). Brain activation modulated by sentence comprehension. *Science, 274*(5284), 114–116.

Kaplan, J. A., Brownell, H. H., Jacobs, J. R., & Gardner, H. (1990). The effects of right hemisphere damage on the pragmatic interpretation of conversational remarks. *Brain and Language, 38*(2), 315–333.

Keller, I., Schlenker, A., & Pigache, R. M. (1995). Selective impairment of auditory attention following closed head injuries or right cerebrovascular accidents. *Cognitive Brain Research, 3*(1), 9–15.

Kelly, M., McDonald, S., & Kellett, D. (2014). Development of a novel task for investigating decision making in a social context following traumatic brain injury. *Journal of Clinical and Experimental Neuropsychology, 36*, 897–913.

Kempler, D. Y., & Van Lancker, D. (1986). *The Familiar and Novel Language Comprehension Test (FANL-C)*. Unpublished protocol.

Kessels, R. P. C., van den Berg, E., Ruis, C., & Brands, A. (2008). The backward span of the Corsi Block-Tapping Task and its association with the WAIS-III digit span. *Assessment, 15*(4), 426–434.

Kessels, R. P. C., van Zandvoort, M. J. E., Postma, A., Kappelle, L. J., & de Haan, E. H. F. (2000). The Corsi Block-Tapping Task: Standardization and normative data. *Applied Neuropsychology, 7*(4), 252–258.

Klepousniotou, E., & Baum, S. R. (2005). Processing homonymy and polysemy: Effects of sentential context and time-course following unilateral brain damage. *Brain and Language, 95*(3), 365–382.

Klepousniotou, E., Gracco, V. L., & Pike, G. B. (2014). Pathways to lexical ambiguity: fMRI evidence for bilateral fronto-parietal involvement in language processing. *Brain and Language, 131*(1), 56–64.

Klepousniotou, E., Pike, G. B., Steinhauer, K., & Gracco, V. (2012). Not all ambiguous words are created equal: An EEG investigation of homonymy and polysemy. *Brain and Language, 123*(1), 11–21.

Klonoff, P. S., Sheperd, J. C., O'Brien, K. P., Chiapello, D. A., & Hodak, J. A. (1990). Rehabilitation and outcome of right-hemisphere stroke patients: Challenges to traditional diagnostic and treatment methods. *Neuropsychology, 4*(3), 147–163.

Knight, C., Alderman, N., & Burgess, P. W. (2002). Development of a simplified version of the Multiple Errands Test for use in hospital settings. *Neuropsychological Rehabilitation, 12*(3), 231–255.

Kuperberg, G. R., Lakshmanan, B. M., Caplan, D. N., & Holcomb, P. J. (2006). Making sense of discourse: An fMRI study of causal inferencing across sentences. *NeuroImage, 33*(1), 343–361.

Langer, S. L., Pettigrew, L. C., & Blonder, L. X. (1998). Observer liking of unilateral stroke patients. *Neuropsychiatry, Neuropsychology, and Behavioral Neurology, 11*(4), 218–224.

Lee, S. S., & Dapretto, M. (2006). Metaphorical vs. literal word meanings: fMRI evidence against a selective role of the right hemisphere. *NeuroImage, 29*, 536–544.

Lee, T. M. (2003). *Normative data: Neuropsychological measures for Hong Kong Chinese*. Hong Kong, China: University of Hong Kong Neuropsychology Laboratory.

Lehman, M. T., & Tompkins, C. A. (1998). Reliability and validity of an auditory working memory measure: Data from elderly and right-hemisphere damaged adults. *Aphasiology, 12*(7–8), 771–785.

Leibovitch, F. S., Vasquez, B. P., Ebert, P. L., Beresford, K. L., & Black, S. E. (2012). A short bedside battery for visuoconstructive hemispatial neglect: Sunnybrook neglect assessment procedure (SNAP). *Journal of Clinical and Experimental Neuropsychology, 34*, 359–368.

Leonard, C. L., & Baum, S. R. (2005). Research note: The ability of individuals with right-hemisphere damage to use context under conditions of focused and divided attention. *Journal of Neurolinguistics, 18*(6), 427–441.

Lezak, M. (1983). *Neuropsychological assessment*. New York, NY: Oxford University Press.

Lezak, M. D., Howieson, D. B., & Loring, D. W. (2004). *Neuropsychological Assessment* (4th ed.). New York, NY: Oxford University Press.

Lindell, A. B., Jalas, M., J., Tenovuo, O., Brunila, T., Voeten, M. J. M., & Hämäläinen, H. (2007). Clinical assessment of hemispatial neglect: Evaluation of different measures and dimensions. *Clinical Neuropsychologist: Neuropsychology, Development and Cognition, 21*(3), 479–497.

Lovseth, K., & Atchley, R. A. (2010). Examining lateralized semantic access using pictures. *Brain and Cognition, 72*(2), 202–209.

Lucas, J. A., Ivnik, R. J., Smith, G. E., Ferman, T. J., Willis, F. B, Petersen, R. C., et al. (2005). Mayo's older African Americans normative studies: Norms for Boston Naming Test, Wrat-3 Reading, Trail Making Test, Stroop Test, and Judgment of Line Orientation. *Clinical Neuropsychologist, 19*(2), 243–269.

Mason, R. A., & Just, M. A. (2007). Lexical ambiguity in sentence comprehension. *Brain Research, 1146*, 115–127.

MacDonald, S. (2005). *Functional Assessment of Verbal Reasoning and Executive Strategies*. Guelph, CA: CCD.

MacDonald, S., & Johnson, C. J. (2005). Assessment of subtle cognitive-communication deficits following acquired brain injury: A normative study of the Functional Assessment of Verbal Reasoning and Executive Strategies (FAVRES). *Brain Injury, 19*, 895–902.

MacGregor, L., Bouwsema, J., & Klepousniotou, E. (2015). Sustained meaning activation for polysemous but not homonymous words: Evidence from EEG. *Neuropsychologia, 68*(1), 126–138.

Mackenzie, C., Begg, T., Lees, K. R., & Brady, M. (1997). *Right hemisphere stroke: Incidence, severity and recovery of language.* Final report to the Stroke Association.

Man, D. W. K., Fleming, J., Hohaus, L., & Shum, D. (2011). Development of the Brief Assessment of Prospective Memory (BAPM) for use with traumatic brain injury populations. *Neuropsychological Rehabilitation, 21*, 884–898.

Marinkovic, K., Baldwin, S., Courtney, M. G., Witzel, T., Dale, A. M., & Halgren, E. (2011). Right hemisphere has the last laugh: Neural dynamics of joke appreciation. *Cognitive, Affective & Behavioral Neuroscience, 11*, 113–130. doi:10.3758/s13415-010-0017-7.

Markowitsch, H. J. (2008). Autobiographical memory: A biocultural relais between subject and environment. *European Archives of Psychiatry and Clinical Neuroscience, 258*(Suppl. 5), 98–103.

Marsh, E. B., & Hillis, A. E. (2008). Dissociation between egocentric and allocentric visuospatial and tactile neglect in acute stroke. *Cortex, 44*(9), 1215–1220.

Mashal, N., Faust, M., Hendler, T., & Jung-Beeman, M. (2007). An fMRI investigation of the neural correlates underlying the processing of novel metaphoric expressions. *Brain and Language, 100*(2), 115–126.

Mason, R. A., & Just, M. A. (2007). Lexical ambiguity in sentence comprehension. *Brain Research, 1146*, 115–127.

Mason, R. A., & Just, M. A. (2009). The role of the Theory-of-Mind cortical network in the comprehension of narratives. *Language and Linguistics Compass, 3*(1), 157–174.

Mattingley, J. B., Bradshaw, J. L., Bradshaw, J. A., & Nettleton, N. C. (1994). Residual rightward attentional bias after apparent recovery from right hemisphere damage. Implications for a multicomponent model of neglect. *Journal of Neurology, Neurosurgery and Psychiatry, 57*(5), 597–604.

McCue, M., Chase, S. L., Dowdy, C., Pramuka, M., Petrick, J., Aitken, S., et al. (1994). *Functional assessment of individuals with cognitive disabilities: A desk reference for rehabilitation.* Pittsburgh, PA: Center for Applied Neuropsychology.

McDonald, S., Flanagan, S., Rollins, J., & Kinch, J. (2003). TASIT: A new clinical tool for assessing social perception after traumatic brain injury. *Journal of Head Trauma Rehabilitation, 18*(3), 219–238.

McDowd, J. M., Filion, D. L., Pohl, P. S., Richards, L. G., & Stiers, W. (2003). Attentional abilities and functional outcomes following stroke. *Journals of Gerontology: Psychological Sciences and Social Sciences, 58*(1), 45–53.

Menon, A., & Korner-Bitensky, N. (2004). Evaluating unilateral spatial neglect post stroke: Working your way through the maze of assessment choices. *Topics in Stroke Rehabilitation, 11*(3), 41–66.

Merten, T. (2002). A short version of the Hooper Visual Organization Test: Development and validation. *Clinical Neuropsychologist, 16*, 136–144.

Meyer, A. M., & Federmeier, K. D. (2008). The divided visual world paradigm: Eye tracking reveals hemispheric asymmetries in lexical ambiguity resolution. *Brain Research, 1222*, 166–183.

Meyers, J. E., & Meyers, K. R. (1995). *Rey Complex Figure Test and Recognition Trial.* Odessa, FL: Psychological Assessment Resources.

Mioni, G., Rendell, P. G., Henry, J. D., Cantagallo, A., & Stablum, F. (2013). An investigation of prospective memory functions in people with traumatic brain injury using Virtual Week. *Journal of Clinical and Experimental Neuropsychology, 35*, 617–630.

Monetta, L., & Joanette, Y. (2003). The specificity of the contribution of the right hemisphere to verbal communication: The cognitive resources hypothesis. *Journal of Speech-Language Pathology, 11*(4), 203–211.

Mueller, J. A., & Dollaghan, C. A. (2013). A systematic review of assessments for identifying executive function impairment in adults with acquired brain injury. *Journal of Speech, Language, and Hearing Research, 56*, 1051–1064.

Murray, L. L. (2002). Cognitive distinctions between depression and early Alzheimer's disease in the elderly. *Aphasiology, 16*(4–6), 573–586.

Murteira, A., & Santos, M. E. (2013). Language processing in right hemisphere stroke patients: Response speed and quality. *Aphasiology, 27*(2), 145–156.

Myers, P. S. (1979). Profiles of communication deficits in patients with right cerebral hemisphere damage. In R. H. Brookshire (Ed.), *Clinical aphasiology: Conference proceedings* (pp. 38–46). Minneapolis, MN: BRK.

Myers, P. S. (2001). Toward a definition of RHD syndrome. *Aphasiology, 15*(10/11), 913–918.

Myers, P. S., & Brookshire, R. H. (1996). Effect of visual and inferential variables on scene descriptions by right-hemisphere-damaged and non-brain-damaged adults. *Journal of Speech and Hearing Research, 39*, 870–880.

Navarro, M.-D., Lloréns, R., Noé, E., Ferri, J., & Alcañiz, M. (2013). Validation of a low-cost virtual reality system for training street-crossing: A comparative study in healthy, neglected and non-neglected stroke individuals. *Neuropsychological Rehabilitation, 23*, 597–618.

Nicholas, L. E., & Brookshire, R. H. (1993a). A system for quantifying the informativeness and efficiency of the connected speech of adults with aphasia. *Journal of Speech and Hearing Research, 36*, 338–350.

Nicholas, L. E., & Brookshire, R. H. (1993b). A system for scoring main concepts in the discourse of non-brain-damaged and aphasic speakers. *Clinical Aphasiology, 21*, 87–99.

Ota, H., Fujii, T., Suzuki, K., Fukatsu, R., & Yamadori, A. (2001). Dissociation of body-centered and stimulus-centered representations in unilateral neglect. *Neurology, 57*, 2064–2069.

Paul, D., Frattali, C., Holland, A., Thompson, C., Caperton, C., & Slater, S. (2004). *Quality of Communication Life Scale (ASHA QCL).* Rockville, MD: American Speech-Language-Hearing Association.

Pell, M. D. (1999). The temporal organization of affective and non-affective speech in patients with right-hemisphere infarcts. *Cortex, 35*(4), 455–477.

Pell, M. D. (2006). Cerebral mechanisms for understanding emotional prosody in speech. *Brain and Language, 96*(2), 221–234.

Pimental, P. A., & Knight, J. A. (2000). *Mini Inventory of Right Brain Injury* (2nd ed.). Austin, TX: Pro-Ed.

Posner, M. I. (1994). Attention: The mechanisms of consciousness. *Proceedings of the National Academy of Sciences of the United States of America, 91*(16), 7398–7403.

Posner, M. I., & Petersen, S. E. (1990). The attention system of the human brain. *Annual Review of Neuroscience, 13,* 25–42.

Poulin, V., & McDermott, A. (2013). *Multiple Errands Test (MET).* http:// http://www.strokengine.ca/assess/met/.

Prutting, C. A., & Kirchner, D. M. (1987). A clinical appraisal of the pragmatic aspects of language. *Journal of Speech, Language, and Hearing Research, 52,* 105–119.

Qualls, C. E., Bliwise, N. G., & Stringer, A. Y. (2000). Short forms of the Benton Judgment of Line Orientation Test: Development and psychometric properties. *Archives of Clinical Neuropsychology, 15*(2), 159–163.

Rand, D., Rukan, S., Weiss, P. L., & Katz, N. (2009). Validation of the Virtual MET as an assessment tool for executive functions. *Neuropsychological Rehabilitation, 19*(4), 583–602.

Randolph, C. (2012). *Repeatable Battery for the Assessment of Neuropsychological Status Update.* San Antonio, TX: Pearson.

Regard, M. (1981). *Cognitive rigidity and flexibility: A neuropsychological study.* Unpublished doctoral dissertation, University of Victoria, Canada.

Renison, B., Ponsford, J., Testa, R., Richardson, B., & Brownfield, K (2012). The ecological and construct validity of a newly developed measure of executive function: The Virtual Library Task. *Journal of the International Neuropsychological Society, 18,* 440–450.

Ribeiro, A. F., Mansur, L. L., & Radanovic, M. (2015). Impairment of inferential abilities based on pictorial stimuli in patients with right-hemisphere damage. *Applied Neuropsychology: Adult.* doi:10.1080/23279095.2014.881367.

Robertson, I. H., Ward, T., Ridgeway, V., & Nimmo-Smith, I. (1994). *Test of Everyday Attention.* Bury St. Edmunds, UK: Thames Valley Test Company.

Rosenbek, J. C., Crucian, G. P., Leon, S. A., Hieber, B., Rodriguez, A. D., Holiway, B., et al. (2004). Novel treatments for expressive aprosodia: A phase I investigation of cognitive linguistic and imitative interventions. *Journal of the International Neuropsychological Society, 10*(5), 786–793.

Ross, D. G. (1986). *Ross Information Processing Assessment.* Austin, TX: Pro-Ed.

Ross, E. D., & Monnot, M. (2011). Affective prosody: What do comprehension errors tell us about hemispheric lateralization of emotions, sex and aging effects, and the role of cognitive appraisal. *Neuropsychologia, 49*(5), 866–877.

Ross-Swain, D. G. (1996). *Ross Information Processing Assessment: Examiner's manual* (2nd ed.). Austin, TX: Pro-Ed.

Roth, R. M., Isquith, P. K., & Gioia, G. A. (2005). *Behavior Rating Inventory of Executive Function-Adult version.* Lutz, FL: Psychological Assessment Resources.

Royle, J., & Lincoln, N. B. (2008). The Everyday Memory Questionnaire–Revised: Development of a 13 item scale. *Disability and Rehabilitation, 30*(2), 114–121.

Ruff, R. M., & Allen, C. C. (1992). *Ruff 2 & 7 Selective Attention Test professional manual.* Odessa, FL: Psychological Assessment Resources.

Scharp, V. L., & Tompkins, C. A. (2013). Suppression and narrative time shifts in adults with right-hemisphere brain damage. *American Journal of Speech-Language Pathology, 22,* S256–S267.

Scharp, V. L., Tompkins, C. A., & Blake, M.T. (2014, May-June). Frequency and co-occurrence of suppression and coarse coding deficits in right hemisphere brain damage. Presented at the Clinical Aphasiology Conference, St. Simons Island, GA.

Schenkenberg, T., Bradford, D. C., & Ajax, E. T. (1980). Line bisection and unilateral visual neglect in patients with neurologic impairment. *Neurology, 30*(5), 509–517.

Schretlen, D. (1997). *Brief Test of Attention professional manual.* Odessa, FL: Psychological Assessment Resources.

Schwartz, M. F., Buxbaum, L. J., Ferraro, M., Veramonti, T., & Segal, M. (2003). *Naturalistic Action Test.* Oxford, UK: Pearson Assessment.

Shallice, T., & Burgess, P. W. (1991). Deficits in strategy application following frontal lobe damage in man. *Brain, 114*(2), 727–741.

Sherratt, S., & Bryan, K. (2012). Discourse production after right brain damage: Gaining a comprehensive picture using a multi-level processing model. *Journal of Neurolinguistics, 25*(4), 213–239.

Sivan, A. B. (1992). *Benton Visual Retention Test* (5th ed.). San Antonio, TX: Psychological Corporation.

Smith, A. (1991). *Symbol Digit Modalities Test.* Los Angeles, CA: Western Psychological Services.

Sohlberg, M. M., & Mateer, C. A. (1989). *Introduction to cognitive rehabilitation: Theory and practice.* New York, NY: Guilford Press.

Spencer, R. J., Wendell, C. R., Giggey, P. P., Seliger, S. L, Katzel, L. I., & Waldstein, S. R. (2013). Judgment of Line Orientation: An examination of eight short forms. *Journal of Clinical and Experimental Neuropsychology, 35,* 160–166.

Strauss, E., Sherman, E. M. S., & Spreen, O. (2006). *A compendium of neuropsychological tests: Administration, norms, and commentary* (3rd ed.). Oxford, UK: Oxford University Press.

Thiel, C. M., Zilles, K., & Fink, G. R. (2004). Cerebral correlates of alerting, orienting and reorienting of visuospatial attention: An event-related fMRI study. *NeuroImage, 21*(1), 318–328.

Titone, D., Wingfield, A., Caplan, D., Waters, G., & Prentice, K. (2001). Memory and encoding of spoken discourse following right hemisphere damage: Evidence from the Auditory Moving Window (AMV) technique. *Brain and Language, 77*(1), 10–24.

Toglia, J. P. (1993). *Contextual Memory Test.* Tucson, AZ: Therapy Skill Builders.

Tompkins, C. A. (1995). *Right hemisphere communication disorders: Theory and management.* San Diego, CA: Singular.

Tompkins, C. A. (2008). Theoretical considerations for understanding "understanding" by adults with right hemisphere brain damage. *Perspectives on Neurophysiology and Neurogenic Speech and Language Disorders, 18,* 45–54.

Tompkins, C. A., & Baumgaertner, A. (1998). Clinical value of online measures for adults with right hemisphere brain damage. *American Journal of Speech-Language Pathology, 7*(1), 68–74.

Tompkins, C. A., Baumgaertner, A., Lehman, M. T., & Fassbinder, W. (2000). Mechanisms of discourse comprehension impairment after right hemisphere brain damage: Suppression in lexical ambiguity resolution. *Journal of Speech, Language, and Hearing Research, 43*(1), 62–78.

Tompkins, C. A., Blake, M. T., Scharp, V. L., Meigh, K. M., & Wambaugh, J. L. (2013, May-June). Implicit treatment of underlying comprehension processes improves narrative comprehension in right hemisphere brain damage. Presented at the Clinical Aphasiology Conference, Tucson, AZ.

Tompkins, C. A., Bloise, C. G. R., Timko, M. L., & Baumgaertner, A. (1994). Working memory and inference revision in brain damaged and normally aging adults. *Journal of Speech and Hearing Research, 37*(4), 896–912.

Tompkins, C. A., Fassbinder, W., Lehman-Blake, M. T., Baumgaertner, A., & Jayaram, N. (2004). Inference generation during text comprehension by adults with right hemisphere brain damage: Activation failure versus multiple activation. *Journal of Speech, Language, and Hearing Research, 47*(6), 1380–1395.

Tompkins, C. A., Fassbinder, W., Scharp, V. L., & Meigh, K. M. (2008). Activation and maintenance of peripheral semantic features of unambiguous words after right hemisphere brain damage in adults. *Aphasiology, 22*(2), 119–138.

Tompkins, C. A., Lehman, M. T., Wyatt, A. D., & Schulz, R. (1998). Functional outcome assessment of adults with right hemisphere brain damage. *Seminars in Speech and Language, 19*(3), 303–321.

Tompkins, C. A., Lehman-Blake, M. T., Baumgaertner, A., & Fassbinder, W. (2001). Mechanisms of discourse comprehension impairment after right hemisphere brain damage: Suppression in inferential ambiguity resolution. *Journal of Speech, Language, and Hearing Research, 44*(2), 400–415.

Tompkins, C. A., Lehman-Blake, M. T, Baumgaertner, A., & Fassbinder, W. (2002). Characterizing comprehension difficulties after right brain damage: Attentional demands of suppression function. *Aphasiology, 16*(4–6), 559–572.

Tompkins, C. A., Lei, C.-M., & Zezinka, A. (2015). The nature and implications of right hemisphere language disorders. In A. Hillis (Ed.), *Handbook of adult language disorders: Integrating cognitive neuropsychology, neurology, and rehabilitation* (2nd ed.). New York, NY: Psychology Press.

Tompkins, C. A., Scharp, V. L., Fassbinder, W., Meigh, K. M., & Armstrong, E. M. (2008). A different story on "theory of mind" deficit in adults with right hemisphere brain damage. *Aphasiology, 22*(1), 42–61.

Tompkins, C. A., Scharp, V. L., Meigh, K. M., Blake, M. L., & Wambaugh, J. L. (2012). Generalization of a novel, implicit treatment for coarse coding deficit in right hemisphere brain damage: A single subject experiment. *Aphasiology, 26*, 689–708.

Tompkins, C. A., Scharp, V. L., Meigh, K. M., & Fassbinder, W. (2008). Coarse coding and discourse comprehension in adults with right hemisphere brain damage. *Aphasiology, 22*(2), 204–223.

Ungerleider, L. G., & Haxby, J. V. (1994). "What" and "where" in the human brain. *Current Opinion in Neurobiology, 4*, 157–165.

Vanhalle, C., Lemieux, S., Joubert, S., Goulet, P., Ska, B., & Joanette, Y. (2000). Processing of speech acts by right hemisphere brain-damaged patients: An ecological approach. *Aphasiology, 14*(11), 1127–1142.

Warrington, E. K., & James, M. (1991). *The Visual Object and Space Perception Battery*. Bury St. Edmunds, UK: Thames Valley Test Company.

Wechsler, D. (2009). Wechsler Memory Scale (4th ed.). San Antonio, Tx: Pearson.

Weed, E., McGregor, W., Nielsen, J. F., Roepstorff, A., & Frith, U. (2010). Theory of Mind in adults with right hemisphere damage: What's the story? *Brain and Language, 113*(2), 65–72.

Weintraub, S., & Mesulam, M. M. (1988). Visual hemispatial inattention: Stimulus parameters and exploratory strategies. *Journal of Neurology, Neurosurgery, and Psychiatry, 51*, 1481–1488.

Whiting, S., Lincoln, N. B., Bhavnani, G., & Cockburn, J. (1985). *The Rivermead Perceptual Assessment Battery*. Windsor, UK: NFER.

Wiig, E. H., & Secord, W. (1989). *Test of Language Competence-Expanded*. San Antonio, TX: Psychological Corporation.

Wilson, B. A., Alderman, N., Burgess, P. W., Emslie, H., & Evans, J. J. (1996). *Behavioural Assessment of the Dysexecutive Syndrome (BADS)*. Bury St. Edmunds, UK: Thames Valley Test Company.

Wilson, B. A., Cockburn, J., & Baddeley, A. D. (1985). *The Rivermead Behavioral Memory Test*. Bury St. Edmunds, UK: Thames Valley Test Company.

Wilson, B. A., Cockburn, J. M., & Halligan, P. (1987). *Behavioural Inattention Test*. Bury St. Edmunds, UK: Thames Valley Test Company.

Wilson, B. A., Emslie, H., Foley, J., Shiel, A., Watson, P., Hawkins, K., et al. (2005). *The Cambridge Prospective Memory Test*. London, UK: Harcourt.

Wilson, B. A., Greenfield, E., Clare, L., Baddeley, A., Cockburn, J., Watson, P., et al. (2008). *The Rivermead Behavioural Memory Test–Third Edition (RBMT-3)*. London, UK: Pearson Assessment.

Wingenfeld, S. A., Holdwick, D. J., Davis, J. L., & Hunter, B. B. (1999). Normative data on computerized Paced Auditory Serial Addition Task performance. *Clinical Neuropsychologist, 13*(3), 268–273.

World Health Organization. (2001). *International classification of functioning, disability, and health: ICF*. Geneva, Switzerland: Author. Retrieved from http://www3.who.int/icf/icftemplate.cfm.

Xu, J., Kemeny, S., Park, G., Frattali, C., & Braun, A. (2005). Language in context: Emergent features of word, sentence, and narrative comprehension. *NeuroImage, 25*(3), 1002–1015.

Yang, Y., Tompkins, C. A., Prat, C. S., & Meigh, K. M. (in press. Voxel-based lesion symptom mapping of coarse coding and suppression deficits in right-hemisphere-damaged patients. *American Journal of Speech-Language Pathology*.

Youngjohn, J. R., Larrabee, G. J., & Crook, T. H. (1993). New adult age- and education-correction norms for the Benton Visual Retention Test. *Clinical Neuropsychologist, 7*, 155–160.

Zaidel, E., Kasher, A., Soroker, N., Batori, G., Giora, R., & Graves, D. (2000). Hemispheric contributions to pragmatics. *Brain & Cognition, 43*(1–3), 438–443.

Zakzanis, K. K., & Azarbehi, R. (2014). Introducing BRAIN*screen*: Web-based real-time examination and interpretation of cognitive function. *Applied Neuropsychology Adult, 21*(2), 77–86).

Zanini, S., Bryan, K., De Luca, G., & Bava, A. (2005). Italian Right Hemisphere Language Battery: The normative study. *Neurological Sciences, 26*(1), 13–25.

Zempleni, M. Z., Renken, R., Hoeks, J. C. J., Hoogduin, J. M., & Stowe, L. (2007). Semantic ambiguity processing in sentence context: Evidence from event-related fMRI. *NeuroImage, 34*, 1270–1279.

Zgaljardic, D. J., Borod, J. C., & Sliwinski, M. (2002). Emotional perception in unilateral stroke patients: Recovery, test stability, and interchannel relationships. *Applied Neuropsychology, 9*(3), 159–172.

Sample Case History Supplement Form

Case History Supplement

Respondent: _____ Date Completed: _____

Relationship to Patient: _____

Respondent's primary concerns and goals regarding communication (please list and rank; 1 = most important)

1.
2.
3.

Daily Surroundings (living/family environment)

Current Location:	Expected Future Location(s):	Notes: (Needs, supports, obstacles outside the patient; specify each)
☐ Home independent	☐	
☐ Home with assistance (e.g., cooking, cleaning, medications)	☐	☐
☐ Living with family member	☐	
☐ Group home environment	☐	
☐ Assisted living	☐	☐
☐ Inpatient rehabilitation facility	☐	
☐ Skilled nursing facility	☐	

Support Network:

	Contact/Phone Number:	Possible Role in Care:	Availability:
Spouse			
Child			
Sibling			
Other family member			
Home health aide/agency			
Nurse			
Therapist(s)			

What resources are available to assist recovery/facilitate future life participation? (For example, has help with medications, money, making appointments, emergency communication; socialization activities such as church groups, bridge club; friends to talk to, go out to dinner with, watch TV or a movie with, etc.)

Social Communication (please note and specify):

☐ Engages in casual conversation

☐ Initiates communication verbally/nonverbally

☐ Communication when TV/radio is on

☐ Manners appropriate for context

☐ Understands "hints" from others

☐ Understands others' emotions

☐ Stays on conversation topic

☐ Contributions are socially appropriate

☐ Understands humor/jokes

☐ Other (specify):

Specify some interests/enjoyable topics for communication:
Changes in communication since brain injury (specify and rank how problematic each is: 1= most important)

    1.

    2.

    3.

Current communication strengths (specify):

Behavior concerns: _____

Can you identify anything that often happens just before a communication or behavior problem? Specify:

Can you identify anything that often happens immediately after a communication/behavior problem? Specify:

Variations in any of the rephrase (if so, specify):

      With different communication partners?

      With more than one person in a communication?

      With different communication topics/demands?

      In different communication environments?

Other comments/questions/concerns about social communication:

Current Skills:	**Desired Skills:**	**Notes:** (e.g., I = independent; A = assisted [describe]; S = spoken cues [describe]; W = written cues [describe]; P = picture cues [describe]; O = other [specify]; OB = obstacles outside the patient [specify]; N = not applicable)

Daily Activities:

☐ Reading/writing ☐

☐ Safety/judgment ☐ ☐

☐ Money management ☐ ☐

☐ Self-care ☐

☐ Telephone use ☐ ☐

☐ Other (specify):

Meals:

☐ At home/living location ☐

☐ Sit-down restaurant ☐ ☐

☐ Fast-food restaurant ☐ ☐

☐ Other (specify):

Shopping:

☐ Food ☐

☐ Clothing ☐ ☐

☐ Pharmacy ☐ ☐

☐ Single store ☐ ☐

☐ Mall environment ☐ ☐

☐ Other (specify):

Transportation:

☐ Public transit ☐ ☐

☐ Drive—independent ☐ ☐

☐ Navigate—walking ☐ ☐

☐ Navigate—driving ☐ ☐

☐ Other (specify):

Safety Concerns:

Social:

☐ Doctor's visit   ☐

☐ Friend/family visit ☐

☐ Church   ☐

☐ Hobbies   ☐   ☐   ☐

☐ Outings   ☐   ☐

☐ Other (specify):

Work/Education/Volunteer Setting:

 Before injury:

 Current:

 Projected:

Existing Skill Sets:

Needed Skill Sets:

A Performance Inventory for Everyday Environments and Tasks

Performance Inventory

Respondent: _____   Date Completed: _____

Relationship to Patient: _____

For each task below either that was important or that remains important to you, please use the rating system to indicate preinjury and current performance.

Rating: I = independent; A = assisted (describe); S = spoken cues (describe);
W = written cues (describe); P = picture cues (describe); O = other (specify);
OB = obstacles outside the patient (specify); U = unknown;
NA = not applicable (e.g., did not do; no longer does)

General	Preinjury Rating:	Current Rating:
Time management		
Make/use schedule		
Read for pleasure		
Read newspaper		

General	Preinjury Rating	Current Rating
Use telephone		
Use calendar		
Make lists		
Use checklists		
Keep track of belongings		
Operate TV, DVD, radio, MP3 player		
Operate computer, read/send e-mail		
Other (specify)		

Medication	Preinjury Rating	Current Rating
Read labels		
Sort pills		
Get refills		
Follow directions, for example, take with food		
Other (specify)		

Money Management	Preinjury Rating	Current Rating
Make budget		
Pay bills		
Write checks		
Handle cash		
Other (specify)		

Family	Preinjury Rating	Current Rating
Socialization		
Interaction with spouse		
Intimate communication		
Conflict resolution		
(Grand) parenting skills		
Other (specify)		

Kitchen	Preinjury Rating	Current Rating
Operate microwave		
Operate stove/oven		
Cleaning		
Other (specify)		
Safety concerns		

Money Management	Preinjury Rating	**Current Rating**
Make budget		
Pay bills		
Write checks		
Handle cash		
Other (specify)		

Bedroom	Preinjury Rating	Current Rating
Make bed		
Put away clothes		
Dressing (appropriate for weather, occasion, activity)		
Other (specify)		

Laundry	Preinjury Rating	Current Rating
Sort clothes		
Operate washer or dryer		
Fold clothes		
Put away clothes		
Other (specify)		

Bathroom	Preinjury Rating	Current Rating
Toileting		
Bathing/showering		
Grooming		
Other (specify)		

Outdoors	Preinjury Rating	Current Rating
Mowing		
Grilling		
Yard work		
Garbage removal		
Other (specify)		

Cleaning	Preinjury Rating	Current Rating
Vacuum		
Dusting		
Light cleaning		
Heavy cleaning		
Other (specify)		

Mail	Preinjury Rating	Current Rating
Sort mail		
File/dispose		
Write/send a card		
Send in bills		
Other (specify)		

Public Transportation	Preinjury Rating	Current Rating
Plan trip		
Check schedule		
Purchase or bring ticket/pass		
Account for weather		
Other (specify)		

Doctor Appointment	Preinjury Rating	Current Rating
Make appointment		
Record appointment		
Arrange transport		
Arrive on time		
Check in and give insurance cards		
Answer questions from doctor/nurse		
Other (specify)		

Church	Preinjury Rating	Current Rating
Arrange transport		
Locate seat		
Attend to service		
Follow procedures (sit, stand, kneel)		
Other (specify)		

Restaurant	Preinjury Rating	Current Rating
Make reservations		
Dress accordingly		
Order meal		
Table manners		
Socialize during meal		
Other (specify)		

OBJECTIVES

The reader will be able to:

1. Describe the kinds of treatment that may be necessary for patients who have anosognosia for the impairments being targeted.

2. Identify two treatments for common right hemisphere disorder (RHD) impairments that have been identified as either practice standards or practice guidelines.

3. Identify two treatments for other deficits that can characterize RHD that have been identified as either practice standards or practice guidelines based on evidence from other population(s).

4. Identify two treatment manipulations suggested by the cognitive resources hypothesis of RHD cognitive–communicative disorders.

5. Identify two types of RHD treatments for which preliminary evidence looks promising.

6. Provide two examples of how a specific deficit can be targeted (a) via a patient's cognitive–communicative strengths and (b) indirectly by addressing obstacles outside the patient.

Treatment of Right Hemisphere Disorders

Connie A. Tompkins and April G. Scott

INTRODUCTION

This chapter focuses on treatment issues, approaches, strategies, and evidence in relation to (a) four primary accounts of cognitive communication deficits in right hemisphere disorders (RHDs), (b) selected language and cognitive domains, and (c) obstacles to goal attainment beyond the patient's deficits. Before addressing treatment per se, we consider in turn some issues involved in focusing treatment, generalization of treatment gains, and evidence-based practice.

FOCUSING TREATMENT

Patient Involvement

Whenever possible, clinicians should look to the patients to (help) formulate treatment goals. Putting patients in the driver's seat invests them in the treatment process.

Approaches to Focusing Treatment

Treatment clinicians adopt various philosophies and approaches. Some clinicians advocate a "relative levels of impairment" approach, in which treatment builds on relative strengths, modalities, or skills; others focus on particular areas of weakness; still others address fundamental abilities, or processes presumed to underlie deficient performances, such as attentional/resource allocation, inferencing, or contextual integration; and others focus solely on functional abilities and activities. Initial treatment targets may address any of the following: (a) obstacles to goal attainment (McCue et al., 1994) that are most distressing to patients or families (e.g., inhibiting profane remarks); (b) areas with potential to make a rapid positive impact on daily living interactions; (c) processes or strategies that are assumed prerequisite to establishing functional interactions; (d) areas of awareness or stimulability; or (e) methods to solidify effective patient-generated strategies or deter emerging bad habits.

Treatment may be oriented more toward restoration early postonset to take advantage of spontaneous recovery processes. Compensation can be the major focus later, although accumulating evidence suggests brain plasticity long postonset as well, which seems to be potentiated by intensive rehabilitation (e.g., Cornelissen et al., 2003; Meinzer et al., 2006). McCue and colleagues (1994) advocate a multidimensional applied cognitive rehabilitation approach that focuses on restoration, accommodation, compensation, or modification of obstacles to patients' attainment of their goals.

Models of Treatment

Just as assessment for cognitive communication disorders typically has followed a medical model, so has treatment. Thus, treatment usually has been *impairment based* and oriented toward restoring function by trying to focus on the patients' disorders. Restorative, deficit-oriented treatment has a central place in the management of RHD cognitive communication disorders (e.g., Tompkins, 1995). In addition, however, the International Classification of Functioning, Disability, and Health (ICF) framework reminds us to consider functional outcomes involving *activity limitations* and *participation restrictions*, along with relevant *contextual factors*. Similarly, McCue and colleagues' (1994) approach points us to the *impact* of deficits and *obstacles* that interfere with patients achieving their goals. In this perspective, (a) impairments may pose obstacles to goal attainment and as such are valid treatment targets if they significantly affect communicative activities and satisfaction; and (b) in addition to treatment to remediate or compensate for impaired cognitive–communicative functioning, we should aim treatment at factors outside the patient, as needed.

As Cherney and Halper (2000) remind us, functionally oriented treatment has several ingredients, including functionally defined outcomes and treatment materials and activities to enhance generalization to a patient's environment. The last may include simulations of goal-relevant activities, group treatment, and treatment outside the clinic room. Whether treatment occurs outside or inside the clinic room, we agree with others (e.g., Brookshire, 2007) that there are many paths to a functional outcome, and that for many patients, treatment does not need to occur in a functional environment to achieve functional goals for many patients.

GENERALIZATION OF TREATMENT GAINS

Achieving meaningful generalization from clinical intervention has remained elusive for most treatments for neurologically based language and cognitive disorders. To some, this problem suggests that treatment should be provided in the natural environment, should use only real-life activities, or should be entirely compensatory in nature. These restrictions may be necessary for patients with limited cognitive skills, but we should not discard remediation-oriented treatments, particularly in light of increasing evidence of neural plasticity and how it can be augmented by treatment.

To enhance the likelihood of generalization, clinicians need to plan for it and program it into treatment. This involves incorporating principles such as those of Stokes and Baer (1977). Among these principles are (a) Treatment should provide a sufficient number of training responses. This refers to targeting many related types of responses, such as different varieties of speech acts, and administering repeated treatment trials to foster overlearning. (b) The next principle is to train responses in a sufficient number of conditions, using a variety of tasks in a variety of contexts (e.g., with familiar and novel partners; in implicit learning or role-playing activities). (c) Treatment involves incorporating aspects of the daily environment by applying natural contingencies (i.e., reactions or responses likely to reinforce target behaviors, such as positive attention) and by various settings and other contextual factors (e.g., purposes and styles of communication, aspects of social interaction). Finally, (d) Treatment should include strategies for mediating generalization, such as teaching self-instruction and verbal mediation, making patients evaluate and modify their own responses, and involving other people in transfer activities. Generalization also may be improved by engaging patients in contexts with higher ecological validity (e.g., group treatment, PACE [promoting aphasics' communicative effectiveness]-like barrier tasks; Davis & Wilcox, 1985, structured conversational exchanges). Such contexts may help patients solidify their self-monitoring and compensation skills as well.

EVIDENCE-BASED PRACTICE

With the exception of unilateral neglect, there is little evidence to guide treatment for RHD. The next portions of this chapter describe treatment approaches and strategies, the existing RHD evidence, and some evidence from

Table 18.1   Potential Variables That Affect Selection and Training of Compensatory Strategies

Environmental–Social Factors

Prestroke social, educational, occupational status and interests

Current functional needs, environmental supports, and obstacles

Perceptual–Cognitive Strengths and Weaknesses

Sensory, perceptual, perceptual–motor, attentional, memory, language abilities

Level of content knowledge and organization of knowledge

Metacognitive abilities: Awareness of strengths, weaknesses, and own strategies; prediction of performance

Spontaneous strategies used and used effectively

Readiness for New Learning

Degree of confusion, disorientation, attentional impairment

Executive Functions

Motivational factors: Presence/appropriateness of goals; perceived need for strategies; attitude toward strategy use

Self-awareness, -initiation, -direction, -monitoring, -evaluation, and -adjustment

Organizing, reasoning, problem solving

Cognitive Style

Impulsive, reflective, persistent, active, passive, flexible, decisive

Personality and Social Control

Shy, aggressive, fearful, confident; attitude toward treatment

Situational Discrimination

Ability to distinguish situations that do or do not call for use of a particular strategy

Data from Tompkins. *Right Hemisphere Communication Disorders*, 1E. © 1995 Delmar Learning, a part of Cengage Learning, Inc.

other populations with similar deficits. To supplement this discussion, readers can consult a number of expert clinical sources, including the work of Blake (2007; Blake, Frymark, & Venedictov, 2013); Ferré, Ska, Lajoie, Bleau, and Joanette (2011); and Mackenzie and Brady (2008). Tompkins (1995) also provides a wealth of information about treatment principles, frameworks, approaches, strategies, and activities. As Blake (2007) notes, much of this expert judgment is based on theories about the nature of cognitive communication impairments.

The bulk of the following material addresses impairment-based treatment, reflecting the current state of the literature. Many of the impairment-based treatments can be made activity based by using material that is relevant to a valued daily activity, as in our neglect treatment with E.A. (see Case Illustration 18.1 at the end of this chapter). Training clients to use compensatory strategies, or training communication partners to prompt the use of strategies or positive behaviors, often focuses on daily activities as well. (See Table 18.1 for a list of general factors that may affect the selection and training of compensatory factors).

TREATMENT FOR COARSE CODING DEFICIT AND RELATED DIFFICULTIES

This section addresses interventions to improve the activation of semantically distant meanings or features of words or to compensate for deficits in this process. It also discusses treatment for deficits in the generation of *inferences* that require integration of features/meanings of words and for the interpretation of *metaphors and other pragmatic forms* because coarse coding has been presumed to underlie these abilities.

Although there is minimal evidence about how to treat a coarse coding deficit, our group (Blake, Tompkins, Scharp, Meigh, & Wambaugh, 2015; Tompkins, Scharp, Meigh, Blake, & Wambaugh, 2012) has early evidence documenting the efficacy of our innovative Contextual Constraint Treatment (CCT). This deficit-oriented treatment is delivered in the auditory modality, and it has a remediation focus. It is implicit and indirect in nature, rather than a more typical metalinguistic treatment. That is, clients are not asked to make explicit judgments or answer questions about the treatment stimuli, to purposely connect them to sentences or pictures, or to discuss their meaning. Rather, in its "coarse coding" version, CCT aims to facilitate the neural underpinnings of the activation of distant meanings and features of words without involving metacognition.

The version of CCT that was designed for coarse coding deficits is built around unambiguous key words like *piano*. For each key word, two context sentences bias a target concept that represents a distant semantic feature (e.g., *song*). A sample stimulus is "She played the melody. She forgot the words. There was a piano"—*song*. Treatment for each key lexical item starts with the strong bias, conveyed by both sentences, then systematically reduces bias one sentence at a time before adding it back in one sentence at a time. On hearing the target (e.g., *song*), the patient responds manually to indicate as quickly as possible whether that target is a real word or not (nonword targets are used in filler stimuli). The overall goal is to reduce response times to the targeted distant features of the key lexical items, increasing the efficiency of coarse coding processes.

Thus far, this treatment appears promising. Treatment-contingent gains have generalized to untrained items, and narrative discourse comprehension has improved for three of four participants while control measures remain stable.

We began this treatment work with a linguistic rather than a visual context because basic linguistic processing is a strength in RHD, it is easier to constrain linguistic context to bias a single interpretation, and the encoding of visual contexts may be impaired in RHD by other visual processing or attentional deficits (e.g., neglect). Nonetheless, some individual patients may benefit from strongly constrained visual contexts.

Other clinical recommendations to target coarse coding impairment have been metalinguistic, such as using tasks that require patients to generate multiple meanings of words. There are two cautions about this approach. First, such tasks are unlikely to target coarse coding unless one or more of the meanings or features are quite distant from the dominant meaning or image of the provided word. In context-free meaning generation tasks, however, people list many meanings or features that are not very distant. Thus, this task may reinforce the activation of dominant-related features or meanings and fail to target a coarse coding deficit. Second, if patients have a suppression deficit instead of a coarse coding deficit, they are already activating and retaining too many meanings or features of words without narrowing to those that are contextually appropriate. A multiple-meaning generation task may reinforce that problem.

We alluded to the focus of other direct treatment approaches. These include activities like discussing the intended meaning or feature of a word, purposely using a provided context to consider what features/meanings are most relevant to it, judging the appropriateness of a given feature/meaning in a given context, or contrasting the appropriateness of several features/meanings.

Whether coarse coding treatment is implicit or explicit and metalinguistic, we recommend tasks that incorporate the desired meaning or feature into some kind of context to improve ecological validity and elicit distant meanings or features of words. Providing a patient with strong contextual bias is likely to be an effective compensatory approach, as well, to help work around coarse coding deficits. As summarized by Tompkins (1995), features of context can range from the external, immediate, and concrete to those that reflect world knowledge and experience.

Clinicians can influence performance by varying the modality of the context, its encoding difficulty, number of cues, consistency of cues, salience of features (related to emphasis, repetition, familiarity, etc.), and the like. Patients who have trouble interpreting or explaining stimuli in light of their own experience can work on associating, organizing, and identifying relationships between treatment stimuli and contextual material. Alternatively, at a more elementary level, they may need to work on identifying, recognizing, or discriminating parts of the stimuli and contexts or even on determining what is most central or relevant.

Inference processes that involve the integration of word features or meanings, such as inference revisions, may be targeted in the same ways. For example, the vignette "Barbara became bored with the history book. She had already spent 5 years writing it" (Brownell, Potter, Bihrle, & Gardner, 1986) requires a comprehender to switch from the initial interpretation that Barbara was reading a book. A biasing context, such as one that emphasizes Barbara's credentials and success as a writer, should help facilitate this process. The same is true for predictive inferences about what may happen next in a story, which can be generated when the linguistic context strongly suggests them (e.g., "He put his rod in the car and drove to the lake" strongly suggests that the "he" in question is going fishing; Lehman-Blake & Tompkins, 2001).

Turning to the *interpretation of metaphor*, one treatment study has been conducted with five adults with RHD (Lundgren, Brownell, Cayer-Meade, Milione, & Kearns, 2011). The quality of spoken interpretations of novel metaphors (of the form "An *X* is a *Y*") improved for all participants, and gains were selective to the metaphor measure for three of the five. One patient made gains on a nonstandard measure of nonliteral language comprehension, and three maintained their gains 3 months later.

The treatment involved structured practice in judging and generating semantic associations between words, using sun diagrams (i.e., a target word takes the position of the sun in the center of an array, and the associated words are arranged at the ends of the sun's rays). Treatment tasks were highly metalinguistic, including steps such as judging connotations of single words and clinician- and self-generated associations between words. The metaphoric associations may well have stimulated coarse coding processes, and it would be interesting to know whether the observed improvements would generalize to other tasks hypothesized to tap coarse coding. Because this treatment is in the early stages of investigation, it is unknown whether the reported gains affected daily life comprehension. We concur with the authors that this visually augmented semantic association approach has potential for other types of RHD communication deficits.

TREATMENT FOR SUPPRESSION DEFICIT AND RELATED DIFFICULTIES

Our group's CCT also has a version for suppression deficit, with promising results for five participants so far (Tompkins, Blake, Scharp, Meigh, & Wambaugh, 2013). The treatment stimuli and task for this version of CCT were derived from our prior investigations of suppression deficit. Treatment stimuli are simple sentences that end in an ambiguous noun and contain a verb that biases the interpretation of that noun toward one of its meanings (e.g., "He dug with a spade"). Target words, presented 1 second after sentence offset, are related to the other, unbiased meaning of the ambiguous noun (e.g., *ace*). The patient responds manually to indicate whether the target word is related to the sentence. The goal is to speed the patient's response ("No," because *ace* is unrelated to the contextually appropriate meaning of *spade*). Otherwise, the treatment is the same as described for coarse coding: Biasing sentences precede each stimulus with an ambiguous noun to implicitly bolster the noun's context-appropriate meaning (the "shovel" interpretation of spade) and rule out the other ("playing card") meaning. For each item, these sentences are systematically removed before being added in again.

Other suggestions for addressing suppression deficit are more highly metalinguistic (see, e.g., Tompkins & Baumgaertner, 1998). These include giving, or priming patients with, alternative meanings (rather than asking patients to generate them) and asking patients to determine contextual relevance or appropriateness in the ways described previously for coarse coding deficit. In addition, the clinician could elicit a client's preferred interpretation of an ambiguous stimulus and then provide the stimulus again with clues toward another interpretation. The client would be asked to indicate whether the first interpretation is still appropriate, why or why not, and what cues influence the decision. In addition, clients could start a conversation or a story and work on sticking to the point while the clinician introduces competing mental activations (e.g., interrupts, diverges from the topic). If needed, topic cue cards can be provided as compensatory supports and faded or continued as necessary.

As noted previously, suppression deficit could account for or contribute to a variety of cognitive–communicative problems in adults with RHD. For instance, it is possible that treatment for suppression deficit would assist in reconciling the multiple perspectives that have to be considered in theory of mind (ToM) tasks or in resolving other conflicting interpretations, in reducing inaccurate inferences, or even in stemming tangential statements or off-topic intrusions.

TREATMENT CONSIDERATIONS RELATED TO THE COGNITIVE RESOURCE HYPOTHESIS

As summarized by Tompkins (1995), the cognitive resource hypothesis underscores performance variations that can be achieved by manipulating presumed demands for processing resources, regardless of the focus or orientation of treatment. For example, adequately acquainting clients with tasks or strategies, providing prestimulation and repeated practice, and promoting overlearning should help habituate some aspects of performance and free up cognitive resources to deal with other elements of a communicative situation. Resource demands also should be lower when treatment tasks exploit a client's expertise, when thematic redundancy is increased, and when inferential complexity, the need to revisit prior context, or requirements to integrate ostensibly disparate information are reduced. Compensations can be implemented, such as assisting clients in chunking units of text or making notes or drawings, to help encode and maintain contextual information or to review previous information and inferences that affect subsequent interpretations, responses, or actions. Table 18.2 lists some other factors to modify the probable ease or difficulty of treatment tasks from the cognitive resources perspective.

Table 18.2 Sample Factors to Modify in Treatment From the Perspective of the Cognitive Resources Hypothesis

Dimension	Attributes
Stimulus characteristics	Perceptual factors (e.g., stimulus clarity, orientation, discriminability, ambiguity)
	Spatial requirements for location, distance, direction, memory; number, arrangement of/attention to elements and arrays
	Central factors (explicitness; redundancy and consistency; predictability; probability, meaningfulness, familiarity, interest, and frequency; computational difficulty)
	Resource factors (requirements for retention, simultaneous processing, coordination, and exact timing in demanding conditions; automatic versus controlled processing; specific demands for selective attention, resisting distraction, differentiating relevant from irrelevant information, and sustaining, dividing, or switching attention)
Stimulus modes	Visual, auditory, tactile, combined (but alert to demands for divided attention)
Task characteristics	Performance criteria; level of processing; demands for metacognition; volitionality
Other facilitators	Procedural factors (practice and demonstration; side from which to deliver treatment). Temporal factors (rate of speech and use of pauses; stimulus–response interval)
	Cues and compensatory strategies

Data from Tompkins. *Right Hemisphere Communication Disorders*, 1E. © 1995 Delmar Learning, a part of Cengage Learning, Inc.www.cengage.com/permissions.

TREATMENT FOR SOCIAL COGNITION DEFICIT

Manly and Murphy (2012) note scant evidence for social cognition treatment in acquired brain injury. For the population with traumatic brain injury (TBI), some benefits have been reported for treatments targeting perception of social/emotional cues (Bornhofen & McDonald, 2008a, 2008b) and for direct training of social skills (e.g., S. McDonald et al., 2008), although it is unknown how these gains translate to daily functioning.

As mentioned, treatment for suppression deficit may improve the reasoning of patients with RHD with ToM. This is possible because adults with RHD may have difficulty with various complex inference processes, whether or not they involve ToM (Tompkins, Scharp, Fassbinder, Meigh, & Armstrong, 2008). Complex social inferences require consideration of multiple factors, such as the relationships between communication partners (e.g., boss versus employee; teacher versus student the number of differing points of view in communicative scenarios; and the purposes of communication (e.g., to instruct, criticize, inform, tease, praise). These factors, together with contextual bias, can be manipulated to address high-level inferencing, including ToM inferences, in activities such as those described previously.

The complexities of social cognition in daily interaction, though, suggest that something more will be needed. For example, clients may need treatment at the same time for problems in their comprehension of prosody, facial expression, and the affect or attitudes conveyed by each.

As suggested by Tompkins (1995), and depending on the client's skills and needs, treatment for social cognition deficits may involve a discussion of social norms or a demonstration that no one's thoughts are transparent (barrier tasks or role-play can be used to demonstrate this). Additional treatment activities may include identification by the client of occasions when the clinician (purposely) provides insufficient information, in light of what the client knows; lists of what is given (known) or assumed by two communication partners in an exchange; or plans on how to make the purpose of an exchange clear. The clinician can manipulate the nature of social relationships or communicative intents in such activities. Clients can also work on identifying what elements or propositions in discourse are essential for different listeners, themes, or communication purposes or work on identifying or listing presuppositions about what a particular type of communication partner knows, needs to know, or considers central to an exchange. Other tasks include having clients establish or verify a shared knowledge base by explicitly introducing referents and background information about people or events to be discussed or by checking a listener's familiarity with background information.

Blake (2007) recommends creating vignettes that manipulate such factors, or using group treatment and discussion, and having clients answer questions such as the following: What did Character *X* mean? How did you figure it out (what cues)? Which clues in the vignette are important/not important? What if *X* was jealous of *Y*? What if *X* and *Y* were competitors, not friends? What is *X*'s (*Y*'s) point of view? Blake also suggests some activities that stem from the hypothesis that social cognition deficits are the result, at least in part, of deficits in executive functioning (see the section, "Executive Functioning Deficits," in this chapter).

Patients with RHD are likely to need ample supports and strategies to succeed in activities like these. Graphic representations of key elements of the text (e.g., diagrams, charts, cue cards) could provide such support, as would reducing demands on cognitive resources. The section, "Treatment of Reading and Writing," in this chapter discusses multimodal compensatory supports that could be pertinent for individual patients.

TREATMENT OF PROSODY

Expressive Aprosodia

Rosenbek and colleagues have provided phase I evidence for two impairment-level treatments for patients with stroke with expressive aprosodia (e.g., Leon & Rodriguez, 2008; Rosenbek et al., 2004). In a cognitive–linguistic treatment, patients are taught how to use features of emotional intonation in their utterances by explaining written descriptions of emotional tones of voice, matching the descriptions to written labels and emotional faces, and reading sentences with prosody. In an imitative–motor treatment, patients work on producing prosody that expresses the emotion conveyed in stimulus sentences, with their productions moving from unison with the clinician to repeating after the clinician to independent productions. The authors report modest to substantial effects in 14 patients, but there has been no generalization to untrained emotions.

Ferré and colleagues (2011) summarize several unpublished case studies that have integrated receptive and expressive tasks. The expressive component of the treatment involves imitation, reading, dialogue, barrier–task interaction, and telephone exchanges. Other recommendations, derived from expert clinical judgment, include using contrastive stress drills, responses to questions, or disambiguation exercises (Tompkins, 1995). Contrastive stress drills start with a simple premise, such as "Noah and Peyton slept late." The clinician makes a statement or asks a question that contradicts the premise (e.g., Did Noah and Peyton stay up late?), and patients are to emphasize the corresponding element of the premise. Query responding is similar. Practice can be accompanied by discussing how emphasis can highlight meaning. If patients are unsuccessful in such tasks, they can be given tasks that require them to identify the target stress location, instruction in how to achieve emphasis (e.g., "Say it louder"), or a variety of visual representations and cues. In disambiguation tasks, patients can work with lexical (e.g., "record" as noun vs. verb), syntactic (e.g., question vs. statement intonation), or semantic/prosodic ambiguities (e.g., sarcasm).

One caution deserves mention. When considering whether to treat expressive aprosodia, we need to keep in mind that this deficit can reflect emotional difficulties such as depression and refer for treatment of the underlying condition when appropriate.

Receptive Aprosodia

Although Ferré et al. (2011) mention several case reports with receptive prosody goals, there is no published evidence on treatment for impaired comprehension of prosody. Tompkins (1995) provides suggestions based on expert clinical opinion. For example, when prosodic comprehension deficits stem from difficulties in judging emotions or attitudes, treatment can focus on determining moods from prosody. Patients can identify moods when linguistic information and prosody are congruent; match emotional prosody to mood labels, to briefly described situations, or to personal experiences; identify discrepancies between prosody and explicit emotional contexts or expected attitudes; or work on reconciling these discrepancies.

Patients also may have prosodic interpretation difficulty for nonemotional signals (e.g., impaired appreciation of emphatic stress, linguistic ambiguity, conversational functions such as inviting responses or closing conversations). Using tasks such as those suggested for prosodic production, patients can be asked to select, associate with different contexts, explain, or contrast the meanings of stimuli; identify central elements on the basis of prosodic emphasis; indicate when it is appropriate for another speaker to take a turn; and so on. If patients have difficulty with contextual tasks such as these, some basic work may be needed in discriminating nonemotional speech patterns.

TREATMENT OF DISCOURSE AND PRAGMATICS

On a general note, we suspect that the implicit CCT approach, described for coarse coding and suppression deficits, could apply broadly across comprehension deficit areas in RHD because a good amount of evidence suggests that adults with RHD do well with semantically consistent, redundant, or strongly biased contexts. For example, contextual bias could be manipulated to facilitate the interpretation of various types of ambiguities in communication, including those conveyed by prosody, emotion, assorted speech acts, humor, headlines, and such or provided as part of a compensatory strategy to aid pragmatic understanding. The previously described treatment for oral metaphor interpretation (Lundgren et al., 2011) also may have potential for various impairment areas. The two types of treatments could be intermixed by using contextual bias implicitly (i.e., without incorporating it directly in the treatment tasks) together with metalinguistic semantic association and evaluation tasks.

As another general note, many of the treatment activities described previously and suggested further in the chapter incorporate elements of extrastimulus context. Adults with RHD have often been described, vaguely, as having difficulty "using context" in cognitive–linguistic processing, although there are quite a few exceptions to this notion in the literature. Regardless, we deem extrastimulus context an important element of treatment activities, across communicative domains, because it is necessary for reducing and resolving the ambiguity that can permeate language production and comprehension in RHD.

Discourse

Narrative production in RHD has been directly targeted in one report of an individual with a right subdural hematoma subsequent to TBI (Cannizzaro & Coelho, 2002). The treatment focused on story retelling, with added analysis of story components, and on story generation, with self-evaluation and cueing to incorporate missing elements. Gains were achieved for the production of targeted story components but were not maintained.

As summarized by Blake and colleagues (2013) and as emphasized previously here, many interventions for discourse and pragmatics revolve around presentation and integration of contextual cues. Tompkins (1995) also provides numerous suggestions for treating discourse production and comprehension that stem from analyses of models of discourse processes. A wide range of variables can be manipulated to influence performance in discourse and conversational treatment tasks. These include participant factors (e.g., extent and awareness of shared knowledge); stimulus factors (e.g., degrees of explicitness and consistency, conventionality); and procedural factors (e.g., orienting tasks/instructions, targeted components/skills; see Tompkins, 1995, for a more

complete list). Clinicians need to remain alert to the likelihood that discourse-level impairments are complicated by, or caused by, other processing deficits (e.g., problems with selective, sustained, divided, or strategic control of attention; working memory; perception; determining what is important or central) or obstacles outside the patient (e.g., conversation partner does not get patient's attention or introduce topic of conversation).

Common tasks to target *macrostructure difficulties* include summarizing, sorting, and explaining stimuli (e.g., by theme or gist, category similarity, or membership), demonstrating appreciation of character motives or story morals, and identifying or explaining contradictions or absurdities. *Microstructure-level difficulties* can be targeted through self-monitoring for typical errors (e.g., unclear/incorrect reference; inadequate lexical reiteration, as when an idea or event is reintroduced after intervening material). Treatment for microlevel ambiguity can proceed like that for other forms of ambiguity. Tasks may include, for example, choosing from among all possible referents; identifying ambiguity in a barrier task when the clinician is purposely inexplicit; discussing when specific reference is important, such as when identifying or reintroducing topics or characters; identifying videotaped examples of ambiguity in others' discourse and in the clients' own; and self-correcting to avoid the confusion such ambiguity entails.

Comprehension of narratives theoretically should be enhanced by treatment for coarse coding or suppression when patients have one of those deficits. Narrative comprehension is often addressed with tasks such as asking patients to synthesize their knowledge of the world with stimulus information to draw inferences or check interpretations; to identify and discard or revise information that is contextually inappropriate or irrelevant; to identify or associate main ideas and salient information; to sort salient from irrelevant information; to identify or sort material relevant to the primary dimensions of a narrative (e.g., protagonist, protagonist's goal, spatial setting, time frame, emotional reactions [e.g., Zwaan, 1999]); or to identify cues in the narrative that signal continuity in these dimensions or a need to shift focus.

Diagrams, charts, note cards, or other visual representations of elements can be used to assist patients in performing these tasks. Performance can likely be improved by focusing on a patient's special knowledge and by keeping inference-supporting elements together in working memory (e.g., foreground them via emphasis; decrease distance or number of propositions or shifts in focus that intervene between them). Inference revisions may be aided via outlines or diagrams of the possibilities that are suggested by discrepant information; by distinguishing plausible versus less likely interpretations, providing reasons if possible; or by making a graphic representation of what is possible or plausible in a specific situation without any reference to a particular stimulus and comparing that representation to crucial parts of the stimulus and to the patient's initial interpretation (see Tompkins, 1995, for expansion of these ideas).

Conversational discourse has been targeted in two individuals with RHD due to TBI-associated hematoma; the purpose was to improve pragmatic communication skills such as conversation initiation and communication partner interaction (Youse & Coelho, 2009). The treatment had a social skills emphasis and used video analysis, coaching, and external strategies, although with minimal effects on conversational output. Several unpublished case studies of conversational intervention for adults with RHD have been reported as well (Ferré et al., 2011). As described, the treatment addressed awareness, then visual or spoken feedback was provided and faded as patients were asked to imagine talking about controversial subjects.

Treatment for conversational discourse can also focus on strategies for topic control, as needed (e.g., call the listener's name; provide an introductory phrase; provide an opener, such as the title of a story). Identifying, monitoring for, and responding to requests for clarification may be another focus (e.g., for requests signaled more or less explicitly, through facial expressions, prosody, or verbalization). In addition, patients could work on identifying various sources of communication breakdown and generating adjustments appropriate to their sources (e.g., reiterating if attention has wandered, repeating louder if not heard, explaining to clear up ambiguity, defining a crucial term). When the trouble source is not clear from a listener's request for clarification, some patients with RHD may be able to learn to ask what the problem is, specifically, or to apply a strategy for repairing their most typical source of difficulty.

In other activities, clients can associate conversational rules with specific settings (e.g., church, poker game) or people (e.g., preacher, poker buddy, grandchild); identify, discuss, or demonstrate the consequences of socially and situationally inappropriate contributions; self-monitor on video or live online; or identify or provide corrective feedback to a clinician who models their problem behaviors. Conciseness can be targeted by asking clients to use as few words as possible or to revise wordy responses or by restricting the time frame for responding. Clients also can learn to identify signals used by others who are ready to take a conversational turn, to establish a new topic, or to end an encounter. Once identified, the client can work on responding appropriately to such signals. Tompkins (1995) elaborates on conversational discourse treatment.

Pragmatics

Cicerone and colleagues' (2000) systematic review endorses treatment for pragmatic communication and conversation in TBI as a *practice standard* (i.e., substantive evidence; this treatment should be considered). Helffenstein and Wechsler (1982) found that 20 hours of analysis of videotaped social exchanges had broad, meaningful outcomes in areas such as self-concept, others' perceptions of the patients' social/interactional abilities, and generalization to social contexts. Effects of self-monitoring training (Gajar, Schloss, Schloss, & Thompson, 1984) and group treatment on interpersonal skills (e.g., Braden et al., 2010; Ehrlich & Sipes, 1985) also have been documented. These approaches have been emphasized along with structured feedback, rehearsal, and modeling in a more recent review of social communication treatment for TBI, as well (Struchen, 2005). Such approaches may be fruitful for adults with RHD and warrant consideration.

Emotion/Nonverbal Processing

Restoration-oriented treatment for emotional and nonverbal deficits could proceed like that for prosody. Compensations might include training communication partners to explicitly state emotions, attitudes, or reactions. For nonverbal communication, Mackenzie and Brady (2008) recommend a familiar sequence of treatment options, such as identifying and building awareness of nonverbal behaviors, what they signal, and how they are signaled (e.g., head nods to indicate interest), and then moving toward identifying instances of and self-monitoring positive and negative nonverbal signals.

Additional Aspects of Pragmatic Functioning

The preceding sorts of tasks and activities are likely to be appropriate for any of the remaining pragmatic areas. In addition, the kinds of *contextually based* identification, selection, interpretation, or self-monitoring tasks we have described thus far, are appropriate for the remaining areas of communicative focus. That said, we skip some deficit areas in subsequent material (e.g., lexical–semantic, addressed in the section, "Treatment for Coarse Coding Deficit and Related Difficulties" previously in this chapter) and touch only briefly on others.

To address *speech acts*, we recommend discourse tasks that involve recognizing, associating, identifying discrepancies, or explaining in relation to the differences between literal and contextually intended meanings of stimuli or between various communicative intentions and purposes. For example, hints could be paired with more direct requests, and different forms of requests could be associated with specific action responses or situations. Factors could be varied to affect the acceptability of direct versus indirect requests, such as the power of the requester, familiarity with requestee, or degree of obligation to reply. Request modifiers also could be identified and trained (e.g., "If it's not too much trouble"; "Would you mind?"; or give reasons for a request). For *figurative meanings*, clients similarly could be asked to express or select appropriate interpretations of figurative utterances for contexts of varying familiarity, with varying types and strength of cues. Other possibilities with very preliminary evidence are provided in the previous section, "Treatment for Coarse Coding Deficit and Related Difficulties." Compensations would include asking communication partners to be direct and literal or to prompt request modifiers or other appropriate behaviors as needed.

TREATMENT OF READING AND WRITING

If reading and writing difficulties are caused by visual processing or attention (e.g., scanning deficits; neglect), impairment-level treatment can focus on remediating or compensating for those areas. For discourse-level problems of comprehension and expression, suggestions in the discourse section are appropriate.

Expert clinical opinion suggests that the choice of whether and how to treat reading and writing will depend on the importance of those skills in patients' lives and the severity of their impairments. Even patients relatively severely affected may profit from basic reading and writing activities so that they can, for instance, read instructions, find something they like on a menu, or write notes on birthday cards. For patients with milder impairments, it may be useful to establish compensatory, organizational guides or structured sets of questions for self-instruction and self-analysis of reading comprehension. One general example of such a guide has five steps: (a) preview the material to be read to identify themes and central ideas; (b) generate questions about the material; (c) read to answer the questions; (d) make note of the answers and summarize; (e) review material to check and verify answers. This kind of strategy can be difficult and tedious to apply, even for college students, so it is certainly not for everyone. More specific examples might cue the patient to look for the who, what, when, where, how/why of a newspaper article or the characters, characters' goals, setting, time frame, complication, and characters' reactions for a narrative. A variety of other compensations may be appropriate: Relevant points or key information can be highlighted or

tape recorded; attention can be focused by covering up portions of text or using a ruler to track the reader's current position; cue cards can be provided to keep themes or topics in focus; or a visual-graphic representation of text can be developed or consulted. For example, an index card that identifies an active topic, character, or location can be placed atop a tree structure, and other information placed on or off other branches of the tree, to represent its current relevance. Tompkins (1995) elaborates on such suggestions.

TREATMENT OF COGNITION

Treatment of impaired cognition is important in its own right and for its potential effects on RHD communication difficulties that stem from cognitive impairments. To preface this section, we note that most often, effects of cognitive treatments on daily life outcomes have not been measured, although that issue has received increasingly more attention. When such measures are included, the effects often have not been achieved. In addition, much of the available research has not provided results or recommendations for RHD adults separate from stroke patients in general. Finally, as a clinical reminder, when considering cognitive treatments we must be mindful of other factors that may contribute to the targeted problems, such as fatigue, medication side effects, anxiety, depression, and pain (e.g., Ponsford et al., 2014).

Anosognosia

Although unawareness of cognitive, emotional, or physical deficits improves with time after RHD, anosognosia remains intractable for some patients. There is insufficient evidence to recommend any particular treatment for self-awareness (Cicerone et al., 2005), but both systematic reviews (Tate et al., 2014) and expert opinion (e.g., Kortte & Hillis, 2011; Sohlberg, 2000) emphasize multifaceted regimens in which various treatment approaches are combined.

Direct approaches generally take one of three forms. In *feedback approaches*, patients receive information about their performance (e.g., observer feedback, self-appraisal, feedback on timing). Video feedback, for example, gained attention after the remission of anosognosia in a 67-year-old patient with RHD (Fotopoulou, Rudd, Holmes, & Kopelman, 2009). Other studies suggest similar gains from direct feedback (e.g., Besharati, Crucianelli, & Fotopoulou, 2014), but more research is needed to determine the efficacy of these approaches. Feedback may be most effective when administered in a multicontextual intervention program (Kortte & Hillis, 2011). *Educational approaches* focus on patients' learning about their deficits and how they affect daily life. These approaches are implemented by, for example, reviewing medical records or comparing ratings of performance, often with video support. In *prediction approaches*, patients predict their performance on specific tasks while considering their own strengths and weaknesses. Overall, these approaches may increase self-regulatory skills, enhance strategy use, and reduce inconsistency between expected and actual performance (Toglia, Johnston, Goverover, & Dain, 2010).

Indirect approaches have also been advocated. It is often assumed that patients must be aware of their deficits to benefit from treatment. This seems obvious for treatments that require an appreciation of how a particular deficit affects daily functioning. Awareness may also be important when treatment requires patient-initiated strategies. However, initiation could be triggered implicitly, instead, by the identification of a cue in the communication environment. For example, patients could be trained to initiate a strategy when a communication partner indicates a need (e.g., by saying, "I didn't understand," lightly tapping the patient's hand, or assuming a quizzical facial expression); to open their memory book every time it is given to them; to refer to a clearly posted checklist every time they begin a daily task.

Indeed, as summarized by Cicerone et al. (2005) in their systematic review, behavior can be improved without self-awareness through treatment that taps implicit learning of a procedure. Such training can take many sessions to consolidate. Some investigators (Sohlberg, Mateer, Penkman, Glang, & Todis, 1998) speculate that a lack of insight may aid compliance in some patients by keeping them from questioning why they need to use a compensatory system. These authors also report, intriguingly, that when patients with TBI targeted behaviors improved without a change in *expression* of self-awareness, caregivers' perceptions of the patients' awareness did not improve, even though the caregivers had selected the target behaviors as indices of awareness. Thus, caregivers may need to be counseled that it is acceptable for patients not to "admit" their deficits.

Feedback may be provided indirectly as well, through experiential exercises. Rather than telling patients they are not able to do something, clinicians support the patients' exploration and experience of subgoals (McCue et al., 1994), with the aim that sufficient awareness emerges for patients to abandon things that are too difficult to achieve. This "supported" or "guided" failure approach can be implemented for a range of concerns, including unrealistic goals.

Attention Deficits

Attention

In a recent Cochrane systematic review, Loetscher and Lincoln (2013) evaluated six randomized control trials of attention treatment that showed immediate effects on divided attention for patients with stroke but no persisting effects on global measures of attention or functional outcomes. An earlier review (Lincoln, Majid, & Weyman, 2000) evaluated two trials that reported benefits on sustained attention and alertness. Both reviews conclude that there is insufficient evidence to recommend for or against direct treatment of post-stroke attention deficits. Focusing on controlled trials for acute, moderate-to-severe stroke, a task force report by the European Federation of Neurological Societies (Cappa et al., 2005) recommends against direct attention training, noting that its effects are indistinguishable from those of spontaneous recovery or general cognitive rehabilitation. However, systematic reviews focused largely on TBI report the greatest improvements in attention deficits when direct training is combined with metacognitive strategy training (Cicerone et al., 2011; Cicerone & Maestas, 2014). Combining these two approaches encourages the development of compensatory strategies, which supports generalization to activities of daily living.

Based on evidence other than that in controlled trials, several reviewers (Cicerone et al., 2000; Duncan et al., 2005) endorse early identification and treatment of post-stroke attention deficits as a clinical *practice guideline* (i.e., evidence of probable effectiveness; this treatment should be considered). The European Federation guidelines (Cappa et al., 2005) and Cicerone and colleagues (2011) suggest that the greatest gains occur from treatment during the postacute recovery stages, although it should be noted that these conclusions are based on data, including patients with TBI. Cicerone and colleagues (2000) strongly recommend against decontextualized computer-based attention drills without a treating clinician, arguing that such treatment has minimal generalizability outside the clinic setting and disregards emotional or behavioral concerns of patients.

A prospective, single-blind trial (Barker-Collo et al., 2009) may tip the scales toward the "recommended" column for patients with stroke who are not very impaired (i.e., with a "deficit" defined as performance one standard deviation below the mean on any attention assessment). In this trial, patients received Attention Process Training (APT; Sohlberg & Mateer, 1986), an intervention based on a theoretical analysis of attention functions and the assumption that distinct cognitive deficits can be improved by specifically targeted activities. The program purports to target sustained, selective, alternating, and divided attention. At a follow-up 5 weeks posttreatment, performance on a test of subtle selective attention problems was better in 38 patients with stroke than in 40 control group patients. Barco-Collo and colleagues also report a trend toward greater improvement on a cognitive failures questionnaire for the treated group.

The latest version of APT (APT-III; Sohlberg & Mateer, 2010) emphasizes the use of compensatory strategies to enhance attention. Cicerone et al. (2005) endorse *strategy training* as a *practice standard* for adults with TBI in the postacute period (i.e., substantive evidence; this treatment should be considered). Benefits have come primarily from complex tasks that require attentional control and regulation. For example, a time-pressure management treatment improved both attention and self-management strategies. Some potential compensations for attention problems are outlined in Table 18.3.

Neglect

There are many published reviews of the neglect treatment literature, and numerous controlled trials have been conducted (e.g., Bowen, Hazelton, Pollock, & Lincoln, 2013; Kerkhoff & Schenk, 2012; Kortte & Hillis, 2011). One systematic review (Luauté, Halligan, Rode, Rossetti, & Boisson, 2006) identifies 18 intervention approaches, many of which address viewer-centered neglect. Of these, Cicerone et al. (2005) endorse only visual scanning treatment (VST) as *a practice standard* (i.e., substantive evidence; this treatment should be considered).

Visual scanning treatment is thought to work by increasing right brain activation or directing spatial attention. It involves consciously scanning the environment and has several components: (a) stimuli or tasks compelling enough to elicit a head turn to the left; (b) a visual anchor, typically a vertical line in the left margin with or without sequential numbering of each horizontal line; (c) slow pacing; and (d) repetition to turn the strategy into a habit. The treatment has been shown to improve performance on impairment-level neglect measures and on some functional measures of motor, reading, or writing tasks. In a few reports, gains have been maintained for as much as a year. Up to 40 treatment sessions, for at least 5 hours per week, may be required to yield such durable gains. Kerkhoff and Schenk (2012) argue that such intense therapy is time consuming for both the patient and the clinician and may be inappropriate for patients with concurrent anosognosia. Kortte and Hillis (2011) echo these sentiments for patients with severe cognitive impairment. The generalization effects of VST to unrelated tasks also remain unclear. Cicerone et al. (2000, 2005) indicate that extending training to more complex stimuli seems to improve the effects, particularly on generalization of treatment.

Cicerone et al. (2005) recommend the inclusion of electronic technologies for VST as a *practice option* (i.e., evidence of possible effectiveness; consider this treatment). Another *practice option* endorsed by these authors is a combination of VST and forced limb activation (LA), a treatment for motor-intentional neglect. Limb activation takes two forms. In active LA, patients with RHD consciously initiate movements of the designated left limb (usually the arm) into left space while performing workbook-type activities. In the passive version, when the limb is paretic, it is moved into left space, by either the patient or someone else. In some cases, patients are asked to locate the moved limb. Active LA appears

---

Table 18.3 Potential Compensations for Attention Deficits

Many of these strategies are appropriate for multiple kinds of attention deficits (sustained, selective, alternating, divided, strategic control).

- Train patients to develop or practice using checklists or charts to track progress.
- Train patients to implement brief periods of compensatory effort and arousal and to list activities or situations that call for it.
- Train communication partners to use spoken alerters (e.g., "I have an idea about that" or simply saying a patient's name) to signal when attention should be switched or as a way to increase task-relevant arousal.
- Enhance alertness and arousal temporarily with novel/unexpected stimuli, salient stimuli, performance incentives, other alerting signals (a touch on the arm, a tap on a table).
- Have patients write down distracting thoughts and set them aside.
- Have patients wear a headset or earplugs.
- Have patients go to a quieter place or modify the environment (e.g., close the door).
- Schedule breaks as necessary.

to have better effects than passive. Even patients with severe neglect may benefit from LA training. For one such patient, lasting gains were achieved in a version that incorporated an alerting device (with a loud buzzer and red light) that the patient had to disable with his left arm (Robertson, Mattingley, Rorden, & Driver, 1998). This device was later reported effective in a randomized controlled trial (Robertson, MacMillan, MacLeod, Edgeworth, & Brock, 2002). To date, however, evidence of functional gains has been elusive.

Virtual reality is a novel approach that is gaining interest for the assessment and treatment of neglect (for reviews, see Fasotti & van Kessel, 2013; Kortte & Hillis, 2011; Tsirlin, Dupierrix, Chokron, Coquillart, & Ohlmann, 2009). Patients view and interact with computer-generated realistic environments in a multimodal three-dimensional world. The virtual environment can be manipulated by both the user and clinician. Preliminary findings are positive, in that improvements have been noted on neglect measures and virtual tasks simulating real life (e.g., Kim, Chun, Yun, Song, & Young, 2011). The use of applications on smart devices (e.g., iPad, iPhone) has also taken hold in the treatment of neglect, despite the lack of evidence on efficacy or effectiveness. Some provide visual scanning assessment and training exercises.

Other treatments have been tried for patients who cannot voluntarily and actively engage with the environment or material to be scanned. Many of these treatments involve technologies to alter the neglect-associated rightward orientation bias back to midline. Generally, the effects of these treatments have been quite brief (Luauté et al., 2006), with one possible exception: prism adaptation (PA). Prism adaptation is a sensorimotor treatment that induces procedural learning. Neglect patients wear special prism glasses that shift the left visual field to the right and perform tasks such as reaching toward a target or throwing a ball. Twenty sessions (20 minutes each, twice daily over a 2-week period) have been sufficient to reduce neglect substantially across sensory modalities, even in some functional tasks (e.g., Frassinetti, Angeli, Meneghello, Avanzi, & Ladavas, 2002). Frassinetti and colleagues also report maintenance of gains for 5 weeks posttreatment for six of seven patients with chronic neglect. Serino, Bonifazi, Pierfederici, and Ladavas (2007) measured gains out to 6 months posttreatment and reported that improvement in the first week of training may be critical to long-lasting amelioration of neglect.

If continued research supports PA treatment, it has the benefit of brevity. It is also possible that combining PA with VST would result in better functional outcomes (Arene & Hillis, 2008). Arene and Hillis suggest that patients with right cerebellar damage may not be good candidates for PA treatment.

Other nonbehavioral stimulation treatments have been studied, including right half-field patching, optokinetic stimulation, and transcranial stimulation (see Kortte & Hillis, 2011, for review). Both transcranial magnetic simulation and transcranial direct current stimulation are potentially viable treatment options that need to be explored further (e.g., Kerkhoff & Schenk, 2012).

No current treatments have worked for stimulus-centered neglect, but Arene and Hillis (2008) propose that attaching irrelevant information to the left of a stimulus may be effective (e.g., a "pseudoprefix" + word, such as *xxx*swarm), reasoning that this manipulation may shift the meaningful stimulus rightward. These authors also suggest that separate treatment may be needed for nonspatial components of neglect (i.e., vigilance, reorienting in viewer-centered space). Currently, the latter seems intractable, but pharmaceutical interventions may be beneficial in the future (Arene & Hillis, 2008). These authors warn against eye patching or other approaches that block part of the visual field for patients with neglect with coexisting hemianopsia.

In extremely severe or intractable cases of neglect, environmental modifications may be the only option. These may serve varied purposes, from reducing the risk of injury or harm to increasing patients' interactions with their environments (by, e.g., approaching from, sitting on, or putting materials on the "good" side of patients' bodies).

Visuoperceptual/Visuospatial Deficits

Visual–perceptual and visuospatial problems can be treated in reading and writing activities, in conjunction with neuropsychologists or occupational therapists when possible. Typical perceptual activities involve discrimination and matching, figure–ground differentiation, and visual integration; spatial activities include asking patients to describe markers along a route (such as street signs), draw and label floor plans, or connect scattered stimulus elements (words, sentences, phrases) to form meaningful larger units.

Memory Deficits

According to a Cochrane systematic review (das Nair & Lincoln, 2007), there are too few randomized controlled trials to make recommendations about poststroke memory treatment. Nonetheless, after reviewing the current literature, an international group of clinicians and experts has developed algorithms to prioritize recommendations and guidelines for best practices in treating memory deficits in patients with TBI (Velikonja et al., 2014). Other types of evidence have supported various approaches for memory training as considered here: the use of external memory aids, acquisition of particular skills or information, and varied instructional methods. Treatment for working memory is addressed briefly as well.

In a systematic review focused on memory impairments with various etiologies, Piras, Borella, Incoccia, and Carlesimo (2011) conclude that direct memory training involving internal memory strategies, such as verbal elaboration, mental imagery, and face–name associations, improves performance only on the trained tasks. Velikonja et al. (2014), focusing on the TBI literature, are more positive about internal compensations, including self-instructional strategies, but agree that memory restoration approaches, such as computer-based treatments, are not well supported by evidence.

The evidence for the effectiveness of *external memory aids* for patients with both focal (Piras et al., 2011; Velikonja et al., 2014) and diffuse lesions (Velikonja et al., 2014), however, is much stronger. For example, a randomized controlled trial targeting prospective memory in TBI demonstrated larger effects on test scores and strategy generalization from a compensatory intervention targeting habitual use of devices or low-tech compensations (e.g., diaries), and integrating time management and organizational strategies, than from a remediation-based approach (Shum, Fleming, Gill, Gullo, & Strong, 2011). Strategy training in a group format has also been found to increase memory test scores and self-reported strategy use for patients with chronic stroke with memory complaints (Miller & Radford, 2014).

Indeed, for relatively mild memory impairments resulting from stroke or TBI, training the use of external memory aids, including technological devices, has been endorsed as a *practice standard* (i.e., substantive evidence; this treatment should be considered) by Cicerone et al. (2005). Effects seem to be optimal when patients function relatively independently, identify their own target problems, and are able and motivated to use trained strategies over time. Reports of daily memory problems have been reduced with training to use a memory notebook protocol, even 2 years postinjury (Schmitter-Edgecombe, Fahy, Whelan, & Long, 1995). Patients also have benefited from a paging system (e.g., Wilson, Emslie, Quirk, Evans, & Watson, 2005), from cellular phone features such as reminders with alarms and text messaging (Culley & Evans, 2009), and from the use of web-based capacities such as Google Calendar, an electronic application that enables users to sync their calendars online with their mobile devices while receiving active reminders from both (A. McDonald et al., 2011. Charters, Gillett, and Simpson (2015) conclude that the evidence for electronic reminder systems is sufficient only to recommend a practice guideline for patients with acquired brain injury, but their review included people with more than mild memory impairments. Jamieson, Cullen, McGee-Lennon, Brewster, and Evans (2014) report medium-to-large effects for technologies to support prospective memory, memory for plans, and task organization for people with acquired brain injury. These authors emphasize, though, that it is not clear that technological systems are better than nontechnological options.

For individuals with moderate-to-severe memory and planning deficits, treatment to achieve functional goals with external compensations (including assistive technology) has been endorsed as a *practice guideline* (i.e., evidence of probable effectiveness; this treatment should be considered; Cicerone et al., 2005; Sohlberg et al., 2007). As one example, Sohlberg and Mateer (1989) describe a comprehensive, three-stage memory notebook training. The continued use and perceived benefit of memory notebooks may be better when practice in self-management is incorporated in treatment (see "Executive Functioning Deficits"). As another example, Svoboda, Richards, Leach, and Mertens (2012) report gains in everyday functioning for individuals with moderate-to-severe memory deficits after an intervention involving errorless acquisition and structured application of smartphone or personal digital assistant technology. Impressively, the gains were maintained up to 19 months posttreatment (Svoboda, Richards, Yao, & Leach, 2015). Again, when possible, training of external compensations should focus on patient-identified needs. Extensive structured treatment may be necessary to establish declarative and procedural memory skills when memory impairments are more severe, and to be useful, compensations likely have to be socially acceptable for the client.

Treatment to acquire particular skills or information is considered a *practice option* (i.e., evidence of possible effectiveness; consider this treatment; Cicerone et al., 2005) for people with moderate-to-severe memory problems. In one study, Todd and Barrow (2008) taught touch typing to patients with severe declarative memory impairments, using an errorless learning approach. Sohlberg, Fickas, Ehlhardt, and Todis (2005) similarly taught patients with severe deficits in memory, attention, or executive functioning to use an adapted e-mail system (see http://www.think-and-link.org for protocol). *Spaced retrieval* practice is one instructional method for improving declarative memory and functional task performance, especially for patients with more severe memory impairments. Also known as expanded rehearsal, this treatment is often used in progressive dementias and involves practicing the recall or performance of target information or procedures over increasing time intervals.

Spaced retrieval may be a useful approach for adults with RHD who need to recall and reproduce important information easily or who need support in daily tasks. Ehlhardt and colleagues (2008) are more positive about this approach than Piras and colleagues (2011), who indicate that the available evidence has not yet convincingly documented amelioration of daily life difficulties.

In relation to other *instructional methods*, systematic reviews (Ehlhardt et al., 2008; Piras et al., 2011) and expert recommendations (Velikonja et al., 2014) summarize support for errorless learning techniques for a range of etiologies, severities, tasks and goals, and memory targets (e.g., declarative information and procedural skills). Memory aids can be integrated with this approach. To foster deeper encoding of target information or procedures, Tailby and Haslam (2003) recommend using meaningful stimuli and building in active participation (self-generated responses, elaboration, using drilled information in a sentence). Errorless learning is often combined with other techniques, so it can be difficult to separate their effects.

In a randomized controlled trial to train skilled use of a personal digital assistant, Powell and colleagues (2012) also demonstrated the value of systematic instruction over a conventional trial-and-error approach. Generalization to other communication partners and skill maintenance were superior for participants given systematic instruction, a comprehensive and well-researched package that incorporates error-reducing methods in the acquisition stage, distributed practice to enhance maintenance, and various techniques to facilitate generalization.

Research on *treatment for working memory* is in its infancy. Nordvik et al. (2012) reported benefits of computerized working memory training for a lawyer with acute RHD. For a patient with chronic stroke, Vallat-Azouvi, Pradat-Diehl, and Azouvi (2014) designed treatments to focus sequentially on different subdomains of working memory (i.e., phonological look, visuospatial sketchpad, central executive) and found gains in each treatment phase specific to the aspects that were trained. And, in a randomized pilot study with a small sample of patients with chronic stroke, Westerberg et al. (2007) reported improvements on test scores and self-reported cognitive function after computerized training on working memory tasks. The results, however, may be confounded by between-group differences on factors like lesion location. Working memory treatment could also follow the procedures and strategies described previously in relation to the cognitive resources hypothesis. As summarized by Manly and Murphy (2012), though, large-scale studies with healthy adults raise significant concerns about generalization of working memory training.

Executive Functioning Deficits

Numerous systematic reviews, some with accompanying meta-analysis, have analyzed executive functioning interventions (e.g., Boelen, Spikman, & Fasotti, 2011; Chung, Pollock, Campbell, Durward, & Hagen, 2013; Cicerone et al., 2011; Kennedy et al., 2008). Tate and colleagues (2014) examined seven such reviews and some new literature to develop practice recommendations for executive function (and self-awareness). Most of the recommendations described here pertain specifically to patients with TBI, but adults with RHD may have many of the same deficits.

Corroborating previous reviews, strong evidence supports the use of metacognitive strategy instruction as a *practice standard* for TBI patients who have difficulties with daily life planning, organization, problem solving, and multitasking (e.g., Kennedy et al., 2008; Tate et al., 2014). When combined with other cognitive strategies (e.g., personal goal setting, external cueing) Goal Management Training is the preferred metacognitive approach (see Krasny-Pacini, Chevignard, & Evans, 2014, for a review), as it is the only one that has been replicated by independent investigators (Tate et al., 2014).

Once endorsed as a *practice guideline* for adults with stroke or TBI (i.e., evidence of probable effectiveness; this treatment should be considered; Cicerone, 2000, 2005), interventions targeting problem solving are still highly recommended (Tate et al., 2014). This kind of treatment typically involves defining daily life problems and possible solutions. The problem-solving process is broken into manageable steps, and patients are trained to refer to a structured diagram or guide (see Table 18.4 for an example).

Previously suggested as a *practice option* (Kennedy et al., 2008), intervention to improve reasoning skills has gained support (Tate et al., 2014; Vas, Chapman, Cook, Elliott, & Keebler, 2011). Recommendations include focusing on strategies that enhance the analysis and synthesis of complex information (Tate et al., 2014). Vas and colleagues (2011) reported significant improvements in reasoning in participants with chronic TBI who completed a Strategic Memory and Reasoning Training (SMART) program versus those in an information-based "Brain Healthy Workshop." The SMART program trains "gist reasoning," constructing generalized meanings versus remembering explicit facts. Vas et al. also found generalization to other executive measures at 6 months posttreatment, including working memory span and self-reported community functioning.

Based on studies of anger management, self-control, and psychosocial function, Cicerone et al. (2000, 2005) recommend treatment to foster self-regulation as a

Table 18.4 A Possible Format for an Organized Approach to Problem Solving

1. **Problem Identification:** Briefly, what is the problem?

   What do you need to accomplish?

   What are some of the differences between the result you want and your current situation? (perhaps diagrammed as Points A and B)

2. **Problem Classification:** What kind of problem is this?

   Is it similar to other situations you have faced?

3. **Goal Identification:** What will you gain by solving the problem?

4. **Identification of Relevant Information:** Do you have any experience with problems like this that could be helpful?

   What do you need to know about, or to count on, or to use, to solve this problem?

5. **Identification of Possible Solutions:** What things could you possibly do to solve this problem?

6. **Evaluation of Solutions:** What is good or bad about each possibility?

   CONSIDER: Effective? Able to do it? Enough time? Like to do it? Break any rules? Worked in the past? Effects on others? Effects on yourself? Effects on the environment?

7. **Decision:** What is the smartest thing to do?

8. **Formulation of a Plan:** How do you plan to accomplish this?

   CONSIDER: Steps, sequence, potential barriers.

9. **Monitoring and Evaluating the Outcome:** Did your plan work?

   Are you satisfied?

   Any new problems encountered?

Data from TOMPKINS. *Right Hemisphere Communication Disorders: Theory and Management*, 1E. © 1995 Delmar Learning, a part of Cengage Learning, Inc. Reproduced by permission. www.cengage.com/permissions.

practice option for TBI (i.e., evidence of possible effectiveness; consider this treatment). One example that reduced expressions of anger used self-instruction and -monitoring to help patients recognize thoughts, emotions, and physical reactions in situations that make them angry (Medd & Tate, 2000). Group treatment for self-awareness and -regulation has also been effective. Cicerone and colleagues underscore the benefits of self-instruction as an element of treatment in other domains as well, including attention, neglect, and memory.

Optimal benefits for most executive function interventions hinge on the patient's awareness of the need to use the strategies (Tate et al., 2014). Although there is scant evidence of its effectiveness, behavioral management of antecedents and consequents may be appropriate in some cases, as well, to deal with troubling behaviors such as disinhibition or impaired social perception. Implementing components of the behavioral approach is useful in any treatment, but it may be heavily emphasized for clients who exhibit particularly disruptive, dangerous, or embarrassing behaviors or for clients whose impairments prevent them from participating in or benefiting from metacognitive strategy instruction.

TREATMENT TARGETING OTHER OBSTACLES TO GOAL ATTAINMENT

To address obstacles outside a patient, clinicians must consider the interaction of the patient's cognitive and behavioral characteristics with environmental and task demands. For example, goal demands should be assessed (e.g., what does a desired hobby or job require), along with situational demands (e.g., who, what, where, when); environmental characteristics (e.g., noisy, busy, crowded); time constraints; the level of complexity required in pertinent activities; the degree of environmental flexibility; and the attitudes/expectations of others. A few potential treatment targets are provided here.

Expectations of others can be particularly problematic obstacles. For instance, people who interact with a client who has significant pragmatic (attention, memory, etc.) problems may think the client is purposely rude (does not listen, is lazy, etc.) and may benefit from education otherwise. Also, as noted previously, Sohlberg et al. (1998) indicate that counseling may be needed to emphasize that patients' behavior can change without patients admitting their deficits. Overprotection is common in aphasia and can also be observed for patients with RHD. Communication partners of patients with strokes also commonly give too much information, too quickly, without other supports for patients' cognitive problems. Demonstrating these problems to communication partners is more likely to have an impact than simple counseling, and in some cases, the pertinent individuals will have to be trained, specifically, to interact in ways that reduce obstacles created by their communicative attitudes or styles. For example, they can be trained to state explicitly the emotions they want to express or to provide a cue card with the appropriate label, instead of expecting patients to infer their moods. Or, they can learn to prompt appropriate responses or to explain background information, as needed, to assist with social cognition.

Regarding *environmental characteristics* that may create obstacles to attaining their goals, patients can work on organizing and labeling items in their desks or closets, using a compensatory chart or list to maintain the organizational scheme. Organizational applications can be downloaded on a patient's smartphone or computer. For crowded, unorganized aisles and setups in stores, patients can be taught to read signs or ask clerks for help and to carry a card to remind themselves to do so. Or, if there is construction on their regular route, patients can use GPS on their cell phone to find an alternate route or keep alternate route information on a card or a map in their purse, wallet, or car.

Considering *situational demands*, patients can be counseled to let phone calls go to an answering machine or voice mail, so they can listen repeatedly later without time pressure. Similarly, friends and family can be encouraged to use text messaging on the phone or instant messaging on the computer to reach patients rather than calling. If family members have inconsistent or variable schedules, a schedule board or calendar can be created to lay out daily routines in a way that is clear and easy for a patient's reference. A shared electronic calendar for the patient and family members may alleviate a patient's stress for remembering dates of important events.

The general principle, again, is to think beyond patients' deficits to identify other factors that may create obstacles to attaining their goals. We consider it both legitimate and necessary to address such obstacles in treatment, although the effects of doing so remain to be demonstrated experimentally.

FUTURE DIRECTIONS

Much work remains. We envision continued expansion of the neglect treatment literature, particularly for noninvasive, nonbehavioral treatments like transcranial direct current stimulation. We foresee the increased use of digital devices as therapy tools, with increasingly larger subsets of patients receiving services virtually and via telerehabilitation (Cherney & van Vuuren, 2012). Another major development we hope for is a more consistent clinical focus on obstacles to goal attainment beyond a patient's deficits. Finally, there is a glaring need for evidence of the efficacy and effectiveness of treatments for nearly all aspects of RHD communication and cognition, including treatments that target obstacles to goal attainment for patient-oriented, daily life functions and goals.

Case Illustration 18.1

E.A. was a 62-year-old man who ran his own landscaping business with his son-in-law. He was referred to us 10 days postonset of right hemisphere stroke. The goal of client E.A. was to return to his landscaping business. After the initial assessment, we implemented a version of VST because of E.A.'s clear neglect, our hypothesis that neglect dyslexia accounted for much of his difficulty with reading comprehension, and the fact that VST is one of the few practice standards for the RHD population. We did a number of things to enhance the likelihood of generalization, including providing treatment five times per week; incorporating real-life stimuli (landscape design sketches, invoices, order forms, poker or rummy hands); mixing complex stimuli with simpler ones; and various conditions by interweaving the various tasks during the treatment session. We added to the traditional VST cueing hierarchy a step in which we provided tactile cues to the elements of the stimuli that were omitted (stick-on Velcro dots). We incorporated social interaction and natural contingencies by interrupting the structured scanning tasks periodically to play several hands of cards with E.A., an activity that he had chosen as a reinforcer. Note that many of these task manipulations are also consistent with the aim of reducing demands on cognitive resources.

(continues)

We also inserted into the VST some activities to target E.A.'s anosognosia and other aspects of executive functioning. For example, we asked him to predict his performance before each trial (how many elements of the stimulus he would omit). We provided tangible feedback by asking him to compare stacks of poker chips (which were even before each trial) after removing from our stack one chip per item omitted. We also used experiential exercises designed to stimulate more insight about his ability to return to work. Specifically, we assigned home practice activities such as preparing a bid for a garden design or locating the best trees for specified environmental conditions in a part of the country with which he was unfamiliar.

Additional treatment activities focused on compensations for daily tasks, including organizing the mail and taking medications independently. We worked with E.A. and his wife to develop compensatory systems they were willing and able to use. They developed a color-coding scheme for dealing with mail (e.g., put in green folder if it needs immediate attention), and we helped them design a simple checklist (with only the numerals 1–5 on it, to check as completed) and audio record the five steps needed to use the scheme. We used the same checklist and audio-recording approach for medications. E.A. kept the recorder in his pocket and listened to it through ear buds. For poker playing, the recorded steps were to "count your cards" and "sort your cards." Initially, we worked with E.A. for about 20 minutes per session to help him habituate these systems. We incorporated the performance prediction/poker chip feedback and added a self-instruction component, in which E.A.'s task was to remind himself to initiate the activities (e.g., get the tape recorder, turn it on, get the mail, get the checklist).

We instructed and observed E. A.'s wife using the compensatory systems with him one to two times a week as well, asking him to provide feedback for her. In the first 2 weeks of treatment, he took a poker chip away from her with some regularity when she rushed him. By the third week of treatment, they had developed a rhythm that seemed to work for both of them; he took no more poker chips from her stack.

E.A.'s performance on other treatment tasks improved over 4 weeks of treatment. He never completed the assignments we sent with him. His wife indicated that he told her he was too tired to begin them. After about 3 weeks, E.A. volunteered that his son-in-law was doing a great job with the business, and he had decided to step back from it, indicating good insight into his present circumstances. E.A.'s neglect improved on all the tasks we had administered before treatment, and he reminded himself three times during the assessments to "check again." His wife reported that he was using the compensatory systems, for the most part independently or after a minor prompt from her. She also told us that he had just begun to go along with his son-in-law to see former clients and suppliers and had recently enjoyed a poker game with a close friend.

We asked E.A's wife and daughter to look over a Case History Supplement and Performance Inventory and mark anything that had changed for better or worse since treatment began and to complete the Dysexecutive Questionnaire again. Both respondents noted improvements in previously problematic areas and indicated that they were providing more assistance in the form of prompting compensations. They also identified some difficulties in tasks that E.A. had not tried yet when they first completed the forms, such as budgeting, but indicated that E.A.'s wife had taken over financial management for the household. E.A. and his family expressed satisfaction with his progress and, when asked, reported that they felt they knew how to deal with difficulties that might come up later.

STUDY QUESTIONS

1. What do you see as the two most significant unmet needs in the area of treatment for RHD cognitive–communicative disorders? What needs to be done first to address each of these needs? Could you begin to address them with your clients? Why or why not? And how?

2. External memory aids or organizing systems are often crucial in cognitive–communicative treatment and for generalization of gains outside treatment. Think of three different cognitive–communicative problems that can affect adults with RHD and three different kinds of external cues/organizers/structures you could create to (begin to) address them.

3. Consider the typical clinical practice of giving a patient an external memory aid, with only a few training sessions, if any. How likely is it that this patient will habituate the use of the aid and use it effectively? Identify three factors that may affect this likelihood.

4. Investigate pragmatic aspects of communication in two cultures other than your own. What are two ways in which pragmatic communication targets might differ from those in your own culture?

5. Choose any three of the objectives at the beginning of this chapter and read the chapter so that you can achieve them. To challenge yourself even further, read to achieve five or all of these outcomes.

REFERENCES

Arene, N. U., & Hillis, A. E. (2008). Rehabilitation of unilateral spatial neglect and neuroimaging. *Europa Mediphysica, 43*(2), 255–269.

Barker-Collo, S. L., Feigin, V. L., Lawes, C. M. M., Parag, V., Senior, H., & Rodgers, A. (2009). Reducing attention deficits after stroke using attention process training: A randomized controlled trial. *Stroke, 40*(10), 3293–3298.

Besharati, S., Crucianelli, L., & Fotopoulou, A. (2014). Restoring awareness: A review of rehabilitation in anosognosia for hemiplegia. *Revista Chilena de Neuropsicologia, 9*(1), 31–37.

Blake, M. L. (2007). Perspectives on treatment for communication deficits associated with right hemisphere brain damage. *American Journal of Speech-Language Pathology, 16*(4), 331–342.

Blake, M. L., Frymark, T., & Venedictov, R. (2013). An evidence-based systematic review on communication treatments for individuals with right hemisphere brain damage. *American Journal of Speech-Language Pathology, 22*(1), 146–160.

Blake, M. L., Tompkins, C. A., Scharp, V. L., Meigh, K. M., & Wambaugh, J. (2015). Contextual Constraint Treatment for coarse coding deficit in adults with right hemisphere brain damage: Generalisation to narrative discourse comprehension. *Neuropsychological Rehabilitation, 25*(1), 15–52.

Boelen, D. H. E., Spikman, J. M., & Fasotti, L. (2011). Rehabilitation of executive disorders after brain injury: Are interventions effective? *Journal of Neuropsychology, 5*(1), 73–113.

Bornhofen, C., & McDonald, S. (2008a). Comparing strategies for treating emotion perception deficits in traumatic brain injury. *The Journal of Head Trauma Rehabilitation, 23*(2), 103–115.

Bornhofen C., & McDonald, S. (2008b). Treating deficits in emotion perception following traumatic brain injury. *Neuropsychological Rehabilitation, 18*(1), 22–44.

Bowen, A., Hazelton, C., Pollock, A., & Lincoln, N. B. (2013). Cognitive rehabilitation for spatial neglect following stroke. *Cochrane Database of Systematic Reviews, 7*, CD003586. doi.10.1002/14651858.CD003586.pub3

Braden, C., Hawley, L., Newman, J., Morey, C., Gerber, D., & Harrison-Felix, C. (2010). Social communication skills group treatment: A feasibility study for persons with traumatic brain injury and comorbid conditions. *Brain Injury, 24*(11), 1298–1310.

Brookshire, R. H. (2007). *Introduction to neurogenic communication disorders* (7th ed.). St. Louis, MO: Mosby.

Brownell, H. H., Potter, H. H., Bihrle, A. M., & Gardner, H. (1986). Inference deficits in right brain-damaged patients. *Brain and Language, 27*(2), 310–321.

Cannizzaro, M. S., & Coelho, C. A. (2002). Treatment of story grammar following traumatic brain injury: A pilot study. *Brain Injury, 16*(12), 1065–1073.

Cappa, S. F., Benke, T., Clarke, S., Rossi, B., Stemmer, B., & van Heugten, C. M. (2005). Task force on cognitive rehabilitation, European federation of neurological societies. EFNS guidelines on cognitive rehabilitation: Report of an EFNS task force. *European Journal of Neurology, 12*(9), 665–680.

Charters, E., Gillett, L., & Simpson, G. K. (2015). Efficacy of electronic portable assistive devices for people with acquired brain injury: A systematic review. *Neuropsychological Rehabilitation, 25*(1), 82–121.

Cherney, L. R., & Halper, A. S. (2000). Assessment and treatment of functional communication following right hemisphere damage. In L. E. Worrall & C. M. Frattali (Eds.), *Neurogenic communication disorders: A functional approach* (pp. 276–292). New York, NY: Thieme.

Cherney, L. R., & van Vuuren, S. (2012). Telerehabilitation, virtual therapists, and acquired neurologic speech and language disorders. *Seminars in Speech and Language, 33*(3), 243–257.

Chung, C., Pollock, A., Campbell, T., Durward, B., & Hagen, S. (2013). Cognitive rehabilitation for executive dysfunction in adults with stroke or other adult nonprogressive acquired brain damage. *Stroke, 44*(7), e77–e78.

Cicerone, K. D., Dahlberg, C., Kalmar, K., Langenbahn, D. M., Malec, J. F., Bergquist, T. F., et al. (2000). Evidence-based cognitive rehabilitation: Recommendations for clinical practice. *Archives of Physical Medicine and Rehabilitation, 81*(12), 1596–1615.

Cicerone, K. D., Dahlberg, C., Malec, J., Langenbahn, D., Felicetti, T., Kneipp, S., et al. (2005). Evidence-based cognitive rehabilitation: Updated review of the literature from 1998 through 2002. *Archives of Physical Medicine and Rehabilitation, 86*(8), 1681–1692.

Cicerone, K. D., Langenbahn, D. M., Braden, C., Malec, J. F., Kalmar, K., Fraas, M., et al. (2011). Evidenced-based cognitive rehabilitation: Updated review of the literature from 2003 through 2008. *Archives of Physical Medicine and Rehabilitation, 92*(4), 519–530.

Cicerone, K. D., & Maestas, K. L. (2014). Rehabilitation of attention and executive function impairments. In A. M. Sander & M. Sherer (Eds.), *Handbook on the neuropsychology of traumatic brain injury* (pp. 191–211). New York, NY: Springer.

Cornelissen, K., Laine, M., Tarkiainen, A., Järvensivu, T., Martin, N., & Salmelin, R. (2003). Adult brain plasticity elicited by anomia treatment. *Journal of Cognitive Neuroscience, 15*(3), 444–461.

Culley, C., & Evans, J. J. (2009). SMS text messaging as a means of increasing recall of therapy goals in brain injury rehabilitation: A single-blind within-subjects trial. *Neuropsychological Rehabilitation, 20*(1), 103–119.

das Nair, R., & Lincoln, N. (2007). Cognitive rehabilitation for memory deficits following stroke. *Cochrane Database of Systematic Reviews, 3*, CD002293.

Davis, G. A., & Wilcox, M. J. (1985). *Adult aphasia rehabilitation: Applied pragmatics.* San Diego, CA: Singular.

Duncan, P. W., Zorowitz, R., Bates, B., Choi, J. Y., Glasberg, J. J., Graham, G. D., et al. (2005). Management of adult stroke rehabilitation care: A clinical practice guideline. *Stroke, 36*(9), 100–143.

Ehlhardt, L. A., Sohlberg, M. M., Kennedy, M., Coelho, C., Ylvisaker, M., Turkstra, L., et al. (2008). Evidence-based practice guidelines for instructing individuals with neurogenic memory impairments: What have we learned in the past 20 years. *Neuropsychological Rehabilitation, 18*(3), 300–342.

Ehrlich, J. S., & Sipes, A. L. (1985). Group treatment of communication skills for head trauma patients. *Cognitive Rehabilitation, 3*(1), 32–37.

Fasotti, L., & van Kessel, M. (2013). Novel insights in the rehabilitation of neglect. *Frontiers in Human Neuroscience, 7*, 1–8.

Ferré, P., Ska, B., Lajoie, C., Bleau, A., & Joanette, Y. (2011). Clinical focus on prosodic, discursive and pragmatic treatment for right hemisphere damaged adults: What's right? *Rehabilitation Research and Practice, 2011*, 131820.

Frassinetti, F., Angeli, V., Meneghello, F., Avanzi, S., & Ladavas, E. (2002). Long-lasting amelioration of visuospatial neglect by prism adaptation. *Brain, 125*, 608–623.

Fotopoulou, A., Rudd, A., Holmes, P., & Kopelman, M. (2009). Self-observation reinstates motor awareness in anosognosia for hemiplegia. *Neuropsychologia, 47*(5), 1256–1260.

Gajar, A., Schloss, P. J., Schloss, C. N., & Thompson, C. K. (1984). Effects of feedback and self- monitoring on head trauma youths' conversational skills. *Journal of Applied Behavior Analysis, 17*(3), 353–358.

Helffenstein, D. A., & Wechsler, F. S. (1982). The use of interpersonal process recall (IPR) in the remediation of interpersonal and communication skill deficits in the newly brain injured. *International Journal of Clinical Neuropsychology, 4*(3), 139–142.

Jamieson, M., Cullen, B., McGee-Lennon, M., Brewster, S., & Evans, J. J. (2014). The efficacy of cognitive prosthetic technology for people with memory impairments: A systematic review and meta-analysis. *Neuropsychological Rehabilitation, 24*, 419–444.

Kennedy, M. R. T., Coelho, C., Turkstra, L., Ylvisaker, M., Sohlberg, M. M., Yorkston, K., et al. (2008). Intervention for executive functions after traumatic brain injury: A systematic review, meta-analysis and clinical recommendations. *Neuropsychological Rehabilitation, 18*(3), 257–299.

Kerkhoff, G., & Schenk, T. (2012). Rehabilitation of neglect: An update. *Neuropsychologia, 50*, 1072–1079.

Kim, Y. M., Chun, M. H., Yun, G. J., Song, Y. J., & Young, H. E. (2011). The effect of virtual reality training on unilateral spatial neglect in stroke patients. *Annals of Rehabilitation Medicine, 35*(3), 309–315.

Kortte, K. B., & Hillis, A. E. (2011). Recent trends in rehabilitation interventions for visual neglect and anosognosia for hemiplegia following right hemisphere stroke. *Future Neurology, 6*(1), 33–43.

Krasny-Pacini, A., Chevignard, M., & Evans, J. (2014). Goal Management Training for rehabilitation of executive functions: A systematic review of effectiveness in patients with acquired brain injury. *Disability & Rehabilitation, 36*(2), 105–116.

Lehman-Blake, M. T., & Tompkins, C. A. (2001). Predictive inferencing in adults with right hemisphere brain damage. *Journal of Speech, Language and Hearing Research, 44*, 639–654.

Leon, S. A., & Rodriguez, A. D. (2008). Aprosodia and its treatment. *SIG 2 Perspectives on Neurophysiology and Neurogenic Speech and Language Disorders, 18*(2), 66–72.

Lincoln, N., Majid, M., & Weyman, N. (2000). Cognitive rehabilitation for attention deficits following stroke. *Cochrane Database of Systematic Reviews, 4*, CD002842.

Loetscher, T., & Lincoln, N. B. (2013). Cognitive rehabilitation for attention deficits following stroke. *Cochrane Database of Systematic Reviews, 5*, CD002842. doi:10.1002/14651858. CD002842.pub2

Luauté, J., Halligan, P., Rode, G., Rossetti, Y., & Boisson, D. (2006). Visuo-spatial neglect: A systematic review of current interventions and their effectiveness. *Neuroscience and Biobehavioral Reviews, 30*(7), 961–982.

Lundgren, K., Brownell, H. H., Cayer-Meade, C., Milione, J., & Kearns, K. P. (2011). Treating metaphor interpretation deficits subsequent to right hemisphere brain damage: Preliminary results. *Aphasiology, 25*(4), 456–474.

Mackenzie, C., & Brady, M. (2008). Communication difficulties following right-hemisphere stroke: Applying evidence to clinical management. *Evidence-Based Communication Assessment and Intervention, 2*(4), 235–247.

Manly, T., & Murphy, F. C. (2012). Rehabilitation of executive function and social cognition impairments after brain injury. *Current Opinion in Neurology, 25*(6), 656–661.

McCue, M., Chase, S. L., Dowdy, C., Pramuka, M., Petrick, J., Aitken, S., et al. (1994). *Functional assessment of individuals with cognitive disabilities: A desk reference for rehabilitation.* Pittsburgh, PA: Center for Applied Neuropsychology.

McDonald, A., Haslam, C., Yates, P., Gurr, B., Leeder, G., & Sayers, A. (2011). Google Calendar: A new memory aid to compensate for prospective memory deficits following acquired brain injury. *Neuropsychological Rehabilitation, 21*(6), 784–807.

McDonald, S., Tate, R., Togher, L., Bornhofen, C., Long, E., Gertler, P., et al. (2008). Social skills treatment for people with severe, chronic acquired brain injuries: A multicenter trial. *Archives of Physical Medicine and Rehabilitation, 89*(9), 1648–1659.

Medd, J., & Tate, R. L. (2000). Evaluation of an anger management therapy programme following acquired brain injury: A preliminary study. *Neuropsychological Rehabilitation, 10*(2), 185–201.

Meinzer, M., Flaisch, T., Obleser, J., Assadollahi, R., Djundja, D., Barthel, G., et al. (2006). Brain regions essential for improved lexical access in an aged aphasic patient: A case report. *BMC Neurology, 6*(28), 1–10.

Miller, L. A., & Radford, K. (2014). Testing the effectiveness of group-based memory rehabilitation in chronic stroke patients. *Neuropsychological Rehabilitation, 24*(5), 721–737.

Nordvik, J. E., Schanke, A. K., Walhovd, K., Fjell, A., Grydeland, H., & Landrø, N. I. (2012). Exploring the relationship between white matter microstructure and working memory functioning following stroke: A single case study of computerized cognitive training. *Neurocase, 18*(2), 139–151.

Piras, F., Borella, E., Incoccia, C., & Carlesimo, G. A. (2011). Evidenced-based practice recommendations for memory rehabilitation. *European Journal of Physical and Rehabilitation Medicine, 47*, 149–175.

Ponsford, J., Bayley, M., Wiseman-Hakes, C., Togher, L., Velikonja, D., McIntyre, A., et al. (2014). INCOG recommendations for management of cognition following traumatic brain injury, part II: Attention and information processing speed. *Journal of Head Trauma Rehabilitation, 29*(4), 321–337.

Powell, L. E., Glang, A., Ettel, D., Todis, B., Sohlberg, M. M., & Albin, R. (2012). Systematic instruction for individuals with acquired brain injury: Results of a randomised controlled trial. *Neuropsychological Rehabilitation, 22*(1), 85–112.

Robertson, I. H., MacMillan, T. M., MacLeod, E., Edgeworth, J., & Brock, D. (2002). Rehabilitation by limb activation training reduces left-sided motor impairment in unilateral neglect patients: A single-blind randomised control trial. *Neuropsychological Rehabilitation, 12*(5), 439–454.

Robertson, I. H., Mattingley, J. B., Rorden, C., & Driver, J. (1998). Phasic alerting of neglect patients overcomes their spatial deficit in visual awareness. *Nature, 395*, 169–172.

Rosenbek, J. C., Crucian, G. P., Leon, S. A., Hieber, B., Rodriguez, A. D., Holiway, B., et al. (2004). Novel treatments for expressive aprosodia: A phase I investigation of cognitive linguistic and imitative interventions. *Journal of the International Neuropsychological Society, 10*(5), 786–793.

Schmitter-Edgecombe, M., Fahy, J. F., Whelan, J. P., & Long, C. J. (1995). Memory remediation after severe closed-head injury: Notebook training versus supportive therapy. *Journal of Consulting and Clinical Psychology, 63*(3), 484–489.

Serino, A., Bonifazi, S., Pierfederici, L., & Ladavas, E. (2007). Neglect treatment by prism adaptation: What recovers and for how long. *Neuropsychological Rehabilitation, 17*(6), 657–687.

Shum, D., Fleming, J., Gill, H., Gullo, M. J., & Strong, J. (2011). A randomized controlled trial of prospective memory rehabilitation in adults with traumatic brain injury. *Journal of Rehabilitation Medicine, 43*(3), 216–223.

Sohlberg, M. M. (2000). Assessing and managing unawareness of self. *Seminars in Speech and Language, 21*(2), 135–151.

Sohlberg, M. M., Fickas, S., Ehlhardt, L., & Todis, B. (2005). The longitudinal effects of accessible email for individuals with severe cognitive impairments. *Aphasiology, 19*(7), 651–681.

Sohlberg, M. M., Kennedy, M. R. T., Avery, J., Coelho, C., Turkstra, L., Ylvisaker, M., et al. (2007). Evidence-based practice for the use of external aids as a memory rehabilitation technique. *Journal of Medical Speech Pathology, 15*(1), xv–li.

Sohlberg, M. M., & Mateer, C. A. (1986). *Attention Process Training (APT)*. Puyallup, WA: Association for Neuropsychological Research and Development.

Sohlberg, M. M., & Mateer, C. A. (1989). Training use of compensatory memory books: A three stage behavioral approach. *Journal of Clinical and Experimental Neuropsychology, 11*(6), 871–891.

Sohlberg, M. M., & Mateer, C. A. (2010). *APT-III: Attention process training: A direct attention training program for persons with acquired brain injury*. Youngville, NC: Lash & Associates.

Sohlberg, M. M., Mateer, C. A., Penkman, L., Glang, A., & Todis, B. (1998). Awareness intervention: Who needs it? *Journal of Head Trauma Rehabilitation, 13*(5), 62–78.

Stokes, T. F., & Baer, D. M. (1977). An implicit technology of generalization. *Journal of Applied Behavior Analysis, 10*, 349–367.

Struchen, M. (2005). Social Communication interventions for persons with traumatic brain injury. In W. M. High, A. M. Sander, M. A. Stuchen, & K. A. Hart (Eds.), *Rehabilitation interventions following traumatic brain injury: State of the science* (pp. 88–117). New York, NY: Oxford University Press.

Svoboda, E., Richards, B., Leach, L., & Mertens, V. (2012). PDA and smartphone use by individuals with moderate-to-severe memory impairment: Application of a theory-driven training programme. *Neuropsychological Rehabilitation, 22*(3), 408–427.

Svoboda, E., Richards, B., Yao, C., & Leach, L. (2015). Long-term maintenance of smartphone and PDA use in individuals with moderate to severe memory impairment. *Neuropsychological Rehabilitation, 25*(3), 353–373.

Tailby, R., & Haslam, C. (2003). An investigation of errorless learning in memory-impaired patients: Improving the technique and clarifying theory. *Neuropsychologia, 41*(9), 1230–1240.

Tate, R., Kennedy, M., Ponsford, J., Douglas, J., Velikonja, D., Bayley, M., et al. (2014). INCOG recommendations for management of cognition following traumatic brain injury, part III: Executive function and self-awareness. *The Journal of Head Trauma Rehabilitation, 29*(4), 338–352.

Todd, M., & Barrow, C. (2008). Teaching memory-impaired people to touch type: The acquisition of a useful complex perceptual-motor skill. *Neuropsychological Rehabilitation, 18*(4), 486–506.

Toglia, J., Johnston, M. V., Goverover, Y., & Dain, B. (2010). A multi-context approach to promoting transfer of strategy use and self regulation after brain injury: An exploratory study. *Brain Injury, 24*(4), 664–677.

Tompkins, C. A. (1995). *Right hemisphere communication disorders: Theory and management*. San Diego, CA: Singular.

Tompkins, C. A., & Baumgaertner, A. (1998). Clinical value of online measures for adults with right hemisphere brain damage. *American Journal of Speech-Language Pathology, 7*(1), 68–74.

Tompkins, C. A., Blake, M. T., Scharp, V. L., Meigh, K. M., & Wambaugh, J. L. (2013, May 28–June 2). *Implicit treatment of underlying comprehension processes improves narrative comprehension in right hemisphere brain damage.* Presented at the 43rd Clinical Aphasiology Conference 2013, Tucson, AZ.

Tompkins, C. A., Scharp, V. L., Fassbinder, W., Meigh, K. M., & Armstrong, E. M. (2008). A different story on "theory of mind" deficit in adults with right hemisphere brain damage. *Aphasiology, 22*(1), 42–61.

Tompkins, C. A., Scharp, V. L., Meigh, K. M., Blake, M. L., & Wambaugh, J. L. (2012). Generalization of a novel, implicit treatment for coarse coding deficit in right hemisphere brain damage: A single subject experiment. *Aphasiology, 26*, 689–708.

Tsirlin, I., Dupierrix, E., Chokron, S., Coquillart, S., & Ohlmann, T. (2009). Uses of virtual reality for diagnosis, rehabilitation and study of unilateral spatial neglect: Review and analysis. *Cyberpsychology & Behavior, 12*(2), 175–181.

Vallat-Azouvi, C., Pradat-Diehl, P., & Azouvi, P. (2014). Modularity in rehabilitation of working memory: A single-case study. *Neuropsychological Rehabilitation, 24*(2), 220–237.

Vas, A. K., Chapman, S. B., Cook, L. G., Elliott, A. C., & Keebler, M. (2011). Higher-order reasoning training years after traumatic brain injury in adults. *The Journal of Head Trauma Rehabilitation, 26*(3), 224–239.

Velikonja, D., Tate, R., Ponsford, J., McIntyre, A., Janzen, S., & Bayley, M. (2014). INCOG recommendations for management of cognition following traumatic brain injury, part V: Memory. *The Journal of Head Trauma Rehabilitation, 29*(4), 369–386.

Westerberg, H., Jacobaeus, H., Hirvikoski, T., Clevberger, P., Östensson, M. L., Bartfai, A., et al. (2007). Computerized working memory training after stroke: A pilot study. *Brain Injury*, *21*(1), 21–29.

Wilson, B. A., Emslie, H., Quirk, K., Evans, J., & Watson, P. (2005). A randomised control trial to evaluate a paging system for people with traumatic brain injury. *Brain Injury*, *19*, 891–894.

Youse, K. M., & Coelho, C. A. (2009). Treating underlying attention deficits as a means for improving conversational discourse in individuals with closed head injury: A preliminary study. *Neurorehabilitation*, *24*(4), 355–364.

Zwaan, R. A. (1999). Five dimensions of narrative comprehension: The event-indexing model. In S. R. Goldman, A. C. Graesser, & P. van den Broek (Eds.), *Narrative comprehension, causality, and coherence: Essays in honor of Tom Trabasso* (pp. 93–110). Mahwah, NJ: Erlbaum.

OBJECTIVES

The reader will be able to:

1. **Describe the mechanisms of traumatic brain injury (TBI) and associated neurobehavioral outcomes.**
2. **Describe the stages of TBI recovery and overall rehabilitation objectives.**
3. **Explain the general principles of TBI assessment and treatment.**
4. **Apply therapeutic principles of cognitive assessment for patients with TBI.**

Traumatic Brain Injury in Adults

Fofi Constantinidou and Mary Kennedy

INTRODUCTION

Traumatic brain injury (TBI) is defined as a blow (or jolt) to the head or a penetrating head injury that disrupts the function of the brain. The severity of a TBI may vary in range from "mild" (i.e., a brief change of mental status or transient loss of consciousness) to "severe" (i.e., a loss of consciousness or amnesia that lasts more than 24 hours). TBI is distinguished from other brain pathologies such as cerebral vascular accidents, space-occupying tumors, and viral or bacterial encephalopathies. Primary causes of brain injury include motor vehicle accidents, falls, and sports-related injuries in nonmilitary, civilian incidents.

According to the US Centers for Disease Control and Prevention, TBI is the primary cause of disability in adults younger than the age of 34 years (Langlois, Rutland-Brown, & Thomas, 2006; Thurman, Alverson, Dunn, Guerrero, & Sniezek, 1999). The young TBI survivor may be left with significant neuropsychological deficits that encompass not only cognitive abilities such as attention, categorization, memory, and executive dysfunction, but also personality, behavioral, and emotional problems relating to disability adjustment, self-awareness, and coping difficulties. Some of these effects may be evident immediately or within days after the injury or may develop over the course of weeks or even months following the injury. Consequently, the patient may be unable to resume preinjury levels of functioning in the home, work, social, or educational settings (Benedictus, Spikman & van der Naalt, 2010; Langlois et al., 2006; Roozenbeek, Maas, & Menon, 2013; Thurman et al., 1999).

The social and economic ramifications of TBI are significant and long lasting. Currently, an estimated 5.3 million Americans live with brain injury–related disabilities, and approximately 57 million individuals worldwide have been hospitalized with one or more TBIs (Langlois et al., 2006). TBI affects approximately 235 individuals per 100,000 in Europe; of these, approximately 10% are moderate or severe cases (J. F. Kraus, Servadei, Korsic, Compagnone, & Tagliaferri, 2005). However, the rate of hospitalization among countries varies significantly as well as the quality of the surveillance systems for accurate and uniform epidemiological data (Roozenbeek et al., 2013). The loss of productivity, as well as direct and indirect medical costs, totaled an estimated $60 billion in the United States alone in 2000 (Finkelstein, Corso, & Miller, 2006). Almost 15% of persons employed full time before a head injury will not have returned to work 4 years later. The unemployment rate rises to 69% for survivors of moderate-to-severe head injury. According to Corrigan, Whiteneck, and Mellick (2004), at least 40% of patients who were hospitalized as a result of TBI have one or more unmet neuropsychological needs at 1 year postinjury. Needs range from cognitive difficulties (such as memory and problem-solving deficits) to emotional–psychosocial difficulties (such as irritability and inability to cope with stress) to difficulties relating to performing job-related tasks successfully (Benedictus et al., 2010; Corrigan et al., 2004).

Traumatic brain injury is also a source of significant disability in older adults over 65 (Haring et al., 2015). While in younger adults the primary cause of injury is motor vehicle accidents, the primary cause in older adults is falls, and that risk increases with each decade over 65. Health outcomes are poorer in older adults due to the presence of other chronic conditions and comorbidities. Furthermore, the normal aging process results in declines in cognitive performance (Giogkaraki, Michaelides, & Constantinidou, 2013), and the presence of injury increases the burden to an already vulnerable system.

The severity and persistence of the neuropsychological deficits following TBI correlate with the severity of the injury, existing health comorbidities, and injury-related sequelae that follow the injury. These injury-related sequelae include cell death and diffuse axonal injury (DAI), brain swelling, anoxia, autoregulating and metabolic problems, the development of posttraumatic seizures, posttraumatic hydrocephalus, and other complications (Constantinidou, Thomas, & Best, 2004).

The purpose of this chapter is to provide an overview of the neuropathology of TBI, the neurological and cognitive sequelae, and directions for assessment and rehabilitation. While this chapter focuses on adult moderate-to-severe TBI, information on mild TBI and sports concussion management is also provided.

The chapter begins with a description of the mechanisms of TBI, neuropathology, and neurological effects of the injury, including brain reorganization. It proceeds to include neurobehavioral recovery and a presentation of the continuum of rehabilitation care. Assessment and rehabilitation principles are presented in the context of the World Health Organization's (WHO's) International Classification of Functioning, Disability, and Health (ICF) model. The chapter concludes with evidence-based practice for the treatment of cognitive communication disorders associated with TBI.

NEUROLOGY AND NEUROPATHOLOGY OF TRAUMATIC BRAIN INJURY

There are two primary types of TBI: *open head injury* and *closed head injury* (CHI). This distinction refers to the primary neuropathology and biomechanics of the injury. In open head injury, the primary biomechanics of the injury cause penetration of the skull and meningeal layers of the brain, as in the case of a gunshot wound. Damage is caused along the path of the penetrating object, resulting in focal brain damage and disruption of networks associated with the locus of the injury.

Closed head injury, the most frequent cause of TBI, is described as a blunt blow to the head associated with acceleration or deceleration forces applied to the skull that result in generalized cerebral dysfunction (Adamovich, Henderson, & Auerbach, 1985; Levin, Benton, & Grossmann, 1982; McAllister, 2011). Although CHI may result in focal lesions (such as hemorrhage and lacerations) resulting from a depressed skull fracture (with bone fragments penetrating the brain parenchyma), the primary neuropathology of a CHI results from the acceleration–deceleration forces applied to the skull. Inertial loading (caused by acceleration or deceleration forces) causes linear and rotational acceleration, which typically coexist or follow each other in CHI (Katz, 1992; Levin et al., 1982; McAllister, 2011) and may cause greater impairment than focal injuries at the site of impact. Rotational acceleration forces may have more devastating effects than linear forces because rotational forces lead to greater strain on the axons. The strain rate is of particular importance in TBI because a particular group of axons will suffer more damage if strained (or displaced) with more intensity and longer duration than if the same axons were strained at a lower rate of intensity and shorter amount of time. The straining of the axon fibers is one mechanism leading to microscopic damage affecting the soma and the axon and subsequently leading to DAI (Blennow, Hardy, & Zetterberg, 2012; Constantinidou & Thomas, 2010; McAllister, 2011).

Cell Function and Cell Death

On contact, the individual may sustain a focal injury at the site of the lesion (coup) or at a site distant to the lesion (countercoup) and inertial loading caused by acceleration–deceleration forces, resulting in multifocal and diffuse lesions (Katz, 1992; McAllister, 2011; Povlishock & Katz, 2005). The higher the velocity at the time of impact, as in the case of high-speed motor vehicle accidents, the stronger the inertia forces applied to the skull. The frontal and temporal lobes of the brain, which include systems critical for language, attention, categorization, strategy building, memory, and learning, are often compromised as a result of coup or countercoup lesions in CHI. These lesions include contusions resulting from hemorrhagic lesions that can lead to cell death (Blennow et al., 2012; Povlishock & Katz, 2005).

Diffuse Axonal Injury

There is a gradient of injury that occurs both at the axonal level and grossly at the distribution of DAI. The distribution of DAI follows a gradient from peripheral hemispheres to deeper parts of the cerebrum in more severe injuries. On magnetic resonance imaging (MRI) scans, DAI is often associated with macroscopic petechial hemorrhages in the area of the corpus callosum and dorsolateral midbrain.

Some of the effects of DAI can be immediate, and some axonal phenomena are delayed and occur 12 to 24 hours postinjury. The delayed effects include autodestructive cellular phenomena linked to surges of the excitatory neurotransmitter glutamate, especially at N-methyl-D-aspartate (NMDA) receptors (see information that follows on metabolic imbalance). These intracellular surges impede neuronal function. Areas of the brain with large numbers of NMDA receptors, such as the hippocampus, are vulnerable to the aforementioned autotoxic changes (Blennow et al., 2012; Katz, 1992; Povlishock & Katz, 2005).

Reactive delayed axonal changes can have devastating effects on neuronal function and on the neuropsychological impact of TBI. Because these effects are delayed, there would be great benefit in determining how to prevent them. In fact, results from experimental animal research suggest that axonal swellings (resulting from the degeneration of axons) in some cases result in neuronal sprouts in the brain stem area of cats (where axonal swellings once occurred) at about a month postinjury that continued to grow and gain access to the rest of the brain 2 to 3 months postinjury (Blennow et al., 2012; Verity, Povlishock, & Cheung, 1988). However, the actual functionality of these neuroplastic changes is still unclear (Blennow et al., 2012; Povlishock & Katz, 2005). Identifying the role of these neuroplastic changes and of neurotrophic growth factors that could promote neuronal regrowth may provide significant benefits to survivors of brain injury.

Gliosis

Brain function is dependent on neuronal networks. Most of the structural support of the brain, however, is provided by glial cells. Immediately following the injury, phagocytes infiltrate the area and dispose of the nonfunctioning tissue. Frequently, glial cells then infiltrate the area vacated by the dead neurons. They either provide nutrients for regenerating axons or form scar tissue that retards functional reconnection between remaining cells. Areas of gliosis are observable in MRI scans of survivors of severe TBI taken several months or years after the trauma (Constantinidou & Thomas, 2010).

Metabolic Dysfunction

The mechanical and cellular changes described can lead to a wide array of metabolic changes. Similar to the changes mentioned, the metabolic cascade can also be focal, multifocal, or diffuse. The metabolic cascade has become a major concern in brain injury management because it can lead to further tissue damage and contribute more extensively to the neurobehavioral outcomes following TBI than the initial mechanical damage does (Henry et al., 2011; Hillered, Vespa, & Hovda, 2005; Hovda, 1998; Yakolev & Faden, 1995). Even persons with mild brain injury are extremely sensitive to slight changes in cerebral blood flow (CBF), increases in intracranial pressure, and apnea. Advances in technology such as positron emission tomography (PET), diffusion tensor imaging (DTI), nuclear magnetic resonance (NMR) spectroscopy, and microdialysis studies have been extremely helpful in understanding the metabolic effects of TBI. However, the exact mechanism of this injury-induced vulnerability is not fully understood, and it appears that this metabolic imbalance is heterogeneous and affects brain areas differently.

Experimental research paradigms and studies with human patients have been used to study the metabolic effects of TBI that render the brain in a vulnerable metabolic state. This vulnerable state seems to be a result of interactive neurochemical and metabolic events that include excitotoxicity, hypoperfusion, oxidation, hyperglycolysis, and disregulation. Table 19.1 provides explanations for each of these mechanisms.

Table 19.1 Dynamic Metabolic and Neurochemical Cascade Following Traumatic Brain Injury

1. *Excitotoxicity.* A massive release of the excitatory neurotransmitter glutamate leads to excitotoxicity and to an increase in glucose metabolism (hyperglycolysis). Areas with NMDA receptors, such as the medial temporal lobe and hippocampal areas, are particularly vulnerable to the glutamate surges (Bergsneider et al., 1997; Povlishock & Katz, 2005; Verity et al., 1988).

2. *Hypoperfusion.* Elevation in extracellular calcium (Ca^{2+}) has been shown to increase vasoconstriction, which may account for the reduction in CBF and may also activate destructive lipases and proteases (Bergsneider et al., 1997; Hall, Mohlberg, & Poole, 1998).

3. *Oxidation.* Production of reactive forms of oxygen species cause damage via the induction of lipid and oxygen oxidation.

4. *Hyperglycolysis.* Ionic fluctuations such as increased levels of extracellular potassium (K^+). The increase in K^+ activates the ATP-dependent sodium–potassium pumps and results in considerable metabolic stress and possibly hyperglycolysis.

5. *Disregulation and metabolic depression.* Loss of autoregulation, as evidenced by increased demand for glucose (hyperglycolysis), lasts from immediately after and up to 1 week following the injury (Bergsneider et al., 1997; Blennow et al., 2012; Yoshino, Hovda, Kawamata, Katayama, & Becker, 1991) and a reduction in CBF. The acute period of hyperglycolysis is followed by a period of metabolic depression and reduction in glucose utilization (i.e., hypoglycolysis) that lasts for up to 10 days in experimental TBI (Yoshino et al., 1991). During this period of time, there is a decrease in protein synthesis and oxidative metabolism, which suggests that the glycolysis is not the only metabolic pathway affected in brain injury (Povlishock & Katz, 2005).

Note: ATP, adenosine triphosphate; CBF, cerebral blood flow.

Data from Constantinidou, F., & Thomas, R. D. (2010). Principles of cognitive rehabilitation in TBI: An integrative neuroscience approach. In M. J. Ashley (Ed.), *Traumatic brain injury: Case management and rehabilitation* (3rd ed., pp. 549–582). Boca-Raton, FL: CRC Press.

Neurological Recovery

Brain Mechanisms of Recovery

Extensive discussion regarding brain plasticity is the focus elsewhere. The focus of the present chapter is to relate the information on brain plasticity to TBI and how these recovery mechanisms are associated with the neurobehavioral outcomes and patient recovery postinjury.

A marked conceptual difference between brain reorganization at birth and brain reorganization in adulthood or following damage lies in the notion of formation of new synapses. During development, changes in brain function and organization are attributed to the formation of new synapses between cells that did not previously interact. However, theories of the changes in cell interaction induced by experience or recovery following brain damage focus on changes in the properties of existing synapses or the sprouting of new synapses between cells that already have direct synaptic contact. Similarly, despite the remarkable behavioral and cognitive changes that accompany adult learning and memory, or recovery of function, most cellular models of neural plasticity do not consider these changes to be accompanied by synaptogenesis between previously noncommunicating neurons.

Experimental research with primates and humans in the past two decades provide evidence for adult neurogenesis (Cameron, Woolley, McEwin, & Gould, 1993; Erickson et al., 1998; Gould & Gross, 2002; Gould, Reeves Graziano, & Gross, 1999; Kernie & Parent, 2010). This process results in continual influx of neurons that are (temporarily) immature and therefore structurally plastic. The hope is that the immature cells can take on functions of mature, adult cells. This, of course, challenges the current theoretical models of neuronal plasticity in the adult brain that generally assume that the new synapses being formed during learning or recovery only strengthen (or weaken) communication between already-interacting neurons (Aimone, Deng, & Gage, 2010; Constantinidou & Thomas, 2010; Kernie & Parent, 2010).

Neurobehavioral Recovery

Neurobehavioral recovery from TBI follows a predictable pattern. The Rancho Los Amigos scale (RLA; Hagen, Malkmus, & Durham, 1979) was developed to document changes in the acute recovery phase (Appendix 19A is the RLA scale). The scale consists of eight levels[1] from no response (Level I) to purposeful, appropriate responses (Level VIII). Level IV indicates that the patient is alert, disoriented, and agitated. These symptoms result from the effects of posttraumatic amnesia (PTA),[2] difficulty processing internal and external stimuli, and inability to regulate responses. Cognitive-based therapy during

Level IV focuses on improving orientation, attention, and response consistency. Level VI signifies the resolution of PTA and improved orientation to time, place, and person, which allows for reliable formal testing and more intense systematic cognitive retraining. It should be mentioned that some patients never reach Level VIII. Residual cognitive deficits as well as depression may be evident at the final stages of recovery (Levels VII and VIII) when patients become more self-aware of their deficits and try to cope with changes brought on by their injury. Patients vary in the rate by which they move from one RLA stage to the next. A patient with a severe TBI may remain in a coma for several days, whereas a patient with a mild injury may be at Level IV (agitated and confused) by the time he or she arrives at the emergency room. Even though plateaus may occur at any given point on the recovery continuum, they occur more frequently at Levels II (persistent vegetative stage) and VII (automatic, appropriate response).

As the patient progresses from the acute phases of recovery to the more chronic phases, the residual cognitive and language sequelae of the injury can be determined. The diagnosis of long-term effects is achieved more effectively when clinicians on a rehabilitation team integrate results from formal tests and informal observations. For example, both speech–language clinicians and neuropsychologists assess aspects of cognition such as memory but follow different theoretical approaches to the assessment (Wertheimer, Roebuck, Constantinidou, Turska, & Pavol, 2008). Hence, clear communication and coordination of the assessment efforts among professionals can result in more valid test results and avoid redundancy.

Cognitive and language effects after TBI can be a direct result of the injury and also a secondary effect of other injury-related complications and their pharmacological outcomes, such as posttraumatic epilepsy and antiepileptic drugs, neuroendocrine problems, and sleep disturbances. These chronic conditions also hamper overall neuropsychological function in patients recovering from TBI.

CONTINUUM OF REHABILITATION IN TRAUMATIC BRAIN INJURY

Research demonstrates that comprehensive rehabilitation following TBI is a worthwhile effort as measured by improvement in performance on neuropsychological tests and functional outcome measures. Table 19.2 is a list of international websites where evidence-based practice recommendations and systematic reviews can be located.[3] Different models of brain injury rehabilitation exist worldwide. In most well-developed healthcare systems, TBI rehabilitation follows a continuum of care starting with emergency trauma care followed by intensive acute and postacute rehabilitation. Survivors of TBI typically require comprehensive rehabilitation services, including speech–language, cognitive, (neuro)psychological, physical, occupational, and vocational treatment. The quality of rehabilitation, including

Table 19.2 Websites with evidence-based practice statements on topics related to traumatic brain injury or cognitive rehabilitation listed alphabetically.

Organization	Website
American Congress of Rehabilitation Medicine	www.acrm.org
American Speech-Language Hearing Association	http://ncepmaps.org/ http://www.asha.org/members/ebp/compendium/
Academy of Neurologic Communication Disorders and Sciences	https://ancds.memberclicks.net/evidence-based-clinical-research
Agency for Healthcare Research and Quality	http://www.ahrq.gov/research/findings/evidence-based-reports/index.html
American Academy of Neurology	https://www.aan.com/Guidelines/
Cochrane Library	http://www.cochranelibrary.com/
National Center for the Dissemination of Disability Research	http://www.ncddr.org/tf/se/
Psychological Database for Brain Impairment Treatment Efficacy	www.psycbite.com/
Speech Pathology Database for Best Interventions and Treatment Efficacy	www.speechbite.com/
Ontario Neurotrauma Foundation	www.onf.org/our-programs/acquired-brain-injury/systematic-reviews-guidelines-and-measurements

intensity, frequency, and length of treatment, varies widely among health-care systems within countries and among countries depending on availability and funding for services.

The continuum of care for the patient with moderate-to-severe TBI typically begins with emergency trauma care and the neurological intensive care unit. More often than not, patients with severe TBI also sustain injuries to other organs and systems (such as respiratory, gastrointestinal, and orthopedic systems). Therefore, during trauma care the medical team focuses on rendering the patient medically stable while reducing further complications (from the injury), including serious neurological sequelae.

In the neurological intensive care unit, intracranial pressure, brain swelling, seizure activity, and the patient's level of consciousness are closely monitored. Once the patient is medically stable and demonstrates improvements in consciousness, he or she is transferred to acute hospital rehabilitation for inpatient rehabilitation. During this phase, the patient's medical progress is closely monitored by medical staff and medically oriented rehabilitation therapists. During this acute phase of recovery, primary cognitive problems result from changes in consciousness, alertness difficulties, and sensory (dys)regulation. The patient typically exhibits slowness in information processing and significant mental/cognitive fatigue. Basic cognitive processes such as attention can be significantly affected. The patient may be unable to concentrate effectively to complete a cognitive (or physical) task or may have difficulty blocking out irrelevant information (resulting from internal or external stimuli) to focus on the task at hand (selective attention and executive control). During the acute phase, the patient may be in PTA and unable to recall day-to-day information. In addition, the patient may be experiencing motor speech, swallowing, and voice difficulties. The Galveston Orientation and Amnesia Test (GOAT; Levin, O'Donnell, & Grossman, 1979) or the Westmead PTA Scale (WPTAS; Marosszeky, Ryan, Shores, Batchelor, & Marosszeky, 1997) can be used to assess a patient's orientation during the acute and subacute stages. These scales can be administered several times during the day until recovery of orientation and PTA resolution are demonstrated (Levin et al., 1979; Tate et al., 2006). However, even after the resolution of PTA, the TBI survivor will sustain periods of confusion resulting from fatigue and increased task demands. Categorization and decision-making problems are also evident during this phase of recovery as well as problems in social cognition and pragmatics. The patient typically uses simplified and concrete language with the primary area of difficulty in word finding and auditory comprehension (because of

reduction in information processing and speed of thinking). Psychosocially, emotional discontrol manifested by inappropriate verbal and physical outbursts and self-injurious behavior are common sequelae. Cognitive rehabilitation during this phase focuses on environmental manipulation and control to improve information processing and reduce overstimulation as well as in activities to improve orientation and improve cognitive stamina to render the patient able to benefit from more intense cognitive treatment.

The length of inpatient rehabilitation varies depending on injury severity and health-care practices and typically ranges from a few days to 2 to 4 weeks. Discharge from acute rehabilitation does not imply that the patient has returned to preinjury levels of functioning. Whereas in many cases the patient may be able to perform some basic activities of daily living (such as self-care tasks) independently or with some supervision, most patients will continue to experience persistent neuropsychological problems. In fact, if the patient has sustained significant trauma to require inpatient rehabilitation, then more than likely he or she will continue to have persistent problems in several areas, such as executive functioning, memory, attention, categorization, abstract reasoning, and self-awareness (Constantinidou, 2008).

Postacute rehabilitation follows inpatient acute rehabilitation. Models of postacute rehabilitation include residential comprehensive treatment programs, day programs, or outpatient treatment. Typically, day treatment and residential programs provide intensive treatment. The patient may have up to 4 to 6 hours of treatment each day that includes cognitive/linguistic treatment, occupational therapy (OT), physical therapy (PT), counseling and psychological services, therapeutic recreation, vocational treatment, and educational services. In the day treatment model, the patient returns home after the therapies are over. Residential treatment programs offer supervised residential accommodations. The level of assistance and supervision during activities of daily living (such as doing the laundry, meal preparation) and during recreational activities decreases as the patient improves and demonstrates readiness to return to the home environment. This additional dimension in the rehabilitation process ensures higher probability of success in community reintegration. One of the many benefits of the day treatment and residential programs is the collaboration among professionals. Typically, patient progress is discussed in weekly or biweekly team meetings. Ideally, a consulting physiatrist monitors the patient's progress in all areas to ensure that the patient goals are being met. Issues such as pain, substance abuse, depression, and behavioral problems, along with the cognitive and physical complications resulting from the injury, are being monitored by the entire team. The length of residential or day treatment rehabilitation can vary from 1 week to 12 weeks (or more) depending on the severity of the injury and the length of treatment authorized by the patient's insurance plan. Comprehensive day treatment and residential rehabilitation have been shown to be effective in improving functional performance in patients with TBI (Constantinidou et al., 2005; Malec, 2001).

Another type of postacute rehabilitation is outpatient rehabilitation. Traditionally, outpatient rehabilitation incorporates speech–language pathology (for speech, cognitive–communication deficits, and residual swallowing problems), PT, and OT. The patient receives each of these services one to three times per week. The patient does not receive the same amount or variety of treatment services as in residential/day treatment programs. This model is more conducive during later stages of recovery when the patient's rehabilitation program can be modified according to his or her needs.

During the postacute phase, as the patient's orientation improves and PTA resolves, clinicians are able to determine the chronic effects of the injury on cognition. Typically, patients who sustain moderate-to-severe TBI will demonstrate impairment in various cognitive abilities, such as information processing, attention, learning and memory, categorization, and executive function. As mental stamina improves, cognitive rehabilitation task demands increase, while support systems are implemented to facilitate learning. During this phase of recovery, the patient may continue to exhibit deficits in judgment and awareness; hence, supervision may still be necessary in the home setting to ensure patient safety. As the patient's abilities improve, cognitive rehabilitation also targets job-specific skills to help the patient reintegrate his or her previous work/educational setting.

Across the rehabilitation continuum, a team approach (often referred to as interdisciplinary or transdisciplinary) to managing the cognitive and communication disorders is a best practice standard (Joint Committee on Interprofessional Relations Between the American Speech-Language-Hearing Association [ASHA] and Division 40 of the American Psychological Association [APA], 2007). Teams of professionals provide specific expertise based on their respective disciplines to provide optimal, individualized services. Depending on the stage of recovery and the service delivery setting, the members of the team will vary. For example, the team serving individuals who have recovered physically but who have lingering disorders of executive functions, working memory, and slowed processing would receive services from the speech–language clinician and the occupational therapist based on each discipline's assessment as well as the assessment findings of the neuropsychologist. The Joint Committee on Interprofessional Relations Between ASHA and APA Division 40 (2007) has published documents that detail the recommended best practice collaboration for speech–language pathology and neuropsychology. In general, speech–language clinicians provide intervention for cognitive disorders as the basis of communication, language, and behavior, whereas neuropsychologists provide more detailed assessment of the cognitive and memory impairments (Wertheimer et al., 2008).

CONCEPTUALIZING COGNITIVE REHABILITATION

In the late 1960s and early 1970s, rehabilitation professionals started to conceptualize the assessment and therapy provided to individuals with TBI as distinctly different from that provided to individuals with other kinds of acquired cognitive and language impairments. In speech–language pathology, this comparison was made to individuals with aphasia. To the clinician in the 21st century, this comparison may seem inappropriate because most individuals with TBI have preserved language structure, but at that time there were few assessment tools available to speech–language clinicians that adequately captured the cognitive-based communication changes after TBI. Thus, many speech–language clinicians used assessment batteries designed to identify communication disorders associated with aphasia. Even so, during acute recovery when individuals are minimally conscious or still confused, performance on such aphasia batteries can mimic the language impairment associated with aphasia even though the basis for the communication problems is impaired cognition. Individuals with TBI can of course have aphasia, with the estimates ranging up to 30% (Code & Petheram, 2011; Sarno, 1980, 1984; Sarno, Buonaguro, & Levita, 1986). When it occurs after TBI, it is associated with concomitant focal injury to the left hemisphere of the brain.

In the past 20 years, there has been a proliferation of tools designed to assess cognitive and communication disorders associated with TBI. The outcomes from these assessments can guide clinicians to identify treatment goals and objectives. Yet, how clinicians conceptualize cognitive rehabilitation dictates the kinds of assessment tools they select and the approach to remediating cognitive and communication disorders after TBI. These conceptualizations are discussed in the following section, followed by a summary of evidence-based practice, both for assessment (formal and informal) and intervention.

Cognitive Rehabilitation and Speech–Language Pathology

The unique role of speech–language clinicians in managing cognitive and communication disorders associated with TBI started in the 1970s (Hagen et al., 1979) when cognitive rehabilitation emerged in the United States. Terms such as *cognitive–language* or *cognitive-linguistic therapy* were used extensively by clinicians and researchers (e.g., Adamovich et al., 1985; Barwood & Murdoch, 2013; Hagen et al., 1979; Kennedy & DeRuyter, 1991) but did not adequately reflect the view that most behaviors (verbal and nonverbal) involve communication. Speech–language pathologists are knowledgeable about normal and abnormal cognitive, language, and speech development across the life span after brain injury. The

> *educational and clinical background prepares speech-language pathologists to assume a variety of roles related to the habilitation and rehabilitation of individuals with cognitive-communication disorders . . . [that] include but are not limited to . . . identification, assessment, intervention, counseling, collaboration, case management, education, prevention, advocacy and research. (ASHA, 2005)*

Emphasizing Executive Functions

The neuropathology of TBI results in a preponderance of symptoms associated with frontal lobe pathology that distinguish TBI from other kinds of brain injury (e.g., stroke, dementia, tumor, and anoxia). The interconnections between the frontal lobes and other brain structures are vulnerable to diffuse and focal neuropathologies. Decades of autopsy and now neuroimaging evidence indicate that neuropathology in the frontal lobes, anterior portions of the temporal lobes, hippocampi, and white matter connections are a hallmark of TBI (e.g., Adams, Graham, Murray, & Scott, 1982; Courville, 1937; M. F. Kraus et al., 2007; Newcombe et al., 2011; Rugg-Gunn, Symms, Barker, Greenwood, & Duncan, 2001; Strich, 1961). In particular, recent evidence shows a lack of integrity in white matter connections after TBI during acute (e.g., Newcombe et al., 2007) and chronic stages of recovery (e.g., Kennedy et al., 2009; Kinnunen et al., 2011), even in those with mild injuries (Lipton et al., 2009; Wilde et al., 2008).

Thus, cognitive rehabilitation includes both the remediation and compensation for lost function of more basic "posterior" brain functions or underlying processing networks *in conjunction with emphasis on the executive monitoring (self-assessment) and control (selection and use*

of strategies) of those underlying systems. Indeed, many have proposed that the interaction between basic systems (e.g., attention, short-term memory) and prefrontal executive functions that best describes the most common symptoms after TBI should be the theoretical basis of cognitive rehabilitation (Chen, Abrams, & D'Esposito, 2006; Chen & D'Esposito, 2010). Executive functions supported by frontal lobe structures and networks are a part of most contemporary theoretical models of attention, memory and learning, decision making, reasoning, and categorization (Constantinidou, Wertheimer, Tsanadis, Evans, & Paul, 2012).

With direct application to TBI, Stuss (1991; 2011) provides a hierarchical model of these relationships where monitoring and control provide self-generated feedback, which over time allows individuals to update their self-perceptions or awareness of abilities and disabilities. Using memory impairment as an example of this, Kennedy and Coelho (2005) distinguish between self-monitoring and -control that occur *while* learning versus the *autobiographical beliefs or self-awareness* that change over time as a result of this updating system. Unfortunately, then, many TBI survivors have dual disabilities: a disability of a more basic, posterior system (e.g., short-term memory) and a disability of executive function (e.g., metamemory). Indeed, Vakil (2005) concludes, "The most common vulnerable memory processes following TBI very much resemble the memory deficits reported in patients from frontal lobe damage, e.g., difficulties in applying active or effortful strategy in the learning or retrieval process" (p. 977). Thus, the therapeutic emphasis on executive monitoring and control of basic processes is fundamental to cognitive rehabilitation.

Speech–Language Pathology in Sports Concussion Management

The majority of TBIs are mild injuries, and a large percentage of those are a result of sports. Rehabilitation professionals have gained a better understanding in the past 20 years on the cumulative effects of sports-related brain injuries. Recent figures estimate that approximately 50% of the 3.8 million cases of sports- and recreation-related TBIs occurring each year in the United States go unreported (Harmon et al., 2013). While a single concussion has been considered less severe compared to other forms of TBI and symptoms are expected to resolve within 7–10 days, a second impact to the head prior to brain recovery may result in greater or more prolonged neurocognitive dysfunction (Harmon et al., 2013). In addition, athletes may incur a cumulative range of mild head impacts over the course of their athletic careers, which can increase the risk of future concussions or long-standing chronic neurocognitive effects resulting in chronic traumatic encephalopathy (CTE; Dashnaw, Petraglia, & Bailes, 2012; Harmon et al., 2013; McCrory, Davis, & Makdissi 2012).

Chronic traumatic encephalopathy results in a neurodegenerative condition with a cascade of cognitive, behavioral, psychiatric, and motor (pyramidal and extrapyramidal) symptoms (Blennow et al., 2012). While the exact incidence of CTE is not established, the majority of reported cases result from sports injuries. Participation in sports such as boxing, American football, soccer, hockey, or professional wrestling increases the risk of CTE due to the frequent opportunities for concussion. The length of participation in the sport and previous history of concussion as well as the age of the previous history (younger or over 65) increase the risk for CTE. Other risk factors include presence of apolipoprotein E4 (APOE4) and APOE4 allele, history of epilepsy, history of domestic abuse, and military blast injuries (Saulle & Greenwald, 2012).

Cognitive and neurobehavioral effects of sports-related concussion can vary in extent, severity, and duration (Harmon et al., 2013; McCrea, Iverson, Echemendia, Makdissi, & Raftery, 2013). Some symptoms can be observed physically on the field by the athletic trainer or team physician (such as alteration in consciousness, confusion, irritability), while others can be carefully revealed through formal neurocognitive testing by the speech–language clinician or the neuropsychologist.

Common cognitive deficits include reductions in verbal and visual memory (immediate and delayed recall), speed of information processing, impulse control, orientation, attention, and executive function; the most common persistent deficits occur in verbal memory, speed of processing (i.e., reaction time), and attention (Bruce & Echemendia, 2009; Covassin, Stearne, & Elbin, 2008; Macciocchi, Barth, Alves, Rimel, & Jane, 1996; McCrea et al., 2013; Schatz, Pardini, Lovell, Collins, & Podell, 2006; Webbe & Barth, 2003). Athletes who have a history of more than three concussions are at a greater risk for lingering deficits in verbal memory and reaction time (Covassin, Moran, & Wilhelm, 2013). Therefore, these athletes are at risk for academic and lingering neurobehavioral deficits and should be monitored closely. In addition, academic modifications and provisions could be made depending on the outcome of the assessment to ensure academic success.

In 2013, the National Collegiate Athletic Association (NCAA) established that all college athletic departments must have detailed concussion management policies in place (NCAA Sports Medicine Handbook, 2012–2013). The effective management of concussion requires an interdisciplinary team approach, with trained professionals (e.g., team physician, athletic trainer, speech–language pathologist, neuropsychologist) observing and analyzing symptoms and behaviors in a variety of scenarios and settings to make the best return-to-play decisions (Harmon et al., 2013). Sports concussion protocols include preseason baseline testing of neurocognitive and psychosocial functioning of all athletes on the sports team. Computerized and paper-and-pencil neurocognitive batteries that are sensitive to the effects of sports concussion are being implemented in athletic testing.

If an athlete sustains a concussion, then that athlete is referred by the team physician for a postconcussion neurocognitive and neurobehavioral assessment at 24 or 48 hours postinjury to determine if the athlete's performance deviates from the baseline. The athlete is educated on the symptoms of concussion, the recovery process, and potential education modifications to assist with his academic performance during the period of recovery. If the athlete's performance deviates 1 standard deviation or more for at least one measure on the battery, then he or she is retested at 5–7 days postinjury and weekly afterward until he or she is symptom free and all test scores have returned to baseline. In parallel to neurocognitive testing, the injured athlete is monitored by the athletic trainer for physical symptoms, and decisions about the athlete's ability to return to physical activity are made by the athletic trainer and team physician in conjunction with the neurocognitive test results and subjective symptomatology. Refer to the work of Knollman Porter, Constantinidou, and Hutchinson Marron (2014) for a description of an interdisciplinary long-standing sports concussion management program at Miami University in the United States.

WHO INTERNATIONAL CLASSIFICATION FRAMEWORK: ASSESSMENT AND TREATMENT OF COGNITIVE AND COMMUNICATION DISORDERS

The ICF framework developed by WHO (2001) provides clinicians with a practical framework to guide assessment and therapy decisions. Table 19.3 provides assessment and therapy examples at each level, including body structure/function, activity, and participation. Appendix 19B organizes tests according to WHO's ICF

Table 19.3 ICF Conceptual Framework for Assessing and Treating Cognitive and Communication Disorders Following TBI

	Body Function and Structure		Activity	Participation
	Pathophysiology	**Impairment**	**Limitation**	**Restriction**
Level of deficit	Damage to cortical and subcortical brain regions, most likely frontal and temporal lobes and hippocampi	Reductions in executive functions, memory, language, and other cognitive systems directly and indirectly associated with the injury	Reduced effectiveness under typical circumstances (home, restaurants, school, work, social settings, etc.) or efficiency under ideal circumstances in functional, contextualized tasks as a result of impaired cognitive or communication abilities	Changes in roles with community, family, work, school, and so forth relative to cognitive or communication performance; can include public or employer policy

framework. In addition, personal and environmental factors influence performance at all levels of deficit, although they are more easily conceptualized at the activity and participation levels.

Why is the distinction between levels of deficit important? Historically, there were two general approaches to cognitive rehabilitation, both of which are reflected in levels of deficit by the WHO ICF. Impairment-based assessment and treatment were characterized by a process-specific, decontextualized approach that assumes that cognitive processes can be isolated and treated somewhat independently from each other (Adamovich et al., 1985; Sohlberg & Mateer, 1989). However, the past two decades of evidence provide support for functional, contextualized therapy in part because of the lack of generalization effects from process-specific, decontextualized therapy (Hartley, 1995; Hughes & Orange, 2007; Ylvisaker & Feeney, 1998). In reality, clinicians use a combination of these approaches based on the state of the evidence, the client's own goals and values, and the clinician's level of expertise. Sohlberg and Mateer (2001) acknowledge this and conclude the following:

> It is increasingly acknowledged that functional changes must be the goal of treatment, and that there are many ways to go about facilitating those functional changes. If we have learned anything, it is that a cookie-cutter approach will not work. Individuals and families respond differently to different interventions, in different ways, and at different times after injury. (p. 4)

The WHO framework provides a common language for various levels of deficits. These levels of deficit may or may not be related to each other. A cognitive rehabilitation focus on cognitive impairments results in improved impairments, but these do not necessarily generalize to activities that may in turn have an effect on the ability to carry out societal and familial roles at the participation level. For example, a family member may wonder why working at the impairment level does not result in functional changes and may be disappointed when this does not happen. Education about addressing the underlying processes as a foundation for future functional change could clarify this. Thus, the WHO framework provides specific language for researchers and clinicians to describe specific changes from various approaches and at various points in recovery to clients and families. ASHA embraces the WHO classification and extends the definition of cognitive rehabilitation to include assessment and intervention directed at activities and participation levels:

> Within a flexible and contextualized approach to rehabilitation, the broad goal is to help individuals with cognitive disabilities achieve functional objectives and participate in chosen activities that are at least temporarily blocked by the impairment. . . . This approach may include . . . context-oriented interventions designed to lessen the impact of cognitive disability on real-world status and functioning by engineering the individual's environment . . . and by modifying the expectations and supportive behavior of people in the individual's everyday life. (Ylvisaker, Hanks, & Johnson-Greene, 2003, p. 61)

NEUROBEHAVIORAL ASSESSMENT IN TRAUMATIC BRAIN INJURY

Formal testing of neurobehavioral functioning requires that the patient has recovered to the point at which he or she is able to comprehend and follow task instructions and sustain attention long enough to complete the test task reliably. Therefore, *formal* cognitive and communication assessment typically begins after the resolution of PTA (RLA Level VI or higher). Typically, assessment is designed to meet the following primary objectives:

- Evaluate strengths and weaknesses and how these affect return to premorbid levels of functioning.
- Guide the development and implementation of treatment goals.
- Guide the development of remedial and compensatory strategies.
- Steer the discussions with patients and family members regarding challenges after discharge.
- Serve as a baseline for future changes resulting from recovery and treatment.

To achieve these objectives, clinicians implement a variety of standardized tests. However, the ecological validity of these tests has been brought into question (Sanders, Nakase-Thomson, Constantinidou, Wertheimer, & Paul, 2007; Silverberg & Millis, 2009). It appears that the ability of standardized tests to predict how the patient will function in daily activities is limited. Hence, clinicians worldwide are encouraged to consider the WHO ICF framework (WHO, 2001) when selecting assessment and treatment methodologies. According to the ICF model, assessment should incorporate the individual's functioning and the context. Sanders et al. (2007) explain that the context aspect of the ICF includes

> *environmental factors (e.g., work, cultural beliefs, social support, and attitudes of others) and personal factors (e.g., age, gender, race, and education level) that shape an individual's life activities and influence treatment outcomes. Environmental and personal factors may serve as barriers to or facilitators of health outcomes, so that there is not a linear translation of impairments in body structures and functions into limitations in activities or participation in meaningful life roles. (p. 322)*

Appendix 19B lists common tests used by speech–language clinicians; these tests are organized according to the WHO ICF framework.

Assessing Cognitive and Communication Disorders

To obtain a comprehensive picture of the patient's neurobehavioral status, assessment following TBI should follow a team approach. Combined data from the neuropsychological and the speech–language assessments provide information regarding the following areas of function, which are typically affected secondary to TBI:

- Intelligence (current and premorbid estimates of intellect)
- Judgment, reasoning, and problem solving
- Executive functioning, decision making, organization, speed and efficiency of information processing
- Attention (attentional control, selective, alternating, and divided attention)
- Memory, learning, and recall capacity for verbal and nonverbal information
- Language abilities relating to expressive and receptive oral and written language skills
- Communication abilities, including pragmatics, discourse organization, and communication effectiveness
- Affect, emotional control, and psychosocial functioning
- Self-awareness and metacognitive abilities
- Impact of cognitive and communication disorders on quality of life

The assessment identifies levels of strengths and weaknesses and also determines patient performance profiles. For instance, a patient may exhibit difficulty in learning a list of seven items, but the underlying cause of the difficulty could be attention problems rather than an impaired short-term memory span per se. Table 19.4 lists the various divisions of human memory.

Typically, most standardized cognitive–linguistic testing addresses only the structure/function by measuring the level of impairment, which may not translate directly to how the patient will perform in specific activities at home or work or in the community. For that reason, it is important to identify the interplay between formal test performance along with environmental parameters that can affect performance, such as personality traits and demographic characteristics (e.g., age, gender, and education level). This interplay can also affect therapy compliance and rehabilitation success in general.

The ecological validity, or the degree to which a measure represents everyday behavior, of impairment-level testing has recently been challenged by many experts in cognitive rehabilitation. Turkstra et al. (2005) review the psychometric properties of 69 tests that speech–language clinicians use to test cognitive, language, and speech disorders after TBI and find that most tests lack ecological validity (see Turkstra et al., 2005, for details; for the technical report, see http://www.ancds.org/assets/docs/EBP/turkstra_standardized_tests_for_individuals.pdf). Indeed, these authors recommend that impairment-level testing be used to obtain baseline information on underlying cognitive processes, but that questionnaires, clinical observation, and other dynamic assessment procedures, such as interviews, be used to obtain information on how the cognitive processes interface with real-life activities in everyday situations.

Table 19.4 Human Memory Systems

System	Subsystems	Divisions	Function	Brain Structure
Working memory	Central executive		Attention control and monitoring of the "slave systems": visual–spatial sketchpad and phonological loop	Bilateral frontoparietal regions Prefrontal lobes
	Visual–spatial sketchpad	Nonverbal visual–spatial store	Holds visual (such as spatial or pictorial) information	Right occipital/parietal
	Phonological loop	Phonological store	Holds acoustic information (typically linguistic)	Left temporal–parietal Left supramarginal gyrus
		Subvocal rehearsal	Refreshes store content	Broca's area Cerebellum
	Buffer	Integration of information from visual–spatial and phonological systems	Use of strategy to guide learning	Frontal lobe
Long-term memory	Explicit	Semantic	Knowledge of general facts	Left MTL Left cerebellum
		Episodic	Autobiographical experiences and events	Left MTL Diencephalon Amygdala
	Implicit	Procedural	Motor and cognitive skill (such as brushing teeth and playing checkers)	Basal ganglia Motor cortex
		Perceptual representation encoding	Priming/perceptual	Occipital lobes Stimulus-dependent primary sensory areas MTL
		Simple associative/classical conditioning		Throughout CNS Cerebellum

Note: CNS, central nervous system; MTL, medial temporal lobe.

Source: Adapted from Constantinidou, F., & Thomas, R. D. (2010). Principles of cognitive rehabilitation in TBI: An integrative neuroscience approach. In M. J. Ashley (Ed.), Traumatic brain injury: Case management and rehabilitation (3rd ed., pp. 549–582). Boca-Raton, FL: CRC Press.

PRINCIPLES OF COGNITIVE REHABILITATION

Even though cognitive rehabilitation is only four decades old, several principles have emerged that should inform clinicians *on how to instruct* individuals with TBI to use strategies that can improve or compensate for a skill or behavior. These principles are based on intact learning processes while emphasizing the real challenges of cognitive rehabilitation. Most of these principles are successfully implemented after the resolution of PTA, when the patient is able neurologically to benefit from intense training and repetition.

Striving for Effortless Behavior

Effortless behavior requires few mental resources whereas effortful behavior requires many mental resources. This theoretical dichotomy is referred to as *automatic* versus *controlled* processing (Schmitter-Edgecombe, 2006). Examples of effortless or automatic behavior include daily routines such as brushing teeth, conversational greetings, the sequence of steps for checking e-mail on a personal digital assistant (PDA), and so forth. These are behaviors that have been over-learned to such a level of automaticity that individuals do not explicitly think or even pay attention to carrying out the skill; indeed, these are carried out with little explicit thought or conscious awareness. Yet, there is a relationship between these automatic and controlled processes: "Controlled processing reevaluates the situation and may inhibit an automatic strategy and initiate a new response. It is possible for some controlled operations to become automatized with experience or extensive practice" (Schmitter-Edgecombe, 2006, p. 132).

It is well documented that individuals with TBI, regardless of severity, suffer impairments in effortful attention, memory, complex problem solving, and reasoning (e.g., Cicerone & Wood, 1986; Crosson, Novack, Trenerry, & Craig, 1998; Haut, Petros, Frank, & Lamberty, 1990; Millis et al., 2001; Schmitter-Edgecombe, 1996; Serino et al., 2006; Vakil, 2005; Varney & Menefee, 1993). These impairments are likely the result of impaired attention processes, working memory, and slow processing, and they become worse as the complexity of the activity increases. However, after TBI, many automatic processes that were learned prior to the injury are preserved in individuals with TBI. For example, Schmitter-Edgecombe and Nissley (2000) manipulated attention (automatic or controlled) to determine its effects on memory for word lists. Although the memory performance of individuals with TBI was worse than those without brain injury, their memory was similarly moderated by the attention condition. Furthermore, the ability to acquire or learn tasks to an automatic, effortless level appears to be preserved after TBI even though it may take longer and require more practice. Thus, there is ample evidence that striving for effortless and accurate performance is a realistic goal of cognitive rehabilitation. Descriptions of how this can be achieved are provided in the examples of instruction approaches further in this chapter.

Capitalizing on Implicit Processes Through Errorless Learning

Effortless performance is only useful when coupled with errorless learning (EL). Habitual routines that are implicitly learned result in the desired outcome (e.g., using a daily planner to get to appointments on time). Ideally, EL occurs when errors are severely constrained or eliminated by providing individuals with correct responses before they make errors during the acquisition phase of a strategy or skill. By doing so, incorrect responses are not allowed, thereby avoiding the neural activation of erroneous search and retrieval processes (Baddeley & Wilson, 1994) while reinforcing the activation of desirable search and retrieval processes. Errorless learning is typically compared to errorful learning (EF), in which errors are not constrained and individuals learn from their mistakes.

The method of vanishing cues (MVC) is another instruction approach commonly used during the acquisition phase of a new skill or strategy. Initially described by Glisky and colleagues (Glisky, Schacter, & Tulving, 1986a, 1986b), cues are either added or removed as the individual makes errors (EF) or responds correctly to a predetermined criterion (EL), respectively. Kessels and de Haan (2003) conducted a meta-analysis that compared the outcomes of MVC to EL in adults with memory impairment; studies that employed the MVC were included in which cues were withdrawn after a criterion was reached. Effect sizes were obtained from 11 studies. Outcomes from EL resulted in statistically significant large effect sizes, whereas the MVC resulted in small and insignificant effect sizes. Thus, the research evidence favors EL over the MVC, even when cues are removed after reaching a criterion.

Ehlhardt and colleagues (2008) conducted a systematic review of instructional practices used in cognitive rehabilitation after acquired brain injury (including TBI), schizophrenia/schizoaffective disorder, and dementia. They searched peer-reviewed journals up to 2006 and found 11 studies that had compared EL to EF instruction techniques with individuals with brain injury. In general, EL results in favorable outcomes for remembering information and procedures.

Person-Centered Rehabilitation

Intuitively, it makes sense that the more actively involved the individual is in the therapy process, the more likely he or she will learn, value, adapt, and maintain strategies over time. Indeed, evidence-based practice includes the values and preferences of the client. But, how should this be done and to what extent? First and foremost, a collaborative partnership should be established between clinicians and clients. This means that goals are decided on together, including their prioritization, which can be accomplished by finding out the clients' functional goals and then educating clients in how larger goals are broken down into smaller ones (Kennedy, O'Brien, & Krause, 2012). For individuals who remain confused, this kind of relationship must wait until further cognitive recovery occurs.

Person-centered therapy also means that therapeutic strategies, supports, cues, and prompts are determined collaboratively with clinicians respectful of clients' preferences. When clients' preferences are ignored, the likelihood of its long-term success is unlikely. Having clients recall and explicitly generate responses themselves while constraining errors appears to be an important feature to obtain optimal outcomes as well. To find out clients' preferences and goals, speech–language pathollogists can conduct interviews. Motivational interviewing techniques can be used to explore how clients view their abilities and disabilities, to identify the strategies (both internal and external compensatory strategies), and to determine why the client is seeking therapy (McFarland, 2012).

Individuals with TBI have additional knowledge or information that is unique to them, and clinicians who partner with clients can use this information to enhance client performance, particularly with recall. A phenomenon called the *generation effect* has been used in this way. The generation effect is said to occur when adults with or without brain injury are more likely to recall information that they overtly or covertly retrieved correctly (Lengenfelder, Chiaravalloti, & DeLuca, 2007; O'Brien, Chiaravalloti, Arango-Lasprilla, Lengenfelder, & DeLuca, 2007). Kennedy, Carney, and Peters (2003) demonstrated this by having adults with TBI restudy word pairs that they had self-selected and had predicted that they would not remember, in addition to restudying items selected by the computer (with low prediction ratings as well). After restudying, adults with TBI remembered more of the items that they themselves had selected than the items the computer had selected. The authors concluded that adults with TBI have idiosyncratic knowledge that is unique to them, and that this should be accessed if possible.

Awareness of Deficits

The importance of being aware of one's abilities and disabilities is obvious; if an individual does not know that a problem exists, then there is no motivation or reason to change the behavior (Kennedy & Coelho, 2005). Individuals with either diffuse TBI or focal frontal lobe injury can display a lack of "awareness" of their cognitive and communication disability (Giacino & Cicerone, 1998). The self–other reports from interviews and questionnaires are the means for determining self-awareness, although there are many drawbacks to comparing these reports directly. For example, this method assumes that the "others'" (e.g., care provider, therapist, and family member) reports are valid. Regardless, numerous studies have validated the following findings about self-awareness after TBI that have important implications for cognitive rehabilitation (e.g., Allen & Ruff, 1990; Hart, Giovannetti, Montgomery, & Schwartz, 1998; Newman, Garmoe, Beatty, & Ziccardi, 2000; Prigatano & Altman, 1990):

- Awareness of physical disability emerges first, followed by awareness of cognitive disabilities.
- Individuals with PTA are less likely to be aware of their disabilities, presumably because of the inability to lay down new memories from day to day.
- There is a positive relationship between awareness and time since the injury; that is, the longer the individual lives with a TBI-related disability, the more self-aware that person becomes.
- Self-awareness after TBI is heterogenic. Some individuals overestimate, some underestimate, and some are very "self-aware."

- Self-awareness varies across domains. Disinhibited individuals may believe that their ability to approach conversational topics is adequate, whereas they may be aware of their difficulty remembering appointments.

Self-awareness can have a direct impact on the success of cognitive rehabilitation and is a strong predictor of rehabilitation outcomes (Constantinidou, 2008). Individuals aware of a disability are more motivated and understand the need for remediation or compensation. Very few intervention studies have targeted awareness explicitly, and those that have addressed it lack adequate experimental control. The reader is directed to the work of Kennedy and Coelho (2005) for a detailed summary.

Self-awareness as a therapeutic goal is not warranted in the early, spontaneous recovery phase or for individuals in PTA, except for awareness of physical disability. Once individuals are out of PTA, self-awareness as a therapeutic goal is more appropriate as long as the goal is domain specific, that is, clinicians should not expect improved self-awareness in one domain to generalize to awareness of disability in other domains (Kennedy, 2004). Early in the rehabilitation process, Prigatano (2003) suggests that various therapists can ask the patient to predict performance on certain activities based on feedback from the therapist. These activities can serve as precursors to more systematic self-awareness training. In addition, exercise to interpret others' intentions and feelings might be helpful in developing perspectives on others' feelings and facilitating critical thinking and judgment abilities. Vectors around awareness that were originally developed by Zeman (2001) describe the stages of consciousness and self-awareness after TBI (Prigatano, 2003):

- Vector 1. Consciousness such as wakefulness. Impairment can lead to loss of consciousness and coma.
- Vector 2. Self-awareness of "me" and "now." Impairment can lead to denial of deficits and lack of awareness and poor rehabilitation outcomes.
- Vector 3. Consciousness as a mental state of theory of "me" and "others" (theory of mind). Impairment can result in impaired perceptions of others and their intentions and subsequently in lack of judgment (Constantinidou, 2008).

Self-monitoring (e.g., predicting and comparing performance) and self-control (making strategy decisions) during or shortly after an activity create the feedback that can be used to update the "sense of self" described previously in the discussion on executive functioning (Kennedy & Coelho, 2005; Stuss, 1991). Even though individuals with focal frontal lobe injury are less accurate at predicting their recall than those without frontal lobe injury (Kennedy & Yorkston, 2004), the link between self-monitoring and self-control remains intact after TBI, that is, individuals can use self-generated feedback from self-monitoring to make strategy decisions (Kennedy et al., 2003). This intact link means that once a strategy is learned and once the individual makes accurate assessments of his or her performance, the individual should be able to quickly learn to implement the strategy in those conditions. And, the more opportunities to self-assess and make strategy decisions, the more likely the person will be to revise his or her "sense of self." Unfortunately, the relationship between self-awareness and the updating needed from self-monitoring and self-control is currently not well understood. Indeed, a common frustration of clinicians is that, too often, individuals with TBI do not use strategies spontaneously when faced with situations in which the conditions are different from those in which they were taught (i.e., lack of generalization).

The Challenge of Generalization

Even though individuals with TBI learn less and do so at a lower rate than those without brain injury, they can and do learn new information and skills. Yet, they do not spontaneously adapt the newly learned skills to new situations (Sohlberg & Mateer, 2001; Vakil, 2005). Once individuals acquire and apply a strategy to trained tasks in ideal contexts, getting them to adapt that strategy to different tasks and under less-than-ideal contexts remains challenging (Kennedy et al., 2008).

There are several reasons for this lack of generalization. First, injury to the frontal, temporal, and hippocampal lobes likely contributes to this phenomenon. These brain regions account not only for new learning but also for the self-monitoring and self-control that are needed to adapt newly acquired information to new situations. For example, individuals with poor attention and self-monitoring may not notice the opportunity to use a newly acquired skill. Second, individuals with TBI appear to have reduced mental resources so that tasks that were once effortless and automatic now require effortful and explicit processing (Constantinidou, 1999; Sohlberg, Ehlhardt, & Kennedy, 2005). Using newly learned strategies in trained situations may still be effortful for individuals with TBI until the effects of large amounts of practice make it effortless or automatic; at this point, generalization would not be expected, yet this is often the point at which therapy ends (i.e., before the adaptation phase begins). Finally, there is strong evidence that TBI results in a reduced ability to be mentally flexible; in general, these are individuals whose learning is stimulus bound. That is, mental flexibility that was effortless prior

to being injured requires effort and explicit control after the injury, the very kinds of processing that are impaired after TBI.

Unfortunately, there is limited published evidence from the cognitive rehabilitation research literature about generalization. Although this trend is changing in more recently published intervention studies, few studies to date include measures that validate the primary outcomes (e.g., care provider reports) or differ in important ways (e.g., the stimulus, the context) (e.g., Constantinidou et al., 2008; Kennedy et al., 2008; Sohlberg et al., 2003; Ylvisaker et al., 2007). Regardless, clinicians and clients expect to see real change in everyday life as the result of cognitive rehabilitation. What can clinicians do to facilitate generalization? The principles discussed in this section provide some answers. Clinicians and clients can establish realistic goals with appropriate time frames (to allow for acquisition, application, and adaptation) based on neuropsychological and speech–language profiles, preinjury intellectual and cognitive status, and client values. Once a skill is acquired and applied through EL, clinicians should do the following:

1. Vary the stimulus (e.g., change from verbal to written, systematically remove cues) and change the context (e.g., from therapy room to doctor's waiting room, from distraction free to distracting environment).
2. Explicitly discuss when, where, why, and how the skill can be used in everyday living and have the client track skill use on a regular basis.
3. Practice the skill in everyday living situations and reevaluate and modify the skill based on client's self-assessment tracked using daily or weekly logs.
4. Using "bridging" statements to explicitly discuss other activities and contexts in which the client could apply the strategy that was learned for a specific purpose. For example, the speech–language clinician could state, "Now that you are using LiveScribe to take notes and record meetings at work, let us list other situations where this tool could be useful."

INSTRUCTIONAL APPROACHES IN COGNITIVE REHABILITATION

The three instructional approaches discussed in this section are based on the cognitive rehabilitation principles just described and have emerged in the past two decades. Selecting the right approach for an individual depends on (a) the phase of recovery (i.e., acute medical, acute rehabilitation, postacute) and assessment of cognitive and communication strengths and weaknesses; (b) clinical recommendations based on the research evidence and the degree to which the individual is demographically similar to the participants on which the research is based; (c) the goals and values of the individual as they pertain to expected treatment outcomes; (d) the knowledge and skills of the clinician; and (e) the required kinds of outcomes for third-party reimbursement. Most likely, clinicians use a combination of approaches to address a wide variety of skills rather than using only one approach and assuming that one size fits all.

Spaced Retrieval

Spaced retrieval therapy (SRT) is an instructional approach that capitalizes on preserved implicit memory processes through EL and large amounts of practice. Individuals are provided with maximum supports initially to retrieve and produce the correct behavior or answer. Timed intervals of interference double as long as the individual is accurate; when the individual makes an error, the clinician models the correct answer and reduces the length of interference by 50% until the correct answer is provided. Initially, SRT was described in 1978 by Landauer and Bjork, but since then variations of the approach have been found to be effective for learning a wide range of information and procedures, such as names, personal information, schedules, activities of daily living, techniques for dysphagia, and the use of daily planners and alternative communication devices (e.g., Brush & Camp, 1998; Cherry, Simmons, & Camp, 1999; Clare et al., 2000). A systematic review of the effectiveness of SRT with adults with dementia provides strong evidence from 15 studies for its use (Hopper et al., 2005).

There is also evidence on the effectiveness SRT with adults with memory impairment with TBI (Bourgeois, Lenius, Turkstra, & Camp, 2007; Hillary et al., 2003; Melton & Bourgeois, 2005; Turkstra & Bourgeois, 2005). Smaller, initial studies provide preliminary evidence that when delivered over the phone, injured individuals with memory impairment not only reached their memory goals but also reported the transfer of these skills to other functional activities that had not been trained (Melton & Bourgeois, 2005). In a single case study, an adult with very severe anterograde amnesia received SRT by phone to improve memory for specific daily activities (taking medication on time, checking e-mail, checking his daily planner) (Turkstra & Bourgeois, 2005). It took 7 days for him to recall the first goal in a 24-hour span, 5 days for the second goal, and 3 days for the third goal. With caregiver training, he was able to quickly learn

procedures or actions; this improvement reduced the level of supervision and care he needed on a daily basis. In a randomized controlled trial, 38 adults with chronic memory impairment received SRT or strategy instruction by phone. The SRT group reported higher level goal mastery immediately after therapy and at follow-up 1 month later than the strategy instruction group did. Some transfer or generalization to untrained tasks was reported by both groups, although there were no group differences, including in the reports by care providers.

The absence of generalization from SRT warrants further discussion. Spaced retrieval therapy uses large amounts of practice to teach individuals very specific actions or information. Responses tend to be bound to the stimuli used in training and are bound to the context in which the skill was trained. It is possible that errorless performance may result in a cost: less flexibility in learning (Turkstra & Bourgeois, 2005). However, with modifications to the SRT procedure, clinicians may be able to incidentally alter the stimulus to improve the chances of generalization. For example, once the individual is accurate over long periods of timed interference (days or weeks depending on the complexity and automaticity of the skill), the stimulus as well as supports, prompts, and cues could be systematically faded until a criterion is reached with the least restrictive stimulus/supports.

Direct and Metacognitive Instruction

Two instructional approaches, direct and metacognitive instruction, came from educational psychology, special education, and neuropsychology and incorporate several cognitive rehabilitation principles. Direct instruction (DI) was originally described by Engelmann and Carnine (1991) to include the following actions: analyzes content for ideas, rules, and generalizable strategies; identifies needed skills and sequences skills hierarchically; performs task analysis; identifies, sequences generalizable examples; simplifies instruction, including scripts; identifies simple learning objectives; establishes high levels of criteria; focuses on prerequisite skills first and immediate feedback through modeling, prompts, and cues to an EL level; provides large amounts of massed, then distributed practice; provides individualized instruction to target weaknesses and identify strengths; engages in cumulative review; and provides ongoing assessment (for further discussion, see Sohlberg et al., 2005).

A systematic review and meta-analysis by Swanson and colleagues reveal that four types of instruction (DI, strategy instruction, combined model [direct and strategy instruction], nondirect/nonstrategy instruction) emerge from 180 empirical studies of children and adults with learning disabilities (Swanson, 1999, 2001; Swanson & Hoskyn, 1998). The combined model resulted in the largest effect sizes, followed by strategy instruction only, then DI only, and last nondirect/nonstrategy instruction. Importantly, a factor analysis revealed that explicit practice, direction to the task, teacher presentation of new material, modeling and sequencing of steps, and systematic feedback were critical features of effective instructional practice. Applied to students with brain injury, Glang, Singer, Cooley, and Tish (1992) demonstrated individualized DI that targets a variety of academic areas using self-management strategies. Ehlhardt, Sohlberg, Glang, and Albin (2005) demonstrated a DI approach when training four individuals with memory and executive dysfunction to use e-mail.

Metacognitive strategy instruction (MSI) is similar to DI but with an additional emphasis on instructing individuals to self-monitor (i.e., self-assess) and to engage in self-control (i.e., make strategy decisions) during strategy acquisition. This is particularly important for individuals with TBI who are likely to have frontal lobe injury and executive dysfunction; they have difficulty carrying out "skill sets that include: (1) setting goals; (2) comparing performance with goals or outcomes (i.e., self-monitoring); (3) making decisions to change one's behavior in order to reach the desired outcome (i.e., self-control) (e.g., selecting an alternative solution); and (4) executing the change in behavior (e.g., implementing an alternative solution)" (Kennedy et al., 2008, p. 259). The research evidence is strong on the effectiveness of MSI with adults with TBI. Sohlberg et al. (2003) found that when intervention included self-evaluation to direct attention training, individuals were likely to maintain attention strategies over time and generalize strategy use to other contexts. Unfortunately, they found that these strategies must be practiced in a variety of contexts to be used in those contexts, again highlighting the lack of generalization without explicit instruction. Kennedy et al. (2008) found that when MSI was included in various intervention approaches for solving complex problems and performing complex activities, treatment effect sizes were significantly large.

Creating Positive Routines

Ylvisaker and Feeney (1998) advocate that by creating contextualized, collaborative positive routines, individuals with TBI would be more likely to implement taught behaviors or strategies in everyday living. At the core of this approach are identifying antecedent behaviors, situations, or tasks that could be used to prevent the occurrence of erroneous responses (procedures or declarative information) or maladaptive behaviors and replacing these behaviors with positive ones. Many

cognitive rehabilitation principles are incorporated into this approach: Clients collaborate with clinicians in determining goals and supports; errorless performance/learning is obtained using spaced retrieval or MVC; large amounts of practice in varied contexts and conditions to promote generalization are provided; and ongoing self-evaluation occurs so that goals and supports can be modified. There is substantial support for this approach from intervention studies that have addressed social skills and behaviors, as described in the following section.

REVIEWING THE EVIDENCE FOR COGNITIVE REHABILITATION

Systematic reviews, meta-analyses, and evidence-based recommendations now provide clinicians with comprehensive summaries and critiques of the effectiveness of cognitive rehabilitation. The goals of reviews vary, however, and clinicians need to be aware that the methods used, such as establishing inclusion and exclusion criteria, can differ dramatically across reviews (Kennedy, 2007). For example, Cicerone and colleagues reviewed all areas of cognitive rehabilitation but included intervention studies for adults with stroke or TBI (Cicerone et al., 2000, 2005, 2011). Conversely, Kennedy and colleagues used a more focused approach to critiquing specific areas of cognitive rehabilitation, including attention training, the use of external memory aids, therapy for behavioral and social problems, and therapy targeting executive functions, and included studies of children or adults with TBI (Kennedy et al., 2002).

Understanding the methodology and the purpose of a review is critical to interpret the results and to attempt to answer a clinical question. And, given the sheer number of published reviews, speech–language clinicians can easily find reviews and be ensured that some bias has been controlled.

> Since clinicians often go to colleagues first [for advice about how to proceed with a client], it is likely that colleagues will recommend a study that reported results based on their own bias. Additionally, clinicians who select a single study to review without examining other studies on the topic run the risk of ignoring studies that may have found dissimilar results. … The assumption here is that the authors of peer-reviewed systematic reviews engaged in methodological processes that protected against their own biases" (Kennedy, 2013, p. 289).

Direct Attention Training

Therapy for attention-based disabilities is critically important for individuals with TBI. Historically, attention deficits after TBI have been characterized as hierarchical from "sustaining attention over time (vigilance), capacity for information, shifting attention, speech of processing, and screening out distractions" (Sohlberg et al., 2003, p. xxii). This characterization of attention was the basis for the Attention Process Training (APT) program (Sohlberg, Johnson, Paule, Raskin, & Mateer, 1994), a process-specific intervention approach in which attention is systematically improved by having individuals respond to increasingly challenging paper/pencil and computer-based tasks presented auditorily and visually.

Several intervention studies have been reviewed to document the efficacy of this approach for improving function-/impairment-level outcomes under ideal conditions (Cicerone et al., 2005, 2008, 2011; Sohlberg et al., 2003). However, improved attention skills during functional activities appear to be dependent on the use of individualized metacognitive or self-evaluation strategies that must be explicitly trained (Sohlberg et al., 2003). Indeed, Ponsford et al. (2014) concluded "metacognitive strategy training focused on functional everyday activities is appropriate" when instructing individuals regarding specific attention strategies (p. 321).

Thus, even though there is strong evidence for the use of direct attention training for impairment-level outcomes, clinicians should not expect generalization to untrained functional activities; explicit instruction and self-evaluation on the use of these attention strategies in everyday situations appear to be necessary.

Categorization Training

Constantinidou and associates developed a hierarchical rehabilitation program, the Categorization Program (CP), beginning with basic levels of categorization (e.g., feature identification), with the ultimate goal to target higher processes such as abstract thought, decision making, and problem solving (Constantinidou et al., 2005). The theoretical model is based on the concept that even the most minimal cognitive act from input to output involves recognition and categorization (Constantinidou et al., 2004). The CP integrates principles of cognitive theory and models of category learning (Rosch & Mervis, 1975; Rosch, Simpson, & Miller 1976), language theory (Braisby & Dockrell, 1999; Younger & Fearing, 1999), and rehabilitation (Adamovich et al., 1985; Parente & Herrmann, 1996) for the design of hierarchical tasks to treat the two aspects of categorization described previously: (a) recognition and categorization of everyday objects and (b) recognition and categorization of novel situations.

As the individual reaches criterion at each of the various levels of CP, the next level becomes increasingly demanding, requiring more cognitive effort. The stimuli begin with concrete objects (to minimize cognitive distance) and progress gradually to abstract ideas.

Abstract reasoning, mental flexibility, and problem-solving abilities are the targets of the higher levels of this systematic perceptual training program (Constantinidou et al., 2004). A preliminary study (Constantinidou et al., 2005) and follow-up randomized controlled trial (Constantinidou et al., 2008) show that CP was effective in improving categorization abilities in individuals with TBI who are enrolled in postacute rehabilitation. Patients who were treated with the CP demonstrated greater gains on neuropsychological tests than those patients who received the standard treatment. Furthermore, the CP facilitated the generalizability of skills into new tasks that required the application of high-level categorization abilities, including mental flexibility. Research with patients with TBI who received this protocol during their postacute rehabilitation phase indicates that the CP helps patients improve their cognitive performance during neuropsychological tests, categorization tasks, and functional outcome measures (Constantinidou et al., 2005, 2008). Although identifying "active ingredients" in complex behavioral treatments is a challenging task, the authors conclude that the following factors contribute to its success:

- The CP is based on neurobiological principles of cognitive skill acquisition. It begins with *concrete* tasks and proceeds to incorporating high levels of *abstraction*.
- The *redundancy* of stimuli and the *cueing levels* provide support and facilitate learning. Consequently, patients are able to learn *strategies* and improve their classification skills.
- In addition, the CP incorporates *episodic memory* during all of the levels and facilitates *executive functioning* abilities such as divergent thinking, problem solving, and decision making.

Therapy for Impaired Memory

Therapy for impaired memory after TBI is characterized by training the use of tools that improve remembering and the use of tools that compensate for remembering. Even though both kinds of tools have been found to be effective, each tool is intended for specific kinds of information and situations. For example, an individual who is returning to college after TBI may need several tools that will improve encoding and retention of academic information and will also need tools and strategies to compensate for everyday memory failures.

Several strategies that improve the encoding or retention of information in individuals with mild-to-moderate memory impairment include the following:

- Visual imagery improves the retention of information when it is taught at an EL level and when individuals generate their own images, such as name–face associations (Hux, Manasse, Wright, & Snell, 2000; Kalla, Downes, & van den Broek, 2001; Kaschel et al., 2002; Lewinsohn, Danaher, & Kikel, 1977). However, visual imagery may not be that effective when used to retain individuals' names with whom they have daily contact (Manasse, Hux, & Snell, 2005).
- Semantic elaboration occurs when explicit semantic associations are made that would otherwise occur spontaneously. For example, if trying to learn the definition of *trellis*, the individual reviews its use (to prop up plants), its shape (like a ladder), and its location (outdoor gardens). This technique has been shown to be effective in improving retention in individuals with and without brain injury (Oberg & Turkstra, 1998). Answering who, what, when, where, why, and how questions is a form of semantic elaboration that improves retention of specific kinds of information, such as learning text-based material or stories.
- Approaches that include metacognitive processing have also been found to be effective in improving retention of text-based information for individuals with and without brain injury. Preview-Question-Read-Summary-Test (PQRST) is an approach to reading and remembering text that includes the principles of direct and metacognitive instruction. Dunlosky, Hertzog, Kennedy, and Thiede (2005) describe a variation of this that emphasizes self-evaluation for use with college students, healthy older adults, and adults with brain injury. Regardless of the specific approach used, having individuals with TBI elaborate on the to-be-remembered information, self-assess their performance, and change their elaboration based on their own feedback appears to be an important feature for improving retention. The degree to which these elaboration sequences generalize to other kinds of information is yet to be documented.

The Brain Injury Association of New York (created by Mark Ylvisaker) provides the following list of steps that are useful during encoding and modified to fit the individual (http://www.projectlearnet.org/tutorials/memory_problems.html):

- Tell myself, "Pay attention; focus."
- Highlight the information that seems most important.
- Organize the information into natural groups.
- Create association links to information that I already know.
- Generate my own examples.
- Think about how I might apply this information.
- Repeat the information.
- Summarize and review.
- Take notes.
- Speak the information out loud; tell or explain it to some other person.
- Create visual images of the new information.
- Create diagrams or flowcharts of the information.
- Test myself on the information.
- Take in reasonably small amounts of information at a time.

External tools used to compensate for prospective memory or the inability to recall and carry out future events/actions include daily planners, notes, alarms, voice and text messages, calendars, and so forth. There is strong evidence that, in general, compensatory tools improve the likelihood that individuals in the chronic stages of TBI will carry out the activity (Cicerone et al., 2000, 2005, 2011; Sohlberg et al., 2007). In a systematic review, Sohlberg and colleagues (2007) reviewed 21 studies published through 2003 that evaluated the use of external memory aids. Seven kinds of aids were identified: memory notebooks or planners, electronic devices, prompting systems, pagers, cell phones, and a guidance system. The outcomes were generally positive, but few studies described the amount and type of instruction and maintenance and generalization effects.

Numerous studies have documented the positive effects of assistive technology on individuals with TBI (Hart, Buchhofer, & Vaccaro, 2004; Stapleton, Adams, & Atterton, 2007; Van Hulle & Hux, 2006; Wilson, Emslie, Quirk, Evans, & Watson, 2005). For example, PDAs were found to improve the likelihood that individuals with severe TBI will carry out specific activities and improve the level of participation as corroborated by care providers (Gentry, Wallace, Kvarfordt, & Bodisch-Lynch, 2008). Recently, DePompei et al. (2008) compared the use of two different PDAs to daily planners in individuals with TBI and with intellectual disabilities. Responses to PDAs were higher than responses to daily planners for all participants, including children and adults, and individuals with TBI responded at higher rates than did adults with intellectual disability.

Last, restorative, computerized therapy programs (e.g., Lumosity) have gained public popularity over the last several years. Unfortunately, there is little scientific evidence that these programs do anything more than train the individual to the task that is being practiced. This is not surprising since we know that practicing can improve accuracy and speed, yet there is no evidence that these improvements generalize to any functional everyday skill. Thus, the "evidence for efficacy of these techniques remains weak and the choice in using these should be guided by special considerations" (Velikonja et al., 2014, p. 369).

Intervention for Social Communication Skills and Behavior

A variety of poor social skills can occur after TBI, including the inability to organize, to inhibit or initiate, and to modify a message according to context and communication partner. Changes in social skills are related to social isolation, vocational status, and depression after TBI (Dahlberg et al., 2006; Douglas & Spellacy, 2000; Wehman et al., 1993). Hartley (1995) proposes that social behavioral problems occur after TBI because of the inability to self-regulate in social situations, that is, the ability to monitor, inhibit/initiate, and modify behavior within social contexts. McDonald (1993) proposes that individuals with TBI have impaired theory of mind, the ability to consider another's perspective. Kennedy and DeRuyter (1991) describe how social skills recovery is related to recovery of attention, memory, and inhibition. Some examples of poor social skills are inappropriate laughing, unpredictable behavior, introduction of topics that are irrelevant to the context, and excessive talking.

How have social skills been remediated? Most intervention studies of social skills have used explicit training techniques with modeling and feedback. For example, in a recent randomized controlled trial, Dahlberg et al. (2007) assigned adults with TBI to a treatment group or a deferred treatment group. Treatment was delivered for 3 months in small groups and included education, self-assessment, collaborative goal setting, focused generalization, homework, and family/friends involvement. The treated group improved in 7 of 10 discrete behaviors on a communication questionnaire, although there were no group differences in communication participation.

Indeed, it is possible to change discrete communication behaviors in individuals with brain injury; however, getting the individual to use newly learned behaviors at the right time, in the right context, and with the right communication partners has proven to be challenging. Why does explicit training for social skills have such limited effects on everyday communication? Although the reasons for this are unclear, some have proposed that implicit and automatic rather than explicit processing accounts for most everyday conversation. Like other implicit processes, everyday conversation skills may not be amenable to being dissected and treated in their component parts. For example, the consequence of artificially addressing eye contact may be awkward staring rather than the dynamic use of eye contact as it occurs while taking conversational turns (Turkstra, 2005).

Creating positive behavior routines, as described previously, is based on implicit processes achieved through EL and large amounts of practice in which the client and clinician collaborate to identify the most appropriate conversational supports. Recently, Ylivsaker et al. (2007) systematically reviewed 51 intervention studies for problem social behavior in children and adults with TBI. They compared the outcomes from studies using positive behavioral routines to studies using reward-based traditional behavioral approaches. Studies that used the positive routines approach had better outcomes (i.e., maintenance and generalization of desired behavior in functional settings) than did more traditional behavioral approaches.

A consensus group recently published five recommendations for managing communication disorders worldwide (Togher et al., 2014):

1. Rehabilitation staff should recognize that levels of communication competence and communication characteristics may vary as a function of communication partner, environment, communication demands, communication priorities, fatigue, and other personal factors (p. 355).
2. A person with TBI who has a cognitive–communication disorder should be offered an appropriate treatment program by a speech–language clinician (p. 358).
3. A cognitive–communication rehabilitation program should take into account the person's premorbid native language, literacy, and language proficiency; cognitive abilities; and communication style, including communication standards and expectations in that individual's culture (p. 359).
4. A cognitive–communication rehabilitation program should provide the opportunity to rehearse communication skills in situations appropriate to the context in which the individual will live, work, study, and socialize (p. 359).
5. A cognitive–communication rehabilitation program should provide education and training of communication partners (p. 360).

Intervention for Complex Activities and Solving Problems

In a review of the research literature, Kennedy et al. (2008) found that three kinds of instructional approaches were used to improve outcomes in complex activities or solving problems: MSI to address the specific aspect of problem solving in which the individual was impaired (e.g., goal setting, identifying alternative solutions, organizing the task, identifying and prioritizing the steps); instruction in strategic thinking for verbal reasoning; and instruction in multitasking. Ten of the 15 studies used aspects of MSI; of the studies that used MSI, five were randomized controlled trials and five were case studies. Outcomes were classified using the WHO ICF categories: body structure and function that measure impairments, activities that measure limitations, and participation that measures restrictions. A meta-analysis found that MSI resulted in significantly larger effect sizes than control interventions but only for activity and participation outcomes, whereas both interventions resulted in statistically significant effect sizes for impairment-level outcomes. Thus, MSI is effective for training a variety of functional activities or skill sets and for obtaining changes in process-specific impairment outcomes, whereas the control interventions were less effective for training functional skill sets. Strategic thinking and multitasking intervention resulted in positive outcomes as well, although more research is needed.

Recently, the MSI standard of practice recommendation was corroborated by an international review of published systematic reviews of intervention for executive functions and self-awareness (Tate et al., 2014). The authors recommended that clinicians use MSIs when addressing functional, self-identified goals with clients who possess sufficient attention and recall abilities that would support generating and selecting goals, identifying and selecting strategies, predicting performance using such strategies, executing the strategies, comparing performance with the original goal, and making goal or strategy adjustments if needed.

While the evidence in favor of therapy for managing self-awareness did not fare as well, recommendations emerged that education and experiential learning could result in positive changes in self-awareness of deficits.

CONCLUSIONS AND FUTURE DIRECTIONS

Rehabilitation after TBI is a highly complex and lengthy process requiring significant resources; cognitive rehabilitation is at the epicenter of such efforts. Therapy methodologies that improve cognitive systems and reduce impairment coupled with activities that improve function in specific cognitive domains have been incorporated successfully during cognitive rehabilitation efforts. In the past 10 years, brain injury researchers have made significant contributions and produced scientific findings that support the effectiveness of cognitive rehabilitation after TBI. As technology continues to develop, researchers can identify more reliably the effects of successful treatment methodologies on neuronal reorganization and determine which patients may benefit from certain types of treatment.

Questions such as effectiveness versus efficacy of cognitive rehabilitation methodologies continue to challenge researchers and will be the focus of future research. The Task Force on Promotion and Dissemination of Psychological Procedures (1995) and the WHO (2001) define *efficacy research* as the examination of an intervention's effect under highly controlled experimental conditions, whereas *effectiveness research* examines the effects of interventions in those settings or conditions in which the intervention will ultimately be delivered. Furthermore, quantifying the optimal "dose" of certain cognitive rehabilitation methodologies is of both research and practical interest in light of challenges posed by third-party payers and the reduction in authorized days of treatment for TBI survivors.

Access to resources and services is of primary importance to survivors and their families. The brain injury community (i.e., survivors, family members, and professionals dedicated to brain injury management) has made significant progress in increasing awareness and systematic education of health-care professionals, legal community, third-party payers, and policy makers regarding the effects of TBI and the necessary components of successful rehabilitation. However, more systematic and intensified efforts are needed to improve the funding and allocation of resources required for successful rehabilitation, support, and reintegration of brain injury survivors into society.

Case Illustration 19.1

Reading about the efficacy and effectiveness of cognitive rehabilitation is certainly easier than incorporating the research evidence in clinical practice. Individuals with TBI have unique cognitive and communication strengths and weaknesses, as well as goals and values. Therefore, the following scenario is meant to be an *example* of how best clinical practice can be applied over the course of recovery.

Teresa was a right-handed 35-year-old warehouse employee who was airlifted to the Level I trauma center in a large urban area after sustaining a severe TBI when she was hit while on her bicycle. She sustained DAI that included portions of the dorsal- and orbital-frontal lobes and had a Glasgow Coma Scale[4] (GCS) score of 5 in the emergency room. Initially, an MRI showed brain swelling with a left-to-right midline shift related to a large sub-dural hematoma. The hematoma was evacuated, and a portion of her skull was removed to manage swelling. She was in a coma for 7 days. By week 2, she was at RLA cognitive functioning Level V, confused, inappropriate, and nonagitated, at which time she was transferred to an inpatient rehabilitation unit.

Teresa spent 4 weeks on the inpatient rehabilitation unit receiving comprehensive interdisciplinary therapy. The rehabilitation team included physiatry, OT, speech–language pathology, PT, social services, and nursing. Initial assessment of her cognition, behavior, and communication was performed using rating scales such as the Functional Independence and Functional Assessment Measures (FIM and FAM; Wright, 2000) and the Disability Rating Scale (DRS; Rappaport, Hall, Hopkins, Belleza, & Cope, 1982); systematic observation during various tasks across settings; and short, formal tests depending on her fluctuating attention. The GOAT (Levin et al., 1979) revealed that Teresa was still in PTA. The Western Aphasia Battery–Revised (WAB-R; Kertesz, 2007), the Boston Naming Test (Kaplan, Goodglass, & Weintraub, 2007), the Repeatable Battery for the Assessment of Neuropsychological Status (RBANS; Randolph, 1998), and the Neurobehavioral Status Examination (Kiernan, Meuller, & Langston, 1995) were administered by the speech–language clinician as soon as Teresa could maintain sufficient attention with some redirection. Although no aphasia or anomia were detected, she was unable to repeat lengthy sentences accurately and carry out three-step verbal instructions relative to her inability to stay on task. Immediate and delayed verbal recall were more severely impaired than visual recall. Naming abilities were intact, but verbal fluency was reduced. Observation by all disciplines revealed that Teresa was very confused on the rehabilitation unit, often repeating herself, confabulating in response to open-ended questions, and unable to navigate within the hospital without getting lost.

Initial inpatient intervention goals primarily focused on improving her sustained attention to the environment and specific tasks while reducing her disorientation and confusion and improving her ability to retain new information. Environmental changes were made to her hospital room by reducing noise, limiting the number of visitors at one time, and providing short, quiet breaks between therapy sessions and other appointments. The speech–language pathologist also taught Teresa to use a simple daily planner that was initially used to keep track of her schedule (appointments, mealtimes), remind Teresa of important dates, and record questions that she had throughout the day. Use of the simple planner was learned to a near-errorless level using spaced retrieval within therapy sessions, and its use was reinforced by all team members. As confusion dissipated and recognition memory improved, the planner was upgraded to include more detailed information and more categories.

To improve sustained and selective attention while listening and reading, the speech–language pathologist had Teresa listen and read very short stories (e.g., three sentences in length) and write down as much as she could immediately after. Then, based on her written notes, she would recall as much of the story as possible. By comparing her recall of stories with and without taking notes, Teresa was able to see how her recall improved when she took notes. With the assistance of the speech–language pathologist, Teresa graphically displayed her performance at the end of each treatment session, which served as positive reinforcement. The OT and speech–language pathologist created a self-assessment form for Teresa to predict and report her own performance for therapy sessions across various disciplines as well. Thus, the routine of self-checking was started early in the rehabilitation process and provided a reason for clinicians and Teresa to discuss the need for alternative strategies. Family members, including her parents, two brothers, and nieces and nephews, were very supportive and engaged in the rehabilitation, visiting and watching therapy as much as possible.

(continues)

Teresa was discharged from the inpatient rehabilitation unit to her parents' home until it was determined that she would be safe to live independently in her own home. She made good progress during inpatient rehabilitation: Her sustained and selective attention improved, her ability to use a daily planner became more consistent, and she emerged from PTA with residual delayed memory impairment but good recognition memory.

Teresa had worked for a large discount retail store chain. Her employer promised to hold her job in inventory and stocking shelves until she could return, knowing that reasonable accommodations were likely going to be needed. Teresa was anxious to return to work and to her own home; however, the rehabilitation team recommended that she first continue to receive outpatient rehabilitation for her remaining attention problems, short-term memory impairment, and executive dysfunction (e.g., planning and organizing steps in complex activities).

When Teresa started outpatient rehabilitation, she underwent more comprehensive neuropsychological and speech–language pathologist evaluations to determine specific strengths and weaknesses that could interfere with her ability to return to work. Impairment-level testing by the neuropsychologist included the California Verbal Learning Test, second edition (Delis, Kramer, Kaplan, & Ober, 2000); the Delis-Kaplan Executive Function System (DKEFS; Delis, Kaplan, & Kramer, 2001); and the Weschler Memory Scale, third edition (WMS-III; Wechsler, 1997). Impairment testing by the speech–language pathologist included portions of the Woodcock-Johnson Tests of Cognitive Abilities–III (Woodcock, McGrew, & Mather, 2001); the Benton Controlled Word Association Test (Spreen & Benton, 1969); the Boston Naming Test (Kaplan et al., 2007); and the National Adult Reading Test, second edition (NART; Nelson & Willison, 1991).

Test results revealed that her recognition memory was better than her ability to recall details from stories and lists of words, and immediate recall was better than delayed recall. Impairment-level testing of executive functions revealed a low-normal ability to switch when drawing designs and the tendency to repeat items during a verbal fluency task. Estimates of her preinjury verbal IQ (from the NART) were in the low-normal range and actually corresponded to her ability to generate words in verbal fluency tasks, revealing that her word-finding skills matched her word knowledge.

Furthermore, picture naming was within normal limits. Activity and participation testing was conducted by the entire rehabilitation team using measures such as the Mayo Portland Adaptability Inventory 4 (MPAI-4; Malec, 2005) and the Community Integration Questionnaire (CIQ; Dijkers, 2000). Speech–language pathology assessment incorporated the Rivermead Behavioral Memory Test, second edition (Wilson, Cockburn, & Baddeley, 2003); the Functional Assessment of Verbal Reasoning and Executive Strategies (FAVRES; MacDonald, 2005); self- and other- version of the LaTrobe Communication Questionnaire (Douglas, Bracy, & Snow, 2000); and a structured awareness interview.

These revealed a variety of functional limitations. She had difficulty remembering names, faces, and appointments. When given a complex problem to solve, she was unable to identify alternative solutions when the first solution failed and did not take into consideration all of the details for determining the best solution. In a structured awareness interview, Teresa demonstrated depth of awareness in her memory problems but could not identify the other challenges she experienced in carrying out complex activities. She believed that the memory problems were preventing her from returning to her home and work; therefore, her self-identified goals focused on ways to improve her memory. According to her family, her social communication skills postinjury were unchanged from preinjury. Teresa had none of the conversation problems that some individuals with TBI have.

Outpatient rehabilitation goals of the speech–language pathologist and OT focused on improving high-level attention abilities, retaining new material, compensating for poor recall of daily events, and organizing and carrying out complex, functional activities that occurred at home and could occur at work. The speech–language pathologist worked on improving divided and alternating attention skills using APT (Sohlberg & Mateer, 2001) and integrated metacognitive assessment by having her predict her performance on these structured attention tasks, compare performance with her prediction, and discuss strategies for improving attention on subsequent tasks. Application of attention strategies was discussed and practiced during complex, functional activities as well. Visual imagery was used to improve retention of name–face associations of new individuals she was meeting, such as the office staff at the outpatient clinic and individuals in her parents' neighborhood. Later, when she transitioned back to work, she was instructed to use imagery when learning new coworkers' names. Several external memory devices were used to help her compensate for keeping track and following through with her daily routine.

(continues)

Now that she had several appointments and family activities to keep track of, she decided to switch from the daily planner to a smartphone. Two weeks of explicit instruction and DI were needed before she could independently access and use the various features that helped her organize her schedule, including timed reminders, keeping track of schedule changes, and making notes of to-be-remembered items.

To prepare Teresa for returning to work, the clinicians obtained the new forms, procedures, and equipment that had been introduced since Teresa had left. She was instructed in "plan-do-review" when learning when and how to use the new materials with EL achieved before increasing the complexity of the situation. Role-playing scenarios with increased distractions helped solidify the automaticity of use of these new materials and provided lots of practice.

Teresa returned to work slowly, by increasing her work hours to full time over a year's time. Importantly, new handheld scanning devices had been implemented since her injury, so she received the same explicit training all employees had received. However, the employer allowed her to shadow another employee who used the device proficiently until Teresa was able to use it herself independently. Teresa's awareness of the consequences of her injury continued to improve slowly over the course of several years as she experienced more real-life situations in which she could self-evaluate and reflect on her strengths and weaknesses.

STUDY QUESTIONS

1. What is traumatic brain injury?
2. What are the primary neurobehavioral sequelae of TBI?
3. What are the expected stages of recovery from a TBI?
4. What are the principles of TBI assessment?
5. What types of assessment procedures should be used by speech–language clinicians to assess memory, executive abilities, reasoning, attention, and participation in home and community activities?
6. Which treatment areas are typically addressed by speech–language clinicians working with individuals with TBI?
7. Which cognitive-based therapy techniques (strategies and instructional approaches) have been shown to be effective in TBI rehabilitation?
8. What is the impact of PTA on assessment and treatment?
9. What is the contribution of rehabilitation during the acute phases of recovery?
10. Which variables are used to determine TBI severity?
11. How can speech–language pathologists contribute to the management of sports concussions?

NOTES

1. Hagen and associates subsequently developed a 10-level RLA scale that further differentiates patient recovery beyond the original Level VIII. However, this 10-point scale is not widely implemented, and most clinicians continue to use the original 8-level scale.
2. Posttraumatic amnesia is the period of time when the patient is unable to remember day-to-day information and includes the period of retrograde amnesia (RA) plus the period of anterograde amnesia (AA). The onset of RA is the last memory remembered prior to the injury; the end of AA is the point of complete return to continuous memory after the injury.
3. For a thorough review of cognitive rehabilitation therapy published reviews, readers are referred to the work of Kennedy (2013) and a special series published by the international INCOG group (i.e, an international team of researchers and clinicians) in 2014, *Journal of Head Trauma Rehabilitation*, volume 29, number 4.
4. The GCS is widely used by emergency personnel to classify injury severity (Jennett & Bond, 1975). The GCS assesses three aspects of wakefulness:

(a) stimulus required to induce eye opening, (b) the best motor response, and (c) the best verbal response. Scores range from a minimum of 3 to a maximum of 15 points. Patients who score 13 or higher on the GCS are classified as having a mild brain injury or concussion. Scores between 9 and 12 are an indication of a moderate concussion. Below 8 points indicates the presence of coma and the injury is classified as severe.

REFERENCES

Adamovich, B. B., Henderson, J. A., & Auerbach, S. (1985). *Cognitive rehabilitation of closed head injured patients: A dynamic approach.* San Diego, CA: College-Hill Press.

Adams, J. H., Graham, D. I., Murray, L. S., & Scott, G. (1982). Diffuse axonal injury due to non-missile head injury in humans: An analysis of 45 cases. *Annals of Neurology, 12,* 557–563.

Aimone, J. B., Deng, W., & Gage, F. H. (2010). Adult neurogenesis: Integrating theories and separating functions. *Trends in Cognitive Science, 14*(7), 325–337.

Allen, C. C., & Ruff, R. M. (1990). Self-rating versus neuropsychological performance of moderate versus severe head-injured patients. *Brain Injury, 4*(1), 7–17.

American Speech-Language-Hearing Association. (2005). *Roles of speech-language pathologists in the identification, diagnosis, and treatment of individuals with cognitive-communication disorders: Position statement* [ASHA Supplement, 25]. Rockville, MD: Author. Retrieved November 7, 2015 from http://www.asha.org/policy/PS2005-00110.htm.

Baddeley, A., & Wilson, B. A. (1994). When implicit learning fails: Amnesia and the problem of error elimination. *Neuropsychologia, 32*(11), 53–68.

Barwood, C. H. S., & Murdoch, B. E. (2013). Unravelling the influence of mild traumatic brain injury (MTBI) on cognitive-linguistic processing: A comparative group analysis. *Brain Injury, 27*(6), 1–6.

Benedictus, M. R., Spikman, J. M., & van der Naalt, J. (2010). Cognitive and behavioral impairment in traumatic brain injury related to outcome and return to work. *Archives of Physical Medicine and Rehabilitation, 91,* 1436–1441.

Bergsneider, M., Hovda, D. A., Shalmon, E., Kelly, D. F., Vespa, P. M., Martin, N. A., et al. (1997). Cerebral hyperglycolysis following severe traumatic brain injury in humans: A positron emission tomography study. *Journal of Neurosurgery, 86,* 241–251.

Blennow, K., Hardy, J., & Zetterberg, H. (2012). The neuropathology and neurobiology of traumatic brain injury. *Neuron, 76,* 886–899.

Bourgeois, M. S., Lenius, K., Turkstra, L., & Camp, C. (2007). The effects of cognitive teletherapy on reported everyday memory behaviours of persons with chronic traumatic brain injury. *Brain Injury, 21*(12), 1245–1257.

Braisby, N., & Dockrell, J. (1999). Why is color naming difficult? *Journal of Child Language, 26,* 23–47.

Bruce, J. M., & Echemendia, R. J. (2009). History of multiple self-reported concussions is not associated with reduced cognitive abilities. *Neurosurgery, 64,* 100–106.

Brush, J., & Camp, C. (1998). Using spaced retrieval as an intervention during speech-language therapy. *Clinical Gerontologist, 19,* 51–64.

Cameron, H. A., Woolley, C. S., McEwin, B. S., & Gould, E. (1993). Differentiation of newly born neurons and glia in the dentate gyrus of the adult-rat. *Neuroscience, 56,* 337–344.

Chen, A. J., Abrams, G. M., & D'Esposito, M. (2006). Functional reintegration of prefrontal neural networks for enhancing recovery after brain injury. *Journal of Head Trauma Rehabilitation, 21*(2), 107–118.

Chen, A. J., & D'Esposito, M. (2010). Traumatic brain injury: From bench to bedside to society. *Neuron, 66,* 11–14.

Cherry, K. E., Simmons, S. S., & Camp, C. J. (1999). Spaced retrieval enhances memory in older adults with probable Alzheimer's disease. *Journal of Clinical Geropsychology, 5,* 159–175.

Cicerone, K. D., Dahlberg, C., Kalmar, K., Langenbahn, D. M., Malec, J. F., Bergquist, T., et al. (2000). Evidence-based cognitive rehabilitation: Recommendations for clinical practice. *Archives of Physical Medicine and Rehabilitation, 81,* 1596–1615.

Cicerone, K. D., Dahlberg, C., Malec, J. F., Langenbahn, D. M., Thomas, F., Kneipp, S., et al. (2005). Evidence-based cognitive rehabilitation: Updated review of the literature from 1998 through 2002. *Archives of Physical Medicine and Rehabilitation, 86,* 1681–1692.

Cicerone, K. D., Langenbahn, D. M., Braden, C., Malec, J. F., Kalmar, K., Fraas, M., et al. (2011). Evidence-based cognitive rehabilitation: Updated review of the literature from 2003 through 2008. *Archives of Physical Medicine and Rehabilitation, 92*(4), 519–530.

Cicerone, K. D., Mott, T., Azulay, J., Sharlow-Galella, M., A., Ellmo, W., J., Paradise, S., &. Friel, J. C. (2008). A randomized controlled trial of holistic neuropsychologic rehabilitation after traumatic brain injury. *Archives of Physical Medicine and Rehabilitation, 89,* 2239-2249.

Cicerone, K. D., & Wood, J. C. (1986). Planning disorder after closed head injury: A case study. *Archives of Physical Medicine and Rehabilitation, 68,* 111–115.

Clare, L., Wilson, B. A., Carter, G., Breen, K., Gosses, A., & Hodges, J. R. (2000). Intervening with everyday memory problems in dementia of the Alzheimer type: An errorless learning approach. *Journal of Clinical and Experimental Neuropsychology, 22,* 132–146.

Code, C., & Petheram, B. (2011). Delivering for aphasia. *International Journal of Speech-Language Pathology, 13*(1), 3–10.

Constantinidou, F. (1999). The effects of stimulus modality on interference and recognition performance following brain injury. *Journal of Medical Speech-Language Pathology, 7*(4), 283–295.

Constantinidou, F. (2008). Neuropsychological and psychological rehabilitation after TBI. In G. J. Murray (Ed.), *The forensic evaluation of traumatic brain injury: A handbook for clinicians and attorneys* (2nd ed., pp. 91–118). Boca-Raton, FL: CRC Press.

Constantinidou, F., & Thomas, R. D. (2010). Principles of cognitive rehabilitation in TBI: An integrative neuroscience approach. In M. J. Ashley (Ed.), *Traumatic brain injury: Case management and rehabilitation* (3rd ed., pp. 549–582). Boca-Raton, FL: CRC Press.

Constantinidou, F., Thomas, R. D., & Best, P. (2004). Principles of cognitive rehabilitation: An integrative approach. In M. J. Ashley (Ed.), *Traumatic brain injury rehabilitation: Rehabilitative treatment and case management* (2nd ed., pp. 337–366). Boca-Raton, FL: CRC Press.

Constantinidou, F., Thomas, R. D., & Robinson, L. (2008). Benefits of categorization training in patients with TBI during post acute rehabilitation: Additional evidence from a randomized controlled trial. *Journal of Head Trauma Rehabilitation, 23*(5), 312–328.

Constantinidou, F., Thomas, R. D., Scharp, V. L., Laske, K. M., Hammerly, M. D., & Guitonde, S. (2005). Effects of categorization training in patients with TBI during postacute rehabilitation: Preliminary findings. *Journal of Head Trauma Rehabilitation, 20,* 143–157.

Constantinidou, F., Wertheimer, J. C., Tsanadis, J., Evans, C., & Paul, D. R. (2012). Assessment of executive functioning in brain injury: Collaboration between speech-language pathology and neuropsychology for an integrative neuropsychological perspective. *Brain Injury, 26*(13–14), 1549–1563.

Corrigan, J. D., Whiteneck, G., & Mellick, D. (2004). Perceived needs following traumatic brain injury. *Journal of Head Trauma Rehabilitation, 19,* 205–216.

Courville, C. B. (1937). *Pathology of the central nervous system.* Mountain View, CA: Pacific Press.

Covassin, T., Moran, R., & Wilhelm, K. (2013). Concussion symptoms and neurocognitive performances of high school and college athletes who incur multiple concussions. *The American Journal of Sports Medicine, 41*(12), 2885–2889.

Covassin, T, Stearne, D., & Elbin, R. (2008). Concussion history and postconcussion neurocognitive performance and symptoms in collegiate athletes. *Journal of Athletic Training, 43*(2), 119–124.

Crosson, B., Novack, T. A., Trenerry, M. R., & Craig, P. L. (1998). California Verbal Learning Test (CVLT) performance in severely head injured and neurologically normal males. *Experimental Neuropsychology, 10,* 754–768.

Dahlberg, C., Cusick, B. A., Hawley, L. A., Newman, J. K., Morey, C. E., Harrison-Felix, C. L., et al. (2007). Treatment efficacy of social communication skills training after traumatic brain injury: A randomized treatment and deferred treatment controlled trial. *Archives of Physical Medicine and Rehabilitation, 88,* 1561–1573.

Dahlberg, C., Hawley, L. A., Morey, C. E., Newman, J. K., Cusick, C. P., & Harrison-Felix, C. L. (2006). Social communication skills in persons with post-acute traumatic brain injury: Three perspectives. *Brain Injury, 20*(4), 425–435.

Dashnaw, M. L., Petraglia, A. L., & Bailes, J. E. (2012). An overview of the basic science of concussion and subconcussion: Where we are and where we are going. *Neurosurgery Focus, 33*(6), E5, 1–9.

Delis, D. C., Kaplan, E., & Kramer, J. H. (2001). *Delis-Kaplan Executive Function System.* San Antonio, TX: Psychological Corporation.

Delis, D. C., Kramer, J. H., Kaplan, E., & Ober, B. A. (2000). *California Verbal Learning Test* (2nd ed.). San Antonio, TX: Psychological Corporation.

DePompei, R., Gillette, Y., Goetz, E., Xenopoulos-Oddsson, A., Bryen, D., & Dowds, M. (2008). Practical applications for use of PDAs and smartphones with children and adolescents who have traumatic brain injury. *NeuroRehabilitation, 23*(6), 487–499.

Dijkers, M. (2000). *The Community Integration Questionnaire.* Retrieved from http://www.tbims.org/combi/ciq

Douglas, J. M., Bracy, C., & Snow, P. (2000). *LaTrobe Communication Questionnaire.* Bundoora, Victoria, Australia: School of Human Communication Sciences, La Trobe University.

Douglas, J. M., & Spellacy, F. J. (2000). Correlates of depression in adults with severe traumatic brain injury and their carers. *Brain Injury, 14*(1), 71–88.

Dunlosky, J., Hertzog, C., Kennedy, M. R. T., & Thiede, K. W. (2005). The self-monitoring approach for effective learning. *International Journal of Cognitive Technology, 10*(1), 4–11.

Ehlhardt, L. A., Sohlberg, M. M., Glang, A., & Albin, R. (2005). TEACH-M: A pilot study evaluating an instructional sequence for persons with impaired memory and executive functions. *Brain Injury, 19*(8), 569–583.

Ehlhardt, L., Sohlberg, M. M., Kennedy, M. R. T., Coelho, C., Turkstra, L., Ylvisaker, M., et al. (2008). Evidence-based practice guidelines for instructing individuals with acquired memory impairments: What have we learned in the past 20 years? *Neuropsychological Rehabilitation, 18,* 300–342.

Engelmann, S., & Carnine, D. (1991). *Theory of instruction: Principles and applications* (2nd ed.). New York, NY: Irvington.

Erickson, P. S., Perfilieva, E., Bjork-Eriksson, T., Alborn, A. M., Nordborg, C., Peterson, D. A., et al. (1998). Neurogenesis in the adult human hippocampus. *Nature Medicine, 4,* 1313–1317.

Finkelstein, E. A., Corso, P. S., & Miller, T. R. (2006). *The incidence and economic burden of injuries in the United States.* New York, NY: Oxford University Press.

Gentry, T., Wallace, J., Kvarfordt, C., & Bodisch-Lynch, K. (2008). Personal digital assistants as cognitive aids for individuals with severe traumatic brain injury: A community-based trial. *Brain Injury, 22*(1), 19–24.

Giacino, J. T., & Cicerone, K. D. (1998). Varieties of deficit unawareness after brain injury. *Journal of Head Trauma Rehabilitation, 13,* 1–15.

Giogkaraki, E., Michaelides, M. P., & Constantinidou, F. (2013). The role of cognitive reserve in cognitive aging: Results from the neurocognitive study on aging. *Journal of Clinical and Experimental Neuropsychology, 35*(10), 1024–1035.

Glang, A., Singer, G., Cooley, E., & Tish, N. (1992). Tailoring direct instruction techniques for use with elementary students with brain injury. *Journal of Head Trauma Rehabilitation, 7,* 93–108.

Glisky, E. L., Schacter, D. L., & Tulving, E. (1986a). Computer learning by memory-impaired patients: Acquisition and retention of complex knowledge. *Neuropsychologia, 24*(3), 313–328.

Glisky, E. L., Schacter, D. L., & Tulving, E. (1986b). Learning and retention of computer-related vocabulary in memory-impaired patients: Method of vanishing cues. *Journal of Clinical and Experimental Neuropsychology, 8*(3), 292–312.

Gould, E., & Gross, C. G. (2002). Neurogenesis in adult mammals: Some progress and progress. *Journal of Neuroscience, 22*(3), 619–623.

Gould, E., Reeves, A. J., Graziano, M. S. A., & Gross, C. G. (1999). Neurogenesis in the neocortex of adult primates. *Science, 286*, 548–552.

Hagen, C., Malkmus, D., & Durham, P. (1979). Levels of cognitive functioning. In *Rehabilitation of the head injured adult: Comprehensive physical management.* (pp 87-88) Downey, CA: Professional Staff Association of Rancho Los Amigos National Rehabilitation Medical Center.

Hall, E. D., Mohlberg, D. N., & Poole, R. M. (1998, Spring). Development of novel therapies for acute traumatic brain injury: Pharmaceutical industry perspective. *Brain Injury Source*, 18–21.

Haring, R. S., Narang, K., Canner, J. K., Asemota, A. O., George, B. P., Selvarajah, S., et al. (2015). Traumatic brain injury in the elderly: Morbidity and mortality trends and risk factors. *Journal of Surgical Research, 195*(1), 1–9.

Harmon, K. G., Drezner, J. A., Gammons, M., Guskiewicz, K. M., Halstead, M., Herring, S. A., et al. (2013). American medical society for sports medicine position statement: Concussion in sports. *British Journal of Sports Medicine, 47*, 15–26.

Hart, T., Buchhofer, R., & Vaccaro, M. (2004). Portable electronic devices as memory and organizational aids after traumatic brain injury: A consumer survey study. *Journal of Head Trauma Rehabilitation, 19*(5), 351–365.

Hart, T., Giovannetti, T., Montgomery, M. W., & Schwartz, M. F. (1998). Awareness of errors of naturalistic action after traumatic brain injury. *Journal of Head Trauma Rehabilitation, 13*(5), 16–28.

Hartley, L. L. (1995). *Cognitive-communicative abilities following brain injury: A functional approach.* San Diego, CA: Singular.

Haut, M. W., Petros, T. V., Frank, R. G., & Lamberty, G. (1990). Short-term memory processes following closed head injury. *Archives of Clinical Neuropsychology, 5*(3), 299–309.

Henry, L. C., Tremblay, S., Leclerc, S., Khiat, A., Boulanger, Y., Ellemberg, D., et al. (2011). Metabolic changes in concussed American football players during the acute and chronic post-injury phases. *Neurology, 11*(105), 1–10.

Hillary, F. G., Schultheis, M. T., Challis, B. H., Millis, S. R., Carnevale, G. J., Glashi, T., et al. (2003). Spacing of repetitions improves learning and memory after moderate and severe TBI. *Journal of Clinical and Experimental Neuropsychology, 25*(1), 49–58.

Hillered, L., Vespa, P. M., & Hovda, D. A. (2005). Translational neurochemical research in acute human brain injury: The current status and potential future for cerebral microdialysis. *Journal of Neurotrauma, 22*(1), 1–34.

Hopper, T., Mahendra, N., Kim, E., Azuma, T., Bayles, K. A., Cleary, S. J., et al. (2005). Evidence-based practice recommendations for working with individuals with dementia: Spaced-retrieval training. *Journal of Medical Speech-Language Pathology, 13*(4), xxvii–xxxiv.

Hovda, D. A. (1998, Spring). The neurobiology of traumatic brain injury: Why is the brain so vulnerable after injury? *Brain Injury Source*, 22–25.

Hughes, J., & Orange, J. B. (2007). Mapping functional communication measurements for traumatic brain injury to the WHO-ICF. *Canadian Journal of Speech-Language Pathology and Audiology, 31*(3), 134–143.

Hux, K., Manasse, N., Wright, S., & Snell, J. (2000). Effect of training frequency on face-name recall by adults with traumatic brain injury. *Brain Injury, 14*, 907–920.

Jennett, B., & Bond, M. (1975). Assessment outcome after severe brain damage: Practical scale. *Lancet, 1*, 480–484.

Joint Committee on Interprofessional Relations Between the American Speech-Language-Hearing Association and Division 40 (Clinical Neuropsychology) of the American Psychological Association. (2007). *Structure and function of an interdisciplinary team for persons with acquired brain injury* [Guidelines]. Retrieved from http://www.asha.org/docs/html/GL2007-00288.html.

Kalla, T., Downes, J., & van den Broek, M. (2001). The pre-exposure technique: Enhancing the effects of errorless learning in the acquisition of face-name associations. *Neuropsychological Rehabilitation, 11*(1), 1–16.

Kaplan, E., Goodglass, H., & Weintraub, S. (2007). *Boston Naming Test (BNT).* Philadelphia, PA: Lippincott Williams & Wilkins.

Kaschel, R., Della, S., Cantagallo, A., Fahlbock, A., Laaksonen, R., & Kazen, M. (2002). Imagery mnemonics for the rehabilitation of memory: A randomised group controlled trial. *Neuropsychological Rehabilitation, 12*(2), 127–153.

Katz, D. I. (1992). Neuropathology and neurobehavioral recovery from closed head injury. *Journal of Head Trauma Rehabilitation, 7*(2), 1–15.

Kennedy, M. R. T. (2004). Self-monitoring recall during two tasks after traumatic brain injury: A preliminary study. *American Journal of Speech-Language Pathology, 13*(2), 142–154.

Kennedy, M. R. T. (2007). Evidence-based reviews of cognitive rehabilitation for individuals with traumatic brain injury: What clinical questions do they answer? *Evidence BRIEF, 1*(4), 69–80.

Kennedy, M. R. T. (2013). Evidence-based practice and cognitive rehabilitation therapy. In S. McDonald, L. Togher, & C. Code (Eds.), *Social and communication disorders following traumatic brain injury* (2nd ed., pp. 282–306). New York, NY: Psychology Press.

Kennedy, M. R. T., Avery, J., Coelho, C., Sohlberg, M., Turkstra, L., & Ylvisaker, M. (2002). Evidence-based practice guidelines for cognitive-communication disorders after traumatic brain injury: Initial committee report. *Journal of Medical Speech-Language Pathology, 10*(2), ix–xiii.

Kennedy, M. R. T., Carney, E., & Peters, S. M. (2003). Predictions of recall and study strategy decisions after brain injury. *Brain Injury, 17*, 1043–1064.

Kennedy, M. R. T., & Coelho, C. (2005). Self-regulation after traumatic brain injury: A framework for intervention of memory and problem solving. *Seminars in Speech and Language, 26*, 242–255.

Kennedy, M. R. T., Coelho, C., Turkstra, L., Ylvisaker, M., Sohlberg, M. M., Yorkston, K., et al. (2008). Intervention for executive functions after traumatic brain injury: A systematic review, meta-analysis and clinical recommendations. *Neuropsychological Rehabilitation, 18*, 257–299.

Kennedy, M. R. T., & DeRuyter, F. (1991). Language and cognitive basis for communication disorders following traumatic brain injury. In D. R. Beukelman & K. M. Yorkston (Eds.), *Communication and swallowing disorders of persons with traumatic brain injury* (pp. 123–190). Austin, TX: Pro-Ed.

Kennedy, M. R. T., O'Brien, K., & Krause, M. O. (2012). Bridging person-centered outcomes and therapeutic processes for college students with traumatic brain injury. *Perspectives on Neurophysiology and Neurogenic Speech and Language Disorders, 22*, 143–151.

Kennedy, M. R. T., Wozniak, J. R., Muetzel, R. L., Mueller, B. A., Chiou, H. H., Pantekoek, K., et al. (2009). White matter and neurocognitive changes in adults with chronic traumatic brain injury. *Journal of the International Neuropsychological Society, 15*, 130–136.

Kennedy, M. R. T., & Yorkston, K. M. (2004). The effects of frontal injury on self-monitoring during verbal learning by adults with diffuse brain injury. *Neuropsychological Rehabilitation, 14*(4), 449–465.

Kernie, S. G., & Parent, J. M. (2010). Forebrain neurogenesis after focal ischemic and traumatic brain injury. *Neurobiology of Disease, 37*(2), 267–274.

Kertesz, A. (2007). *Western Aphasia Battery* (2nd ed.). San Antonio, TX: Psychological Corporation.

Kessels, R. C. P., & de Haan, E. H. F. (2003). Implicit learning in memory rehabilitation: A meta-analysis on errorless learning and vanishing cues methods. *Journal of Clinical and Experimental Neuropsychology, 25*, 805–814.

Kiernan, R. J., Meuller, J., & Langston, J. W. (1995). *Cognistat (Neurobehavioral Cognitive Status Examination)*. Lutz, FL: Psychological Assessment Resources.

Kinnunen, K. M., Greenwood, R., Powell, J. H., Leech, R., Hawkins, P. C., Bonnelle, V., et al. (2011). White matter damage and cognitive impairment after traumatic brain injury. *Brain, 134*, 449–463.

Knollman Porter, K., Constantinidou, F., & Hutchinson Marron, K. (2014). Speech-language pathology and concussion management in intercollegiate athletics: The Miami University Concussion Management Program. *American Journal of Speech-Language Pathology, 23*, 507-519.

Kraus, J. F., Servadei, F., Korsic, M., Compagnone, C., & Tagliaferri, F. (2005). A systematic review of brain injury epidemiology in Europe. *Acta Neurochirurgica, 148*(3), 255–268.

Kraus, M. F., Susmaras, T., Caughlin, B. P., Walker, C. J., Sweeney, J. A., & Little, D. M. (2007). White matter integrity and cognition in chronic traumatic brain injury: A diffusion tensor imaging study. *Brain, 130*, 2508–2519.

Landauer, T. K., & Bjork, R. A. (1978). Optimum rehearsal patterns and name learning. In M. M. Gruneberg, P. E. Morris, & R. N. Sykes (Eds.), *Practical aspects of memory* (pp. 625–632). London, UK: Academic Press.

Langlois, J. A., Rutland-Brown, W., & Thomas, K. E. (2006). *Traumatic brain injury in the United States: Emergency department visits, hospitalizations, and deaths 2002–2006*. Atlanta, GA: Centers for Disease Control and Prevention, National Center for Injury Prevention and Control. Retrieved from http://www.cdc.gov/traumaticbraininjury/tbi_ed.html.

Lengenfelder, J., Chiaravalloti, N. D., & DeLuca, J. (2007). The efficacy of the generation effect in improving new learning in persons with traumatic brain injury. *Rehabilitation Psychology, 52*(3), 290–296.

Levin, H. S., Benton, A. L., & Grossmann, R. G. (1982). *Neurobehavioral consequences of closed head injury*. New York, NY: Oxford University Press.

Levin, H. S., O'Donnell, V. M., & Grossman, R. G. (1979). The Galveston Orientation and Amnesia Test: A practical scale to assess cognition after head injury. *Journal of Nervous and Mental Disease, 167*, 675–684.

Lewinsohn, P., Danaher, B., & Kikel, S. (1977). Visual imagery as a mnemonic aid for brain-injured persons. *Journal of Consulting and Clinical Psychology, 45*(5), 717–723.

Lipton, M. L., Gulko, E., Zimmerman, M. E., Friedman, B. W., Kim, M., Gellella, E., et al. (2009). Diffusion-tensor imaging implicates prefrontal axonal injury in executive function impairment following very mild traumatic brain injury. *Radiology, 252*(3), 816–824.

MacDonald, S. (2005). *Functional Assessment of Verbal Reasoning and Executive Strategies (FAVRES)*. Guelph, ON, Canada: CCD.

Macciocchi, S. N., Barth, J. T., Alves, W. M., Rimel, R. W., & Jane, J. A. (1996). Neuropsychological functioning and recovery after mild head injury in collegiate athletes. *Neurosurgery, 39*, 510–514.

Malec, J. F. (2001). Impact of comprehensive day treatment on societal participation for persons with acquired brain injury. *Archives of Physical Medicine and Rehabilitation, 82*, 885–895.

Malec, J. F. (2005). *Introduction to the Mayo Portland Adaptability Inventory*. Center for Outcome Measurement in Brain Injury. Retrieved from http://www.tbims.org/combi/mpai.

Manasse, N., Hux, K., & Snell, J. (2005). Teaching face-name associations to survivors of traumatic brain injury: A sequential treatment approach. *Brain Injury, 19*(8), 633–641.

Marosszeky, N. E. V., Ryan, L., Shores, E. A., Batchelor, J., & Marosszeky, J. E. (1997). The PTA Protocol: Guidelines for using the Westmead Post-Traumatic Amnesia (PTA) Scale. Sydney, Australia: Wild & Wooley.

McAllister, T. W. (2011). Neurobiological consequences of traumaticbrain injury. *Dialogues in Clinical Neurosciences, 13*, 287–300.

McCrea, M., Iverson, G., Echemendia, R., Makdissi, M., & Raftery, M. (2013). Day of injury assessment of sport-related concussion. *British Journal of Sports Medicine, 47*, 272–284.

McCrory, P., Davis, G., & Makdissi, M. (2012). Second impact syndrome or cerebral swelling after sporting head injury. *Current Sports Medicine Reports, 11*, 21–23.

McDonald, S. (1993). Pragmatic language skills after closed head injury: Ability to meet the informational needs of the listener. *Brain and Language, 44*, 28–46.

McFarland, L. (2012). Motivational interviewing: Practical strategies for speech-language pathologists and audiologists. *Canadian Journal of Speech-Language Pathology and Audiology, 36*(1), 8–16.

Melton, A. K., & Bourgeois, M. S. (2005). Training compensatory memory strategies via telephone for persons with TBI. *Aphasiology, 19*(3–5), 353–364.

Millis, S. R., Rosenthal, M., Novack, T. A., Sherer, M., Nick, T. G., Kreutzer, J. S., et al. (2001). Long-term neuropsychological outcome after traumatic brain injury. *Journal of Head Trauma Rehabilitation, 16*(4), 343–355.

NCAA Sports Medicine Handbook (2012–2013). Retrieved September 15, 2013, from http://www.ncaapublications.com/productdownloads/MD12.pdf

Nelson, H. E., & Willison, J. (1991). *National Adult Reading Test* (2nd ed.). Windsor, UK: MFER-Nelson.

Newcombe, V. F. J., Outtrim, J. G., Chatfield, D. A., Manktelow, A., Hutchinson, P. J., Coles, J. P., et al. (2011). Parcellating the neuroanatomical basis of impaired decision-making in traumatic brain injury. *Brain, 134*, 759–768.

Newcombe, V. F. J., Williams, G. B., Nortje, J., Bradley, P. G., Harding, S. G., Smielewski, P., et al. (2007). Analysis of acute traumatic axonal injury using diffusion tensor imaging. *British Journal of Neurosurgery, 21*, 340–348.

Newman, A. C., Garmoe, W., Beatty, P., & Ziccardi, M. (2000). Self-awareness of traumatically brain injured patients in the acute inpatient rehabilitation setting. *Brain Injury, 14,* 333–344.

Oberg, L., & Turkstra, L. S. (1998). Use of elaborative encoding to facilitate learning after adolescent traumatic brain injury. *Journal of Head Trauma Rehabilitation, 13*(3), 44–62.

O'Brien, A., Chiaravalloti, N., Arango-Lasprilla, J. C., Lengenfelder, J., & DeLuca, J. (2007). An investigation of the differential effect of self-generation to improve learning and memory in multiple sclerosis and traumatic brain injury. *Neuropsychological Rehabilitation, 17*(3), 273–292.

Parente, R., & Herrmann, D. (1996). *Retraining cognition: Techniques and applications.* Gaithersburg, MD: Aspen.

Ponsford, J., Bayley, M., Wiseman-Hakes, C., Togher, L., Velikonja, D., McIntyre, A., et al., &. (2014). INCOG recommendations for management of cognition following traumatic brain injury, part II: Attention and information processing speed. *The Journal of Head Trauma Rehabilitation, 29*(4), 321–337.

Povlishock, J. T., & Katz, D. I. (2005). Update on neuropathology and neurological recovery after traumatic brain injury. *Journal of Head Trauma Rehabilitation, 20*(1), 76–94.

Prigatano, G. P. (2003). Challenging dogma in neuropsychology and related disciplines. *Archives of Clinical Neuropsychology, 18,* 811–825.

Prigatano, G. P., & Altman, I. M. (1990). Impaired awareness of behavioral limitations after traumatic brain injury. *Archives of Physical Medicine and Rehabilitation, 71,* 1058–1064.

Randolph, C. (1998). *Repeatable Battery for the Assessment of Neuropsychological Status (RBANS).* San Antonio, TX: Pearson/Psychological Corporation.

Rappaport, M., Hall, K. M., Hopkins, K., Belleza, T., & Cope, D. N. (1982). Disability rating scale for severe head trauma: Coma to community. *Archives of Physical Medicine and Rehabilitation, 63*(3), 118–123.

Rosch, E., & Mervis, C. B. (1975). Family resemblances: Studies in the internal structure of categories. *Cognitive Psychology, 7,* 573–605.

Rosch, E., Simpson, E. J., & Miller, R. S. (1976). Structural bases of typicality effects. *Journal of Experimental Psychology, 2,* 491–502.

Roozenbeek, B., Maas, A. I., & Menon, D. K. (2013). Changing patterns in the epidemiology of traumatic brain injury. *Nature Reviews Neurology, 9*(4), 231–236.

Rugg-Gunn, F. J., Symms, M. R., Barker, G. J., Greenwood, R., & Duncan, J. S. (2001). Diffusion imaging shows abnormalities after blunt head trauma when conventional magnetic resonance imaging is normal. *Journal of Neurology, Neurosurgery, and Psychiatry, 70,* 530–533.

Sanders, A., Nakase-Thomson, R., Constantinidou, F., Wertheimer, J., & Paul, D. (2007). Memory assessment on an interdisciplinary rehabilitation team: A theoretically based framework. *American Journal of Speech-Language Pathology, 16,* 316–330.

Sarno, M. T. (1980). The nature of verbal impairment after closed head injury. *Journal of Nervous and Mental Disease, 168,* 685–692.

Sarno, M. T. (1984). Verbal impairment after closed head injury. *Journal of Nervous and Mental Disease, 172,* 475–479.

Sarno, M. T., Buonaguro, A., & Levita, E. (1986). Characteristics of verbal impairment in closed head injured patients. *Archives of Physical Medicine and Rehabilitation, 67,* 400–405.

Saulle, M., & Greenwald, B. D. (2012). Chronic traumatic encephalopathy: A review. *Rehabilitation Research and Practice, 2012,* 1–9.

Schatz, P., Pardini, J. E., Lovell, M. R., Collins, M. W., & Podell, K. (2006). Sensitivity and specificity of the ImPACT Test Battery for concussion in athletes. *Archives of Clinical Neuropsychology, 21,* 91–99.

Schmitter-Edgecombe, M. (1996). Effects of divided attention on implicit and explicit memory performance following severe closed head injury. *Neuropsychology, 10,* 155–167.

Schmitter-Edgecombe, M. (2006). Implications of basic science research for brain injury rehabilitation: A focus on intact learning mechanisms. *Journal of Head Trauma Rehabilitation, 21*(2), 131–141.

Schmitter-Edgecombe, M., & Nissley, H. M. (2000). Effects of divided attention on automatic and controlled components of memory after severe closed-head injury. *Neuropsychology, 14,* 559–569.

Serino, A., Ciaramelli, E., Di Santantonio, A., Malagu, S., Servadei, F., & Ladava, E. (2006). Central executive system impairment in traumatic brain injury. *Brain Injury, 20,* 23–32.

Silverberg, N. D., & Millis, S. R. (2009). Impairment versus deficiency in neuropsychological assessment: Implications for ecological validity. *Journal of the International Neuropsychological Society, 15,* 94–02.

Sohlberg, M., Avery, J., Kennedy, M. R. T., Coelho, C., Ylvisaker, M., Turkstra, L., et al. (2003). Practice guidelines for direct attention training. *Journal of Medical Speech-Language Pathology, 11*(3), xix–xxxix.

Sohlberg, M. M., Ehlhardt, L., & Kennedy, M. (2005). Instructional techniques in cognitive rehabilitation: A preliminary report. *Seminars in Speech and Language, 26*(4), 268–279.

Sohlberg, M. M., Johnson, L., Paule, L., Raskin, S. A., & Mateer, C. A. (1994). *Attention process training II: A program to address attentional deficits for persons with mild cognitive dysfunction* [Rehabilitation materials]. Puyallup, WA: Association for Neuropsychological Research & Development.

Sohlberg, M. M., Kennedy, M. R. T., Avery, J., Coelho, C., Turkstra, L., Ylvisaker, M., et al. (2007). Evidence based practice for the use of external aids as a memory rehabilitation technique. *Journal of Medical Speech Pathology, 15*(1), xv–li.

Sohlberg, M. M., & Mateer, C. A. (1989). *Introduction to cognitive rehabilitation: Theory and practice.* New York, NY: Guilford Press.

Sohlberg, M. M., & Mateer, C. A. (2001). *Cognitive rehabilitation: An integrative neuropsychological approach.* New York, NY: Guilford Press.

Spreen, O., & Benton, A. L. (1969). *Neurosensory Center Comprehensive Examination for Aphasia: Manual of directions.* Victoria, BC, Canada: Neuropsychology Laboratory, University of Victoria.

Stapleton, S., Adams, M., & Atterton, L. (2007). A mobile phone as a memory aid for individuals with traumatic brain injury: A preliminary investigation. *Brain Injury, 21*(4), 401–411.

Strich, S. J. (1961). Shearing nerve fibres as a cause of brain damage due to head injury. *Lancet, 2,* 443–448.

Stuss, D. T. (1991). Self, awareness and the frontal lobes: A neuropsychological perspective. In J. Strauss & G. R. Goethals (Eds.), *The self: Interdisciplinary approaches* (pp. 255–278). New York, NY: Springer-Verlag.

Stuss, D. T. (2011). Functions of the frontal lobes: Relation to executive functions. *Journal of the International Neuropsychological Society, 17,* 759–765.

Swanson, H. L. (1999). Instructional components that predict treatment outcomes for students with learning disabilities: Support for the combined strategy and Direct Instruction Model. *Learning Disabilities Research and Practice, 14*(3), 129–140.

Swanson, H. L. (2001). Searching for the best model for instructing students with learning disabilities. *Focus on Exceptional Children, 34*(2), 2–15.

Swanson, H. L., & Hoskyn, M. (1998). A synthesis of experimental intervention literature for students with learning disabilities: A meta-analysis of treatment outcomes. *Review of Educational Research, 68*, 277–322.

Task Force on Promotion and Dissemination of Psychological Procedures. (1995). Training in and dissemination of empirically validated psychological treatments. *Clinical Psychologist, 48*, 13–23.

Tate, R., Kennedy, M. R. T., Bayley, M., Bragge, P., Douglas, J., Kita, M., et al. (2014). INCOG Recommendations for Management of Cognition following Traumatic Brain Injury Part VI: Executive Function and Self-awareness, *Journal of Head Trauma Rehabilitation, 29*(4), 338–352. doi:10.1097/HTR.0000000000000068

Tate, R. L., Pfaff, A., Baguley, I. J., Marosszeky, J. E., Gurka, J. A., Hodgkinson, A. E., et al. (2006). A multicentre, randomised trial examining the effect of test procedures measuring emergence from post-traumatic amnesia. *Journal of Neurology, Neurosurgery, and Psychiatry, 77*(7), 841–849. doi:10.1136/jnnp.2005.074989.

Thurman, D. J., Alverson, C., Dunn, K. A., Guerrero, J., & Sniezek, J. E. (1999). Traumatic brain injury in the United States: A public health perspective. *Journal of Head Trauma Rehabilitation, 14*, 602–615.

Togher, L., Wiseman-Hakes, C., Douglas, J., Stergiou-Kita, M., Ponsford, J., Teasell, R., et al., &. (2014). INCOG recommendations for management of cognition following traumatic brain injury, part IV: Cognitive communication. *The Journal of Head Trauma Rehabilitation, 29*(4), 353–368.

Turkstra, L. S. (2005). Looking while listening and speaking: Eye-to-face gaze in adolescents with and without traumatic brain injury. *Journal of Speech Language & Hearing Research, 48*(6), 1429–1441.

Turkstra, L. S., & Bourgeois, M. S. (2005). Intervention for a modern day HM: Errorless learning of practical goals. *Journal of Medical Speech Language Pathology, 13*(3), 205–212.

Turkstra, L., Ylvisaker, M., Coelho, C., Kennedy, M., Sohlberg, M. M., & Avery, J. (2005). Practice guidelines for standardized assessment for persons with traumatic brain injury. *Journal of Medical Speech-Language Pathology, 13*(2), ix–xxxviii.

Vakil, E. (2005). The effect of moderate to severe traumatic brain injury (TBI) on different aspects of memory: A selective review. *Journal of Clinical & Experimental Neuropsychology, 27*, 997–1021.

Van Hulle, A., & Hux, K. (2006). Improvement patterns among survivors of brain injury: Three case examples documenting the effectiveness of memory compensation strategies. *Brain Injury, 20*(1), 101–109.

Varney, N. R., & Menefee, L. (1993). Psychosocial and executive deficits following closed head injury: Implications for orbital frontal cortex. *Journal of Head Trauma Rehabilitation, 8*(1), 32–44.

Velikonja, D., Tate, R., Ponsford, J., McIntyre, A., Janzen, S., & Bayley, M. (2014). INCOG recommendations for management of cognition following traumatic brain injury, part V: Memory. *The Journal of Head Trauma Rehabilitation, 29*(4), 369–386.

Verity, A. M., Povlishock, J., & Cheung, M. (1988). Brain cellular injury and recovery—Horizons for improving medical therapies in stroke and trauma. *Western Journal of Medicine, 148*(6), 670–684.

Webbe, F. M., & Barth, J. T. (2003). Short-term and long-term outcome of athletic closed head injuries. *Clinics in Sports Medicine, 22*, 577–592.

Wechsler, D. (1997). *The Wechsler Memory Scale–3rd Edition (WMS-III)*. San Antonio, TX: Psychological Corporation.

Wehman, P., Kregel, J., Sherron, P., Nguyen, S., Kreutzer, J., Fry, R., et al. (1993). Critical factors associated with the successful support employment placement of patients with severe traumatic brain injury. *Brain Injury, 7*, 31–44.

Wertheimer, J., Roebuck, T., Constantinidou, F., Turskstra, L., & Pavol, M. (2008). Collaboration between neuropsychologists and speech language pathologists in rehabilitation settings. *Journal of Head Trauma Rehabilitation, 23*(5), 273–285.

Wilde, E. A., McCauley, S. R., Hunter, J. V., Bigler, E. D., Chu, Z., Wang, Z. J., et al. (2008). Diffusion tensor imaging of acute mild traumatic brain injury in adolescents. *Neurology, 70*, 948–955.

Wilson, B. A., Cockburn, J., & Baddeley, A. (2003). *Rivermead Behavioral Memory Tests* (2nd ed.). Bury St. Edmunds, UK: Thames Valley Test Company.

Wilson, B. A., Emslie, H., Quirk, K., Evans, J., & Watson, P. (2005). A randomized control trial to evaluate a paging system for people with traumatic brain injury. *Brain Injury, 19*(11), 891–894.

Woodcock, R. W., McGrew, K. S., & Mather, N. (2001). *Woodcock-Johnson Tests of Cognitive Abilities (WJ III)*. Itasca, IL: Riverside.

World Health Organization. (2001). *International classification of functioning, disability, and health framework*. Retrieved from http://www3.who.int/icf/icftemplate.cfm

Wright, J. (2000). *Introduction to the Functional Assessment Measure*. Center for Outcome Measurement in Brain Injury. Retrieved from http://www.tbims.org/combi/FAM

Yakolev, A. G., & Faden, A. I. (1995). Molecular strategies in central nervous system injury. *Journal of Neurotrauma, 12*(5), 767–777.

Ylvisaker, M., & Feeney, T. (1998). *Collaborative brain injury intervention: Positive everyday routines*. San Diego, CA: Singular.

Ylvisaker, M., Hanks, R., & Johnson-Greene, D. (2003). Rehabilitation of children and adults with cognitive-communication disorders after brain injury. *ASHA Supplement, 23*, 59–72.

Ylvisaker, M., Turkstra, L., Coelho, C., Kennedy, M. R. T., Sohlberg, M. M., & Yorkston, K. M. (2007). Behavioral interventions for individuals with behavior disorders after traumatic brain injury: A systematic review. *Brain Injury, 21*(8), 769–805.

Yoshino, A., Hovda, D. A., Kawamata, T., Katayama, Y., & Becker, D. P. (1991). Dynamic changes in local cerebral glucose utilization following cerebral concussion in rats: Evidence of a hyper-and subsequent hypermetabolic state. *Brain Research, 561*, 106–119.

Younger, B. A., & Fearing, D. D. (1999). Parsing items into separate categories: Developmental changes in infant categorization. *Child Development, 70*(2), 291–303.

Zeman, A. (2001). Consciousness. *Brain, 124*(7), 1263–1289.

Rancho Los Amigos Scale

I. No Response

Patient is in coma and unresponsive to stimuli.

II. Generalized Response

Patient reacts inconsistently and nonpurposefully to stimuli in a nonspecific manner. Reflexes are limited and often undifferentiated, regardless of stimuli presented.

III. Localized Response

Patient responses are specific but inconsistent and are directly related to the type of stimulus presented, such as turning head toward a sound or focusing on a presented object. He may follow simple commands inconsistently and with delay.

IV. Confused-Agitated

Patient is in a heightened state of activity and severely confused, disoriented, and unaware of present events. His behavior is frequently bizarre and inappropriate. He is unable to perform self-care tasks. If not physically disabled, he may perform automatic motor activities such as sitting, reaching, and walking as part of his agitated state, but not necessarily purposefully.

V. Confused-Inappropriate, Nonagitated

Patient appears alert and responds to simple commands. On occasion he is able to respond to more complex commands, however inconsistently and randomly. The patient may show some agitated behavior in response to external stimuli rather than internal confusion. He is highly distractible and generally has difficulty in learning new information. His memory is impaired, and verbalization is often inappropriate. He can manage self-care activities with assistance.

VI. Confused-Appropriate

Patient shows goal-directed behavior but relies on cueing for direction. He can relearn old skills such as activities of daily living, but memory problems interfere with new learning. He has beginning awareness of self and others. Posttraumatic amnesia begins to resolve.

VII. Automatic-Appropriate

Patient goes through daily routines automatically but is robot-like with appropriate behavior and minimal confusion. He has shallow recall of activities and superficial awareness of, but lack of insight to, his condition. He requires at least minimal supervision because judgment, problem solving, and planning skills are impaired.

VIII. Purposeful-Appropriate

Patient is alert and oriented and is able to recall and integrate past and recent events. He can learn new activities and continue in home and living skills, though deficits in stress tolerance; judgment; abstract reasoning; social, emotional, and intellectual capacities may persist.

Source: Adapted from Hagen, C., Malkmus, D., & Durham, P. (1979). Levels of cognitive functioning. In Rancho Los Amigos Hospital, *Rehabilitation of the head injured adult: Comprehensive physical management.* Downey, CA: Professional Staff Association of Rancho Los Amigos National Rehabilitation Medical Center.

Assessment Tools Based on the World Health Organization Model

Function-/Impairment-Based Assessment Tools

Benton Controlled Word Association Test (COWAT). Spreen, O., & Benton, A. L. (1969). Victoria, BC: Neuropsychology Laboratory, University of Victoria. [See also Ruff, R. M., Light, R. H., Parker, S. B., & Levin, H. S. (1996). Benton Controlled Oral Word Association Test: Reliability and updated norms. *Archives of Clinical Neuropsychology, 11*, 329–338.]

Boston Naming Test (BNT). Kaplan, E., Goodglass, H., & Weintraub, S. (2007). Philadelphia, PA: Lippincott Williams & Wilkins.

Brief Test of Head Injury (BTHI). Helm-Estabrooks, N., & Holtz, G. (1991). Austin, TX: Pro-Ed.

Cognistat: Neurobehavioral Cognitive Status Examination. Kiernan, R. J., Mueller, J., & Langston, J. W. (1995). Lutz, FL: Psychological Assessment Resources.

Detroit Test of Learning Aptitude–4 (DTLA-4). Hammill, D. (1998). Austin, TX: Pro-Ed.

Discourse Comprehension Test (2nd ed.). Brookshire, R. H., & Nicholas, L. E. (1997). Retrieved from http://www.picaprograms.com.

Galveston Orientation and Amnesia Test (GOAT). Levin, H. S., O'Donnell, V. M., & Grossman, R. G. (1979). *Journal of Nervous Mental Disorders, 167*(11), 675–684.

Montreal Cognitive Assessment (2015). Retrieved March 18, 2015, from http://www.mocatest.org/

National Adult Reading Test (2nd ed.). Nelson, H. E., & Willison, J. (1991). Windsor, UK: MFER-Nelson.

Repeatable Battery for the Assessment of Neuropsychological Status (RBANS). Randolph, C. (1998). San Antonio, TX: Pearson/Psychological Corporation.

Ross Information Processing Assessment–II. Ross, D. (1996). Austin, TX: Pro-Ed.

Scales of Cognitive Ability for Traumatic Brain Injury (SCATBI). Adamovich, B. B., & Henderson, J. (1992). Chicago, IL: Riverside.

Test of Language Competence–Expanded Edition. Wiig, E., & Secord, W. (1989). San Antonio, TX: Psychological Corporation.

Wechsler Memory Scale–IV Edition (WMS-IV). Wechsler, D. (2009). San Antonio, TX: Pearson.

Western Aphasia Battery (2nd ed.). Kertesz, A. (2007). San Antonio, TX: Psychological Corporation.

Woodcock-Johnson Tests of Cognitive Abilities (WJ III). Woodcock, R. W., McGrew, K. S., & Mather, N. (2001). Chicago IL: Riverside.

Activity/Limitation-Based Assessment Tools

American Speech-Language-Hearing Association Functional Assessment of Communication Skills for Adults (ASHA FACS). Frattali, C. M., Thompson, C., Holland, A., Wohl, A., & Ferketic, M. (1995). Rockville, MD: ASHA.

Behavioral Assessment of the Dysexecutive Syndrome (BADS). Wilson, B. A., Alderman, M., Burgess, P., Emslie, H., & Evans, J. J. (1996). Bury St. Edmunds, UK: Thames Valley Test Company.

Behavioral Inattention Test (BIT). Wilson, B. A., Cockburn, J., & Halligan, P. (1987). Bury St. Edmunds, UK: Thames Valley Test Company.

Communication Activities of Daily Living (2nd ed.). Holland, A., Frattali, C., & Fromm, D. (1999). Austin, TX: Pro-Ed.

Disability Rating Scale (DRS). Rappaport, M., Hall, K. M., Hopkins, K., Belleza, T., & Cope. D. N. (1982). Disability rating scale for severe head trauma: Coma to community. *Archives of Physical Medicine and Rehabilitation, 63*(3), 118–123.

Everyday Memory Questionnaire. Sunderland, A., Harris, J., & Baddeley, A. (1983). Do laboratory tests predict everyday memory? A neuropsychological study. *Journal of Verbal Learning and Verbal Behavior, 22*, 341–357. [See also

Royle, J., & Lincoln, N. B. (2008). The Everyday Memory Questionnaire–revised: Development of a 13-item scale. *Disability & Rehabilitation, 30*(2), 114–121.]

Functional Assessment of Verbal Reasoning and Executive Strategies (FAVRES). MacDonald, S. (2005). Guelph, ON, Canada: CCD.

Rivermead Behavioral Memory Tests (original, 1985; extended version, 1998; 2nd ed., 2003). Wilson, B. A., Cockburn, J., & Baddeley, A. Bury St. Edmunds, UK: Thames Valley Test Company.

Test of Everyday Attention (TEA). Robertson, I. H., Ward, T., Ridgeway, V., & Nimmo-Smith, I. (1994). Bury St. Edmunds, UK: Thames Valley Test Company.

Participation-/Restriction-Based Assessment Tools

Awareness Questionnaire. Sherer, M. (2004). Retrieved April 14, 2010, from http://www.tbims.org/combi/aq

Behavior Rating Inventory of Executive Function (Children and Adult versions). Gioia, G. A., Isquith, P. K., Guy, S. C., & Kenworthy, L. (2000). Odessa, FL: Psychological Assessment Resources.

California Verbal Learning Test (2nd ed.). Delis, D. C., Kramer, J. H., Kaplan, E., & Ober, B. A. (2000). San Antonio, TX: Psychological Corporation.

College Survey for Students With Brain Injury. Kennedy, M. R. T., & Krause, M. O. (2009). Retrieved March 18, 2015, from http://neurocognitivelab.com/wp-content/uploads/2011/12/College-Survey-for-Students-with-Brain-Injury.pdf

Community Integration Questionnaire. Dijkers, M. (2000). Retrieved April 14, 2010, from http://www.tbims.org/combi/ciq

Craig Handicap Assessment and Reporting Technique–Short Form. Mellick, D. (2000). Retrieved April 14, 2010, from http://www.tbims.org/combi/chartsf

Delis-Kaplan Executive Function System. Delis, D. C., Kaplan, E., & Kramer, J. H. (2001). San Antonio, TX: Psychological Corporation. [See also Delis, D. C., Kramer, J. H., Kaplan, E., & Holdnack, J. (2004). Reliability and validity of the Delis-Kaplan Executive Function System: an update. *Journal of the International Neuropsychological Society, 10*(2), 301–303.]

Functional Assessment Measure. Wright, J. (2000). The Center for Outcome Measurement in Brain Injury. Retrieved July 17, 2010, from http://www.tbims.org/combi/FAM

LaTrobe Communication Questionnaire. Douglas, J., Bracy, C., & Snow, P. (2000). Bundoora, Victoria, Australia: School of Human Communication Sciences, La Trobe University.

Mayo-Portland Adaptability Inventory. Malec, J. (2005). The Center for Outcome Measurement in Brain Injury. Retrieved March 23, 2015, from http://tbims.org/combi/mpai.

Patient Competency Rating Scale. Hart, T. (2000). Retrieved April 14, 2010, from http://www.tbims.org/combi/pcrs

Self-Awareness of Deficits Interview (SADI). Fleming, J. M., Strong, J., & Ashton, R. (1996). Self-awareness of deficits in adults with traumatic brain injury: How best to measure? *Brain Injury, 10*, 1–15. [See also Simmond, M., & Fleming, J. (2003). Reliability of the Self-Awareness of Deficits Interview for adults with traumatic brain injury. *Brain Injury, 17*(4), 325–337.]

Self-Regulation Skills Interview (SRSI). Ownsworth, T. L., McFarland, K., & Young, R. (2000). Development and standardization of the Self-Regulation Skills Interview (SRSI): A new clinical assessment tool for acquired brain injury. *Clinical Neuropsychologist, 14*, 76–92.

OBJECTIVES

The reader will be able to:

1. Define the syndrome of dementia and commonly associated diseases.

2. Summarize the impaired and spared cognitive functions associated with different types of dementia.

3. Detail the cognitive communication abilities of individuals with dementia.

4. Discuss the role of speech–language clinicians working with individuals who have dementia.

5. Select appropriate evaluation methods and assessment tools for individuals with dementia.

6. Explain a conceptual framework for interventions for individuals with dementia.

7. Develop intervention programs for individuals with dementia and their caregivers, based on theoretical principles of dementia management and research evidence.

Dementia and Related Cognitive Disorders

Nidhi Mahendra and Tammy Hopper

INTRODUCTION

Global aging has been accurately described as a tipping point that is transforming the world as we know it. Rapid and unprecedented demographic changes in the last few decades have resulted in a rising median age of the world's population and an approximately 20-year increase in the average life span (United Nations, 2002). Between 2000 and 2030, the population of adults aged 65 years and older is projected to increase from 6.9% to 12% worldwide (US Census Bureau, 2001), from 15.5% to 24.3% in Europe, from 12.6% to 20.3% in North America, from 6.0% to 12.0% in Asia, and from 5.5% to 11.6% in Latin America and the Caribbean (Kinsella & Velkoff, 2001). In the United States, the 2010 national census revealed that there were more individuals who were 65 years of age or older than in any prior recorded census (US Census Bureau, 2011). This accelerated global aging brings with it the increased incidence and prevalence of age-related health conditions and neurologic diseases that can cause dementia.

DEFINING THE SYNDROME OF DEMENTIA

Grabowski and Damasio (2004) define dementia as a syndrome characterized by acquired and persistent impairment of multiple cognitive domains that is severe enough to limit competence in activities of daily living, occupation, and social interaction. Affected cognitive domains include memory, language, attention, executive function, and visuospatial abilities. Importantly, cognitive impairments in these domains occur in the absence of delirium, which is an acute but reversible state of confusion associated with temporary impairments of attention, perception, and cognition. Prince and colleagues (2013) have estimated that nearly 35.6 million persons worldwide were living with dementia in 2010.

Dementia may be reversible (e.g., resulting from depression, normal-pressure hydrocephalus, vitamin deficiency, thyroid disease) or irreversible (e.g., resulting from progressive neurodegenerative conditions such as Alzheimer's disease [AD], Parkinson's disease [PD], and frontotemporal lobar degeneration [FTLD]). Alzheimer's disease is the most common cause of irreversible dementia in adults older than age 65 years, accounting for approximately 50% to 70% of cases (Plassman et al., 2007). Recently released facts and figures estimate that 1 in 9 older Americans has AD; that is, AD affects an estimated 5.3 million Americans (Alzheimer's Association, 2015). The vast majority of patients with AD have sporadic or late-onset AD that is diagnosed at or beyond the age of 65 years. Approximately 1% or fewer AD cases develop because of mutations to any of three specific genes with autosomal dominant inheritance, characterized by early onset of AD symptoms, usually when individuals are below age 65 and as early as age 30 (Alzheimer's Association, 2015; Selkoe, 2000). Early-onset AD has been linked to three genetic variations specifically involving genes for the amyloid precursor protein on chromosome 21 and the genes for the presenilin proteins (1 and 2) on chromosomes 1 and 14 (Alzheimer's Association, 2015; Lendon, Ashall, & Goate, 1997). Late-onset AD develops after age 65 and has been associated with one significant genetic risk factor—apolipoprotein E (APOE)—that increases a person's risk for developing AD. Apolipoprotein E is responsible for making a protein that transports cholesterol and other types of fat in the bloodstream and helps with neuronal repair (Jorm, 2000; National Institutes of Health, 2011). This *ApoE* gene found on chromosome 19 has three common alleles: APOE ε2, APOE ε3, and APOE ε4. The APOE ε2 allele is least common and thought to provide some protection against AD; the APOE ε3 allele is the most common in the general population, and neither decreases nor increases the risk of AD. Approximately 10% to 15% of the general population and nearly 40% of persons who develop late-onset AD have the APOE ε4 allele (National Institutes of Health, 2011). Regardless of ethnic group, the e4/e4 genotype specifically is associated with nearly 15 times the risk of AD when compared to persons who have no copies of this allele (Farrer et al., 1997).

Besides AD, other common causes of irreversible dementia are vascular dementia (VaD), accounting for 10% to 17% of cases, and dementia with Lewy bodies (DLB), PD, FTLD, and mixed dementia types; together, these account for approximately 13% of diagnosed cases (Plassman et al., 2007). In this chapter, we focus predominantly on AD because of its much greater prevalence; however, we also summarize recent findings and salient features pertaining to other dementias.

NEUROPATHOLOGY IN ALZHEIMER'S DISEASE

Different types of dementia have distinct cognitive signatures that reflect underlying patterns of neuropathology. Generally, the neuropathology of AD is characterized by a loss of neurons and synapses in the cerebral cortex and select subcortical regions. This neuronal loss gradually results in gross atrophy of affected regions (Figure 20.1) and is especially marked in the medial temporal lobe, the hippocampus and entorhinal cortex (Daulatzai, 2015), parietal lobe, and parts of the frontal cortex and cingulate gyrus (Wenk, 2003). Eventually, this neuronal atrophy spreads through the cortex and encompasses the association cortices of the temporal, parietal, and frontal lobes (Figure 20.2).

The earliest-appearing hallmark neuropathological changes and sine qua non of AD are beta-amyloid plaques and neurofibrillary tangles that are visible on microscopic examination of brain tissue taken from persons with AD (Tiraboschi, Hansen, Thal, & Corey-Bloom, 2004). Plaques are dense, insoluble deposits of the protein beta-amyloid (Figure 20.3), which is a fragment of a larger protein called amyloid precursor protein. In AD, for as yet unknown reasons, the amyloid precursor protein begins to break down into beta-amyloid fragments that aggregate outside neurons to form plaques (Tiraboschi et al., 2004). Neurofibrillary tangles

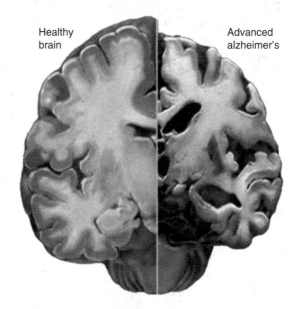

Healthy brain

Advanced alzheimer's

Figure 20.1 Cortical changes in AD.
Source: Copyright 2010. Alzheimer's Association. www.alz.org. All rights reserved. Image credit: Jannis Productions. Stacy Jannis.

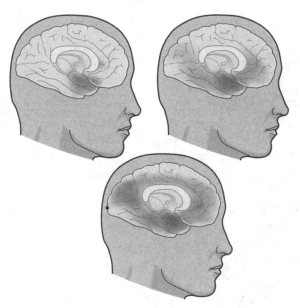

Figure 20.2 Progression of plaque and tangle development in Alzheimer's disease.

Source: Copyright 2010. Alzheimer's Association. www.alz.org. All rights reserved. Image credit: Jannis Productions. Stacy Jannis.

(Figure 20.3) result from abnormalities of another protein called tau, typically associated with microtubules inside neuronal cells. Microtubules are critical elements of a neuron's cytoskeleton, and in AD, the tau protein undergoes chemical changes that lead to disintegration of these microtubules to form tangles that disrupt critical neuronal transport systems (Hernández & Avila, 2007). Plaques and tangles first appear in the hippocampal complex (Braak & Braak, 1991), specifically in the entorhinal cortex (Wang & Zhou, 2002), the subiculum, and primary afferent and efferent pathways of the hippocampus (Albert, 1996). These pathological changes are accompanied by a pronounced decrease in the production of the neurotransmitter acetylcholine, especially important for learning and memory (Hasselmo, 2006).

Glutamate is another important excitatory neurotransmitter that plays a key role in information processing, storage, and retrieval. In AD, excessive deposition of amyloid results in widespread neuronal damage and cell death. Such neuronal degeneration triggers the excessive release of glutamate, which causes overstimulation of the N-methyl-D-aspartate (NMDA) subtype of glutamate receptors (Molinuevo, Ladó, & Rami, 2005). This overactivation of NMDA receptors is referred to as excitotoxicity because it triggers a postsynaptic calcium ion influx into nerve cells, further exacerbating neuronal degeneration (Hynd, Scott, & Dodd, 2004).

The critical role of these neurotransmitters—acetylcholine and glutamate—in the pathophysiology of AD has significantly influenced pharmacological treatment strategies and drug development for AD. The US Food and Drug Administration (FDA) has approved two types of medications to treat the cognitive symptoms of AD. The first approved category of medications is cholinesterase inhibitors, which enhance cholinergic transmission by inhibiting the enzyme acetylcholinesterase (ACE), which hydrolyzes or breaks down acetylcholine (Anand & Singh, 2013). Three ACE inhibitors that are frequently prescribed for persons with AD include donepezil (Aricept), rivastigmine (Exelon), and galantamine (Razadyne). Whereas donepezil has been approved for treating all stages of AD, rivastigmine and galantamine have been approved only for treating mild-to-moderate AD (Alzheimer's Association, 2012a). It is noteworthy that there is recent evidence (Doody et al., 2009) to support using ACE inhibitors for treating the cognitive symptoms associated with *mild cognitive impairment* (MCI)—widely regarded as a prodromal state for dementia (Petersen & Negash, 2008). Further, in one recent study, Lu and colleagues (2009) demonstrated that using donepezil delayed the progression to AD in persons with MCI and concomitant depression. The second class of approved drugs works by regulating glutamate levels at the aforementioned NMDA receptor sites and by preventing the previously described process of excitotoxicity. Currently, there is only one such drug, called memantine (Namenda), for the treatment of cognitive symptoms associated with moderate-to-severe AD. Approved in 2003 by the FDA, memantine is the first NMDA-receptor antagonist medication for AD (Alzheimer's Association, 2012a).

In 2011, McKhann et al. provided updated recommendations for the diagnosis of AD dementia or dementia secondary to AD neuropathology. To be diagnosed with probable AD dementia, an individual has to meet the criteria for dementia, in addition to having (a) an insidious onset (symptoms have a gradual onset over months to years); (b) a clear-cut history of worsening of cognition; and (c) initial and most prominent cognitive deficits that are either amnestic (episodic memory impairments)—the most common type of AD dementia—or nonamnestic (language, visuospatial, or executive function deficits).

DEFINING MILD COGNITIVE IMPAIRMENT

There is widespread consensus that neuropathological changes precede the clinical expression of AD by many years (Bennett et al., 2006; Price & Morris, 1999), and

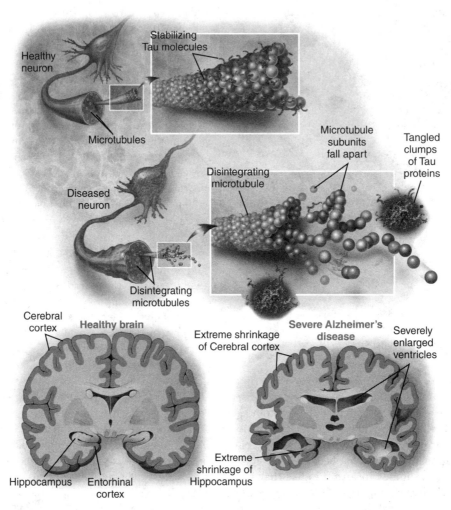

Figure 20.3 How the brain and nerve cells change during Alzheimer's disease.

Source: 2002–2010. Robert F. Morreale.

that subtle cognitive deficits may exist up to 9 years prior to a diagnosis of dementia (Amieva et al., 2005). This situation led researchers to characterize a nosological entity called *mild cognitive impairment*, a term first introduced by Flicker, Ferris, and Reisberg (1991). Petersen and colleagues (1997, 2001) further developed the concept of MCI as a preclinical state and a condition of intermediate symptomatology between the cognitive changes associated with healthy or typical aging and the more pathological changes that accompany AD or another type of dementia (Langa & Levine, 2014; Mariani, Monastero, & Mecocci, 2007; Petersen, 2003).

In concert with the development of updated guidelines for the diagnosis of AD dementia, the National Institute on Aging–Alzheimer's Association work group also developed updated diagnostic criteria for MCI due to AD, also known as the symptomatic predementia phase of AD (Albert et al., 2011). The core clinical criteria proposed by the working group include the following: concern

regarding a change in cognition, impairment in one or more cognitive domains, preservation of independence in functional abilities, and no dementia. Albert and colleagues (2011) also propose clinical research criteria that incorporate the use of biomarkers (imaging data, cerebrospinal fluid) to increase the certainty with which MCI due to AD can be diagnosed.

Distinct subtypes of MCI also have been identified based on the specific aspect of cognition that is most impaired at initial presentation (Petersen, 2004). The most common subtype of MCI is amnestic MCI (a-MCI), which is most likely to be associated with conversion to AD in longitudinal studies and features episodic memory impairment as the most prominent symptom. Another subtype of MCI is single-domain (nonmemory domain) MCI or sd-MCI (Petersen, 2004), characterized by prominent deficits in language ability, executive function, or visuospatial function. Finally, multiple-domain MCI (md-MCI) features involvement of multiple cognitive domains

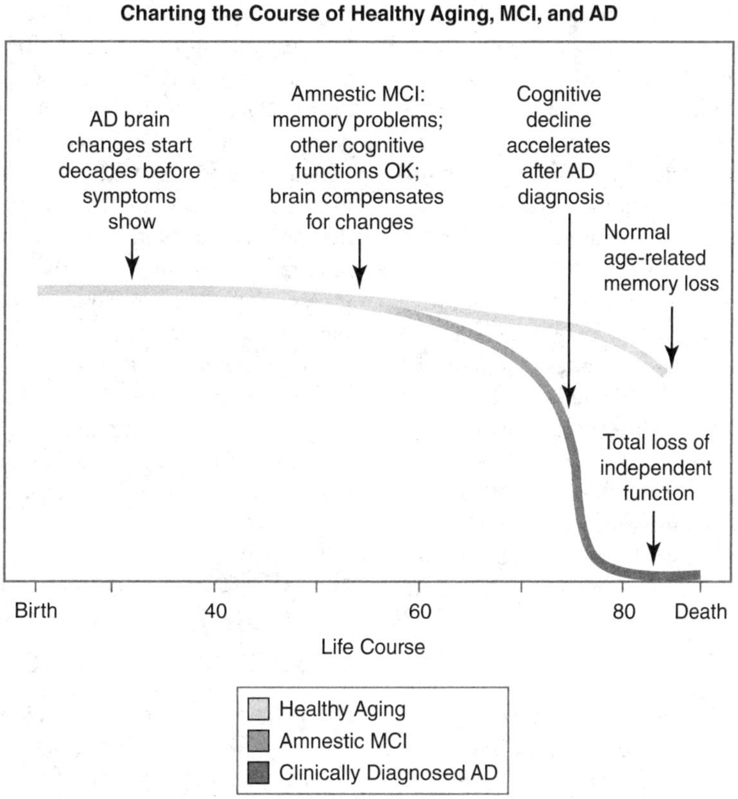

Charting the Course of Healthy Aging, MCI, and AD

Figure 20.4 Charting the course of aging, MCI, and AD.

© National Institute on Aging. *2004–2005 Progress report on Alzheimer's disease*. Available at. progress_report_on_alzheimers_disease_20042005small.pdf. Accessed November 5, 2015.

and may occur with memory impairments (md-MCI +a) or without them (md-MCI –a). Epidemiologic studies reveal that compared to older adults without MCI, those diagnosed with MCI are significantly more likely to develop AD or another dementia within a 5-year period. For example, in one study, 56% of a-MCI participants and 50% of nonamnestic MCI participants converted to AD or another dementia within a 4-year time period (Rountree et al., 2007). Figure 20.4 illustrates contemporary views about the transition from healthy cognitive aging to a-MCI to AD. Next, we discuss how AD affects cognitive functioning in affected persons.

EFFECTS OF ALZHEIMER'S DISEASE ON COGNITION

To understand how AD affects distinct cognitive domains, it is especially useful to understand how this disease affects human memory systems. Human memory comprises multiple components dependent on different yet interdependent neuroanatomical systems. Long-term memory has two foundational systems of stored knowledge: declarative memory and nondeclarative memory. *Declarative memory* refers to stored

knowledge of episodes and conceptual facts that can be consciously recalled and declared (Squire & Zola, 1996). It consists of three related subsystems that store factual knowledge about concepts (semantic memory), events (episodic memory), and words (lexical memory) as well as rules for their use (Baddeley, 2002; Bayles & Kim, 2003). For instance, a healthy adult knows that a lemon is a citrus fruit (concept), can recall that he or she had lemonade at lunch the previous day (episode), and that the word *lemon* is a noun and is spelled *l-e-m-o-n* (lexical knowledge). Declarative memory contrasts with nondeclarative memory; the latter is described as knowing how to do something and is referred as a "heterogeneous collection of unconscious learning capacities that are expressed through performance and do not afford access to any conscious memory content" (Squire & Zola, 1996, p. 13515). Nondeclarative memory consists of motor memory, cognitive skills and strategies, priming, conditioned responses, and reflexes (Bayles & Tomoeda, 2014; Squire & Dede, 2015).

The pattern of neuropathology in AD results in marked and early-appearing impairments in attention (Foldi, Lobosco, & Schaefer, 2002); working memory (Baddeley, Baddeley, Bucks, & Wilcock, 2001); episodic memory

(DeVreese, Neri, Fioravanti, Belloi, & Zanetti, 2001; Salmon & Bondi, 2009); and some aspects of executive function (Salmon & Bondi, 2009) while relatively sparing nondeclarative memory functions until much later in the disease process. Selective and divided attention deficits are notable in AD, resulting from a combination of damage to frontal and parietal association cortices, disconnection of the anterior and posterior attention networks, as well as reduced cholinergic function.

Episodic memory is a component of the declarative system of long-term memory and refers to the ability to consciously recollect events and episodes, with specific information about the time and space constraints in which these events occurred (Squire & Zola-Morgan, 1991; Tulving, 1983). Declarative memory relies on the medial temporal lobe system (Tulving & Markowitsch, 1998)—the hippocampus and surrounding entorhinal, perirhinal, and parahippocampal cortices—significantly affected in AD (Salmon & Bondi, 2009). Thus, episodic memory impairment is the earliest-appearing hallmark symptom of AD (Bäckman et al.,1999; Bayles, 1991; Salmon & Bondi, 2009).

Whereas semantic memory is eventually affected by the middle stages of AD, there is some evidence that multiple aspects of it are better preserved than previously thought, especially in early AD (Bayles, Tomoeda, & Cruz, 1999; Bayles, Tomoeda, & Rein, 1996; Cox, Bayles, & Trosset, 1996). Regarding nondeclarative memory in AD, current evidence and expert opinion reveals that its components remain relatively preserved until the later stages of AD (Sternberg & Sternberg, 2011). This is likely because nondeclarative memory systems are dependent on the integrity of the corticostriatal system (i.e., reciprocal connections between the neocortex and basal ganglia), the amygdala, cerebellum, and reflex pathways (Squire & Kandel, 1999; Squire & Schacter, 2002; Squire & Zola, 1996)—structures that are not critically implicated in the neuropathology of AD.

To highlight how these memory subsystems interact and affect an individual's functioning, we end this section with an example from the book *Searching for Memory* by noted cognitive psychologist and author Daniel Schacter (1996). He describes the behavior and performance of a man with early AD and associated mild dementia during a game of golf. This man had been a very skilled golfer for 30 years and remarkably retained his skill for playing golf (i.e., his procedural memory for the steps involved in playing golf). He had no difficulty with driving, putting, choosing appropriate clubs for his shots, or with using internalized rules and strategies of golf. Further, he demonstrated spared semantic knowledge and correctly used contextual golf-related vocabulary (e.g., birdies, wedge, and par). However, in a classic showcase of the debilitating impact of AD on episodic memory, this man often failed to recall the shot he had hit moments ago and would attempt to hit again. When complimented on a recent shot, he was surprised to have no recollection of hitting such a shot. Shortly after the game, he could not recollect any details of the game he had just played (e.g., with whom he played or that he had played that day at all). To summarize, persons with AD demonstrate early and severe impairments of working and episodic memory that worsen as the disease progresses, initially spared but gradually impaired semantic memory, and relatively preserved nondeclarative memory until the later stages of the disease. It is important to note that these specific memory impairments directly and adversely affect linguistic communication because of the inextricable link between memory and language (Azuma & Bayles, 1997; Bayles & Tomoeda, 2014).

SYMPTOMATOLOGY OF COMMUNICATION DISORDERS IN ALZHEIMER'S DISEASE

The language and communication abilities of individuals with AD have been investigated in longitudinal and cross-sectional studies over the past 20 years. In a seminal study conducted in the early 1980s (Bayles & Boone, 1982), the researchers tested the cognitive and language abilities of 35 individuals with a diagnosis of dementia (presumably AD, based on inclusion criteria). The test battery included multiple cognitive measures and five language tasks (i.e., story retelling, naming, sentence correction, sentence disambiguation, and verbal expression). In addition to finding strong correlations between cognitive and memory/learning and language tasks, Bayles and Boone were among the first to describe a profile of language functioning in AD that was marked by a significant decline in semantic aspects of language, with a relative sparing of phonological and syntactic components. These findings provided the foundation for subsequent research on the nature of communication in AD. In the section that follows, we briefly describe linguistic communication profiles of individuals with AD. Readers are encouraged to review recent summaries of research provided in comprehensive textbooks (Bayles & Tomoeda, 2014; Bourgeois & Hickey, 2009) and writings devoted to the subject (Reilly, Troche, & Grossman, 2011; Taler & Phillips, 2008).

Language Expression

Consistent with the findings of Bayles and Boone (1982), researchers have found that individuals with AD have difficulty with tasks that require the creative, novel generation of language for communication purposes. Anomia is common, even in the early stages of AD, and results in circumlocutions, perseverations, and paraphasias (Martin & Fedio, 1983; Nicholas, Obler, Albert, & Helm-Estabrooks, 1985; Ober, Dronkers, Koss, Delis, & Friedland, 1986) that are apparent in single-word and discourse-level tasks. Across different types of discourse (conversational, descriptive, etc.), individuals with AD produce less content and are increasingly irrelevant and tangential (Bucks, Singh, Cuerden, & Wilcock, 2000; Nicholas et al., 1985; Obler, 1983; Ripich & Terrell, 1988; Tomoeda & Bayles, 1993) and use more formulaic language (e.g., fixed expressions; Bridges & Van Lancker Sidtis, 2013) than healthy age- and education-matched control participants. Syntactic complexity may also be reduced, although the findings on this topic are mixed and vary by discourse type, elicitation method, and language (de Lira, Ortiz, Campanha, Bertolucci, & Minett, 2011).

Despite these deficits, individuals with AD can contribute meaningfully in conversation, with appropriate support (Bourgeois, 1990; Egan, Berube, Racine, Leonard, & Rochon, 2010; Hopper, Bayles, & Kim, 2001); can provide on-topic opinions in response to questions (Arkin & Mahendra, 2001; Mahendra & Arkin, 2003; Mahendra, Fremont, & Dionne, 2013); and may be able to describe those things that they cannot name, at least in the early stages of AD (Bayles & Tomoeda, 1993). Individuals with moderately severe AD present more variability in communication abilities; however, many still retain the ability to correct misinformation, follow one-step commands, and verbally respond to greetings and compliments (Bayles, Tomoeda, Cruz, & Mahendra, 2000). Individuals with AD even in the later stages may continue to demonstrate a desire to communicate with others (Goldfarb, 2006), an important strength, albeit a nonlinguistic one.

Written language is also impaired. Similar to oral expression, individuals with AD demonstrate reduced complexity of written language, and although syntax is relatively well preserved, spelling errors are common early on in the disease course; at the discourse level, common deficits include semantic and phonological paraphasias, reduced number of words, fewer units of information, more empty and indefinite phrases, and shorter and less semantically complex sentences (Forbes-McKay, Shanks, & Venneri, 2014; Groves-Wright, Neils-Strunjas, Burnett, & O'Neill, 2004; Kemper et al., 1993; Rapcsak, Arthur, Bliklen, & Rubens, 1989).

Language Comprehension

Working memory deficits have a significant negative impact on auditory comprehension of language at the discourse level (Kempler, Almor, Tyler, Andersen, & MacDonald, 1998). However, individuals with AD are often able to understand simple directions (two- to three-step commands) and respond appropriately to simple, concrete questions until the middle stages of the disease (Bayles & Tomoeda, 1994; Hopper et al., 2001).

Whereas < auditory comprehension has been studied more extensively than reading comprehension in persons with dementia, reading comprehension is adversely affected as a result of dementia. Indeed, the ability to draw inferences from discourse-level written material and to answer questions based on content have been shown to be impaired in dementia (Creamer & Schmitter-Edgecombe, 2010; Small, Kemper, & Lyons, 1997). In studying single-word reading in AD, several investigators have demonstrated retained ability to read aloud single words without comprehension in moderate and even severe stages of cognitive decline (Bayles & Tomoeda, 1994; Raymer & Berndt, 1996). Also, findings from other investigators have revealed that reading comprehension of single words (Strain, Patterson, Graham, & Hodges, 1998), particularly those that are personally relevant, may remain somewhat spared into moderate stages of the disease (Bourgeois, 1990).

ROLE OF SPEECH–LANGUAGE CLINICIANS WORKING WITH INDIVIDUALS WHO HAVE DEMENTIA

Speech–language pathologists have important roles in the clinical management of individuals with degenerative dementia. The American Speech-Language-Hearing Association (ASHA, 2005b, 2005c) published a technical report and position statement outlining these various roles as follows: (a) identification, through screening, of individuals who are at risk for developing dementia or who have cognitive communication disorders suggestive of dementia; (b) assessment of cognitive communication disorders of dementia, using formal, standardized and informal, nonstandardized evaluation tools; (c) intervention for cognitive communication disorders of dementia, using evidence-based techniques provided to individuals with dementia and their caregivers; (d) counseling, for both individuals with dementia and their caregivers, about the nature of dementia and its course; (e) collaboration, with individuals with dementia and their personal and professional caregivers to develop intervention plans for maintaining cognitive communication and other functional abilities at their highest level throughout the disease course; (f) case management, acting as case manager, coordinator, or team leader to ensure the development of a comprehensive intervention plan; (g) education, developing curricula, teaching and supervising speech–language pathologistss, and educating caregivers, families, other professionals, and the public regarding the communication needs of individuals with dementia; (h) advocacy for individuals with dementia; and (i) research, advancing the knowledge base about communication disorders of dementia and their management. Speech–language pathologists may adopt one or more of these roles depending on various factors, including work environment, patient and caregiver needs, and clinician competencies in different domains. Clinicians who lack the requisite knowledge and skills for working with people who have dementia may view intervention as a fruitless endeavor, unlikely to have a significant impact on the functioning of a person with a degenerative disease. In recent electronic listserv discussions by members of ASHA's Special Interest Group 2 (Neurophysiology and Neurogenic Speech and Language Disorders), speech–language pathologists debated the ethics of providing cognitive communication interventions to long-term care (LTC) residents with dementia. Decisions about ethical and quality practice must be made by each clinician, within the context of his or her professional organization's code of ethics and scope of practice (ASHA, 2005a, 2007) (e.g., in the United States, ASHA; in Canada, the Canadian Association of Speech-Language Pathologists and Audiologists). Indeed, not all individuals with dementia will benefit from participation in speech–language pathologist interventions; however, clinicians should not make a determination of candidacy for treatment based merely on the presence of a diagnosis of dementia. A comprehensive evaluation of communication abilities and needs has many purposes for planning care, including determining potential of a client to benefit from a specific intervention program.

EVALUATION OF COMMUNICATION IN CLIENTS WITH ALZHEIMER'S DISEASE AND OTHER DEMENTIAS

At the outset of this section on evaluation, we present the diagnostic categories of mild neurocognitive disorder and major neurocognitive disorder (NCD), as detailed in the recently released fifth edition of the *Diagnostic and Statistical Manual of Mental Disorders* (*DSM-5*; American Psychiatric Association, 2013). Per these new criteria, persons with dementia could fall into any of these two categories of NCDs, depending on severity of symptoms. Whereas MCI has not been specifically mentioned as a category in the *DSM-5*, most persons with MCI by definition would likely fall into the mild NCD category. For an individual to meet the

DSM-5 diagnostic criteria for major NCD, there must be evidence of significant cognitive decline (e.g., in memory or language/communication), and this observed cognitive decline must be severe enough to disrupt independence in activities of daily living (Ganguli et al., 2011). For an individual to meet the *DSM-5* criteria for mild NCD, an individual must demonstrate modest cognitive decline from prior performance levels that *does not* interfere with completion of everyday activities. Usually, persons with a mild NCD are able to perform tasks requiring money management or taking their medications but will report that these tasks are more demanding for them. In both categories of major and mild NCD, noted cognitive declines should not occur only during delirium or be attributable to another mental disorder (e.g., schizophrenia). One explicit advantage of these newer *DSM-5* criteria are the psychometric specifications to help identify major NCD as indicative of test performance two or more standard deviations below appropriate norms (or below the third percentile). Similarly, the *DSM-5* criteria benchmark mild NCD as test performance between one and two standard deviations below norms (or between the 3rd and 16th percentiles). Another advantage is that when identifying major NCD, physicians are required to be specific about the cause of dementia: whether it is AD, VaD, FTLD, DLB, or dementia from another cause.

Screening

A brief screening often precedes assessment of a client with dementia and serves to (a) determine the need for a comprehensive evaluation, (b) provide direction regarding the main purposes of a subsequent evaluation, and (c) identify comorbid conditions. Screenings for older adults with suspected dementia should ideally include the components described in the following sections.

Medical History

Current and past medical history should be reviewed with emphasis on active medical diagnoses, chronic health conditions, current medications, recent history of illness, surgeries or hospitalizations, physical or psychological trauma, behavioral problems, and cognitive symptoms (e.g., word retrieval impairments, memory loss, and disorientation). Information from medical records, client self-report, caregiver report, and direct observations may be used to obtain a Hachinski Ischemia Score (HIS; Hachinski et al., 1975). The HIS provides a quick and precise means for clinicians to screen for the possibility of VaD. The HIS consists of 13 clinical features that are determined to be present or absent based on the client's medical history. Original criteria proposed by Hachinski and colleagues (1975) suggest that a score of four or less is consistent with a clinical diagnosis of probable or possible AD, whereas a score of seven or greater suggests the possibility of VaD. These same cutoff scores were subsequently validated in a meta-analysis of the HIS in pathologically verified dementias (Moroney et al., 1997).

Hearing and Vision Impairments

Hearing loss is the third most prevalent chronic health condition affecting older adults (Yueh, Shapiro, MacLean, & Shekelle, 2003), with an estimated 37% of adults older than age 70 years presenting with hearing loss (Desai, Pratt, Lentzner, & Robinson, 2001). Hearing loss negatively affects communication, socialization, and quality of life in older adults and often mimics early signs of dementia. Per current guidelines suggested by ASHA (2005c), a hearing screening for older adults with probable or possible dementia should include otoscopy, pure-tone audiometric screening, hearing aid inspection (when applicable), and a cursory check of word recognition ability. More recently, Jupiter (2009) has demonstrated that using distortion product otoacoustic emissions (DPOAEs) may be useful for screening hearing in healthy older adults and those with dementia. Use of DPOAEs has the advantage of not requiring a voluntary response as is the case in pure-tone audiometry.

Vision impairments also occur frequently in older adults and should be addressed during screening. One practical method of screening for visual impairments is to administer tasks that require letter or number scanning, reading aloud, and object or picture identification. It is noteworthy that hearing and vision problems, if undetected, can easily confound the reliable and valid screening and assessment of cognitive status in older adults.

Depression

Depression is common in persons with dementia and often contributes to poorer performance on testing (ASHA, 2005c). Depression may adversely affect a client's willingness to participate in assessment and treatment and may hinder outcomes of intervention programs. Depression is a medical condition that requires appropriate referral and medical management. Therefore, screening for depression is warranted using a client or caregiver report measure, such as the Geriatric Depression Scale–Short Form (GDS-SF; Sheikh & Yesavage, 1986). The GDS-SF has multiple advantages, including brevity and ease of administration, multiple language availability, and now free availability as iPhone and Android apps. If depression is suspected, speech–language clinicians should consult with psychologists, social workers, and other health-care professionals with expertise in mental health disorders.

Subjective Report of Memory Problems

Client or caregiver statements detailing memory problems reveal awareness of cognitive changes. Some researchers have suggested that subjective memory complaints are predictive of a greater risk for developing dementia, even when clients' objective performance data reveal cognitive functioning within the normal range for age (Wang et al., 2004). Also, as mentioned, subjective report of memory complaints is one of the required criteria for identifying MCI (Petersen, 2003). Information about memory problems may be elicited during a brief interview with the client or the client's caregiver.

Cognitive Function

By definition, dementia is marked by cognitive impairment, most often of episodic memory and, including other domains, such as attention, executive function, language, and praxis. Further, a *DSM-5*-supported diagnosis of mild or major NCD now requires objective evidence of cognitive impairment. Therefore, screening cognitive status is a critical component in the process leading to identification of dementia. Although it is not within speech–language pathologists' scope of practice to formally diagnose dementia, speech–language pathologists can screen for cognitive impairment and trigger referrals or provide results that support a physician's eventual diagnostic evaluation. In this section, we discuss five common options for cognitive screening tests: the Mini-Mental State Examination (MMSE; Folstein, Folstein, & McHugh, 1975); the Clock Drawing Test (CDT; Agrell & Dehun, 1998, Sunderland et al., 1989); the Short Portable Mental Status Questionnaire (SPMSQ; Pfeiffer, 1975); the Montreal Cognitive Assessment (MoCA©); and the Veterans Affairs Medical Center Saint Louis University Mental Status Exam (SLUMS; Tariq, Tumosa, Chibnall, Perry, & Morley, 2006). Although several others exist, we selected these five as exemplars for discussion based on their psychometric properties and clinical utility.

Mini-Mental State Examination The MMSE has 11 items (worth a total of 30 points) and can be administered within 10 minutes. It has been shown to have high sensitivity and specificity for screening cognitive status after correcting for age and number of years of education

(Crum, Anthony, Bassett, & Folstein, 1993; Harvan & Cotter, 2006). Administering the MMSE involves asking clients to perform simple tasks designed to test orientation, memory, verbal fluency, visuospatial skills, and reading/writing. Examples of items include asking clients to state the year/season/month, repeat a phrase, name and recall names of objects, copy a figure of intersecting pentagons, write a sentence, and follow directions. Although other global cognitive screening instruments exist, the MMSE (now MMSE-2) remains widely used in many countries, is now available in brief and extended versions, comes in many non-English languages, and is well known among health-care professionals.

Clock Drawing Test Administering the CDT requires clients to draw a clock showing a specific time or to draw the face of a clock and its hands given a circle already drawn. Performance on the CDT worsens as dementia severity increases and enables distinguishing healthy aging from mild, moderate, or severe dementia. The CDT has low sensitivity for distinguishing very mild dementia from healthy aging; however, when CDT performance is used in conjunction with MMSE scores (Powlishta et al., 2002), the combined sensitivity and specificity are superior to either screening measure alone.

Short Portable Mental Status Questionnaire The SPMSQ is a 10-item test with questions related to orientation, memory, attention, and executive function (e.g., What is the date? Who is the current president? What was your mother's maiden name? Can you count backward from 20 by 3s?). Scoring is based on the number of errors made by respondents, with three or more errors indicative of cognitive impairment (performance can be adjusted based on education—grade school or less; high school or beyond; Pfeiffer, 1975). It has been shown to have good reliability and validity in identification of dementia in various settings, including hospitals and LTC facilities (Erkinjuntti, Sulkava, Wikstrom, & Autio, 1987; Pfeiffer, 1975).

Montreal Cognitive Assessment The MoCA (Nasreddine et al., 2005) is a 12-item test that screens across multiple cognitive domains and yields a maximum score of 30. Notably, this test was particularly designed to help distinguish between healthy aging, AD, and MCI. Advantages of the MoCA include its easy availability, fully developed versions in many languages, and alternate versions to reduce the odds of test–retest effects; a tablet-based version (the eMoCA) is currently in development.

Saint Louis University Mental Status Exam The SLUMS is similar to the MMSE and features 11 items on a 30-point test. Advantages of using the SLUMS over the MMSE are that the former includes measures of forward and backward digit span, story recall, and clock drawing. In addition, the SLUMS provides education-corrected scores and is available in multiple languages.

The tests mentioned are presented as recommended components of screening for clients with dementia. These types of screening tools often may be part of a comprehensive, standardized, or nonstandardized assessment of cognitive and communicative function for persons with dementia. For example, as part of a diagnostic evaluation, clinicians may use the MMSE-2 or the MoCA to quantify severity of cognitive impairment in persons with suspected or known dementia.

Comprehensive Assessment

A comprehensive assessment for a person with dementia is best conceptualized as an interdisciplinary, collaborative process in which speech–language pathologists play a central role. Other key members of the interdisciplinary team are primary care physicians, geriatricians, neurologists, radiologists, neuropsychologists, clinical psychologists, social workers, and caregivers. There are myriad approaches to assessing individuals with dementia. As a starting point, clinicians must consider the key reasons for assessing a client with a suspected or established dementia, which include the following:

- Early identification of dementia and determination whether a clinical diagnosis of dementia is appropriate
- Identification of significantly impaired versus relatively spared neuropsychological capacities
- Prediction of skills that are most vulnerable to future decline and using this information for educating and counseling caregivers (Tomoeda, 2001)
- Establishment of baseline cognitive and communicative function prior to implementing pharmacologic or nonpharmacologic or behavioral intervention
- Use of dynamic assessment approaches (Lidz, 1991) to document a client's restorative potential or candidacy for specific therapeutic interventions and the ability to benefit from such interventions

A thorough assessment of cognitive and communicative function in dementia must be evidence based and least biased. As best as possible, data must be obtained to address three recommended levels of functioning per the International Classification of Functioning, Disability, and Health (ICF; World Health Organization [WHO], 2001), namely, Body Functions and Structures, Activity/Participation, and Environmental and Personal factors (Hopper, 2007). Further, clinicians need to be mindful of the increasing diversity of patients with dementia with regard to cultural, linguistic, and educational backgrounds. For assessment to be least biased, clinicians should know which tests are available in non-English languages (e.g., the MMSE-2, the MoCA [Nasreddine et al., 2005], the Arizona Battery for Communication Disorders of Dementia [ABCD; Bayles & Tomoeda, 1993]) as well as those that provide age- and education-corrected normative scores (e.g., the MMSE-2, the Dementia Rating Scale [DRS-2; Mattis, Jurica, & Leitten, 1982], the Repeatable Battery for the Assessment of Neuropsychological Status [RBANS; Randolph, Tierney, Mohr, & Chase, 1998], and the SLUMS). Also, developing skills in working with trained interpreters and using ethnographic interviewing techniques contribute significantly to reducing bias when testing culturally and linguistically diverse clients. Finally, greater attention is needed to competently convey the results of assessment of cognitive or communicative function to clients and their families, given recent data revealing that approximately 50% of individuals with dementia have no documentation of a diagnosis in their medical record (Alzheimer's Association, 2012b).

An important consideration for assessment of LTC residents with dementia is the Minimum Data Set (MDS; Morris et al., 1990), a comprehensive rating scale used to evaluate the functional status of LTC residents. The MDS is part of the Resident Assessment Instrument (RAI) that is used to evaluate and plan care for all residents in Medicare-funded LTC facilities in the United States (Centers for Medicare and Medicaid Services, 2001; http:// www.cms.gov) and is used in many other countries. The prior version of the MDS (2.0) included 74 items in 16 assessment domains, one of which was Hearing and Communication Patterns. Appropriate care plans, including necessary referrals to rehabilitation professionals, were generated from ratings on the MDS. A new version of the MDS (3.0) is now used in the United States (Wisely, 2010). This new version features 115 items in 17 assessment domains and "requires determination of a patient's ability to be a reliable informant (including the patient's ability to communicate) prior to completion of the first full assessment" (pp. 8–9). The most significant change in this newly implemented version of the MDS is the use of direct interview items to elicit the perceptions and preferences of LTC residents. The involvement of communication professionals remains integral to accurate and timely completion of the MDS by providing screening and evaluation results on relevant domains (e.g., Section B on Hearing, Speech, and Vision or Section C on Cognitive Patterns) to nurse case managers, who generally coordinate full completion of the MDS.

Specific Approaches to Comprehensive Assessment

Clinicians and researchers have many choices of measures to use for standardized and nonstandardized assessment of clients with dementia. The choice of specific measures depends primarily on the purpose of the evaluation, a client's type and severity of dementia, and the nature of information desired most from an evaluation. Several approaches to comprehensive assessment may be considered. First, individual standardized measures of overall neuropsychological status such as the RBANS (Randolph et al., 1998) or the DRS-2 (Mattis et al., 1982) may be used to profile functioning across multiple cognitive domains. Second, a clinician may evaluate a patient to assess distinct cognitive domains in more depth after a diagnosis of dementia has already been established. For example, speech–language pathologists interested in quantifying linguistic communication may use the ABCD (Bayles & Tomoeda, 1993). The ABCD was designed for individuals with mild AD and consists of vision and hearing screening subtests as well as 14 subtests designed to assess aspects of linguistic expression and comprehension, verbal episodic memory, visuospatial construction, and mental status. Similarly, the Rivermead Behavioral Memory Test–III (RBMT-3; B. A. Wilson et al., 2008), the fourth edition of the Wechsler Memory Scale (WMS-IV; Wechsler, 2009), or select subtests of these batteries may be used to assess various aspects of everyday memory functioning. Alternatively, a clinician may want to administer a brief test to quantify overall severity of cognitive impairment followed by nonstandardized testing using specific subtests from full-length batteries. For example, the MMSE or the MoCA (Nasreddine et al., 2005) may be used for screening, with follow-up testing using the Auditory Verbal Comprehension subtest from the Western Aphasia Battery–Revised (WAB-R; Kertesz, 2006b).

Because the focus of cognitive communication intervention for individuals with dementia is primarily on functional needs in everyday contexts, clinicians must evaluate functional communication. The ICF provides a framework for holistic assessment of an individual's level of activity/participation in life and environmental variables that hinder or facilitate functioning. Few standardized tests are designed for assessment of functional communication of individuals with dementia. One useful test is the Functional Linguistic Communication Inventory (FLCI; Bayles & Tomoeda, 1994), which contains 10 subtests that evaluate greeting and naming, question answering, writing, sign comprehension, object–picture matching, word reading and comprehension, ability to reminisce, following commands, pantomime, gesture, and conversation. The FLCI was designed for individuals in the moderate-to-later stages of AD. The test yields a total score and subtest scores that can be used to develop a profile of functioning across communication activities. The Communication Activities of Daily Living (CADL-2; Holland, Frattali, & Fromm, 1998) is another well-designed measure of communication performance across various activities; however, it was designed primarily for people with aphasia and may be most appropriate for individuals in the mild stages of AD. In Table 20.1, eight patient-centered questions are presented with recommendations for specific tests and measures that will allow clinicians to answer each question. These recommendations are not exhaustive but intended to be representative of some available options for assessment.

Beyond standardized tests, a comprehensive evaluation should include informal yet systematic observations of individuals with dementia as they go about their daily lives (Bourgeois, 1998; Hopper, 2007). Clinicians may be reticent to adopt observational assessment techniques because they assume that they will have to transcribe and analyze language samples, a difficult task in clinical settings. However, data gleaned from observations do not have to be qualitative in nature. Rating scales can yield quantitative data (e.g., frequency or severity scores) and provide structure and efficiency in naturalistic assessment (Bourgeois, 1998; Bourgeois & Hickey, 2009). The Communication/Environment Assessment and Planning Guide (Lubinski, 1995) is a valuable resource for clinicians working in LTC and could be adapted for use in other settings. The guide contains more than 40 questions related to the physical environment as well as the psychosocial environment. Similar to this guide, a more recently developed tool is the Environment and Communication Toolkit (ECAT) for Dementia Care (Brush, Calkins, Bruce, & Sanford, 2012). The ECAT was developed to evaluate client performance using yes/no questions, to assess the environment and barriers in it, and to select and customize interventions for persons with dementia. This test provides clinicians with over 300 specific recommendations to intervene or modify the environment to facilitate communication and positive behaviors from persons with dementia during activities of daily living.

Rating scales and questionnaires may be used as the basis for caregiver interview, an important component of a holistic evaluation. Individuals with dementia may be unable to participate in structured testing, and caregivers provide necessary information on communication activity/participation limitations and restrictions. Measures such as the SAILR (Sonies, 1997) comprise a combination of functional independence checklists, client and caregiver interview protocols, and language and recall tasks.

All of the previously mentioned assessment strategies help the clinician determine a client's current level of functioning or, in the language of the ICF (WHO, 2001), "capacity without assistance." Also known as static assessment (Lidz, 1987; Olswang & Bain, 1991, 1996), these types of evaluations are designed to minimize contextual support and to assess "already learned products" (Lidz, 1991, p. 4). In contrast, the term *dynamic assessment* is used to describe procedures that focus on identifying "learning processes" (Lidz, 1991, p. 4) or "potential level of performance" (Olswang & Bain, 1996, p. 415) and that measure a person's abilities given specific support through cues and manipulations of test procedures (Ylvisaker & Feeney, 1998).

Bourgeois and Hickey (2009) recently discussed the application of dynamic assessment procedures for use with individuals who have dementia. Such procedures have been used for decades with children with developmental and learning disabilities and communicative disorders. Importantly, determining treatment potential through "trial therapy" is conceptually somewhat similar to dynamic assessment and is used with adults who have neurogenic communication disorders (Bourgeois & Hickey, 2009; Coelho, Ylvisaker, & Turkstra, 2005). Specific examples of implementing dynamic assessment for clients with dementia include presenting stimuli multiple times using fixed or spaced repetition to assess effects on recall, presenting information in different modalities (e.g., as printed text or pictures versus verbally), administering tasks without time limits, and including multiple practice trials prior to assessing task performance. The data from such dynamic assessment procedures are particularly important in determining readiness/ability to learn and selecting appropriate treatment techniques.

COGNITIVE COMMUNICATION INTERVENTIONS IN DEMENTIA: CHALLENGES AND OPPORTUNITIES

In the past, progressive worsening of the cognitive impairment that defines dementia meant that treatment approaches were typically limited to pharmacological therapy early in the syndrome course and palliative measures in the later stages of decline. In the latter part of the 20th century, however, a paradigm shift occurred. Within the discipline of speech–language pathology, Bourgeois

Table 20.1   Choice of Assessment Measures by Key Questions and Client Dementia Severity

Clinicians' Questions Guiding Assessment	Dementia Severity	
	Mild to Moderate Dementia	**Moderately Severe to Severe Dementia**
1. What critical data do I have access to in the medical records of a person with dementia?	Medical record data[a]: Current/admitting *ICD-10* diagnostic codes, performance on ADLs, list of current medications, recent medical history, MDS ratings, and related resident assessment protocols[b]	Medical record data[a]: Current/admitting *ICD-10* diagnostic codes, performance on ADLs, list of current medications, recent medical history, MDS, and related resident assessment protocols[b]
2. What brief/quick tests may be used to quantify overall dementia severity?	Global Deterioration Scale (GDS), age- and education-corrected Mini-Mental State Examination (MMSE) or MMSE-Extended version scores, Montreal Cognitive Assessment (MoCA), the SLUMS, the Cognitive Linguistic Quick Test (CLQT; Helm-Estabrooks, 2001)	Functional Assessment Stages (FAST—extension of the GDS), age- and education-corrected MMSE scores, education-corrected SLUMS score
3. What in-depth tests may be used to quantify overall dementia severity and obtain a profile of impairment across multiple cognitive domains?	Clinical Dementia Rating Scale (CDR), Dementia Rating Scale (DRS-2), Repeatable Battery for the Assessment of Neuropsychological Status (RBANS)	In-depth tests not appropriate; nonstandardized assessment approaches recommended
4. What is the profile of memory impairment?	Rivermead Behavioral Memory Test (RBMT-3), Wechsler Memory Scale (WMS-4), CLQT to some extent	Nonstandardized assessment recommended
5. What is the profile of linguistic communication?	Arizona Battery for Communication Disorders of Dementia (ABCD), Western Aphasia Battery–Revised (WAB-R), Progressive Aphasia Severity Scale for PPA (PASS; Sapolsky, Domoto-Reilly, & Dickerson, 2014); nonstandardized assessment	Severe Impairment Battery (SIB); observational data
6. What tests may be used to assess functional communication in dementia?	Communication Activities of Daily Living (CADL-2); Scales of Adult Independence, Language, and Recall (SAILR); nonstandardized discourse measures	Functional Linguistic Communication Inventory (FLCI), nonstandardized assessment, conversational discourse measures
7. What is the level of executive function impairment?	Clock Drawing Test (CDT); Delis Kaplan Executive Function System (D-KEFS)—select subtests	Not usually recommended for this severity of dementia
8. Which tests can be used to track progression of dementia or cognitive impairments over time?	GDS, CDR Tests with alternate forms: RBANS, DRS-2, RBMT-3	GDS Observational data Physical status markers (ambulation, continence, feeding behaviors)

Note: ADLs, activities of daily living; GDS, Global Deterioration Scale; *ICD-10, International Classification of Diseases, Ninth Revision*; MDS, Minimum Data Set.

[a] Medical record data vary in format and detail by client's place of residence (home, assisted living, dementia unit, etc.).

[b] Minimum Data Set information is available only in Medicare-certified facilities in the United States.

Source: Adapted/expanded with permission from Mahendra, N., & Apple, A. (2007, November 27). Human memory systems: A framework for understanding dementia. *ASHA Leader*, 12(16), 8–11.

(1991), Bayles and Tomoeda (1993), Lubinski (1995), and others proposed cognitive communication interventions to maximize quality of life for individuals with dementia. Since then, researchers worldwide have studied treatments to improve functioning of individuals with dementia. Theoretically motivated, evidence-based cognitive communication interventions are appropriate for use with individuals who have AD or related dementias (Bayles et al., 2005; see http://www.ancds.org for practice guidelines and evidence tables; Hopper et al., 2013), and clinicians are increasingly aware of the potential of individuals with dementia to benefit from behavioral interventions. In a survey of speech–language pathologists in Canada, Hopper, Cleary, Donnelly, and Dalton (2007) found that the majority of respondents agreed that individuals with dementia could learn functional information (78.6%) and have strengths that can be capitalized on in intervention programs (88.8%). Importantly, in the United States, Medicare fiscal intermediaries cannot deny payment for rehabilitation services based on dementia diagnosis alone (Centers for Medicare and Medicaid Services, 2001), a decision that reflects a shift in perceptions of dementia and rehabilitation.

To ensure that interventions are effective, speech–language pathologists must focus beyond the progressively worsening impairment in cognition, which defines most common types of dementia. In the following sections, we discuss a conceptual framework for interventions in dementia, theoretical principles of management, selected cognitive communication intervention strategies and research evidence to support their use, and the role of the speech–language pathologist in working with individuals who have dementia.

Conceptual Framework for Interventions in Dementia

The ICF (WHO, 2001) is a conceptual framework well suited to classify and describe interventions for cognitive–communication disorders of dementia (see Figure 20.5). Within this framework, and specific to dementia, the health condition of AD causes impairments in cognition, language, and behavior. These impairments limit one's ability to engage in communication activities that range from describing physical discomfort to engaging in social conversation. In turn, these limitations may exacerbate behavior impairments. For example, inability to communicate about physical discomfort may result in the person with dementia

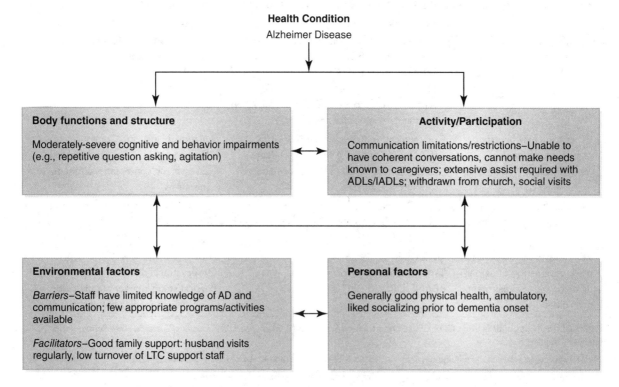

Figure 20.5 Application of the ICF to individuals with dementia (Assessment focus).

Source: World Health Organization. (2001). *International classification of functioning, disability, and health.* Geneva, Switzerland: Author, p. 18.

becoming agitated if techniques to manage such discomfort are not effective.

Bidirectional influences also exist between functioning and disability components (impairments, activity limitations/participation restrictions) and contextual environmental and personal factors. Environmental factors include physical, social, and attitudinal aspects of settings in which people live and work (WHO, 2001). Lawton (1980) views the environment as an active contributor, rather than a passive backdrop, to the lives of older adults, and this conceptualization of the environment is a key component of the ICF model. Environmental factors may have a particularly strong effect on the functioning of individuals with dementia. Specifically, individuals with dementia may be less able to adapt to changes in their environments (Lawton, 1980; Lubinski, 1995).

The ability to adapt to changes in the environment (e.g., different care partners and residences) as well as everyday demands (e.g., under- or overstimulation from external sources) is related to competence (Lawton, 1980). Individuals with dementia have cognitive impairments that affect their competence; consequently, they often express negative affect and behavior in response to environmental demands (Calkins, 2003; Cohen-Mansfield, 2001; Weisman & Moore, 2003). These impairments, referred to as behavioral and psychological symptoms, or more recently as "responsive" behaviors, are a set of complex symptoms manifesting as agitation, disinhibition, physical or verbal aggression, anxiety, depression, and delusions (Alzheimer Society of Canada, 2010). The term *responsive* makes explicit the recognition that, through such behaviors, the person with dementia is responding to something negative, frustrating, or confusing in his or her environment, that the reasons for challenging behaviors may be external rather than within the individual, and that problems in the social or physical environment can be addressed and changed (Alzheimer Society of Ontario, n.d.).

Although neurobiological changes associated with AD certainly contribute to responsive behaviors, factors in the environment such as care partners' attitudes and communication patterns also exert strong influences. Indeed, communication dysfunction has been linked to the occurrence of verbal and physical aggression among individuals with dementia (Talerico, Evans, & Strumpf, 2002), a finding that underscores the importance of interventions that address environmental factors influencing impairments, limitations, and participation.

Personal factors are idiosyncratic and include demographic factors (e.g., age, cultural/linguistic background, education, and socioeconomic status) as well as personality traits (e.g., coping styles). These personal factors have a profound effect on health (Threats, 2008) and are important to consider when designing person-centered interventions for individuals with dementia. According to Howe (2008), personal factors can be divided into mutable and more difficult to change or immutable factors. Potentially changeable factors include other health conditions, fitness level, lifestyle, habits, and coping styles, whereas ones that are unchangeable are age, race/ethnicity, nationality, upbringing, and past experiences (Howe, 2008). However, the variability in these factors makes them difficult to study in systematic ways, and there is a limited literature body devoted to their influence in dementia and communication disorders.

The complex interaction among different levels of functioning and contextual factors makes holistic assessment and intervention of communication a necessity for people with dementia. Rarely is cognition or communication treated in isolation from the context of everyday life, and most interventions should be used in combination as part of a comprehensive dementia care program.

Theoretical Principles of Cognitive–Communicative Interventions

Cognitive–communication interventions in dementia should be based on several principles as outlined by Bayles and Tomoeda (2014). First, treatment should capitalize on spared cognitive abilities and reduce demands on impaired ones. Second, treatment should include stimuli that evoke positive emotion, action, and fact memory. Specific treatment stimuli and activities should be individualized to ensure meaningfulness. Third, treatment should focus on strengthening knowledge and processes that have the potential to improve. It is important to highlight that interventions also need to be culturally and linguistically appropriate. Bourgeois and Hickey (2009) stress the overarching philosophy of intervention for dementia as one in which quality of life is maintained through supported participation and engagement in tasks that are personally relevant and likely to be used daily.

In this chapter, the emphasis is on intervention strategies that foster effective communication with individuals who have dementia. Specifically, we discuss creating opportunities for social interaction through activities and caregiver training and addressing specific cognitive communication limitations through direct interventions.

Intervention Strategies: Creating Opportunities for Social Interaction

Social interaction is integral to the emotional and physical health of all people and is particularly important for older adults with dementia. In LTC settings, communication for social purposes can be lacking (Kaakinen,

1995; Lubinski, 1995). Kaakinen (1995) notes that residents often do not initiate communication with each other, and Burgio and associates (1990) and Lubinski (1995) report that most communication interactions they observed between care partners and residents in LTC settings were related to caregiving tasks. This type of "task talk" comprises language that is basic and functional and is used to get individuals with dementia to do something (Santo Pietro & Ostuni, 2003).

Task talk is not confined to LTC settings. Even in the home, personal care partners may limit social interactions with individuals who have dementia because of increasingly negative perceptions of the individual's ability to engage in social conversations. Implicit in social interaction is recognition of personhood: Each person is a unique individual, with "a history, personality, likes, dislikes, abilities, interests, beliefs, values and commitments" (Kitwood, 1997, p. 10). Personhood can only be acknowledged through relationships in which there is a bond or emotional tie (Kitwood, 1997). This bond cannot be created through task talk; rather, social interaction must be the bedrock of person-centered care for individuals with dementia. The creation of a shared context for conversations is the crux of the first intervention we describe: reminiscence therapy (RT).

Reminiscence Therapy

Reminiscence therapy (RT) is discussion of the past that is meant to stimulate recall. Many individuals with dementia of the Alzheimer's type have the ability to access salient remote life memories, to recognize objects they cannot accurately recall, to perform well-known procedures, and to answer simple questions with meaningful responses (Bayles & Tomoeda, 2014; Bourgeois & Hickey, 2009; Hopper et al., 2001). Thus, reminiscing about the past may facilitate conversation that reveals ability rather than disability (e.g., difficulty recalling and talking about recent events).

Harris (1997) discusses the importance of RT as an intervention that has personal relevance for healthy older adults, many of whom are from culturally and linguistically diverse backgrounds. The heterogeneity represented by the older adult demographic requires an intervention that can be individualized, such as RT.

Reminiscence therapy discussion groups are commonly used in day respite programs and LTC centers. In general, the purpose of these groups is to facilitate social engagement related to a topic meant to elicit positive emotions and fact memory. Groups must be conducted by a trained facilitator who asks specific questions to stimulate recollection. Topics are illustrated using pictures, clothing, props, and so on that are associated with meaningful life themes (Hellen, 1992). Themes may be based on famous events from a specific era (e.g., man walking on the moon) or personal events of significance to each person (e.g., wedding) (Bayles & Tomoeda, 1997). Any tangible stimulus that evokes positive recollections may be used (e.g., stuffed animals; Hopper, Bayles, & Tomoeda, 1998). Music is also a potent stimulus for reminiscence (Ashida, 2000) and for facilitating language in persons with dementia (Brotons & Koger, 2000).

Kim et al. (2006) reviewed the literature on group RT for individuals with AD and other types of dementia. The authors included the results of one randomized controlled trial (Tadaka & Kanagawa, 2004) as well as the results of a Cochrane Systematic Review. Kim and colleagues reported generally positive overall outcomes related to affect, cognition, and engagement, all of which are related to successful communication interactions. In addition, when LTC residents participated in group and individual RT sessions, staff members' perceptions of residents' communication abilities improved (Gibson, 1994; Hopper, Cleary, Baumback, & Fragomeni, 2007). Similarly, speech–language pathology graduate students had enhanced impressions of the ability of persons with dementia to recall information and to express it verbally when using reminiscence paired with sensory stimuli (Mahendra et al., 2013). Consistent with these findings, Cotelli, Manenti, and Zanetti (2012) found generally positive outcomes of RT for improving cognitive and mood among individuals with AD and VaD.

The reviewed studies have highlighted beneficial effects of RT on mood, cognition, and behavior of individuals with dementia. More research is necessary; however, regarding the effects of RT on communication outcomes and on methods of implementation. Reminiscence therapy is inherently an intervention that relies heavily on communication. Thus, the format of the RT session should include consideration of language and communication strategies that are tailored to the individual needs of participants.

Memory Books

Written and graphic cues are the basis for memory books and wallets, as developed by Bourgeois (1990). The original purpose of memory books was to use written words and pictures to stimulate recall of personal information necessary to have a meaningful conversation (Bourgeois & Hickey, 2009). Memory books contain factual information that is personally relevant, important, and likely to be used regularly by the individual with dementia. The information is presented with pictures and written words and helps individuals with dementia reduce demands on impaired episodic and working memory systems while recruiting recognition memory and the ability to read aloud.

Memory books take many forms and can be individualized with various topics. Bourgeois (2007) provides a complete guide to memory books and other graphic cueing systems to improve communication and engagement in daily life activities. Memory books are also well suited for use in reminiscence therapy when developed with sections related to topics about the individual's past.

A solid line of research evidence supports the use of these aids to improve conversations with individuals who have AD and other types of dementia. When individuals with AD used memory books, researchers reported positive outcomes, including improved topic maintenance, decreased repetitiveness, and fewer ambiguous statements (Bourgeois, 1990, 1992; Hoerster, Hickey, & Bourgeois, 2001). In a recent review, Egan et al. (2010) report that among several methods to improve verbal communication among individuals with dementia, memory aids demonstrated the clearest effectiveness in improving on-topic discourse and enhancing topic maintenance, as exhibited by improvement in time on topic, words per topic, and fewer topic changes made by individuals with dementia across several studies.

Environmental Considerations: Creating Opportunities for Social Interaction

An individual's surroundings can facilitate or hinder social interaction. Social, attitudinal, and physical characteristics of the environment of the individual with dementia are important factors to consider when speech–language pathologists and other health-care professionals work to create communication opportunities.

Much has been written about the impact of the physical environment on the functioning of individuals with dementia. Calkins (2009) reviewed the literature on the effects of the built environment on the emotional, cognitive, and physical functioning of individuals with dementia in LTC settings. Although the results of the review on factors such as lighting, home-like design, and dining room configuration were positive with respect to outcomes such as safety (falls), way finding, food and fluid intake, and general well-being of individuals with dementia, the complexity of the settings and methodological limitations of the studies "make it difficult to come up with definitive or unquestionable results" (p. 152). Of importance to speech–language pathologists, none of the studies reviewed included a focus on quality or quantity of communication as a function of the built environment. Despite gaps in the evidence base, there is a growing body of research to support environmental

modifications to promote quality of life for individuals with dementia.

Multisensory Stimulation Programs

Creating positive, stimulating activities is another form of environmental modification designed to capitalize on relatively intact cognitive abilities of individuals with dementia and to promote engagement and meaningful communication with others. Two multisensory stimulation programs that were originally developed for children and later adapted for individuals with dementia have garnered much attention in recent years: Montessori-based interventions and Snoezelen® therapy/multisensory stimulation environments (MSSEs).

Montessori-Based Interventions Montessori activities were developed in the early part of the 20th century by Maria Montessori, a teacher, to create structured, stimulating environments that facilitate self-paced learning and independence in children (Mahendra et al., 2006). Mahendra and colleagues summarize the conceptual framework for Montessori programs for individuals with dementia as follows:

- Design of a prepared environment, adapted for persons with dementia, with the intent of providing meaningful stimulation and purposeful activities
- Progression of activities from simple and concrete to more complex and abstract
- Segmentation of tasks/activities into component parts, with individuals learning each component in sequence with external cues to reduce errors and minimize the risk of failure
- Facilitation of participants' learning of tasks/activities in stages, first through observation and recognition, then through recall and demonstration
- Use of real-life, tangible materials that are functional and aesthetically pleasing
- Emphasis on multisensory stimulation (auditory, visual, and tactile) in all activities

As applied to individuals with dementia, Montessori programming promotes learning through procedural memory processes, utilizes concrete everyday stimuli to facilitate action and memory, and reduces demands on episodic and working memory by using structured tasks and repetition (Hopper & Bayles, 2007).

Cameron Camp was the first researcher to study the effects of Montessori-based activities on the functioning of individuals with AD, and several other researchers have conducted studies over the past decade. Mahendra et al. (2006) conducted a systematic review of the literature on Montessori techniques conducted individually and in groups for individuals with dementia. Five original intervention articles met criteria for inclusion in the review. Across the five studies, individuals with mild-to-severe dementia participated in different types of Montessori activities, in group, one-on-one, and intergeneration (with young children) formats. Outcome measures were focused on affect and engagement (attention to task) and cognition. Findings were positive for affect and engagement, with variable findings related to changes in cognition (Vance & Johns, 2002; Vance & Porter, 2000). In addition, Camp and Skrajner (2004) demonstrate that individuals with mild AD could function as group leaders of Montessori activities for individuals with more severe cognitive impairments. The four individuals who were taught to lead the activities reported much satisfaction in their leadership roles. This finding is particularly important as it relates to social independence and skills and the opportunity for individuals with dementia to play a meaningful role in their environment (Mahendra et al., 2006). In summary, Montessori activities have the potential to improve well-being of individuals with dementia. Future research should include a focus on the effects of Montessori activities on the communication abilities of individuals with dementia.

Snoezelen® Therapy Snoezelen® therapy is another type of multisensory stimulation program that was originally developed to create a calm, controlled environment for children with multiple disabilities. For individuals with dementia, the purpose of Snoezelen® or MSSE is to provide "sensory stimuli to stimulate the primary senses of sight, hearing, touch, taste and smell, through the use of lighting effects, tactile surfaces, meditative music and the odor of relaxing essential oils" (Chung & Lai, 2002, p. 2). This approach is similar in theoretical motivation to Montessori in that it reduces demands on impaired cognitive abilities of individuals with dementia and capitalizes on more intact ones (sensorimotor skills).

Researchers have conducted several studies on the effects of MSSE on mood and behaviors of individuals with AD. In a Cochrane Systematic Review conducted by Chung and Lai (2002), the researchers report limited data to support claims about the efficacy of MSSE as related to improved behavior, mood, or interactions of individuals with dementia. However, the Cochrane reviews are limited to randomized controlled trials. Studies using different designs (single-subject, quasi-experimental group designs) have yielded positive outcomes in mood, behaviors, and interactions among individuals with dementia (see Sanchez, Millan-Calenti, Lorenzo-Lopez, & Maseda, 2011; Ward-Smith, Llanque, & Curran, 2009, for examples and reviews). Although little information exists on the effects of MSSE on communication abilities of individuals with AD, speech–languagepathologists should be aware of MSSE approaches and their potential for use in therapeutic programs designed to maximize the overall functioning of individuals with dementia.

Caregiver Education in Effective Communication Techniques

Any intervention aimed at improving opportunities for social conversation must be paired with use of effective communication strategies. Personal and professional care partners must be included in communication strategies training to support the use of such techniques in the everyday environments of individuals with dementia. Commonly recommended strategies are those that compensate for cognitive impairments through linguistic modifications such as slowing speech rate, simplifying syntax, limiting the number of propositions per utterance, repeating and paraphrasing, summarizing what has been said, using yes/no and choice questions instead of open-ended ones, and using written cues instead of verbal presentation to facilitate recall (Bayles & Tomoeda, 1993, 2014; Mahendra, Bayles, & Harris, 2005; Orange & Colton-Hudson, 1998; Ripich, Ziol, Fritsch, & Durand, 1999; Ripich, Ziol, & Lee, 1998; Small & Gutman, 2002). However, the effectiveness of some of these strategies continues to be the topic of investigation. Small, Gutman, Makela, and Hillhouse (2003) found that certain strategies (e.g., speaking more slowly) were associated with increased frequency of communication breakdowns between caregivers and individuals with dementia. Others, such as using simple sentences, were associated with positive communication outcomes. Savundranayagam and Orange (2014) also note that care partners' perceptions of the effectiveness of specific communication strategies may not always match evidence of effectiveness. Thus, continued research in this area is necessary.

One of the first evidence-based caregiver communication training programs was the FOCUSED program (Ripich, 1994). FOCUSED is an acronym for the specific communication strategies recommended for use by caregivers: F, functional and face to face; O, orient to topic; C, continuity of topic, concrete topics; U, unstick any communication blocks; S, structure with yes/no and choice questions; E, exchange conversation, encourage interaction; and D, direct, short, simple sentences (Ripich, 1994; Ripich et al., 1998, 1999). Positive outcomes related to caregiver knowledge of these strategies were found in the initial study and replicated in others. Further, Zientz and colleagues (2007) performed a systematic review of multicomponent communication training programs and noted overwhelmingly positive outcomes on caregiver knowledge and perceptions of communication success.

However, outcomes of communication training programs on the language and communication of individuals with dementia are still unclear. A notable exception is with regard to caregiver training in the use of memory books, which has been shown to have positive effects on communication of care partners and individuals with dementia (Dijkstra, Bourgeois, Burgio, & Allen, 2002; Egan et al., 2010). However, as noted by Egan et al., most other programs designed to be used by care partners to improve verbal communication of individuals with dementia in fact lack data on language and social interaction outcomes of the participants with dementia. In addition, Savundranayagam and Orange (2014) note that much of the research on the topic of effective communication strategies has been conducted in the context of task completion procedures and outcomes of these, rather than in a context of social interaction (see R. Wilson, Rochon, Leonard, & Mihailidis, 2012, 2013, for examples). This issue is an important one, as Small and Perry (2013) note that any effective communication enhancement program for individuals with dementia and their care partners should include compensatory (cognitive–linguistic) and connecting (relational) dimensions of communication.

Despite some limitations in the literature on this topic, the knowledge that communication problems are associated with care partner burden in dementia (Savundranayagam, Hummert, & Montgomery, 2005; Watson, Aizawa, Savundranayagam, & Orange, 2012) and may contribute to limited social interaction between care partners and people with dementia necessitates speech–language pathologists involvement in assessment and treatment with care partners.

It is within the scope of practice of speech–language pathologists to counsel caregivers about dementia and its effects on communication, cognition, and swallowing and to provide intervention for care partner communication. However, if speech–language pathologists suspect depression or caregiver stress and burden, they must refer care partners and individuals with dementia to mental health professionals for appropriate assessment and treatment.

Direct Interventions for Common Cognitive Communication Problems

In addition to opportunities for social interaction, some individuals with dementia may be candidates for direct intervention to address specific communication problems, such as anomia or prospective memory limitations (remembering to do something at a future time).

An intervention that has gained popularity because of its ease of use and growing research evidence base is spaced retrieval training (SRT).

Spaced Retrieval Training

Spaced retrieval training is a shaping procedure applied to memory (Brush & Camp, 1998). In SRT, the individual with dementia is asked to recall a piece of information repeatedly after increasingly longer intervals of time. Although the mechanisms of SRT are not completely understood, researchers propose that it exploits relatively intact implicit memory processes, helps strengthen conceptual associations, compensates for impaired episodic memory and learning, requires little cognitive effort on behalf of the person with dementia, and promotes errorless learning (Brush & Camp, 1998; Camp, 1989). As opposed to trial-and-error learning in which individuals' responses are unconstrained, errorless learning involves the elimination or minimization of errors during the learning process (Baddeley, 1992; Clare & Jones, 2008). In SRT, each recall trial should always end with a successful response.

Researchers have published numerous reports on the effectiveness of SRT for teaching various types of information and functional behaviors, and reviews within the context of speech–language pathology are available for interested readers (Creighton, van der Ploeg, & O'Connor, 2013; Hopper et al., 2005, 2013; Oren, Willerton, & Small, 2014). Positive outcomes have been reported across numerous domains of language and memory, with SRT successfully used to teach individuals with dementia names of family members, friends, and medications; techniques for safe swallowing and transfers; and information on routes to important locations.

Questions about clinical application inevitably arise and include issues related to the implementation of SRT, particularly as related to the spacing of the recall intervals and activities used to fill recall intervals. With regard to spacing of the intervals, gradually expanding the intervals may not offer significant benefits to learning as compared to equally spaced intervals. Hochhalter, Overmier, Gasper, Bakke, and Holub (2005) compared gradually expanding intervals to other rehearsal and recall schedules, including random intervals, massed intervals, and uniformly distributed intervals with a small sample of individuals with AD. They found no significant advantage for expanded retrieval as compared to other equally spaced schedules of practice. Balota, Duchek, Sergent-Marshall, and Roediger (2006) continued this line of investigation, examining whether an expanded retrieval schedule as compared to other spacing schedules produced better memory performance in healthy aging adults and those with AD. They found no advantage of the expanded retrieval schedule compared to a comparably spaced equal interval schedule. In summary, preliminary data support the use of both equally spaced intervals and expanding rehearsal intervals to promote learning of information and behaviors by individuals with AD.

How to fill the recall intervals is another important issue because content in the intervals may facilitate or hinder learning. In a recent study, Hopper, Drefs, Bayles, Tomoeda, and Dinu (2010) found that filling the intervals with tasks unrelated to the target face–name association did not adversely affect learning by individuals with mild-to-moderately severe AD. This finding is important in the clinical application of the SRT technique across various contexts because it lends support to the practice of embedding SRT in other activities, such as games, conversation, and physical therapy. Recently, researchers have reported that persons with AD respond positively to computer-assisted SRT and can successfully learn novel and previously familiar (but forgotten) face–name associations (Mahendra, 2011) and novel motor procedures (Mahendra, 2008) using a laptop computer.

Treating Anomia in Individuals With AD and Other Dementias

Anomia is a common symptom in AD and other dementias and may be particularly prominent in individuals with vascular and frontotemporal dementia types. Researchers have used several strategies to address the anomia in semantic dementia (Henry, Beeson, & Rapcsak, 2008; Henry et al., 2013; Jokel, Rochon, & Leonard, 2006) and in individuals with progressive non-fluent aphasia, including cueing hierarchies (McNeil, Small, Masterson, & Fossett, 1995), verb retrieval with sentence modeling (Schneider, Thompson, & Lurhing, 1996), and more recently, noun-retrieval cued naming (Jokel, Cupit, Rochon, & Leonard, 2009).

The crucial variable to consider in these studies is that the participants presented with anomia in relative isolation from the pervasive cognitive deficits that define all dementias in the later stages. Thus, with clients who have dementia, impairment-based treatments should be used judiciously and with a focus on how outcomes of the intervention will affect functioning in daily life activities (Clare, Wilson, Carter, & Hodges, 2003). Clinicians can use the dynamic assessment procedures and trial therapy described previously to help predict learning ability and the ability of a client to benefit from a specific intervention.

Mahendra (2010) recently described the use of semantic feature analysis (SFA; Boyle & Coelho, 1995) in conjunction with SRT to address word retrieval impairments in a person with mild dementia of the Alzheimer type, who presented with relatively preserved semantic memory and notable word retrieval impairments. A functional vocabulary of 30 items was targeted for training (based on standardized testing, observations, and multiple baselines) over 12 sessions (6 weeks) using SFA. After 12 sessions, this individual could name 21 of 30 items spontaneously and correctly answer attribute questions for 27 of 30 items.

Implementing Direct Interventions

Speech–language pathologists have reported challenges to providing direct cognitive communication interventions to individuals with dementia. In the Canadian context, Hopper et al. (2007) found that speech–language pathologists reported that they often do not intervene with individuals who have dementia because patients with more acute concerns have priority (e.g., those with dysphagia or aphasia). Also, speech–language clinicians reported a lack of referrals from other health-care professionals. To overcome such barriers, speech–language clinicians must focus on alternative methods of service delivery as well as education to increase appropriate referrals. Specifically, speech–language clinicians should act as consultants to paraprofessionals or volunteers who can carry out programs designed by the speech–language clinician. Jordan, Worrall, Hickson, and Dodd (1993) created and implemented an intervention program for groups of LTC residents who had specific communication disorders (e.g., dementia, hearing impairment). They taught volunteers to facilitate intervention groups and provided supervision over the course of the program (6 weeks in duration). Outcomes of the program were positive and demonstrated that the use of volunteers may be beneficial to residents, even when the speech–language clinician is not directly involved in providing treatment. With regard to education, a "train-the-trainer" approach may also result in more appropriate referrals. In consultative approach in several LTC facilities in Alberta, Canada, a small number of clinicians have implemented this technique with a focus on training other professionals and nursing assistants to more readily identify LTC residents who need a communication assessment. Although a limited number of speech–language clinicians work in LTC settings in Canada (approximately 3%; Hopper et al., 2007), this type of approach may be a viable one to improve communication care.

Arkin (1995, 1996, 2011) also demonstrated positive language and communication outcomes when community-dwelling individuals with AD were paired with university student volunteers. The Volunteers in Partnership (VIP) program involved people with mild-to-moderate dementia. The university students provided memory and language stimulation (based on activities designed by a clinician) as

Table 20.2 Types of Dementia and Clinical Presentation

Type of Dementia	Onset and Course	Hallmark Features
Alzheimer's disease (AD)	Insidious onset Gradual, slow progression	Most common type of dementia Pervasive episodic memory impairment Relatively spared nondeclarative memory function until later stages
Vascular dementia (VaD)	Abrupt or more gradual onset, temporally related to cerebrovascular event Stepwise progression	Documented evidence of cerebrovascular and cardiovascular disease Long-term memory less impaired than in AD Executive function more impaired than AD Gait disturbances, falls, early onset of incontinence, personality and mood changes
Dementia with Lewy bodies (DLB) and Parkinson's disease with dementia	Insidious onset Relatively rapid progression	Rapid fluctuations in cognitive function Recurrent visual hallucination Parkinsonian features Worse visuospatial and executive function impairments than AD Better memory function than AD early on
Mixed dementia	Variable onset Variable progression	Combination of features of AD and VaD (most common) Combination of features of AD and DLB (less common)
Frontotemporal lobar degeneration (FTLD)	Early onset (usually well before age 65 years) Rapid progression	Early appearance of changes in behavior, social function, language, and personality Episodic memory relatively spared in the early stages

well as helped with weekly volunteer activities. Outcomes were positive, with 8 of the 11 participants with AD showing improvement on language and memory tasks during the program. In addition, the students and patient participants expressed satisfaction with their roles.

In summary, the evidence base for cognitive communication interventions for individuals with dementia is growing rapidly. Clinicians can use this evidence, in combination with clinical expertise and client and care partner input, to develop appropriate behavioral management plans. At a minimum, interventions for individuals with dementia should be based on theory and evidence and should be tailored to individual needs. Most available research evidence is based on studies with individuals who have AD. More research is necessary to examine the extent to which these research findings can be generalized to individuals with non-Alzheimer dementia or with a combination of AD and another type of dementia. Because of advances in the accurate diagnosis of other types of dementia, speech–language clinicians should know about similarities and differences in the clinical presentation of the most common of these dementia types. In the next section of the chapter, we present salient features of other dementias beyond AD. Readers also are referred to excellent, in-depth reviews on these other dementias (Boeve, 2006; Knopman, 2001; Knopman, Boeve, & Petersen, 2003; Reilly, Rodriguez, Lamy, & Neils-Strunjas, 2010). In Table 20.2, the different

types of dementia (AD and other dementias) are listed with a summary of characteristics pertaining to onset, progression, and salient clinical features.

OTHER DEMENTIAS

Vascular Dementia

Vascular dementia, formerly referred to as multi-infarct or poststroke dementia, by itself accounts for about 10% of dementia cases (Alzheimer's Association, 2015). New data suggest that VaD is quite common in older adults with dementia, with approximately 50% demonstrating pathologic evidence of VaD (e.g., infarcts). Further, in many cases of mixed dementia, neuropathologic changes associated with VaD may coexist with those typically seen in AD (Roman, 2004). Vascular dementia results from ischemic changes to the brain, and the onset of VaD can be sudden because of an acute event or more chronic as caused by ongoing ischemia. Further, VaD is classically characterized by a stepwise deterioration in cognitive function; clients remain relatively stable between consecutive ischemic events and then suffer a sudden, significant loss of function with recurrent strokes or other vascular events.

Like AD, the pathophysiology of VaD involves the loss of cholinergic neurons (Erkinjuntti, Roman, & Gauthier, 2004), and both AD and VaD share common risk factors such as hypertension, hypercholesterolemia, atrial fibrillation, diabetes mellitus, and cigarette smoking (Iadecola & Gorelick, 2003; National Institutes of Health, 2013). More recently, with the release of the *DSM-5* (American Psychiatric Association, 2013), the term *vascular cognitive impairment* or VCI is preferred as it better captures the spectrum of cognitive impairment from MCI of vascular origin to a definite VaD (Gorelick et al., 2011; National Institutes of Health, 2013). Per current guidelines, a diagnosis of probable VaD requires evidence of:

- A decline in cognitive function, from the client's prior baseline and documented cognitive impairment (on testing) in two or more domains of cognition (e.g., executive function, language).
- Imaging evidence of cerebrovascular disease (e.g., on computed tomographic or magnetic resonance imaging scans).
- Impairments in performing activities of daily living, independent of the motor or sensory consequences of vascular disease.
- A clear temporal relationship between occurrence of a vascular event (e.g., a stroke) and the subsequent onset of cognitive deficits.
- A clear relationship in severity and pattern of cognitive impairment and the presence of diffuse, cortical, or subcortical cerebrovascular disease.

- No history of gradually progressive cognitive deficits before or after the stroke that might suggest a non-vascular neurodegenerative condition.

The clinical presentation of VaD has both similarities to and some notable differences from that of AD. Although memory impairments are the earliest reported concern by persons with AD and VaD, these are more severe in AD than in VaD. Persons with VaD are more likely to present with gait disturbances, unsteadiness, falls, earlier onset of incontinence (especially in case of subcortical lesions), and more significant mood and personality changes than typically observed in persons with AD (e.g., earlier onset of apathy than seen in AD). Table 20.3 highlights clinical features that facilitate accurate differential diagnosis of VaD from AD.

Regarding assessment, it is important to keep in mind that scientists' understanding of VaD has come a long way in the last decade and is continuing to evolve rapidly. Currently, few psychometric tests of cognition or linguistic communication include VaD patients in their standardization samples. This is largely because when these tests were developed mostly in the mid- to late 1990s, patients seldom presented with a diagnosis of VaD. However, the absence of tests specifically normed on VaD patients should not deter clinicians from conducting a thorough assessment of spared and impaired cognitive and communicative aspects

Table 20.3 Clinical Features That Facilitate Differential Diagnosis of VaD From AD

Clinical Feature	VaD	AD
Onset and progression	Abrupt onset; stepwise progression in classic VaD	Insidious onset; gradual progression
Neuroimaging findings	Evidence of multiple ischemic lesions, hemorrhagic events, and white matter lesions required for diagnosis per *DSM-5* guidelines	Evidence of hypoperfusion of the medial temporal lobe areas, including the hippocampus, subiculum, entorhinal and perirhinal cortices, and parahippocampal gyrus No evidence of a cerebrovascular event for probable AD diagnosis per DSM-5 guidelines
Focal neurological signs	Present	Usually absent
Hachinski Ischemia Scores (HIS)	Score of 7 or greater	Score of 4 or lower
Attention	Worse performance than AD, especially on complex attention and processing speed measures	Better performance than VaD
Episodic memory impairment	Better performance on immediate and delayed verbal memory measures compared to persons with AD	Cardinal, early appearing, severe deficit on delayed episodic recall
Gait alterations	Present early and are more common; balance issues	May present later; not common in AD early on
Personality changes	More likely; tend to occur earlier in the course (e.g., apathy)	Less likely than in VaD; tend to present in the middle-to-late stages

using the screening and assessment considerations mentioned previously. Tests that provide scores and percentile ranks for patients with VaD are especially useful for clinicians and researchers. For example, the RBANS reports mean scores for groups of patients with VaD, as well as for mixed AD and VaD. For a detailed discussion of assessing cognitive communication impairments in VaD and to learn about the effects of VaD on linguistic communication over time, readers are referred to a recently published case study (Mahendra & Engineer, 2009).

In treating the cognitive communication impairments of VaD, much can be learned from the rich and burgeoning literature on treating similar impairments in AD. In addition, important themes in treating patients with VaD are facilitating auditory comprehension, word retrieval, discourse cohesion, and topic maintenance and targeting attention and executive function impairments. In addressing these cognitive–communicative aspects, clinicians also should strongly consider extending validated aphasia treatment strategies to designing interventions for VaD. For example, specific approaches such as SFA (Boyle & Coelho, 1995), conversational coaching strategies (Hopper, Holland, & Rewega, 2002), and reciprocal scaffolding treatment (Avent & Austerman, 2003) all are relevant in managing the cognitive–communication impairments in VaD.

Dementia With Lewy Bodies and Parkinson's Disease With Dementia

Dementia with Lewy bodies and Parkinson's disease dementia (PDD) are both neurodegenerative disorders characterized by a combination of cognitive impairments and extrapyramidal signs and symptoms (Knopman, 2001). Researchers believe that DLB and PDD have many similarities (Weisman & McKeith, 2007)

and represent the same pathological process on a spectrum (Hanson & Lippa, 2009). Pathophysiologically, DLB and PDD differ significantly from AD and VaD in that the former two are characterized by abnormal intracellular structures called *Lewy bodies,* balloon-like structures composed of the alpha-synuclein protein accumulating inside nerve cells (National Institutes of Health, 2013; Pollanen, Dickson, & Bergeron, 1993). These Lewy bodies are distinctly different from the plaques and tangles typical in AD. Interestingly, many older patients diagnosed with DLB or PDD present with both neuritic plaques and Lewy bodies; however, tangles are unusual in both these types of dementia (Neef & Walling, 2006). In DLB, Lewy bodies are present in the frontotemporal cortex and in subcortical areas, but in PDD, these remain concentrated mainly in the substantia nigra (Neef & Walling, 2006).

Dementia with Lewy bodies is typified by fluctuating cognitive impairments, recurring and detailed visual hallucinations, and Parkinsonian features—tremors, rigidity, and bradykinesia (Weisman & McKeith, 2007). Additional features that may help to establish a diagnosis of DLB include sleep disturbances, repeated falls and syncope, unexplained transient loss of consciousness, severe neuroleptic sensitivity, delusions, and hallucinations in other modalities (olfactory, auditory, or tactile). Patients with DLB usually present with worse visuospatial and executive impairments than do patients with AD, with relative sparing of memory function in the early stages. Overall, it is critical to note that many experts believe that the relationship among DLB, PDD, and AD is complex, still evolving, and incompletely understood (Ince, Perry, & Morris, 1998). Clinical features that allow accurate differential diagnosis of DLB and PDD from AD are presented in Table 20.4.

Table 20.4 Clinical Features That Facilitate Differential Diagnosis of DLB and PD From AD

Clinical Feature	DLB and PDD	AD
Onset and progression	Insidious onset; relatively rapid progression	Insidious onset; gradual progression
Histopathology	Hallmark: Abnormal intracellular inclusion bodies called Lewy bodies, composed of alpha-synuclein protein Neuritic plaques may be present; neurofibrillary tangles are rarely present	Hallmark: Neurofibrillary tangles and neuritic plaques, composed of beta-amyloid
Extrapyramidal signs and Parkinsonian features	Present (tremors, rigidity, bradykinesia)	Rare but possible
Visuospatial impairments	Impairments more pronounced than in AD	Impairments exist; not as pronounced as in DLB/PDD
Executive function impairments	Worse than AD	Better than DLB and PDD
Visual hallucinations and fluctuations in consciousness	Present early and are more common	Not common in typical presentation of AD

Frontotemporal Lobar Degeneration

Frontotemporal lobar degeneration is an umbrella term for a constellation of neurodegenerative diseases or conditions that result from progressive, circumscribed degeneration of the frontal and anterior temporal lobes of the brain (Cairns et al., 2007; Wittenberg et al., 2008). It is well established that the human frontal lobes are associated with decision making and control of behavior and the temporal lobes with language and emotional processing. As expected, given the progressive degeneration of the frontal and anterior temporal lobes in FTLD, this type of dementia is accompanied by disturbing changes in behavior, personality, judgment, social function, and language with a relatively young age of onset.

This type of dementia used to be considered rare but is now known to account for 10 to 15% of all dementia cases. Further, the Association for Frontotemporal Degeneration (2011) recognizes FTLD as among the most common dementias affecting younger individuals. Often diagnosed in their 50s or early 60s, persons with FTLD experience much faster decline and disease progression than that seen in AD. Also, FTLD has a stronger genetic component than reported in AD, with 30–40% of patients presenting with a positive family history of FTLD or related neurodegenerative dementia (Josephs, 2007). Genetic linkage studies have identified an association between FTLD and a locus on chromosome 18 in the gene encoding the tau protein and another locus on chromosome 3 (Nestor & Hodges, 2000).

It is particularly important for speech–language pathologists to note that isolated speech and language impairments are often the earliest-appearing symptoms of FTLD (Gorno-Tempini et al., 2004). The distinct types of FTLD include a behavioral variant (bvFTLD) and three language variants (Kertesz, 2006a). The three language variants are typically placed in the category of primary progressive aphasias or PPAs (Gorno-Tempini et al., 2004, 2011; Harciarek & Kertesz, 2011). Technically, the use of the term PPA is appropriate when speech and language impairments have been the primary complaint for at least a period of two years (Mesulam, 1982). Next, we describe these four variants.

Behavioral Variant of FTLD

The behavioral variant of FTLD is characterized by bilateral frontal lobe atrophy with more right hemisphere atrophy than left and early appearance of neuropsychiatric as opposed to neuropsychological deficits. These patients exhibit executive function impairments and significant behavioral changes marked by an overall disinhibition, including stereotypical or repetitive behaviors (e.g., hand rubbing or humming the same tune repeatedly), inappropriate sexual behavior or compulsive overeating, apathy, loss of empathy, lack of interest in grooming and personal appearance (Kertesz, 2006a) despite having relatively spared episodic memory function early on in the disease. Persons with frontal variant FTLD are described as distractible, impulsive, unmotivated, and socially disinhibited (Nestor & Hodges, 2000).

Language Variants of FTLD

Three major language variants or PPA subtypes have been identified in the last 5 to 10 years (Sapolsky et al., 2011). These variants are discussed next.

Semantic Variant of PPA The semantic PPA variant (SV-PPA) has been described as "a fluent aphasia syndrome characterized by a gradual deterioration of conceptual knowledge" (Henry et al., 2008, p. 60). Individuals with SV-PPA demonstrate severe, early appearing, semantic memory deficits and loss of word and object meanings despite reasonably well-functioning episodic memory. Bilateral anterior temporal lobe atrophy is distinctly associated with this semantic variant (Wittenberg et al., 2008). Early in the disease, the symptoms include a prominent anomia (Sapolsky et al., 2011) with circumlocutions and marked impairment on confrontation naming and category fluency tasks. Errors on confrontation naming tasks are often semantically related, being either superordinate (*food* for *orange*) or coordinate errors (e.g., *horse* for *zebra*) and not phonemic errors. Consequently, patients with SV-PPA do not benefit from phonemic cueing (Hodges, Patterson, Oxbury, & Funnell, 1992). As the disease progresses, the severity of anomia increases and significantly affects conversational ability, resulting in frequent pauses, empty speech, and numerous semantic paraphasias. Eventually, the rapid erosion of semantic knowledge begins to present as language comprehension deficits.

Recently, one of our clients with SV-PPA was observed to have significant difficulty in explaining the meaning of common objects (e.g., a nail, a pencil). She was unable to consistently answer questions about physical attributes (What does it look like?) and functions of these objects (What do you use this object for?). For some low-frequency exemplars, when she was provided the label of an object she was unable to name (e.g., harmonica), she would appear confused and ask, "Harmonica . . . huh . . . what's that?" On another task in the assessment, she was asked to name some common colors and was able to identify five basic colors. However, when asked to color common fruits "in their usual colors" to assess her semantic associations, she presented with a stark inability to relate colors to common objects and colored a banana in blue and an orange in black. She also presented with a near-complete loss of her factual knowledge about famous personalities (e.g., Marilyn Monroe, President John F. Kennedy) and historical facts. Yet, she recalled several salient details of her son's wedding from six months ago.

In a review on the treatment of anomia in SV-PPA (Henry et al., 2008), the authors provide evidence that new lexical learning is possible in patients with various severity of SV-PPA. However, newly learned information is acquired rigidly and not easily accessed in varied contexts (Snowdon, Griffiths, & Neary, 1996). Specifically, it is suggested that learning is more feasible and successful early in the disease process prior to excessive deterioration of semantic memory. Further, important features of interventions designed to facilitate lexical relearning in SV-PPA are capitalizing on spared recognition memory and episodic memory (e.g., deriving cues or stimuli from recent experience), consistent rehearsal, using autobiographical and personally relevant stimuli (Snowdon & Neary, 2002), and implementing errorless learning approaches (Frattali, 2004; Jokel et al., 2006).

Progressive Nonfluent Aphasia In direct contrast to the fluent language disorder of SV-PPA, progressive nonfluent aphasia (PNFA) is characterized as a nonfluent, agrammatic variant marked by preserved ability on semantic tasks, early and dramatic reduction of expressive speech, impaired repetition, impaired syntactic processing (e.g., reduced ability to conjugate verbs, errors in appropriate use of prepositions), and caregiver report of affected persons with deteriorating linguistic expression. Nestor and Hodges (2000) have appropriately described the language production impairment in PNFA

as "Broca-like aphasia" (p. 441) that eventually progresses to a state of mutism. It is also not uncommon for PNFA to be accompanied by a frank motor speech disorder such as apraxia of speech (AOS) or a combination of AOS and dysarthria (Ogar, Dronkers, Brambati, Miller, & Gorno-Tempini, 2007; Sapolsky et al., 2011). Neuroimaging evidence reveals that PNFA is marked by atrophy of the left inferior frontal regions and of the insula (Wittenberg et al., 2008).

It remains to be established what specific treatment strategies for improving speech and language production are most beneficial for persons with PNFA. It is very likely that many aphasia treatment strategies for facilitating linguistic expression as well as the application of low-tech and high-tech augmentative and alternative communication (AAC) devices or apps will prove useful for PNFA.

Logopenic Variant Logopenic variant PPA (LV-PPS) (Gorno-Tempini et al., 2008, 2011; Mahendra, 2012) was characterized most recently. It has a unique profile distinct from SV-PPA and PNFA. Persons with LV-PPA present with overall reduced verbal output (Kertesz, Davidson, McCabe, Takagi, & Munoz, 2003), reduced speech rate with frequent pauses (Sapolsky et al., 2011), grammatically simpler but correct sentence structure, impaired auditory comprehension (Henry & Gorno-Tempini, 2010), and routine word-finding difficulty (Gorno-Tempini et al., 2004). Also present are impaired repetition (Gorno-Tempini et al. 2004, 2008) and impaired reading (Brambati, Ogar, Neuhaus, Miller, & Gorno-Tempini, 2009) and spelling ability (Sepelyak et al., 2011). Table 20.5 provides a quick comparison of the speech and language characteristics across the three language variants of PPA.

Table 20.5 Comparison of Speech and Language Characteristics Across Variants of PPA

	Semantic (Fluent) Variant (SV-PPA)	Progressive Nonfluent Aphasia (PNFA)	Logopenic Variant (LV-PPA)
Speech sound distortions	Absent	Common; frequent paraphasias	Absent; phonological paraphasias may be present
Rate of speech	Faster rate of speech than other two variants	Significantly reduced rate of speech; effortful, halting speech	Reduced rate of speech overall, but greater than nonfluent PPA
Frank syntactic errors	Absent	Common; agrammatic output common; comprehension of grammatically complex sentences also impaired	Absent
Lexical retrieval	Severe impairment of lexical retrieval; impaired confrontation naming and poor object knowledge	Impaired word finding; spared object knowledge	Impaired lexical retrieval; able to use low-frequency nouns and some pronouns
Repetition	Spared repetition	Impaired repetition	Impaired repetition

Table 20.6 Clinical Features That Facilitate Differential Diagnosis of FTLD From AD

Clinical Feature	FTLD	AD
Onset and progression	Early onset prior to age 65 years; onset most common in the 50s Rapid progression	Insidious onset Gradual progression
Neuroimaging	Progressive atrophy of the frontal and anterior temporal lobes **SV-PPA:** Bilateral anterior temporal lobe atrophy **PNFA:** Atrophy of the left perisylvian area (insula, Broca's area, motor and premotor cortices) **LV-PPA:** Focal neuronal degeneration of the frontal lobes; may have overlap with early-onset AD **Behavioral variant:** Orbitomedial and frontal lobe atrophy	Hypoperfusion of the medial temporal lobe, including the hippocampus, entorhinal and perirhinal cortices, and parahippocampal gyrus
Histopathology	Prominent neuronal loss with microvacuolar or spongiform changes, severe gliosis, inclusion bodies (Pick bodies) in some cases	Neurofibrillary tangles and neuritic plaques, composed of beta-amyloid
Episodic memory	Relatively spared, especially in early stages	Severely impaired in early stages
Social disinhibition	Early appearing and marked deterioration in socially appropriate behavior	Not the cardinal symptom in early stages; when present, social disinhibition is not as marked as in FTLD
Language deficits	Variable depending on type of FTLD **SV-PPA:** Semantic associations and conceptual knowledge are dramatically affected **PNFA:** Agrammatism, apraxia of speech, dysarthria, verbal perseveration, mutism **LV-PPA:** Impaired naming ability, auditory comprehension, and phrase and sentence repetition **Behavioral variant:** Possible echoing of another individual's speech, verbal disinhibition, sparse language	Subtle in early stages; more pronounced in middle stages Language deficits stem from episodic memory impairment

Beyond these three language variants, there exist other types of FTLD, including corticobasal degeneration, progressive supranuclear palsy, and Pick's disease. Clinical features that facilitate differential diagnosis of these FTLD variants from AD are presented in Table 20.6.

FUTURE DIRECTIONS

In the near future, our nation will continue to age rapidly and with a rising prevalence of AD and related dementias. There will be a much greater awareness of dementia, more emphasis on building cognitive reserve prior to onset of MCI and dementia, implementation of multifaceted pharmacological treatments in combination with cognitive and lifestyle interventions to slow cognitive decline in AD, and concerted efforts to control modifiable risk factors (e.g., vascular system functioning, diabetes, hypertension, brain injury). The key to the success

of these preventive approaches will be implementing them as early as possible in the disease process, preferably in preclinical stages. Early identification of AD and other dementias has been the target of much current research, with cognitive scientists and neuroimaging experts developing screening instruments that are sensitive to the presence of the earliest neurologic, neuropsychological, and neuropsychiatric deficits in dementia. Basic science research is also being conducted to better identify the presence of genetic risk factors and physiologic biomarkers in the blood or cerebrospinal fluid of individuals at risk for developing AD.

Whereas, these are promising ongoing avenues for research, millions of individuals worldwide already live or will be living with AD or another dementia over the next decade. For these affected individuals and their families, the focus will continue to be on maintaining function, optimizing communication and cognition, and improving quality of life through person-centered interventions and environmental modifications. More research will involve the use of personal technology for a variety of purposes. Indeed, there is a growing body of literature on using personalized cognitive training programs in interventions for persons with MCI and AD. Also, sophisticated technological applications are being developed to provide prompting and assistance for completion of activities of daily living, to use sensors for fall prevention, to design smart homes and facilities with improved safety features that promote aging in place, and to employ global positioning systems to assist with way finding.

In speech–language pathology, researchers will continue to test interventions to improve cognitive communication abilities of individuals with different types of dementia. Speech–language pathologists will work in concert with other health and rehabilitation professionals to develop theoretically sound, evidence-based programs that target multiple levels of function (body structures/function, activities/participation) and address associated barriers and facilitators to optimal functioning (environmental and personal factors). Although there is not yet a cure for AD, the next decade will yield robust advances in prevention, identification, and management of dementia across the continuum of disease severity.

We conclude this chapter with a case study of a woman with dementia due to AD and a profile of her cognitive–communicative functioning as well as recommendations for interventions.

Case Illustration 20.1

As a speech–language pathologist working in a large continuum-of-care facility, you receive a referral for a comprehensive evaluation of the cognitive communication functioning of a high-functioning patient with dementia, Mrs. K. To prepare for evaluating Mrs. K., you begin by carefully reviewing her complete medical record. Data contained in her medical record reveal that she is a 76-year-old woman who lives in an assisted living facility, is right handed, monolingual (in English), and of Caucasian descent; she has 12 years of education. Active medical diagnoses include hyponatremia, peripheral vestibulopathy, bilateral high-frequency hearing loss, and probable AD with onset 2 years prior to the time of your evaluation. Mrs. K. has been prescribed a daily 10-mg dose of Namenda (memantine) for AD and also is taking Antivert (meclizine) (for dizzy spells). Next, you plan a comprehensive assessment for Mrs. K. that includes naturalistic observations and interview with staff or professional caregivers, followed by administration of standardized test batteries and dynamic assessment.

Your observations reveal that Mrs. K is polite, pleasant, and well groomed. She wears hearing aids and bifocal lenses. Per data contained in her chart, she is able to perform activities of daily living with minimal or no assistance; however, she required mild-to-moderate assistance with instrumental activities of daily living (IADLs), such as using the telephone and the microwave oven in her apartment or shopping for simple items at the facility convenience store. She appeared to be embarrassed by her inability to remember things and often made negative comments about her impairments (e.g., "My mind is like a black hole now"). Some staff members who care for Mrs. K. report that she routinely forgets information (e.g., timings for meals and activities, accounts of recent events) and placement of her belongings and occasionally loses her way around the facility. Per the staff, Mrs. K. reacts to these situations with high frustration and, occasionally, tearful outbursts. She becomes particularly upset when she cannot answer basic biographical questions about herself.

Based on this background information, you decide to conduct a short screening in which you administer the MMSE, the GDS-SF to quickly screen for depression, and you use a speech discrimination screening measure to screen for significant hearing loss in a one-on-one interaction. You do this by presenting a phonemically balanced list of words and asking Mrs. K. to repeat each word after you. Following this screening, you decide to conduct an assessment consisting of the DRS-2, the ABCD, and the RBMT-3. It is important to point out that administering the DRS-2 requires an advanced degree (PhD), and this test allows you to profile multiple cognitive domains and obtain age- and education-corrected scaled scores for each domain. The RBANS is an equally good alternative for profiling Mrs. K.'s performance across cognitive domains. Next, you administer the ABCD to obtain a measure of linguistic communication and the RBMT-3 to assess how this patient's dementia is affecting memory processes for everyday tasks (e.g., recalling a short story, recognizing faces that were viewed, remembering the location of a personal belonging). Table 20.7 provides a summary of Mrs. K.'s results on these aforementioned screening and assessment measures, along with their interpretation.

(continues)

Table 20.7 Assessment Data for Clinical Case Illustration

Screening Measures

Mini-Mental State Exam (MMSE)	Score: 16/30. *Interpretation:* Moderate cognitive impairment
GDS–Short Form	Score: 0/15. *Interpretation:* Passed (i.e., not reporting depressed mood)
Speech Discrimination Screening	Able to repeat 14 of 20 spoken words presented face to face at conversational loudness

Assessment Measures

Dementia Rating Scale (DRS-2)	*Domain Range*	*Age-Corrected Scaled Score*	*Percentile*
	Attention	13	72–81
	Initiation/Perseveration	2	1
	Construction	10	41–59
	Conceptualization	4	3–5
	Memory	2	<1

Total DRS-2 raw score = 9; age- and education-corrected scaled score: 1

Interpretation: Significantly impaired overall cognition
Spared abilities: Attention: average/intact performance
   Construction: Below average but intact performance
Impaired abilities: Initiation/perseveration, memory, and conceptualization
   (semantic memory): severe impairment

Arizona Battery for Communication Disorders of Dementia (ABCD)	*Construct Summary Score*	*Average Construct*
	Mental Status	2.0
	Episodic Memory	2.0
	Linguistic Expression	2.5
	Linguistic Comprehension	2.8
	Visuospatial Construction	3.0

Total overall score = 12.3 (maximum = 25)

Interpretation: Cognitive communication impairments consistent with
   moderate severity of dementia

Rivermead Behavioral Memory Test (RBMT-3)	Sum of scaled scores = 49
	General Memory Index: Below the second percentile
	Interpretation: Moderately impaired memory function

Findings across screening, observation, interview, and static and dynamic testing yield information on impairment, activity and participation levels of functioning, as well as personal and environmental factors contributing to her cognitive communication abilities. You confirm that Mrs. K. had an overall moderate severity of cognitive impairment marked by preserved attention and mild impairment of visuospatial and constructional abilities. She presented with mild-to-moderate impairments on semantic memory tasks requiring her to state differences and similarities between exemplars of the same category or to identify which of three exemplars did not belong to a semantic category (on the DRS-2). Performance on episodic memory tasks across tests (e.g., being able to retell a short story after a delay [ABCD]; recalling a sentence she had just read or constructed [DRS-2]; being able to recall where an item of hers had been placed [RBMT-3]) and on prospective memory tasks (e.g., remembering to request her belonging back from the examiner at the end of testing [RBMT-3]) was particularly impaired. Also, you noticed

(continues)

that she demonstrated significant impairments on tasks requiring initiation (e.g., naming as many items as she could find in a supermarket [DRS-2]) and linguistic expression (e.g., generative naming of transportation items, describing an object, and defining concepts [ABCD]).

On the ABCD, some of her cognitive–communicative strengths were as follows: She was able to follow one- and two-step commands, repeat simple stimuli, read and comprehend single words and simple sentences, and recognize words presented on a list-learning task with 70% accuracy. Similarly, on the RBMT-3 Mrs. K. did fairly well on immediate and delayed recognition of presented photographs as well as immediate and delayed recall of a route. During the evaluation, she appeared motivated (albeit nervous), demonstrated good awareness of her performance (e.g., making comments like, "Now that is hard" or "I think I nailed that one"), and spontaneously self-corrected her responses on multiple occasions. Staff input corroborated that she was often aware of her problems and the impact of her impairment on functioning in the assisted living environment (episodes of frustration and forgetfulness).

On completing testing, you conduct a short dynamic assessment to determine if Mrs. K. would benefit from SRT. Mrs. K. responded accurately to repeated, spaced recall of the answer to a question ("What is your apartment number?"), which she had been unable to answer initially.

In summary, the primary purpose of this assessment was to evaluate Mrs. K.'s episodic and prospective memory impairments and determine the appropriateness of cognitive intervention. Her level of impairment; the positive aspects of her living environment (e.g., good staff support); facilitative personal factors (e.g., awareness, motivation); and dynamic assessment results (e.g., ability to learn) suggest that she has the potential to benefit from direct intervention using a technique such as SRT. This strategy should be used consistently and across behaviors to facilitate learning of important information (e.g., her apartment); procedures (e.g., remembering to take her keys on a wristband with her before she left her apartment or how to call her son using her phone); and routes (e.g., from her room to the dining room or recreational room and back). Staff education should be included as part of the intervention, with a focus on how and when to use SRT. Staff members also may need general information about communication strategies to help in the case of communication breakdowns and to ensure Mrs. K. has adequate opportunities for social interaction.

Further intervention would be determined based on need. Observational data suggest that it would be important to capitalize on her reading ability to help with orientation in her surroundings (using a large, easy-to-read calendar and visual schedule in her apartment as well as a schedule she could carry in her purse). Also, creating a memory wallet about Mrs. K.'s basic biographical information and teaching her to use it might reduce her episodes of frustration at being unable to recall personally meaningful details of her life that she would like to share with others.

The assessment techniques used with Mrs. K., and the proposed interventions, were guided by her needs and abilities within the framework of the ICF. The aim of the interventions is to facilitate functional communication through direct training and caregiver education. Focusing on specific activity limitations, increasing opportunities for successful communication, and capitalizing on preserved abilities are integral aspects of this and any treatment program for individuals with dementia.

STUDY QUESTIONS

1. Define the dementia syndrome.
2. What is the effect of AD on cognition?
3. Explain language and communication deficits associated with AD.
4. What roles do speech–language pathologists have when working with individuals who have dementia?
5. Define MCI and discuss its relationship to AD.
6. What are three cognitive screening tests appropriate for individuals with dementia?
7. Discuss the components of a thorough cognitive communication assessment for individuals with dementia.
8. Differentiate between static assessment and dynamic assessment strategies for individuals with dementia.
9. What is one conceptual framework for developing interventions and measuring outcomes for individuals with dementia?

10. Discuss three theoretical principles of interventions for people with dementia-associated cognitive communication disorders.

11. What are two intervention strategies to increase social communication opportunities for individuals with dementia?

12. Explain SRT and why it is appropriate for use with some individuals who have dementia.

13. What are some methods to treat anomia among individuals with dementia? How might treatment goals differ from those designed for people with aphasia?

14. Describe other causes of dementia besides AD.

15. Discuss similarities and differences in cognition and communication among VaD, DLB, and frontotemporal dementia variants.

ACKNOWLEDGMENT

1. Preparation of this chapter was partly supported, by a grant from The California Wellness Foundation (TCWF) Grant 2012-048 awarded to the first author.

REFERENCES

Agrell, B., & Dehun, O. (1998). Review: The Clock Drawing Test. *Age and Ageing*, 27, 399–403.

Albert, M. S. (1996). Cognitive and neurobiologic markers of early Alzheimer's disease. *Proceedings of the National Academy of Sciences of the United States of America*, 93, 13547–13551.

Albert, M. S., DeKosky, S. T., Dickson, D., Dubois, B., Feldman, H. H., Fox, N. C., et al. (2011). The diagnosis of mild cognitive impairment due to Alzheimer's disease: Recommendations from the National Institute on Aging-Alzheimer's Association workgroups on diagnostic guidelines for Alzheimer's disease. *Alzheimer's and Dementia*, 7, 270–279.

Alzheimer's Association. (2012a). *FDA-approved treatment for Alzheimer's*. Retrieved from http://www.alz.org/national/documents/topicsheet_treatments.pdf.

Alzheimer's Association. (2012b). *Increasing disclosure of dementia diagnosis*. Retrieved from http://www.alz.org/documents_custom/inbrief_disclosure.pdf.

Alzheimer's Association. (2015). 2015 Alzheimer's disease facts and figures. *Alzheimer's and Dementia: The Journal of the Alzheimer's Association*, 11(3), 1–83.

Alzheimer Society of Canada. (2010). *Rising tide: The impact of dementia on Canadian society*. Retrieved from http://www.alzheimer.ca/ ~ /media/Files/national/Advocacy/ASC_Rising_Tide_Full_Report_e.pdf.

Alzheimer Society of Ontario. (n.d). *What are responsive behaviors*. Retrieved from http://u-first.ca/understanding-dementia/what-are-responsive-behaviours/.

American Psychiatric Association. (2013). *Diagnostic and Statistical Manual of Mental Disorders* (5th ed.). Arlington, VA: Author.

American Speech-Language-Hearing Association. (2005a). *Health care issues brief—Long term care*. Rockville, MD: Author. Retrieved from http://www.asha.org/slp/healthcare/long_term.htm.

American Speech-Language-Hearing Association. (2005b). *The roles of speech-language pathologists working with individuals with dementia: Position statement*. Rockville, MD: Author. Available from http://www.asha.org/docs/html/PS2005-00118.html.

American Speech-Language-Hearing Association. (2005c). *The roles of speech-language pathologists working with individuals with dementia: Technical report*. Rockville, MD: Author. Retrieved from http://www.asha.org/docs/html/TR2005-00157.html.

American Speech-Language-Hearing Association. (2007). *Scope of practice in speech-language pathology*. Rockville, MD: Author. Retrieved from http://www.asha.org/docs/html/SP2007-00283.html

Amieva, H., Jacqmin-Gadda, H., Orgogozo, J.-M., Le Carret, N., Helmer, C., Letenneur, L., et al. (2005). The 9-year cognitive decline before dementia of the Alzheimer type: A prospective population based study. *Brain*, 128(5), 1093–1101.

Anand, P., & Singh, B. (2013). A review on cholinesterase inhibitors for Alzheimer's disease. *Archives of Pharmacological Research*, 36(4), 375–399. doi:10.1007/s12272-013-0036-3.

Arkin, S. (1996). Volunteers in partnership: An Alzheimer's rehabilitation program delivered by students. *American Journal of Alzheimer's Disease*, 11, 12–22.

Arkin, S., & Mahendra, N. (2001). Discourse analysis of Alzheimer's patients before and after intervention: Methodology and outcomes. *Aphasiology*, 15(6), 533–569.

Arkin, S. M. (1995). Volunteers in partnership: A rehabilitation program for Alzheimer's patients [Videotape]. In C. K. Tomoeda (Producer) & J. Chitwood (Director), *Telerounds*. Tucson, AZ: University of Arizona.

Arkin, S. M. (2011). Service learning students as Alzheimer treatment providers. *Topics in Geriatric Rehabilitation*, 27(4), 253–311.

Ashida, S. (2000). The effect of reminiscence music therapy sessions on changes in depressive symptoms in elderly persons with dementia. *Journal of Music Therapy*, 37(3), 170–182.

Association for Frontotemporal Degeneration (2011). *Fast facts about frontotemporal degeneration*. Retrieved from http://www.theaftd.org/wpcontent/uploads/2009/05/Fast-Facts-Final-11-12.pdf.

Avent, J. R., & Austerman, S. (2003). Reciprocal scaffolding: A context for communication treatment in aphasia. *Aphasiology*, 17(4), 397–404.

Azuma, T., & Bayles, K. A. (1997). Memory impairments underlying language difficulties in dementia. *Topics in Language Disorders, 18*(1), 58–71.

Bäckman, L., Andersson, J. L., Nyberg, L., Winblad, B., Nordberg, A., & Almkvist, O. (1999). Brain regions associated with episodic retrieval in normal aging and Alzheimer's disease. *Neurology, 52*(9), 1861–1870.

Baddeley, A. D. (1992). Implicit memory and errorless learning: A link between cognitive theory and neuropsychological rehabilitation? In L. R. Squire & N. Butters (Eds.), *Neuropsychology of memory* (2nd ed., pp. 309–314). New York, NY: Guilford Press.

Baddeley, A. D. (2002). The concept of episodic memory. In A. Baddeley & M. A. Conway (Eds.), *Episodic memory: New directions in research* (pp. 1–10). Oxford, UK: Oxford University Press.

Baddeley, A. D., Baddeley, H. A., Bucks, R. S., & Wilcock, G. K. (2001). Attentional control in Alzheimer's disease. *Brain, 124*, 1492–1508.

Balota, D. A., Duchek, J. M., Sergent-Marshall, S., & Roediger, H. L., III. (2006). Does expanded retrieval produce benefits over equal-interval spacing? Explorations of spacing effects in healthy aging and early stage Alzheimer's disease. *Psychology and Aging, 21*(1), 19–31.

Bayles, K. A. (1991). Alzheimer's disease symptoms: Prevalence and order of appearance. *Journal of Applied Gerontology, 10*(4), 419–430.

Bayles, K. A., & Boone, D. R. (1982). The potential of language tasks for identifying senile dementia. *Journal of Speech and Hearing Disorders, 47*, 210–217.

Bayles, K. A., & Kim, E. (2003). Improving the functioning of individuals with Alzheimer's disease: Emergence of behavioral interventions. *Journal of Communication Disorders, 36*(5), 327–343.

Bayles, K. A., Kim, E. S., Azuma, T., Bond-Chapman, S., Cleary, S., Hopper, T., et al. (2005). Developing evidence-based practice guidelines for speech language pathologists serving individuals with dementia. *Journal of Medical Speech Language Pathology, 13*(4), xiii–xxv.

Bayles, K. A., & Tomoeda, C. K. (1993). *The Arizona Battery for Communication Disorders of Dementia.* Tucson, AZ: Canyonlands.

Bayles, K. A., & Tomoeda, C. K. (1994). *Functional Linguistic Communication Inventory.* Tucson, AZ: Canyonlands.

Bayles, K. A., & Tomoeda, C. K. (1997). *Improving function in dementia and other cognitive-linguistic disorders.* Tucson, AZ: Canyonlands.

Bayles, K. A., & Tomoeda, C. K. (2014). *Cognitive–communication disorders of dementia: Definition, diagnosis and treatment* (2nd ed.). San Diego, CA: Plural.

Bayles, K. A., Tomoeda, C. K., & Cruz, R. (1999). Performance of Alzheimer's disease patients in judging word relatedness. *Journal of the International Neuropsychological Society, 5*, 668–675.

Bayles, K. A., Tomoeda, C. K., Cruz, R. F., & Mahendra, N. (2000). Communication abilities of individuals with late-stage Alzheimer disease. *Alzheimer Disease and Associated Disorders, 14*(3), 176–181.

Bayles, K. A., Tomoeda, C. K., & Rein, J. A. (1996). Phrase repetition in Alzheimer's disease: Effect of meaning and length. *Brain & Language, 54*(2), 246–261.

Bennett, D. A., Schneider, J. A., Arvanitakis, Z., Kelly, J. F., Agarwal, N. T., Shah, R. C., et al. (2006). Neuropathology of older persons without cognitive impairment from two community-based studies. *Neurology, 66*(12), 1837–1844.

Boeve, B. F. (2006). A review of the non-Alzheimer dementias. *Journal of Clinical Psychiatry, 67*, 1985–2001.

Bourgeois, M. S. (1990). Enhancing conversation skills in patients with Alzheimer's disease using a prosthetic memory aid. *Journal of Applied Behavior Analysis, 23*(1), 29–42.

Bourgeois, M. S. (1991). Communication treatment for adults with dementia. *Journal of Speech and Hearing Research, 34*, 831–844.

Bourgeois, M. S. (1992). Evaluating memory wallets in conversations with patients with dementia. *Journal of Speech and Hearing Research, 35*, 1344–1357.

Bourgeois, M. S. (1998). Functional outcome assessment of adults with dementia. *Seminars in Speech and Language, 19*, 261–279.

Bourgeois, M. S. (2007). *Memory books and other graphic cuing systems: Practical communication and memory aids for adults with dementia.* Baltimore, MD: Health Professions Press.

Bourgeois, M. S., & Hickey, E. (2009). *Dementia from diagnosis to management: A functional approach.* New York, NY: Psychology Press.

Boyle, M., & Coelho, C. A. (1995). Application of semantic feature analysis as a treatment for aphasic dysnomia. *American Journal of Speech Language Pathology, 4*, 94–98.

Braak, H., & Braak, E. (1991). Neuropathological staging of Alzheimer-related changes [Review]. *Acta Neuropathologica, 82*, 239–259.

Brambati, S. M., Ogar, J., Neuhaus, J., Miller, B. L., & Gorno-Tempini, M. L. (2009). Reading disorders in primary progressive aphasia: A behavioral and neuroimaging study. *Neuropsychologia, 47*(8–9), 1893–1900.

Bridges, K. A., & Van Lancker Sidtis, D. (2013). Formulaic language in Alzheimer's disease. *Aphasiology, 27*(7), 799–810. doi:10.1080/02687038.2012.757760.

Brotons, M., & Koger, S. M. (2000). The impact of music therapy on language functioning in dementia. *Journal of Music Therapy, 37*(3), 183–195.

Brush, J., Calkins, M., Bruce, C., & Sanford, J. (2012). *Environment and Communication Assessment Toolkit (ECAT) for Dementia Care.* Baltimore, MD: Health Professions Press.

Brush, J., & Camp, C. (1998). *A therapy technique for improving memory: Spaced-retrieval.* Beachwood, OH: Menorah Park Center for the Aging.

Bucks, R. S., Singh, S., Cuerden, J. M., & Wilcock, G. K. (2000). Analysis of spontaneous, conversational speech in dementia of Alzheimer type: Evaluation of an objective technique for analysing lexical performance. *Aphasiology, 4*(1), 71–91.

Burgio, L., Engel, B. T., Hawkins, A., McCormick, K., Scheve, A., & Jones, L. T. (1990). A staff management system for maintaining improvements in continence with elderly nursing home residents. *Journal of Applied Behaviour Analysis, 23*, 111–118.

Cairns, N. J., Bigio, E. H., Mackenzie, I. R., Neumann, M., Lee, V. M., Hatanpaa, K. J., et al. (2007). Neuropathologic diagnostic and nosologic criteria for frontotemporal lobar degeneration: Consensus of the Consortium for Frontotemporal Lobar Degeneration. *Acta Neuropathologica, 114*(1), 5–22.

Calkins, M. P. (2003). Powell Lawton's contributions to long-term care settings. In R. Scheidt & P. Windley (Eds.), *Physical environments and aging* (pp. 67–84). London, UK: Haworth Press.

Calkins, M. P. (2009). Evidence-based long term care design. *NeuroRehabilitation, 25*, 145–154.

Camp, C. J. (1989). Facilitation in learning of Alzheimer's disease. In G. Gilmore, P. Whitehouse, & M. Wykle (Eds.), *Memory and aging: Theory, research, and practice.* (pp. 212–225). New York, NY: Springer.

Camp, C. J., & Skrajner, M. J. (2004). Resident Assisted Montessori Programming (RAMP): Training persons with dementia to serve as group activity leaders. *Gerontologist, 44*(3), 426–431.

Centers for Medicare and Medicaid Services. (2001, September 25). *Medical review of services for patients with dementia (Program Memorandum Intermediaries/Carriers: Transmittal AB-01-135).* Washington, DC: US Department of Health and Human Services. Retrieved from http://www.cms.gov/Transmittals/downloads/AB-01-135.pdf.

Chung, J., & Lai, C. (2002; updated 2009). Snoezelen for dementia. *Cochrane Database of Systematic Reviews, 4*, Art. No. CD003152. doi:10.1002/14651858.CD003152.

Clare, L., & Jones, R. S. P. (2008). Errorless learning in the rehabilitation of memory impairment: A critical review. *Neuropsychology Review, 18*, 1–23.

Clare, L., Wilson, B. A., Carter, G., & Hodges, J. R. (2003). Cognitive rehabilitation as a component of early intervention in Alzheimer's disease: A single case study. *Aging & Mental Health, 7*(1), 15–21. doi:10.1080/1360786021000045854.

Coelho, C., Ylvisaker, M., & Turkstra, L. (2005). Nonstandardized assessment approaches for individuals with traumatic brain injuries. *Seminars in Speech & Language, 26*(4), 223–241.

Cohen-Mansfield, J. (2001). Nonpharmacologic interventions for inappropriate behaviors in dementia: A review, summary, and critique. *American Journal of Geriatric Psychiatry, 9*(4), 361–381.

Cotelli, M., Manenti, R., & Zanetti, O. (2012). Reminiscence therapy in dementia: A review. *Maturitas, 72*(3), 203–205. doi:10.1016/j.maturitas.2012.04.008.

Cox, D. M., Bayles, K. A., & Trosset, M. W. (1996). Category and attribute knowledge deterioration in Alzheimer's disease. *Brain and Language, 52*(3), 536–550.

Creamer, S., & Schmitter-Edgecombe, M. (2010). Narrative comprehension in Alzheimer's disease: Assessing inferences and memory operations with a think-aloud procedure. *Neuropsychology, 24*(3), 279–290.

Creighton, A. S., van der Ploeg, E .S., & O'Connor, D. W. (2013). A literature review of spaced-retrieval interventions: A direct memory intervention for people with dementia. *International Psychogeriatrics, 25*(11), 1743–1763. doi:10.1017/S1041610213001233.

Crum, R. M., Anthony, J. C., Bassett, S. S., & Folstein, M. F. (1993). Population-based norms for the Mini-Mental State Examination by age and education level. *Journal of the American Medical Association, 269*(18), 2386–2391.

Daulatzai, M. A. (2015). Olfactory dysfunction: Its early temporal relationship and neural correlates in the pathogenesis of Alzheimer's disease. *Journal of Neural Transmission.* E-pub ahead of print. doi:10.1007/s00702-015-1404-1406.

de Lira, J. O., Ortiz, K. Z, Campanha, A. C., Bertolucci, P. H. F., & Minett, T. S. C. (2011). Microlinguistic aspects of the oral narrative in patients with Alzheimer's disease. *International Psychogeriatrics, 23*(3), 404–412.

Desai, M., Pratt, L. A., Lentzner, H., & Robinson, K. N. (2001). *Trends in vision and hearing among older Americans.* Hyattsville, MD: National Center for Health Statistics.

DeVreese, L. P., Neri, M., Fioravanti, M., Belloi, L., & Zanetti, O. (2001). Memory rehabilitation in Alzheimer's disease: A review of progress. *International Journal of Geriatric Psychiatry, 16*(8), 794–809.

Dijkstra, K., Bourgeois, M., Burgio, L., & Allen, R. (2002). Effects of a communication intervention on the discourse of nursing home residents with dementia and their nursing assistants. *Journal of Medical Speech Language Pathology, 2*(10), 143–157.

Doody, R. S., Ferris, S. H., Salloway, S., Sun, Y., Goldman, R., Watkins, W. E., et al. (2009). Donepezil treatment of patients with MCI: A 48-week, randomized, placebo-controlled trial. *Neurology, 72*(18), 1555–1561.

Egan, M., Berube, D., Racine, G., Leonard, C., & Rochon, E. (2010). Methods to enhance verbal communication between individuals with Alzheimer's disease and their formal and informal caregivers: A systematic review. *International Journal of Alzheimer's Disease, 2010*, 1–12. doi:10.4061/2010/906818.

Erkinjuntti, T., Roman, G., & Gauthier, S. (2004). Treatment of vascular dementia—Evidence from clinical trials with cholinesterase inhibitors. *Journal of the Neurological Sciences, 226*(1–2), 63–66.

Erkinjuntti, T., Sulkava, R., Wikstrom, J., & Autio, L. (1987). Short Portable Mental Status Questionnaire as a screening test for dementia and delirium among the elderly. *Journal of the American Geriatrics Society, 35*(5), 412–416.

Farrer, L. A., Cupples, L., Haines, J. L., Hyman, B., Kukull, W. A., Mayeux, R., et al. (1997). Effects of age, sex, and ethnicity on the association between apolipoprotein E genotype and Alzheimer disease. *Journal of the American Medical Association, 278*, 1349–1356.

Flicker, C., Ferris, S. H., & Reisberg, B. (1991). Mild cognitive impairment in the elderly: Predictors of dementia. *Neurology, 41*, 1006–1009.

Foldi, N. S., Lobosco, J. J., & Schaefer, L. A. (2002). The effect of attentional dysfunction in Alzheimer's disease: Theoretical and practical implications. *Seminars in Speech and Language, 23*(2), 139–150.

Folstein, M. F., Folstein, S. E., & McHugh, P. R. (1975). Mini-Mental State: A practical method for grading the cognitive state of patients for the clinician. *Journal of Psychiatric Research, 12*, 189–198.

Forbes-McKay, K., Shanks, M., & Venneri, A. (2014). Charting the decline in spontaneous writing in Alzheimer's disease: A longitudinal study. *Acta Neuropsychiatrica, 26*(4), 246–252.

Frattali, C. (2004). An errorless learning approach to treating dysnomia in frontotemporal dementia. *Journal of Medical Speech Language Pathology, 12*, 11–24.

Ganguli, M., Blacker, D., Blazer, D. G., Grant, I., Jeste, D. V., Paulsen, J. S., et al. (2011). Classification of neurocognitive disorders in *DSM-5*: A work in progress. *American Journal of Geriatric Psychiatry, 19*(3), 205–210.

Gibson, F. (1994). What can reminiscence contribute to people with dementia? In J. Bornat (Ed.), *Reminiscence reviewed: Perspectives, evaluations, achievements* (pp. 46–60). Buckingham, UK: Open University Press.

Goldfarb, R. (2006). Differential diagnosis of adults with neurogenic communication disorders In E. M. Welsh (Ed.), *Topics in Alzheimer's disease* (pp. 89–109). New York, NY: Nova Science.

Gorelick, P. B., Scuteri, A., Black, S. E., DeCarli, C., Greenberg, S. M., Iadecola, C., et al. (2011). Vascular contributions to cognitive impairment and dementia—A statement for healthcare professionals from the American Heart Association/ American Stroke Association. *Stroke, 42*, 2672–2713. doi:10.1161/STR.0b013e3182299496.

Gorno-Tempini, M. L., Brambati, S. M., Ginex, V., Ogar, J., Dronkers, N. F., Marcone, A., et al. (2008). The logopenic/ phonological variant of primary progressive aphasia. *Neurology, 71*(16), 1227–1234.

Gorno-Tempini, M. L., Dronker, N. F., Rankin, K. P., Ogar, J. M., Phengrasamy, L., Rosen, H. J., et al. (2004). Cognition and anatomy in three variants of primary progressive aphasia. *Annals of Neurology, 55*(3), 335–346.

Gorno-Tempini, M. L., Hillis, A. E., Weintraub, S., Kertesz, A., Mendez, M., Cappa, S. F., et al. (2011). Classification of primary progressive aphasia and its variants. *Neurology, 76*, 1–9.

Grabowski, T. J., & Damasio, A. R. (2004). Definition, clinical features, and neuroanatomical basis of dementia. In M. Esiri, V. Lee, & J. Trojanowski (Eds.), *Neuropathology of dementia* (2nd ed.) (pp. 1–10). Cambridge, UK: Cambridge University Press.

Groves-Wright, K., Neils-Strunjas, J., Burnett, R., & O'Neill, M. J. (2004). A comparison of verbal and written language in Alzheimer's disease. *Journal of Communication Disorders, 37*(2), 109–130.

Hachinski, V. C., Iliff, L. D., Zilhka, E., DuBoulay, G. H., McAlister, V. L., Marshall, J., et al. (1975). Cerebral blood flow in dementia. *Archives of Neurology, 32*(9), 632–637.

Hanson, J. C., & Lippa, C. F. (2009). Lewy body dementia. *International Review of Neurobiology, 84*, 215–228.

Harciarek, M., & Kertesz, A. (2011). Primary progressive aphasias and their contribution to the contemporary knowledge about the brain-language relationship. *Neuropsychology Review. 21*, 271–278.

Harris, J. (1997). Reminiscence: A culturally and developmentally appropriate language intervention for older adults. *American Journal of Speech Language Pathology, 6*(3), 19–26.

Harvan, J. R., & Cotter, V. (2006). An evaluation of dementia screening in the primary care setting. *Journal of the American Academy of Nurse Practitioners, 18*(8), 351–360.

Hasselmo, M. E. (2006). The role of acetylcholine in learning and memory. *Current Opinion in Neurobiology, 16*(6), 710–715.

Hellen, C. (1992). *Alzheimer's disease: Activity-focused care.* Stoneham, MA: Butterworth-Heinemann.

Helm-Estabrooks, N. (2001). *Cognitive Linguistic Quick Test (CLQT).* San Antonio, TX: Pearson.

Henry, M. L., Beeson, P. M., & Rapcsak, S. Z. (2008). Treatment for anomia in semantic dementia. *Seminars in Speech and Language, 29*, 60–70.

Henry, M. L., & Gorno-Tempini, M. L. (2010). The logopenic variant of primary progressive aphasia. *Current Opinion in Neurology, 23*(6), 633–637.

Henry, M. L., Rising, K., DeMarco, B. L., Miller, M. L, Gorno-Tempini, M. L., & Beeson, P. M. (2013). Examining the value of lexical retrieval treatment in Primary Progressive Aphasia: Two positive cases. *Brain and Language, 127*(2), 145–156. doi:10.1016/j.bandl.2013.05.018.

Hernández, F., & Avila, J. (2007). Tauopathies. *Cellular and Molecular Life Science, 64*(17), 2219–2233.

Hochhalter, A. K., Overmier, J. B., Gasper, S. M., Bakke, B. L., & Holub, R. J. (2005). A comparison of spaced retrieval to other schedules of practice for people with dementia. *Experimental Aging Research, 31*, 101–118.

Hodges, J. R., Patterson, K., Oxbury, S., & Funnell, E. (1992). Semantic dementia: Progressive fluent aphasia with temporal lobe atrophy. *Brain, 115*, 1783–1806.

Hoerster, L., Hickey, E., & Bourgeois, M. (2001). Effects of memory aids on conversations between nursing home residents with dementia and nursing assistants. *Neuropsychological Rehabilitation, 11*, 399–427.

Holland, A. L., Frattali, C., & Fromm, D. (1998). *Communicative Abilities in Daily Living (CADL 2).* Austin, TX: Pro-Ed.

Hopper, T. (2007). The ICF and dementia. *Seminars in Speech and Language, 28*, 273–282.

Hopper, T., & Bayles, K. A. (2007). Management of neurogenic communication disorders associated with dementia. In R. Chapey (Ed.), *Language intervention strategies in aphasia and related neurogenic communication disorders* (5th ed., pp. 988–1008). New York, NY: Lippincott Williams & Wilkins.

Hopper, T., Bayles, K. A., & Kim, E. (2001). Retained neuropsychological abilities of individuals with Alzheimer's disease. *Seminars in Speech and Language, 22*(4), 261–273.

Hopper, T., Bayles, K. A., & Tomoeda, C. K. (1998). Using toys to stimulate communicative function in individuals with Alzheimer's disease. *Journal of Medical Speech Language Pathology, 6*(2), 73–80.

Hopper, T., Bourgeois, M., Pimentel, J., Qualls, C. D., Hickey, E., Frymark, T., et al. (2013). An evidence-based systematic review on cognitive interventions for individuals with dementia. *American Journal of Speech-Language Pathology, 22*, 126–145. doi:10.1044/1058–0360(2012/11-0137).

Hopper, T., Cleary, S., Baumback, N., & Fragomeni, A. (2007). Table fellowship: Mealtime as a context for conversation with individuals who have dementia. *Alzheimer's Care Quarterly, 8*(1), 34–42.

Hopper, T., Cleary, S., Donnelly, M. J., & Dalton, S. (2007). Service delivery for older Canadians with dementia: A survey of speech language pathologists. *Canadian Journal of Speech Language Pathology and Audiology, 31*(3), 114–126.

Hopper, T., Drefs, S., Bayles, K. A., Tomoeda, C. K, & Dinu, I. (2010). The effects of modified spaced-retrieval training on learning and retention of face-name associations by individuals with dementia. *Neuropsychological Rehabilitation, 20*(1), 81–102.

Hopper, T., Holland, A., & Rewega, M. (2002). Conversational coaching: Treatment outcomes and future directions. *Aphasiology, 16*(7), 745–761.

Hopper, T., Mahendra, N., Kim, E., Azuma, T., Bayles, K. A., Cleary, S., et al. (2005). Evidence-based practice recommendations for individuals working with dementia: Spaced retrieval training. *Journal of Medical Speech Language Pathology, 13*(4), xxvii–xxxiv.

Howe, T. J. (2008). The ICF Contextual Factors related to speech-language pathology. *International Journal of Speech-Language Pathology, 10*(1/2), 27–37. doi:10.1080/14417040701774824

Hynd, M. R., Scott, H. L., & Dodd, P. R. (2004). Glutamate-mediated excitotoxicity and neurodegeneration in Alzheimer's disease. *Neurochemistry International, 45*(5), 583–595.

Iadecola, C., & Gorelick, P. B. (2003). Converging pathogenic mechanisms in vascular and neurodegenerative dementia. *Stroke, 34,* 335–337.

Ince, P. G., Perry, E. K., & Morris, C. M. (1998). Dementia with Lewy bodies: A distinct non-Alzheimer dementia syndrome? *Brain Pathology, 8*(2), 299–324.

Jokel, R., Cupit, J., Rochon, E., & Leonard, C. (2009). Relearning lost vocabulary in nonfluent progressive aphasia with MossTalk Words®. *Aphasiology, 23*(2), 175–191.

Jokel, R., Rochon, E., & Leonard, C. (2006). Treating anomia in semantic dementia: Improvement, maintenance, or both? *Neuropsychological Rehabilitation, 16,* 241–256.

Jordan, F. M., Worrall, L. E., Hickson, L. M. H., & Dodd, B. J. (1993). The evaluation of intervention programs for communicatively impaired elderly people. *European Journal of Disorders of Communication, 28,* 63–85.

Jorm, A. (2000). Risk factors for Alzheimer's disease. In J. O'Brien, D. Ames, & A. Burns (Eds.), *Dementia* (2nd ed., pp. 383–388). New York, NY: Oxford University Press.

Josephs, K. A. (2007). Frontotemporal lobar degeneration. *Neurologic Clinics, 25*(3), 683–696.

Jupiter, T. (2009). Screening for hearing loss in the elderly using distortion product otoacoustic emissions, pure tones, and a self-assessment tool. *American Journal of Audiology, 18,* 99–107.

Kaakinen, J. (1995). Talking among elderly nursing home residents. *Topics in Language Disorders, 15*(2), 36–46.

Kemper, S., LaBarge, E., Farraro, R., Cheung, H., Cheung, H., & Storandt, M. (1993). On the preservation of syntax in Alzheimer's disease. *Archives of Neurology, 50,* 81–86.

Kempler, D., Almor, A., Tyler, L. K., Andersen, E. S., & MacDonald, M. E. (1998). Sentence comprehension deficits in Alzheimer's disease: A comparison of off-line vs. on-line sentence processing. *Brain and Language, 64,* 297–316.

Kertesz, A. (2006a). *The banana lady and other stories of curious behavior and speech.* Victoria, BC, Canada: Trafford.

Kertesz, A. (2006b). *Western Aphasia Battery–Revised.* San Antonio, TX: Pearson.

Kertesz, A., Davidson, W., McCabe, P., Takagi, K., & Munoz, D. (2003). Primary progressive aphasia: Diagnosis, varieties, evolution. *Journal of the International Neuropsychological Society, 9*(5), 710–719.

Kim, E., Cleary, S., Hopper, T., Bayles, K. A., Mahendra, N., Azuma, T., et al. (2006). Evidence-based practice recommendations for working with individuals with dementia: Group reminiscence therapy. *Journal of Medical Speech Language Pathology, 14*(3), xxiii–xxxiv.

Kinsella, K., & Velkoff, V. (2001). *An aging world: 2001* (Series P95/01–1). Washington, DC: US Government Printing Office.

Kitwood, T. (1997). The concept of personhood and its relevance for a new culture of dementia care. In B. M. L. Miesen (Ed.), *Caregiving in dementia: Research and applications* (Vol. 2, pp. 3–13). New York, NY: Routledge.

Knopman, D. S. (2001). An overview of common non-Alzheimer dementias. *Clinics in Geriatric Medicine, 17*(2), 281–301.

Knopman, D. S., Boeve, B., & Petersen, R. (2003). Essentials of the proper diagnoses of mild cognitive impairment, dementia, and major subtypes of dementia. *Mayo Clinic Proceedings, 78,* 1290–1308.

Langa, K. M., & Levine D. (2014). The diagnosis and management of Mild Cognitive Impairment: A clinical review. *Jama-Journal of the American Medical Association, 312*(23), 2551-2561.

Lawton, M. P. (1980). *Environment and aging.* Belmont, CA: Brooks/Cole.

Lendon, C. L., Ashall, F., & Goate, A. M. (1997). Exploring the aetiology of Alzheimer disease using molecular genetics. *Journal of the American Medical Association, 277,* 825–831.

Lidz, C. S. (1987). *Dynamic assessment: An interactional approach to evaluating learning potential.* New York, NY: Guilford Press.

Lidz, C. S. (1991). *Practitioner's guide to dynamic assessment.* New York, NY: Guilford Press.

Lu, P. H., Edland, S. D., Teng, E., Tingus, K., Petersen, R. C., & Cummings, J. L. (2009). Donepezil delays progression to AD in MCI subjects with depressive symptoms. *Neurology, 72*(24), 2115–2121.

Lubinski, R. (Ed.). (1995). *Dementia and communication.* Philadelphia, PA: Decker.

Mahendra, N. (2008, October). *Computerized cognitive interventions for persons with Alzheimer's disease: Facts, surprises, and challenges.* Paper presented at the Everyday Technology for Alzheimer Care (ETAC) Consortium Conference, Hillsboro, OR.

Mahendra, N. (2010). An adult with dementia of the Alzheimer type: Screening, assessment, and cognitive-linguistic interventions. In S. Chabon & E. Cohn (Eds.), *The communication disorders casebook: Learning by example* (pp. 410–421). Boston, MA: Allyn & Bacon.

Mahendra, N. (2011). Computer-assisted spaced retrieval training of faces and names for persons with dementia. *Nonpharmacological Therapies for Dementia, 1*(3), 1–21.

Mahendra, N. (2012). The logopenic variant of primary progressive aphasia: Effects on linguistic communication. *Perspectives on Gerontology, 17*(2), 50–59. doi:10.1044/gero17.2.50

Mahendra, N., & Apple, A. (2007, November 27). Human memory systems: A framework for understanding dementia. *ASHA Leader, 12*(16), 8–11.

Mahendra, N., & Arkin, S. M. (2003). Effect of four years of exercise, language, and social interventions on Alzheimer discourse. *Journal of Communication Disorders, 36*(5), 395–422.

Mahendra, N., Bayles, K. A., & Harris, F. P. (2005). Effect of presentation modality on immediate and delayed recall in individuals with Alzheimer's disease. *American Journal of Speech Language Pathology, 14*(2), 144–155.

Mahendra, N., & Engineer, N. (2009). Effects of vascular dementia on cognition and linguistic communication: A case study. *Perspectives—ASHA Special Interest Division 2: Neurogenic and Neurophysiologic Disorders, 19*(4), 106–115.

Mahendra, N., Fremont, K., & Dionne, E. (2013). Teaching future providers about dementia: The impact of service learning. *Seminars in Speech and Language, 34*(1), 5–17.

Mahendra, N., Hopper, T., Bayles, K., Azuma, T., Cleary, S., & Kim, E. (2006). Evidence-based practice recommendations for working with individuals with dementia: Montessori-based interventions. *Journal of Medical Speech Language Pathology, 14*(1), xv–xxv.

Mariani, E., Monastero, R., & Mecocci, P. (2007). Mild cognitive impairment: A systematic review. *Journal of Alzheimer's Disease, 12,* 23–35.

Martin, A., & Fedio, P. (1983). Word production and comprehension in Alzheimer's disease: The breakdown of semantic knowledge. *Brain and Language, 19,* 124–141.

Mattis, S., Jurica, P., & Leitten, C. (1982). *Dementia Rating Scale (DRS-2)*. Lutz, FL: Psychological Assessment Resources.

McKhann, G., Knopman, D. S., Chertkow, H., Hyman, B. T., Jack, C. R., Kawas, C. H., et al. (2011). The diagnosis of dementia due to Alzheimer's disease: Recommendations from the National Institute on Aging and the Alzheimer's Association workgroup. *Alzheimers & Dementia, 7*(3), 263–269.

McNeil, M. R., Small, S. L., Masterson, R. J., & Fossett, T. R. D. (1995). Behavioral and pharmacological treatment of lexical-semantic deficits in a single patient with primary progressive aphasia. *American Journal of Speech Language Pathology, 4*, 76–87.

Mesulam, M. M. (1982). Slowly progressive aphasia without generalized dementia. *Annals of Neurology, 11*(6), 592–598.

Molinuevo, J. L., Ladó, A., & Rami, L. (2005). Memantine: Targeting glutamate excitotoxicity in Alzheimer's disease and other dementias. *American Journal of Alzheimer's Disease and Other Dementias, 20*(2), 77–85.

Moroney, J. T., Bagiella, E., Desmond, D. W., Hachinski, V. C., Molsa, P. K., Gustafson, L., et al. (1997). Meta-analysis of the Hachinski Ischemia Score in pathologically verified dementias. *Neurology, 49*, 1096–1105.

Morris, J. N., Hawes, C., Fries, B. E., Phillips, C. D., Mor, V., Katz, S., et al. (1990). Designing the national resident assessment instrument for nursing homes. *Gerontological Society of America, 30*(3), 293–302.

Nasreddine, Z. S., Phillips, N. A., Bédirian, V., Charbonneau, S., Whitehead, V., Collin I., et al. (2005). The Montreal Cognitive Assessment (MoCA): A brief screening tool for mild cognitive impairment. *Journal of the American Geriatric Society, 53*, 695–699.

National Institutes of Health. (2011). *Alzheimer's disease genetics* (NIH Publication No. 11-6424, 1–8). Retrieved from http://www.nia.nih.gov/sites/default/files/alzheimers_disease_genetics_fact_sheet_0.pdf

National Institutes of Health. (2013). *The dementias: Hope through research* (NIH Publication No. 13-2252). Retrieved from http://www.ninds.nih.gov/disorders/dementias/the-dementias.pdf

Neef, D., & Walling, A. D. (2006). Dementia with Lewy bodies: An emerging disease. *American Family Physician, 73*, 1223–1229.

Nestor, P., & Hodges, J. (2000). Non-Alzheimer dementias. *Seminars in Neurology, 20*(4), 439–446.

Nicholas, M., Obler, L., Albert, M., & Helm-Estabrooks, N. (1985). Empty speech in Alzheimer's disease and fluent aphasia. *Journal of Speech and Hearing Research, 28*, 405–410.

Ober, B., Dronkers, N., Koss, E., Delis, D., & Friedland, R. (1986). Retrieval from semantic memory in Alzheimer type dementia. *Journal of Clinical and Experimental Neuropsychology, 8*, 75–92.

Obler, L. (1983). Language and brain dysfunction in dementia. In S. Segalowitz (Ed.), *Language functions and brain organization* (pp. 267–282). New York, NY: Academic Press.

Ogar, J. M., Dronkers, N. F., Brambati, S. M., Miller, B. L., & Gorno-Tempini, M. L. (2007). Progressive nonfluent aphasia and its characteristic motor speech deficits. *Alzheimer's Disease and Associated Disorders, 21*(4), S23–S30.

Olswang, L., & Bain, B. (1991). When to recommend intervention. *Language, Speech, and Hearing Services in Schools, 22*, 255–263.

Olswang, L., & Bain, B. (1996). Assessment information for predicting upcoming change in language production. *Journal of Speech Language Hearing Research, 39*(2), 414–423.

Orange, J. B., & Colton-Hudson, A. (1998). Enhancing communication in dementia of the Alzheimer's type. *Topics in Geriatric Rehabilitation, 14*(2), 56–75.

Oren, S., Willerton, C., & Small, J. (2014). Effects of spaced retrieval training on semantic memory in Alzheimer's disease: A systematic review. *Journal of Speech, Language, and Hearing Research, 57*, 247–270. doi:10.1044/1092-4388(2013/12-0352)

Petersen, R. C. (Ed.). (2003). *Mild cognitive impairment: Aging to Alzheimer's disease*. New York, NY: Oxford University Press.

Petersen, R. C. (2004). Mild cognitive impairment as a diagnostic entity. *Journal of Internal Medicine, 256*, 183–194.

Petersen, R. C., & Negash, C. (2008). Mild cognitive impairment: An overview. *CNS Spectrums, 13*(1), 45–53.

Petersen, R. C., Smith, G. E., Waring, S. C., Ivnik, R. J., Kokmen, E., & Tangalos, E. G. (1997). Aging, memory, and mild cognitive impairment. *International Psychogeriatry, 9*, 65–69.

Petersen, R. C., Stevens, J. C., Ganguli, M., Tangalos, E. G., Cummings, J. L., & DeKosky, S. T. (2001). Practice parameter: Early detection of dementia: Mild cognitive impairment (an evidence-based review). Report of the quality standards subcommittee of the American Academy of Neurology. *Neurology, 56*, 1133–1142.

Pfeiffer, E. (1975). A short portable mental status questionnaire for the assessment of organic brain deficit in elderly patients. *Journal of American Geriatrics Society, 23*(10), 433–441.

Plassman, B. L., Langa, K. M., Fisher, G. G., Heeringa, S. G., Weir, D. R., Ofstedal, M. B., et al. (2007). Prevalence of dementia in the United States: The Aging, Demographics, and Memory Study (ADAMS). *Neuroepidemiology, 29*, 125–132.

Pollanen, M. S., Dickson, D. W., & Bergeron, C. (1993). Pathology and biology of the Lewy body. *Journal of Neuropathology and Experimental Neurology, 52*, 183–191.

Powlishta, K. K., Von Dras, D. D., Stanford, A., Carr, B. B., Tsering, C., Miller, J. P., et al. (2002). The clock drawing test is a poor screen for very mild dementia. *Neurology, 59*, 898–903.

Price, J. C., & Morris, J. L. (1999). Tangles and plaques in nondemented aging and "preclinical" Alzheimer's disease. *Annals of Neurology, 45*, 358–368.

Prince, M., Bryce, R., Albanese, E., Wimo, A., Ribeiro, W., & Ferri, C. P. (2013). The global prevalence of dementia: A systematic review and metaanalysis. *Alzheimer's and Dementia, 9*(1), 63–75.

Randolph, C., Tierney, M., Mohr, E., & Chase, T. (1998). The Repeatable Battery for the Assessment of Neuropsychological Status (RBANS"): Preliminary clinical validity. *Journal of Clinical and Experimental Neuropsychology, 20*, 310–319.

Rapcsak, S., Arthur, S., Bliklen, D., & Rubens, A. (1989). Lexical agraphia in Alzheimer's disease. *Archives of Neurology, 46*, 65–68.

Raymer, A. M., & Berndt, R. S. (1996). Reading lexically without semantics: Evidence from patients with probable Alzheimer's disease. *Journal of the International Neuropsychological Society, 2*(4), 340–349.

Reilly, J., Rodriguez, A. D., Lamy, M., & Neils-Strunjas, J. (2010). Cognition, language, and clinical pathological features of non-Alzheimer's dementias: An overview. *Journal of Communication Disorders, 43*(5), 438–452.

Reilly, J., Troche, J., & Grossman, M. (2011). Language processing in dementia. In A. E. Budson & N. W. Kowall (Eds.), *The handbook of Alzheimer's disease and other dementias* (pp. 336–368). Malden, MA: Wiley-Blackwell.

Ripich, D. N. (1994). Functional communication with Alzheimer's disease patients: A caregiver training program. *Alzheimer's Disease and Associated Disorders, 8*(Suppl. 3), 95–109.

Ripich, D. N., & Terrell, B. (1988). Patterns of discourse cohesion and coherence in Alzheimer's disease. *Journal of Speech and Hearing Disorders, 53,* 8–15.

Ripich, D. N., Ziol, E., Fritsch, T., & Durand, E. J. (1999). Training Alzheimer's disease caregivers for successful communication. *Clinical Gerontologist, 21*(1), 37–56.

Ripich, D. N., Ziol, E., & Lee, M. (1998). Longitudinal effects of communication training on caregivers of persons with Alzheimer's disease. *Clinical Gerontologist, 19*(2), 37–55.

Roman, G. C. (2004). Facts, myths, and controversies in vascular dementia. *Journal of Neurological Sciences, 226,* 49–52.

Rountree, S. D., Waring, S. C., Chan, W. C., Lupo, P. J., Darby, E. J., & Doody, R. S. (2007). Importance of subtle amnestic and non-amnestic deficits in mild cognitive impairment: Prognosis and conversion to dementia. *Dementia and Geriatric Cognitive Disorders, 24*(6), 476–482.

Salmon, D. P., & Bondi, M. W. (2009). Neuropsychological assessment of dementia. *Annual Review of Psychology, 60,* 257–282.

Sanchez, A., Millan-Calenti, J. C., Lorenzo-Lopez, L., & Maseda, A. (2011). Multisensory stimulation for people with dementia. *American Journal of Alzheimer's Disease and Other Dementias, 28*(17), 7–14.

Santo Pietro, M. J., & Ostuni, E. (2003). *Successful communication with persons with Alzheimer's disease: An in-service manual.* St. Louis, MO: Butterworth-Heinemann.

Sapolsky, D., Domoto-Reilly, K., & Dickerson, B. C. (2014). Use of the Progressive Aphasia Severity Scale (PASS) in monitoring speech and language status in PPA. *Aphasiology, 28*(8–9), 993–1003. doi:10.1080/02687038.2014.931563

Sapolsky, D., Domoto-Reilly, K., Negreira, A., Brickhouse, M., McGinnis, S., & Dickerson, B. C. (2011). Monitoring progression of primary progressive aphasia: current approaches and future directions. *Neurodegenerative Disease Management, 1,* 43–55.

Savundranayagam, M. Y., Hummert, M. L. and Montgomery, R. J. V. (2005). Investigating the effects of communication problems on caregiver burden. *Journals of Gerontology Series B—Psychological Sciences and Social Sciences, 60*(1), S48–S55.

Savundranayagam, M. Y., & Orange, J. B. (2014). Matched and mismatched appraisals of the effectiveness of communication strategies by family caregivers of persons with Alzheimer's disease. *International Journal of Language and Communication Disorders, 49*(1), 49–59. doi:10.1111/1460-6984.12043.

Schacter, D. L. (1996). *Searching for memory.* New York, NY: Basic Books, Harper Collins.

Schneider, S. L., Thompson, C. K., & Lurhing, B. (1996). Effects of verbal plus gestural matrix training on sentence production in a patient with primary progressive aphasia. *Aphasiology, 10,* 297–317.

Selkoe, D. J. (2000). The genetics and molecular pathology of Alzheimer's disease: Roles of amyloid and the presenelins. *Neurologic Clinics, 18,* 903–922.

Sepelyak, K., Crinion, J., Molitoris, J., Epstein-Peterson, Z., Bann, M., Davis, C., et al. (2011). Patterns of breakdown in spelling in primary progressive aphasia. *Cortex, 47*(3), 342–352.

Sheikh, J. I., & Yesavage, J. A. (1986). Geriatric Depression Scale (GDS): Recent evidence and development of a shorter version. *Clinical Gerontologist, 5*(1–2), 165–173.

Small, J., & Gutman, G. (2002). Recommended and reported use of communication strategies in Alzheimer caregiving. *Alzheimer's Disease & Associated Disorders, 16*(4), 270–278.

Small, J., Gutman, G., Makela, S., & Hillhouse, B. (2003). Effectiveness of communication strategies used by caregivers of persons with Alzheimer's disease during activities of daily living. *Journal of Speech Language and Hearing Research, 46,* 353–367.

Small, J., Kemper, S., & Lyons, K. (1997). Sentence comprehension in Alzheimer's disease: Effects of grammatical complexity, speech rate and repetition. *Psychology & Aging, 12,* 3–11.

Small, J., & Perry, J. A. (2013). Training family care partners to communicate effectively with persons with Alzheimer's disease: The TRACED program. *Canadian Journal of Speech-Language Pathology and Audiology, 36*(4), 332–350.

Snowdon, J. S., Griffiths, H. L., & Neary, D. (1996). Semantic-episodic memory interactions in semantic dementia: Implications for retrograde memory function. *Cognitive Neuropsychology, 13,* 1101–1137.

Snowdon, J. S., & Neary, D. (2002). Relearning of verbal labels in semantic dementia. *Neuropsychologia, 40*(10), 1715–1728.

Sonies, B. C. (1997). *Scales of adult independence, language, and recall.* Austin, TX: Pro-Ed.

Squire, L. R., & Dede, J. O. (2015). Conscious and unconscious memory systems. *Cold Spring Harbor Perspectives in Biology, 7,* 1–15. doi:10.1101/cshperspect.a021667.

Squire, L. R., & Kandel, E. R. (1999). *Memory: From mind to molecules.* New York, NY: Scientific American Library.

Squire, L. R., & Schacter, D. L. (2002). *Neuropsychology of memory* (3rd ed.). New York, NY: Guilford Press.

Squire, L. R., & Zola, S. M. (1996). Structure and function of declarative and nondeclarative memory systems. *Proceedings of the National Academy of Sciences, 93,* 13515–13522.

Squire, L. R., & Zola-Morgan, S. (1991). The medial temporal lobe memory system. *Science, 253,* 1380–1386.

Sternberg, R. J, & Sternberg, K. (2011). *Cognitive Psychology* (6th ed.). Belmont, CA: Wadsworth Cengage Learning.

Strain, E., Patterson, K., Graham, N., & Hodges, J. R. (1998). Word reading in Alzheimer's disease: Cross-sectional and longitudinal analyses of response time and accuracy data. *Neuropsychologia, 36*(2), 155–171.

Sunderland, T., Hill, J. L., Mellow, A. M., Lawlor, B. A., Gundersheimer, J., Newhouse, P. A., et al. (1989). Clock drawing in Alzheimer's disease: A novel measure of dementia severity. *Journal of the American Geriatrics Society, 37*(8), 725–729.

Tadaka, E., & Kanagawa, K. (2004). A randomized controlled trial of a group care program for community-dwelling elderly people with dementia. *Japan Journal of Nursing Science, 1,* 19–25.

Taler, V., & Phillips, N. A. (2008). Language performance in Alzheimer's disease and mild cognitive impairment: A comparative review. *Journal of Clinical and Experimental Neuropsychology, 30,* 501–556.

Talerico, K., Evans, L., & Strumpf, N. (2002). Mental health correlates of aggression in nursing home residents with dementia. *The Gerontologist, 42,* 169–177.

Tariq, S. H., Tumosa, N., Chibnall, J. T., Perry, M. H., & Morley, J. E. (2006). Comparison of the Saint Louis University Mental Status Examination and the Mini-Mental State Examination for detecting dementia and mild neurocognitive disorder: A pilot study. *American Journal of Geriatric Psychiatry, 14,* 900–910.

Threats, T. T. (2008). Use of the ICF for clinical practice in speech-language pathology. *International Journal of Speech-Language Pathology, 10*(1–2), 50–60.

Tiraboschi, P., Hansen, L. A., Thal, L. J., & Corey-Bloom, J. (2004). The importance of neuritic plaques and tangles to the development and evolution of AD. *Neurology, 62*(11), 1984–1989.

Tomoeda, C. K. (2001). Comprehensive assessment for dementia: A necessity for differential diagnosis and management. *Seminars in Speech and Language, 22*(4), 275–289.

Tomoeda, C. K., & Bayles, K. A. (1993). Longitudinal effects of AD on discourse production. *Alzheimer Disease and Associated Disorders, 7*(4), 223–236.

Tulving, E. (1983). *Elements of episodic memory*. New York, NY: Oxford University Press.

Tulving, E., & Markowitsch, H. J. (1998). Episodic and declarative memory: Role of the hippocampus. *Hippocampus, 8*(3), 198–204.

United Nations. (2002). *Report of the Second World Assembly on Aging*. Madrid, Spain: Author.

US Census Bureau. (2001). *International database. Table 094. Midyear population by age and sex*. Retrieved from http://www.census.gov/population/www/projections/natdet-D1A.html.

US Census Bureau. (2011). *The older population: 2010*. 2010 Census Briefs. Retrieved from http://www.census.gov/prod/cen2010/briefs/c2010br-09.pdf

Vance, D. E., & Johns, R. N. (2002). Montessori improved cognitive domains in adults with Alzheimer's disease. *Physical and Occupational Therapy in Geriatrics, 20*(3/4), 19–36.

Vance, D. E., & Porter, R. (2000). Montessori methods yield cognitive gains in Alzheimer's daycares. *Activities, Adaptation, & Aging, 24*(3), 1–21.

Wang, L., van Belle, G., Crane, P. K., Kukull, W. A., Bowen, J. D., McCormick, W. C., et al. (2004). Subjective memory deterioration and future dementia in people aged 65 and older. *Journal of the American Geriatrics Society, 52*, 2045–2051.

Wang, Q., & Zhou, J. N. (2002). Retrieval and encoding of episodic memory in normal aging and patients with mild cognitive impairment. *Brain Research, 924*, 113–115.

Ward-Smith, P., Llanque, S. M., & Curran, D. (2009). The effect of multisensory stimulation on persons residing in an extended care facility. *American Journal of Alzheimer's Disease and Other Dementias, 24*, 450–455.

Watson, B., Aizawa, L. D., Savundranayagam, M. Y., & Orange, J. B. (2012). Links among communication, dementia, and caregiver burden. *Canadian Journal of Speech-Language Pathology & Audiology, 36*(4), 276–283.

Wechsler, D. (2009). *Wechsler Memory Scale* (4th ed.). San Antonio, TX: Pearson.

Weisman, D., & McKeith, I. (2007). Dementia with Lewy bodies. *Seminars in Neurology, 27*(1), 42–47.

Weisman, G. D., & Moore, K. D. (2003). Vision and values: M. Powell Lawton and the philosophical foundations of environment-aging studies. In R. Scheidt & P. Windley (Eds.), *Physical environments and aging* (pp. 23–37). London, UK: Haworth Press.

Wenk, G. L. (2003). Neuropathologic changes in Alzheimer's disease. *Journal of Clinical Psychiatry, 64*(Suppl. 9), 7–10.

Wilson, B. A., Greenfield, E., Clare, L., Baddeley, A., Cockburn, J., Watson, P., et al. (2008). *The Rivermead Behavioural Memory Test* (3rd ed.). London, UK: Pearson Assessment.

Wilson, R., Rochon, E., Leonard, C., & Mihailidis, A. (2012). Examining success of communication strategies used by formal caregivers assisting individuals with Alzheimer's disease during an activity of daily living. *Journal of Speech, Language, and Hearing Research, 55*, 328–341. doi:10.1044/1092-4388(2011/10-0206).

Wilson, R., Rochon, E., Leonard, C., & Mihailidis, A. (2013). Quantitative analysis of formal caregivers' use of communication strategies while assisting individuals with moderate and severe Alzheimer's disease during oral care. *Journal of Communication Disorders, 46*(3), 249–263. doi:10.1016/j.jcomdis.2013.01.004

Wisely, J. (2010, May 18). Skilled nursing facility assessment tool focuses on patient communication. *ASHA Leader*, 8–9.

Wittenberg, D., Possin, K. L., Rascovsky, K., Rankin, K. P., Miller, B. L., & Kramer, J. H. (2008). The early neuropsychological and behavioral characteristics of frontotemporal dementia. *Neuropsychology Review, 18*, 91–102.

World Health Organization. (2001). *International classification of functioning, disability and health*. Geneva, Switzerland: Author.

Ylvisaker, M., & Feeney, T. (1998). *Collaborative brain injury intervention: Positive everyday routines*. San Diego, CA: Singular.

Yueh, B., Shapiro, N., MacLean, C. H., & Shekelle, P. G. (2003). Screening and management of adult hearing loss in primary care: Scientific review. *Journal of the American Medical Association, 289*, 1976–1985.

Zientz, J., Rackley, A., Chapman, S. B., Hopper, T., Mahendra, N., Kim, E., et al. (2007). Evidence-based practice recommendations for dementia: Educating caregivers on Alzheimer's disease and training communication strategies. *Journal of Medical Speech Language Pathology, 15*(3), 1iii–1iv.

OBJECTIVES

The reader will be able to:

1. Give a broad definition of acquired apraxia of speech (AoS) and be aware of a number of hurdles standing in the way of a more precise characterization.

2. Recognize the main clinical presenting characteristics of the disorder and how it differs from closely related motor speech disorders.

3. Appreciate various conceptualizations of AoS according to different speech output models and views on the neurological organization of speech control.

4. Describe principles of motor learning (PML) that may be pertinent to the treatment of AoS and recognize the limitations of current data supporting implementation of these principles.

5. Identify weaknesses in the existing AoS evidence base with respect to the World Health Organization (WHO) International Classification of Functioning, Disability, and Health (ICF) (WHO, 2001) levels of functioning.

6. Describe available articulatory–kinematic techniques for treating AoS.

7. Describe available rate/rhythm control strategies for treating AoS.

8. Recognize the existence of the Academy of Neurologic Communication Disorders and Sciences (ANCDS) AoS practice guidelines and understand their recommendations.

Acquired Apraxia of Speech

Nick Miller and Julie Wambaugh

INTRODUCTION

What is acquired apraxia of speech (AoS), and how should it be treated? These are the central themes of this chapter. It starts with an outline definition of the disorder. But, pronouncements on AoS are not without their problems, and we highlight several hurdles along the path toward a more precise definition and delineation of AoS from other speech disorders. The first sections move from a description of clinical presentation, via issues in clinical differential diagnosis and assessment, to a consideration of where speech apraxic breakdown might lie in models of speech output and an outline of lesion sites associated with it. The second half of the chapter focuses on the evidence base for approaches to treatment.

DEFINING APRAXIA OF SPEECH

Apraxia of speech is broadly defined as an acquired disorder of learned volitional actions associated with breakdown in the planning or programming of the movements needed for speech. Persons with AoS are believed to "know" the word(s) they wish to use and what sounds they need for the word, thereby separating AoS from disorders of language or phonology. Individuals have the capability (e.g., range, force, velocity, sustainability) to make the movements of the articulators necessary to produce sounds, thus differentiating AoS from neuromuscular disorders affecting primary sensorimotor functions, as found in various dysarthrias. The problem in AoS is deemed to lie in actually specifying and coordinating the movement parameters required to produce strings of sounds, situating the likely breakdown at a stage of phonetic encoding or control.

Designating apraxia as a disorder of learned actions indicates problems performing actions that have to be consciously or unconsciously developed, in contrast to basic, reflexive, and more automatic movements, which remain intact. The disorder is said to manifest especially in actions where elicitation and control oblige volitional (intentional, propositional) control. As an action problem, breakdowns occur in assembling and controlling more basic movements to produce concerted, goal-directed performance, not in accomplishing the individual, basic movement components themselves.

This appears a straightforward characterization, one that might even receive relatively general agreement. However, the brief definition sidesteps fundamental debates that for more than 150 years have dogged attempts to achieve consensus on what does precisely characterize and underlie speech apraxic breakdown. Some of the key issues surrounding these arguments are highlighted in the course of the chapter, in particular challenges around what exactly is meant by planning versus programming versus execution of speech, whether these are separate or one and the same process; contentions concerning what is planned and programmed precisely in speech output (sound targets, spatiotemporal targets, sounds, syllables, etc.); and views on how speech control relates to language production and to nonspeech motor control. Opposing stances regarding these debates account for the seemingly conflicting definitions and advice found in the literature. Search for enlightenment from theories of phonology, speech output, or brain organization often provide little resolution, partly from the fact that most models of speech motor control and its breakdown remain highly underspecified—few address issues around apraxia directly, partly because the fields of phonology, brain organization, and the like have ample unsettled controversies of their own. Differing solutions to all these conundrums have led to contrasting definitions of AoS, to variability in differential diagnosis procedures, and to differing emphases and targets in treatment.

Indeed, the abundance of theories of how speech control is organized, with consequent divergences of beliefs surrounding AoS, casts a long shadow over endeavors to study the disorder. It is frequently the case that what one person has described as AoS is classed as a different disorder by another researcher. Behaviors one person accepts as core features of AoS are dismissed by others as epiphenomena or features of a co-occurring dysfunction unconnected to the AoS itself. Unfortunately, it is almost certain that individuals included in different studies and labeled as having AoS constitute a highly heterogeneous group. These potentially confounding features sit over and above issues of straightforward clinical complexity. Cases of pure AoS are vanishingly rare; only a few individuals had been described (Odell, McNeil, Rosenbek, & Hunter, 1990; Square-Storer, Darley, & Sommers, 1988). Therefore, the task in clinic more likely is to extricate behaviors resulting from AoS from

symptoms associated with co-occurring aphasic, motor, and other neuropsychological disturbances. These caveats notwithstanding, the following material attempts to simplify the whole matter.

THE NATURE OF APRAXIA OF SPEECH

This section looks at the presenting symptomatology of AoS and how this might differ from other (motor) speech disorders. It contrasts surface appearances with underlying features and suggests some assessment approaches that can prolong these characteristics.

Presenting Picture of Apraxia of Speech

Clearly, the presenting picture in AoS differs according to severity—from complete muteness to more or less fluent output where disruptions may be heard only occasionally on particularly challenging words or when the speaker is under pressure of time, tiredness, or emotions. When output is possible, the auditory perceptual impression is that speech is slowed, even for apparently fluent speech, when compared to unimpaired speakers and even though speakers with AoS can reach movement velocity levels comparable to nondisordered speakers (McNeil, Caliguiri, & Rosenbek, 1989). Speech is dysfluent, interrupted, often repeatedly, by visible and audible struggle to attain targets, by inter- and intraword and syllable pauses. The slowness and struggle may disrupt prosody, but this can also be affected by disruptions of syllable structure (e.g., insertion of a schwa in consonant clusters), altered stress placement, tendency to syllabic speech (Kent & Rosenbek, 1982; Ziegler, 2002), or overreliance on a limited repertoire of prosodic forms. Voice quality in successful speech is normal.

When sounds are derailed, it can seem as if they are distorted (e.g., /bɪt/ is produced with excessive aspiration on the /b/, or an overshortened or prolonged vowel); substituted (/bɪt/ sounds like /pɪt/, /mɪt/, or /beɪt/); or even distorted substitutions (/bɪt/ might sound like /pᶠɪt/). Other sounds appear omitted (/bɪt/ sounds like /ɪt/; /spɪk/ like /sɪk/ or /pɪk/); added (/bɪt/ sounds like /bzɪt/, /spɪk/ like /sprɪk/); transposed (/spɪk/ sounds like /psɪk/; *sitting room* like "ritting soom"); or anticipated or perseverated (/kafi/ sounds like /fkafi/; *telephone* like "teletone" or "felifone").

Whether transpositions and noncontiguous anticipations and perseverations belong to AoS remains disputed (Miller, 1995; Odell et al., 1990). Some assert such derailments represent a phonological, premotoric, nonapraxic breakdown or that the clinician must distinguish between apparent straight transpositions (*telephone* as "felitone"; "skeap" for *speak*) and inertial perseverations/anticipations (e.g., "dedidon" for *telephone*; "bibIb" for *speaking*). This issue is not yet resolved. Disagreements here doubtless arise from the group heterogeneity problem, as a consequence of various interpretations from different speech output models, and whether narrow transcription was utilized in any given study.

Perceptual evaluation, though, only describes surface behaviors. Similar-sounding derailments may stem from diverse underlying disruptions, and perceived derailment types are not unique to AoS. This is amply illustrated in instrumental (acoustic, kinematic, physiological) investigations. For example, studies show that in AoS the variable nature of the voiced–voiceless contrast in word initial position (and perceived substitution of voiced for voiceless sounds) and apparent misselection of nasal for oral sounds rest not on problems of wrong retrieval of sounds, but on the miscoordination of gestural timing between laryngeal and oral, and tongue/lip and velopharyngeal subsystems (Itoh & Sasanuma, 1984; Ziegler & von Cramon, 1986). Perceived substitutions can also arise from application of a closing or opening gesture to the wrong articulatory effector, not just misphasing between gestures. This is addressed thoroughly further in the chapter. In addition, in perceived omissions the underlying target gesture can still be present but not fully realized or is masked by competing misdirected gestures (e.g., Hardcastle & Edwards, 1992; Pouplier & Hardcastle, 2005); conversely, perceived additions can be the result of competing or misdirected gestures both producing an audible outcome.

Perceptual and instrumental studies further exemplify that AoS is characterized by a loss of coarticulatory cohesion (McNeil, Hashi, & Southwood, 1994; Ziegler & von Cramon, 1985, 1986), most probably a reflection of increased problems in transitions between sounds and reduced planning capacity for larger stretches of speech. Compensatory slowing and syllabification may in part reflect an attempt to surmount this difficulty.

Examining whether or not a sound derailment is accommodated to the new phonetic environment has been taken as a marker that betrays a phonological versus motoric source of a slip—for instance, when unaspirated /p/ in "spot" in English is adjusted to an aspirated /pʰ/ when the /s/ is omitted. Buchwald and Miozzo (2012) provide a recent example of argumentation in this direction. Such an interpretation stems from a view of strict separation of phonological and phonetic control. Within more unified, interactive models, where phonetic "knowledge" is part of phonology, the same phenomenon is accounted for by the absence of any learned motor program that would permit /pot/ with an unaspirated /p/ or through the extremely low transitional probability

that such sequences would occur. In an examination of whether accommodation occurred or not in initial consonant cluster slips (in healthy speakers), Pouplier, Marin, and Waltl (2014) found no results that would support (a lack of) accommodation as a diagnostic pointer for the processing level at which an error occurred. Rather, their findings support speech production models that allow for an integrated view of phonological and phonetic processing.

The preceding remarks point to possible characteristics to listen and look for in identifying AoS. The following section looks at some tasks and materials that clinicians might employ to elicit these features.

CLINICAL ASSESSMENT AND DIFFERENTIAL DIAGNOSIS

To provide the data to triangulate clusters of symptoms that point (more) to one underlying disorder than another, materials should include words of contrasting length and complexity and number of gestural adjustments required to say them (see the discussion that follows) and words varying by frequency, lexicality, and phonotactic probability (how likely one sound will follow another in a particular language; e.g., the word initial sequence <*sf*> in English has a low phonotactic probability, whereas the sequence <*sp*> has a high probability). It is also relevant to compare performance on the same or closely matched words in contexts of greater versus lesser automaticity (e.g., counting 1–5 versus 5–1; salt and pepper versus salt and paper, or in Britain, fish and chips versus fish and chicks) and the same word produced spontaneously (e.g., in picture naming or picture description; describing how to carry out an activity) versus on a reading tasks versus elicited by repetition. Focus can be on segmental accuracy but not to the exclusion of syllable, prosodic, and metrical integrity.

Where, how, which, and why derailments occur is as important, if not more important, than whether they arise, given that no one error type, length effect, and so forth is pathognomonic of AoS. Readily available instrumental techniques can supplement naked ear and eye judgments, but careful narrow phonetic transcription is always invaluable in identifying key differences in perceived distortions versus substitutions versus distorted substitutions and in pinpointing transitional difficulties (problems moving from one sound target to the next) and alterations to stress and rhythmic patterns. A good deal of past confusion regarding AoS and its differentiation from other disorders has ensued from studies that misguidedly relied on broad phonemic analyses.

Several assessment batteries or checklists claim to differentially diagnose AoS on the basis of whether speakers succeed or not on their range of tasks (Dabul, 2000; Feiken, Jonkers, Lettinga, & Stuive, 2012; Strand, Duffy, Clark, & Josephs, 2014). Given that there is no agreed-on unique profile of apraxic breakdown, such aspirations still need to be treated with some skepticism. Unfortunately, it has happened that test devisers have acted as judge and jury, with reasoning subject to circularity of argument. A set of features has been assembled allegedly characterizing AoS. The test has been administered to speakers whom the test devisers consider to have AoS, but based of course on their preconceived notion of what counts as AoS and not on independently verifiable criteria. Alternatively, the test is administered to groups of people with neurological impairment, some of whom may have AoS. Those who fail on the battery are deemed apraxic. Both approaches employ the false logic of choosing a premise to prove a conclusion but then using that conclusion to prove the original premise. Such risks will remain until speech features can be identified that are independently indicative of AoS versus other disorders. Such features might, for instance, be based on predictions from speech output models (see the discussion of models that follows). Difficulties in differential diagnosis will also remain until ways are developed of assessing characteristics of speech output that achieve desirable levels of rater agreement and discriminability (Haley, Jacks, de Riesthal, Abou-Khalil, & Roth, 2012). These reservations notwithstanding, there are clinical procedures with some degree of agreement.

A speech motor examination plays a role in differentiation of dysarthric from apraxic and paraphasic breakdown. Diadochokinetic tasks (Bohland & Guenther, 2006; Deger & Ziegler, 2002; Gadesmann & Miller, 2008; Hurkmans, Jonkers, Boonstra, Stewart, & Reinders-Messelink, 2012; Nishio & Niimi, 2006; Ziegler, 2002) provide an economic means of gaining multiple insights. They provide measures of single (/pa.pa.pa.pa/) and alternating (/pa.ta.pa.ta/) syllable rates; rhythm (e.g., duration, stress); and stability (ability to remain on target and how accurately on target, e.g., on, then off, then on the target; gradually losing the target over the repetitions). They can be tailored to examine coordination between different gestural subsystems (e.g., alternations of *pie-buy* for voiced–voiceless stability, *my-buy* for oral-nasal coordination, *die-guy* for tongue tip–dorsum performance, *sigh-tie* for control over degree of closure). Repeated trials tasks can be used to gauge variability and struggle, both not only as possible diagnostic markers, but also as therapy outcome measures. Speech that is less variable and exhibits less disruptive struggle can be associated with benefits to intelligibility and acceptability, independent of gains (or not) on particular sounds or sound contrasts (Haley & Martin, 2011).

Pure AoS is not associated with changes to tone and power in the muscles of articulation, whereas in spastic and flaccid dysarthria, articulatory derailments are linked to the degree and site of neuromuscular changes. In hypokinetic dysarthria, the picture is of underscaling of movement parameters (Sapir, 2014), and in ataxic dysarthria one of dysmetria and dysrhythmia (Lowit, Kuschmann, & Kavanagh, 2014; Spencer & Slocomb, 2007). Seldom does AoS occur in isolation, so more likely than not a degree of muscle weakness, slowed movements, and reduced range of articulatory excursions is present. The task, then, is to disentangle dysarthric sound distortions arising from neuromuscular disruption from derailments due to disruption at stages prior to movement initiation. As a rule of thumb, the less the pattern of sound derailments corresponds in type (e.g., labial, tongue tip) to the site of muscle weakness and the more disparity exists between the relative mildness of physical dysfunction and severity of speech derailments, the more likely it is that apraxic or paraphasic breakdown underlies the changes.

In terms of perceived error types, dysarthrias (at least of the flaccid, spastic, and hypokinetic types and when occurring in isolation) are more likely to be characterized by predominantly perceived distortions, omissions, and some perceived substitutions, with no displacements (noncontiguous transpositions, perseverations, anticipations) (Haley, Bays, & Ohde, 2001; Miller, 1995). Constant hypernasality is likely to indicate a dysarthria. A profile of predominantly displacements and apparent frank substitutions typifies phonemic paraphasia, especially if perceived substitutions seem to involve multiple changes of place and manner of articulation (e.g., *beat* sounds like *cheat*), and these derailments are linked mainly to content words, and when errors are absent, there is normal speech rate and prosody. Apraxia of speech gives predominantly distortions, followed by substitutions and distorted substitutions, and additions (with arguments over whether some of these are better classified as suppressed displacements or struggle behavior) and omissions (Haley, Bays, et al., 2001; Mauszycki, Wambaugh, & Cameron, 2010a; Miller, 1995; Odell et al., 1990), although proportions may vary according to target phoneme and severity.

Periodically, the claim arises that in AoS only consonants and not vowels are affected, and that this distinguishes it from dysarthric speech. Jacks, Mathes, and Marquardt (2010) have recently resurrected this claim, based on repetitions of six English vowels by seven speakers with Broca's aphasia and AoS produced in a uniform /hCV/ context. Their study depended on single-word citations without a direct comparison group (they employed general norms from other studies) and on analyses of vowel formants, with no other variables (e.g., articulatory timing) that may be predicted as disordered in AoS. Other investigators have found evidence of vowel distortions and substitutions in AoS both acoustically and perceptually, and without a doubt speakers with more severe AoS struggle to produce target vowels, even in isolation; even when they succeed, this may be highly unstable (Haley, Ohde, & Wertz, 2001). Thus, differential impairment of consonant versus vowel impairment cannot be taken as a pathognomonic feature or a differential diagnosis marker in assessment.

The fact that vowels appear less impaired may stem from the greater perceptual leeway for distortion permitted in English before a derailment is heard. Vowels require less fine motor adjustment compared to consonants, and this may also play a role. It may stem from differences in processing between place and manner of articulation and feedforward control (Lotte et al., 2015; Maas, Mailend, & Guenther, 2015). In languages with more complex vowel systems, one would predict that this relative immunity would be correspondingly diminished (Miller & Lowit, 2014). Others may have classed vowel derailments as prosodic disturbance or as the result of neighboring consonantal distortion, coarticulatory incoherence, or altered accent, especially in mild AoS.

What may be diagnostically telling is the profile of error types and ways in which the profile alters according to elicitation mode; where derailments occur (in the syllable, word, phrase); and clues to the underlying reasons why breakdown occurred. For instance, in dysarthrias the likelihood of errors remains relatively uniform across matched reading, repetition, and spontaneous speech elicitation contexts (on formal reading and repetition tasks, even healthy speakers tend to be more precise). In comparison, speakers with AoS improve on "watch and listen to me" repetition or unison elicitation and may find that the written word facilitates production. People with conduction aphasia perform markedly more poorly on repetition tasks than they do on spontaneous speech. Apraxia of speech and phonemic paraphasia, in contrast to dysarthrias, are characterized by higher error probability on nonsense words, lower-frequency words/ syllables, or words with lower phonotactic probability (Cholin, Levelt, & Schiller, 2006; Lallini, Miller, & Howard, 2007; Staiger & Ziegler, 2008).

People with dysarthria show little variation between relatively automatic (e.g., overlearned sequences, asides) output and more propositional speech, or high- versus low-frequency words, compared to speakers with AoS. People with AoS are not necessarily error free on overlearned sequences and high-frequency words; rather, they are proportionately better on more automatic compared to matched less overlearned tasks (count

1–5; count 5–1) compared to speakers with dysarthria. Where the dissociation point falls between automatic–propositional is closely tied to overall severity (van der Merwe, 2007; van Lancker, 1987).

A debate concerns whether people with AoS versus phonemic paraphasia vary in their error consistency in comparison to people with flaccid, spastic, and hypokinetic dysarthrias (Haley, Jacks, & Cunningham, 2013; Haley & Martin, 2011; Mauszycki, Dromey, & Wambaugh, 2007; Mauszycki et al., 2010a; McNeil, Odell, Miller, & Hunter, 1995; Miller, 1992; Seddoh et al., 1996; Shuster & Wambaugh, 2008; Staiger, Finger-Berg, Aichert, & Ziegler, 2012). Speakers with dysarthria are said to show relatively stable error types, in keeping with the site and severity of the underlying neuromuscular picture. The profile in ataxic dysarthria may differ (Lowit et al., 2014; Spencer & Slocomb, 2007) and present greater variability of production. For speakers with apraxia, there may be consistency in which words/syllables/sound sequences they find difficult, the proportion of perceived error types (e.g., distortions versus substitutions) may remain constant, and the hierarchy of sounds within a language that are more likely to be derailed may be relatively stable (Mauszycki, Wambaugh, & Cameron, 2010b). This can give an impression of consistency. However, the precise derailment that surfaces for a given sound (or sound sequence) can be highly variable, whether this is on immediate repetition of a particular word, repetition on different occasions, or realization of a particular sound in different words or syllable contexts (Staiger et al., 2012).

Some research findings (Haley et al., 2012; Staiger et al., 2012) emphasize the need to avoid floor and ceiling effects in elicitation. If items are too easy (for a given speaker), everything is consistently correct; if too difficult, speakers are unable to produce sufficient sound differentiation. Indeed, some speakers with motor speech disorders make a strategic choice to utter words with specific sound derailments; for example, /st/ is consistently realized as /d/. They find this enables them to remain fluent and be predictable for the listener, rather than attempt the full target word and know they will fail. Miller, Lowit, and O'Sullivan (2006) described a speaker with AoS who, among other strategies, regularly split up consonant clusters with a schwa. This led to fluent, but foreign-sounding, speech. If she was obliged to attempt the full target cluster and eliminate the schwa, her speech became markedly dysfluent and sounded disordered.

McNeil et al. (1995) claimed there is high consistency in apraxic speech. They compared four speakers with "pure" AoS with speakers with "pure" conduction aphasia and concluded that people with AoS are consistent in the locus and type of errors, in contrast to the participants with conduction aphasia. They also concluded that repeated attempts at target were more likely to end in success for speakers with phonemic paraphasias than for the ones with apraxic errors. To date, these findings have not been replicated, while other works mentioned here have confirmed the presence of variability of target realization.

Debate continues regarding whether different motor speech disorders display unique struggle behaviors. If struggle is present in dysarthria, it is typically to achieve articulatory ranges and velocities in the face of underlying weakness, fatigue, or general underscaling of movements. In AoS and phonemic paraphasias (i.e., *conduites d'approche*), struggle is manifest as repeated false starts and midflow repeated self-corrections to reach a target, where sounds realized in the stream of attempts clearly demonstrate the problem is not one of range or sustainability of articulatory movement, but of gaining the desired articulatory configuration. Preparatory trial-and-error efforts may be silent but visible or clearly audible. Whether there is a distinction between AoS and conduites d'approche in success at arriving at a target, the number of trials to reach it and the nature of the repeated attempts remain unsettled (Buchwald & Miozzo, 2012; Joanette, Keller, & Lecours, 1980; Kohn, 1984; Liss, 1998; McNeil et al., 1995).

Considering error location, articulatory derailments in AoS are generally deemed more probable in word or syllable initial position, especially on consonant clusters (Riecker, Brendel, Ziegler, Erb, & Ackermann, 2008). It is currently unresolved whether the predilection represents the exaggeration of a normal effect also present in healthy speakers, a by-product of initial stressed syllables being more prominent in the languages studied in AoS (and people with AoS having more problems with stressed syllables), a transcriber perceptual bias, or some other factor(s). Error location in phonemic paraphasia is less clear, with unsettled claims for a more equal spread across the word or even a tendency to occur later in the word (Canter, Trost, & Burns, 1985). In dysarthria, word or phrase final production is more prone to disturbance overall, based on increasing difficulties sustaining rate, range, and force of movements, but this has not been systematically investigated.

Increasing likelihood of derailments on longer and more complex words has been listed as a feature of AoS. Length of words has been shown to be a strong predictor of inaccuracies (Nickels & Howard, 2004). However, length and complexity effects, slowness, and dysfluencies are not unique to an apraxic etiology. Speakers with dysarthria or paraphasias also experience added problems on longer, more complex words. Furthermore, numerous studies illustrate that a simple linear additive

model of speech planning and organization misses a deeper appreciation of the relationship between length and complexity and error prediction. Alternative views point to nonlinear conceptualizations as providing more fruitful insights (Aichert & Ziegler, 2004a; Cholin, 2008; Cholin & Levelt, 2009; Perret, Schneider, Dayer, & Laganaro, 2012; Staiger & Ziegler, 2008; Ziegler, 2009). In general, nonlinear models propose a view of speech output planning, and phonetic plan organization in particular, where articulatory gestures arise and are organized not in an undifferentiated straight line (plan for /t/ + plan for /o/ + plan for /p/ to arrive at *top*), but in nonlinear hierarchically nested tiers of control (e.g., laryngeal versus oral control subsystems; within the oral control tier, subsystems of jaw versus lip versus tongue control) (Browman & Goldstein, 1992; Ziegler, 2009). Following this conceptualization, probability of derailment in a planning disorder would be predicted to increase more in keeping with gestural complexity, the number of adjustments required to produce a syllable or word or move from one sound to the next, rather than simple additive length. Some examples illustrate this.

Not all consonant clusters are equal. Clusters vary in likelihood of derailment and in which element is affected (Romani & Galluzzi, 2005). Syllable frequency plays a part and can interact with cluster accuracy (Aichert & Ziegler, 2004b; Perret et al., 2012). High frequency of words and syllables may confer a degree of immunity to disruption compared to low-frequency words, where the cluster effect can be especially strong (Ziegler, 2009).

The gestural complexity effect is illustrated where syllables may have a matched surface structure (e.g., both CVC) and word frequency yet diverge in the number of articulator adjustments that need to be controlled to produce the syllable. One would predict greater likelihood of derailment for someone with a speech-planning disorder on the more complex gesture. *Maim* and *tame* are simple CVC structures consisting of high-frequency sounds for English and comparable word frequency. However, in saying *maim* adjustments entail only a velopharyngeal gesture (nasality switch) and a single close-open-close lip gesture. Conversely, in *tame* adjustment demands switches in oral–nasal, voiceless–voiced, stop–continuant, and alternation between lip and tongue tip closure. Such observations suggest incorporating measures of gestural complexity and bi- or triphone predictability when analyzing apraxic breakdown and devising therapy materials.

The integration of gestures into the metrical, rhythmic structure of utterances is also emphasized (Boucher, 2006; Boucher, Garcia, Fleurant, & Paradis, 2001; Brendel & Ziegler, 2008; Janßen & Domahs, 2008; Ziegler, 2013), especially given the prominent prosodic disturbance present in AoS. Stress patterns that depart from the predominant type for a language are more likely to provoke errors in people with AoS. Hence one would predict greater likelihood of derailment for an English speaker, other variables being equal, on saying an unstressed–stressed syllable (e.g., settee) versus stressed–unstressed (city), the latter being the canonical stress pattern for two-syllable words in English. Ziegler (2009) finds that the degree to which speech gestures are integrated into metrical feet reduces workload in phonetic planning and in turn the likelihood of errors.

Taking the points presented, the general tenor of clinical distinctions between dysarthric speech due to neuromuscular impairment and speech associated with disruptions at higher levels of organization (AoS, phonemic paraphasia) is summarized in Table 21.1.

Less consensus exists for whether and how one might distinguish AoS from phonemic paraphasia (Haley et al., 2013; Laganaro, 2012; Perret et al., 2012). Contending claims are inextricably entwined with the debates over output models of speech (see further discussion) and views on the nature of and relation between phonology and phonetics. The story over the past decades has been strongly influenced by a categorical dichotomy that differentiates between the presence of intact articulation (no motor problems) but with disorders of phonological access or phonological representations, which lead to phonemic paraphasia, versus translating well-formed phonological specifications into commands for articulatory execution (i.e., presence of motor problems) said to characterize AoS (Darley, Aronson, & Brown, 1975; van der Merwe, 2008). The quest therefore has been to pinpoint linguistic, phonological (sound selection and ordering) problems versus motor realization (e.g., timing difficulties) on a variety of tasks.

Based on this dichotomy, the general direction of reasoning has been that output from a phonological output lexicon proceeds to phonological assembly. Breakdown there is typified by (depending on severity) more or less persistent phonemic paraphasic slips, with wrong sounds selected (beach sounds like peach; camel like bamel) or right sounds in the wrong order (teapot sounds like peatot). In milder cases, the clinician hears clearly target-oriented word attempts, but in more severe cases, neologistic phonological jargon may predominate. The difficulty affects all spoken output (reading, spontaneous, repetition). Indeed, conduction aphasia is diagnosed when repetition is significantly more impaired than

Table 21.1 Rules of Thumb for Distinguishing Between Apraxic and Paraphasic Speech Versus Dysarthric Speech

Variable	Apraxic and Paraphasic Speech	Dysarthric Speech
Muscle control impairment	None or degree insufficient to explain speech status	Present
Speech–physical status relationship	Pattern of speech errors inconsistent with site and severity of any underlying neuromuscular deficit	Close coupling between nature and site of neuromuscular changes and type and degree of speech problem
Muscle control on casual observation of articulators when not involved in speech	Breath control, phonation, resonance, range of movement of articulators all normal	Similar degree of impairment as seen when asked to engage in conscious action
Vegetative function of articulators	Spontaneously performed nonlanguage functions of the articulators normal (e.g., coughing, laughing, clearing throat, sucking, licking lips)	Dysfunction in keeping with the pattern of physical impairment
Propositionality effect	Present—the more the person has to think about what he or she says, the less frequent the word, the greater the speech problem	Absent—type and degree of severity similar across word classes and nonconscious versus conscious control
Struggle	Visible and audible trial-and-error groping, self-correction to get to and maintain target	Struggle only commensurate with effort to overcome weakness problems
Variability	Wide variations in realization of target segments on repeated trials, diadochokinetic (DDK) tasks and spontaneous speech	Variability clearly linkable to increasing fatigue, waning breath support; cerebellar dysarthria tends to give variable production
Phonation, resonance	Apart from occasional apraxic mutism, normal; or only intermittent dysfunction linked to instances of articulatory breakdown	Constantly affected in keeping with the site and degree of neuromuscular impairment

spontaneous speech. Because the speaker knows what target they are aiming for, output may contain repeated run-ups to a target (conduites d'approche). Longer, phonologically more complex words are more problematic. Repetition and reading of nonsense words are poorer than for real words, ostensibly because the speaker is not able to rely on intact lexical knowledge to aid output, or alternatively, there is impairment of phonological input to output conversion.

This contrasts with AoS, for which lexical processing and phonological assembly are said to be intact, and the problem lies instead in translating the intact frameworks into movements for speech sounds. The expectation would be targets are apparent but segments and transitions are typified by mistiming and misplacement of articulatory movements and not misselection of phonemes.

Alas, these neat divisions have not proved to be so neat (Haley et al., 2013; Laganaro, 2012; Ziegler, Aichert, & Staiger, 2012). It continues to be problematic to identify specific features of phonemic paraphasia/phonological assembly versus AoS problems to secure a differential diagnosis. Similar issues arise in differentiating apraxic from dysarthric sources of mistiming or distortion. For instance, cerebellar lesions lead to dysmetric and dysrhythmic incoordinations very similar or indistinguishable from apraxic distortions.

The reasons for this are numerous. Reliance on surface perceptual characteristics fails to discriminate between diverse underlying etiologies. Even where instrumental analyses have sought to bypass perceptual biases, elements of motor dysfunction are apparent in ostensibly intact phonological strings, and phonological breakdown signs are seen alongside motoric disruption. Conflicting definitions of disorders and divergent predictions concerning error (profiles) based on contrasting models of speech control have further led to contradictory diagnostic claims. The heterogeneous composition of groups that have been compared to settle arguments around unique markers clouds the picture. As elucidated in the following material, because of the essentially interactive nature of speech output control, it is likely that "pure" cases of AoS or phonemic paraphasia are the exception, and that the general rule is that speakers will evidence a mixture of markers of the two extremes. The distinguishable characteristics are outlined in Table 21.2.

Based on the premise that phonology is intact in AoS and disordered in phonemic paraphasia, some authors recommend the use of assessments that purport to tap (internal) phonology but not motor aspects of processing.

Table 21.2 Rules of Thumb for Differentiating Between Paraphasic and Apraxic Type Speech

More to Speech Apraxia	More to Phonemic Paraphasia
Perceived errors are predominantly distortions and substitutions that differ in one (place/manner) feature from the target. Presence of distorted substitutions.	Higher proportion of displacement errors and apparent distant substitutions (multiple feature changes).
On DDK tasks, difficulties are apparent already on single-syllable (/'ta'ta'ta/) repetitions (rhythm, drifting on and off target, effortfulness).	On DDK tasks, the individual performs normally on single-syllable repetition once the individual has latched on to the correct target, but falls down on alternating tasks (e.g., /'pa'ta'ka/).
On alternating tasks, the individual is more likely to have perseveration errors (stuck on one target). /pataka/ may be produced as /papapa/.	Alternating tasks tend to be disrupted by sequence errors or distant substitutions. /pataka/ may be produced as /tapaka/ or /kraftakap/.
Perceptually tends to involve all word classes.	Perceptually tends to be restricted to content words.
Performance on reading or repetition may be better than spontaneous speech.	Speakers with reproduction conduction aphasia are significantly worse on repeating words and sentences compared to spontaneous speech.
Slow rate even in on-target utterances.	(Near) normal rate in on-target utterances.
Inability to increase rate while maintaining phonemic integrity.	Variable ability to increase rate and maintain phonemic accuracy, but rate within normal limits.
Variable, but overall prolonged movement transitions.	Variable, but within normal limits movement transition durations.
Variable, but abnormally long vowels in multisyllable utterances.	Variable, but within normal limits for vowel duration in multisyllable utterances.
Variable, but increased movement durations for individual speech gestures in connected speech.	Variable, but durations within normal limits.

If the phonological, nonmotor tasks fail, then the disorder must be paraphasia. Thus, individuals with phonemic paraphasia are said to fail and people with AoS to succeed on sound and syllable segmentation ("What's the first/last sound in *nose*?" "What's *become* without *be*?"); rhyme judgment ("Do *sign* and *pine* rhyme with each other?") and lexicality tasks ("Is *stelk* a real word?"). Sound and syllable segmentation, though, show wide variation even in the non–brain-damaged population (Nickels & Cole-Virtue, 2004) and can be strongly influenced by literacy acquisition methods and skills (Colaço, Mineiro, & Castro Caldas, 2014; Pattamadilok, Morais, Colin, & Kolinsky, 2014). People with AoS do fail rhyme and lexicality judgments and same–different tasks ("Are these two words the same or different? *pait–pite, face–phase*").

This suggests that the distinction between intact and disordered phonology is not a valid or watertight diagnostic feature. The reason may be because the dichotomy phonology/phonetics and language/motor are not precisely circumscribed (see section on models) or surface production analyses are not sensitive enough to detect different underlying reasons for failing such tasks. A prime candidate for why people with AoS find such tasks difficult is a working memory impairment. There is little doubt that the tasks mentioned tax working memory and that people with AoS display a working memory deficit (Hickok et al., 2014; Rochon, Caplan, & Waters, 1990). Working memory capacity may be diminished by brain damage (to key areas shared with speech and language); AoS may interfere with the rehearsal and refreshing necessary to maintain material in working memory, including prosodic chunking (Boucher, 2006); or probably there is some interaction of the two. Whichever reason, it means reliance on such tests is not productive for differential diagnosis.

Solutions to decisions concerning whether someone is presenting with an apraxic or paraphasic disturbance go beyond clinical assessment techniques. As intimated, the whole controversy may be traced to disputes over models of speech production and arguments surrounding the relationship of phonology and phonetics. For those who uphold a strict division between AoS and phonemic paraphasia, the resolution of how to clinically differentiate between them is merely awaiting *the* key diagnostic features to be recognized. For others, striving to achieve separation based on the dichotomous criteria mentioned is misguided because it remains unclear what the precise underlying impairment(s) is/are in disordered speech programming; by extension, therefore, it remains unclear what one would listen to or look for to distinguish between the disorder types. The following section takes a brief look at some issues regarding models of speech output and their implications for understanding speech motor (dys)function.

Before leaving assessment issues, though, one must underline that while the focus here was on impairment features, this should not preclude equal attention to activity and participation evaluation in terms of how the AoS might affect speech intelligibility, work and leisure pursuits, and impact on self and others.

SPEECH OUTPUT MODELS AND APRAXIA OF SPEECH

Numerous models of speech production exist. Most have been seriously underspecified vis-à-vis what precisely happens within or between their components. Frequently, they are restricted to one domain (e.g., linguistics, physiology). They may lack consideration of how postulated processes relate to neuropsychological and neurophysiological processes in the brain. Within these models, views on the relationship of phonology and phonetics or how motor and sound components relate to each other are diverse, often contradictory, and commonly fudged—for example, covered by statements such as "abstract phonological strings are mapped onto motor commands" without regard to what the phonological strings are or how this mapping occurs or what motor commands might be. Past decades saw the dominance of discrete point, serial order, hierarchical models (Miller, 2000) rooted in a categorical phonology–phonetics split, with feedback limited to external feedback loops (e.g., Darley et al., 1975).

Ultimately these models have failed to produce a viable account of speech output control or its breakdown. How abstract phoneme specifications converted into concrete, physical movements was never convincingly demonstrated. Evidence of phonological influences on movement and motor influences in phonology spoke against the strict separation of phonological and phonetic processes in output and emphasized more interactive processing (Laganaro, 2012; Miller, 2000). Perturbation studies illustrated how control cannot be based exclusively on fixed, top-down, central commands (Mitsuya, MacDonald, Purcell, & Munhall, 2011; Munhall, Lofqvist, & Kelso, 1994; Shaiman & Gracco, 2002). The saliency of the phoneme as the (sole) unit of control could not be sustained (Cholin, 2008; Cholin & Levelt, 2009; Janßen & Domahs, 2008; Ziegler, 2009). The independence of input and output is challenged by findings indicating interaction between perception and production (Hickok, 2012a, 2012b; Nozari, Dell, & Schwartz, 2011). Poeppel, Emmorey, Hickok, and Pylkkänen (2012, p. 14125) summed up the situation with the conclusion that the "era of the classical model is over," asserting that "the model is incorrect along too many dimensions for new research to be considered mere updates" (p. 14126). This discussion largely confirms this, where the search for features derived from these models that might be unique to AoS or aid differentiation of AoS from other disorders has been largely unsuccessful.

It is beyond the scope of this chapter to offer a detailed exposition of models of speech output (see e.g., Hickok, 2012a, 2013b; Houde & Nagarajan, 2011; Ziegler, 2013). The following paragraphs sketch some developments, drawing out how revised conceptualizations of speech control have reshaped our view of AoS and its differentiation from other clinical entities.

Recent approaches to speech output modeling emphasize the unification of phonological and motor dimensions. Speech is movement, but movement constrained by the sound system of a language (Miller, 2000; Ziegler & Ackermann, 2013). A task of output is to produce movements that achieve auditory goals. There are thus, sound and movement targets, but these must be matched through ongoing monitoring to achieve congruence between the two. This suggests auditory–phonological and motor–phonological components are key aspects of such models, with ongoing interaction between them in production (Guenther & Hickok, 2015; McMillan, Corley, & Lickley, 2009; Nozari et al., 2011). A pivotal role is accorded to internal feedback and feedforward mechanisms to provide sensory-guided control to achieve the interaction and matching (Hickok, 2012b; Houde & Nagarajan, 2011; Poeppel et al., 2012). Speech sound (contrasts) are dependent on selecting and ordering the correct configuration and sequence of opening and closing gestures across the whole vocal tract while ensuring tight adjustment of relative timing, phasing, and placement between and within gestures. This argues for elements of production oriented to selection and others to ordering (Goldenberg, 2013), but not necessarily as envisaged in serial, discrete point models as operating independently and sequentially to each other. Rather, they are applied in tandem and in interaction with each other. Furthermore, in contrast to the exclusively cortical focus conjectured in previous models of speech motor control, more active participation is assigned to subcortical structures, most notably the cerebellum and cerebellar-cortical circuits (Dick, Bernal, & Tremblay, 2014; Hickok, 2012a; Kotz & Schwartze, 2010), well in keeping with frequent observations of parallels between ataxic and apraxic disruption to segmental timing and prosodic disturbance.

This represents the tenor of more recent models that are proving successful in accounting for speech acquisition, performance, and breakdown and have opened new avenues for the understanding of AoS and phonemic

paraphasia. Arguments concerning the finer detail of models are ongoing (see, e.g., discussion papers following Hickok, 2013a). The following models illustrate the overall direction of scholarship: the hierarchical state feedback control (HSFC) model of Hickok and others (Guenther & Hickok, 2015; Hickok, 2012a, 2012b, 2013a); the DIVA/GODIVA (gradient order directions into velocities of articulators) model (Bohland, Bullock, & Guenther, 2010; Guenther & Hickok, 2015; Guenther & Vladusich, 2012); and the ACT (short for ACTion) model (Kröger, Miller, & Lowit, 2011; Kröger, Kannampuzha, & Neuschaefer-Rube, 2009). The principles of articulatory/gestural phonology (Browman & Goldstein, 1992) reflect the notions of unification of and transparency between sound and movement control and elements of output responsible for relationships between overall gestures versus internal regulation of gestures. Ziegler and Ackermann (2013) underline that speech control is unique to speech, and though other activities may employ the same effector muscles, functionally different tasks such as oral–nonverbal movements and swallowing entail functionally different control frameworks.

Hickok (2012a) summarizes the HSFC model as comprising lexical–conceptual versus phonological components. The latter incorporate a motor and a sensory system that both receive inputs from the lexical–conceptual system. Activation of an auditory speech form, whether from the lexical–conceptual system or from the external environment, activates a corresponding motor program. The model hypothesizes that higher-level auditory targets encode vocal tract open–close cycles roughly corresponding to syllable-level units. A lower level of control encodes information related to articulatory features for local adjustments of open–close cycle parameters that can be decomposed into somatosensory targets roughly corresponding to phoneme-level units. Central to the model is an internal forward prediction system and feedback control loop. This operates integrally in motor selection and planning from the start rather than merely serving post hoc correction evaluation of motor execution errors (Hickok, 2012b; Houde & Nagarajan, 2011).

DIVA (Guenther & Hickok, 2015; Guenther & Vladusich, 2012), illustrated in Figure 21.1, is a computationally derived model that drives an articulatory synthesizer. GODIVA (Bohland et al., 2010) is an extension to DIVA that incorporates an explicit parallel representation of upcoming utterances that interfaces with learned speech sensorimotor programs. DIVA simulates the acquisition, control, and production of speech sounds but goes beyond other models in claiming empirically supported transparency between computations and activity in specified regions of brain. The model "learns" sounds and lays down speech sound maps through a system of matching

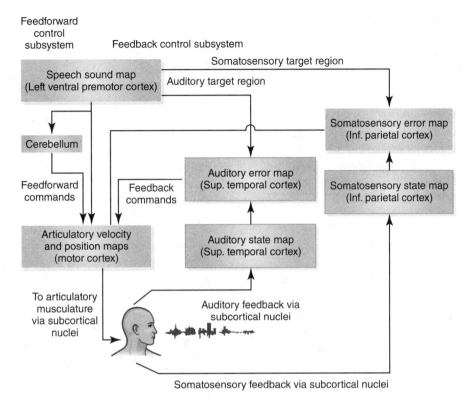

Figure 21.1 The DIVA model.

Figure reproduced by kind permission of Frank Guenther, Boston University, USA, http://www.bu.edu/speechlab/files/2013/05/DIVA. jpg (accessed 31 March 2015).

input to output. Initial coarse distinctions and approximations are gradually refined in childhood via auditory and somatosensory feedback and feedforward loops.

Based on this information, the model learns an auditory target for each sound. Importantly, these are associated not with fixed target points, but target regions that encode permitted movement/signal variability. Somatosensory targets are also learned through repeated production of sounds. During speech development, the feedforward control evolves over time until, eventually, when fully automatized, it can serve alone as the stimulus for sound production under normal circumstances.

According to DIVA, projections from the left frontal operculum (inferior and posterior portion of Broca's area), supplemented by cerebellar connections, reach the primary motor cortex, and these form feedforward motor commands, or an efferent copy as this has sometimes been termed. Error detection and correction circuits (posited to reside in temporal–parietal brain regions) monitor and fine-tune performance. The speech sound maps that form the basis of articulatory activity, following the principles of mirror neurons (Guenther & Vladusich, 2012), are activated when sounds are both heard and produced (for discussion concerning mirror neuron function in speech, see Hickok, 2010).

Kröger et al. (2011) employed ACT (Kröger et al., 2009), a model similar to DIVA, to simulate apraxic errors. The model shows how perceived aspects of AoS such as trial-and-error groping, and consonant and vowel distortions could arise from errors in temporal–gestural coordination linked to particular defects in mappings (e.g., phonetic to motor plan) or processing (e.g., the motor-planning module itself).

Support for these classes of models has come from computer modeling, but more crucially from imaging and experimental investigations and from case reports with speakers with and without brain damage, which, in contrast to earlier models, provides support that proposed components and processes are compatible with neurophysiological activity during speech (Dick et al., 2014; Guenther & Vladusich, 2012; Hickok, 2012a, 2012b; Lotte et al., 2015; Perret et al., 2012).

The ways in which these mechanisms may be impaired, and what the sound and movement consequences might be, provides new insights into the bases of motor speech disorders and their characteristics. Based on the models mentioned, AoS and phonemic paraphasia arise from disruptions within a single mechanism but to different processes within the overall scheme. Derailments could arise from a variety of nodes in the model, such as:

- a misselection of gestural scores (i.e., the overall "plans," such as wrong opening or closing settings and sequences);
- a problem of access to or degradation of scores (Aichert & Ziegler, 2004a, 2004b; Mailend & Maas, 2013);
- an unresolved or erroneously resolved competition within the system between competing scores and gesture internal adjustments can lead to a perceived sound change (Nozari et al., 2011) (e.g., unresolved competition between the tongue tip versus dorsum raising in target *take* may lead to what the listener hears as *cake*, or /ceɪk/, or /tʃeɪk/);
- a correct sequence of opening–closing may be applied to the wrong articulator (e.g., closing gesture to tongue dorsum instead of lips)

One consequence of this is that for most patients, the error picture will result in both selection and ordering derailments, and pure forms of these will be rare (Laganaro, 2012; Perret et al., 2012). Perturbation of the adjustments themselves and (failure of) detection and correction of errors during output may serve as further possible sources of breakdown (Hickok, 2012b; Maas et al., 2015).

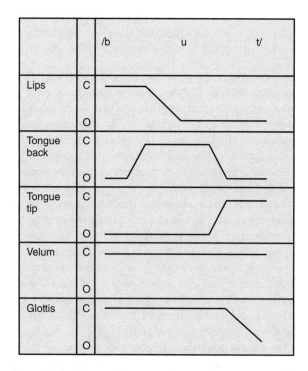

Figure 21.2 Schematic representation of the movement and phasing of main articulators to produce the word 'boot', /but/. C = closed, O = open.

Source: Based on figure from Miller N (2000). Changing ideas in apraxia of speech. In I Papathanasiou (Ed.), Acquired neurogenic communication disorders (p. 182). London, UK: Whurr. Reproduced for this volume with permission of Wiley Publishers, Hoboken, NJ, USA. Not for further reproduction.

Deger and Ziegler (2002) concluded that, in AoS, a prime difficulty may be integrating syllables into a single motor program (and incidentally the authors thereby provide an account for the tendency to syllabification in AoS). In their study, people with AoS succeeded in production of syllable strings of different lengths, which entailed simple repetition of the same syllable (e.g., dada versus dadada), but failed when alternating between syllables was demanded (e.g., daba). Other evidence points to sequential integration as a possible locus of breakdown, contrasting with impairment of plan internal adjustments (e.g. tongue height, grooved versus flattened tongue). For instance, Klapp (2003) put forth a model that involves an element that retrieves and unpacks separate motor programs or speech sound maps in their assigned sequence versus processes that prepare the internal spatiotemporal properties for a program. In keeping with this, Maas, Robin, Wright, and Ballard (2008) and Wright et al. (2009) uncovered dissociations between a process responsible for organizing the internal features of a programmed unit versus a process involved in organizing sequences of programmed units for output. Maas and Mailend (2012) and Mailend and Maas (2013) lent further support to this direction through their review of reaction time studies with people with AoS and delayed picture–word interference tasks.

Hickok (e.g., 2012a), within his HSFC model, has proposed that conduction aphasia arises from the role of the sensory system in production. Specifically, the latter defines the targets and online monitoring of speech actions. In conduction aphasia, there is an interruption of the system that serves at the interface between auditory targets and the motor speech actions to achieve them. Without clear targets, output will be derailed, in particular for more complex and less automated targets. Articulatory parameters are intact in pure conduction aphasia since frontal motor circuits are unaffected, hence normal prosody and undistorted derailments. In AoS, access to motor phonological codes is affected. However, because the whole system is interactive and speech is emergent from this interaction, phonetic derailments can still arise from competing activation of lexical items and their sound patterns and between open–close cycle specifications and their phonetic timing adjustments (Laganaro, 2012).

Based on a schematic representation of the chief opening and closing gestures and their relative timing in producing the word *boot* (Figure 21.2), Miller (2000) illustrated possible sources of breakdown within the ACT model that, along with similar models, envisages gestural cycle selection and ordering and fine-tuning within and between sequences.

Failure of selection of a tongue back closing gesture would result in hearing /baːt/ or /bʌt/ instead of /but/.

Failure to perform the syllable final glottis opening gesture would lead to /bud/ being heard, while applying an open–close glottal sequence instead of close–open would give what sounds like /pud/. Applying the initial closing gesture to the tongue tip rather than lips would bring about /dut/. Mis- or unresolved competition between the gestural scores of, for example, boot-loot-shoot may result in frank substitution with /lut/ or /ʃut/ or apparent distorted substitution such as /bˡut/.

At the more local level, perturbation of spatiotemporal fine-tuning and resolution could lead to both perceived substitutions and distortions. If the timing of the glottal opening gesture is delayed, the auditory outcome would sound like /bud/; incomplete lip closing may be heard as /wut/, /vut/, or /ut/. Delayed or prolonged offset of the final tongue tip closure may result in what sounds like /buts/ or /butʃ/. As has been illustrated in other studies (Pouplier & Hardcastle, 2005), mistimings may cause one (misdirected) gesture to mask another, resulting in perceived omissions, so premature tongue tip raising may mask the tongue dorsum raising to sound like /bit/ or a distorted vowel midway between /u/ and /i/. Masking of tongue tip raising by a delayed tongue dorsum raising gesture in *clean* may give the impression of an omitted /l/, or the initial cluster sounds like a lateral fricative. Conversely, overseparation of gestures may have the effect of leading to perceived additions. Unlinking the tongue tip and velum gestures at the end of *clean* may produce what sounds like *cleaned*.

What is underlined here is that sound derailments are not the result of misselected sound targets but of movement patterns. Producing /kaɪməl/ for Michael may sound like a substitution of /k/ for /m/ or transposition of sounds, but the impairment is due to misselection or misordering of articulatory gestures associated with the underlying apraxia. Hearing *pear* for *bear* may sound like a substitution of one phoneme for another, but the origin in speech-planning breakdown is likely to be mistiming between the oral and laryngeal voice onset time (VOT) gestures.

This section has drawn attention to how new conceptualizations of speech output control have attempted to move beyond the mutually exclusive division between premotor and motor, phonological and phonetic, sensory and motor, frameworks that ultimately have not succeeded in producing viable accounts of clinical pictures. More recent endeavors to describe or account for aspects of speech output have emphasized the interactive nature of output control, interaction between top-down and bottom-up influences, and the importance of online feedforward and feedback monitoring. Moves have been toward solving the mental–physical divide conundrum, where abstract plans by some sleight of hand turned into concrete movements. Solutions offered have been in the direction of unitary models where more abstract specifications, that is, gestural scores, are already in terms of parameters that can be directly related to overall goal-directed actions and the individual movements (opening and closing gestures, phasing between gestures) required to achieve them. They have also been in the direction of models that have sought to be transparent in the relationship between speech motor control parameters and underlying neurophysiological processes, a topic now briefly addressed.

LESION SITES ASSOCIATED WITH APRAXIA OF SPEECH

Which part(s) of the brain one believes is/are associated with AoS depends very much on what one considers to be impaired in apraxic speech and the location(s) of that process in the brain. Hence, many different sites have been suggested. An earlier claim (Dronkers, 1996) declaring the left/dominant anterior insula a sole seat of speech apraxic breakdown and therefore, the location to search for the nature of the disorder has not been accepted based on various criticisms of the studies and counterexamples (Hillis et al., 2004; Robin, Jacks, & Ramage, 2008). Dronkers's (1996) inclusion and exclusion criteria for AoS meant that individuals with dysarthria and with aphasia (and phonemic paraphasia) were highly likely to have been included. Although the speakers may well have had overlapping lesions in the insular region, many studies report people with lesions or hypoperfusion in the insula who are free of speech output disorders, who have AoS associated with lesions not implicating the insula, or whose insular lesion is associated with phonemic paraphasias and not AoS (Ballard, Tourville, & Robin, 2014; Deutsch, 1984; Graff-Radford et al., 2014; Hillis et al., 2004; Peach & Tonkovich, 2004; Trupe et al., 2013). Recent studies (e.g., Oh, Duerden, & Pang, 2014) support a role of parts of the left and right insulae in speech production but stress that the role may be one of a functional hub integrating or relaying messages from a distributed system rather than performing a unique or primary function in speech production.

It is not hard to see why the situation regarding lesion sites is unclear. Recall previous comments regarding varying inclusion criteria for studies of AoS. Given the apparent rarity of pure cases of AoS, it can be problematic (especially in studies that did not have available to them some of the more sophisticated functional imaging techniques developed recently) to sift out which part of the lesion or symptom picture might be associated with AoS and which with co-occurring disruptions (therefore the indispensability of detailed aphasia, motor, and broader neuropsychological assessments alongside speech assessments). Some earlier studies lacked the benefits of control speakers with other identified disorders or free of neurological disruption or did not control for variations such as habitual versus slowed speech. The variety of speech tasks employed across studies also clouds comparisons. Activation and output in AoS and other speech disorders vary according to speaking task and materials (e.g., reading, repetition, naming versus imagining saying the word; nonsense versus real words; single words versus connected speech).

Others argue that pursuing a reductionist quest for *the* site of AoS will always prove fruitless. Speech is not a one-dimensional phenomenon that operates in isolation and that is likely to be located in a single site or circuit. Speech is based on sounds, sounds are linked to meaning, but sounds are produced from movements. Movements are not random. They are tightly tied to the system of sound contrasts, phonotactic possibilities, and syllabic and rhythmic structure of a language (Miller & Lowit, 2014). Differentiation between sounds relies on contrasting movements geared to auditory ends. Contrasts arise out of variations in timing and phasing between movements and shaping of articulators. Movements are shaped by targets of production, be they auditory memories, space–time targets, gestural codes, or whatever. Speech also interacts with language variables (e.g., lexicon, sentence stress, affective content) and, importantly, also with other cognitive neuropsychological variables (e.g., attention, short- and long-term memory; Hickok et al., 2014; Rochon et al., 1990; Sidiropoulos, de Bleser, Ackermann, & Preilowski, 2008).

Recent models (DIVA, HSFC, ACT; see previous discussion) see control represented in a complex network of sites and pathways, with brain areas involved well beyond the traditional Wernicke's–Broca's axis (Ballard et al., 2014; Dick et al., 2014; Lotte et al., 2015; Price, 2012). Just as intelligibility is not the property of any one articulator (Miller, 2013), speech sound production is not encapsulated in any one location. It emerges from the interaction of all the components, with the possibility that disruption may stem from the very act of interaction and integration, not dysfunction in any particular component part. In HSFC, Poeppel et al. (2012) posit and offer evidence for an early (prelinguistic) decoding, largely bilaterally organized ventral stream processing input for comprehension, and a strongly left-dominant dorsal stream mapping acoustic speech signals directly to frontal articulatory networks.

The role of mirror neurons in (among other things) acquisition of motor control, perception and production of speech, and cross-modal transitions and meaning-sound-movement associations underscores the interactive nature of speech processing (Guenther & Vladusich, 2012; Hickok, 2010). Mirror neurons provide a framework for solutions to issues surrounding the relationship between phonological specifications and motor commands insofar as they present hypotheses for seamless links between input and output and between meaning and sound representations and mappings between sound and movement targets without having to create additional, discrete stages of processing to translate intention into articulation.

Ideally, we desire complete transparency between descriptions of brain functioning and models of speech motor control. Solutions await the development of models that permit this convergence. Currently, this situation does not pertain, although studies concerning the DIVA, ACT, and HSFC models offer firm claims based on empirical evidence that can be further refined.

TREATMENT

Lessons From Theoretical Frameworks

Given the preceding reflections on the assumed underlying mechanisms of breakdown in AoS, what pointers might this give toward intervention strategies covered in the following sections? Apraxia of speech represents a disorder of manipulation of planning and control units in output, not a disorder of primary sensorimotor parameters. This points to following PML to reestablish underlying programs (Ludlow et al., 2008). Motor programs and intelligibility, though, are built up/defined within systems of contrasts (Miller, 2013). This suggests a role for minimal pair therapies. Given the importance of feedforward and feedback in this process, there is a need to emphasize self-monitoring. The role of mirror neurons suggests watch-and-listen/imitation therapies will assist (re)acquisition. Speech is dynamic; it arises from supraglottic movements modifying an underlying airstream and phonation. Hence, practice of static postures or isolated elements of movements divorced from the overall gesture, from breathing and phonation and adjustment of the articulators, which includes arbitrary nonspeech movements, should have no place. Because sounds only ever occur in context, this advocates whole-syllable/word/utterance-level units in practice. Because AoS is associated with difficulties in transitions between sounds, practice of sounds or part movements in isolation and then endeavoring to piece them together again is likely to prove counterproductive. Because metrical, stress/rhythm properties of utterances are integral to speech motor plans and intelligibility, incorporation of rhythmic variation or contrasts is warranted from the start. Because difficulty of sound sequences appears to be linked closely to the number of adjustments to the vocal tract that are required from point to point, then (especially in more severe cases) syllables and contrasts are built up from minimal to gradually more and more degrees of freedom in control. Slowing speech appears to improve output in AoS, most likely for a variety of reasons. How far, though, are such notions and predictions borne out in practice? The chapter now turns to the topic of specific interventions for AoS.

Treatment Approaches

Knowledge concerning treatment for AoS has increased significantly since the first published investigation of a therapy for AoS in 1973 (Rosenbek, Lemme, Ahern, Harris, & Wertz, 1973). Many therapeutic approaches have been developed, and a growing evidence base supporting behavioral interventions for AoS now exists. Converging evidence from AoS treatment investigations, the motor learning literature (Schmidt & Lee, 2005), neuroscience (Kleim & Jones, 2008), and models of speech motor control (Guenther, 2006) may allow realization of the development of a principled technology of AoS treatment in the near future.

The ANCDS AoS Treatment Guidelines Writing Committee provided the first evidence-based AoS treatment guidelines report; this report became available in 2006 (Wambaugh, Duffy, McNeil, Robin, & Rogers, 2006a, 2006b). The committee reviewed and critically evaluated the extant English language literature pertaining to treatment for AoS published through 2003. On the basis of evaluation of 59 published investigations, they reported that although the evidence base for AoS treatment was relatively sparse and lacking in many respects, there was sufficient support for the statement that "individuals with AoS can be expected to make improvements in speech production as a result of treatment, even when AoS is chronic" (Wambaugh et al., 2006b, p. lxiii). The ANCDS AoS Treatment Guidelines Writing Committee recently completed a systematic review of AoS treatment publications that is intended as an update of the original guidelines report (Ballard et al., 2015). The committee identified and evaluated 26 AoS treatment reports published from 2004 through 2012. They reported that the body of AoS treatment evidence has been substantially strengthened through the addition of these more recent reports.

The AoS studies that comprised the original AoS guidelines reports were described as falling into one of four categories of general approaches to AoS remediation.

These categories were based on similarities across therapeutic rationale, treatment targets, and treatment techniques: (a) articulatory-kinematic treatments, (b) rate/rhythm control treatments, (c) intersystemic facilitation/reorganization treatments, and (d) alternative augmentative communication (AAC) approaches (Wambaugh et al., 2006b). At the time of the 2006 guidelines report, the majority of AoS treatment studies were characterized as "articulatory–kinematic" (29 of 59 studies), with the remaining studies distributed across the other categories. Ballard et al. (2015) found that 24 of the 26 studies included in their recent systematic review were articulatory–kinematic in nature. The remaining two investigations were rate/rhythm control approaches. The four AoS guidelines categories of treatments are used as an organizational framework for the following discussion of AoS treatments. The discussion includes information from treatment studies summarized in the guidelines report and associated systematic review as well as from more recent reports.

Articulatory–Kinematic Approaches

The majority of the evidence base for treatment of AoS consists of reports of therapies that are considered to be articulatory–kinematic in nature (Ballard et al., 2015; Wambaugh et al., 2006b). Articulatory–kinematic techniques aim to improve speech production through facilitating spatial targeting, movement, or coordination of the articulators. The ANCDS AoS guidelines committee provided an effectiveness rating of "probably effective" and recommended "that articulatory-kinematic approaches be utilized with individuals with moderate to severe AoS who demonstrate disrupted communication due to disturbances in the spatial and temporal aspects of speech production" (Wambaugh et al., 2006b, p. lxii).

A variety of techniques have been used to promote improved articulation in speakers with AoS. There have been no direct comparisons of specific articulatory–kinematic techniques, and in most treatment investigations, a combination of techniques has been used. The following discussion addresses techniques included across all investigations considered to be articulatory–kinematic.

Repeated, motoric practice has been included as an important ingredient of almost all articulatory–kinematic treatments. Repeated practice is likely one of the most potent treatment factors and is in keeping with findings from the limb motor learning literature (Schmidt & Lee, 2005), principles of experience-dependent neural plasticity (Kleim & Jones, 2008), and neural models of speech production (Guenther, 2006). As noted by Ludlow and colleagues (2008), "Changes in neural substrates will occur only as a result of extensive and prolonged practice and . . . neural changes may not become consolidated until later in the training process" (p. S243). Wambaugh, Nessler, Cameron, and Mauszycki (2012) examined the effects of a treatment consisting of repeated practice with minimal performance feedback with 10 speakers with chronic AoS and aphasia. They found that repeated practice alone (with no other therapy techniques employed) resulted in substantial improvements in articulation for 8 of the 10 participants. This study highlighted the potential benefits of repeated practice as a key therapeutic ingredient in AoS treatment.

Modeling–repetition has been a frequently used method for eliciting productions in AoS treatments. A variation of modeling–repetition, *integral stimulation* (i.e., watch me, listen to me, say it with me) has also often been included in AoS therapies (LaPointe, 1984; Rosenbek et al., 1973; Wambaugh, Kalinyak-Fliszar, West, & Doyle, 1998). The use of modeling–repetition and integral stimulation is consistent with the theorized importance of the development of sound target regions through sensory information associated with speech (Guenther, 2006) and the hypothesized role of mirror neurons in speech production (Ahlsen, 2008).

As discussed by Wambaugh and Shuster (2008), "Integral stimulation attempts to bring to a conscious level of awareness the 'look' and 'sound' of the movement pattern, while combining this awareness with simultaneous practice" (p. 1022). Many other articulatory–kinematic techniques also are designed to augment the individual's own auditory and somatosensory feedback by focusing on various sensory aspects of speech production.

Speech-generating AAC devices have been used by Lasker and colleagues (Lasker, Stierwalt, Hageman, & LaPointe, 2008; Lasker, Stierwalt, Spence, & Cavin-Root, 2010) to provide opportunities for practice with an auditory model. That is, the AAC device was used in place of the clinician to provide an auditory-only model for use in repeated practice. This practice strategy was employed with practice at home (Lasker et al., 2008, 2010) and was also paired with webcam interactive technology for remote delivery of treatment (Lasker et al., 2010). Because the focus of treatment was on improving articulation of speech rather than on use of the device to augment or replace speech, the studies by Lasker and colleagues were considered to represent articulatory–kinematic approaches to treatment (Ballard et al., 2015).

Articulatory cueing entails the provision of descriptions of how sounds are produced with respect to *what* (which articulators), *where* (positioning or location), and *how* (manner and voicing) the articulators should be behaving. Articulatory cueing may take the form of verbal instructions (e.g., /p/: "put your lips together and make a popping sound"), visual modeling, drawings, videotaped depictions, or manipulation of the orofacial musculature by the clinician. Ideally, articulatory cueing should occur within the context of the target utterance and not in isolation. *Phonetic derivation, key word,* or other shaping techniques (Wertz, LaPointe, & Rosenbek, 1984) may be combined with articulatory cueing. A production that is already in the patient's repertoire (e.g., speech sound, nonspeech verbalization or movement, or well-learned word or phrase) is used as the basis for shaping a new production. For example, if a patient can produce /i/ but not /ɝ/, the patient may be instructed to produce /i/ and then move his or her tongue posteriorly along the palate to approximate /ɝ/.

Instrumental feedback approaches have received increased attention, as noted by Ballard and colleagues (Ballard et al., 2015). Data from several different areas of study indicate that persons with AoS may benefit from instrumentally generated biofeedback.

Electropalatography (EPG) is a method that provides a real-time visual display of the tongue's position relative to the palate. It involves the speaker wearing a custom-fitted pseudopalate, which is an acrylic plate embedded with a varying number of electrodes that fits tightly against the hard palate. The electrodes detect tongue-to-palate contacts, and signals are directed to an external processor via a lead-out wire that attaches to a computer, enabling the timing and location of tongue-to-palate contacts to be recorded, stored, and displayed. The clinician and patient can each wear a pseudopalate so that the clinician's display may serve as a model for target productions. Thus, visual targets are possible, as is real-time visual feedback. Electropalatography has been used successfully to treat different types of speech production disorders, including those associated with hearing disorders, cleft palate, glossectomy, and dysarthria (Gibbon, 2006). Limited research has been conducted to date with respect to EPG and treatment of AoS. Howard and Varley (1995) described improvements in articulation in a case study with an individual with AoS. Recently, Mauszycki and colleagues applied EPG in the context of single-subject multiple baseline designs with two persons with chronic AoS and aphasia; positive changes in articulation were found for both participants (Mauszycki, Wambaugh, & Aikyama, 2015). Increasing availability of this technology is likely to lead to increased research and application with patients with AoS.

Electromagnetic articulography (EMA) has also been used to provide visual biofeedback of the articulators. Electromagnetic articulography provides online tracking of articulator movements through the use of magnetic fields and small receiver coils that are affixed to the articulators. Katz, Bharadwaj, and Carstens (1999) were the first to demonstrate use of EMA with a speaker with AoS and reported improved /s/-/ʃ/ contrasts in response to treatment. Katz, McNeil, and colleagues (Katz, McNeil, & Garst, 2010; McNeil et al., 2010) completed a series of single-subject experimental studies investigating the utility of EMA in the treatment of AoS. The investigators found that AoS speakers benefited from EMA-augmented feedback, with improvements found for production of various speech targets. At the current time, the relatively high cost of EMA would be prohibitive for most clinical use.

Ballard, Maas, and Robin (2007) employed spectrographic displays to treat voicing with two speakers with AoS. Spectrographic feedback was used along with articulatory cues during prepractice instruction to facilitate production of continuous voicing and appropriate VOT. Both speakers demonstrated improvements in continuous voicing, and one speaker displayed improvements in VOT.

Preliminary evidence is available for the use of ultrasound visual feedback in the treatment of AoS. Improved production of rhotics was noted for a speaker with chronic AoS with provision of ultrasound visual feedback, verbal instruction and feedback, and repeated practice (Preston & Leaman, 2014).

Specific AoS treatment protocols that utilize a combination of articulatory–kinematic techniques have been developed. Most published AoS treatment investigations have used a combination of articulatory–kinematic techniques. However, only a few unified treatments have received systematic study such that their effects have been replicated (Wambaugh, 2002). The ANCDS AoS Treatment Guidelines Writing Committee is in the process of describing and evaluating synthesized evidence associated with specific therapy protocols or techniques. Several treatment protocols for which treatment effects have been studied repeatedly are discussed briefly in the following sections.

Rosenbek and colleagues (1973) were the first to describe and provide evidence for an AoS treatment protocol (Rosenbek et al., 1973). Their eight-step continuum included steps that progressed from imitation of target utterances with maximal clinician cueing to production of target utterances in role play, with clinician support being reduced systematically. Evidence for improved production of target words, phrases, and sentences with application of the eight-step continuum is available from several case study reports (Deal & Florance, 1978; Rosenbek et al., 1973; Simmons, 1978).

Prompts for Restructuring Oral and Muscular Phonetic Targets (PROMPT; Square, Martin, & Bose, 2001) is a well-developed therapy approach for delivering tactile–kinesthetic cues concerning articulation (i.e., place of articulation, timing, transitioning, and amount and type of contraction) to enhance sensory feedback. The therapy can be tailored to meet individual patient needs and has been used to improve levels of speech production ranging from movement parameters such as jaw opening to sentence productions. This treatment approach requires training for appropriate application (www.promptinstitute.com). The reader is referred to the work of Square et al. (2001) for a more complete description.

Sound production treatment (SPT; Wambaugh et al., 1998) consists of a response-contingent hierarchy that is directed toward specific sound targets in words, phrases, or sentences. The steps, which increase in the amount of clinician instruction, are as follows: (a) verbal modeling with repetition; (b) graphemic cueing (letter representing target sound) with modeling and repetition; (c) integral stimulation; and (d) articulatory cueing. Sound production treatment has received relatively extensive, systematic study, with findings indicating (a) consistent gains in articulatory accuracy of treated sounds in trained word/phrase/sentence contexts, (b) consistent generalization to untrained exemplars of trained items, and (c) limited generalization to untrained, unrelated sounds. The findings from 24 participants across multiple SPT investigations have recently been synthesized using meta-analytic procedures; effect sizes for SPT are now available that provide an indication of the magnitude of changes expected with treated and untreated items (D. Bailey, Eatchel, & Wambaugh, in press). Effect sizes were mostly positive and large, with benchmarks for untreated items slightly smaller than those for treated items.

Comparison of articulatory–kinematic techniques has rarely occurred. Rose and Douglas (2006) compared three modes of delivering articulatory instructions in an investigation with a single AoS speaker. They used a simultaneous treatment design with multiple baselines to examine the effects of three treatments on accuracy of naming. The three treatments all entailed contrasting imitation, target, and error productions; providing information about manner and place of production; and providing reinforcement. One treatment delivered articulatory instructions via gesturally cued articulation, a second treatment provided verbal phoneme placement cueing, and the third treatment combined both methods. Rose and Douglas found large effect sizes for all of the treatments with no clinically relevant differences among treatments. Thus, their findings suggested that, for their patient, the type of information provided (i.e., articulatory instruction contrasting target with error) was more important than the way in which the information was delivered.

Rate and Rhythm Control Approaches

Treatments that control either the rate or the rhythm of speech production during practice have been demonstrated to have positive effects for persons with AoS (Ballard et al., 2015; Wambaugh et al., 2006b). Techniques have included metronomic pacing (Dworkin & Abkarian, 1996; Dworkin, Abkarian, & Johns, 1988; Mauszycki & Wambaugh, 2008; Wambaugh & Martinez, 2000); computer pacing of oral reading (Southwood, 1987); metrical frame pacing (Brendel & Ziegler, 2008; Brendel, Ziegler, & Deger, 2000); and use of a pacing board (McHenry & Wilson, 1994).

The evidence base supporting the use of rate and rhythm treatments for AoS consists of case studies, several single-subject experimental investigations, and a small-group experimental investigation. The ANCDS AoS guidelines committee provided a likelihood rating of "possibly effective," indicating that such treatments may have positive outcomes for AoS patients. With respect to recommendations for use, the committee indicated that rate and rhythm approaches should be considered treatment "options" (Wambaugh et al., 2006b).

The general rationale underlying the use of rate and rhythm treatments is that AoS is characterized by disturbances in the timing of speech production and rhythm is a fundamental component of the speech production process. Specific mechanisms for the effects of rate and rhythm treatments remain speculative. It has been suggested that rhythm control treatments for AoS may help reestablish temporal patterning (or metrical processing; Brendel & Ziegler, 2008; Brendel et al., 2000). In addition, it has been theorized that central pattern generators (CPGs) are involved in speech production (Barlow, Finan, & Park, 2004) and may be disrupted in AoS (Dworkin & Abkarian, 1996). Rhythmic treatments are a form of entrainment (phase locking of movements/rhythms) that may facilitate functioning of CPGs (Wambaugh & Martinez, 2000). Although speakers with AoS typically exhibit reduced rate, further slowing of speech production through pacing is thought to provide additional time for motor planning or programming as well as for processing of sensory feedback.

Metronomic pacing treatments involve repeatedly practicing the treatment targets in time with the beat of a metronome. Selection of rate of production has varied across investigations. Dworkin and colleagues (Dworkin & Abkarian, 1996; Dworkin et al., 1988) began treatment at very low rates of production (i.e., 15 and 30 beats per minute [bpm], respectively) and increased to 120 bpm over the course of the investigations. Wambaugh and Martinez (2000) calculated the patient's average word durations and selected a metronome rate (93 bpm)

that would result in word durations being increased by 50%. They also increased rate over the course of the investigation and eventually introduced a syncopated rhythm to approximate a more natural speech rhythm. Mauszycki and Wambaugh (2008) also used their patient's habitual utterance durations to determine metronome settings and systematically increased durations 10%, and then decreased durations in 10% increments. For clinical purposes, it is suggested that the patient's typical rate of production be considered in selecting a practice rate. Also, trial therapy employing different metronome settings may be utilized to determine appropriate practice rates.

Behaviors targeted for treatment have also varied across and within investigations. For example, Dworkin and colleagues (Dworkin & Abkarian, 1996; Dworkin et al., 1988) developed a treatment that progressed from raising and lowering the tongue to the beat of the metronome, to alternate motion rate production, to multisyllabic word production, and finally to sentence production. Dworkin and Abkarian (1996) focused on improving voicing control and devised a treatment in which isolated vowels and vowel plus /h/ sequences were practiced. Wambaugh and Martinez (2000) trained multisyllabic words with differing stress patterns, and Mauszycki and Wambaugh (2008) trained multisyllabic words and phrases.

The way in which practice with a metronome is organized and applied has not been systematically investigated. It is likely that the patient will initially require instruction or modeling to be able to produce target items in time with the metronome. The reader is referred to the work of Wambaugh and Martinez (2000) for an example of a treatment protocol in which clinician participation is gradually withdrawn.

Metronomic pacing has not been directly compared to other treatment approaches. However, Wambaugh et al. (2012) applied metronomic rate/rhythm treatment following repeated practice treatment (discussed previously). In addition, modest gains were found for several participants with application of rate/rhythm treatment.

The use of metrical pacing is closely related to metronomic pacing but goes a step beyond in that the metrical form or rhythm of the target utterance is imposed (Brendel & Ziegler, 2008; Brendel et al., 2000). The investigators devised "metrical templates" for target utterance based on syllable onset times derived from waveforms of the utterances produced with natural prosody at a normal rate. The templates were used to ensure that the pacing tones could be presented at different rates while keeping the natural, *relative distances* of the syllables of the utterance constant. That is, the pacing tones reflect the natural rhythm of the utterances, regardless of rate of production (this is in contrast to metronome pacing, which does not take into account the natural rhythm of the utterance).

Brendel and Ziegler (2008) compared metrical pacing therapy (MPT) to a control treatment with 10 speakers with AoS ranging from mild to severe. Approximately 15 target items were individually devised for each patient. The patients were provided with repeated models of the target utterances and were familiarized with the pacing signal. They were instructed to produce the target in synchrony with the pacing rhythm and to maintain fluent articulation while not attending closely to articulation. Treatment also included hand tapping to stress syllable onsets and choral speaking, with clinician participation fading as needed. Rates of production were determined by baseline rates and were reduced and increased as needed. The control treatment included use of a variety of articulatory kinematic techniques (e.g., phonetic placement, gestural facilitation, integral stimulation, minimal pair contrast, word derivation), but with no focus on rhythm or metrical features. The investigators reported that both treatments were associated with significantly reduced numbers of sound errors, but only MPT resulted in a reduced proportion of dysfluencies and changes in duration.

Brendel and Ziegler's (2008) finding that pacing resulted in improved articulation, without any specific articulation treatment, was consistent with findings from metronomic pacing treatments that included no articulatory training (Mauszycki & Wambaugh, 2008; Wambaugh & Martinez, 2000). Improved articulatory accuracy without specific instruction has also been reported with the use of prolonged speech and computer-controlled slow rate (Southwood, 1987).

Other methods are available for slowing rate but have received limited study. A pacing board (i.e., a board with regularly spaced, raised crosspieces) is a device used to slow rates by having the patient move the hand/finger along the board in time to the production of syllables. McHenry and Wilson (1994) provide a case study report in which a pacing board is one component of a treatment regime for an individual with severe AoS and dysarthria. Finger counting (e.g., raising one finger at a time in conjunction with syllable production) has also been reported in one investigation with a patient with severe AoS and aphasia (Simmons, 1978).

Intersystemic Facilitation/Reorganization Approaches

Intersystemic facilitation/reorganization refers to the use of a relatively intact system to facilitate functioning of a more impaired system (Rosenbek, Collins, & Wertz, 1976). Gestures have been used to facilitate speech production in speakers with AoS (Code & Gaunt, 1986; Raymer & Thompson, 1991; Simmons, 1978). Different types of gestures have been used and include meaningful gestures (Code & Gaunt, 1986; Raymer & Thompson, 1991); nonmeaningful gestures such as hand tapping or finger counting (Simmons, 1978; Wertz et al., 1984); and cued articulation gestures (Rose & Douglas, 2006; Square et al., 2001). In the 2006 ANCDS AoS guidelines report, intersystemic treatments included relatively few investigations, were rated as being possibly effective, and were recommended to be considered a treatment option. Ballard et al. (2015) found that no recent treatment studies utilized treatment techniques that were described as intersystemic facilitation/reorganization.

Gestural stimulation has been paired with articulatory–kinematic techniques in several investigations. For example, Simmons (1978) incorporated finger counting in the Rosenbek et al. (1973) eight-step continuum. Rose and Douglas (2006) used gestures as an instructional mode for providing articulatory cuing. Similarly, PROMPT (Square et al., 2001) employs tactile–kinesthetic cues to provide information concerning articulatory-kinematics.

Melodic intonation therapy (MIT) was developed in the early 1970s as a behavioral therapy for severe nonfluent aphasia. Its developers theorized that MIT's effects derived from the right cerebral hemisphere's dominance for musical abilities and speech prosody (Sparks, Helm, & Albert, 1974). Thus, MIT could be considered to represent an intersystemic facilitation/reorganization approach to the treatment of aphasia. The treatment paradigm includes repeated practice of target utterances using a slowed rate of speech production with musical intoning. Verbal productions are accompanied by hand tapping. Melodic intonation therapy entails a gradual progression through multiple levels of practice wherein the clinician's modeling and participation are systematically reduced. In addition to promoting improved language production, MIT has the potential to positively impact the symptoms of AoS. Elements of MIT, such as modeling, repeated practice, hand tapping, and slowing the rate of speech production have all been shown to improve articulation in AoS (Wambaugh et al., 2006b).

However, the effects of MIT on AOS have received little research attention. There were early anecdotal reports of improvement in articulation following MIT (Sparks & Holland, 1976), and Sparks (2008) reported that clinicians have been using a "phonological" form of MIT (no data provided). Zumbansen, Peretz, and Hébert (2014) have cautioned that what some clinicians carry out under the label of MIT is not as originally envisaged by Sparks et al. (1974). They underline that it remains to be determined what the precise mechanisms of operation might be in those speakers for whom MIT does appear successful. Merrett, Peretz, and Wilson (2014) argue for effects on several interrelated levels. Recent work (van der Meulen, van de Sandt-Koenderman, Heijenbrok-Kal, Visch-Brink, & Ribbers, 2014) has suggested some improvements in repetition and overall communication associated with MIT in individuals with chronic nonfluent aphasia, some of whom may be considered to have had AoS. However, as stated, beyond anecdotal reports, there remain minimal empirical data regarding the effects of MIT specifically in relation to AoS symptoms.

Augmentative and Alternative Communication Approaches

Augmentative alternative communication has been utilized with individuals with AoS in efforts to improve communication by supplementing inadequate speech production or replacing speech. In addition, AAC has been used as a means for improving speech production in AoS (Lasker et al., 2008, 2010). Reported AAC approaches have included use of symbol systems (S. Bailey, 1983; Lane & Samples, 1981); utilization of voice output communication aids (Lasker & Bedrosian, 2001; Rabidoux, Florance, & McCauslin, 1980); development of comprehensive or total communication systems (Fawcus & Fawcus, 1990; Yorkston & Waugh, 1989); and implementation of strategies to circumvent AoS maladaptive behavior (Lustig & Tompkins, 2002).

The AAC AoS treatment literature consists primarily of case study reports, with the exception of a few single-subject experimental investigations. Consequently, there was insufficient evidence for the ANCDS AoS guidelines committee to make a determination regarding the likelihood of benefit of AAC treatments for individuals with AoS. In terms of recommendations for use, the committee indicates that AAC approaches should be considered treatment options (Wambaugh et al., 2006b).

It is likely that the clinical use of AAC to treat AoS is more widespread than the sparse treatment literature indicates. Published cases have typically involved chronic cases of AoS in which a relatively permanent AAC solution is considered necessary. However, AAC may serve as a temporary means of communication, particularly in acute, improving cases of AoS. Currently, no data suggest negative (e.g., maladaptive) effects on speech recovery of early use of AAC in the acute phase. However, clinicians should bear in mind Kleim and Jones's (2008) first principle of experience-dependent plasticity: "Use it or lose it." The acute phase of recovery appears to require a careful balance between training the patient to utilize AAC to provide essential communication and therapy aimed at regaining speech skills.

The AAC approaches should be tailored to the individual's needs. A comprehensive communication system may provide maximum flexibility for communication (Yorkston & Waugh, 1989). Comprehensive systems must be multimodal and may include any usable speech, a gestural system, a drawing/writing system, a communication book/aid, or trained communication partners.

Most individuals who have AoS that is severe enough to warrant consideration of an AAC system will also have significant aphasia. The language disruption may be the major determinant in the development of an AAC system. Language strengths and weaknesses associated with the aphasia (e.g., auditory comprehension skills, reading skills, writing skills) will be important considerations in AAC planning with persons with AoS.

Beyond aphasia, other considerations in selecting an AAC system include adequate motor skills to employ an AAC device/system. Limb apraxia may interfere with use of devices or gestural systems. However, Code and Gaunt (1986) demonstrated successful acquisition of gestural skills with a patient with limb apraxia. Sufficient visual perceptual skills are also requisite for various AAC systems.

Perhaps the most important factor in the choice of an AAC system is the individual's motivation to use such a system. AAC users may not optimally utilize AAC options if they have issues with acceptance of AAC as part of their communication system. Counseling and treatment focused on utilization in functional settings are likely to be necessary with many AoS AAC users. For example, Lasker and Bedrosian (2001) report a case in which an individual with chronic aphasia and AoS was averse to using an AAC device in functional communication situations outside the speech and language clinic. The researchers successfully implemented a community-based therapy approach entailing role play and practice during planned outings.

A reluctance to accept AAC options may stem from an unwillingness to "give up on speech." Recent findings by Lasker et al. (2008) suggest that an AAC device may provide a means for improving speech. The investigators report a case study of an individual with chronic, profound AoS and moderate, nonfluent aphasia who demonstrated clinically significant improvements in intelligibility with treatment utilizing an AAC device (digitized device and synthesized voice output device). The device was used in the context of "motor learning guided" treatment that entailed repeated practice with and without modeling and knowledge of results (KR) provided on a 30% schedule. Treatment progressed from functional, one-syllable words (e.g., *hi, no*) to multisyllabic words and phrases (e.g., patient's name, *Holy Ghost*). Treatment sessions were conducted one time per week at a university speech and language clinic, and home practice was also completed. Intelligibility ratings for trained and untrained items improved to 75% (from near 0%) with positive generalization to untrained items reported (although at lower levels than trained items). In a subsequent investigation, Lasker and colleagues successfully paired use of an AAC device as a practice tool with webcam interactive technology to provide therapy remotely (Lasker et al., 2010).

A desire to communicate via speech, even when speech is extremely difficult, may lead to the development of unproductive behaviors. Lustig and Tompkins (2002) devised a treatment for an individual with moderate-to-severe AoS and aphasia who had developed a maladaptive pattern of persistent verbal struggle behavior. When the patient experienced breakdowns in verbal speech/language, she produced excessive verbal reattempts that interfered with communication. The treatment required the patient to identify her verbal struggle behavior and employ a written response instead of persisting with the unsuccessful verbal attempts. Practice in employing the strategy was conducted in the context of conversations with the clinician and then with unfamiliar partners. Positive findings were reported in terms of improved conversation.

Other Approaches to Treatment of Apraxia of Speech

Conversational abilities have been the focus of a few AOS treatment reports. Florance and Deal (1979) provide a case study report of an individual with chronic, moderate AoS who had an extremely limited verbal repertoire. The patient practiced verbal sentence production with audiovisual cues and then practiced those sentences in the context of pseudoconversations. Treatment progressed to practice in generating novel sentences in pseudoconversations. Conversational practice was then extended to card games, phone calls, and home treatments with the spouse. Substantial increases in spontaneous productions in the home environment were reported.

Florance, Rabidoux, and McCauslin (1980) also focus on conversational skills in a report of three cases with individuals with severe AoS. In this investigation, however, the emphasis was on training significant other persons in clinical interviewing tactics. One participant received training in self-monitoring, self-regulation, and pseudoconversation. The authors report large increases in mean length of utterance and "communicative success" with corresponding improvements in life

management. Unfortunately, the lack of a controlled design and the time postonset of the patients (i.e., 5–6 months) limit the utility of the findings.

Brain stimulation therapies have received increasing attention in the treatment of aphasia and have also been recently directed toward treatment of AoS. Marangolo and colleagues examined the effects of transcranial direct current stimulation (tDCS; Marangolo et al., 2011, 2013) with speakers with chronic AoS and aphasia. In their initial investigation, Marangolo et al. (2011) applied anodic tDCS over the left Broca's area in conjunction with behavioral speech/language therapy with three participants. In a subsequent investigation, Marangolo et al. (2013) paired bihemispheric anodic ipsilesional and cathodic contralesional stimulation with speech/language therapy with eight participants. A sham condition was included in both investigations. Results from both investigations indicated that tDCS combined with behavioral therapy resulted in substantial, lasting changes in speech that exceeded the benefits achieved from the sham condition.

Considerations in Structuring Treatments

As noted previously, principles from the nonspeech motor learning literature have possible relevance to the treatment of AoS (Maas, Robin, Austermann Hula, et al., 2008). The reader is cautioned that there are currently limited data in the area of AoS treatment and motor learning, and it should not be assumed that principles of limb motor learning will necessarily apply to speech motor learning (or in the case of AoS, relearning). Bislick and colleagues completed a systematic review of evidence associated with PML applied to speech motor learning (Bislick, Weir, Spencer, Kendall, & Yorkston, 2012). The reviewers concluded those data supporting the use of PML in the treatment of motor speech disorders are limited, albeit promising. The following sections include discussions of various PML that may have applicability to the treatment of AoS.

Variability of Practice

Variable practice involves structuring practice on different variations of a movement, whereas *constant* practice involves only one version of the movement (Schmidt & Lee, 2005). As summarized by Maas, Robin, Austermann Hula, et al. (2008), variable motoric practice is likely to result in a more reliable schema and better transfer of learned behaviors, but constant practice may have benefits early in the learning process. Both types of practice may interact with other variables, such as amount and structure of practice. Currently, there are no data concerning the relative merits of variable versus constant practice in the treatment of AoS. However, contrastive practice has long been advocated and employed successfully in the treatment of AoS (Wertz et al., 1984). In addition, contrastive practice is consistent with models of speech production/learning that stress the importance of refining target regions through contrastive somatosensory feedback (Guenther, 2006).

Wertz and colleagues (1984) discuss beginning contrastive practice of syllables by pairing the target sound with different vowels (e.g., /be/–/bi/–/bu/). After successful completion of this level, they recommend practice in contrasting the target sound with dissimilar sounds (e.g., /be/–/fe/; /bi/–/si/). They then suggest increasing the difficulty of the contrasts by practicing sounds that are more similar to the target (e.g., /pi/–/bi/) or employing a more difficult production environment for the target sound (e.g., *pike–pint*). Other investigators have also used contrastive practice successfully in the form of minimal pair words, with the target sound paired with the patient's error sound (Howard & Varley, 1995; Square-Storer & Hayden, 1989; Wambaugh et al., 1998).

As remarked previously, there is a lack of evidence to guide selection of constant or variable practice in the treatment of AoS. However, the clinician should keep in mind these issues when selecting targets for treatment.

Organization of Practice

The organization of practice has been demonstrated to have important ramifications for nonspeech motor learning with *blocked* stimulus presentation practice resulting in more rapid acquisition of motor behaviors during treatment, but *random* stimulus presentation practice promoting better retention and transfer (Schmidt & Lee, 2005). Blocked stimulus presentation practice entails practicing the same behavior repeatedly with no intervening trials of other behaviors. Random stimulus presentation practice involves alternating practice on different behaviors randomly. The terms *retention* and *transfer* are used in the motor learning literature to refer to maintenance and generalization, respectively. Knock, Ballard, Robin, and Schmidt (2000) were the first to investigate the effects of blocked and random stimulus presentation practice on production of stops and fricatives with two participants with AoS. Their findings did not coincide with the limb motor learning literature with respect to acquisition during treatment (i.e., blocked and random acquisition rates were similar). However, their findings did suggest that,

for one participant, random stimulus presentation practice may have resulted in superior retention and transfer. Wambaugh and colleagues provided two reports of the effects of blocked and random practice on outcomes associated with SPT (Wambaugh, Nessler, Cameron, & Mauszycki, 2013; Wambaugh, Nessler, Wright, & Mauszycki, 2014). They reported that, although all participants benefited from both forms of SPT (blocked and random), a few participants appeared to have slightly better maintenance associated with the random SPT condition.

Practice Distribution

Practice distribution concerns how a specific amount of treatment (e.g., 16 sessions) is dispensed over time (e.g., 4 hours per day for 4 days versus 1 hour per day for 16 days). Distribution has been described as being "massed," with little intervening time between sessions, or "distributed," with more time between sessions (Maas, Robin, Austermann Hula, et al., 2008). As discussed by Maas, Robin, Austermann Hula, and associates (2008), distributed practice has been found to be superior to massed practice for both immediate learning and retention for nonspeech tasks. Aspects of intensity of treatment relate to the concepts of practice distribution (Warren, Fey, & Yoder, 2007). Specifically, dose frequency (how often sessions are administered within a given time period) and intervention duration can be manipulated to evaluate massed versus distributed practice.

Wambaugh and colleagues (2013) conducted a pilot investigation of the effects of treatment intensity on outcomes associated with SPT with four speakers with chronic AOS and aphasia. They compared the effects of SPT administered with an intense dose frequency (4 hours per day for 4 days per week) to a traditional dose frequency (1 hour per day, 3 days per week), while holding number of total treatment sessions constant. Treatment intensity did not result in different outcomes within participants in this preliminary study (Wambaugh et al., 2013).

Administration of Feedback

Clinician-provided feedback is an important aspect of most AoS treatments but has received relatively little attention. The motor learning literature differentiates between feedback that provides KR and knowledge of performance (KP). Knowledge of results is used to provide the learner with information concerning the outcome of the motor act relative to the target (e.g., correct or incorrect); KP is used to provide qualitative information concerning the nature of the movement (e.g., "your lips need to be rounded") (Maas, Robin, Austermann Hula, et al., 2008). No data are available concerning the value of KR or KP in the treatment of AOS.

Recently, Austermann Hula, Robin, Maas, Ballard, and Schmidt (2008) studied both the frequency and timing of administration of feedback (KR) in the treatment of AoS. The effects of administration of high-frequency feedback (HFF; clinician feedback provided for 100% of trials) and low-frequency feedback (LFF; clinician feedback provided for 60% of trials) were compared within four individual speakers with AoS using single-subject experimental designs. For two participants, LFF may have enhanced retention of trained behaviors. However, for those two participants, superior performance with LFF was observed for only one of two treatment phases. For one of the remaining two participants, better performance was observed under HFF conditions in one treatment phase, and for the other participant, performance was always associated with specific sounds regardless of feedback condition.

Two of the participants in the feedback frequency investigation were then studied in a second study in which HFF was provided under two conditions: immediate feedback (IF; no delay between production and clinician feedback) and delayed feedback (DF; 5-second delay between production and provision of feedback). Results were equivocal, with one participant demonstrating better performance with HFF in one phase and LFF in the second phase. For the other participant, superior maintenance was associated with LFF for one phase but not the other phase.

Overall, these studies suggest that consideration of administration of feedback may be important for some speakers with AoS. Unfortunately, results may have been confounded with stimulus difficulty in some cases, which may have obscured effects.

Complexity of Practice Stimuli

Skill level or difficulty appears to be important in cortical motor reorganization (Kleim & Jones, 2008). In the treatment of aphasia, systematic research has led to the development of the *complexity account of treatment efficacy* (CATE; Thompson, Shapiro, Kiran, & Sobecks, 2003). This treatment postulates that treatment generalization will occur from more complex behaviors to less complex behaviors that are closely related linguistically (and that the reverse type of generalization does not occur). Such generalization has been observed for different language behaviors in the areas of syntax (Thompson & Shapiro, 2007), phonology (Gierut, 2007), and word retrieval (Kiran, 2007).

Of course, AoS is not considered to result from disruptions at a linguistic level. However, a few researchers have investigated the potential application of CATE to AoS treatment (Maas, Barlow, Robin, & Shapiro, 2002; Schneider & Frens, 2005). Maas et al. trained nonwords containing three-sound clusters (e.g., spreeze) or singletons (e.g., reeze). They found that one participant demonstrated partial generalization from three-sound clusters to untrained two-sound clusters and singletons but did not demonstrate generalization from singletons to clusters. The other participant did not demonstrate generalization in either direction.

Schneider and Frens (2005) trained multisyllabic nonwords of various complexity (e.g., Level 1: /bobobobo/, Level 4: /bonatig/) with three participants with AoS. They predicted, based on CATE, that training of more complex levels would generalize to untrained less complex levels. For two participants, training of less complex utterances did not generalize to more complex utterances. However, for one participant, training at Level 3 resulted in improvements in Level 4. In addition, in only one instance (of four training opportunities) did training of more complex utterances generalize to less complex utterances.

Support for CATE has been equivocal across both investigations focused on this issue with AoS speakers. Furthermore, generalization from more simple to more complex utterances has been demonstrated (albeit not consistently) with some AoS speakers (Wambaugh, 2004; Wambaugh et al., 1998, Wambaugh, Nessler, Mauszycki, & Cameron, 2014). Also, findings from facilitation studies with AoS speakers (analogous to very short duration treatment studies) indicate that generalization can occur from less complex to more complex syllables (Aichert & Ziegler, 2008; Schoor, Aichert, & Ziegler, 2012). More research is certainly warranted in this area of study. At the current time, it may be best for clinicians to use their judgment and perhaps trial therapy to determine at what level of complexity patients may best learn.

Principles of Experience-Dependent Neural Plasticity

Advances in the understanding of neural plasticity have begun to inform rehabilitation. "By understanding the basic principles of neural plasticity that govern learning in both the intact and damaged brain, identification of the critical behavioral and neurobiological signals that drive recovery can begin" (Kleim & Jones, 2008, p. S225). Kleim and Jones highlight 10 general principles of experience-dependent neural plasticity that pertain to rehabilitation following brain damage. These principles, such as "use it or lose it," "use it and improve it," and "salience matters," may be extremely important considerations in the treatment of motor speech disorders such as AoS. As discussed by Ludlow and colleagues (2008), these principles have received limited study relative to rehabilitation of motor speech disorders to date but are certainly deserving of attention.

The principles of experience-dependent neural plasticity coincide with several well-developed PML (Schmidt & Lee, 2005). For example, the principles of "repetition matters" and "intensity matters" have been demonstrated to be important factors in the behavioral motor learning literature. As discussed previously, inroads are being made relative to our understanding of PML, some of which relate directly to principles of neural plasticity.

Application of the WHO ICF to AoS Treatment

To date, no published, formalized attempts have been made to structure treatment or outcome measures for AoS using the framework of the ICF. As discussed by Threats (2009), the ICF framework provides a structure for describing functioning but does not provide any directions specifying how measurement should occur. Thus, the ICF framework is "more of a challenge than an answer" (Threats, 2009, p. 13).

Wambaugh and Mauszycki (2010a) reviewed the AoS treatment literature to determine how levels of the ICF have been addressed. They found that the vast majority of AOS treatments and outcome measures have focused at the level of the ICF's Body Functions construct. Consequently, many challenges remain for incorporating the concepts of the ICF into AoS management. Specifically, the constructs of Activity/Participation and Contextual Factors require significant attention. The following sections briefly describe ways in which AoS treatment and outcome measures have related to the ICF and highlight areas that are deserving of future clinical and research consideration.

The preponderance of treatments for AoS has been directed toward improving the spatial and timing accuracy of the articulators during speech production (Wambaugh et al., 2006b; Wambaugh & Mauszycki, 2010b). The dependent measures used to quantify the effects of such treatments have most often taken the form of phonetic transcription, ratings of accuracy or quality, or qualitative descriptions of speech. Therefore, the majority of therapies and corresponding outcome measures for AoS would be considered to reflect the levels of "articulation function" or "fluency and rhythm of speech functions" according to the WHO ICF.

In only a few reports have treatments or outcome measures focused on ICF concepts other than Body Functions. As described previously, AAC approaches have intended to improve global communication behaviors. As such, they would be considered to address the ICF construct of Activity/Participation. A few functional, conversational approaches to AoS treatment have also targeted communicative success by training conversational skills (Florance & Deal, 1979) or training communication partners (Florance et al., 1980).

The only instance in which the ICF construct of Contextual Factors has been addressed with AoS treatment is an investigation by Lustig and Tompkins (2002), in which they trained an individual with AoS to use an alternative communication strategy when verbal speech–language breakdowns occurred. They included pre- and posttreatment measures of psychosocial well-being (i.e., Communication Attitude Inventory [Andrews & Cutler, 1974]; Recovery Locus of Control Scale [Partridge & Johnson, 1989]; and Rosenberg Self-Esteem Scale [Rosenberg, 1965]). These measures reflect the ICF's concept of Personal Factors. In addition, Lustig and Tompkins obtained ratings from unaffiliated raters of different aspects of videotaped pre- and posttreatment conversational exchanges, which constitutes measurement of Activity/Participation factors.

The lack of treatments and outcome data that pertain to the ICF constructs of Activity/Participation and Contextual Factors does not equate to inadequate treatments. That is, insufficiency of measurement is not synonymous with lack of treatment effect. It is quite possible that current treatments may have positive outcomes on patients' functioning beyond the level of Body Functions, but clinicians should not assume that this is the case. Researchers and clinicians should keep in mind that measurement tools are available for use in determining the effects of treatment in terms of Activity/Participation. Specifically, measures of speech intelligibility and ratings of functional communication (e.g., American Speech-Language-Hearing Association Functional Assessment of Communication Skills for Adults [ASHA FACS]; Frattali, Holland, Thompson, Wohl, & Ferketic, 1995) may be used as outcome measures. Unfortunately, the sensitivity of functional communication measures for documenting changes in speech in persons with AoS has not been documented. Overall, there is a shortage of valid and reliable tools to measure the effects of motor speech treatments in comprehensive ways. Clinicians should be encouraged not to let the paucity of measurement tools deter incorporation of ICF levels beyond Body Functions into assessment and treatment. However, those who wish to measure the impact of their treatment with respect to participation and contextual factors may need to look to psychosocial measures such as those employed by Lustig and Tompkins (2002) or devise individually relevant measures such as self-ratings, observations, or behavioral inventories. Of course, any clinician-developed measure carries with it the caveat that reliability may be less than optimal.

FUTURE DIRECTIONS

Considering that the label AoS was only coined and linked to a particular model of speech output in the late 1960s (Darley et al., 1975), even though the disorder had been discussed previously under other labels, such as apraxia of the glosso-labio-pharyngeal structures, aphemia, syndrome of phonetic disintegration, or verbal apraxia, it should be apparent that significant progress has been made in describing its symptoms and understanding its nature. It should also be evident that treatment of AoS has advanced considerably. However, much remains to be learned about virtually all aspects of AoS.

As described in the first portions of this chapter, many unanswered questions remain concerning the underlying nature of AoS as well as the behaviors that should be considered characteristic of the disorder. Technological advances in areas such as functional neuroimaging, physiological measurement, and neural network modeling will certainly add to our understanding of this disorder.

Improved understanding of the nature of AoS should translate to improved treatment. Although there is now sufficient evidence to assert that AoS treatments can be expected to result in improved production of speech, much remains unknown about treatment efficacy, and no data exist concerning treatment effectiveness. As noted previously, little attention has been given to examination of the effects of treatment on activities and participation. Valid and reliable measures of activities and participation should be developed and incorporated into AoS treatment research.

Technological advances can be expected to extend directly to the treatment of AoS. Technologically sophisticated adjuvant therapies such as tDCS (Marangolo et al., 2011, 2013) appear to have promise for enhancing behavioral treatments; additional cortical stimulation therapies will eventually be tested with AoS behavioral treatments. Other adjuvants, such as aerobic exercise, are likely to be evaluated in the treatment of AoS and may also prove to be beneficial. Progress in neurorehabililitation will certainly affect management of AoS. Regardless of the treatment technologies, systematic study of treatment effects, including comparative studies, will be required to allow clinicians and patients to make informed, evidence-based decisions.

Case Illustration 21.1

As a home health speech–language clinician, you receive a referral for a new client, Mr. X. Mr. X.'s medical records and history forms indicate that 12 months ago he had a single, left hemisphere ischemic stroke involving the entire left middle cerebral artery distribution. He received inpatient rehabilitation services (speech–language therapy, occupational therapy, and physical therapy) followed by approximately 1 month of outpatient rehabilitation. His speech therapy records report a diagnosis of acquired AoS and Broca's aphasia. The records concerning speech–language therapy are brief and nonspecific and suggest that treatment included therapy in the following areas: word retrieval, phrase production, communication notebook use, and auditory comprehension.

Mr. X. resides at home with his wife and two college-age children, all of whom are reportedly very supportive of Mr. X. Mr. X. has limited ambulation as a result of right-sided hemiparesis and has reduced stamina because of cardiovascular problems and diabetes. He is scheduled for three 45-minute sessions per week of speech–language therapy.

You complete formal aphasia testing, and the results confirm a diagnosis of Broca's aphasia of moderate severity. You also complete a screening for AoS that includes the following: mono- and multisyllabic word productions, productions of words of increasing length, repeated productions of multisyllabic words, sentence repetition, alternate motion rates, sequential motion rates, counting, naming the days of the week, and singing (Duffy, 2005). These speech samples combined with those produced during the aphasia testing confirm a diagnosis of AoS. Specifically, the behaviors considered necessary for AoS diagnosis (McNeil, Robin, & Schmidt, 2009; Wambaugh et al., 2006a) were present: slow rate of speech production (increased segment durations and time between syllables), sound errors that were predominantly distortions, and disrupted prosody.

(continues)

You meet with Mr. X. and his family members to review the test results, obtain additional history information, and discuss participation level issues (e.g., restrictions and desired areas of increased participation). After reviewing various participation domains, Mr. X. and his family indicate that they would like therapy to facilitate personal communication for an upcoming event (i.e., specific phrases for a wedding) and requests for food and assistance in the home. They express little interest in AAC and indicate a desire to improve speech production. They convey dissatisfaction with a lack of emphasis on speech production in previous therapy. They acknowledge that Mr. X.'s speech production skills will likely remain quite limited but feel that improvements can be made.

You complete additional assessments to plan therapy. Specifically, it is necessary to determine Mr. X.'s strengths and weaknesses in terms of sound production. In the preceding assessments, Mr. X.'s spontaneous productions were limited to a few stereotypies and perseverations, all containing an approximation of the word *water*. This appeared to be related to reports from the family that early in the therapy process, a misguided clinician had Mr. X. repeatedly practice the phrase "I want water" to the exclusion of any other speech practice. You conduct an inventory of sound production at the monosyllabic word level by asking Mr. X to repeat an extensive set of words, representing five exemplars of all consonants in the word-initial and word-final positions. The results indicate that Mr. X. has an extremely limited phonetic repertoire, with only the sounds /w, n, b/, and /m/ being produced correctly at least 50% of the time. Most of his errors were productions of distorted /w/ for the target sounds. It appears that Mr. X.'s early therapy experiences served to limit differentiated sound production. Mr. X. was able to consistently determine correct and incorrect productions (approximating his errors) when produced by the clinician. He could not judge correct versus incorrect productions in his own speech.

Mr. X.'s verbal production difficulties appear to be both motoric and linguistic in nature. However, his AoS appears to be the main limiting factor, which is consistent with the observation that written language skills (e.g., word retrieval, sentence construction) are notably superior to verbal language skills. Given that the client and his family wish to improve speech production and that the client received limited therapy directed toward speech, articulatory–kinematic therapy appears to be warranted.

Expansion of Mr. X.'s sound production repertoire through the development of (or facilitation of access to) a system of contrasts is selected as an overarching goal. You and the client and his family select words that are functional in nature and that represent selected target sounds. You have decided to employ a modified version of SPT (Wambaugh & Nessler, 2004) in which several target sounds will be practiced in the context of words. Sound production treatment combines minimal contrast practice, integral stimulation (modeling and unison production), and articulatory placement instructions. It also employs blocked and randomized practice schedules in keeping with PML. The treatment relies heavily on auditory and visual modeling and repeated practice, which is consistent with theories of speech acquisition/production (e.g., Guenther, 2006) and of mirror neurons. Because Mr. X. displays great difficulty in self-monitoring his errors, SPT will be modified to require self-judgments. That is, at the point in the SPT hierarchy when Mr. X. is required to repeat a correct production five times, he will be asked to determine whether each production is correct or incorrect, with clinician feedback/correction used as needed.

The SPT requires treatment of 8 to 10 words per sound target. Consequently, you and the family develop the appropriate number of treatment items, and you devise minimal pair words to match those treatment items. In addition, you select five different words per target sound that will not be treated but will be used for measuring response generalization. You will also use the techniques employed in SPT to facilitate production of utterances selected by Mr. X. and his family to address issues of participation (e.g., "I love you," "I'm thirsty," "more ice," etc.).

Prior to starting treatment, you conduct measures to be used to document the outcomes of the treatment. You measure the treatment and generalization words repeatedly in probes so that you can understand and document Mr. X.'s normal production variability. In addition, you obtain a speech sample to be used to rate speech intelligibility (by another clinician), and you ask Mr. X.'s spouse to complete the Communication Effectiveness Index (Lomas et al., 1989). You also ask Mr. X.'s family members to keep a log of his spontaneous utterances over a period of a week. You plan to repeat these measures at the completion of treatment.

Mr. X. has expressed interest in practicing between treatment sessions. You use this interest as an opportunity to introduce an AAC device (synthesized voice output device). You train Mr. X. and his family in the operation of the device and program his treatment items into the device. You then instruct Mr. X. and his family in methods

(continues)

for using the AAC device to practice the target words. You hope that familiarity with the AAC device as a practice tool may lead to eventual acceptance of the device for purposes of communication (i.e., not just practice).

You plan to provide SPT for a minimum of 10 sessions, along with the home-based practice, to determine if gains may be achieved. If progress is evident, you will continue treatment with the first set of items until maximal improvements have been achieved (ideally, this would be clearly differentiated sound productions). You then plan to select another set of words representing different sounds to continue expanding Mr. X.'s sound repertoire and will continue in this fashion until he achieves a level of intelligibility that satisfies his and his family's day-to-day needs in communication. Extension of the number of functional phrases that are practiced also targets his ability to resume his roles within his community. In the event that progress is not made via SPT, you plan to pursue other speech facilitation approaches and perhaps AAC.

STUDY QUESTIONS

1. A patient with AoS has difficulty in production of consonant clusters in monosyllabic words. Develop a set of outcome measures reflecting the WHO ICF's levels of Body Functions and Activity/Participation for a treatment that targets production of clusters.

2. Discuss how a rate control treatment could be combined with an articulatory–kinematic treatment.

3. No measures currently exist for rating perceived speaking effort for use with patients with AoS. Discuss how such a rating would fit into the WHO ICF scheme. Devise a set of perceived effort scales that a clinician might be able to use as a self-report measure.

4. Discuss how different PML could be implemented with a published AoS treatment protocol (i.e., a treatment described in the literature).

5. Discuss how an AoS treatment that targets activity/participation levels of functioning may or may not affect the underlying neuropathophysiological deficit in AoS. Consider theoretical models discussed in this chapter as part of this discussion.

6. What are the challenges faced in selecting participants for a study on AoS, and what solutions offer themselves for these challenges?

7. What are the four categories of AoS treatments identified in the ANCDS AoS treatment guidelines report?

8. What is the difference between blocked and randomized schedules of practice?

9. What are three articulatory–kinematic techniques that may be used with speakers with AoS?

10. In what ways do more recent interactive models of speech motor control and breakdown differ from earlier hierarchical, discrete point models?

11. Which of these words involves the greatest number of articulatory adjustments in production: *name, save, same*?

12. A patient experiences predominantly no responses and a "feeling of knowing" on a picture naming task but articulatorily has good repetition performance. Where does this suggest the possible breakdown in speech output lies?

13. Why might people with AoS fail on such tasks as rhyme judgment, syllable segmentation, and lexical decision despite having intact phonology?

14. Which of the following perceived error types would you expect to hear in someone with AoS but not in someone with dysarthria: additions, distorted substitutions, omissions, distortions?

15. Give an articulatory, gestural coordination explanation of the apparent misproduction of *tea* for *Dee* and *nose* for *doze*.

REFERENCES

Ahlsen, E. (2008). Embodiment in communication—Aphasia, apraxia and the possible role of mirroring and imitation. *Clinical Linguistics & Phonetics, 22*(4–5), 311–315.

Aichert, I., & Ziegler, W. (2004a). Segmental and metrical encoding in aphasia: Two case reports. *Aphasiology, 18*(12), 1201–1211.

Aichert, I., & Ziegler, W. (2004b). Syllable frequency and syllable structure in apraxia of speech. *Brain and Language, 88*(1), 148–159.

Aichert, I., & Ziegler, W. (2008). Learning a syllable from its parts: Cross-syllabic generalization effects in patients with apraxia of speech. *Aphasiology, 22,* 1216–1229.

Andrews, G., & Cutler, J. (1974). Stuttering therapy: The relation between changes in symptom level and attitudes. *Journal of Speech and Hearing Disorders, 39*, 312–319.

Austermann Hula, S., Robin, D., Maas, E., Ballard, K., & Schmidt, R. (2008). Effects of feedback frequency and timing on acquisition, retention, and transfer of speech skills in acquired apraxia of speech. *Journal of Speech, Language, and Hearing Research, 51*, 1088–1113.

Bailey, D., Eatchel, K., & Wambaugh, J. (2015). Sound production treatment: Synthesis and quantification of outcomes. *American Journal of Speech-Language Pathology.* 2015 Jul 1. doi:10.1044/2015_AJSLP-14-012.

Bailey, S. (1983). Blissymbols and aphasia therapy: A case study. In C. Code & D. Müller (Eds.), *Aphasia therapy* (pp. 178–186). London, UK: Arnold.

Ballard, K., Maas, E., & Robin, D. (2007). Treating control of voicing in apraxia of speech with variable practice. *Aphasiology, 21*(12), 1195–1217.

Ballard, K., Tourville, J., & Robin, D. (2014). Behavioural, computational, and neuroimaging studies of acquired apraxia of speech. *Frontiers in Human Neuroscience, 8.* Retrieved from http://dx.doi.org/10.3389/fnhum.2014.00892.

Ballard, K., Wambaugh, J., Duffy, J., Layfield, C., Maas, E., Mauszycki, S., et al. (2015). Updated treatment guidelines for acquired apraxia of speech: A systematic review of intervention research between 2004 and 2012. *American Journal of Speech-Language Pathology, 24*, 316–337.

Barlow, S., Finan, D., & Park, S. (2004). Sensorimotor entrainment of respiratory and orofacial systems in humans. In B. Massen, R. Kent, H. Peters, P. van Lieshout, & W. Hulstijn (Eds.), *Speech motor control in normal and disordered speech* (pp. 211–224). Oxford, UK: Oxford University Press.

Bislick, L., Weir, P., Spencer, K., Kendall, D., & Yorkston, K. (2012). Do principles of motor learning enhance retention and transfer of speech skills. A systematic review. *Aphasiology, 26*(5), 709–728.

Bohland, J., Bullock, D., & Guenther, F. (2010). Neural representations and mechanisms for the performance of simple speech sequences. *Journal of Cognitive Neuroscience, 22*(7), 1504–1529.

Bohland, J., & Guenther, F. (2006). An fMRI investigation of syllable sequence production. *NeuroImage, 32*(2), 821–841.

Boucher, V., Garcia, L., Fleurant, J., & Paradis, J. (2001). Variable efficacy of rhythm and tone in melody-based interventions: Implications for the assumption of a right-hemisphere facilitation in non-fluent aphasia. *Aphasiology, 15*(2), 131–149.

Boucher, V. J. (2006). On the function of stress rhythms in speech: Evidence of a link with grouping effects on serial memory. *Language and Speech, 49*(4), 495–519.

Brendel, B., & Ziegler, W. (2008). Effectiveness of metrical pacing in the treatment of apraxia of speech. *Aphasiology, 22*(1), 1–26.

Brendel, B., Ziegler, W., & Deger, K. (2000). The synchronization paradigm in the treatment of apraxia of speech. *Journal of Neurolinguistics, 13*, 241–327.

Browman, C. P., & Goldstein, L. (1992). Articulatory phonology—An overview. *Phonetica, 49*(3–4), 155–180.

Buchwald, A., & Miozzo, M. (2012). Phonological and motor errors in individuals with acquired sound production impairment. *Journal of Speech, Language, and Hearing Research, 55*(5), S1573–S1586.

Canter, G., Trost, J., & Burns, M. (1985). Contrasting speech patterns in apraxia of speech and phonemic paraphasia. *Brain and Language, 24*(2), 204–222.

Cholin, J. (2008). The mental syllabary in speech production: An integration of different approaches and domains. *Aphasiology, 22*(11), 1127–1141.

Cholin, J., & Levelt, W. (2009). Effects of syllable preparation and syllable frequency in speech production: Further evidence for syllabic units at a post-lexical level. *Language and Cognitive Processes, 24*(5), 662–684.

Cholin, J., Levelt, W., & Schiller, N. (2006). Effects of syllable frequency in speech production. *Cognition, 99*(2), 205–235.

Code, C., & Gaunt, C. (1986). Treating severe speech and limb apraxia in a case of aphasia. *British Journal of Disorders of Communication, 21*(1), 11–20.

Colaço, D., Mineiro, A., & Castro Caldas, A. (2014). Phonological and speech output in adult nonliterate groups. In N. Miller & A. Lowit (Eds.), *Motor speech disorders: A cross language perspective* (pp. 105–124). Clevedon, UK: Multilingual Matters.

Dabul, B. (2000). *Apraxia battery for adults* (2nd ed.). Austin, TX: Pro-Ed.

Darley, F., Aronson, A., & Brown, J. (1975). *Motor speech disorders.* Philadelphia, PA: Saunders.

Deal, J., & Florance, C. (1978). Modification of the eight-step continuum for treatment of apraxia of speech in adults. *Journal of Speech and Hearing Disorders, 43*, 89–95.

Deger, K., & Ziegler, W. (2002). Speech motor programming in apraxia of speech. *Journal of Phonetics, 30*(3), 321–335.

Deutsch, S. (1984). Prediction of site of lesion from speech apraxic error patterns. In J. Rosenbek, M. McNeil, & A. Aronson (Eds.), *Apraxia of speech* (pp. 113–133). San Diego, CA: College Hill.

Dick, A. S., Bernal, B., & Tremblay, P. (2014). The language connectome: New pathways, new concepts. *The Neuroscientist, 20*(5), 453–467.

Dronkers, N. F. (1996). A new brain region for coordinating speech articulation. *Nature, 384*(6605), 159–161.

Duffy, J. (2005). *Motor speech disorders.* St. Louis, MO: Elsevier Mosby.

Dworkin, J., & Abkarian, G. (1996). Treatment of phonation in a patient with apraxia and dysarthria secondary to severe closed head injury. *Journal of Medical Speech-Language Pathology, 2*, 105–115.

Dworkin, J., Abkarian, G., & Johns, D. (1988). Apraxia of speech: The effectiveness of a treatment regime. *Journal of Speech and Hearing Disorders, 53*, 280–294.

Fawcus, M., & Fawcus, R. (1990). Information transfer in four cases of severe articulatory dyspraxia. *Aphasiology, 4*(2), 207–212.

Feiken, J., Jonkers, R., Lettinga, A., & Stuive, I. (2012). DIAS: Diagnostisch instrument voor apraxie van de spraak. *Logopedie en Foniatrie, 4*, 112–119.

Florance, C., & Deal, J. (1979). Treatment for apraxia of speech: A conversational program. *Ohio Journal Speech and Hearing, 14*, 184–191.

Florance, C., Rabidoux, P., & McCauslin, L. (1980). An environmental manipulation approach to treating apraxia of speech. In R. H. Brookshire (Ed.), *Clinical Aphasiology Conference proceedings* (pp. 285–293). Minneapolis, MN: BRK.

Frattali, C., Holland, A., Thompson, C., Wohl, C., & Ferketic, M. (1995). *American Speech-Language-Hearing Association functional assessment of communication skills for adults.* Rockville, MD: American Speech-Language-Hearing Association.

Gadesmann, M., & Miller, N. (2008). Reliability of speech diadochokinetic test measurement. *International Journal of Language & Communication Disorders, 43*(1), 41–54.

Gibbon, F. (2006). *Bibliography of electropalatographic (EGP) studies in English (1957–2006).* Retrieved from http://www.qmu.ac.uk/ssrc/pubs/EPG_biblio_2006_june.pdf

Gierut, J. (2007). Phonological complexity and language learnability. *American Journal of Speech-Language Pathology, 16,* 6–17.

Goldenberg, G. (2013). *Apraxia: The cognitive side of motor control.* Oxford, UK: Oxford University Press.

Graff-Radford, J., Jones, D., Strand, E., Rabinstein, A., Duffy, J., & Josephs, K. (2014). The neuroanatomy of pure apraxia of speech in stroke. *Brain and Language, 129,* 43–46.

Guenther, F. (2006). Cortical interactions underlying the production of speech sounds. *Journal of Communication Disorders, 39*(5), 350–365.

Guenther, F., & Hickok, G. (2015). Role of the auditory system in speech production. *Handbook of Clinical Neurology, 129,* 161–175.

Guenther, F., & Vladusich, T. (2012). A neural theory of speech acquisition and production. *Journal of Neurolinguistics, 25*(5), 408–422.

Haley, K., Bays, G., & Ohde, R. (2001). Phonetic properties of aphasic-apraxic speech: A modified narrow transcription analysis. *Aphasiology, 15*(12), 1125–1142.

Haley, K., Jacks, A., & Cunningham, K. (2013). Error variability and the differentiation between apraxia of speech and aphasia with phonemic paraphasia. *Journal of Speech, Language, and Hearing Research, 56*(3), 891–905.

Haley, K., Jacks, A., de Riesthal, M., Abou-Khalil, R., & Roth, H. (2012). Toward a quantitative basis for assessment and diagnosis of apraxia of speech. *Journal of Speech, Language, and Hearing Research, 55*(5), S1502–S1517.

Haley, K., & Martin, G. (2011). Production variability and single word intelligibility in aphasia and apraxia of speech. *Journal of Communication Disorders, 44*(1), 103–115.

Haley, K., Ohde, R., & Wertz, R. (2001). Vowel quality in aphasia and apraxia of speech: Phonetic transcription and formant analyses. *Aphasiology, 15*(12), 1107–1123.

Hardcastle, W., & Edwards, S. (1992). EPG-based description of apraxic speech errors. In R. Kent (Ed.), *Intelligibility in speech disorders* (pp. 287–328). Amsterdam, the Netherlands: Benjamins.

Hickok, G. (2010). The role of mirror neurons in speech perception and action word semantics. *Language and Cognitive Processes, 25*(6), 749–776.

Hickok, G. (2012a). Computational neuroanatomy of speech production. *Nature Reviews. Neuroscience, 13*(2), 135–145.

Hickok, G. (2012b). The cortical organization of speech processing: Feedback control and predictive coding the context of a dual-stream model. *Journal of Communication Disorders, 45*(6), 393–402. doi:10.1016/j.jcomdis.2012.06.004

Hickok, G. (2013a). The architecture of speech production and the role of the phoneme in speech processing. *Language, Cognition and Neuroscience, 29*(1), 2–20.

Hickok, G. (2013b). Towards an integrated psycholinguistic, neurolinguistic, sensorimotor framework for speech production. *Language, Cognition and Neuroscience, 29*(1), 52–59.

Hickok, G., Rogalsky, C., Chen, R., Herskovits, E., Townsley, S., & Hillis, A. (2014). Partially overlapping sensorimotor networks underlie speech praxis and verbal short-term memory: Evidence from apraxia of speech following acute stroke. *Frontiers in Human Neuroscience, 8.* doi:10.3389/fnhum.2014.00649.

Hillis, A., Work, M., Barker, P., Jacobs, M., Breese, E., & Maurer, K. (2004). Re-examining the brain regions crucial for orchestrating speech articulation. *Brain, 127*(7), 1479–1487.

Houde, J. F., & Nagarajan, S. (2011). Speech production as state feedback control. *Frontiers in Human Neuroscience, 5,* 82. doi:10.3389/fnhum.2011.00082.

Howard, S., & Varley, R. (1995). Using electropalatography to treat severe acquired apraxia of speech. *European Journal of Disorders of Communication, 30*(2), 246–255.

Hurkmans, J., Jonkers, R., Boonstra, A., Stewart, R., & Reinders-Messelink, H. (2012). Assessing the treatment effects in apraxia of speech: Introduction and evaluation of the Modified Diadochokinesis Test. *International Journal of Language & Communication Disorders, 47*(4), 427–436.

Itoh, M., & Sasanuma, S. (1984). Articulatory movements in apraxia of speech. In J. Rosenbek, M. McNeil, & A. Aronson (Eds.), *Apraxia of speech* (pp. 135–165). San Diego, CA: College Hill.

Jacks, A., Mathes, K., & Marquardt, T. (2010). Vowel acoustics in adults with apraxia of speech. *Journal of Speech, Language, and Hearing Research, 53*(1), 61–74.

Janßen, U., & Domahs, F. (2008). Going on with optimised feet: Evidence for the interaction between segmental and metrical structure in phonological encoding from a case of primary progressive aphasia. *Aphasiology, 22*(11), 1157–1175.

Joanette, Y., Keller, E., & Lecours, A. (1980). Sequences of phonemic approximations in aphasia. *Brain and Language, 11*(1), 30–44.

Katz, W., Bharadwaj, S., & Carstens, B. (1999). Electromagnetic articulography treatment for an adult with Broca's aphasia and apraxia of speech. *Journal of Speech, Language, and Hearing Research, 42*(6), 1355–1366.

Katz, W., McNeil, M., & Garst, D. (2010). Treating apraxia of speech with EMA-supplied visual augmented feedback. *Aphasiology, 24*(6–8), 826–837.

Kent, R., & Rosenbek, J. (1982). Prosodic disturbance and neurologic lesion. *Brain and Language, 15*(2), 259–291.

Kiran, S. (2007). Complexity in the treatment of naming deficits. *American Journal of Speech-Language Pathology, 16,* 18–29.

Klapp, S. (2003). Reaction time analysis of two types of motor preparation for speech articulation: Action as a sequence of chunks. *Journal of Motor Behavior, 35*(2), 135–150.

Kleim, J., & Jones, T. (2008). Principles of experience-dependent neural plasticity: Implications for rehabilitation after brain injury. *Journal of Speech, Language, and Hearing Research, 51,* S225–S239.

Knock, T., Ballard, K., Robin, D., & Schmidt, R. (2000). Influence of order of stimulus presentation on speech motor learning: A principled approach to treatment for apraxia of speech. *Aphasiology, 14*(5/6), 653–668.

Kohn, S. (1984). The nature of the phonological disorder in conduction aphasia. *Brain and Language, 23*(1), 97–115.

Kotz, S., & Schwartze, M. (2010). Cortical speech processing unplugged: A timely subcortico-cortical framework. *Trends in Cognitive Sciences, 14*(9), 392–399.

Kröger, B., Kannampuzha, J., & Neuschaefer-Rube, C. (2009). Towards a neurocomputational model of speech production and perception. *Speech Communication, 51*(9), 793–809.

Kröger, B., Miller, N., & Lowit, A. (2011). Defective neural motor speech mappings as a source for apraxia of speech: Evidence from a quantitative neural model of speech processing. In A. Lowit & R. Kent (Eds.), *Assessment of motor speech disorders* (pp. 325–346). San Diego, CA: Plural.

Laganaro, M. (2012). Patterns of impairments in AOS and mechanisms of interaction between phonological and phonetic encoding. *Journal of Speech, Language, and Hearing Research, 55*(5), S1535–S1543.

Lallini, N., Miller, N., & Howard, D. (2007). Lexical influences on single word repetition in acquired spoken output impairment: A cross language comparison. *Aphasiology, 21*(6), 617–631.

Lane, V. W., & Samples, J. M. (1981). Facilitating communication skills in adult apraxics: Application of blissymbols in a group setting. *Journal of Communication Disorders, 14*, 157–167.

LaPointe, L. (1984). Sequential treatment of split lists: A case report. In J. Rosenbek, M. McNeil, & A. Aronson (Eds.), *Apraxia of speech: Physiology, acoustics, linguistics, management* (pp. 277–286). San Diego, CA: College Hill.

Lasker, J., & Bedrosian, J. (2001). Promoting acceptance of augmentative and alternative communication by adults with acquired communication disorders. *Augmentative & Alternative Communication, 17*(3), 141–153.

Lasker, J., Stierwalt, J., Hageman, C., & LaPointe, L. (2008). Using motor learning guided theory and augmentative and alternative communication to improve speech production in profound apraxia: A case example. *Journal of Medical Speech-Language Pathology, 16*(4), 225–233.

Lasker, J., Stierwalt, J., Spence, M., & Cavin-Root, C. (2010). Using webcam interactive technology to implement treatment for severe apraxia: A case example. *Journal of Medical Speech-Language Pathology, 18*(4), 71–76.

Liss, J. M. (1998). Error-revision in the spontaneous speech of apraxic speakers. *Brain and Language, 62*(3), 342–360.

Lomas, J., Pickard, L., Bester, S., Elbard, H., Finlayson, A., & Zoghaib, C. (1989). The communicative effectiveness index: Development and psychometric evaluation of a functional communication measure for adult aphasia. *Journal of Speech and Hearing Disorders, 54*, 113–124.

Lotte, F., Brumberg, J. S., Brunner, P., Gunduz, A., Ritaccio, A. L., Guan, C., et al. (2015). Electrocorticographic representations of segmental features in continuous speech. *Frontiers in Human Neuroscience, 9.* doi:10.3389/fnhum.2015.00097.

Lowit, A., Kuschmann, A., & Kavanagh, K. (2014). Phonological markers of sentence stress in ataxic dysarthria and their relationship to perceptual cues. *Journal of Communication Disorders, 50*, 8–18.

Ludlow, C., Hoit, J., Kent, R., Ramig, L. O., Shrivastav, R., Strand, E., et al. (2008). Translating principles of neural plasticity into research on speech motor control recovery and rehabilitation. *Journal of Speech, Language, and Hearing Research, 51*(1), S240–S258.

Lustig, A., & Tompkins, C. (2002). A written comprehension strategy for a speaker with aphasia and apraxia of speech: Treatment outcomes and social validity. *Aphasiology, 16*(4/5/6), 507–521.

Maas, E., Barlow, J., Robin, D., & Shapiro, L. (2002). Treatment of sound errors in aphasia and apraxia of speech: Effects of phonological complexity. *Aphasiology, 16*(4/5/6), 609–622.

Maas, E., & Mailend, M.-L. (2012). Speech planning happens before speech execution: Online reaction time methods in the study of apraxia of speech. *Journal of Speech, Language, and Hearing Research, 55*(5), S1523–S1534.

Maas, E., Mailend, M.-L., & Guenther, F. (2015). Feedforward and feedback control in apraxia of speech: Effects of noise masking on vowel production. *Journal of Speech, Language, and Hearing Research, 58*(2), 185–200.

Maas, E., Robin, D. A., Austermann Hula, S. N., Wulf, G., Ballard, K., & Schmidt, R. (2008). Principles of motor learning in treatment of motor speech disorders. *American Journal of Speech-Language Pathology, 17*, 277–298.

Maas, E., Robin, D., Wright, D., & Ballard, K. (2008). Motor programming in apraxia of speech. *Brain and Language, 106*(2), 107–118.

Mailend, M.-L., & Maas, E. (2013). Speech motor programming in apraxia of speech: Evidence from a delayed picture-word interference task. *American Journal of Speech-Language Pathology, 22*(2), S380–S396.

Marangolo, P., Fiori, V., Cipolari, S., Campana, S., Razzano, C., DiPaola, M., et al. (2013). Bihemispheric stimulation over left and right inferior frontal region enhances recovery from apraxia of speech in chronic aphasia. *Cognitive Neuroscience, 38*, 3370–3377.

Marangolo, P., Marinelli, C., Bonifazi, S., Fiori, V., Ceravolo, M., Provinciali, L., et al. (2011). Electrical stimulation over the left inferior frontal gyrus (IFG) determines long-term effects in the recovery of speech apraxia in three chronic aphasics. *Behavioral Brain Research, 225*, 498–502.

Mauszycki, S., Dromey, C., & Wambaugh, J. (2007). Variability in apraxia of speech: A perceptual, acoustic, and kinematic analysis of stop consonants. *Journal of Medical Speech-Language Pathology, 15*, 223–242.

Mauszycki, S., & Wambaugh, J. (2008). The effects of rate control treatment on consonant production accuracy in mild apraxia of speech. *Aphasiology, 22*(7), 906–920.

Mauszycki, S., Wambaugh, J., & Aikyama, N. (2015, May). *The use of electropalatography in the treatment of apraxia of speech.* Poster presentation at the annual Clinical Aphasiology Conference, Monterey, CA.

Mauszycki, S., Wambaugh, J., & Cameron, R. (2010a). Apraxia of speech: Perceptual analysis of bisyllabic word productions across repeated sampling occasions. *Journal Medical Speech-Language Pathology, 18*(4), 89–98.

Mauszycki, S., Wambaugh, J., & Cameron, R. (2010b). Variability in apraxia of speech: Perceptual analysis of monosyllabic word productions across repeated sampling times. *Aphasiology, 24*(6–8), 838–855.

Merrett, D., Peretz, I., & Wilson, S. (2014). Neurobiological, cognitive, and emotional mechanisms in melodic intonation therapy. *Frontiers in Human Neuroscience, 8*, 401. doi:10.3389/fnhum.2014.00401

McHenry, M., & Wilson, R. (1994). The challenge of unintelligible speech following traumatic brain injury. *Brain Injury, 8*(4), 363–375.

McMillan, C., Corley, M., & Lickley, R. (2009). Articulatory evidence for feedback and competition in speech production. *Language and Cognitive Processes, 24*(1), 44–66.

McNeil, M., Caliguiri, M., & Rosenbek, J. (1989). Comparison of labiomandibular kinematic durations, displacements, velocities and dysmetrias in apraxic and normal adults. *Clinical Aphasiology, 17*, 173–193.

McNeil, M., Hashi, M., & Southwood, H. (1994). Acoustically derived perceptual evidence for coarticulatory errors in apraxic and conduction aphasic speech production. *Clinical Aphasiology, 22,* 203–218.

McNeil, M., Katz, W., Fossett, T., Garst, D., Szuminsky, N., Carter, G., et al. (2010). Effects of online augmented kinematic and perceptual feedback on treatment of speech movements in apraxia of speech. *Folia Phoniatrica et Logopedica, 62*(3), 127–133.

McNeil, M., Odell, K., Miller, S., & Hunter, L. (1995). Consistency, variability, and target approximation for successive speech repetitions among apraxic, conduction aphasic, and ataxic dysarthric speakers. *Clinical Aphasiology, 23,* 39–55.

McNeil, M., Robin, D., & Schmidt, R. (2009). Apraxia of speech. In M. McNeil (Ed.), *Clinical management of sensorimotor speech disorders* (pp. 249–268). New York, NY: Thieme.

Miller, N. (1992). Variability in speech dyspraxia. *Clinical Linguistics & Phonetics, 6*(1–2), 77–85.

Miller, N. (1995). Pronunciation errors in acquired speech disorders: The errors of our ways. *European Journal Disorders of Communication, 30*(3), 346–361.

Miller, N. (2000). Changing ideas in apraxia of speech. In I. Papathanasiou (Ed.), *Acquired neurogenic communication disorders* (pp. 173–202). London, UK: Whurr.

Miller, N. (2013). Measuring up to speech intelligibility. *International Journal of Language and Communication Disorders, 46*(6), 613–624.

Miller, N., & Lowit, A. (Eds.). (2014). *Motor speech disorders: A cross language perspective.* Clevedon, UK: Multilingual Matters.

Miller, N., Lowit, A., & O'Sullivan, H. (2006). What makes acquired foreign accent syndrome foreign? *Journal of Neurolinguistics, 19*(5), 385–409.

Mitsuya, T., MacDonald, E. N., Purcell, D. W., & Munhall, K. (2011). A cross-language study of compensation in response to real-time formant perturbation. *Journal of the Acoustical Society of America, 130*(5), 2978–2986. doi:10.1121/1.3643826.

Munhall, K., Lofqvist, A., & Kelso, J. (1994). Lip-pharynx coordination in speech: Effects of mechanical perturbations to the lower lip. *Journal of the Acoustical Society of America, 95*(6), 3605–3616.

Nickels, L., & Cole-Virtue, J. (2004). Reading tasks from PALPA: How do controls perform on visual lexical decision, homophony, rhyme, and synonym judgements? *Aphasiology, 18*(2), 103–126.

Nickels, L., & Howard, D. (2004). Dissociating effects of number of phonemes, number of syllables, and syllabic complexity on word production in aphasia: It's the number of phonemes that counts. *Cognitive Neuropsychology, 21*(1), 57–78.

Nishio, M., & Niimi, S. (2006). Comparison of speaking rate, articulation rate and alternating motion rate in dysarthric speakers. *Folia Phoniatrica et Logopaedica, 58*(2), 114–131.

Nozari, N., Dell, G., & Schwartz, M. (2011). Is comprehension necessary for error detection? A conflict-based account of monitoring in speech production. *Cognitive Psychology, 63*(1), 1–33.

Odell, K., McNeil, M., Rosenbek, J., & Hunter, L. (1990). Perceptual characteristics of consonant production by apraxic speakers. *Journal of Speech and Hearing Disorders, 55*(2), 345–359.

Oh, A., Duerden, E., & Pang, E. (2014). The role of the insula in speech and language processing. *Brain and Language, 135,* 96–103.

Partridge, C., & Johnson, M. (1989). Perceived control of recovery from physical disability: Measurement and prediction. *British Journal of Clinical Psychology, 28,* 53–59.

Pattamadilok, C., Morais, J., Colin, C., & Kolinsky, R. (2014). Unattentive speech processing is influenced by orthographic knowledge: Evidence from mismatch negativity. *Brain and Language, 137,* 103–111.

Peach, R., & Tonkovich, J. (2004). Phonemic characteristics of apraxia of speech resulting from subcortical hemorrhage. *Journal of Communication Disorders, 37*(1), 77–90.

Perret, C., Schneider, L., Dayer, G., & Laganaro, M. (2012). Convergences and divergences between neurolinguistic and psycholinguistic data in the study of phonological and phonetic encoding: A parallel investigation of syllable frequency effects in brain-damaged and healthy speakers. *Language, Cognition and Neuroscience, 29*(6), 714–727.

Poeppel, D., Emmorey, K., Hickok, G., & Pylkkänen, L. (2012). Towards a new neurobiology of language. *The Journal of Neuroscience, 32*(41), 14125–14131.

Pouplier, M., & Hardcastle, W. (2005). A re-evaluation of the nature of speech errors in normal and disordered speakers. *Phonetica, 62*(2–4), 227–243.

Pouplier, M., Marin, S., & Waltl, S. (2014). Voice onset time in consonant cluster errors: Can phonetic accommodation differentiate cognitive from motor errors? *Journal of Speech, Language, and Hearing Research, 57*(5), 1577–1588.

Preston, J., & Leaman, M. (2014). Ultrasound visual feedback for acquired apraxia of speech: A case report. *Aphasiology, 28*(3), 278–295.

Price, C. (2012). A review and synthesis of the first 20 years of PET and fMRI studies of heard speech, spoken language and reading. *NeuroImage, 62*(2), 816–847.

Rabidoux, P., Florance, C., & McCauslin, L. (1980). The use of a Handi Voice in the treatment of a severely apractic nonverbal patient. In R. H. Brookshire (Ed.), *Clinical Aphasiology Conference proceedings* (pp. 294–301). Minneapolis, MN: BRK.

Raymer, A., & Thompson, C. (1991). Effects of verbal plus gestural treatment in a patient with aphasia and severe apraxia of speech. In T. E. Prescott (Ed.), *Clinical aphasiology* (Vol. 20, pp. 285–298). Austin, TX: Pro-Ed.

Riecker, A., Brendel, B., Ziegler, W., Erb, M., & Ackermann, H. (2008). The influence of syllable onset complexity and syllable frequency on speech motor control. *Brain and Language, 107*(2), 102–113.

Robin, D., Jacks, A., & Ramage, A. (2008). The neural substrates of apraxia of speech as uncovered by brain imaging: A critical review. In R. Ingham (Ed.), *Neuroimaging in communication sciences and disorders* (pp. 129–154). San Diego, CA: Plural.

Rochon, E., Caplan, D., & Waters, G. (1990). Short-term memory processes in patients with apraxia of speech. *Journal of Neurolinguistics, 5,* 2–3.

Romani, C., & Galluzzi, C. (2005). Effects of syllabic complexity in predicting accuracy of repetition and direction of errors in patients with articulatory and phonological difficulties. *Cognitive Neuropsychology, 22*(7), 817–850.

Rose, M., & Douglas, J. (2006). A comparison of verbal and gesture treatments for a word production deficit resulting from acquired apraxia of speech. *Aphasiology, 20*(12), 1186–1209.

Rosenbek, J., Collins, M., & Wertz, R. (1976). Intersystemic reorganization for apraxia of speech. In R. H. Brookshire (Ed.),

Clinical Aphasiology Conference proceedings (pp. 255–260). Minneapolis, MN: BRK.

Rosenbek, J., Lemme, M., Ahern, M., Harris, E., & Wertz, R. (1973). Treatment for apraxia of speech in adults. *Journal of Speech and Hearing Disorders, 38*(4), 462–472.

Rosenberg, M. (1965). *Society and the adolescent self-image.* Princeton, NJ: Princeton University Press.

Sapir, S. (2014). Multiple factors are involved in the dysarthria associated with Parkinson's disease: A review with implications for clinical practice and research. *Journal of Speech, Language, and Hearing Research, 57*(4), 1330–1343.

Schmidt, R., & Lee, T. (2005). *Motor control and learning: A behavioral emphasis.* Champaign, IL: Human Kinetics.

Schneider, S., & Frens, R. (2005). Training four-syllable CV patterns in individuals with acquired apraxia of speech: Theoretical implications. *Aphasiology, 19*(3/4/5), 451–471.

Schoor, A., Aichert, I., & Ziegler, W. (2012). A motor learning perspective on phonetic syllable kinships: How training effects transfer from learned to new syllables in severe apraxia of speech. *Aphasiology, 26,* 880–894.

Seddoh, S., K., Robin, D., Sim, H., Hageman, C., Moon, J., & Folkins, J. (1996). Speech timing in apraxia of speech versus conduction aphasia. *Journal of Speech and Hearing Research, 39*(3), 590–603.

Shaiman, S., & Gracco, V. (2002). Task-specific sensorimotor interactions in speech production. *Experimental Brain Research, 146*(4), 411–418.

Shuster, L., & Wambaugh, J. (2008). Token-to-token variability in adult apraxia of speech: A perceptual analysis. *Aphasiology, 22*(6), 655–669.

Sidiropoulos, K., de Bleser, R., Ackermann, H., & Preilowski, B. (2008). Pre-lexical disorders in repetition conduction aphasia. *Neuropsychologia, 46*(14), 3225–3238.

Simmons, N. (1978). Finger counting as an intersystemic reorganizer in apraxia of speech. In R. H. Brookshire (Ed.), *Clinical Aphasiology Conference proceedings* (pp. 174–179). Minneapolis, MN: BRK.

Sparks, R., Helm, N., & Albert, M. (1974). Aphasia rehabilitation resulting from melodic intonation therapy. *Cortex, 10*(4), 303–316.

Sparks, R., & Holland, A. (1976). Melodic intonation therapy. *Journal of Speech and Hearing Disorders, 41,* 287–297.

Sparks, R. W. (2008). Melodic intonation therapy. In R. Chapey (Ed.). *Language intervention strategies in aphasia and related neurogenic communication disorders* (5th ed., pp. 837–851). Philadelphia, PA: Lippincott, Williams, & Wilkins.

Spencer, K., & Slocomb, D. (2007). The neural basis of ataxic dysarthria. *The Cerebellum, 6*(1), 58–65.

Southwood, H. (1987). The use of prolonged speech in the treatment of apraxia of speech. In R. H. Brookshire (Ed.), *Clinical Aphasiology Conference proceedings* (pp. 277–287). Minneapolis, MN: BRK.

Square, P., Martin, R., & Bose, A. (2001). Nature and treatment of neuromotor speech disorders in aphasia. In R. H. Chapey (Ed.), *Language intervention strategies in adult aphasia* (4th ed., pp. 847–884). Baltimore, MD: Williams & Wilkins.

Square-Storer, P., Darley, F., & Sommers, R. (1988). Nonspeech and speech processing skills in patients with aphasia and apraxia of speech. *Brain and Language, 33*(1), 65–85.

Square-Storer, P., & Hayden, D. (1989). PROMPT treatment. In P. Square-Storer (Ed.), *Acquired apraxia of speech in aphasic adults* (pp. 190–219). Hove, UK: Erlbaum.

Staiger, A., Finger-Berg, W., Aichert, I., & Ziegler, W. (2012). Error variability in apraxia of speech: A matter of controversy. *Journal of Speech, Language, and Hearing Research, 55*(5), S1544–S1561.

Staiger, A., & Ziegler, W. (2008). Syllable frequency and syllable structure in the spontaneous speech production of patients with apraxia of speech. *Aphasiology, 22*(11), 1201–1215.

Strand, E., Duffy, J., Clark, H., & Josephs, K. (2014). The apraxia of speech rating scale: A tool for diagnosis and description of apraxia of speech. *Journal of Communication Disorders, 51*(0), 43–50.

Thompson, C., & Shapiro, L. (2007). Complexity in treatment of syntactic deficits. *American Journal of Speech-Language Pathology, 16,* 30–42.

Thompson, C., Shapiro, L., Kiran, S., & Sobecks, J. (2003). The role of syntactic complexity in treatment of sentence deficits in agrammatic aphasia: The complexity account of treatment efficacy (CATE). *Journal of Speech, Language, and Hearing Research, 46,* 591–607.

Threats, T. T. (2009). Severe aphasia: Possible contributions of using the ICF in assessment. *Perspectives on Neurophysiology and Neurogenic Speech and Language Disorders, 19,* 7–14.

Trupe, L., Varma, D., Gomez, Y., Race, D., Leigh, R., Hillis, A., et al. (2013). Chronic apraxia of speech and Broca's area. *Stroke, 44*(3), 740–744.

van der Merwe, A. (2007). Self-correction in apraxia of speech: The effect of treatment. *Aphasiology, 21*(6), 658–669.

van der Merwe, A. (2008). Theoretical framework for the characterisation of pathological speech sensorimotor control. In M. McNeil (Ed.), *Clinical management of sensorimotor speech disorders* (2nd ed., pp. 3–18). New York, NY: Thieme.

van der Meulen, I., van de Sandt-Koenderman, W., Heijenbrok-Kal, M., Visch-Brink, E., & Ribbers, G. (2014). The efficacy and timing of melodic intonation therapy in subacute aphasia. *Neurorehabilitation and Neural Repair, 28*(6), 536–544.

van Lancker, D. (1987). Nonpropositional speech. In A. W. Ellis (Ed.), *Progress in the psychology of language* (Vol. 3, pp. 49–118). Hillsdale, NJ: LEA.

Wambaugh, J. (2002). A summary of treatments for apraxia of speech and review of replicated approaches. *Seminars in Speech and Language, 23*(4), 293–308.

Wambaugh, J. (2004). Stimulus generalization effects of sound production treatment for apraxia of speech. *Journal of Medical Speech-Language Pathology, 12*(2), 77–97.

Wambaugh, J., Duffy, J., McNeil, M., Robin, D., & Rogers, M. (2006a). Treatment guidelines for acquired apraxia of speech: A synthesis and evaluation of the evidence. *Journal of Medical Speech-Language Pathology, 14*(2), xv–xxxiii.

Wambaugh, J., Duffy, J., McNeil, M., Robin, D., & Rogers, M. (2006b). Treatment guidelines for acquired apraxia of speech: Treatment descriptions and recommendations. *Journal of Medical Speech-Language Pathology, 14*(2), xxxv–lxvii.

Wambaugh, J., Kalinyak-Fliszar, M., West, J., & Doyle, P. (1998). Effects of treatment for sound errors in apraxia of speech and aphasia. *Journal of Speech, Language, and Hearing Research, 41,* 725–743.

Wambaugh, J., & Martinez, A. (2000). Effects of rate and rhythm control treatment on consonant production accuracy in apraxia of speech. *Aphasiology, 14*(8), 851–871.

Wambaugh, J., & Mauszycki, S. (2010a). Application of the WHO ICF to management of acquired apraxia of speech. *Journal of Medical Speech-Language Pathology, 18*(4), 133–140.

Wambaugh, J., & Mauszycki, S. (2010b). Sound production treatment: Application with severe apraxia of speech. *Aphasiology, 24*(6–8), 814–825.

Wambaugh, J., & Nessler, C. (2004). Modification of sound production treatment in AoS: Acquisition and generalisation effects. *Aphasiology, 18*, 407–427.

Wambaugh, J., Nessler, C., Cameron, R., & Mauszycki, S. (2012). Acquired apraxia of speech: The effects of repeated practice and rate/rhythm control treatments on sound production accuracy. *American Journal of Speech-Language Pathology, 21*(2), s5–s27.

Wambaugh, J., Nessler, C., Cameron, R., & Mauszycki, S. (2013). Treatment for acquired apraxia of speech: Examination of treatment intensity and practice schedule. *American Journal of Speech-Language Pathology, 22*, 84–102.

Wambaugh, J., Nessler, C., Mauszycki, S., & Cameron, R. (2014). Stimulus generalization effects of treatment for acquired apraxia of speech. *Journal of Medical Speech-Language Pathology, 21*(3), 195–233.

Wambaugh, J., Nessler, C., Wright, S., & Mauszycki, S. (2014). Sound production treatment: Effects of blocked and random practice. *American Journal of Speech-Language Pathology, 23*, s225–s245

Wambaugh, J., & Shuster, L. (2008). The nature and management of neuromotor speech disorders accompanying aphasia. In R. Chapey (Ed.), *Language intervention strategies in aphasia and related neurogenic communication disorders* (5th ed., pp. 1009–1042). Philadelphia, PA: Lippincott Williams & Wilkins.

Warren, S., Fey, M., Yoder, P. (2007). Differential treatment intensity research: A missing link to creating optimally effective communication interventions. *Mental Retardation and Developmental Disabilities Research Reviews, 13*, 70–77.

Wertz, R., LaPointe, L., & Rosenbek, J. (1984). *Apraxia of speech in adults: The disorder and its management.* Orlando, FL: Grune & Stratton.

World Health Organization. (2001). *International classification of functioning, disability, and health.* Geneva, Switzerland: Author.

Wright, D., Robin, D., Rhee, J., Vaculin, A., Jacks, A., Guenther, F., et al. (2009). Using the self-select paradigm to delineate the nature of speech motor programming. *Journal of Speech, Language, and Hearing Research, 52*(3), 755–765.

Yorkston, K., & Waugh, P. (1989). Use of augmentative communication devices with apractic individuals. In P. Square-Storer (Ed.), *Acquired apraxia of speech in aphasic adults* (pp. 267–283). Hove, UK: Erlbaum.

Ziegler, W. (2002). Task-related factors in oral motor control: Speech and oral diadochokinesis in dysarthria and apraxia of speech. *Brain and Language, 80*(3), 556–575.

Ziegler, W. (2009). Modelling the architecture of phonetic plans: Evidence from apraxia of speech. *Language and Cognitive Processes, 24*(5), 631–661.

Ziegler, W. (2013). The rhythmic organisation of speech gestures and the sense of it. *Language, Cognition and Neuroscience, 29*(1), 38–40.

Ziegler, W., & Ackermann, H. (2013). Neuromotor speech impairment: It's all in the talking. *Folia Phoniatrica et Logopaedica, 65*(2), 55–67.

Ziegler, W., Aichert, I., & Staiger, A. (2012). Apraxia of speech: Concepts and controversies. *Journal of Speech, Language, and Hearing Research, 55*(5), S1485–S1501.

Ziegler, W., & von Cramon, D. (1985). Anticipatory coarticulation in a patient with apraxia of speech. *Brain and Language, 26*(1), 117–130.

Ziegler, W., & von Cramon, D. (1986). Disturbed coarticulation in apraxia of speech: Acoustic evidence. *Brain and Language, 29*(1), 34–47.

Zumbansen, A., Peretz, I., & Hébert, S. (2014). The combination of rhythm and pitch can account for the beneficial effect of melodic intonation therapy on connected speech improvements in broca's aphasia. *Frontiers in Human Neuroscience, 8*, 592. doi:10.3389/fnhum.2014.00592.

OBJECTIVES

The reader will be able to:

1. Discuss contemporary directions in the computational modeling of speech production.

2. Identify issues pertaining to a life-span perspective on dysarthria.

3. List the different types of dysarthria and discuss current issues in terms of dysarthria classification.

4. Describe how dysarthria can affect an individual at each level of functioning within the International Classification of Functioning, Disability, and Health (ICF; World Health Organization [WHO], 2001) model.

5. Identify relevant assessment procedures for evaluating speech impairment and its consequences in individuals with dysarthria.

6. Summarize major approaches for direct and indirect treatment of communication difficulties associated with dysarthria and be aware of their evidence base.

Management of Dysarthria

A. Lowit and R. D. Kent

INTRODUCTION

Dysarthria is a disturbance in the sensorimotor processes of speech production associated with damage to the central or peripheral nervous system. Together with apraxia of speech (AoS), the dysarthrias comprise the motor speech disorders. In their classic text, Darley, Aronson, and Brown (1975) defined dysarthria as a speech disorder resulting from a weakness, paralysis, or incoordination of the speech musculature that is of neurological etiology. As discussed further in this chapter, this definition does not align completely with current concepts in neurology, especially in regard to the various syndromes in the category of movement disorders. Many dysarthrias are not accompanied by obvious weakness or paralysis, and incoordination is difficult to assess clinically.

A more contemporary definition is from Duffy (2013): "A group of neurologic speech disorders resulting from abnormalities in the strength, speed, range, steadiness, tone, or accuracy of movements, required for control of the respiratory, phonatory, resonatory, articulatory, and prosodic aspects of speech production" (p. 4). Duffy expands this definition to indicate etiology (abnormalities of the central or peripheral nervous system) and associated motor signs or symptoms (weakness, spasticity, incoordination, involuntary movements, or excessive, reduced, or variable muscle tone). An alternative definition is given in a further section of this chapter following discussion of several background issues.

Traditionally, dysarthria has been regarded as a problem in motor execution, that is, difficulty in carrying out a motor plan or program, which itself is assumed to be intact. However, van der Merwe (1997) proposed a different perspective in which dysarthrias are classified as either a disorder of programming–execution or a disorder of execution, depending on the type of dysarthria. Support for the concept of motor programming dysfunction in dysarthria comes from a priming study by Spencer and Rogers (2005), who interpreted their data as evidence that some individuals with dysarthria may have difficulties in maintaining a motor program or in switching between programs. More recent reports have confirmed the principle that the dysarthrias should be understood as more than disorders of execution (Melle & Gallego, 2012; Sapir, 2014). Aspects of motor programming may be interwoven with aspects of motor execution, an idea that is consistent with the task sensitivity of speech production in individuals with dysarthria (Kempler & Van Lancker, 2002; Kent, Kent, Rosenbek, Vorperian, & Weismer, 1997; Spencer & Slocomb, 2007; Ziegler, 2002). The idea that movement disorders are not solely disorders of execution also has been raised in the neurological literature, especially with respect to issues of motor preparation (Ho, Bradshaw, & Iansek, 2008), selection and inhibition of competing motor programs (Mink, 1996), integration of somatosensory information (Kaňovský, 2002), and executive functions such as planning and set-shifting (i.e., adjustments in the mode of response to handle changing circumstances) (Monchi, Petrides, Strafella, Worsley, & Doyon, 2006).

As discussed in the next section, this conception of motor control is consistent with recent neurocomputational modeling of speech production.

MODELS OF SPEECH PRODUCTION AND SPEECH MOTOR CONTROL

Progress in understanding dysarthria comes not only from studies of dysarthria per se but also from studies of normal motor processes in speech, particularly advances in neural models and neuroimaging. Integrating the knowledge from different methods of study is not always straightforward, as D. V. L. Sidtis (2007) discusses with respect to reconciling results from functional brain imaging and traditional lesion studies. But, a notable convergence can be seen in neuroimaging studies of normal speech production, neuroimaging, and other lesion studies of dysarthria and computational modeling of speech production. This convergence may signal a new era in the study of dysarthria.

Activation studies have helped define the essential neural network of speech production. This network includes mesiofrontal structures (supplementary motor area and anterior cingulate gyrus); bilateral precentral and postcentral convolutions, extending rostrally into posterior parts of the inferior frontal gyrus; the left anterior insula as well as bilateral components of the basal ganglia (notably the putamen, caudate, and globus pallidus); the cerebellum (notably lobule VI, including the declive); the thalamus; and the superior temporal gyrus (Bohland & Guenther, 2006; S. Brown et al., 2009; Golfinopoulos, Tourville, & Guenther, 2010; Hickok, 2012; Price, 2012; Riecker, Brendel, Ziegler, Erb, & Ackermann, 2008; Sörös et al., 2006). Many of the same neural structures have been identified in lesion studies of the dysarthrias (Duffy, 2013; Kent, Duffy, Slama, Kent, & Clift, 2001). The neural network determined from studies of adult speakers also seems to apply in general respects to the speech production network in children, although vulnerability to neural damage is not equivalent in developing and mature individuals (Liegeois & Morgan, 2012).

The results of studies of functional activation have contributed to the development of computational neural network models of speech production, including directions into velocities of the articulators (DIVA; Guenther & Vladusich, 2012); state feedback control (SFC; Houde & Nagarajan, 2011); hierarchical state feedback control (HSFC; Hickok, 2012); and the neurocomputational model developed by Kröger and colleagues (Kröger, Schnitker, & Lowit, 2008). Common to these models is the use of feedback and feedforward signals that enable predictive and adaptive control over articulatory movements in speech. Feedback signals are critically important in the development of speech motor control, and it is often assumed that auditory feedback is used to establish an initial set of motor programs that are eventually refined through somatosensory feedback. Children who are learning speech are highly dependent on feedback, but adults use feedback only intermittently and rely instead on feedforward signals to control speech movements. Modern conceptions of the neural systems involved in speech production are an important foundation for advances in the understanding of dysarthria in children and adults.

LIFE-SPAN PERSPECTIVES ON DYSARTHRIA

Dysarthria can arise because of congenital conditions (as in genetic disorders or cerebral palsy) or can be acquired at any age as the result of neurologic injury or disease. Motor speech disorders (dysarthria and apraxia of speech) in children often have been viewed through the lens of motor speech disorders in adults, reversing the adage that "the child is father (mother) to the man (woman)." But, there is good reason to believe that the disorders in children are different from those acquired by adults who had premorbidly normal speech. A lifespan perspective on motor speech disorders must contend with the developmental processes of speech that pertain to children versus the mature maintenance processes that apply in adults.

Recent research on the neural correlates of childhood speech disorders indicates that persistent and severe disorders are associated with bilateral neurological damage, whereas adult speech disorders often result from unilateral damage (Liegeois & Morgan, 2012). In a review of studies of the speech features in acquired childhood dysarthria, van Mourik, Catsman-Berrevoets, Yousef-Bak, and van Dongen (1997) remarked that definite similarities to adult dysarthria were not evident, although there was some similarity to acquired childhood dysarthria due to basal ganglia lesions. They concluded that "acquired childhood dysarthria requires its own classification" (p. 299). Now, more than 15 years later, no such classification is widely adopted. Especially in the case of a dysarthria with infantile onset, it cannot be assumed that the child ever develops age-typical motor programs for speech production.

Life-span perspectives also can be important for acquired dysarthria in adults, especially when the dysarthria is stable or progressive, in which case the original pathophysiology of the dysarthria may interact with processes of aging. Studies of healthy older adults evince changes in voice, articulatory precision, and speaking rate (Amerman & Parnell, 1990; Gorham-Rowan & Laures-Gore, 2006; Hartman & Danhauer, 1976; L. A. Ramig, 1983; Ryan & Burk, 1974), which often are features descriptive of dysarthria. Especially in older adults with dysarthria, it is likely that aging processes may contribute to the speech disorder. For example, Amerman and Parnell (1990) found that the speech of several normal elderly speakers was judged as dysarthric by a group of speech–language clinicians. It is therefore important to be mindful of the effects of normal aging when diagnosing a person with a suspected speech disorder in order not to misinterpret symptoms of natural speech deterioration as evidence of speech impairment.

ISSUES OF DYSARTHRIA CLASSIFICATION

As a first step in considering the classification of the dysarthrias, we propose the following definition: *The dysarthrias are a group of speech disorders resulting from neurologic disease or damage affecting the sensorimotor processes of speech production, typically associated with hypokinesia, hyperkinesia, spasticity, weakness, or disturbances of tone.* This definition departs from most others in two respects. First, it emphasizes that speech production is based on sensorimotor processes, that is, on the integration of sensory information in the planning and execution of movements. Second, it

aligns with contemporary patterns in neurologic classifications relevant to dysarthria. Both of these points are elaborated in the following material.

Sensory factors, rather neglected in considerations of dysarthria, are coming into view. As discussed in the section on models of speech production and speech motor control, current efforts to develop computational models of speech assign a critical role to sensory processes. Perhaps more than any other motor system, speech generates plurimodal sensory information, including auditory, barometric, kinesthetic, and tactile signals that are fundamental to the development of speech in children and to its maintenance in adults. Although sensory testing may not be routine or standardized in the clinical examination of dysarthria, there are indications that sensory processing may be disrupted, to the detriment of speech motor control. For example, sensory dysfunction has been reported in Parkinson's disease (PD; Hammer & Barlow, 2010; Trail et al., 2005). It is becoming clear that damage to some of the neural structures that are implicated in dysarthria have important roles in sensory function related to motor control. Disturbances of sensorimotor integration have been linked to movement disorders resulting from damage to the basal ganglia (Abbruzzese & Berardelli, 2002). In addition, the cerebellum, which receives considerable sensory input, appears to play a role in predicting the sensory consequences of action (Blakemore, Frith, & Wolpert, 2001).

One example of evolving classifications in neurology is the group of movement disorders. These disorders have been defined as "neurological syndromes in which there is either an excess of movement or a paucity of voluntary and automatic movements, unrelated to weakness or spasticity" (Fahn, 2011, p. 948). Current thinking is that movement disorders are better conceptualized in terms of clinical phenomenology rather than on anatomic location. Fahn (2011) pointed out that a term such as *extrapyramidal* to describe the anatomic basis of movement disorders is misleading because "the basal ganglia have intimate connections with the pyramidal tract system, and therefore, the basal ganglia are not truly extrapyramidal" (p. 947). He also notes that some disorders of abnormal movement, such as ataxia and myoclonus, are not associated with pathology of the basal ganglia and would more appropriately be considered in a general category of movement disorders. Dysarthria is associated with many, but not all, movement disorders recognized by Fahn, Jankovic, and Hallett (2011). Table 22.1 lists the most relevant movement disorders in the two general categories of hypokinesias and hyperkinesias. Dysarthrias also result from other neurological conditions, such as weakness and spasticity.

Table 22.1 Movement Disorders (Following Fahn, Jankovic, & Hallett, 2011) Most Likely to Be Associated With a Motor Speech Disorder

Hypokinesia	Hyperkinesia
Akinesia/bradykinesia (parkinsonism)	Ataxia
Apraxia	Athetosis
Rigidity	Chorea
	Dystonia
	Hemifacial spasm
	Myoclonus
	Stereotypy
	Tics
	Tremor

Having established that all dysarthrias are associated with underlying sensorimotor impairments, the classification of the disorder into distinct types needs to be considered next. In medicine, diseases are classified primarily by etiology, pathogenesis, or symptomatology. In the case of dysarthria, taxonomy is usually based on perceptual features (symptomatology) or by underlying neuropathology (etiology or pathogenesis). Classification of dysarthrias by perceptual features is reasonable given that dysarthria is defined as a speech disorder and most speech disorders historically have been characterized according to their perceptual attributes. Classification by neuropathology assumes the availability and validity of a neurologic diagnosis. Darley, Aronson, and Brown (1969a, 1969b) distinguished the dysarthrias by their auditory–perceptual features but concluded that the resulting classifications were consonant with neurological diagnoses. The dysarthria classifications defined by Darley, Aronson, and Brown (often called the Mayo system, as we do here), or similar classifications such as that in the Frenchay Dysarthria Assessment (FDA; Enderby, 1983), are the predominant nosologies of dysarthria.

The dysarthria classifications in the Mayo system are summarized in Table 22.2, which shows the dysarthria types, associated neurologic lesions, and commonly associated injuries or diseases. The dysarthria types in Table 22.2 often occur in combinations, such as flaccid–spastic dysarthria in amyotrophic lateral sclerosis (ALS). Table 22.3 lists several neurologic diseases that are typically associated with such mixed dysarthrias. Darley et al. (1969a, 1969b) regarded their dysarthria classifications as hypotheses, and they were quite reasonable proposals given the state of knowledge and technology at the time. As Morgan (2013) commented, "The sub classifications were based on relatively gross anatomical distinctions such as the cerebellum (ataxic dysarthria) or the basal ganglia (hyper or hypokinetic dysarthria), arguably using a locationist approach" (p. 251). But, as mentioned in the first section of this chapter, speech production is accomplished with a large network of neural structures.

Table 22.2 Perceptual Types of Dysarthria in the Mayo System With Associated Neurologic Lesions and Commonly Associated Injuries or Diseases

Dysarthria Type	Common Lesion Site	Common Associated Injury or Disease
Flaccid	Lower motor neuron (cranial or spinal nerve) (lower motor neuron syndrome)	Peripheral nervous system trauma, myasthenia gravis, amyotrophic lateral sclerosis
Spastic	Pyramidal motor system (upper motor neuron syndrome)	Stroke (especially bilateral), amyotrophic lateral sclerosis, progressive supranuclear palsy, traumatic brain injury
Ataxic	Cerebellum and its outflow tracts; cerebellar damage usually bilateral or generalized; focal lesions typically right sided, involving posteromedial or paravermal regions or lateral hemisphere	Friedreich's ataxia and other spinocerebellar syndromes, cerebellar degeneration, multiple sclerosis, multiple system atrophy, posterior fossa surgery (especially in children)
Hypokinetic	Basal ganglia: nigrostriatal pathways	Parkinson's disease, progressive supranuclear palsy, corticobasal degeneration, striatonigral degeneration, multiple system atrophy
Hyperkinetic–choreic	Basal ganglia	Sydenham's chorea, Huntington's disease, tardive dykinesia, stroke
Hyperkinetic–dystonic	Basal ganglia	Spasmodic torticollis

Table 22.3 Examples of Neurologic Diseases Typically Associated With Mixed Dysarthrias

Neurologic Disease	Type of Dysarthria	Main Lesion Sites	Comments
Amyotrophic lateral sclerosis (also known as Lou Gehrig's disease, Charcot disease, or especially in the United Kingdom, motor neuron disease)	Flaccid–spastic	A progressive, invariably fatal neurological disease that attacks the motor neurons in the brain, brain stem, and spinal cord	A distinction often is made between limb-onset and bulbar-onset disease, with speech and swallowing difficulties characterizing the latter.
Multiple sclerosis (also known as disseminated sclerosis or encephalomyelitis disseminate)	Spastic–ataxic + others possible	Variable among patients	Inflammatory disease that damages the myelin covering of nerve cells in the brain and spinal cord.
Multiple-system atrophy–C (also called sporadic olivopontocerebellar atrophy)	Ataxic–spastic	Cerebellar features; cerebellar ataxia predominates	Adult-onset, sporadic, rapidly progressive, multisystem, neurodegenerative, fatal disease.
Multiple-system atrophy–P (also called striatonigral degeneration, parkinsonian variant)	Hypokinetic–spastic	Extrapyramidal features predominate; parkinsonism	Adult-onset, sporadic, rapidly progressive, multisystem, neurodegenerative, fatal disease.
Progressive supranuclear palsy	Spastic–hypokinetic (sometimes ataxic)	Especially affected are the basal ganglia, substantia nigra, subthalamus, and brain stem	Neurodegenerative disease characterized by supranuclear, initially vertical, gaze dysfunction, along with extrapyramidal symptoms and cognitive dysfunction.
Traumatic brain injury	Highly variable, depending on location and severity of neural damage. Flaccid dysarthria is typical of damage to the cranial nerves. Central nervous system damage often is associated with a mixed dysarthria.	Focal and diffuse pathologies can occur independently or concurrently, with focal effects, including contusion and hematoma formation, and diffuse effects, including diffuse axonal injury and diffuse microvascular damage. These pathologies can be accompanied by more generalized pathologies, such as widespread neuroexcitation and heterogeneous as well as global metabolic changes.	Lesions are highly variable across individuals, and the dysarthria may be accompanied by a number of cognitive and personality disorders.
Wilson's disease	Spastic–ataxic–hypokinetic	Diffuse damage, especially to dentorubrothalamic, pontocerebellar, and corticospinal tracts	Rare autosomal recessive inherited disorder of copper metabolism that results in excessive deposition of copper in the liver, brain, and other tissues.

To give Darley et al. (1969a, 1969b) their due, it should be emphasized that their work accomplished a major systematization of brain–behavior relationships in the understanding of dysarthria, helping to bridge between speech and language pathology and neurology. But, the effort should not end there, especially with the capability of current neuroimaging tools to depict regional activations in the neural network of speech production in both healthy and disordered speakers.

The Mayo system rests largely on auditory perceptual ratings of speech. Since the publication of the seminal papers on this system, studies on the reliability of the perceptual classification of the dysarthrias have yielded mixed results. Modest or poor reliability has been reported in several studies. Fonville et al. (2008) wrote that, "Neurological trainees as well as experienced neurologists have great difficulty in identifying specific types of dysarthria on the basis of perceptual analysis alone" (p. 1545). Similarly, van der Graaf et al. (2009) cautioned that, "Neurologists should be aware of the unreliability of identifying the dysarthria type without the use of additional validated instruments or rating scales in a clinical setting" (p. 295).

A more positive conclusion on the reliability of auditory ratings of dysarthria comes from the study of Bunton, Kent, Duffy, Rosenbek, and Kent (2007), who reported that agreement between judges for auditory perceptual dimensions of dysarthria was within 1 scale value or less for 67% of the pairwise comparisons. Whether this level of agreement is satisfactory for clinical application depends on the purpose(s) of clinical assessment. If the goal is to construct an overall profile of the speech disturbance, then this level of agreement probably suffices. But, if the goal is to detect subtle changes in speech, such as might be related to an ongoing treatment or to disease progression, then this level of agreement may not be satisfactory. For example, in an investigation of the optimal settings for deep brain stimulation in individuals with PD, Chenausky, MacAuslan, and Goldhor (2011) concluded that, "It would not be possible to identify either compromise or optimal single-purpose settings without consideration of acoustic measures of speech such as the ones used here, because perceptual differences are not always fine or reliable enough to accurately assess small differences in speech" (p. 12).

Bunton et al. (2007) concluded that the perceptual fingerprint of dysarthria was generally expressed in a speech sample duration of 40 seconds. In a study involving quantitative acoustic analysis, it was reported that hypokinetic dysarthria could be distinguished from healthy speech with a sample of 2 minutes (Rosen, Kent, Delaney, & Duffy, 2006). These studies show that essential properties of dysarthria may be evident in relatively short samples of speech.

Poor reliability in the perceptual classification of dysarthria type for a corpus of mixed dysarthrias does not necessarily mean that classification is unreliable for all types of dysarthria and for all judges who make perceptual ratings. Some types may have greater perceptual salience than others. It also is likely that reliability of classification is affected by listener training and experience with dysarthric speech samples representing a range of severity and diverse types of dysarthria. Rather than discard perceptual classification altogether, an alternative is to assign a confidence rating to the classification for an individual speaker.

The perceptual features associated with particular type of dysarthria may vary with the severity of the dysarthria and with differences in underlying pathophysiology. Taking ataxic dysarthria as an example, it has been reported that perceptual speech characteristics vary with lesions in different cerebellar nuclei (Vandana & Manjula, 2014), among three genotypes of ataxia (J. J. Sidtis, Ahn, Gomez, & Sidtis, 2011), and among individuals with Friedreich's ataxia (Folker et al., 2010). Ataxic dysarthria may be a convenient rubric for speech disturbances associated with damage to the cerebellum and its efferent tracts, but it does not imply an invariant constellation of perceptual features. Ataxic dysarthria probably is not unique in this respect. Given the multidimensionality of the acoustic speech signal, the complexity of the neural network serving speech production, and the large and variegated muscular system by which speech is produced, it is not surprising to observe individual variation in the auditory–perceptual features of a given dysarthria. Adding to the complexity are the possibilities of individual compensations to dysarthria and the presence of concomitant disorders such as hearing loss, apraxia of speech, or aphasia.

Even if the perceptual classification of dysarthria is not always reliable for a given judge or group of judges, the identification of atypical perceptual dimensions (e.g., disorders of voice quality, rhythm, speech sound production) can have value in describing the profile of the dysarthria for purposes such as assessing disease progression or planning treatment. Classification of type of dysarthria is not necessarily critical to the development of a treatment plan, especially if such a plan is based on factors such as subsystem integrity (e.g., the functionality of the respiratory, phonatory, articulatory, and resonatory systems of speech production). The approach to perceptual evaluation of dysarthria may be evolving. For example, the seminal studies of dysarthria by Darley et al. (1969a, 1969b) at the Mayo Clinic in the United States involved the rating of 38 perceptual dimensions on a 7-point equal-appearing interval scale. But, current practice at the Mayo Clinic is to make ratings on a 5-point scale, with each scale value having a verbal descriptor (normal, mild, moderate, marked, severe) (Duffy, 2013). In addition, some dimensions (e.g., pitch level, overall loudness, and speaking rate) are rated simply with a plus or minus. Typically, ratings are made for the most salient perceptual dimensions rather than the full list of 38 dimensions used in the earlier Mayo Clinic studies. The selection of a clinicometric tool is a balance of several factors, including validity, sensitivity, reliability, efficiency, and general applicability. Rating of 38 perceptual dimensions probably is too cumbersome for routine clinical applications, but rating of a few select dimensions runs the risk of providing incomplete information.

The potential for classification of dysarthria is not only in the mind of a human listener but also in the processing capability of computers. Several efforts have been made to design and test computer-based systems for the assessment of dysarthria in terms of severity level (Kadi, Selouani, Bourdraa, & Boudraa, 2013) and dysarthria type (Guerra & Lovely, 2003; Mujumdar & Kubichek, 2010; Stylios, Georgopoloulos, Malandraki, & Chouliara, 2008). The results are promising and may lead to the development of automatic and objective assessments that can complement and, in some instances even replace, judgments from humans. Perhaps the most interesting lesson to be drawn from applications of computational algorithms is that machines can replicate with moderate-to-good success the classifications performed by expert human judges. Such results usually assume that human perceptual judgments are in fact the gold standard for the identification of dysarthria types, which leaves open the question whether all judges are capable of gold standard expertise. One step toward evaluation of computer-based approaches is the use of dysarthric speech samples from openly accessible databases, as such resources provide opportunities to compare various approaches to the assessment of dysarthria. Unfortunately, only a few modest-size databases exist (H. Kim et al., 2008; Menendez-Pidal, Polikoff, Peters, Leonzjo, & Bunnell, 1996; Rudzicz, Namasivayam, & Wolff, 2012).

The classification of dysarthria can have a role in neurologic diagnosis (Auzou et al., 2000; Duffy, 2010), but classification has not emerged as a particularly potent factor in recent studies of muscle tone (Dietsch et al., 2014), acoustic correlates of dysarthria (Y. Kim, Kent, & Weismer, 2011), and auditory free-classification of dysarthric speech samples (Lansford, Liss, & Norton, 2014). Weismer and Kim (2010) called for a taxonomic approach to research in dysarthria, including a relaxation, if not outright rejection, of demands that type of dysarthria be specified in research articles and research grant applications.

With respect to clinical applications other than neurologic diagnosis, the primary question is whether knowing the type of dysarthria is an important variable in designing treatment. We turn to this issue in the next section.

ASSESSMENT OF DYSARTHRIA

The answer to the question of whether knowing the dysarthria type is an important variable in treatment design in many cases is no. Instead, effective management of dysarthria depends on a thorough consideration of the nature of the communication problem and how it affects the person's quality of life (QOL). This follows the ideas of the ICF (WHO, 2001) framework, which has moved our thinking away from considering patients in terms of their impairments and paying closer attention to how impairments limit their activity and participation in communication.

Unfortunately, this approach is not reflected in many of the published dysarthria tests, which were developed at a time when Darley et al.'s (1975) medical model was the primary approach applied to assessment of the disorder. Darley et al.'s (1975) own procedure, as well as other variants such as the FDA (Enderby, 1983), FDA-2 (Enderby & Palmer, 2008), the Robertson Dysarthria Profile (Robertson, 1982), or the Dysarthria Examination Battery (Drummond, 1993), all focus heavily on the body level of the ICF and include tasks, mostly of a nonspeech nature, that determine the functioning of the various speech subsystems, that is, respiratory, laryngeal, and velopharyngeal systems as well as oral musculature. The intelligibility section of these tests is often the only part that can inform on activity limitation, and little consideration is given to participation in any formal sense.

Some of these assessments, such as the FDA, also attempt to match a patient's performance to a specific diagnostic category, such as ataxic or spastic dysarthria. The issues regarding the validity of these concepts have already been discussed in this chapter. In addition, heavy emphasis on assessment of underlying physiological functions based on nonspeech tasks can lead to a number of problems in clinical decision making:

1. There is a question regarding the reliability of such data. In particular, maximum performance tests (maximum phonation time [MPT], alternating motion rate [AMR], sequential motion rate [SMR], and maximum force or pressure) have been criticized as patient performance might vary due to practice effects and other factors (Kent, Kent, & Rosenbek, 1987). In addition, tasks looking at movement force in particular are prone to poor reliability of scoring unless instrumental

techniques are available. Maximum performance tasks are summarized further in this chapter.

2. Impairments of physiological function do not necessarily relate directly to the observed speech problems. Although there is an ongoing argument whether there might be at least some relationship between certain aspects of speech and nonspeech performance (Ballard, Robin, & Folkins, 2003; Ziegler, 2002, 2003), no study to date has been able to show a strong correlation between individual physiological assessments and connected speech intelligibility. This is because speech is produced through a complex interaction of phonetic features that cannot be represented by individual or a series of individual movement tasks. In addition, our articulators serve more basic functions for eating, drinking, and the like, and nonspeech tasks often tend to tap into those vegetative functions rather than movement control for speech purposes.

3. The resulting information, even if it were reliable and valid, does not provide sufficient information to the clinician to make clinical decisions that are tailored to an individual's needs.

We therefore suggest that to arrive at a holistic assessment of patients with motor speech disorders, the clinician should start by identifying the status of the individual's current level of communication participation and to what degree he or she is affected by the communication disorder. This will determine whether the patient should be offered treatment and whether the speech and language clinician is the most appropriate person to deliver it. Often, the prominent underlying reason impacting communication ability will be a reduction in intelligibility and naturalness. In this case, these features should be assessed in different contexts and speaking tasks, with a focus on segmental articulation as well as prosodic aspects of speech production. Finally, the clinician can assess physiological functioning of the patient with maximum performance tasks to understand which impairments in motor function and control might have an impact on intelligibility and naturalness. Maximum performance tasks can hold clinical value in determining if neurologic disease has affected physiological strength or capacity, even when speech is not impaired. Reduced maximum performance has been reported for ALS (Langmore & Lehman, 1994; Weikamp, Schelhaas, Hendriks, de Swart, & Geurts, 2012); traumatic brain injury (Goozee, Murdoch, & Theodoros, 2001; Theodoros, Murdoch, & Stokes, 1995); myasthenia gravis (Weijnen et al., 2000); and PD (Solomon, Robin, & Luschei, 2000).

The following sections cover each of these levels in detail. It should be noted that the discussion of assessment techniques is primarily based on English language resources and considerations. More information on cross-linguistic differences and how these might affect assessment can be found in Miller and Lowit (2014).

Assessment of Impact and Participation

Assessment of impact should consider to what degree a communication disorder affects a person's QOL and participation in communicative activities. These concepts are difficult to define given the individualized nature of people's communication environments and needs. To gain better understanding of impact, recent research explored patients' feelings and perceptions following acquired motor speech disorders (Bloch, Beeke, & Miller, 2011; Brady, Clark, Dickson, Paton, & Barbour, 2011; Dickson, Barbour, Brady, Clark, & Paton, 2008; Hartelius, Elmberg, Holm, Lövberg, & Nikolaidis, 2008; Miller, Andrew, Noble, & Walshe, 2011; Miller, Noble, Jones, & Burn, 2006; Walshe & Miller, 2011). Results suggest that feelings of isolation and loneliness, depression, and a negative self-image as well as a fear of communication are common consequences of motor speech disorders and frequently result in avoidance of particular speaking contexts or complete withdrawal from communication.

Another focus of researchers was to investigate how such feelings could be quantified to develop assessments that could capture the level of impact and participation. Before the development of dysarthria-specific measures, the only tools available to clinicians were questionnaires designed for more generic issues, such as QOL, or other related communication disorders. A review of these can be found in the work of Thomas (2010) or Walshe (2011). Since then, Walshe, Peach, and Miller (2009) have published the dysarthria impact profile, and Baylor, Yorkston, and coworkers (Baylor, Burns, Eadie, Britton, & Yorkston, 2011; Baylor, Yorkston, Bamer, Britton, & Amtmann, 2010; Baylor, Yorkston, Eadie, Miller, & Amtmann, 2009; Yorkston et al., 2006, 2008) have been validating their communicative participation item bank across a number of speech disorders (see also Barnish, Horton, Butterfint, & Deane, 2013), as well as refining the question set to produce a shorter version (Baylor et al., 2013). While the applicability of these tools as outcome measures to monitor success of treatment still needs to be determined further, the information they provide will aid the clinician in focusing treatment more appropriately.

Assessment of Impairment: Intelligibility and Naturalness

Intelligibility

Intelligibility relates to how well the acoustic signal is understood by a listener. It reflects the effects of impairments at the physiological level of speech production and is one of the most frequently employed measures of the severity of a speech disorder. It is therefore an important aspect to consider when deciding on the best management pathway. In addition, the fact that the concept can be quantified makes it suitable to function as an outcome measure for treatment.

Comprehensibility of speech or communication effectiveness are related measures that look beyond the acoustic signal to consider how nonverbal aspects of speech production as well as contextual cues contribute to understanding and allow patients to get their message across. In terms of clinical assessment, the latter aspects are more useful in characterizing the communicative performance of an individual; however, intelligibility can be valuable in terms of assessing the impact of underlying physiological deficits on speech.

The focus of assessment will determine what assessment materials are chosen. Intelligibility assessment requires the removal of contextual factors, thus requiring single-word lists or sentences of unpredictable content (e.g., McHenry & Parle's 2006 Unpredictable Sentence Test). In addition, scorer familiarity with the material needs to be avoided. Published assessments such as the Assessment of Intelligibility of Dysarthric Speech (AIDS or ASSIDS) single-word intelligibility section (Yorkston, Beukelman, & Traynor, 1984), or the most recent edition of the FDA, the FDA-2 (Enderby & Palmer, 2008) offer a pool of items to choose from to address this issue. A further issue to consider when performing an intelligibility assessment is whether the purpose is simply to quantify the severity of the problem or to guide clinical management. In the latter case, care needs to be taken to structure the word list in such a way that it highlights which sound categories and phonetic contrasts are affected, as is the case, for example, for the Multi-Word Intelligibility Test (MWIT; Kent, Weismer, Kent, & Rosenbek, 1989).

To gain a better picture of a speaker's functional level, and thus their comprehensibility or communication effectiveness, contextual speech needs to be assessed. Common tasks are sentence or passage reading, as well as conversation or monologue. Validated sentence-level tests include the sentence section of the ASSIDS (Yorkston et al., 1984) or the FDA-2 (Enderby & Palmer, 2008), which provide clinicians a choice from a pool of sentences. The most commonly applied reading passages in dysarthria assessments are the Grandfather Passage (Darley et al., 1975) or the Rainbow Passage (Fairbanks, 1960). Others have been developed over the years in an attempt to include more prosodic variation into the text to elicit more naturalistic performance from the patient and allow the clinician to assess certain prosodic features from the same task (A. Brown & Docherty, 1995; Lowit, Brendel, & Howell, 2006; Patel et al., 2013).

An important issue to take into consideration in spontaneous speech assessment is the comparability of different samples. Fluency, rate, and pausing behavior are affected by the cognitive load of the task, and they in turn can have a considerable impact on the comprehensibility of the speaker. Any comparisons with individuals against norms or between pre- and posttreatment performance should thus ensure that results are not affected by the nature of the task. Another issue to consider is whether to use a monologue task or more natural conversation. Monologue tasks have the advantage that the cognitive load as well as topic and vocabulary can be controlled to some extent, but conversations can produce more natural speech output and allow the clinician to observe other factors, such as turn-taking skills, topic maintenance and shifts, and so on. Some forms of controlled dialogue have been proposed in the literature, such as the map task (Anderson et al., 1991), in which both the patient and the clinician have to provide instructions to each other on how to reach a particular point on a map, or Diapix (Bradlow, Bakes, Choi, Kim, & van Engen, 2007), for which conversational partners discuss differences of two versions of the same picture.

One other factor to consider is that observing patients during isolated speech tasks in quiet clinical surroundings might not truly reflect their functional communication. More natural speaking contexts can be approximated by asking individuals to perform concurrent tasks, such as manipulating objects while talking (e.g., Dromey & Bates, 2005; Dromey & Benson, 2003). Listening conditions can also be altered, such as performing evaluations under noisy conditions (Adams, Dykstra, Jenkins, & Jog, 2008).

In addition to having to choose from a range of elicitation tasks, clinicians will have to think carefully about their evaluation methods. Interval scaling, by which the patient's performance is judged on a 5-point scale, for example, with one end indicating no impairment and the other severe impairment, is a popular method that has also been incorporated into some published assessment batteries, such as the Robertson Dysarthria Profile (Robertson, 1982) or the FDA-2 (Enderby & Palmer, 2008). Unfortunately, this method is associated with relatively poor interrater reliability for some severity levels; that is, although there is generally good agreement at the extreme ends of the scale, scores can vary a great deal in the midrange. There is also an issue whether the distance between points is too great to be sufficiently sensitive to small differences in performance. On the other hand, the variability issues mentioned are exacerbated if the points of the scales are extended. Although a number of different rating methods have been published in assessment protocols and research papers over the years, there is no agreed format to date that is widely accepted as the gold standard of intelligibility assessment.

Another common method is percentage scoring. This can reflect a global estimate of how much the listener understood or a quantification of how much of the output was identified or transcribed correctly. The latter technique is more reliable if the target is known and thus, is more difficult to apply to spontaneous speech. Where performance scores are global estimates, Kent and Kim (2011) suggest an alternative to percentage scoring in the form of visual analogue scales, where the listener places a mark on a line to show how much they thought they understood. This can then be turned back into a percentage mark for quantification purposes. A further evaluation method used in research studies is direct magnitude estimation; a speech sample is compared to a standard speech sample (Weismer & Laures, 2002; Whitehill, Lee, & Chun, 2002). However, this can be impractical in the clinical context owing to the difficulty of the procedure.

Irrespective of the choice of evaluation method, assessment of intelligibility or comprehensibility needs to go beyond estimates of severity and also serve a diagnostic purpose; that is, it should allow the clinician to identify the reasons for the deficit and suggest appropriate pathways to effective treatment (Miller, 2013). This will require further analysis of the segmental and suprasegmental aspects that are having an impact on the clarity of speech. In addition, listener factors need to be taken into account to draw a clear picture of functionality. For example, is the person mainly conversing with familiar or unfamiliar listeners, in face-to-face situations or over the telephone, and so on? There are a number of environmental changes or behavioral strategies that can improve comprehensibility without directly addressing the patient's articulatory deficits (see management section), and a clear picture of potential changes in comprehensibility depending on the communication environment should thus, be gained at the assessment stage.

Naturalness/Prosody

The second area to address at the level of impairment is the naturalness of speech output. Unlike intelligibility, it is rarely quantified in terms of percentage grades, although a scalar judgment might be applied at times. Generally, clinicians will simply state whether naturalness is affected or not. A decline in naturalness has traditionally been attributed to deviations in prosody, such as unnatural speaking rate or inappropriate pause placement, rhythm, or intonation patterns. In actual fact, the division between intelligibility and naturalness and their relationship to segmental and prosodic articulation is not as clear cut. It has been recognized for some time that prosodic changes can have a significant impact on intelligibility (Weismer & Martin, 1992), and it is also possible that segmental deviations could affect the perception of naturalness. Given the impact of prosody on both intelligibility and naturalness, it is important to conduct a detailed assessment of its functionality to evaluate its impact and potential role in treatment.

Prosody forms part of the suprasegmental aspects of speech, that is, parameters that apply to structures larger than segments. At the phonetic level, these consist of pitch, loudness, duration, silence, and voice quality. At the phonological level, these aspects are used to express linguistic meaning through the manipulation of tempo, pause, intonation, stress, and rhythm. Production of prosody is achieved through the same underlying physiological functions as for segments, that is, the respiratory and laryngeal system, as well as the oral musculature, again underlining the fact that the contribution of segmental and suprasegmental aspects to effective communication should always be considered jointly rather than regarding them as separate, unrelated entities.

Both levels of prosodic production, that is, phonetic as well as phonological, need to be assessed. Only the latter is covered in this section, as the phonetic aspects are part of the physiological assessment discussed further in the chapter.

As mentioned, the phonological level includes tempo, pause, intonation, stress, and rhythm. Of these, speech tempo/rate and its phonetic counterpart, articulation rate, are the most commonly reported features in dysarthria research. They also play an important part in the management of intelligibility problems and are thus, a frequent focus of assessment. Nevertheless, the terminology and measurement of these concepts is often confused. Tempo is a purely perceptual concept that primarily depends on the speed of articulatory movement but is also influenced by the amount, length, and location of pauses, as well as other factors such as voice quality or articulatory clarity. Tempo cannot be quantified but only judged as appropriate, too fast, or too slow. To obtain an objective measure, speech/articulation rate needs to be measured by quantifiable means, such as instrumental analysis. This involves taking counts of words or syllables and dividing them by the time taken for production. In the clinical context, speech rate is the more feasible measure, as the articulation rate requires the removal of pause time from the signal.

While the assessment of tempo and speech/articulation rate can provide information on the severity of the presenting disorder, it does not necessarily point the clinician to the most appropriate path for treatment. In addition to assessing habitual performance, patients should therefore, be asked to decrease their rate and to do so in different ways, such as using longer pauses, inserting more pauses, prolonging phonemes, and so on. This can provide the clinician with information on whether rate changes have any impact on the patient's communication effectiveness and what degree and technique of rate reduction leads to the best results.

It would furthermore, be beneficial to consider pauses in their own right and determine whether pausing behavior alone might be at the center of the communication deficit; for example, reducing inappropriate pause placement can have a more beneficial effect on listener understanding than improving the production of individual phonemes.

Rhythm should also be considered part of a prosody assessment. Rhythm relates to the regularity of speech timing, which can be a difficult concept to evaluate perceptually. It is often confounded by rate and pausing behavior, and irregular pitch and loudness modulation and articulatory errors can also lead to the perception of distorted rhythm in the absence of actual speech timing problems (Lowit, 2014). Therefore, it is important to look closely at these aspects if rhythm is judged inappropriate to identify how best to address the problem. In addition, it is important to assess patients across a number of tasks, as rhythm problems might only show themselves in particular contexts. Henrich, Lowit, Schalling, and Mennen (2006), for example, found that speakers with ataxic dysarthria performed close to healthy controls in the highly rhythmic Limerick task but differed significantly in a spontaneous speech task.

A classic task for assessing intonational modulation is by asking the patient to signal different illocutionary acts, for example, "She is coming for dinner" expressed as a statement or question or to disambiguate different syntactic structures, for example, the Cognitive Linguistic Quick Test, "Tim said | the teacher was very clever" versus "Tim | said the teacher | was very clever"; $2 \times (3 + 4)$ versus $(2 \times 3) + 4$; or chocolate, biscuits, and cake (three items) versus chocolate biscuits and cake (two items) (see Profiling Elements of Prosody in Speech-Communication [PEPS-C]; Peppé & McCann, 2003). Further disambiguation tasks can include different stress placement, both at lexical (**con**duct versus con**duct**) or sentence (Tom scored a **goal** versus **Tom** scored a goal) level.

It is important to remember that the correct functional use of any of the prosodic features mentioned depends not only on adequate speech production skills but also on higher-order processing, such as deciding which word to stress in an utterance or selecting an appropriate intonation contour to express a particular syntactic or pragmatic meaning. As the effect on speech production can be similar, patients' performance needs to be observed across a range of tasks and communication contexts to identify whether motor, cognitive, or language problems have an impact on their speech production.

A number of dedicated prosodic assessments have been published over the years; unfortunately, none of these cover all the aspects of prosody mentioned previously at a sufficiently detailed level. Examples are the Prosody-Voice-Screening Profile (Shriberg, Kwiatkowski, & Rasmussen, 1990) and the Profile of Prosody (Crystal, 1992) (see Patel, 2011, for a more detailed review of procedures). There have been some more recent developments in the pediatric field (PEPS-C; Peppé & McCann, 2003), which could potentially also be used with adults. Otherwise, research papers outlining assessments of particular prosodic functions can be consulted for further indications of suitable tasks and normative data. Dysarthria assessments also cover prosody to some degree; however, they tend to focus on the phonetic level described in the next section.

Physiological Level

Following assessment of the areas discussed, the clinician should have an overview of the level of functioning of his or her patient and how this has an impact on communication participation and well-being. The clinician should also have information on what aspects of speech production are impaired. However, further analysis might be required to tease apart the degree that individual subsystems are affected and contributing to the reduction in communication effectiveness, thus relating to the structure/function components of the ICF model. Such assessment of the physiological level of speech production is commonly performed via nonspeech tasks and maximum performance tests. The drawbacks of these tasks in relation to reliability and validity have already been discussed. On the other hand, they have been shown to highlight differences in underlying motor pathology (Kent & Kent, 2000; Kent, Kent, Duffy, & Weismer, 1998;

Kent & Kim, 2003). And, while we would not promote the use of these findings to classify the neurological type of dysarthria, a description of which subsystem is affected (i.e., respiratory, phonatory, resonatory, or articulatory function) can aid treatment planning.

A detailed investigation of motor speech physiology will be aided by the use of instrumental measures to derive aerodynamic, acoustic, or kinematic information to improve accuracy and facilitate data storage and transfer (see Murdoch, 1998, 2011, for a comprehensive review of available systems). However, many of these are not routinely available to clinicians, with the exception of tools to measure respiratory function and voice quality. For other aspects of speech production, clinicians therefore tend to rely on maximum performance tasks, as these can often be conducted with little or no specialized equipment. The following outline summarizes some of the most commonly used observations and tasks:

A. Respiratory system
   1. Observation of the patient at rest, noting posture, type of breathing (diaphragmatic versus clavicular), as well as depth and rate of breathing (Duffy, 2013).
   2. Examination of diaphragm (Hixon & Hoit, 1998), abdominal wall (Hixon & Hoit, 1999), and rib cage wall (Hixon & Hoit, 2000).
   3. Determination of respiratory driving pressure (Hixon, Hawley, & Wilson, 1982).
   4. Measurement of MPT (Kent et al., 1987; Solomon, Garlitz, & Milbrath, 2000).
   5. Loudness modulation during prolonged vowel, counting, and so on (Duffy, 2013).
B. Laryngeal system
   1. Observation of breathing at rest, particularly in relation to presence of inhalatory stridor (Duffy, 2013).
   2. Differentiation between respiratory and laryngeal problems by observation of strength of cough versus glottal coup (sharp glottal stop) (Duffy, 2013).
   3. Measurement of laryngeal AMR (also called laryngeal diadochokinesis, L-DDK, or vocal fold diadochokinesis, VFDDK) (Ptacek, Sander, Maloney, & Jackson, 1966; Renout, Leeper, Bandur, & Hudson, 1995). The goal of the task is to examine the maximum repetition rate of a syllable typically composed of a glottal consonant (such as /h/) and a vowel.
   4. Measurement of MPT (see respiratory system).
   5. Observation of extent of pitch modulation in pitch glides on prolonged vowels (Duffy, 2013).
C. Oral articulatory system
   1. Observation of articulator range (e.g., moving tongue from side to side) and strength (e.g., maintaining lip closure to blow up the cheeks).
   2. Measurement of diadochokinesis (DDK; speed and coordination of articulators)
      a. Nonspeech (Duffy, 2013; Kent, 2015).
      b. Syllable AMR (repetition of a syllable; used as an index of motor control in various dysarthrias) (Ackermann, Hertrich, & Hehr, 1995; Konstantopoulos, Charalambous, & Veroeven, 2011; Masaki & Seiji, 2002; Nishio & Niimi, 2000; Wang, Kent, Duffy, Thomas, & Weismer, 2004; Ziegler, 2002). Usually, AMR is determined for consonant–vowel syllables where the consonant is a bilabial, alveolar, or velar stop.
      c. SMR (repetition of two or more syllables differing in vowel or consonant composition).
   3. Maximum force, such as maximum compression force developed by the lips or tongue (Kent et al., 1987).
D. Velopharynx
   1. Observation of velum for symmetry, elevation as well as myoclonus (spontaneous movements of the palate).
   2. Repetition of a series of /a/ sounds while observing the symmetry and movement of the velum.
   3. Differentiation of oral versus nasal stop contrasts (e.g., "may–bay") (Duffy, 2013).

Recent studies indicate that the value of tasks such as DDK or MPT can be enhanced by examining the responses to derive information on the regularity of performance. For example, AMR responses can be analyzed with acoustic methods to determine temporal or energy variability among items in a train. The DDK profiles have been described for the dysarthrias secondary to cerebellar disease (Wang, Kent, Duffy, & Thomas, 2008); PD (Skodda, Lorenz, & Schlegel, 2013; Tjaden & Watling, 2003); multiple sclerosis (Tjaden & Watling, 2003); progressive supranuclear palsy (Skodda, Grönheit, & Schegel, 2012); and stroke (Kent, Duffy, Kent, & Vorperian, 1999).

Some of the techniques described are included in dysarthria assessment protocols such as Darley et al.'s motor speech examination (1975), the FDA-2 (Enderby & Palmer, 2008), or the Robertson Dysarthria Profile (Robertson, 1982). In such cases, normative values or grading scales are provided to allow clinicians to judge not only the presence but also the severity of the symptoms. However, given the subjectivity of some of the evaluations and, consequently, the qualitative nature of the severity descriptors, there can be issues in terms of interrater reliability, as well as how well a patient's performance fits the descriptors of a scale. This should be borne in mind when making clinical decisions on the basis of these assessment protocols.

INTERVENTIONS FOR DYSARTHRIA

Having performed a comprehensive assessment of the patient, the clinician is faced with the task of devising an appropriate management plan. This section reviews methods suggested in the literature to address the various components and features of speech production. However, we begin with a brief discussion of factors that need to be considered irrespective of the individual presentation of the patient.

The most important principle to keep in mind when planning treatment is to look beyond the speech impairment. This applies to the symptom complex of the patient, that is, any comorbidity with other problems that can affect treatment progress (e.g., cognitive or language problems) or other health issues that might have an impact on fatigue levels, motivation, and ability to participate in treatment. In addition, those in the patient's immediate surroundings (i.e., spouse, other family members, carers, etc.) should not be ignored, both in relation to how they can help the patient improve his or her communication and in terms of what their own support needs might be. Any of these issues are likely to warrant the involvement of other professionals, such as medical specialists, physio- and occupational therapists, clinical psychologist or counselors, and a multidisciplinary approach to the treatment of dysarthria is thus, desirable.

Focusing on the treatment of specific speech problems, the use of the aforementioned nonspeech tasks requires careful consideration. Although these methods might be unavoidable in assessment to gain information on subcomponents of speech production in the absence of sophisticated measurement tools and procedures, they should not be used unquestioningly in the treatment of a patient's communication deficit given the evidence that different motor control circuits are used in nonspeech versus speech movements (Hodge, 2004; Ziegler, 2002, 2003). If nonspeech tasks are considered, their purposes should be weighed in terms of the patient's physiological status and their relevance to speech motor capabilities. Kent (2015) developed a taxonomy of nonspeech tasks that may be helpful in this regard. The primary objective of the taxonomy is to categorize various nonspeech oral tasks in terms of their constituent motor patterns.

Another factor influencing the choice of management approach is whether the patient presents with a progressive or stable disorder. Both types of disorder might present with similar functional deficits, such as reduced respiratory support, slower articulatory movements, and so on; however, the treatment goals and follow-up procedures will differ considerably. A patient with dysarthria after stroke might thus present with similar levels of intelligibility deficit than another diagnosed with multiple system atrophy (MSA) or ALS/motor neuron disease (MND). However, while it is realistic to expect to see some long-term treatment benefits in the stroke patient with appropriately planned therapy, this is unlikely for the patient with MSA or ALS/MND due to the fast progression of their disorder. Instead, it would be more appropriate to focus on maximizing current speech functionality while preparing the patient for the future by, for example, familiarizing him or her with augmentative or alternative communication possibilities.

As noted in this chapter, determination of type of dysarthria does not necessarily dictate treatment strategy. Often, treatment is designed with consideration of other factors, such as intelligibility, subsystem impairments, and response to manipulation of speaking rate, stress, or other prosodic variables. Some interventions, such as LSVT (Lee Silverman Voice Treatment), may originally have been developed for patients with a particular neurologic disease or a particular type of dysarthria, but it is often the case that they are used with other patient groups as well. That is, many interventions are not specific to the perceptual type of dysarthria. Mixed dysarthrias present a special challenge in this regard, as one may well ask if treatment is determined by the predominant type of dysarthria or by some other strategy. Our impression is that intervention usually is planned according to goals such as prosodic modification (e.g., slow speaking rate), subsystem improvement (e.g., enhanced respiratory support), or increased intelligibility (e.g., overarticulation). There are instances in which the predominant type of dysarthria may be important to consider. For example, the therapeutic plan for a patient with multiple system atrophy – parkinsonian (MSA-P) subtype may be different from that for a patient with multiple system atrophy – cerebellar dysfunction (MSA-C) subtype if the former presents with accelerated speech and the latter with scanning speech. The two patients may respond quite differently to manipulation of prosodic patterns.

Once the decision has been made regarding which aspects should be treated in a patient, it is important to decide on the optimum treatment schedule and delivery style. Some significant work was undertaken in the 1980s and 1990s on motor learning, which has an impact on how speech therapy should be delivered to achieve effective retention of skills developed during treatment (see Maas et al., 2008, for a comprehensive discussion of this topic). Maas et al.'s (2008) review highlights that there is insufficient systematic evidence to advocate specific feedback and practice conditions to treat motor speech disorders. However, there is evidence that people with motor impairment are affected by similar issues as nonimpaired learners (Adams, Page, & Jog, 2002; Croce, Horvat, & Roswal, 1996; Jordan & Sagar, 1994; Knock, Ballard, Robin, & Schmidt, 2000; Roy, Saint-Cyr, Taylor, & Lang, 1993; Schulz, Dingwall, & Ludlow, 1999). Clinicians therefore need to be aware of the general principles of motor learning to plan an appropriate treatment schedule, to evaluate whether their therapy provision is achieving its goals, and to indicate which aspects to change if progress does not follow the anticipated path. These include the importance of prepractice, which relates to the fact that patients should be sufficiently motivated to complete the treatment block, have a good understanding of what tasks they are required to perform, and show a sufficient degree of stimulability (i.e., at least some ability to reach the set target; see the stimulability test included in the LSVT assessment).

Maas et al. (2008) also conclude that investigations into the effects of amount of practice on skills retention suggest that larger amounts are more beneficial, as long as they are presented in a variable rather than constant practice paradigm (e.g., practicing rate reduction across different sentences rather than the same sentence over again). Furthermore, if several tasks are to be focused on in a session, a random rather than block presentation of these can lead to better retention by the learner (Schmidt & Bjork, 1996).

A further aspect that is thought to influence the effectiveness of any chosen treatment approach is the frequency of task presentation or treatment. There is a perception among clinicians that a higher frequency of treatment results in better outcomes than the traditional schedule of one session a week. In most cases, the success of the highly intensive LSVT is cited in support. However, Spielman, Ramig, Mahler, Halpern, and Gavin (2007) report similar outcomes when frequency of LSVT was reduced by half; that is, two rather than four sessions per week were provided over a longer period of time. Studies into motor learning in fact suggest that distributed practice over a longer period of time should result in better retention than massed practice of skill; however, this could so far only be demonstrated for nonspeech tasks (Maas et al., 2008).

In addition to manipulations of how tasks are presented, the type and frequency of feedback on performance can also affect how well a speaker learns and retains new skills. For example, it has become clear that while feedback is beneficial to aid patients' recovery, too frequent feedback can prevent them from developing their self-monitoring skills and in turn lead to poorer retention (Salmoni, Schmidt, & Walter, 1984; Schmidt

& Bjork, 1996; Schmidt, Young, Swinnen, & Shapiro, 1989). Another factor affecting performance is whether feedback is very general, indicating only whether the target was reached or not (i.e., Knowledge of Results), or whether specific performance errors are pointed out to the individual (i.e., Knowledge of Performance) (e.g., you did not close your lips sufficiently). Furthermore, learning can be affected by the timing of feedback, that is, whether it is presented immediately after performing the task or with some delay. As was the case for task presentation, there are yet no clear indications of which type and scheduling of feedback is optimal for speech tasks. In addition, there are indications that all of the variables discussed are highly interdependent; for example, a particular task presentation schedule will only work better than another if provided with a particular frequency of task or feedback. Furthermore, the type of task and desired goal can affect which presentation method is optimal; for example, patients might respond differently when practicing nonspeech tasks versus speech tasks.

In summary, there are a number of aspects that need to be taken into consideration when planning treatment; however, no clear guidance can be given at this point on which is the best method, and no such indications are likely to emerge in the future given the complexity and varied nature of learning tasks employed for motor speech disorders. A further issue to consider is that treatment needs to consider patients holistically, not just their motoric impairment. For example, despite indications that withholding feedback might encourage better retention, this principle should not be enforced if it is clear that individuals require frequent feedback on their performance to engage them in the task due to cognitive issues or to motivate them while they are trying to come to terms with the changes affecting their communication. The best course of action therefore, is to be aware of the factors that can affect the effectiveness of treatment provision and to monitor the patient's progress closely to make necessary adjustments as and when required and tailor treatment to the individual's needs.

A final consideration in the process of deciding on an appropriate course of treatment for an individual is to ensure that the chosen methods have a good evidence base. This remains a problem across most rehabilitation disciplines, including motor speech disorders. Despite relative agreement among clinicians about how particular problems can be addressed, evidence for the effectiveness of most of these approaches relies on clinician opinion rather than properly controlled treatment studies. To provide clinicians with information on treatment efficacy, a number of professional bodies have commissioned reports that review the evidence base for published therapeutic techniques.

The largest number of these were instigated by the Academy of Neurological Communication Disorders and Sciences (ANCDS), resulting in reviews of treatment studies for spasmodic dysphonia, velopharyngeal and respiratory deficiency, as well as the use of speech supplementation (Duffy & Yorkston, 2003; Yorkston, Hakel, Beukelman, & Fager, 2007; Yorkston, Spencer, & Duffy, 2003; Yorkston, Spencer, Duffy, Beukelman, Golper, Miller, et al., 2001; Yorkston, Spencer, Duffy, Beukelman, Golper, Miller, Strand, et al., 2001). Furthermore, the American Speech-Language-Hearing Association has focused on the management of speaking rate (Hammen, 2004), nonspeech exercises in treatment (Hodge, 2004), as well as issues relating to the use of augmentative and alternative communication (AAC; Mathy, 2004). In the United Kingdom, a number of Cochrane reviews have been undertaken, two on PD (Deane et al., 2001a, 2001b; Herd et al., 2012a, 2012b) and one on nonprogressive dysarthria as a consequence of stroke (Sellars, Hughes, & Langhorne, 2005). In addition, the evidence base for treatment of ataxic dysarthria has been reviewed recently (Vogel, Folker, & Poole, 2014). A further resource are the guidelines collated by the Royal College of Speech and Language Therapists (RCSLT); these guidelines are based on the findings of the ANCDS and Cochrane reviews to provide an evidence base of dysarthria treatment (RCSLT, 2009).

Unfortunately, the conclusion of most of these reviews indicates that there is insufficient evidence available for the majority of treatments described in the literature. This of course does not necessarily mean that the therapy is not effective; it just has not been demonstrated yet by sufficiently rigorous research studies. In the absence of evidence for which treatment technique is most appropriate, clinicians will need to exercise their own judgment regarding whether the chosen method is producing the desired outcomes by monitoring behavioral changes carefully, using the methods described in the assessment section.

We now proceed with a brief overview of treatment approaches that have been proposed in the literature for the various speech subsystems, as well as factors affecting impairment and participation. In line with the structure followed in the assessment section, we commence with how to address issues of communication participation, followed by impairment and finally the various speech subsystems.

Participation

There is no treatment as such that addresses communication participation. Given the fact that tools to measure this aspect were only published over the last 5 years, (e.g., Baylor et al.'s work; see "Assessment of Impact and Participation"), their use has not yet translated into analyses of treatment efficacy. The general assumption here would be that improvements at the physiological and impairment levels will improve communication effectiveness and thus, result in the patient participating more widely in communication. However, it is highly likely that other factors will also be important to address to maximize functioning at this level.

One of these will be patient attitude and confidence. It is not uncommon to see some speakers with relatively mild problems withdraw from communication to a greater degree than others who face much more difficult issues. This will be largely due to differences in how the patients perceive themselves and their environment. Raising their awareness of the real extent of their problem or ensuring a supportive communication environment could thus, improve participation as much as directly working on intelligibility. Previous work on conversation analysis in people with aphasia (e.g., Milroy & Perkins, 1992) has demonstrated how conversational partner behavior can inhibit as well as support communication exchanges, and the most recent work by Bloch and colleagues (e.g., Bloch, Saldert, & Ferm, 2015; Bloch & Wilkinson, 2009; Saldert, Ferm, & Bloch, 2014) demonstrates that similar issues apply to speakers with motor speech disorders. Involvement of the communication partner should thus, be an integral part of treatment when possible. In addition, changes to the environment can make a difference, such as reducing background noise, ensuring adequate hearing levels in both conversational partners, highlighting the importance of visual cues during conversation and thus, good visibility, and so on.

Impairment

As already discussed in the assessment section, impairment in dysarthria relates to deficits in intelligibility and naturalness of speech, which requires consideration of both segmental and suprasegmental features. The latter achieve this by facilitating listener perception, such as guiding the listener to the important content in the speech output (through intonation and stress placement), providing information on the grammatical structure through intonational phrasing, as well as signaling lexical boundaries, thus helping the listener to segment the speech signal into meaningful units. In relation to the segmental features, articulatory precision is often regarded as the most direct correlate of how well a speaker can be understood, and a range of treatment techniques have been described in the literature to address this. Interestingly, some of those also involve the manipulation of prosody instead of purely segmental issues, thus again highlighting the importance of prosody for a speaker's intelligibility.

Some patients, particularly those with greater degrees of severity, might require work on individual phonemes to increase articulatory clarity. This is covered here in the speech subsystems section. As a more indirect strategy to improve intelligibility, the concept of clear speech can be helpful. The individual should be asked to overarticulate speech sounds, with the aim to achieve greater clarity and precision of articulatory gestures. This technique has had some success in increasing intelligibility compared to the patient's habitual conversational speech style (Beukelman, Fager, Ullman, Hanson, & Logemann, 2002; Kennedy, Strand, & Yorkston, 1994). In addition, Lam and Tjaden (2011) investigated whether effects differed in relation to asking patients to speak more loudly, more clearly, or as if talking to someone with a hearing impairment. They found that individuals showed the greatest intelligibility improvements for the last instruction, suggesting that this would be an appropriate concept to use in treatment.

The overarticulation arising from clear speech will not only have an impact on articulatory gestures but also will reduce speaking rate to some degree. Reduced rate in itself is a commonly applied prosodic technique to improve intelligibility (Blanchet & Snyder, 2009). It allows the speaker more time to execute articulatory gestures, which can compensate for reduced movement speed. It also helps listeners because they will have more time to process what the speaker is saying, particularly as word boundaries might be more clearly delineated. A wide range of rate reduction strategies have been described in the literature, including rigid techniques such as pacing boards, metronomes, or ABC boards and methods that retain the rhythmicity of the speech signal and result in more natural speech (Blanchet & Snyder, 2010; Hammen, 2004; Yorkston, Beukelman, Strand, & Bell, 1999; Yorkston, Hammen, Beukelman, & Traynor, 1990). The two main methods of achieving rate reduction are either a modification of pause time and frequency or phoneme prolongation. As already discussed in the assessment section, it is important to identify which is most beneficial to the patient and then choose the cueing method accordingly.

There is further evidence that modulation of other prosodic components, in particular pitch and loudness,

can have a secondary effect on speech rate (see the next section for treatment strategies for these components). This was first observed by Simmons (1983), who noted that exercises focusing on greater loudness and pitch variation resulted in reduced rate, presumably to allow for more time to execute the required prosodic modulations. Dromey (2000) later replicated these results in an instrumental study in which he observed that speaking with a louder voice resulted in changes in the velocity and displacement of articulatory movements in both disordered and healthy speakers. The results are also consistent with the rate reduction reported for LSVT (L. O. Ramig, Countryman, Thompson, & Horii, 1995).

As a word of caution, despite the many reports highlighting the beneficial effects of rate reduction, the strategy should not be regarded as a panacea for intelligibility deficits. For example, Turner, Tjaden, and Weismer (1995) found that not all of their participants with ALS improved with rate reduction, and van Nuffelen, De Bodt, Vanderwegen, van de Heyning, and Wuyts (2010) and van Nuffelen, De Bodt, Wuyts, and van de Heyning (2009) observed similar results across a wider range of dysarthria types and rate reduction techniques. It is therefore essential that the effects of rate reduction are assessed in detail before this is suggested as a strategy. In addition, a variety of reduction techniques should be trialed to identify which one is most effective.

In contrast to intelligibility, there have been few studies investigating treatment strategies for reduced naturalness of speech. This is most likely due to the fact that this can be caused by a multitude and combination of factors; therefore, no single treatment technique will be able to address this issue. The clinician will have to perform a careful evaluation of which segmental or suprasegmental aspects contribute to the perception of naturalness and address these as best as possible. Clinicians should also be aware that certain treatments might benefit intelligibility but have a negative effect on naturalness, rate reduction being a typical example. It is therefore essential that such secondary effects be monitored and discussed with the patient to ensure that the treatment strategies suggested by the clinician are acceptable and will be generalized into everyday speech production. A study of the effect of vocal exercises and singing concluded that such a treatment program may lead to improved intelligibility and naturalness (Tamplin, 2008), but more research is needed to determine which patients are good candidates for this type of intervention.

While the methods discussed so far have the potential to improve communication effectiveness considerably, it is likely that most patients will benefit from additional work addressing the underlying subsystems responsible for speech production.

Treatment of Speech Subsystems

There are two areas that need to be considered when addressing any of the subcomponents of speech production. The first is the muscular movement itself, that is, its speed, range, and force. The second is the control of this movement and its coordination with other articulatory systems during speech. Treatment will differ according to the origin of the observed deficits, and clinicians therefore need to have performed a detailed assessment of the patient identify how best to address the impairment. The logic of a speech subsystem approach to treatment has been described for adults (Netsell & Daniel, 1979) and children (Pennington, Miller, Robson, & Steen, 2010). The following summary addresses the subsystems of respiration, phonation, articulation, resonance, and prosody (the last of these is not a physiological subsystem per se but rather reflects the combined use of the other listed subsystems).

Respiratory System

Good respiratory support is essential to speech production, and there are few patients with motor speech disorders who do not require work in this area. It is therefore important to ensure their awareness of the role of respiration and how it coordinates with other speech production mechanisms.

One of the first aspects clinicians should consider is whether the patient's posture affects respiratory support. A slumped posture impedes the expansion of the diaphragm during inspiration, thus limiting the volume of air that can be inhaled. A multidisciplinary approach involving physiotherapy and other relevant professionals might be required to address such postural issues. More radical adjustments, such as placing patients in a supine position to let gravity aid expiration, have been suggested in the past. However, besides the impractical nature of such adjustments, there is no evidence for their effectiveness (Spencer & Yorkston, 2004; Yorkston et al., 2003).

In addition to adjusting posture where necessary, the clinician should ensure that the patient is using optimal breathing patterns, that is, diaphragmatic as opposed to clavicular breathing.

To improve muscle strength as well as control, patients can be asked to breathe against resistance, such as exhaling through a water manometer (Hixon et al., 1982; Netsell & Daniel, 1979). The voice literature includes further detail of behavioral methods to increase respiratory support as well as control (e.g., Sapienza & Hoffman-Ruddy, 2009; Schwartz, 2004). One important difference between patients with motor speech disorders and voice disorders is that the former will have a physiological limitation to how much they can improve. It is therefore also important to address speech patterns to make adjustments to the reduced respiratory support that remains once breathing behavior has been optimized. This will mostly focus on pause placement and requires careful consideration by the clinician on the optimal utterance length that will allow the patient to maintain adequate breath support for speech.

Phonatory System

While many types of motor speech disorder can all result in reduced breath support, the nature of phonatory dysfunction is more closely linked to the underlying physiology. Spastic or hyperkinetic dysarthria, for example, lead to hyperadduction of the vocal folds due to the spasticity of the muscle tone, whereas flaccid or hypokinetic dysarthria are characterized by hypoadduction. Each of these requires different management approaches, and an accurate diagnosis is thus essential. To improve hypoadduction, the patient needs to focus on increasing effort during voice production. The LSVT achieves this by cueing the patient to speak louder. This might not be successful in all individuals, however, and increasing overall muscle tension such as clasping hands during phonation can be successful in such cases, although this strategy also has limitations, as discussed by Solomon and Charron (1998). Other techniques include postural adjustments or manipulation of the thyroid cartilage (Spencer & Yorkston, 2004).

Treatment of hyperadduction needs to focus on reducing instead of increasing tension. In line with treatment of voice disorders, whole-body relaxation and the use of biofeedback to monitor vocal fold tension was advocated at one point. However, there is limited evidence for effectiveness of such methods. On the other hand, some success has been recorded for effort-reducing strategies, such as easy onset of phonation, yawning, and so on (Dworkin & Johns, 1980; Murry & Woodson, 1995), although the number of studies in this area is limited.

Articulatory System

Reductions in articulatory accuracy are due to limitations in the strength, range, precision, and speed of muscular movements. It thus seems to follow that exercises to improve these aspects should have a beneficial effect on sound production. However, as already discussed, there is no evidence that the oromotor exercises frequently proposed for this have demonstrated benefit for intelligibility (see Hodge, 2004, for a review). Articulation is a major contributor to speech intelligibility in dysarthria (DeBodt, Hernandez-Diaz Huici, & van de Heyning, 2002), but there are surprisingly few studies on the nature of the articulation errors in various types and severities of the disorder. For Korean speakers with dysarthria, Lee, Sung, Sim, Han, and Song (2012) concluded that omissions, substitutions, and nonspeech sounds were significant predictors of speech intelligibility. For American-English adult individuals with cerebral palsy, H. Kim, Martin, Hasegawa-Johnson, and Perlman (2010) reported that phonemes with high articulatory complexity were most often misarticulated, and that manner errors were more frequent for speakers with mid and low levels of intelligibility. There are few studies reporting on the effectiveness of articulation exercises in dysarthria. However, if practice of individual phonemes is deemed necessary, it would appear sensible to design such exercises in terms of the phonetic contrasts identified as deficient during assessment. In addition, material should be constructed at syllable rather than individual segment level to incorporate practice of both the articulatory movement and the aspect of coordination that is necessary for the production of larger lexical units.

Resonatory System

Velopharyngeal dysfunction is relatively prevalent in certain types of dysarthria, with hypernasality being more prevalent than hyponasality. Hypernasality has more serious effects on intelligibility as it filters out the higher frequencies of a sound's acoustic signature and thus makes it more difficult to distinguish from others.

No effective behavioral treatment for velopharyngeal incompetence has been identified to date. There is a lack of evidence for strength training in nonspeech tasks, but Kuehn and Wachtel (1994) and Cahill et al. (2004) report improvements from resistance training against air pressure in speech tasks for a small number of patients. In addition, reduced rate and clear speech or overarticulation can have some beneficial effects (Yorkston, Spencer, Duffy, Beukelman, Golper, Miller, Strand, et al., 2001). Biofeedback on nasal airflow can help patients monitor their performance. In severe cases, clinicians might want to resort to prosthetic devices, such as palatal lifts or nasal obturators to block nasal airflow. This will render the patient hyponasal but might improve their intelligibility. There is little evidence for the effectiveness of surgical procedures to improve velopharyngeal dysfunction (Yorkston, Spencer, Duffy, Beukelman, Golper, Miller, Strand, et al., 2001).

Prosody

Not many treatment studies have considered prosodic aspects with the exception of modifications to speaking rate and loudness. Rate reduction has already been covered in this chapter. In terms of loudness, most of the evidence comes from evaluations of LSVT (see Yorkston et al., 2007, for a review). These studies have largely focused on speakers with PD; however, a small number of other populations, such as those with traumatic brain injury (Solomon, McKee, & Garcia-Barry, 2001; Wenke, Cornwell, & Theodoros, 2010; Wenke, Theodoros, & Cornwell, 2008, 2010) and multiple sclerosis (Sapir et al., 2001) have also been investigated. The LSVT studies appear to suggest that the treatment is more likely to result in communication benefits than a range of other treatments such as working only on respiratory support (Baumgartner, Sapir, & Ramig, 2001; Borrie et al., 2007; L. O. Ramig et al., 1995; Sapir et al., 2002) and can retain these effects long term (L. O. Ramig et al., 2001; Sapir et al., 2002). Clinicians who are not LSVT trained but plan to work on loudness need to consider that treatment will need to go hand in hand with establishing adequate respiratory support. In addition, it is important to monitor adverse effects on the patient's voice quality.

Another area of common focus is stress production; tasks typically consist of emphatic stress exercises, either on particular syllables in a word (lexical stress) or on a word within a phrase or sentence (sentence stress). Such tasks are designed to work on the coordinated control of pitch, loudness, and duration. For the remaining prosodic aspects, little information is available. Intonation is often addressed by practicing different contours, such as contrasting statements from questions. In addition, patients are sometimes encouraged to widen their pitch range using glides on prolonged vowels. The effectiveness of this nonspeech task is again doubtful. Proposed techniques for impaired rhythm include stress tasks as outlined previously, as well as reading of rhythmical materials such as limericks. Yorkston et al. (2007) reviewed the available literature and concluded that current evidence does not support the effectiveness of prosodic treatment with the exception of the treatment of loudness in speakers with PD.

Instrumentation and Alternative Augmentative Communication Devices

There is a long history of instrumental methods being used to support the treatment of dysarthria by providing biofeedback to the patient. In addition, technology has been developed to function as AAC. Biofeedback systems provide visual or tactile feedback to patients about an aspect of their speech behavior, and evidence generally suggests that they are effective means of supporting the treatment of speech disorders (e.g., Austermann

Hula, Robin, Maas, Ballard, & Schmidt, 2008). They are most commonly based on acoustic measures and provide information on features such as phonation, nasality, pitch, loudness, or duration (e.g., the Kay Pentax Voice Games, nasometers, the lingWAVES TheraVox from Wevosys, as well as a growing number of apps available for aspects such as breath support, voice quality, rate, etc.). In addition, other systems that measure air pressure and airflow or muscle force (e.g., the Iowa Performance Instrument; Robin, Goel, Somodi, & Luschei, 1992) can be useful in treatment.

For example, recent work by Johansson, Fredrikson, Hartelius, and Schalling (2012) reported positive effects of expiratory muscle training with the aid of a positive expiratory pressure threshold trainer in people with multiple sclerosis. Devices that breach the gap between a training aid and AAC are systems that remind patients to maintain particular behaviors or induce desired effects through manipulation of parameters. Examples include the Voxlog™ (Schalling, Bulukin-Wilen, Gustafson, & Södersten, 2012), which emits a stimulus when a speaker's voice drops below a certain loudness level.

A different approach to achieving loudness is taken by the Speechvive™ (Huber et al., 2012), which induces the Lombard effect through providing a masking noise. Such systems can be advantageous in patients who find it difficult to voluntarily increase their loudness. A similar effect is achieved through altered auditory feedback, which can either delay the auditory signal (delayed auditory feedback) or alter its pitch (frequency shifted feedback). Although not successful in all speakers, it has shown positive effects in reducing rate and increasing intelligibility in a subset of patients with PD (Lowit, Dobinson, Timmins, Howell, & Kröger, 2010).

If biofeedback tools are implemented during treatment, clinicians should be cautious about the timing, type, and frequency of biofeedback, as overreliance on externally provided feedback can lead to poorer internalization of the new behavior and thus less carryover into natural speech behavior. While these tools are thus helpful at the start to increase awareness of the therapy target, they should be withdrawn as the patient progresses lest they become maladaptive. In addition, systems such as altered feedback or the Speechvive should only be introduced if patients fail to manipulate the desired speech aspects on their own accord.

If an individual is so severely impaired that speech is not a viable communication option all of the time, then AAC should be considered. The literature describes a wide variety of low- and high-tech aids for people with motor speech disorders (see Hanson, Yorkston, & Beukelman, 2004, and Mathy, 2004 for reviews). Important considerations in choosing the right AAC are the patient's cognitive and language skills, as well as his or her visual and fine motor abilities. Furthermore, acceptability to the user and potential communication partners are important factors to consider.

Alternative augmentative communication aids are divided into two main categories: speech supplementation and speech replacement techniques. The latter furthermore is divided into high- and low-tech aids. The alphabet board is the most common supplementation system used in dysarthria. It can be used to completely spell out the message or to provide additional cues to the speech output to facilitate listener understanding (Hanson & Beukelman, 2006; Hanson, Beukelman, Heidemann, & Shutts-Johnson, 2010; Hustad & Garcia, 2005). Speech replacement systems can be as low tech as pen and paper, whereas at the high-tech end, they can speak for the patient. Given the costs associated with the latter, it is important to determine the communication needs of the patients and their ability to use the various systems offered. More detailed information on choosing the right AAC for individuals with motor speech disorders can be found in texts such as that of Beukelman, Garrett, and Yorkston (2007).

FUTURE DIRECTIONS

It is possible that dysarthria will be reconceptualized through empirical research and computational modeling of speech production. Particular aspects of this new perspective are that the motor disorder in some, if not many, dysarthrias will be considered to involve a programming disorder as well as an execution disorder and a component related to sensory processing or sensorimotor integration. The perceptual classification of type of dysarthria has come into question, especially as it relates to the reliability of listener judgments, its application to childhood and adult dysarthrias, and its relationship to neurologic diagnosis. Whatever may unfold regarding the classification of dysarthria types, there is a need for the development of sensitive methods, perceptual or instrumental, to determine the combination of sensorimotor dysfunctions that result in the dysarthria of an individual patient. This information is essential to diagnosis and assessment, treatment planning, and monitoring of change related to treatment or disease progression. Advances in research are likely given the ongoing development of tools and databases for the study of dysarthria, increased efforts to describe dysarthrias in different languages, integration of normal and disordered behavior in models of speech production and motor control, and emphasis on evidence-based practice for motor speech disorders in children and adults.

Especially within the last two decades, research on dysarthria has gone beyond issues in impairment to focus on communication impact and participation. This broader view of the disorder sheds new light on how dysarthria affects the lives of individuals. Progress also has been made in the understanding of impairments and how assessment and treatment procedures can be enhanced to guide more effective clinical services. However, it is clear that a great deal more work is required to guide clinicians in both of these areas. As discussed, current assessment methods have some reliability issues that are yet to be resolved. In addition, we lack large normative data sets to evaluate patients' performance against. A significant amount of effort has gone into and continues to go into developing automated, instrumental measures to address reliability issues, but these can be fraught with problems of their own, mainly in relation to validity and clinical applicability. Further consolidation of existing and new evidence would thus be welcome in order to arrive at an agreed set of tasks and analysis methods to assess body function and impairment in dysarthria that is supported by an appropriate normative database.

An important step forward in assessment practice was made by the recent establishment of impact and participation measures, and it is hoped that their use will become more established in coming years. However, more work is required in this area to establish a clearer link between assessment findings and appropriate intervention methods to address the issues identified as limiting a patient's participation.

In addition, there remains a significant research need for studies of clinical effectiveness to widen the evidence base for the management of this disorder. However, this is also inextricably linked to having the right tools available to measure the outcomes of the treatment we provide, irrespective of whether we evaluate treatment regimens with appropriately designed randomized controlled trials or by collecting evidence from a multitude of small-group or case studies.

Case Illustration 22.1

Diane is 34 years old and was diagnosed with multiple sclerosis 7 years ago. She lives with her husband, David, and her two young children, Tommy (4) and Amy (2). Both her and David's parents live about 2 hours away. David travels extensively and for long periods for his work. Diane has been employed full time as a primary schoolteacher for the last 10 years. However, she recently took the decision to stop working as the pressures of bringing up the children and her job were having an adverse effect on her health.

Diane's deteriorating health has had an impact on her communication. Since her most recent relapse, she reports that her speech has remained mildly dysarthric, and she finds it difficult to participate in conversations, particularly when she is tired. Her neurologist has referred her to speech and language therapy to assess her needs and provide intervention if appropriate.

Considering the fact that Diane is a young woman who recently had to come to terms with the fact that her progressive illness is starting to have a serious impact on her life, it was important for the clinician to start by establishing the psychosocial issues surrounding this case. It emerged that Diane did feel low as a consequence of her deteriorating symptoms, in particular her speech problems, which had surfaced for the first time at the last relapse. She indicated that these were the main reason for discontinuing work, as she felt that she could not communicate as clearly as was necessary for her to be efficient in her job. Leaving work created additional problems, as the family was no longer able to afford the full-time day care for the two children, and Diane has to look after them by herself at home, which significantly increases her fatigue and exacerbates her speech problems.

Diane reported some withdrawal from communication situations as she found it difficult to participate in group conversations in noisy environments and thus no longer joined her friends on social outings. She was also more apprehensive to speak on the phone to strangers as there had been some occasions of communication breakdown that left her feeling embarrassed. Furthermore, she indicated that it could be difficult at times to assert herself in front of her children as she could not raise her voice as much as before.

Having established that the communication problems had a significant impact on Diane's QOL, the clinician proceeded to assess the level of communication impairment. The Assessment of Intelligibility of Dysarthric Speech (Yorkston, Beukelman, & Traynor, 1984) showed 100% intelligibility for single words, although some sound distortions were evident, such as weak release for plosives and a mild level of hypernasality. These features persisted

(continues)

in the sentence intelligibility test (Unpredictable Sentence Test; McHenry & Parle, 2006) and the reading passage (Grandfather Passage; Darley et al., 1975), for which she also scored 100%. Additional features emerging from the reading passage were mildly reduced articulation rate, occasional misplacement of breath pauses, and ambiguous stress placement; however, these did not yet affect the overall naturalness of the sample. Given her professional background these errors could be attributed to the speech problem rather than unfamiliarity with the reading task. There was also no noticeable difference between the reading and a natural speech sample (spontaneous monologue), suggesting that cognitive load did not have a significant impact on speech output.

As Diane had reported difficulties in raising her voice, the clinician also asked her to read a passage over background noise (a radio playing in the background). While she managed to maintain an appropriate level of loudness during reading, she reported that she found this task more difficult than the previous ones. The reduced stress placement was further investigated in single-word and sentence contrastive stress tasks. Diane performed well on the words but revealed difficulties stressing items toward the end of the sequence at sentence level.

The speech distortions observed in the connected speech samples suggested a mild weakening of the articulatory musculature. This finding was confirmed by the physiological assessment, which revealed reduced ability to maintain lip closure and to elevate the velum. Performance on DDK rates indicated a slower repetition rate of around 3 syllables/second, combined with some irregularity in syllable length, and again weak plosives. There was also a marked reduction in respiratory volume, as Diane could only hold a prolonged vowel for 8 seconds, which explained the inappropriately placed pauses observed in the reading sample to some degree. Reduced breath support also appeared to have an impact on her performance on loudness glides, which were better going from loud to quiet than quiet to loud, where she appeared to have insufficient breath available to produce a loud voice at the end of the glide. Further problems with loudness control became evident in this task as she did not start off on a sufficiently quiet voice. Laryngeal function appeared normal in relation to pitch variation as well as voice quality, although the latter showed some signs of breathiness when Diane was raising her voice.

In addition to the speech assessment, the clinician performed a language and cognitive assessment (Cognitive Linguistic Quick Test; Helm-Estabrooks, 2001) to establish whether any of these might also contribute to the communication problem, particularly as Diane reported problems in participating in group conversations. She scored within normal limits in all sections of the test, suggesting that her current problems are primarily caused by motoric consequences of her multiple sclerosis. The clinician also assessed Diane's swallow. Although lip seal showed some weakness during speech, it was still functional during swallowing, as were all other components of the process.

In summary, the assessment revealed that Diane was experiencing mild effects of muscular weakness on her speech, that is, predominantly flaccid signs of dysarthria, which were not yet having an impact on her intelligibility or naturalness. However, she did show signs of withdrawal from communication situations as a result and experienced a worsening of symptoms when tired or in more demanding contexts.

Despite the relatively low level of impairment, the clinician decided that treatment was appropriate considering the high impact this was having on Diane's well-being. The approach focused on self-management skills as well as exercises to improve articulation. Direct intervention thus included awareness raising of the strengths and weaknesses of Diane's communication ability to allow for effective self-monitoring. In addition, she was given exercises to improve clarity of articulation through clear speech (Beukelman et al., 2002; Kennedy, Strand, & Yorkston, 1994; Lam & Tjaden, 2011). Breath support was targeted, largely by optimizing posture to allow her to take in a maximum amount of air and practicing appropriate breathing patterns. In addition, appropriate phrase length was established for normal and loud speech contexts. Use of LSVT was discussed as a potential treatment in the future should her loudness level become a more significant factor in her communication problems (Sapir et al., 2001). Diane was also familiarized with some apps that would allow her to practice some of these aspects without further clinician input when she felt the need.

Indirect measures to improve Diane's communication ability included a reduction of unnecessary background noise at home (TV, radio) to facilitate communication with the family. In addition, it was suggested to establish a behavioral rule system for the children that could be supported with external aids (e.g., a whistle) to avoid Diane having to raise her voice to gain their attention or establish order. Similar measures were agreed with the rest of

(*continues*)

the family and friends to allow Diane to use nonverbal signals to indicate a desire to contribute something without having to fight for the floor, thus facilitating contributions to group conversations.

Diane was also referred to physiotherapy and occupational therapy to manage her fatigue; in addition, social services were contacted to see what help could be provided to relieve Diane from child care. Diane also visited a counselor to help her come to terms with the increasing impact of her multiple sclerosis and to improve her mental health. Joint efforts between the counselor and the clinician managed to change her attitude toward her communication difficulty and give her the confidence to look for alternative areas of employment that relied less on oral communication. Furthermore, she joined a local multiple sclerosis support group, which helped her come to terms with the changes she was experiencing in her daily life.

Finally, Diane was provided with information on what changes might still lay ahead of her in relation to speech deterioration, language and cognitive skills, and in particular swallowing difficulties to facilitate effective self-referral at a later stage should she feel the need for further support.

The 6-month follow-up suggested a successful outcome of this multidisciplinary approach. Although there was no noticeable change in her communication patterns, Diane generally felt more confident about her abilities and had regained her previous level of socialization with family and friends. In addition, she had approached her old employer and managed to obtain a part-time position as an educational support worker that allowed her to use her teaching experience without having to deal with whole-classroom situations, thus avoiding the need to retrain for a new skill set.

STUDY QUESTIONS

1. What are the main components of computational models of speech production?
2. Discuss why a life-span perspective is needed for clinical practice related to the dysarthrias.
3. What are the different types of dysarthria, and how closely do they relate to the lesion site?
4. Discuss the benefits and potential issues with using nonspeech tasks in the assessment and treatment of dysarthria.
5. Explain what areas should be included in a comprehensive assessment of an individual with dysarthria.
6. How can treatment of prosodic functions improve intelligibility?
7. List three treatment approaches for speech subsystems that would be appropriate for an individual with spastic dysarthria.

REFERENCES

Abbruzzese, G., & Berardelli, A., (2002). Sensorimotor integration in movement disorders. *Movement Disorders*, *18*, 231–240.

Ackermann, H., Hertrich, I., & Hehr, T. (1995). Oral diadochokinesis in neurological dysarthrias. *Folia Phoniatrica et Logopaedica*, *47*, 15–23.

Adams, S. G., Dykstra, A. D., Jenkins, M., & Jog, M. (2008). Speech-to-noise levels and conversational intelligibility in hypophonia and Parkinson's disease. *Journal of Medical Speech-Language Pathology*, *16*, 165–172.

Adams, S. G., Page, A. D., & Jog, M. (2002). Summary feedback schedules and speech motor learning in Parkinson's disease. *Journal of Medical Speech-Language Pathology*, *10*, 215–220.

Amerman, J. D., & Parnell, M. M. (1990). Auditory impressions of the speech of normal elderly adults. *British Journal of Disorders of Communication*, *25*, 35–43.

Anderson, A. H., Bader, M., Bard E. G., Boyle, E., Doherty, G., Garrod, S., et al. (1991). The HCRC map task corpus. *Language and Speech*, *34*, 351–366.

Austermann Hula, S. N., Robin, D. A., Maas, E., Ballard, K. J., & Schmidt, R. A. (2008). Effects of feedback frequency and timing on acquisition, retention, and transfer of speech skills in acquired apraxia of speech. *Journal of Speech, Language, and Hearing Research*, *51*(5), 1088–1113.

Auzou, P., Ozsancak, C., Jan, M., Menard, J. F., Eustache, F., & Hannequin, D. (2000). Evaluation of motor speech function in the diagnosis of various forms of dysarthria. *Revue Neurologique*, *156*, 47–52.

Ballard, K. J., Robin, D. A., & Folkins, J. W. (2003). An integrative model of speech motor control: A response to Ziegler. *Aphasiology*, *17*, 37–48.

Barnish, M., Horton, S., Butterfint, Z., & Deane, K. (2013). Relationships between cognitive status, speech characteristics and communicative participation in Parkinson's disease. *Movement Disorders*, *28*, S178–S178.

Baumgartner, C. A., Sapir, S., & Ramig, T. O. (2001). Voice quality changes following phonatory-respiratory effort treatment

(LSVT) versus respiratory effort treatment for individuals with Parkinson disease. *Journal of Voice, 15,* 105–114.

Baylor, C., Burns, M., Eadie, T., Britton, D., & Yorkston, K. (2011). A qualitative study of interference with communicative participation across communication disorders in adults. *American Journal of Speech-Language Pathology, 20,* 269–287.

Baylor, C., Yorkston, K., Bamer, A., Britton, D., & Amtmann, D. (2010). Variables associated with communicative participation in people with multiple sclerosis: A regression analysis. *American Journal of Speech-Language Pathology, 19,* 143–153.

Baylor, C. R., Yorkston, K., Eadie, T., Kim, J., Chung, H., & Amtmann, D. (2013). The Communicative Participation Item Bank (CPIB): Item bank calibration and development of a disorder-generic short form. *Journal of Speech, Language, and Hearing Research, 56,* 1190–1208.

Baylor, C. R., Yorkston, K. M., Eadie, T. L., Miller, R. M., & Amtmann, D. (2009). Developing the Communicative Participation Item Bank: Rasch analysis results from a spasmodic dysphonia sample. *Journal of Speech, Language, and Hearing Research, 52,* 1302–1320.

Beukelman, D., Fager, S., Ullman, C., Hanson, E. K., & Logemann, J. A. (2002). The impact of speech supplementation on the intelligibility of persons with traumatic brain injury. *Journal of Medical Speech-Language Pathology, 10,* 237–242.

Beukelman, D., Garrett, K. L., & Yorkston, K. M. (2007). *Augmentative communication strategies for adults with acute or chronic medical conditions.* Baltimore, MD: Brookes.

Blanchet, P. G., & Snyder, G. J. (2009). Speech rate deficits in individuals with Parkinson's disease: A review of the literature. *Journal of Medical Speech-Language Pathology, 17,* 1–7.

Blanchet, P. G., & Snyder, G. J. (2010). Speech rate treatments for individuals with dysarthria: A tutorial. *Perceptual and Motor Skills, 110,* 965–982.

Blakemore, S. J., Frith, C. D., & Wolpert, D. M. (2001). The cerebellum is involved in predicting the sensory consequences of action. *NeuroReport, 12*(11), 1879–1884.

Bloch, S., Beeke, S., & Miller, N. (2011). Acquired communication disorders: Looking beyond impairment. *Disability and Rehabilitation, 33,* 175–177.

Bloch, S., & Wilkinson, R. (2009). Acquired dysarthria in conversation: Identifying sources of understandability problems. *International Journal of Language & Communication Disorders, 44,* 769–783.

Bloch, S. J., Saldert, C., & Ferm, U. (2015). Problematic topic transitions in dysarthric conversation. *International Journal of Speech-Language Pathology, 17*(4), 373–383.

Bohland, J. W., & Guenther, F. H. (2006). An fMRI investigation of syllable sequence production. *NeuroImage, 32,* 621–841.

Borrie, S., McAuliffe, M. J., Tillard, G., Ormond, T., Anderson, T., & Hornibrook, J. (2007). Effect of the Lee Silverman Voice Treatment (LSVT®) on articulation in speakers with Parkinson's disease. *New Zealand Journal of Speech-Language Therapy, 62,* 29–36.

Bradlow, A. R., Bakes, R. E., Choi, A., Kim, M., & van Engen, K. J. (2007). The Wilcat corpus of native- and foreign-accented English. *Journal of the Acoustical Society of America, 121,* 3072.

Brady, M. C., Clark, A. M., Dickson, S., Paton, G., & Barbour, R. S. (2011). The impact of stroke-related dysarthria on social participation and implications for rehabilitation. *Disability and Rehabilitation, 33,* 178–186.

Brown, A., & Docherty, G. J. (1995). Phonetic variation in dysarthric speech as a function of sampling task. *European Journal of Disorders of Communication, 30,* 17–35.

Brown, S., Laird, A. R., Pfordresher, P. O., Thelen, S. M., Turkeltaub, P., & Liotti, M. (2009). The somatotopy of speech: Phonation and articulation in the human motor cortex. *Brain and Cognition, 70,* 31–41.

Bunton, K., Kent, R. D., Duffy, J. R., Rosenbek, J. C., & Kent, J. (2007). Listener agreement for auditory-perceptual ratings of dysarthria. *Journal of Speech, Language & Hearing Research, 50,* 1481–1495.

Cahill, L. M., Turner, A. B., Stabler, P. A., Addis, P. E., Theodoros, D. G., & Murdoch, B. E. (2004). An evaluation of continuous positive airway pressure (CPAP) therapy in the treatment of hypernasality following traumatic brain injury: A report of 3 cases. *Journal of Head Trauma Rehabilitation, 19,* 241–253.

Chenausky, K., MacAuslan, J., & Goldhor, R. (2011). Acoustic analysis of PD speech. *Parkinson's Disease,* Volume 2011, Article ID 435232.

Croce, R., Horvat, M., & Roswal, G. (1996). Augmented feedback for enhanced skill acquisition in individuals with traumatic brain injury. *Perceptual and Motor Skills, 82,* 507–514.

Crystal, D. (1992). *Profiling linguistic disability* (2nd ed.). London, UK: Whurr.

Darley, F. L., Aronson, A. E., & Brown, J. R. (1969a). Clusters of deviant speech dimensions in the dysarthrias. *Journal of Speech and Hearing Research, 12,* 462–496.

Darley, F. L., Aronson, A. E., & Brown, J. R. (1969b). Differential diagnostic patterns of dysarthria. *Journal of Speech and Hearing Research, 12,* 246–269.

Darley, F. L., Aronson, A. E., & Brown, J. R. (1975). *Motor speech disorders.* Philadelphia, PA: Saunders.

Deane, K. H., Whurr, R., Playford, E. D., Ben-Shlomo, Y., & Clarke, C. E. (2001a). A comparison of speech and language therapy techniques for dysarthria in Parkinson's disease. *Cochrane Database of Systematic Reviews, 2,* CD002814.

Deane, K. H., Whurr, R., Playford, E. D., Ben-Shlomo, Y., & Clarke, C. E. (2001b). Speech and language therapy versus placebo or no intervention for dysarthria in Parkinson's disease. *Cochrane Database of Systematic Reviews, 2,* CD002812. doi:10.1002/14651858.CD002812

DeBodt, M. S., Hernandez-Diaz Huici, M. E., & van de Heyning, P. H. (2002). Intelligibility as a linear communication of dimensions in dysarthric speech. *Journal of Communication Disorders, 35,* 283–292.

Dickson, S., Barbour, R. S., Brady, M., Clark, A. M., & Paton, G. (2008). Patients' experiences of disruptions associated with post-stroke dysarthria. *International Journal of Language and Communication Disorders, 43,* 135–153.

Dietsch, A. M., Solomon, N. P., Sharkey, L. A., Duffy, J. R., Strand, E. A., & Clark, H. M. (2014). Perceptual and instrumental assessments of orofacial muscle tone in dysarthric and normal speakers. *Journal of Rehabilitation Research & Development, 51,* 1127–1142.

Dromey, C. (2000). Articulatory kinematics in patients with Parkinson disease using different speech treatment approaches. *Journal of Medical Speech-Language Pathology, 8,* 155–161.

Dromey, C., & Bates, E. (2005). Speech interactions with linguistic, cognitive, and visuomotor tasks. *Journal of Speech, Language and Hearing Research, 48,* 295–305.

Dromey, C., & Benson, A. (2003). Effects of concurrent motor, linguistic, or cognitive tasks on speech motor performance.

Journal of Speech, Language and Hearing Research, 46, 1234–1246.

Drummond, S. (1993). *Dysarthria Examination Battery.* Tucson, AZ: Communication Skill Builders.

Duffy, J. R. (2010). Distinguishing among motor speech disorders is important: The role of speech pathology in neurologic diagnosis. In B. Maassen & P. van Lieshout (Eds.), *Speech motor control: New developments in basic and applied research* (pp. 271–281). Oxford, UK: Oxford University Press.

Duffy, J. R. (2013). *Motor speech disorders: Substrates, differential diagnosis, and management.* St. Louis, MO: Elsevier Health Sciences.

Duffy, J. R., & Yorkston, K. M. (2003). Medical interventions for spasmodic dysphonia and some related conditions: A systematic review. *Journal of Medical Speech-Language Pathology, 11*(4), ix–lviii.

Dworkin, J. P., & Johns, D. F. (1980). Management of velopharyngeal incompetence in dysarthria: A historical review. *Clinical Otolaryngology & Allied Sciences, 5,* 61–74.

Enderby, P. (1983). *Frenchay Dysarthria Assessment.* Austin, TX: Pro-Ed.

Enderby, P., & Palmer, R. (2008). *Frenchay Dysarthria Assessment* (2nd ed.). Austin, TX: Pro-Ed.

Fahn, S. (2011). Classification of movement disorders. *Movement Disorders, 26,* 947–957.

Fahn, S., Jankovic, J., & Hallett, M. (2011). *Principles and practice of movement disorders* (2nd ed.). Philadelphia, PA: Elsevier.

Fairbanks, G. (1960). *Voice and articulation drillbook* (2nd ed., pp. 124–139). New York: Harper & Row.

Folker, J., Murdoch, B., Cahill, L., Delatycki, M., Corben, L., & Vogel, A. (2010). Dysarthria in Friedreich's ataxia: A perceptual analysis. *Folia Phoniatrica et Logopaedica, 62,* 97–103.

Fonville, S., van der Worp, H., Maat, P., Aldenhoven, M., Algra, A., & van Gijn, J. (2008). Accuracy and inter-observer variation in the classification of dysarthria from speech recordings. *Journal of Neurology, 255,* 1545–1548.

Golfinopoulos, E., Tourville, J. A., & Guenther, F. H. (2010). The integration of large-scale neural network modeling and functional brain imaging in speech motor control. *NeuroImage, 52,* 682–874.

Goozee, J. V., Murdoch, B. E., & Theodoros, D. G. (2001). Physiological assessment of tongue function in dysarthria following traumatic brain injury. *Logopedics, Phoniatrics, Vocology, 26,* 51–65.

Gorham-Rowan, M. M., & Laures-Gore, J. (2006). Acoustic-perceptual correlates of voice quality in elderly men and women. *Journal of Communication Disorders, 39,* 171–184.

Guenther, F. H., & Vladusich, T. (2012). A neural theory of speech acquisition and production. *Journal of Neurolinguistics, 25,* 408–422.

Guerra, E. C., & Lovely, D. F. (2003). Suboptimal classifier for dysarthria assessment. In A. Sanfeliu & J. Ruize-Schulcloper (Eds.), *Progress in pattern recognition, speech and image analysis* (pp. 314–321). Berlin, Germany: Springer.

Hammen, V. L. (2004). Managing speaking rate in dysarthria. In E. Strand (Ed.), *Treatment of dysarthria: Evidence-based practice* (pp. 19–24). Rockville, MD: American Speech-Language-Hearing Association.

Hammer, M. J., & Barlow, S. M. (2010). Laryngeal somatosensory deficits in Parkinson's disease: Implications for speech respiratory and phonatory control. *Experimental Brain Research, 201,* 401–409.

Hanson, E. K., & Beukelman, D. R. (2006). Effect of omitted cues on alphabet supplemented speech intelligibility. *Journal of Medical Speech-Language Pathology, 14,* 185–196.

Hanson, E. K., Beukelman, D. R., Heidemann, J. K., & Shutts-Johnson, E. (2010). The impact of alphabet supplementation and word prediction on sentence intelligibility of electronically distorted speech. *Journal of Speech Communication, 52,* 99–105.

Hanson, E. K., Yorkston, K. M., & Beukelman, D. R. (2004). Speech supplementation techniques for dysarthria: A systematic review. *Journal of Medical Speech-Language Pathology, 12*(2), ix–xxix.

Hartelius, L., Elmberg, M., Holm, R., Lövberg, A.-S., & Nikolaidis, S. (2008). Living with dysarthria: Evaluation of a self-report questionnaire. *Folia Phoniatrica et Logopedica, 60,* 11–19.

Hartman, D. E., & Danhauer, J. L. (1976). Perceptual features of speech for males in four perceived age decades. *Journal of the Acoustical Society of America, 59,* 713.

Helm-Estabrooks, N. (2001). *Cognitive Linguistic Quick Test.* London, UK: Pearson Assessment.

Henrich, J., Lowit, A., Schalling, E., & Mennen, I. (2006). Rhythmic disturbance in ataxic dysarthria: A comparison of different measures and speech tasks. *Journal of Medical Speech-Language Pathology, 14,* 291–296.

Herd, C. P., Tomlinson, C. L., Deane, K. H. O., Brady, M. C., Smith, C. H., Sackley, C. M., et al. (2012a). Comparison of speech and language therapy techniques for speech problems in Parkinson's disease. *Cochrane Database of Systematic Reviews, 8,* 1-CD002814. doi:http://dx.doi.org/10.1002/14651858.CD002814.pub2.

Herd, C. P., Tomlinson, C. L., Deane, K. H. O., Brady, M. C., Smith, C. H., Sackley, C. M., et al. (2012b). Speech and language therapy versus placebo or no intervention for speech problems in Parkinson's disease. *Cochrane Database of Systematic Reviews, 8,* 1-CD002812. doi:http://dx.doi.org/10.1002/14651858.CD002812.pub2

Hickok, G. (2012). The cortical organization of speech processing: Feedback control and predictive coding the context of a dual-stream model. *Journal of Communication Disorders, 45,* 393–402.

Hixon, T. J., Hawley, M. S., & Wilson, J. M. (1982). An around-the-house device for the clinical determination of respiratory driving pressure. *Journal of Speech & Hearing Disorders, 47,* 413–415.

Hixon, T. J., & Hoit, J. D. (1998). Physical examination of the diaphragm by the speech-language pathologist. *American Journal of Speech-Language Pathology, 7,* 37–45.

Hixon, T. J., & Hoit, J. D. (1999). Physical examination of the abdominal wall by the speech-language pathologist. *American Journal of Speech-Language Pathology, 8,* 335–346.

Hixon, T. J., & Hoit, J. D. (2000). Physical examination of the rib cage wall by the speech-language pathologist. *American Journal of Speech-Language Pathology, 9,* 179–196.

Ho A. K., Bradshaw, J. L. & Iansek, R. (2008) For better or worse: The effect of levodopa on Parkinsonian speech. *Movement Disorders, 23*(4), 574–580.

Hodge, M. (2004). Nonspeech oral motor treatment approaches for dysarthria: Perspectives on a controversial clinical practice. In E. Strand (Ed.), *Treatment of dysarthria: Evidence-based practice* (pp. 25–32). Rockville, MD: American Speech-Language Hearing Association.

Houde, J. F., & Nagarajan, S. S. (2011). Speech production as state feedback control. *Frontiers in Human Neuroscience, 5,* 82.

Huber, J., Stathopoulos, E., Sussman, H., Darling, M., Snyder, S., & Richardson, K. (2012, February 28–March 4). *Changes to physiology as a result of a new treatment, Speechvive for individuals with Parkinson's disease*. Paper presented at the Conference on Motor Speech, Santa Rosa, CA.

Hustad, K. C., & Garcia, J. M. (2005). Aided and unaided speech supplementation strategies: Effect of alphabet cues and iconic hand gestures on dysarthric speech. *Journal of Speech, Language and Hearing Research, 48*, 996–1012.

Johansson, K., Fredrikson, S., Hartelius, L., & Schalling, E. (2012, February 28–March 4). *Effects of EMST (expiratory muscle strength training) on speech and respiration in individuals with multiple sclerosis*. Paper presented at the Conference on Motor Speech, Santa Rosa, CA.

Jordan, N., & Sagar, H. J. (1994). The role of the striatum in motor learning: Dissociations between isometric motor control processes in Parkinson's disease. *International Journal of Neuroscience, 77*, 153–165.

Kadi, K. L., Selouani, S.-A., Bourdraa, B., & Boudraa, M. (2013, July 3–5). *Discriminative prosodic features to assess the dysarthria severity levels*. Proceedings of the World Congress on Engineering, WCE 2013, Vol. III, London.

Kaňovský, P. (2002). Dystonia: A disorder of motor programming or motor execution? *Movement Disorders, 17*, 1143–1147.

Kempler, D., & Van Lancker, D. (2002). Effect of speech task on intelligibility in dysarthria: A case study of Parkinson's disease. *Brain and Language, 80*, 449–464.

Kennedy, M. R. T., Strand, E. A., & Yorkston, K. M. (1994). Selected acoustic changes in the verbal repairs of dysarthric speakers. *Journal of Medical Speech-Language Pathology, 2*, 263–279.

Kent, R. D. (2015, June 29). Nonspeech oral movements and oral motor disorders: A narrative review. *American Journal of Speech-Language Pathology*. [Epub ahead of print] doi:10.1044/2015_AJSLP-14-0179.

Kent, R. D., Duffy, J., Kent, J. F., & Vorperian, H. K. (1999). Quantification of motor speech abilities in stroke: Time-energy analyses of syllable and word repetition. *Journal of Medical Speech-Language Pathology, 7*, 83–90.

Kent, R. D., Duffy, J. R., Slama, A., Kent, J. F., & Clift, A. (2001). Clinicoanatomic studies in dysarthria: Review, critique, and directions for research. *Journal of Speech, Language and Hearing Research, 44*, 535–551.

Kent, R. D., & Kent, J. F. (2000). Task-based profiles of the dysarthrias. *Folia Phoniatrica et Logopaedica, 52*, 48–53.

Kent, R. D., Kent, J. F., Duffy, J., & Weismer, G. (1998). The dysarthrias: Speech-voice profiles, related dysfunctions, and neuropathology. *Journal of Medical Speech-Language Pathology, 6*, 165–211.

Kent, R. D., Kent, J. F., & Rosenbek, J. C. (1987). Maximum performance tests of speech production. *Journal of Speech and Hearing Disorders, 52*, 367–387.

Kent, R. D., Kent, J. F., Rosenbek, J. C., Vorperian, H. K., & Weismer, G. (1997). A speaking task analysis of the dysarthria in cerebellar disease. *Folia Phoniatrica et Logopaedica, 49*, 63–82.

Kent, R. D., & Kim, Y. (2011). The assessment of intelligibility in motor speech disorders. In A. Lowit & R. D. Kent (Eds.), *Assessment of motor speech disorders* (pp. 21–38). San Diego, CA: Plural.

Kent, R. D., & Kim, Y. J. (2003). Toward an acoustic typology of motor speech disorders. *Clinical Linguistics and Phonetics, 17*, 427–445.

Kent, R. D., Weismer, G., Kent, J. F., & Rosenbek, J. C. (1989). Toward phonetic intelligibility testing in dysarthria. *Journal of Speech and Hearing Disorders, 54*, 482–499.

Kim, H., Hasegawa-Johnson, M., Perlman, A., Gunderson, J., Huang, T., Watkin, K., et al. (2008, September 22–26). *Dysarthric speech database for universal access research*. INTERSPEECH 2008—9th Annual Conference of the International Speech Communication Association, Brisbane, Australia, pp. 1741–1744. ISCA Archive, http://www.isca-speech.org/archive/interspeech_2008.

Kim, H., Martin, K., Hasegawa-Johnson, M., & Perlman, A. (2010). Frequency of consonant articulation errors in dysarthric speech. *Clinical Linguistics & Phonetics, 24*, 759–770.

Kim, Y., Kent, R. D., & Weismer, G. (2011). An acoustic study of the relationships among neurologic disease, dysarthria type, and severity of dysarthria. *Journal of Speech, Language, and Hearing Research, 54*, 417–429.

Knock, T. R., Ballard, K. J., Robin, D. A., & Schmidt, R. A. (2000). Influence of order of stimulus presentation on speech motor learning: A principled approach to treatment for apraxia of speech. *Aphasiology, 14*, 653–668.

Konstantopoulos, K., Charalambous, M., & Veroeven, J. (2011, August 17–21). Sequential motion rates in the dysarthria of multiple sclerosis: A temporal analysis. In W.-S. Lee & E. Zee (Eds.), *Proceedings of the International Congress of Phonetic Sciences (ICPhS) XVII*, Hong Kong.

Kröger, B. J., Schnitker, R., & Lowit, A. (2008). The organization of a neurocomputational control model for articulatory speech synthesis. In A. Esposito, N. Bourbakis, N. Avouris, & I. Hatzilygeroudis (Eds.), *Verbal and nonverbal features of human–human and human–machine interaction* (pp. 126–141). Berlin. Germany: Springer.

Kuehn, D. P., & Wachtel, J. M. (1994). CPAP therapy for treating hypernasality following closed head injury. In J. A. Till, K. M. Yorkston, & D. Beukelman (Eds.), *Motor speech disorders: Advances in assessment and treatment*. (pp 207–212) Baltimore, MD: Paul H. Brooks.

Lam, J., & Tjaden, K. (2011, June 8–11). *Intelligibility of clear speech: Effect of instruction*. Paper presented at the 6th International Conference on Speech Motor Control, Groningen, the Netherlands.

Langmore, S. E., & Lehman, M. E. (1994). Physiologic deficits in the orofacial system underlying dysarthria in amyotrophic lateral sclerosis. *Journal of Speech, Language, and Hearing Research, 37*, 28–37.

Lansford, K. L., Liss, J. M., & Norton, R. E. (2014). Free-classification of perceptually similar speakers with dysarthria. *Journal of Speech, Language, and Hearing Research, 57*, 2051–2064.

Lee, Y. M., Sung, J. E., Sim, H. S., Han, J. H., & Song, H. N. (2012). Analysis of articulation error patterns depending on level of speech intelligibility in adults with dysarthria. *Communication Sciences and Disorders, 17*, 130–142.

Liegeois, F. J., & Morgan, A. T. (2012). Neural bases of childhood speech disorders: Lateralization and plasticity for speech functions during development. *Neuroscience and Biobehavioral Reviews, 36*, 439–458.

Lowit, A. (2014). Quantification of rhythm problems in disordered speech: A re-evaluation. *Philosophical Transactions of the Royal Society B: Biological Sciences, 369*(1658).

Lowit, A., Brendel, B., & Howell, P. (2006, March 22–26). *The relationship between cognitive ability and speech performance under AAF conditions*. Paper presented at the Conference on Motor Speech: Motor Speech Disorders & Speech Motor Control, Austin, TX.

Lowit, A., Dobinson, C., Timmins, C., Howell, P., & Kröger, B. (2010). The effectiveness of traditional methods and altered auditory feedback in improving speech rate and intelligibility in speakers with Parkinson's disease. *International Journal of Speech-Language Pathology*, 12, 426–436.

Maas, E., Robin, D. A., Austermann Hula, S. N., Freedman, S. E., Wulf, G., Ballard, K. J., et al. (2008). Principles of motor learning in treatment of motor speech disorders. *American Journal of Speech-Language Pathology*, 17, 277–298.

Masaki, N., & Seiji, N. (2002). A study of oral diadochokinesis in dysarthric speakers [Japanese]. *Japan Journal of Logopedics and Phoniatrics*, 43, 9–20.

Mathy, P. (2004). Augmentative and alternative communication intervention in neurogenic disroders with acquired dysarthria. In E. Strand (Ed.), *Treatment of dysarthria: Evidence-based practice* (pp. 33–41). Rockville, MD: American Speech-Language and Hearing Association.

McHenry, M. A., & Parle, A. M. (2006). Construction of a set of unpredictable sentences for intelligibility testing. *Journal of Medical Speech-Language Pathology*, 14, 269–272.

Melle, N., & Gallego, C. (2012). Differential diagnosis between apraxia and dysarthria based on acoustic analysis. *The Spanish Journal of Psychology*, 15, 495–504.

Menendez-Pidal, X., Polikoff, J. B., Peters, S. M., Leonzjo, J. E., & Bunnell, H. (1996). The Nemours database of dysarthric speech. In H. T. Bunnell & W. Idsardi (Eds.), *Proceedings of the Fourth International Conference on Spoken Language Processing* (Volume 3; pp. 1962–1965). New York, NY: IEEE.

Miller, N. (2013). Measuring up to intelligibility. *International Journal of Language and Other Communication Disorders*, 48, 601–612.

Miller, N., Andrew, S., Noble, E., & Walshe, M. (2011). Changing perceptions of self as a communicator in Parkinson's disease: A longitudinal follow-up study. *Disability and Rehabilitation*, 33(3), 204–210. doi:10.3109/09638288.2010.508099.

Miller, N., & Lowit, A. (2014). *Motor speech disorders: A cross-language perspective*. Clevedon: Multilingual Matters.

Miller, N., Noble, E., Jones, D., & Burn, D. J. (2006). Life with communication changes in PD. *Age and Ageing*, 35, 235–239.

Milroy, L., & Perkins, L. (1992). Repair strategies in aphasic discourse: Towards a collaborative model. *Clinical Linguistics & Phonetics*, 6, 27–40.

Mink, J. W. (1996). The basal ganglia: Focused selection and inhibition of competing motor programs. *Progress in Neurobiology*, 50, 381–425.

Monchi, O., Petrides, M., Strafella, A. P., Worsley, K. J., & Doyon, J. (2006). Functional role of the basal ganglia in the planning and execution of actions. *Annals of Neurology*, 59, 257–264.

Morgan, A. (2013). Speech-language pathology insights into genetics and neuroscience: Beyond surface behavior. *International Journal of Speech-Language Pathology*, 15, 245–254.

Mujumdar, M. V., & Kubichek, R. F. (2010, March 14–19). *Design of a dysarthria classifier using global statistics of speech features.* Paper presented at the IEEE International Conference on Acoustics, Speech and Signal Processing (ICASSP), Dallas, TS.

Murdoch, B. E. (Ed.). (1998). *Dysarthria: A physiological approach to assessment and treatment.* Cheltenham, UK: Thornes.

Murdoch, B. E. (2011). Physiological assessment. In A. Lowit & R. D. Kent (Eds.), *Assessment of Motor Speech Disorders* (pp. 39–74). San Diego, CA: Plural.

Murry, T., & Woodson, G. E. (1995). Combined-modality treatment of adductor spasmodic dysphonia with botulinum toxin and voice therapy. *Journal of Voice*, 9, 460–465.

Netsell, R., & Daniel, B. (1979). Dysarthria in adults: Physiologic approach to rehabilitation. *Archives of Physical Medicine & Rehabilitation*, 60, 502–508.

Nishio, M., & Niimi, S. (2000). Changes over time in dysarthric patients with amyotrophic lateral sclerosis (ALS): A study of changes in speaking rate and maximum repetition rate (MRR). *Clinical Linguistics & Phonetics*, 14, 485–497.

Patel, R. (2011). Assessment of prosody. In A. Lowit & R. D. Kent (Eds.), *Assessment of motor speech disorders* (pp. 75–96). San Diego, CA: Plural.

Patel, R., Connaghan, K., Franco, D., Edsall, E., Forgit, D., Olsen, L., et al. (2013). "The Caterpillar": A novel reading passage for assessment of motor speech disorders. *American Journal of Speech-Language Pathology*, 22, 1–9.

Pennington, L., Miller, N., Robson, S., & Steen, N. (2010). Intensive speech and language therapy for older children with cerebral palsy: A systems approach. *Developmental Medicine & Child Neurology*, 52, 337–344.

Peppé, S., & McCann, J. (2003). Assessing intonation and prosody in children with atypical language development: The PEPS-C test and the revised version. *Clinical Linguistics & Phonetics*, 17, 345–354.

Price, C. J. (2012). A review and synthesis of the first 20 years of PET and fMRI studies of heard speech, spoken language and reading. *Neuroimage*, 62, 816–847.

Ptacek, P. H., Sander, E. K., Maloney, W. H., & Roe Jackson, C. C. (1966). Phonatory and related changes with advanced age. *Journal of Speech, Language, and Hearing Research*, 9, 353–360.

Ramig, L. A. (1983). Effects of physiological aging on vowel spectral noise. *Journal of Gerontology*, 38, 223–225.

Ramig, L. O., Countryman, S., Thompson, L. L., & Horii, Y. (1995). Comparison of two forms of intensive speech treatment for Parkinson disease. *Journal of Speech and Hearing Research*, 38, 1232–1251.

Ramig, L. O., Sapir, S., Countryman, S., Pawlas, A. A., O'Brien, C., Hoehn, M., et al. (2001). Intensive voice treatment (LSVT) for patients with Parkinson's disease: A 2 year follow up. *Journal of Neurology, Neurosurgery, and Psychiatry*, 71, 493–498.

Renout, K. A., Leeper, H. A., Bandur, D. L., & Hudson, A. J. (1995). Vocal fold diadochokinetic function of individuals with amyotrophic lateral sclerosis. *American Journal of Speech-Language Pathology*, 4, 73–80.

Riecker, A., Brendel, B., Ziegler, W., Erb, M., & Ackermann, H. (2008). The influence of syllabic onset complexity and syllable frequency on speech motor control. *Brain and Language*, 107, 102–113.

Robertson, S. J. (1982). *Dysarthria Profile*. Tucson, TX: Communication Skill Builders.

Robin, D. A., Goel, A., Somodi, L. B., & Luschei, E. S. (1992). Tongue strength and endurance: Relation to highly skilled movements. *Journal of Speech and Hearing Research*, 35, 1239–1245.

Rosen, K. M., Kent, R. D., Delaney, A. L., & Duffy, J. R. (2006). Parametric quantitative acoustic analysis of conversation produced by speakers with dysarthria and healthy speakers. *Journal of Speech, Language, and Hearing Research, 49,* 395–411.

Roy, E. A., Saint-Cyr, J., Taylor, A., & Lang, A. (1993). Movement sequencing disorders in Parkinson's disease. *International Journal of Neuroscience, 73,* 183–194.

Royal College of Speech and Language Therapists. (2009). *RCSLT resource manual for commissioning and planning services for SLCN: Dysarthria.* London, UK: Author.

Rudzicz, F., Namasivayam, A. K., & Wolff, T. (2012). The TORGO database of acoustic and articulatory speech from speakers with dysarthria. *Language Resources & Evaluation, 46,* 523–541.

Ryan, W. J., & Burk, K. W. (1974). Perceptual and acoustic correlates of aging in the speech of males. *Journal of Communication Disorders, 7,* 181–192.

Saldert, C., Ferm, U., & Bloch, S. J. (2014). Semantic trouble sources and their repair in conversations affected by Parkinson's disease. *International Journal of Language and Communication Disorders, 49,* 710–721.

Salmoni, A. W., Schmidt, R. A., & Walter, C. B. (1984). Knowledge of results and motor learning: A review and critical reappraisal. *Psychological Bulletin, 95,* 355–386.

Sapienza, C., & Hoffman-Ruddy, B. (2009). *Voice disorders* (2nd ed.). San Diego, CA: Plural.

Sapir, S. (2014). Multiple factors are involved in the dysarthria associated with Parkinson's disease: A review with implications for clinical practice and research. *Journal of Speech, Language, and Hearing Research, 57,* 1330–1343.

Sapir, S., Pawlas, A. A., Ramig, L., Seeley, E., Fox, C., & Corboy, J. (2001). Effects of intensive phonatory-respiratory treatment (LSVT) on voice in two individuals with multiple sclerosis. *Journal of Medical Speech-Language Pathology, 9,* 141–151.

Sapir, S., Ramig, L. O., Hoyt, P., Countryman, S., O'Brien, C., & Hoehn, M. (2002). Speech loudness and quality 12 months after intensive voice treatment (LSVT) for Parkinson's disease: A comparison with an alternative speech treatment. *Folia Phoniatrica et Logopaedica, 54,* 296–303.

Schalling, E., Bulukin-Wilen, F., Gustafson, J., & Södersten, M. (2012, February 28–March 4). *Voice use and effects of biofeedback in Parkinson's disease, studied with a newly developed portable voice accumulator, VoxLog.* Paper presented at the Conference on Motor Speech, Santa Rosa, CA.

Schmidt, R. A., & Bjork, A. B. (1996). New conceptualizations of practice: Common principles in three paradigms suggest new concepts for training. In D. A. Robin, K. M. Yorkston, & D. R. Beukelman (Eds.), *Disorders of motor speech: Assessment, treatment and clinical characterization* (pp. 3–23). Baltimore, MD: Brooks.

Schmidt, R. A., Young, D. E., Swinnen, S., & Shapiro, D. C. (1989). Summary knowledge of results for skill acquisition: Support for the guidance hypothesis. *Journal of Experimental Psychology: Learning, Memory and Cognition, 15,* 352–359.

Schulz, G. M., Dingwall, W. O., & Ludlow, C. L. (1999). Speech and oral motor learning in individuals with cerebellar atrophy. *Journal of Speech, Language and Hearing Research, 42,* 1157–1175.

Schwartz, S. K. (2004). *The source for voice disorders: Adolescent & adult.* East Moline, IL: LinguiSystems.

Sellars, C., Hughes, T., & Langhorne, P. (2005). Speech and language therapy for dysarthria due to non-progressive brain damage. *Cochrane Database of Systematic Reviews, 3,* CD002088. doi:10.1002/14651858.CD002088.pub2

Shriberg, L., Kwiatkowski, J., & Rasmussen, C. (1990). *The Prosody-Voice Screening Profile.* Tucson, AZ: Communication Skill Builder.

Sidtis, D. V. L. (2007). Reprint of "Does functional neuroimaging solve the questions of neurolinguistics?" [Brain and Language 98 (2006) 276–290]. *Brain and Language, 102,* 200–214.

Sidtis, J. J., Ahn, J. S., Gomez, C., & Sidtis, D. (2011). Speech characteristic associated with three genotypes of ataxia. *Journal of Communication Disorders, 44,* 478–492.

Simmons, N. N. (1983). Acoustic analysis of ataxic dysarthria: An approach to monitoring treatment. In W. Berry (Ed.), *Clinical dysarthria* (pp. 283–294). Austin, TX: Pro-Ed.

Skodda, S., Grönheit, W., & Schegel, U. (2012). Instability of syllable repetition in progressive supranuclear palsy. *Journal of Neural Transmission, 119,* 457–462.

Skodda, S., Lorenz, J., & Schlegel, U. (2013). Instability of syllable repetition in Parkinson's disease—Impairment of automated speech performance? *Basal Ganglia, 3,* 33–37.

Solomon, N. P., & Charron, S. (1998). Speech breathing in able-bodied children and children with cerebral palsy: A review of the literature and implications for clinical intervention. *American Journal of Speech-Language Pathology, 7,* 61–78.

Solomon, N. P., Garlitz, S.J., & Milbrath, R. L. (2000). Respiratory and laryngeal contributions to maximum phonation duration. *Journal of Voice, 14,* 331–340

Solomon, N. P., McKee, A., & Garcia-Barry, S. (2001). Intensive voice treatment and respiration treatment for hypokinetic-spastic dysarthria after traumatic brain injury. *American Journal of Speech and Language Pathology, 10,* 51–64.

Solomon, N. P., Robin, D. A., & Luschei, E. S. (2000). Strength, endurance, and stability of the tongue and hand in Parkinson disease. *Journal of Speech, Language and Hearing Research, 43,* 256–267.

Sörös, P., Sokoloff, L. G., Bose, A., McIntosh, A. R., Graham, S. J., & Stuss, D. T. (2006). Clustered functional MRI of overt speech production. *Neuroimage, 32,* 376–387.

Spencer, K. A., & Rogers, M. A. (2005). Speech motor programming in hypokinetic and ataxic dysarthria. *Brain and Language, 94,* 347–366.

Spencer, K. A., & Slocomb, D. (2007). The neural basis of ataxic dysarthria. *The Cerebellum, 6,* 58–65.

Spencer, K. A., & Yorkston, K. M. (2004). Evidence for the treatment of respiratory/phonatory dysfunction from dysarthria. In E. Strand (Ed.), *Treatment of dysarthria: Evidence-based practice* (pp. 5–17). Rockville, MD: American Speech-Language Hearing Association.

Spielman, J., Ramig, L. O., Mahler, L., Halpern, A., & Gavin, W. J. (2007). Effects of an extended version of the Lee Silverman Voice Treatment on voice and speech in Parkinson's disease. *American Journal of Speech-Language Pathology, 16,* 95–107.

Stylios, C. D., Georgopoloulos, V. C., Malandraki, G. A., & Chouliara, S. (2008). Fuzzy cognitive map architectures for medical decision support systems. *Applied Soft Computing, 8,* 1243–1251.

Tamplin, J. (2008). A pilot study into the effect of vocal exercises and singing on dysarthric speech. *NeuroRehabilitation, 23,* 207–216.

Theodoros, D. G., Murdoch, B. E., & Stokes, P. (1995). A physiological analysis of articulatory dysfunction in dysarthric speakers following severe closed-head injury. *Brain Injury, 9,* 237–254.

Thomas, S. (2010). Evaluation of anxiety and depression in people with acquired communication impairments. In S. M. Brumfitt (Ed.), *Psychological well-being and acquired communication impairments* (pp. 25–43). Chichester, UK: Wiley-Blackwell.

Tjaden, K., & Watling, E. (2003). Characteristics of diadochokinesis in multiple sclerosis and Parkinson's disease. *Folia Phoniatrica et Logopaedica, 55,* 241–259.

Trail, M., Fox, C., Ramig, L. O., Sapir, S., Howard, J., & Lai, E. C. (2005). Speech treatment for Parkinson's disease. *NeuroRehabilitation, 20,* 205–221.

Turner, G. S., Tjaden, K., & Weismer, G. (1995). The influence of speaking rate on vowel space and speech intelligibility for individuals with amyotrophic lateral sclerosis. *Journal of Speech, Language and Hearing Research, 38,* 1001–1013.

Vandana, V. P., & Manjula, R. (2014). Perceptual speech characteristics of cerebellar dysarthria associated with lesions in different cerebellar nuclei. *Language in India, 14,* 342–349.

van der Graaff, M., Kuiper, T., Zwinderman, A., van de Warrenburg, B., Poels, P., Offeringa, A., et al. (2009). Clinical identification of dysarthria types among neurologists, residents in neurology and speech therapists. *European Neurology, 61,* 295–300.

van der Merwe, A. (1997). A theoretical framework for the characterization of pathological speech sensorimotor control. In M. R. McNeil (Ed.), *Clinical management of sensorimotor speech disorders* (pp. 1–26). New York, NY: Thieme.

van Mourik, M., Catsman-Berrevoets, C. E., Yousef-Bak, E., & van Dongen, H. R. (1997). Acquired childhood dysarthria: Review of its clinical presentation. *Pediatric Neurology, 17,* 299–307.

van Nuffelen, G., De Bodt, M., Vanderwegen, J., Van de Heyning, P., & Wuyts, F. (2010). Effect of rate control on speech production and intelligibility in dysarthria. *Folia Phoniatrica et Logopaedica, 62,* 110–119.

van Nuffelen, G., De Bodt, M., Wuyts, F., & Van de Heyning, P. (2009). The effect of rate control on speech rate and intelligibility of dysarthric speech. *Folia Phoniatrica et Logopaedica, 61,* 69–75.

Vogel, A. P., Folker, J., & Poole, M. L. (2014). Treatment for speech disorder in Friedreich ataxia and other hereditary ataxia syndromes *Cochrane Database of Systematic Reviews, 10,* CD008953. doi:10.1002/14651858.CD008953.pub2

Walshe, M. (2011). The psychological impact of acquired motor speech disorders. In A. Lowit & R. D. Kent (Eds.), *Assessment of motor speech disorders* (pp. 97–122). San Diego, CA: Plural.

Walshe, M., & Miller, N. (2011). Living with acquired dysarthria: The speaker's perspective. *Disability and Rehabilitation, 33,* 195–203.

Walshe, M., Peach, R. K., & Miller, N. (2009). Dysarthria Impact Profile: Development of a scale to measure psychosocial effects. *International Journal of Language & Communication Disorders, 44,* 693–715.

Wang, Y.-T., Kent, R. D., Duffy, J. R., & Thomas, J. E. (2008). Analysis of diadochokinesis in ataxic dysarthria using the Motor Speech Profile Program. *Folia Phoniatrica et Logopaedica, 61,* 1–11.

Wang, Y.-T., Kent, R. D., Duffy, J. R., Thomas, J. E., & Weismer, G. (2004). Alternating motion rate as an index of speech motor disorder in traumatic brain injury. *Clinical Phonetics & Phonetics, 18,* 57–84.

Weijnen, F. G., Kuks, J. B. M., van der Bilt, A., van der Glas, H. W., Wassenberg, M. W. M., & Bosman, F. (2000). Tongue force in patients with myasthenia gravis. *Acta Neurological Scandinavica, 102,* 303–308.

Weikamp, J. G., Schelhaas, H. J., Hendriks, J. C. M., de Swart, B. J. M., & Geurts, A. C. H. (2012). Prognostic value of decreased tongue strength on survival time in patients with amyotrophic lateral sclerosis. *Journal of Neurology, 259,* 2360–2365.

Weismer, G., & Kim, Y. (2010). Classification and taxonomy of motor speech disorders: What are the issues? In B. Maassen & P. van Lieshout (Eds.), *Speech motor control: New developments in basic and applied research* (pp. 229–241). Oxford, UK: Oxford University Press.

Weismer, G., & Laures, J. S. (2002). Direct magnitude estimates of speech intelligibility in dysarthria: Effects of a chosen standard. *Journal of Speech, Language and Hearing Research, 45,* 421–433.

Weismer, G., & Martin, R. E. (1992). Acoustic and perceptual approaches to the study of intelligibility. In R. D. Kent (Ed.), *Intelligibility in speech disorders: Theory, measurement and management* (pp. 67–118). Amsterdam, the Netherlands: Benjamins.

Wenke, R. J., Cornwell, P., & Theodoros, D. G. (2010). Changes to articulation following LSVT® and traditional dysarthria therapy in non-progressive dysarthria. *International Journal of Speech-Language Pathology, 12,* 203–220.

Wenke, R. J., Theodoros, D., & Cornwell, P. (2008). The short- and long-term effectiveness of the LSVT for dysarthria following TBI and stroke. *Brain Injury, 22,* 339–352.

Wenke, R. J., Theodoros, D., & Cornwell, P. (2010). Effectiveness of Lee Silverman Voice Treatment (LSVT)® on hypernasality in non-progressive dysarthria: The need for further research. *International Journal of Language and Communication Disorders, 45,* 31–46.

Whitehill, T. L., Lee, A. S., & Chun, J. C. (2002). Direct magnitude estimation and interval scaling of hypernasality. *Journal of Speech, Language, and Hearing Research, 45,* 80–88.

World Health Organization. (2001). *International classification of functioning, disability, and health.* Geneva, Switzerland: Author.

Yorkston, K. M., Baylor, C. R., Dietz, J., Dudgeon, B. J., Eadie, T., Miller, R. M., et al. (2008). Developing a scale of communicative participation: A cognitive interviewing study. *Disability and Rehabilitation, 30,* 425–433.

Yorkston, K. M., Baylor, C. R., Klasner, E. R., Deitz, J., Dudgeon, B. J., Eadie, T., et al. (2006). Satisfaction with communicative participation as defined by adults with multiple sclerosis: A qualitative study. *Journal of Communication Disorders, 40,* 433–451.

Yorkston, K. M., Beukelman, D., & Traynor, C. D. (1984). *Assessment of intelligibility of dysarthric speech* Austin, TX: Pro-Ed.

Yorkston, K. M., Beukelman, D. R., Strand, E. A., & Bell, K. R. (1999). *Management of motor speech disorders in children and adults.* Austin, TX: Pro-Ed.

Yorkston, K. M., Hakel, M., Beukelman, D. R., & Fager, S. (2007). Evidence for effectiveness of treatment of loudness, rate, or prosody in dysarthria: A systematic review. *Journal of Medical Speech-Language Pathology, 15*(2), xi–xxxvi.

Yorkston, K. M., Hammen, V. L., Beukelman, D. R., & Traynor, C. D. (1990). The effect of rate control on the intelligibility and naturalness of dysarthric speech. *The Journal of Speech and Hearing Disorders, 55*(3), 550–560.

Yorkston, K. M., Spencer, K. A., & Duffy, J. R. (2003). Behavioral management of respiratory/phonatory dysfunction from dysarthria: A systematic review of the evidence. *Journal of Medical Speech-Language Pathology, 11*(2), xiii–xxxviii.

Yorkston, K. M., Spencer, K. A., Duffy, J. R., Beukelman, D. R., Golper, L. A., Miller, R. M., et al. (2001). Evidence-based medicine and practice guidelines: Application to the field of speech-language pathology. *Journal of Medical Speech-Language Pathology, 9,* 243–256.

Yorkston, K. M., Spencer, K. A., Duffy, J. R., Beukelman, D. R., Golper, L. A., Miller, R. M., Strand, E., et al. (2001). Evidence-based practice guidelines for dysarthria: Management of velopharyngeal function. *Journal of Medical Speech-Language Pathology, 9,* 257–273.

Ziegler, W. (2002). Task-related factors in oral motor control: Speech and oral diadochokinesis in dysarthria and apraxia of speech. *Brain and Language, 80,* 556–575.

Ziegler, W. (2003). Speech motor control is task-specific: Evidence from dysarthria and apraxia of speech. *Aphasiology, 17,* 3–36.

Index

Note: Page numbers followed by *f* or *t* represent figures or tables respectively.